CONTACT LENSES

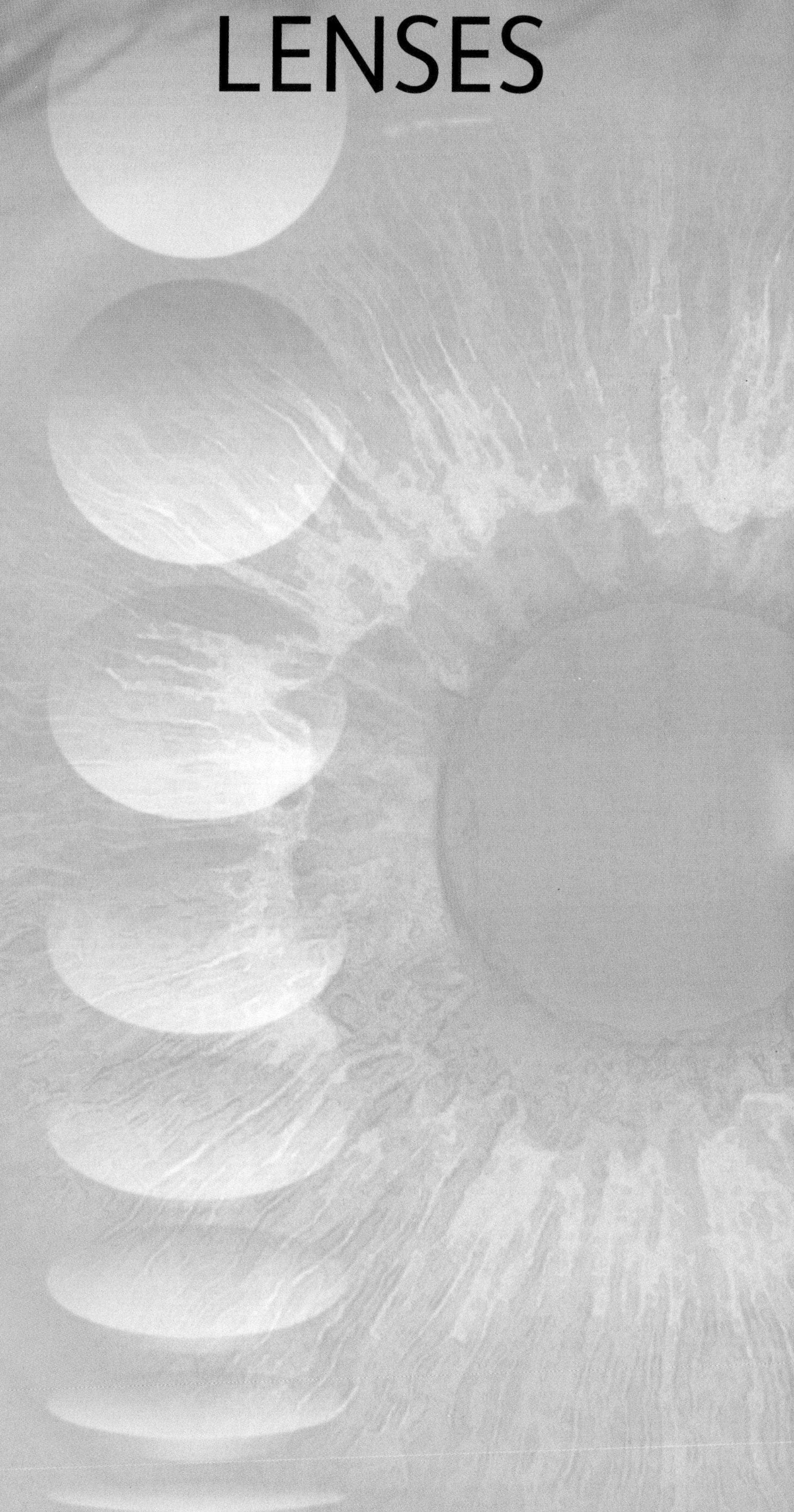

The Editors wish gratefully to acknowledge the help, support and tolerance of their respective spouses, Susan and Colin, in the three years' preparation of this edition.

For Elsevier Butterworth-Heinemann:

Commissioning Editor: Robert Edwards
Development Editor: Kim Benson
Project Manager: Jane Dingwall
Design Direction: George Ajayi
New Illustrations by: David Graham and Ian Ramsden
Illustration Manager: Bruce Hogarth

CONTACT LENSES

FIFTH EDITION

Edited by

Anthony J. Phillips MPhil, FBOA, HD, FCOptom, FAAO, FVCO, DCLP, FCLSA

Department of Ophthalmology, Flinders Medical Centre and The Women's and Children's Hospital, Adelaide, Australia

and

Lynne Speedwell BSc, MSc (Health Psych), FCOptom, DCLP, FAAO

Department of Ophthalmology, Great Ormond Street Hospital for Children and Optometry Department, Moorfields Eye Hospital, London, UK

Consulting editor

Judith Morris MSc, FCOptom, FAAO, FIACLE

Associate Director of Contact Lens Teaching, City University, London and Head of Contact Lenses, Institute of Optometry, London, UK

CD-ROM created by

Tony Hough BA, MBA

Director, CLS Software Limited, UK

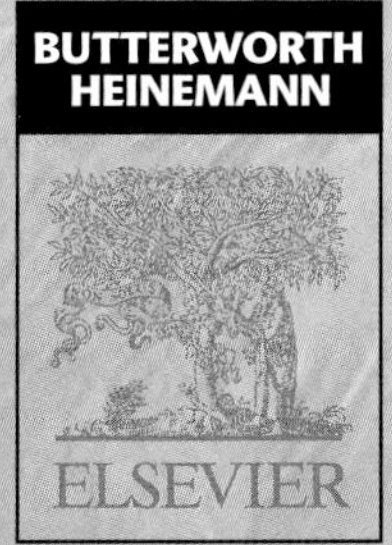

EDINBURGH LONDON NEW YORK OXFORD PHILADELPHIA ST LOUIS SYDNEY TORONTO 2007

BUTTERWORTH
HEINEMANN
ELSEVIER

First published 1972
Reprinted 1976
Second edition (2 vols) 1980, 1981
Combined second edition 1984
Third edition 1989
Fourth edition 1997
Reprinted 2000
Fifth edition 2007

ISBN-13: 978 0 7506 8818 5
ISBN-10: 0 7506 8818 1

British Library Cataloguing in Publication Data
A catalogue record for this book is available from the British Library.

Library of Congress Cataloging in Publication Data
A catalog record for this book is available from the Library of Congress.

Note
Knowledge and best practice in this field are constantly changing. As new research and experience broaden our knowledge, changes in practice, treatment and drug therapy may become necessary or appropriate. Readers are advised to check the most current information provided (i) on procedures featured or (ii) by the manufacturer of each product to be administered, to verify the recommended dose or formula, the method and duration of administration, and contraindications. It is the responsibility of the practitioner, relying on their own experience and knowledge of the patient, to make diagnoses, to determine dosages and the best treatment for each individual patient, and to take all appropriate safety precautions. To the fullest extent of the law, neither the Publisher nor the Editors assumes any liability for any injury and/or damage to persons or property arising out or related to any use of the material contained in this book.

The Publisher

Printed in China

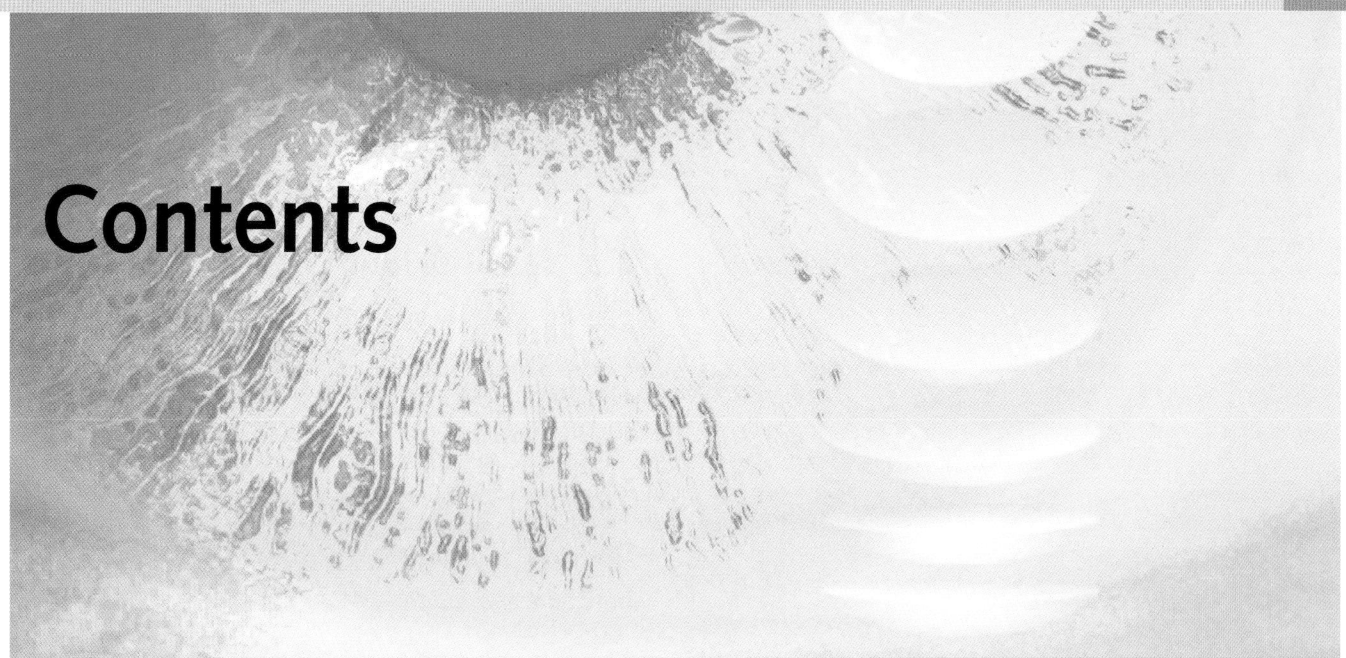

Contents

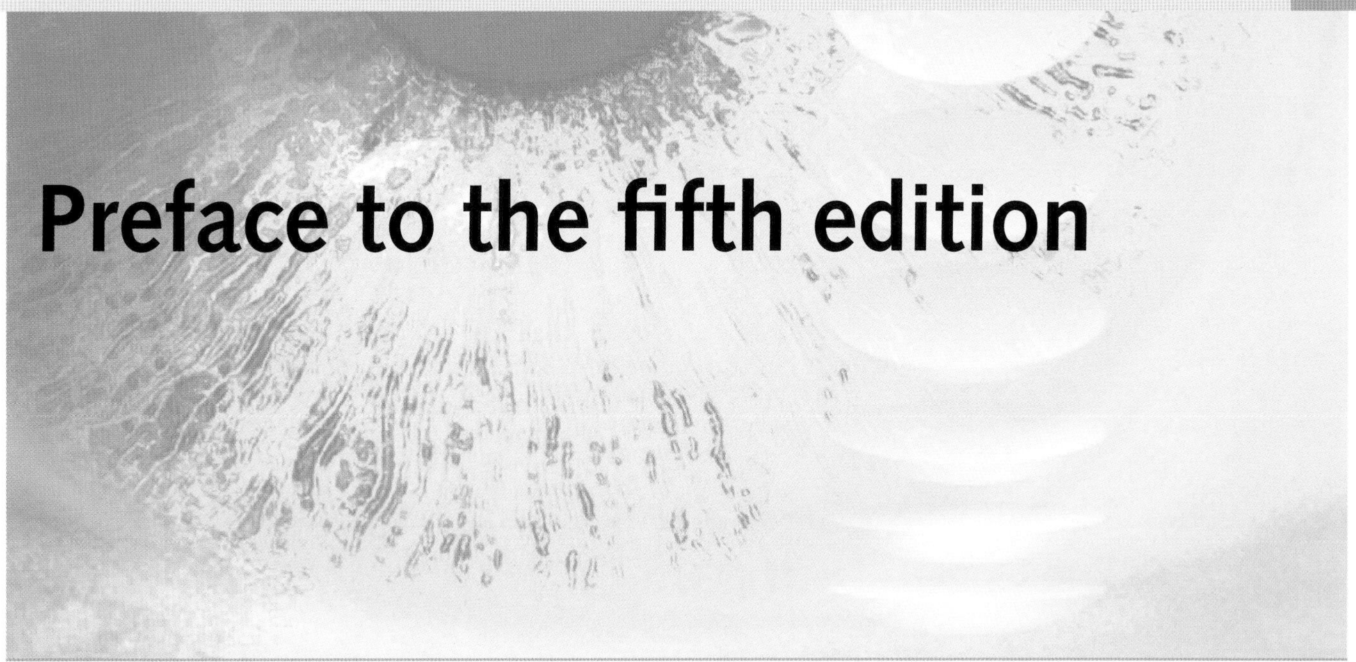

Preface to the fifth edition

It has now been nearly 40 years since work began on the 1st edition of *Contact Lenses*.

Looking back over this period, it is impressive what huge changes have been made in lens materials, design and manufacture, and in practice equipment and practitioner education. Most changes have evolved from technical and academic research over the years while others have resulted from practitioner experience. For these reasons the editors have always selected co-authors who are world renowned for both their academic credentials and (where relevant) their clinical expertise.

As well as improvements in the technology of contact lens practice, the technologies of printing and communication have also leapt forward. In the first edition, diagrams were kept to a minimum and were in black and white as the cost of colour plates was prohibitive. All communication was by post as telephone calls, especially international ones, were rare. Nowadays, colour printing is no restriction, the illustrations are lavish, and the text is much easier to read. Letter writing and telephone calls are used only occasionally as consultation and alterations are made at the click of a mouse.

It is also pertinent to comment on the major developments that have occurred since the 4th edition. At that time it was still beyond the scope of materials science that silicone hydrogel lenses could become a reality. Since then, not only are they in production but they have become a growing part of the armamentarium of the contact lens practitioner. Disposable soft lenses now account for a large proportion of contact lens practice. The chapter on orthokeratology, introduced simply for completeness in the 4th edition, is now a major subject in its own right, thanks very largely to the work of John Mountford.

Since the 1st edition, several co-authors have sadly passed away – Freddie Burnett-Hodd, Gordon Ruskell, Roy Rengstorf, Morley Ford, Peter Marriott and Eddie Proctor. All giants in their field, we acknowledge their great contribution.

This 5th edition is a major revision and update of the previous text covering new areas and bringing in new co-authors, now representing the UK, USA, Australia, Canada, New Zealand and Germany. We are privileged to have these authors and the wealth of knowledge they impart.

It would be remiss of the editors to let the retirement of Janet Stone pass without comment. Her academic record, her work at the Institute of Optometry, and her influence on thousands of contact lens practitioners are testament to the huge contribution she has made towards optometric education. Those who worked with her on the first three editions will recall her being a hard taskmaster, but a perfectionist in achieving a first class result. Her chapters on the Optics of Contact Lenses still serve as classics in their own right.

Our thanks are due to Judith Morris who we welcome on board as consultant editor and of course to the team at Elsevier for their part in the production of this text.

T.P. & L.S.

Preface to the first edition

The writing of this book has been prompted by the need for a current British text embodying the latest thoughts and research for the contact lens practitioner and yet still containing adequate basic information for the student. As the science of contact lenses advances so its many facets become skills within a skill. For this reason, several authors have contributed to this book, each having a particular interest in the subject of the chapter he or she has written. A small amount of duplication between some chapters has been necessary where it serves to stress an important point. The small number of contradictions which appears between one author and another are of minor importance and serve to show the individuality of a clinical skill.

As mentioned above, it is intended that this book will be of clinical and academic value to both practitioner and student. It is assumed that the reader has undergone or is undergoing a course in ophthalmic optics and that clinical tuition will also be available to supplement the written word. For the practitioner who has not graduated in recent years, the chapter on anatomy and physiology will bring him up to date with current knowledge of those parts of the eye and adnexa with which he will be dealing so intimately.

The editors wish gratefully to acknowledge Professor R. J. Fletcher of The City University, London, who conceived the idea of such a book, and F. R. H. 'Budge' Wilmot and Rita Dickins, both of whom acted as original co-coordinators and without whose enthusiasm this book would not have come into being.

We would also like to thank those people who have taken colour photographs for us, especially Michael S. Wilson, as well as the 'subjects' for these photographs. The many people who have assisted with typing and checking, and particularly Mr G. M. Dunn and the Staff of the British Optical Association have our grateful thanks for their help and encouragement.

Finally, we must thank our contributors, whose skill and knowledge has been put into print for the benefit of all.

JANET STONE and TONY PHILLIPS
London and Loughborough 1971

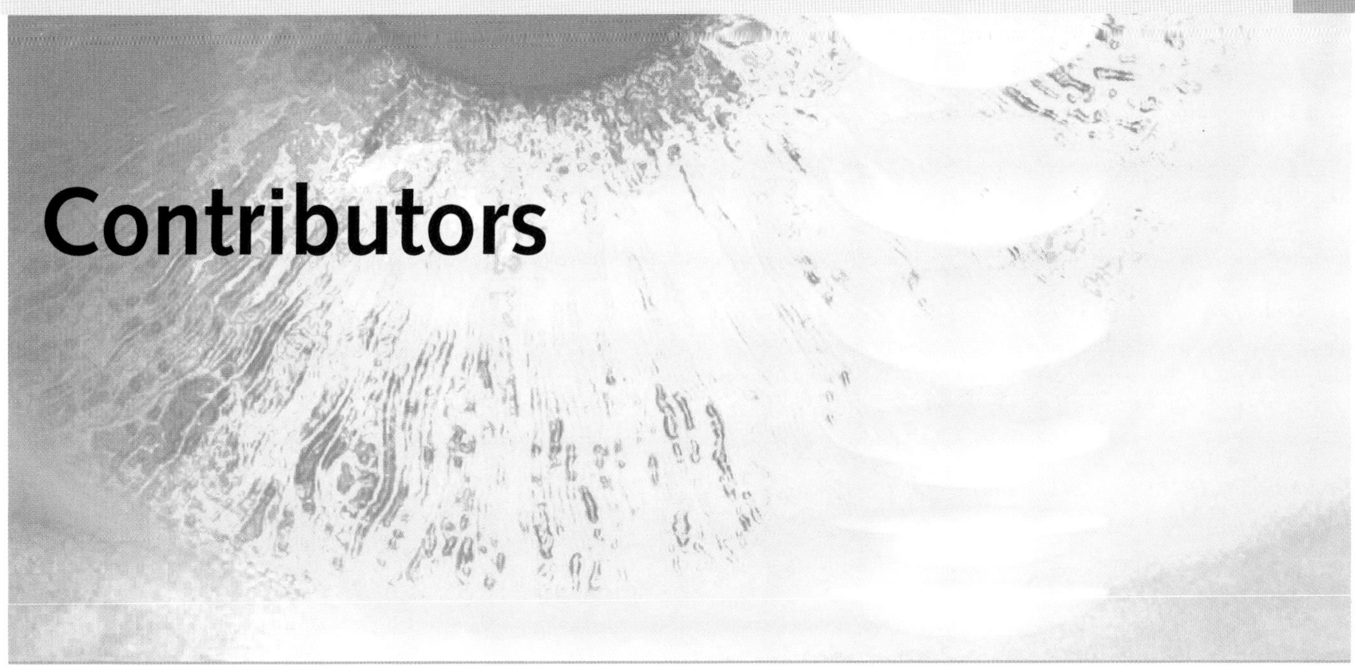

Contributors

Kerry W. Atkinson, BSc, FCOptom, DCLP
Contact Lens Practitioner; Academic Associate and Clinical Associate in Contact Lens Practice, Department of Optometry, University of Auckland, Auckland, New Zealand

Edward S. Bennett, OD, MSEd
Associate Professor of Optometry; Chief, Contact Lens Service; Director of Student Services, College of Optometry, The University of Missouri-St Louis, St Louis, Missouri, USA

Jan P. G. Bergmanson, OD, PhD, FAAO, FCOptom
Director and Professor, Texas Eye Research Technology Center, University of Houston College of Optometry, Houston, Texas, USA

Wolfgang Cagnolati, MS, DSc (Hons), MCOptom, FAAO
Optometrist and Contact Lens Practitioner; Visiting Associate Professor, Pennsylvania College of Optometry (USA); Chairman, European Board of Management in Optometry (ECOO), Institute of Ophthalmic Optics and Optometry, Am Buchenbaum, Germany

Patrick J. Caroline, FAAO
Assistant Clinical Professor, Oregon Health Sciences Unviersity, Department of Ophthalmology, Oregon, USA

Jennifer D. Choo, BSc, OD
Project Director, Institute for Eye Research, Sydney, New South Wales, Australia

John H. Clamp, MS (USA), MCOptom, FAAO
Chief Operating Officer, Ultravision CLPL, Leighton Buzzard, Bedfordshire, UK

Kathy Dumbleton, MSc, MCOptom, FAAO
Faculty Senior Research Associate, Centre for Contact Lens Research, University of Waterloo, Waterloo, Ontario, Canada

Frank Eperjesi, BSc (Hons), PhD, MCOptom, DipOrth, FAAO
Director of Undergraduate Studies, Optometry, School of Life and Health Sciences, Aston University, Birmingham, UK

Desmond Fonn, DipOptom, MOptom, FAAO (DipCL)
Professor, School of Optometry; Centre for Contact Lens Research, University of Waterloo, Waterloo, Ontario, Canada

Morley W. Ford, FCOptom, FAAO, DCLP *(deceased)*
Former Optometrist and Contact Lens Practitioner, North Shields, Tyne and Wear, UK

Bernard Gilmartin, BSc, PhD, FCOptom, FAAO
School of Life and Health Sciences; Professor of Optometry, Aston University, Birmingham, UK

Andrew Godfrey, BAppSc (Optometry) (Hons)
Consultant Optometrist, Centre for Ophthalmology and Vision Science, Lions Eye Institute, Nedlands, Western Australia

Jean-Pierre Guillon, BSc (Optom), PhD
Centre for Ophthalmology and Vision Science, Lions Eye Institute, Nedlands, Western Australia

Sheila B. Hickson-Curran, BSc, MCOptom
Clinical Research, Vistakon Research & Development, Jacksonville, Florida, USA

Brien A. Holden, BAppSc, PhD, DSc, FCLSA, OAM
Scientia Professor; Chief Executive Officer, Institute for Eye Research; Deputy CEO, The Vision Cooperative Research Centre, Sydney, New South Wales, Australia

Tony Hough, MBA, BA
Director, CLS Software Limited, St Neots, Cambridgeshire, UK

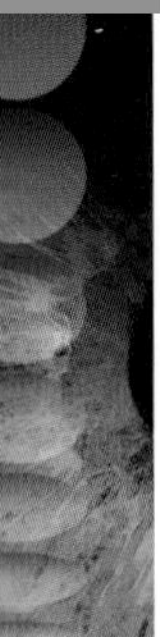

Lyndon W. Jones, PhD, FCOptom, DipCLP, FAAO
Associate Professor, Centre for Contact Lens Research, University of Waterloo, Waterloo, Ontario, Canada

Jacqueline Lamb, BSc, MCOptom, DCLP
Head of Optometry, Birmingham and Midland Eye Hospital, Birmingham, UK

Mark Lazarus, FRANZCO
Head of Contact Lens Clinic, Royal Victorian Eye and Ear Hospital and Senior Fellow, Department of Ophthalmology, University of Melbourne, Melbourne, Victoria, Australia

Richard G. Lindsay, BSc (Optom), MBA, FAAO (DipCL), FCLSA
Senior Fellow, Department of Optometry and Vision Sciences, University of Melbourne, Melbourne, Victoria, Australia

Nicola Logan, BSc, PhD, MCOptom
Lecturer in Optometry, School of Life and Health Sciences, Aston University, Birmingham, UK

Russell Lowe, BSc (Optom), FAAO
Contact Lens Practitioner, Carlton, Victoria, Australia

Charles W. McMonnies, MSc, FAAO, FCLSA
Adjunct Professor, School of Optometry and Vision Science, University of New South Wales, Sydney, New South Wales, Australia

Michael Mihailidis, BOptom, LLM
Contact Lens Practitioner and Barrister at Law, Sydney, New South Wales, Australia

Lalitha C. M. Moodaley, MBBS, DO, MRCOphth
Associate Specialist External Disease and Contact Lens Service, Moorfields Eye Hospital, London, UK

Judith A. Morris, MSc, FCOptom, FAAO, FIACLE
Head of Contact Lenses, Institute of Optometry, London; Associate Director of Contact Lens Teaching, Department of Optometry and Visual Science, City University, London, UK

John Mountford, FAAO, FVCO, FCLSA, Dip App Sc (Optom)
Contact Lens Practitioner, Brisbane, Queensland, Australia

Anthony J. Phillips, MPhil, FBOA, HD, FCOptom, FAAO, FVCO, DCLP, FCLSA
Department of Ophthalmology, Flinders Medical Centre and The Adelaide Women's and Children's Hospital, Adelaide, Australia

Kenneth W. Pullum, BSc, FCOptom, DCLP
Senior Optometrist, Moorfields and Oxford Eye Hospitals, London, UK

Ronald B. Rabbetts, MSc, FCOptom, SMSA, DipCLP
Rabbetts Sight Care, Portsmouth, UK

Martin P. Rubinstein, PhD, FCOptom, FAAO
Head of Optometry Unit, Department of Ophthalmology, University Hospital, Nottingham, UK

Gordon L. Ruskell, MS, PhD, DSc, FCOptom *(deceased)*
Formerly Emeritus Professor, Department of Optometry & Vision Sciences, City University, London, UK

Anthony G. Sabell, MSc, FCOptom, DCLP
Visiting Consulting Specialist in Scleral Lenses, Birmingham and Midland Hospital, Birmingham, UK

Lynne Speedwell, BSc, MSc (Health Psych), FCOptom, DCLP, FAAO
Department of Ophthalmology, Great Ormond Street Hospital for Children, London, UK; Optometry Department, Moorfields Eye Hospital, London, UK

Fiona Stapleton, MSc, PhD, MCOptom, FAAO, DCLP
Associate Professor, Director of Academic Education, The Vision Cooperative Research Centre, University of New South Wales, Sydney, New South Wales, Australia

Christopher F. Steele, BSc (Hons), FCOptom, DCLP, Dip Oc
Head of Optometry, Consultant Optometrist, Sunderland Eye Infirmary, Sunderland, Tyne and Wear, UK

Janet Stone, FBOA, HD, FCOptom, DCLP
Former Contact Lens Practitioner, Shrewsbury, Shropshire, and Lecturer, The Institute of Optometry, London, UK

Helen A. Swarbrick, PhD, MSc, BSc, DipOptom (NZ), FAAO
Associate Professor, School of Optometry and Vision Science, University of New South Wales, Sydney, New South Wales, Australia

Serina Stretton, BSc, PhD
Project Director, The Vision Cooperative Research Centre, Sydney, New South Wales, Australia

Deborah F. Sweeney, BOptom, PhD, FAAO
Associate Professor; Chief Executive Officer, The Vision Cooperative Research Centre, University of New South Wales, Sydney, New South Wales, Australia

Robert Terry, MSc
Principal Research Optometrist, The Vision Cooperative Research Centre, University of New South Wales, Sydney, New South Wales, Australia

Brian J. Tighe, PhD, Chem, FRSC
Professor of Polymer Science, Department of Chemical Engineering & Applied Science, Aston University, Birmingham, UK

Lewis Williams, AQIT (Optom), MOptom, PhD
Tawic Lens Consultants, Sydney, New South Wales, Australia

James S. Wolffsohn, BSc (Hons), PhD, PgDipAdvClinOptom, PgCHE, MCOptom, FAAO, FIACLE, FBCLA
Subject Group Convenor, Optometry, School of Life and Health Sciences, Aston University, Birmingham, UK

E. Geoffrey Woodward, PhD, FCOptom, DCLP
Emeritus Professor, Department of Optometry & Visual Science, City University, London, UK

Graeme Young, MPhil, PhD, FCOptom, DCLP, FAAO
Managing Director, Visioncare Research Ltd, Farnham, Surrey, UK

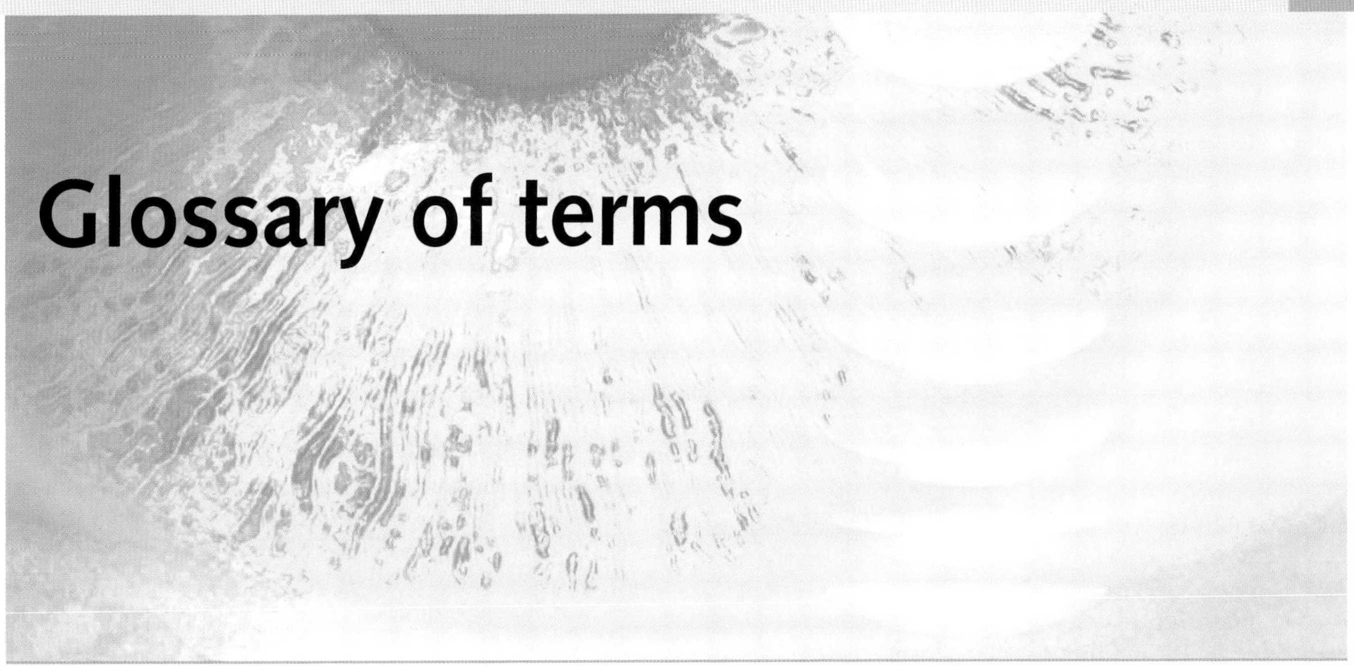

Glossary of terms

The 1995 edition of ISO 8320 has been expanded by the addition of new terms and the omission of ambiguities, and the list below comprises the relevant terms from the 2003 edition. Terms are grouped in sections to enable the reader to find information easily. The list is not complete and only the more commonly used terms are included. The reader is advised to refer to the original document ISO 8320-1: (2003) for the comprehensive list, which can be obtained from BSI Customer Services, 389 Chiswick High Road, London W4 4AL. Tel: +44 (0)20 8996 9001; email: cservices@bsi-global.com

The Table of Symbols is given in its entirety in order to help with the calculations in Chapter 6. The letter *t* indicates thickness and the letter L is no longer used. In France, the abbreviation *e* for épaisseur is used, rather than *t* for thickness.

2 General terms and definitions

2.1.1 **axial edge lift**, l_{EA}: Distance between a point on the back of a lens at the edge and the vertex sphere, measured parallel to the lens axis. NOTE – This is often a value computed by the manufacturer and may be altered by the edging process.

2.2 **back vertex power**, F'_v: Reciprocal of the paraxial back vertex focal length, in metres, of the optic zone of the lens in air.

2.8 **bi-toric lens**: Lens having both front and back optic zones of toroidal form.

2.9 **blending**: Process of forming a polished transition at a junction. NOTE – This does not constitute the formation of an aspheric zone.

2.10 **carrier**: That part of a lenticular lens peripheral to the front optic zone(s). NOTE – The carrier may be negative, positive or parallel in construction but is radially symmetrical.

2.12 **composite lens**: Contact lens composed of two or more different materials. NOTE – For example, a laminated lens, a fused segment lens or a lens with a rigid centre and a flexible periphery.

2.14 **contact shell**: Appliance similar in form to a contact lens but not designed to correct vision.

2.15 **corneal lens**: Contact lens designed to be worn in its entirety on the cornea.

2.16 **cosmetic lens**: Contact lens specifically designed to change or mask the appearance of the eye. NOTE – Cosmetic lenses are devices which may also be used for therapeutic purposes.

2.17 **cosmetic shell**: Contact shell specifically designed to change the appearance of the eye. NOTE – Cosmetic shells are devices which may also be used for therapeutic purposes.

2.18 **disposable lens**: A lens intended for single use. NOTE – The lens is not intended to be re-used and is discarded after removal from the eye.

2.21 **fenestration**: Specified hole which passes from the front surface to the back surface of a contact lens.

2.22 **front vertex power**, F_v: Reciprocal of the paraxial front vertex focal length, in metres, of the optic zone of the lens, in air.

2.23 **geometric centre**, *c*: Centre of the circle containing the lens edge. NOTE – For a scleral lens, the geometric centre is taken as the centre of the optic zone. For a truncated lens, the geometric centre is taken as the centre of the circle that contains the circular portion of the edge.

2.24 **high water content lens**: A lens whose water content is greater than 65%.

2.25 **hydrogel lens**: A contact lens made of water absorbing (hydrophilic) material having an equilibrium water

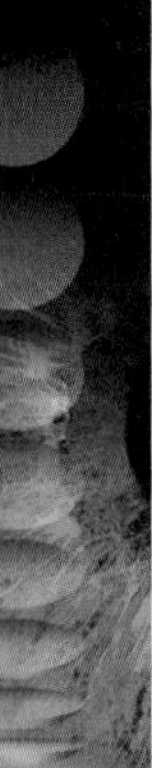

content greater than or equal to 10% in standard saline (ISO 10344) at 20°C.

2.28 **lens axis**: A line passing through the geometric centre, perpendicular to a plane containing the edge of the lens.

2.29 **lenticular lens**: Lens having a front optic zone made smaller than the total diameter. NOTE – This construction is conventionally used to reduce the centre thickness of a positively powered lens or reduce the edge thickness of a negatively powered lens.

2.31 **low water content lens**: A lens whose water content is less than 50%.

2.32 **mid water content lens**: A lens whose water content is between 50 and 65%.

2.35 **multi-curve lens**: A lens whose back surface is composed of more than three intersecting spherical zones.

2.37 **optic zone**: That part of a contact lens which has a prescribed optical effect. NOTE – The term may be qualified by either the prefix 'back' or 'front' in the case of a surface with a single optical component. In the case of an alternating vision bifocal, the term may be qualified by either the prefix 'distance' or 'near'. In the case of a concentric bifocal, the term may be qualified by the prefix 'central' or 'peripheral'.

2.40 **prism ballast**: The use of prism to create a wedge design for lens stabilization. NOTE – The base of the prism is at or near the bottom of the lens.

2.41 **radial lift**, l_R: Distance between a specified point on the back surface of a lens and the vertex sphere measured along a radius of curvature of the latter.

2.42.1 **frequent replacement lens**: A planned replacement lens for which the replacement frequency is 3 months or less.

2.42.2 **planned replacement**: A lens for which the manufacturer has recommended a replacement frequency.

2.43 **rigid lens; hard lens**: Contact lens which, in its final form and under normal conditions, retains its form without support. NOTE – The term 'semi-soft lens' is deprecated.

2.44 **rigid (hard) gas permeable (RGP) lens**: Rigid lens which contains one or more components in sufficient concentration to permit oxygen transmission through the lens.

2.45 **sagitta (sagittal depth, sagittal height)**: The maximum distance from a chord, which is perpendicular to the axis of rotation of a surface, to the curved surface.

2.46 **scleral lens**: Contact lens designed to be worn in front of the cornea and on most of the bulbar conjunctiva.

2.48 **soft lens**: Contact lens which requires support to maintain its form.

2.51 **therapeutic lens**: A lens used to maintain or restore the integrity of ocular tissue and which may have a refractive element. NOTE – some therapeutic lenses are used to deliver drugs to ocular tissues.

2.53 **toric lens**: Lens with front and/or back optic zone of toroidal form.

2.54 **toric periphery lens**: Lens with one or more back peripheral zones of toroidal form which surround a spherical back optic zone.

4 Tinted lenses

4.1 **tinted contact lens**: A contact lens containing some coloration for a specified or an intended use.

4.1.1 **enhancing tint**: A coloration which is added to a contact lens in order to alter the apparent iris colour of the wearer.

4.1.2 **handling (visibility) tint**: A coloration added to a contact lens which is intended to improve the visibility of the lens during handling but which is not intended to have any effect on eye colour.

4.1.3 **opaque tinted lens** (eye masking tint lens): A lens containing sufficient colour in order to mask all or most of the natural iris colour. NOTE – This is a colloquial term and not all such lenses are completely opaque.

5 Material properties

5.2 **gas permeability**: Mathematical product of gas solubility and diffusion coefficients.

Permeability =

$$\frac{\text{amount of gas (cm}^3) \times \text{thickness (cm)}}{\text{area (cm}^2) \times \text{time(s)} \times \text{pressure difference (mmHg)}}$$

5.2.1 **oxygen permeability**, *Dk*: The most commonly used gas permeability for contact lens materials. NOTE -- units are $(cm^2/s)\ (mlO_2/[ml \times mmHg])$, or $cm^3[O_2] \times cm/cm^2 \times s \times mmHg$. For Dk units in terms of hectopascals instead of mmHg the following units are used: $cm^3[O_2] \times cm/cm^2 \times s \times mmHg \times 0.75$.

5.4 **oxygen flux**, *j*: Amount of oxygen (μl), per unit of time(s), which diffuses through a unit area (cm^2) of a contact lens under specified conditions. NOTE – The specified conditions include temperature, thickness of the sample and partial pressure of oxygen on both sides of the sample.

5.5 **oxygen transmissibility**, Dk/*t*: Value for oxygen permeability divided by the thickness (cm) of the measured sample under specified conditions.

5.6 **water content**: Proportion by mass of water retained within a lens under specified conditions.

6 Multifocal and progressive power lenses

6.2 **bifocal lens**: A multifocal lens having two portions, usually for distance and near.

6.5 **centre near (CN) lens**: A multifocal or progressive power lens designed to correct presbyopia where the maximum plus (or minimum minus) power is found in the central optic zone of the lens.

6.6 **concentric bifocal lens**: A lens having two optic zones of different power, each having coincident geometric centres. NOTE – This excludes diffractive bifocal lenses.

6.9 **fused segment lens**: Multifocal lens made from materials of different refractive indices.

6.10 **multifocal lens**: A lens designed to provide two or more visibly divided zones of different corrective powers.

6.11 **peripheral optic zone(s)**: Optic zone(s) surrounding the central optic zone of a concentric multifocal.

6.13 **progressive optical zone**: An aspheric zone designed to provide a continuous change of surface power.

7 Scleral lenses and shells

7.1 **back scleral size**: Maximum internal dimension of the back scleral surface before the sharp edge has been rounded.

7.3 **impression lens**: Scleral lens, the back surface of which has been produced by moulding from a cast of the eye.

7.6 **preformed scleral lens**: Scleral lens, not an impression lens, the back surface of which is of a predetermined form.

7.7 **primary optic diameter**: The diameter of the optic zone before any transition is added. NOTE – In a case where the optic zone is not circular, the longest chord passing through the geometric centre is used.

7.8 **primary optic plane**: Plane perpendicular to the lens axis and containing the primary optic diameter.

7.9 **primary sagitta**: Distance along the lens axis from the back vertex of the optic zone to the primary optic plane.

7.10 **scleral chord**: In a specified meridian, the distance from the optic–scleral junction to the junction of the back scleral surface with the edge.

7.11 **scleral thickness**: Thickness of the scleral zone measured normal to the front scleral surface at any specified point.

7.12 **scleral zone**: That zone of a scleral lens (or shell) designed to lie in front of the sclera.

8 Dimensional terms

8.1 **Radius of curvature (*r*)**: NOTE – Radii relating to zones on the back of the lens are designated by a numerical subscript starting with zero (r_0). The subscript becomes larger from the lens centre to the lens edge. Radii relating to the front surface of the lens have a double subscript, the first part of which is the letter a. The second part is a number from zero upwards, for example, r_{a2}. In the case of an aspheric zone, a mathematical equation or expression may be used to describe the curvature of the zone.

8.1.1 **back optic zone radius (base curve)**, r_0: Radius[1] of curvature of the back optic zone of a surface with a single refractive element.

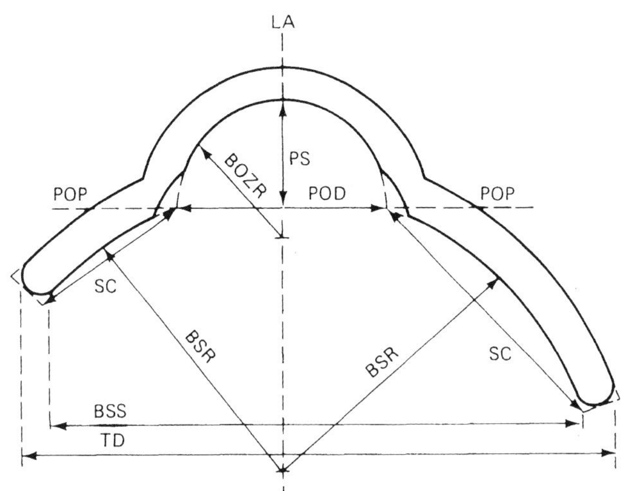

Abbreviation	*Term*
LA	lens axis
BOZR	back optic zone radius
PS	primary sagitta
POD	primary optic diameter
POP	primary optic plane
SC	scleral chord
BSR	back scleral radius
BSS	back scleral size
TD	total diameter
d	displacement

8.1.1.1 **back central optic radius**, r_0: Radius of curvature of the back central optic zone of a multifocal lens.

8.1.1.2 **back peripheral optic radius**: Radius of curvature of a back peripheral optic zone of a multifocal lens.

8.1.2 **back peripheral radius**[2]: Radius[1] of curvature of a back peripheral zone.

8.1.3 **front optic zone radius**: Radius[1] of curvature of the front optic zone of a surface with a single refractive element.

8.1.3.1 **front central optic radius**: Radius of curvature of the front central optic zone of a multifocal lens.

8.1.3.2 **front peripheral optic radius**: Radius of a curvature of a front peripheral optic zone of a multifocal lens.

8.1.4 **front peripheral radius**[2]: Radius[1] of curvature of a front peripheral zone.

8.2 Diameters (Ø)

In cases of elliptical shapes, the maximum and minimum sizes are used for measurement purposes. Elliptical zones which are toroidal, or adjacent to a toroidal zone, have their diameter specified on the flattest meridian. In lenses with concentric posterior surface zones, the zones are qualified by a subscript number from zero starting with the innermost zone ($Ø_0$). On the anterior surface the number is always preceded by the letter a, for example ($Ø_{a0}$).

---

[1] On a toroidal zone there will be two values.
[2] May be preceded by first, second, third, etc.

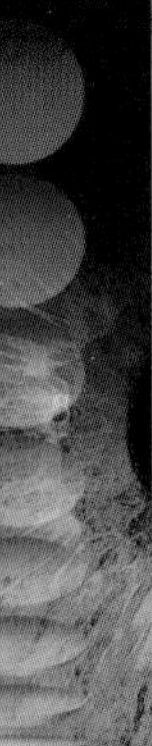

8.2.1 **back optic zone diameter**: Diameter of the back optic zone on a surface with a single optical component[3].

8.2.1.1 **back central optic diameter**: Diameter of the posterior central optic zone of a concentric multifocal lens.

8.2.1.2 **back peripheral optic diameter**[2]: Diameter of a posterior peripheral optic zone of a concentric multifocal lens.

8.2.2 **back peripheral zone diameter**[2]: Diameter of a back peripheral zone.

8.2.3 **displacement of optic** (for lenses other than scleral lenses), *d*: Displacement of the optic zone relative to the lens periphery.

8.2.4 **front optic zone diameter**: Diameter of the front optic zone on a surface with a single refractive element[3].

8.2.4.1 **front central optic diameter**: Diameter of the anterior central optic zone of a multifocal lens.

8.2.4.2 **front peripheral optic diameter**: Diameter of an anterior peripheral optic zone of a multifocal lens.

8.2.5 **front peripheral zone diameter**: Diameter of a front peripheral zone.

8.2.9 **total diameter**, $Ø_T$: Maximum external dimensions of the finished lens or shell. NOTE – In the cases of truncated lenses, the short axis is taken as a line passing through the mid-point of the truncation(s) and the lens axis. The major axis is perpendicular to the short axis and also passes through the lens axis.

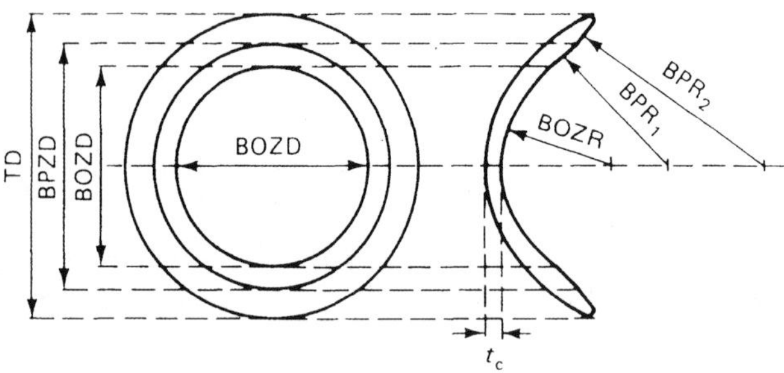

8.3 Thickness

8.3.1 **axial thickness**, t_A: Thickness of the lens, parallel to the lens axis, at a specified position.

8.3.1.1 **axial edge thickness**, t_{EA}: Axial thickness at a defined point from the edge.

8.3.3 **geometric centre thickness**, t_C: Thickness of the lens or shell at its geometric centre.

8.3.4 **harmonic mean thickness**, t_{HM}: Thickness of a radially symmetrical lens calculated from the expression

$$t_{HM} = \frac{h+1}{1/t_0 + 1/t_1 + 1/t_2 + 1/t_3 \ldots\ldots\ldots\ldots 1/t_h}$$

where h + 1 is a series of concentric annuli of equal surface area from the lens geometric centre to the edge of the exposed sample area.

8.3.4 **optical centre thickness**: Thickness of the lens at its optical centre.

8.3.6 **radial thickness**, t_R: The thickness of a lens along a line which passes through the centre of the vertex sphere and intersects the lens at a specified point.

8.3.6.1 **radial edge thickness**, t_{ER}: Thickness of the lens measured normal to the front surface at a specified distance from the edge, for example, $t_{ER(0,2)}$ indicates the radial edge thickness is measured 0.2 mm from the lens edge.

9 Table of symbols

Dimension	Symbols	Reference to text
Back optic zone radius	r_0	8.1.1
Back central optic radius	r_0	8.1.1.1
Back peripheral optic radius	$r_1, r_2, \ldots\ldots$	8.1.1.2
Back peripheral radius	$r_1, r_2, \ldots\ldots$	8.1.2
Front optic zone radius	r_{a0}	8.1.3
Front central optic radius	r_{a0}	8.1.3.1
Front peripheral optic radius	$r_{a1}, r_{a2}, \ldots\ldots$	8.1.3.2
Front peripheral radius	$r_{a1}, r_{a2}, \ldots\ldots$	8.1.4
Back optic zone diameter	$Ø_0$	8.2.1
Back central optic diameter	$Ø_0$	8.2.1.1
Back peripheral optic diameter	$Ø_1, Ø_2, \ldots\ldots$	8.2.1.2
Back peripheral zone diameter	$Ø_1, Ø_2, \ldots\ldots$	8.2.2
Front optic zone diameter	$Ø_{a0}$	8.2.4
Front central optic diameter	$Ø_{a0}$	8.2.4.1
Front peripheral optic diameter	$Ø_{a1}, Ø_{a2}, \ldots\ldots$	8.2.4.2
Front peripheral zone diameter	$Ø_{a1}, Ø_{a2}, \ldots\ldots$	8.2.5
Total diameter	$Ø_T$	8.2.9
Axial thickness	t_A	8.3.1
Axial edge thickness	t_{EA}	8.3.1.1
Carrier junction thickness	t_{CJ}	8.3.2
Geometric centre thickness	t_C	8.3.3
Harmonic mean thickness	t_{HM}	8.3.4
Peripheral junction thickness	t_{PJ}	8.3.5
Radial edge thickness	$t_{ER\ (suffix)}$	8.3.6.1
Axial lift	l_A	2.1
Axial edge lift	l_{EA}	2.1.1
Radial lift	l_R	2.41
Radial edge lift	l_{ER}	2.41.1
Back vertex power	F'_v	2.2
Front vertex power	F_v	2.22
Displacement of optic	d	7.2; 8.2.3
Oxygen permeability	Dk	5.2.1
Oxygen flux	j	5.4
Oxygen transmissibility	Dk/t	5.5

(Reproduced with permission of the British Standards Institution)

[2] May be preceded by first, second, third, etc.
[3] The optic zone of a toric periphery lens is usually elliptical in shape.

Chapter 1

The history of contact lenses

Jacqueline Lamb and Anthony Sabell

CHAPTER CONTENTS

This chapter follows the development of contact lenses from the concept through to the finished article. It is written in chronological order though occasionally, due to the volume of developments, the timeline is split. As you read it, remember that for the original 'contact lens pioneers' both their equipment and the materials available to them were incredibly limited. As the chapter unfolds it is of interest to see the development of materials, designs and the transition of lenses being initially fitted solely by medical doctors, moving to the emergence of the optometrist and contact lens practitioner. As our knowledge of the physiology of the cornea has developed, so too has the success of contact lenses.

THEORIES INTO PRACTICE

One of the earliest references of relevance to this history dates back to 1508 and relates to the development of the basic theories of sight.

1508: Leonardo da Vinci, in his Codex D, folio 3, famously illustrated a man with his head lowered into a large transparent bowl of water (Fig. 1.1). The bowl or globe was intended to represent a model of the human eye and immersing the observer's face in the water resulted in the optical neutralization of his cornea (Ferrero 1952, Hofstetter & Graham 1953, Gasson 1976). This was not a prototype contact lens but the beginning of understanding corneal neutralization (Heinz 2003).

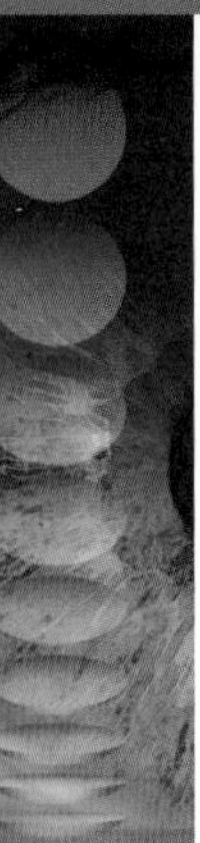

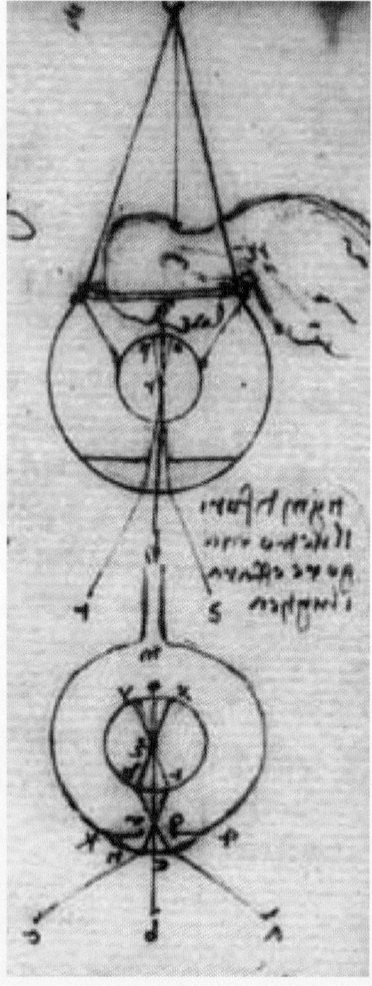

Figure 1.1 Codex D, folio 3 by Leonardo da Vinci (reproduced with permission from Bibliothèque de l'Institut de France – Paris)

It was over 100 years later that the first work involving the eye and a potential lens was published.

1637: René Descartes described in his seventh *Discourse of La Dioptrique* a fluid-filled tube used to enlarge the size of the retinal image (Enoch 1956). The elongated water-filled tube used by Descartes (1637) would have been impossible to wear as an appliance for the correction of vision and appears to be more a theoretical idea. Interestingly, more recently, scientists constructed a contact-tube device according to the diagrams shown by Descartes and placed it on the eye, only to find it functioned as a microscope rather than a telescope.

Theories and experiments about the neutralization of the cornea continued into the 17th and 18th century:

1685: Philip de la Hire, a French mathematician, presented his dissertations on the neutralization of the cornea in 1685 and 1694. He also speculated on the cause of myopia being axial or refractive. Sadly, his theories about accommodation and entoptic phenomenon were considered so controversial that his views on optics were largely ignored (Duke-Elder 1970).

1801: Thomas Young, a physician and physicist, having studied medicine in London and Edinburgh and physics at Gottingen, conducted research into the eye, identifying the cause of astigmatism and publishing a three-colour theory of perception. As a fellow at Cambridge University, he carried out his classic experiment on accommodation using the water-filled lens principle from Leonardo da Vinci, which he placed on the eye to neutralize the refractive effect of the cornea (Young 1801).

1827: George B. Airy, inspired by Thomas Young, colluded with John Herschel at Cambridge University and, experimenting with his own astigmatism, described not only the optical theory of astigmatism but also its correction with a theoretical back surface toric lens. He used the first few days of the moon's crescent (similar to a stenopæic slit) to distinguish the astigmatic axis of his own eye (Airy 1827). He was quoted in John Herschel's dissertation on light (Herschel 1845): 'the ingenious idea of a double concave lens, in which one surface should be spherical, the other cylindrical. The use of the spherical surface was to correct the general defect of a too convex cornea. That of the cylindrical may be thus explained' and he went on to describe its application onto the astigmatic cornea.

It was not until 1845 that the theoretical ideas began developing into clinical experiments:

1845: Sir John F. W. Herschel, in his dissertation on Light as mentioned above, also described the optical correction of malformed and distorted corneas using convex lenses applied to the eye. He suggested correcting 'very bad cases of irregular cornea' by using 'some transparent animal jelly contained in a spherical capsule of glass' and then went on to suggest whether 'an actual mould of the cornea might be taken and impressed on some transparent medium' (Herschel 1845).

1886: Dr Xavier Galezowsky suggested the idea of using a gelatine disc applied to the cornea immediately after cataract extraction. The disc was to be impregnated with cocaine and sublimate of mercury which would provide corneal anaesthesia to relieve postoperative pain and an antiseptic cover to prevent infection (Mann 1938). Despite the horrifying implications of such a procedure, we may see in the proposal not only the first use of a soft and hydrophilic contact appliance but also the forerunner of the hydrophilic lens as a dispenser of ophthalmic medication. Local anaesthesia was widely used by 1886 in the form of cocaine drops. Initially adopted by Karl Koller in 1884, their use in German ophthalmology became almost universal (www.rsm.ac.uk).

Between 1887 and 1889 the forerunners of modern lenses evolved, the stimulus for their development being a need to solve ophthalmic medical problems. Lenses were evolving simultaneously in at least four centres across Europe.

1887: Fredrich A. Müller and **Albert C. Müller**, specialist glassblowers and artificial eye makers, working in their family business in Wiesbaden, made and supplied a protective device for a patient of Dr Theodore Saemisch. The patient had skin cancer, which had resulted in the destruction and removal of the right lower lid and the temporal part of the upper lid, causing entropion and trichiasis of the remaining eyelashes. The right cornea was permanently exposed. It was the man's only useful eye as the left was very myopic and had a cataract. By making a clear glass shell, which encased but did not touch the cornea, fluid was maintained around the cornea preventing its further desiccation. The protective shell was transparent and maintained the vision (Nissel 1965). The patient wrote a letter in 1908 reporting that since 1887 he had worn the lens continuously – day and night for 1½–2 years at a time. Indeed, the lens was successfully worn with good tolerance and no apparent corneal damage for 21 years in total (Müller & Müller 1910, Müller 1920, Mann 1973).

The Müllers continued to produce thin, lightweight blown glass lenses with clear corneal regions and white scleral portions (Fig. 1.2), which were well tolerated. The optic portions were variable and years later it was proposed that the excellent toleration of these sealed glass lenses (and apparent avoidance of corneal oedema) was probably due to the characteristic aspheric shape of their scleral zones, producing loose channels for the free passage of fresh tears, oxygen to the cornea and removal of the waste products of corneal metabolism.

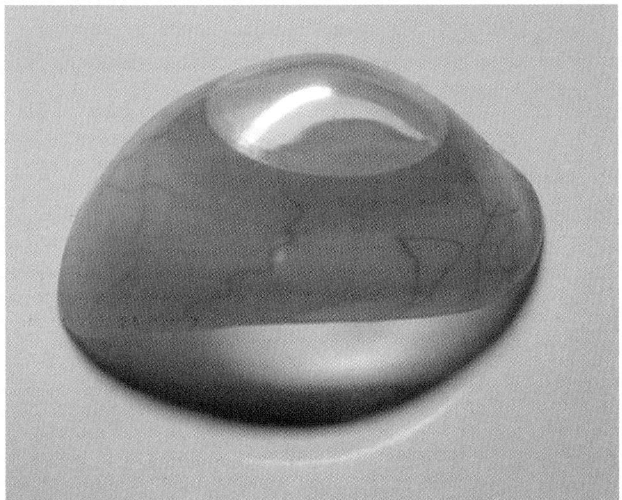

Figure 1.2 Blown glass Müller lens showing the transparent corneal and white scleral portions complete with blood vessels, circa 1900

Meanwhile, in Zurich, only about 185 miles south of the Müller brothers in Wiesbaden, was another pioneer in contact lens development.

1888: Adolf Eugen Fick was a German ophthalmologist who, after returning from South Africa, began work in the Ophthalmic Clinic in Zurich under Professor Haab. He was interested in keratoconus and had been experimenting with rabbits' eyes, making moulds of the cornea and constructing glass shells. He progressed to human cadaver eyes and had glass scleral lenses made by Professor Ernst Abbe at Zeiss Optical in Jena. Fick (1888) described six patients on whom he had tried his lenses: one was keratoconic, the other five having varying degrees of corneal opacity. In the keratoconic eye he improved the vision from 2/60 to 6/36 but at the time of publishing none of these patients was actually wearing the lenses for any length of time.

Fick was very observant and in his article he noted several points not previously documented.

- From plaster casts of human eyes, he observed that the radius of curvature of the cornea was steeper than that of the sclera or globe of the eye, and that the conjunctiva flattened steadily away from the cornea.
- Corneal oedema, later called Fick's phenomenon or Sattler's veil, was observed as clouding in the epithelial layer and Fick recognized that an adaptation process enabled the wearer to become more tolerant to lens usage. He also recognized that air trapped behind the contact lens on insertion retarded the onset of visual clouding.
- Inserting contact lenses disinfected with boiled 2% grape sugar solution gave 8–10 hours wear by his rabbits before corneal clouding developed.
- Cosmetic (prosthetic) contact shells, used when corneal scarring precluded good vision. Fick also suggested an iridectomy to produce an artificial pupil. A contact lens could then be fitted upon which an opaque iris and a black pupil was painted with a clear aperture positioned adjacent to the iridectomy. This he suggested as an alternative to corneal tattooing which often resulted in severe infection.
- Lenses used in aphakia where 'the high degree of hypermetropia could be diminished by increased curvature of the glass cornea'.
- Opaque lenses with pinhole apertures to correct the sight of keratoconic patients and those with irregular corneas.
- Preformed lenses for his rabbit experiments, using glass vesicles 21, 20 and 19 mm in diameter with a separate segment a few millimetres from the equator of the sphere. The lenses, subsequently made by Professor Abbe, had an optic radius of 8 mm, diameter of 14 mm and a scleral band of 3 mm width, with a radius of curvature of 15 mm. This made a total diameter of just less than 20 mm.

Professor Ernst Karl Abbe joined Carl Zeiss' optical works, on the banks of the River Saale in Jena, in 1866 as a research director. He was Professor of Physics and Mathematics at the University of Jena and a prolific inventor and writer of scientific papers on optics.

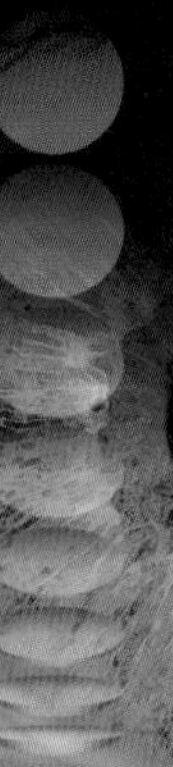

Abbe developed the first Zeiss contact lenses from glass refined and produced by Otto Schott, a glassmaker (www.zeiss.com).

1888: Straub introduced ophthalmological solutions of fluorescein for the investigation of corneal lesions. However, its fluorescent properties under blue light were not recognized for another 50 years (Straub 1888, Obrig 1938a).

1889: Eugene Kalt of Paris investigated corneal contact lenses as 'orthopaedic appliances' in the treatment of keratoconus. He laid the groundwork that led to contact lenses being considered as a means of myopia control and to their use in orthokeratology.

Between 1887 and 1889 another pioneer was working in Germany:

1889: August Müller, a final year medical student, presented his inaugural thesis at the University of Kiel for his doctorate in medicine. The dissertation, entitled 'Spectacle lenses and corneal lenses', was the correction of his own 14 dioptres of myopia with contact lenses. It was the first time a reference had been made to a 'corneal lens'. Müller did not pursue a career in ophthalmology but went into orthopaedics because of his poor sight. However, he did make several interesting observations which might explain why he was unsuccessful with his own lenses:

- The adverse signs and symptoms of lens wear were ascribed to '... a disturbance of nourishment of corneal tissue...'. This astute hypothesis appears to have been overlooked by later historians as a result of poor attempts at translation. It was not possible to validate Müller's hypothesis until the 1950s, when it was demonstrated that the cornea requires atmospheric oxygen, dissolved in tears, to maintain a normal respiratory status (Pearson 1978).
- Lens discomfort arose from pressure on the conjunctiva from the scleral zone of the lens.
- He had difficulty inserting his lenses without air bubbles and avoided this by inserting the lenses under water. This almost certainly limited tolerance because corneal oedema would develop within about 15 minutes.
- Discomfort, caused by marked hypotonicity of the liquid behind the contact lens, accounted for Müller's use of cocaine eye drops prior to lens insertion but the toxicity of cocaine would have further inhibited his success (Müller 1889).
- He thought Plaster of Paris was potentially suitable for taking living eye impressions. However, we now know that the setting characteristics of Plaster of Paris make it unsuitable for reproducing accurately the shape of a mobile living organ. In addition, the absorbent qualities of the drying plaster would create marked disturbance of the epithelial surface and its mucin coating.

1892: Henri Dor, an ophthalmologist in Lyons, Paris, recommended the use of physiological saline solution to insert contact lenses. This remained popular until the early 1940s (Dor 1892).

By 1892 the potential uses of contact lenses were realized. Correction of visual errors, protection of the exposed cornea, remoulding the corneal shape and neutralizing corneal irregularity were possible. Lenses could be used for cosmetic and prosthetic purposes and also as applicators of ophthalmic drugs.

Although the reasons for failure of contact lenses had been recognized, it took another 40 years before the topography and physiology of the anterior segment were understood well enough to predict successful lens wear.

In the early 20th century, lens choice lay between the blown glass lenses produced by the firm of Müllers of Wiesbaden and the ground glass contact lenses such as those made by Carl Zeiss of Jena. The former were inferior in consistency of optical quality, but superior in comfort and duration of wear. Zeiss lenses could correct reasonable amounts of ametropia but their maximum wearing time was between 30 minutes and 2 hours. Poor wearing times did not preclude the use of contact lenses for short-term application.

1900: Dr Louis de Wecker proposed the use of a contact splint to retain a corneal graft in position during healing (Mann 1938).

1911: Allvar Gullstrand of Sweden invented the slit-lamp, facilitating more detailed examination of the cornea.

1912: Carl Zeiss made ground glass 'experimental contact lenses' for Professor H. Erggelet to induce artificial ametropia in order to test 'the optical quality of the corrected curve glasses' (Obrig & Salvatori 1957a). These were actually corneal lenses but were too heavy to wear successfully (von Rohr & Stock 1912, Mann 1938).

1917: Mustard gas was first used in trench warfare in Ypres in July 1917. The official number of non-fatal mustard gas casualties in World War I was 160,526 (the number of fatalities was 4,086) (Tallet 1998).

Mustard gas is soluble in water, making it difficult to wash off. Hydrolysis, the splitting of a compound by water, is rapid and the chemical causes blisters on contact with any damp skin or mucous membrane. The lungs and eyes are acutely targeted. Those surviving the lung effects endured loss of corneal epithelium, stromal opacification and thinning followed by secondary infection and uveitis. Later, abnormalities of the limbal vascular bed, ischaemia and ulceration can occur (Fig. 1.3) (www.dh.gov.uk/PublicationsAndStatistics/fs/en). Fitting contact

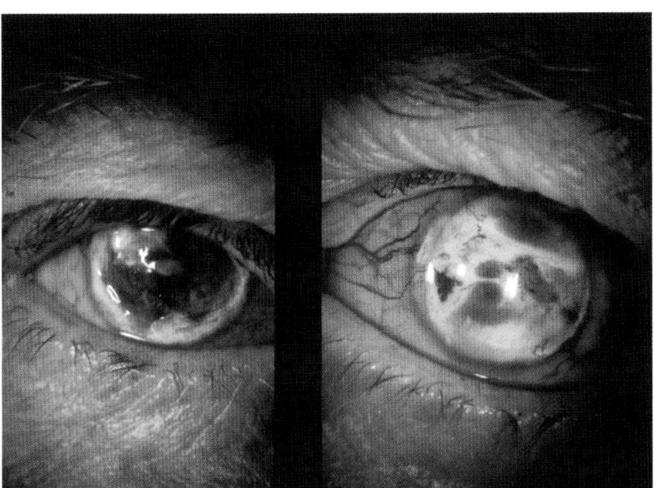

Figure 1.3 Mustard gas injuries from World War I

lenses could help restore optical function but tolerance was still a problem (see p. 10, 1939+: Dallos).

1918: Zeiss lenses were made with small lead pellets embedded in them to assist locating ophthalmic foreign bodies in conjunction with X-ray images.

1918: Dr L. Koeppe described a contact lens for specialist observation of internal features of the eye using a slit-lamp biomicroscope. This type of short-use lens was termed a gonioscope (Koeppe 1918).

1920: Carl Zeiss manufactured a four-lens preformed fitting set primarily for the investigation of keratoconus. It was introduced and developed by Stock (1920) who was a sufferer of the condition. The first lens had a 12 mm back scleral radius but later a full range from 10.0 to 14.0 mm in 0.25 mm steps became available (Dallos 1936).

1927: Adolf Wilhelm Mueller-Welt of Stuttgart, Germany, was descended from a family of artificial glass eye makers. Starting with the experience of making and fitting artificial eyes, Mueller-Welt (1950) described the design of his lenses as having 'a capillary tear layer over the cornea and retaining an air cushion beneath the scleral zone'.

The lenses, made from glass obtained from Schott of Jena, were blown over a series of preformed toric castings, which formed the scleral portion of the lens. These included areas of differing curvature to incorporate the insertions of the recti muscles (Schiller 1969). The unfinished corneal portion was later ground and polished to the desired prescription.

Among those with whom Mueller-Welt worked and sought advice were Professors Heine, Sattler, Siegrist and Stock, as well as with many university eye clinics in Germany and other European countries. His work prospered greatly and he was granted patent DRP.Nr. 553843 in 1932. He understood the stresses produced by working the glass and was able to relax the tension in the structure to improve his lenses (Figs 1.4–1.8).

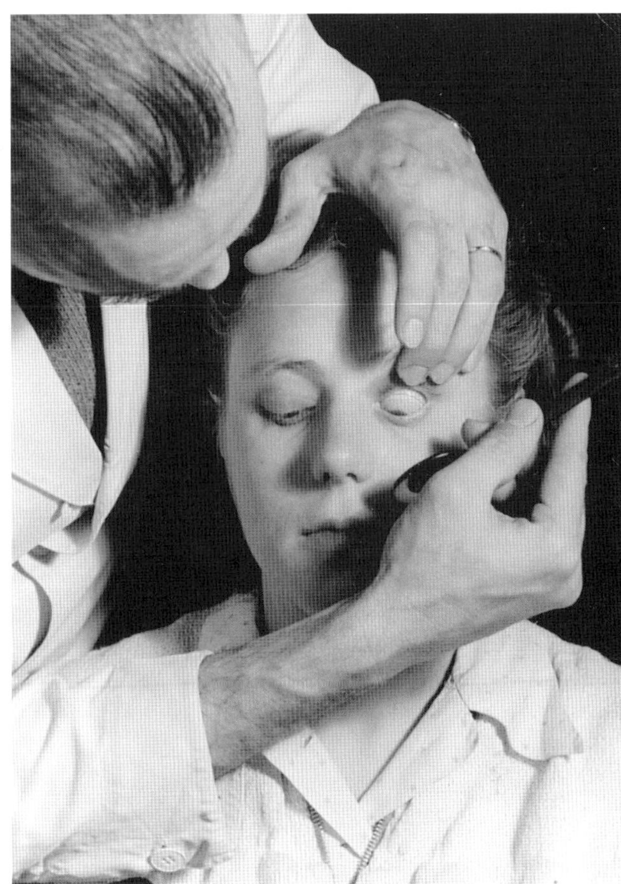

Figure 1.4 Mueller-Welt GmbH lenses being fitted to a patient c.1950 (Courtesy of Brigitte Mueller-Welt Caffrey, daughter of Adolf Mueller-Welt)

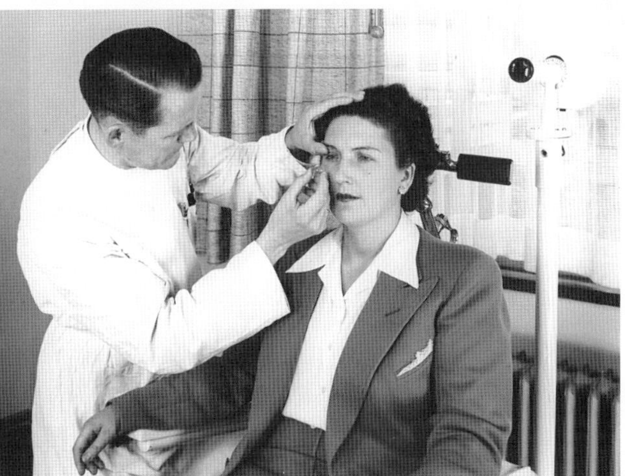

Figure 1.5 Mueller-Welt GmbH lenses being fitted to a patient c.1950 (Courtesy of Brigitte Mueller-Welt Caffrey)

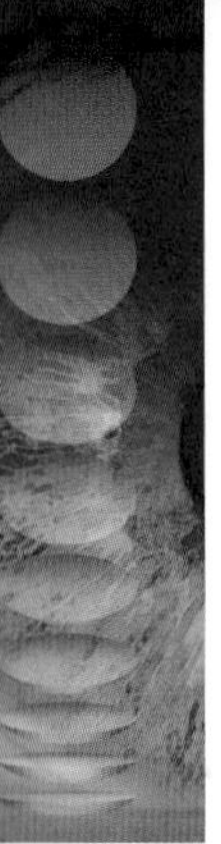

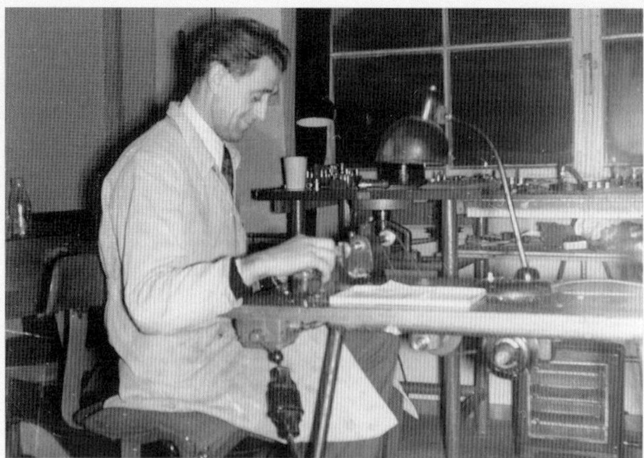

Figure 1.6 Lathing and polishing of Mueller-Welt GmbH lenses (Courtesy of Brigitte Mueller-Welt Caffrey)

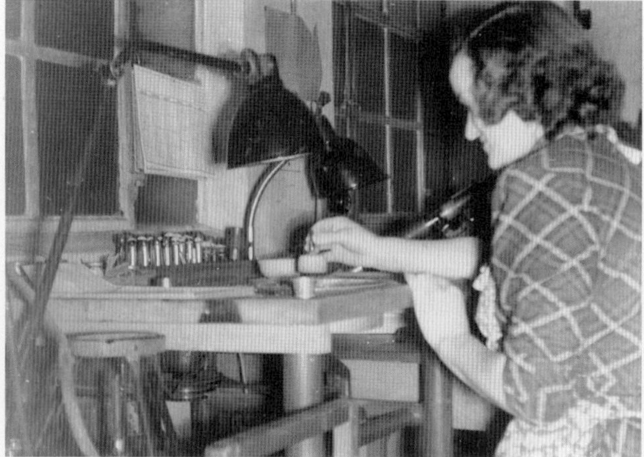

Figure 1.7 Lathing and polishing of Mueller-Welt GmbH lenses (Courtesy of Brigitte Mueller-Welt Caffrey)

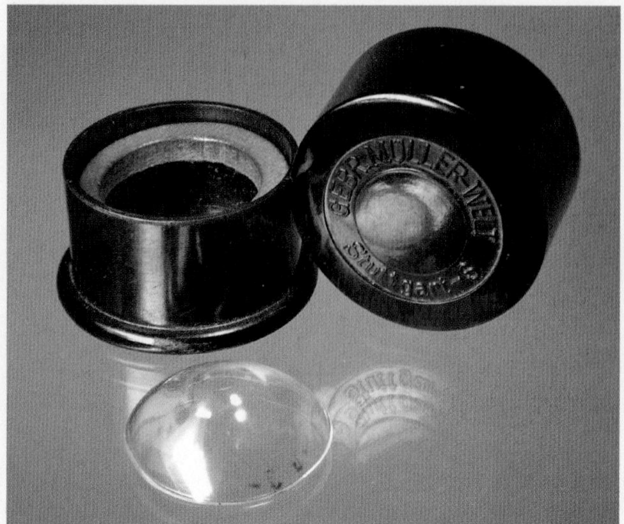

Figure 1.8 Glass scleral Mueller-Welt lens and case (originally Müller-Welt)

From 1930 to 1950, developments were numerous. They are split into three sections although they all evolved simultaneously:

- *Impressions of the eye.*
- *The move from glass to plastics.*
- *Designing and making the lenses.*

IMPRESSIONS OF THE EYE

The ability to reproduce the exact corneal shape was important in the development of successful contact lens wear and this was achieved through accurate impressions made of the eye. Since 1880 there had been many attempts to replicate the surface. After 1930, more information on ocular topography began to emerge as techniques improved.

- **1930: Josef Dallos**, a physician at the No. 1 Eye Clinic at the Royal Hungarian Peter Pazmany University at Budapest (Fig. 1.9), developed an interest in the use of contact lenses for the correction of visual defects. To this end, he investigated various impression materials and used Negocoll (derived from seaweed and described by Dr Alphons Poller of Zurich) on a cadaver face and noted that the corneal surface was reproduced with a smooth polished texture. He prepared a positive cast of this impression in the wax-like substance Hominit and the smooth appearance of the visible corneal segment convinced him that Negocoll would be a suitable medium for ophthalmic impressions (Dallos, J., personal communication; 1977). Dallos used Müller contact lenses as impression trays (Sabell 1980a).
- **1936: Theodore E. Obrig**, an optical technician who later studied medicine, worked for Gall and Lembke in New York. He also used Negocoll to produce corneal impressions in funnel-shaped blown glass shells. These were 22 mm in diameter, 7 mm deep and had a 25 mm long hollow handle plugged with cotton wool to retain the Negocoll. The shells were marked with coloured spots or

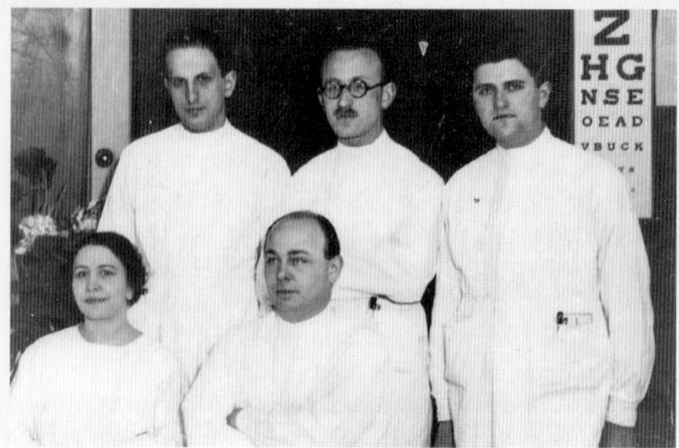

Figure 1.9 Dallos at No. 1 Eye Clinic in Budapest (centre, back row)

lines, red for right and light blue for left, which also indicated the position of the nasal canthus on the otherwise round shell. Some time later, he drilled perforations in the tray for the impression material to key on to and a variety of different sized, oval-shaped impression trays to conform to various eye shapes and sizes (Obrig 1938b). From the measurement of a large number of impression casts Obrig produced a table showing average corneal dimensions, which set the pattern of full corneal clearance fitting during the following decade.

- **1936: C. L. Stevens** in New York described an alternative method of producing eye impressions with Negocoll, using aluminium tubes in the same manner as von Csapody's glass cylinders (von Csapody 1929). These formed the impression trays that rested on the eye surface and held the lids apart. They were about 1 inch (2.5 cm) in length and squeezed to form an oval section corresponding more nearly to the palpebral aperture (Stevens 1936).

Other advances were taking place at this time:

1936: Carl Hubert Sattler, an Austrian ophthalmologist working in Leipzig, investigated the corneal oedema induced by wearing ground spherical contact lenses (Sattler's veil) (Sattler 1938).

Investigation of the cornea was becoming easier by means of improved equipment and techniques:

1938: Theodore E. Obrig accidentally discovered that a blue filter introduced into a slit-lamp beam greatly enhanced the brightness of fluorescein solution. This made limbal pressure from contact lenses more obvious (Obrig 1938a).

While moulding continued to be used as a regular method of initial contact lens fitting, more impression materials were being developed:

- **1939: Maisler** described 'a reversible hydrocolloid gel' introduced some months earlier by a San Francisco dental surgeon. This material – Kerr's hydrocolloid – was manufactured by the Detroit Dental Manufacturing Company and was packaged in collapsible toothpaste-type tubes. The tube was immersed in hot water and kneaded to soften the consistency. It was applied onto the eye at 100–104°F (38–40°C). Maisler found that the blown-glass impression trays as recommended by Obrig (1938b) were too fragile and described his own thin silver trays which were sufficiently malleable to be adjusted for each eye (Maisler 1939).
- **1943: Theodore Obrig**, still working to simplify and improve his eye impressions, introduced Ophthalmic Moldite, the first cold alginate impression material intended specifically for ophthalmic work. By now he was using acrylic impression trays with hollow tubular handles and perforated bowls instead of his earlier blown glass ones (Obrig 1943).
- **1945: Dental Zelex**, a cold setting impression material, was used in the UK. Ophthalmic Zelex was developed by Charles Keeler in Windsor, UK, during World War II (Fig. 1.10).
- **1947: Obrig Laboratories** opened a London branch and Moldite became readily available.
- **1948:** American optometrists were not allowed to use anaesthesia without a physician being present due to the drug laws. An injection method of moulding was developed so that the patient's eye could remain stationary while the impression material was being applied and avoid unseen contact between the cornea and the impression shell (Steele 1948).
- **1949: Drs Newton Wesley and George Jessen** in Chicago produced yet another corneal moulding technique – 'concentric moulding'. It used a contact lens-like impression tray with no handle and the inside surface was 'scored or grooved' for good adhesion of the Moldite. The theory was that, provided the impression tray had the same dimensions and proportions as the finished lens, it would centre itself accurately with its optic zone corresponding to the patient's cornea, so that eye positioning was not critical (Jessen & Wesley 1949).

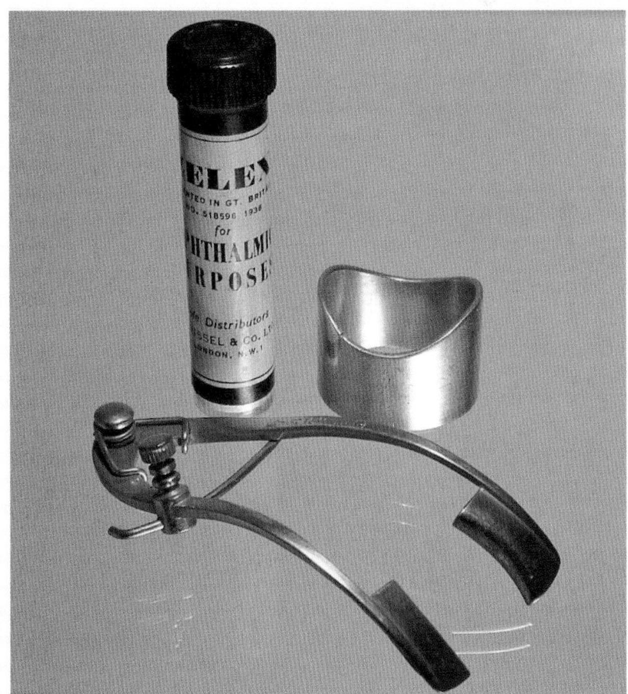

Figure 1.10 Ophthalmic Zelex (1945+), aluminium tubes for impression material applied to the eye (Stevens 1936) and gold-plated lid retractors

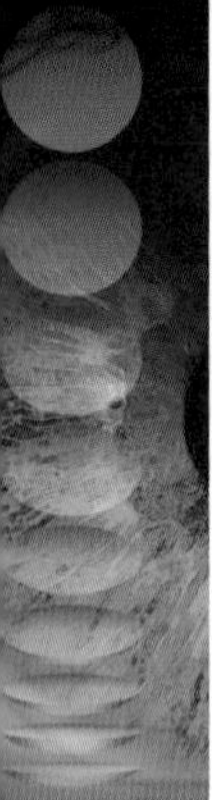

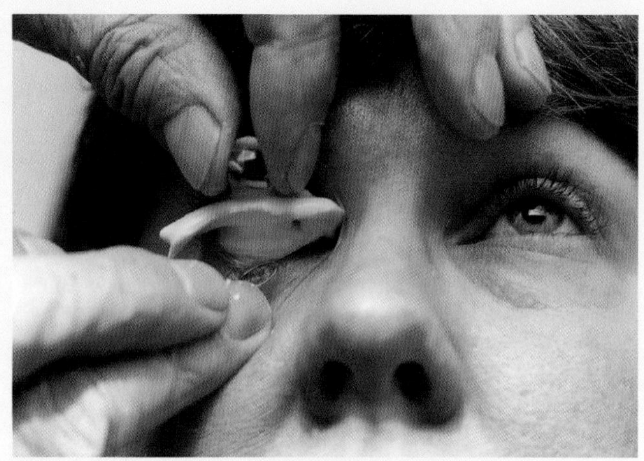

Figure 1.11 Orthoprint impression being removed using a blunt squint hook

- **1950+: Frederick Burnett-Hodd** in London, UK, developed the method of using trays without handles, which, in certain circumstances, was superior to the use of trays with handles.
- **1950: George Nissel**, a contact lens manufacturer, packaged Ophthalmic Zelex into single-dose plastic tubes (Fig. 1.10).
- More recently there has been a return to dental alginates, such as Tissutex, Kromopan and Orthoprint (Fig. 1.11). Storey (1972) published some observations on the possible use of polysulphide rubber impression materials, and silicone rubber impression materials became popular with some practitioners (Silk, A., personal communication; 1982).

THE MOVE FROM GLASS TO PLASTIC

Up until the mid 1930s, all contact lenses had been made of blown or ground glass. Since the mid 20th century, new materials called plastics had been developing.

Originally, these were made of resins derived from vegetable matter such as cellulose (from cotton), furfural (from oat hulls), oils (from seeds) and starch derivatives. Casein (from milk) was a non-vegetable material that was used. More recently, most raw materials are derived from the petrochemical industry.

Plastics – polymers made up of long chains of monomers – went through a developmental evolution as new chemical compounds, solvents and methods of manufacture were invented. They provided new materials for scientific experimentation: cellulose nitrate (celluloid; highly flammable), cellulose acetate (used in spectacle frames), bakelite (made into multiple household objects), polyvinyl acetate (emulsion paint and adhesives), polyacrylates (developed by Otto Rohm and Otto Haas in their factory in Darmstadt and used in paint) and polystyrene (made by Imperial Chemical Industries (ICI) into numerous household electrical items).

1931: Chalmers, in Canada, described a new hard methacrylate polymer. **John Crawford** and **Rowland Hill,** working separately for ICI in the UK, developed polymethylmethacrylate (PMMA), which led to a transformation in contact lens development. The registered trade name was 'Perspex' but it had several other names such as Lucite, Plexiglas and Diakon. The Rohm & Haas Company were licensed to use the ICI process to make Plexiglas sheets in Germany in the mid 1930s. (Anderson 1952; www.plastiquarian.com).

From the mid 1930s plastic contact lenses started to replace glass. One of the authors (Sabell 1980b) described several plastic scleral lenses, which predate the introduction of PMMA. Early plastics used in the USA failed, principally through their unsuitability.

- **1936: William Feinbloom**, a New York optometrist, introduced a scleral lens using a plastic material for the haptic portion and bonded it to a central glass optic zone. In his report he acknowledged Mr George S. Weith, chief of the Research Division of the Bakelite Corporation of America, with having developed this resin (Feinbloom 1936).
- **1938: Theodore E. Obrig** in New York, together with an engineer called Mullen, made the first plastic contact lens using the newly discovered 'Plexiglas'. The material was lightweight, optically clear, non-reactive, easily moulded, ground and polished, and inexpensive. However, Obrig was still using fluid-filled sealed scleral lenses, which meant that the normal saline solution filling the lens had to be changed every few hours to prevent corneal oedema. He set up the Obrig Laboratories in the USA making an all-plastic, moulded scleral lens.
- **1938: Dr Istvan Györffy**, a Hungarian ophthalmologist working in the Maria Street Eye Clinic in Budapest (where Dallos also worked) was the first to use PMMA for contact lenses in Europe. He came across the material during a visit to Germany in 1938 (Györffy 1964) and appreciated its potential. On his return to Budapest he developed a technique for moulding this sheet plastic and grinding the back and front optic surfaces. By late 1938 he had begun to fit acrylic scleral lenses and later went on to fit corneal lenses in this material (Györffy 1940, 1950, 1968, 1980, 1981).
- **1938: C. W. Dixey & Son Ltd** in the UK introduced lathe-turned preformed acrylic scleral lenses, which were easier both to produce and to modify (Dixey 1943, Ridley 1946). Dixeys used a precision lathe to cut contact lenses from solid blocks of ICI Transpex material. The lathe was developed by Harry Birchall, a dispensing optician, and Cyril Winter, an engineer. The process allowed greater variability in dimensions than was readily obtainable from the glass-grinding methods of Zeiss. The lenses could also be made thinner (0.3 mm) than Zeiss lenses without

becoming excessively fragile, saving about 60% on the weight. A glass corneal lens made by Zeiss in 1932 measured 0.6 mm thick, whereas a 1948 acrylic lens measured 0.3 mm thick. The glass lens was at least four times the weight of the plastic one (Graham 1959).

DESIGNING AND MAKING THE LENS

Corneal measurement and reproduction was becoming more precise, leading to a better understanding of contact lens fitting. It was recognized that much intolerance was due to limbal pressure, especially at the nasal and temporal positions.

1929: Professor Leopold Heine, an ophthalmologist at Kiel, Germany, extended the original fitting set of Zeiss lenses to design the 'afocal lens' range (Heine 1929). This developed into a large afocal lens set where the increasing range of back optic zone radii utilized the liquid lens alone to correct the ametropia. Some optical power could be ground onto the Zeiss prescription lens so that the total correction was made up of a combination of the liquid lens and the optical power of the contact lens. This was limited to approximately ±7.00 D.

1930s: Josef Dallos in Budapest was moulding clear, thin glass photographic plates to produce an initial contact shell. He transferred a Negocoll impression, via a Hominit positive cast, to a Plaster of Paris negative cast. Using basic equipment, it was finally converted into a brass die suitable for the glass moulding (Sabell 1980c) (Figs 1.12, 1.13). The heated metal die was secured in the swinging arm of the press and pushed into the softened glass plate at a suitable temperature, as judged by its colour. The heat was then removed and the glass solidified immediately. The central zone of these shells had to be able to be optically ground and polished.

This method of manufacturing lenses could be used, with some minor modifications, for the new acrylic materials introduced some 10 years later. Dallos laid down physiological principles for the fitting of scleral contact lenses. Working on the assumption that the natural body fluid offers the best chance of success, he set out to conserve the tear reservoir and to allow for its interchange by fresh tears.

In 1933, Dallos suggested that if the front optic diameter were restricted to 8 mm, much higher optical values would be achievable, which would reduce lens thickness and weight.

1930+: Theodore Obrig in the USA initiated the full clearance method of fitting scleral lenses by using a large optic zone, improving comfort by reducing corneal pressure. Although it was widely used in the USA and the UK, it had some drawbacks (Dickinson & Hall 1946):

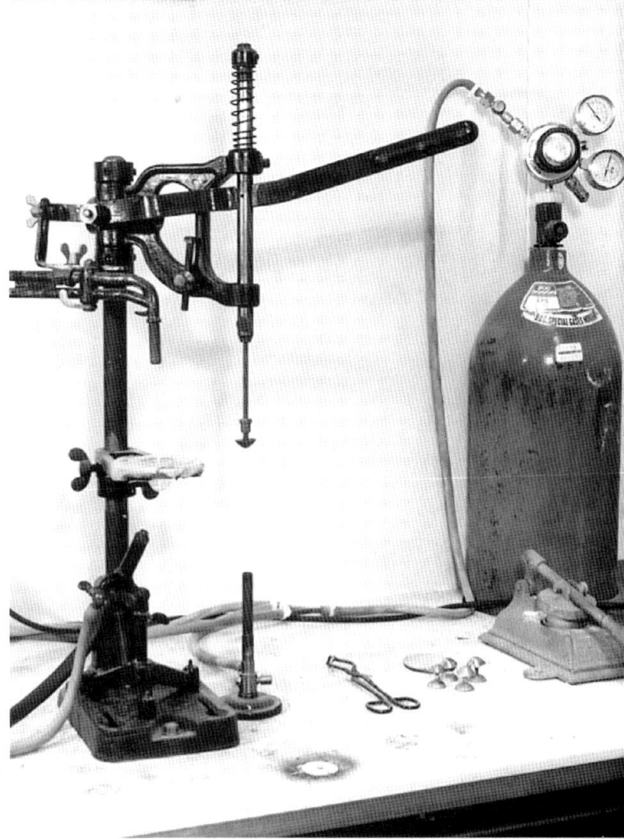

Figure 1.12 Dallos' press for making glass lenses

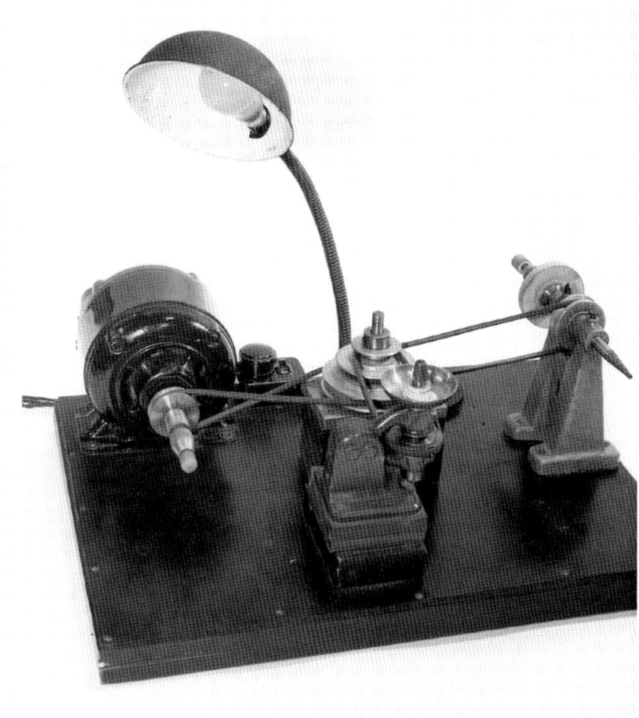

Figure 1.13 Dallos' lens modifying spindles c.1945

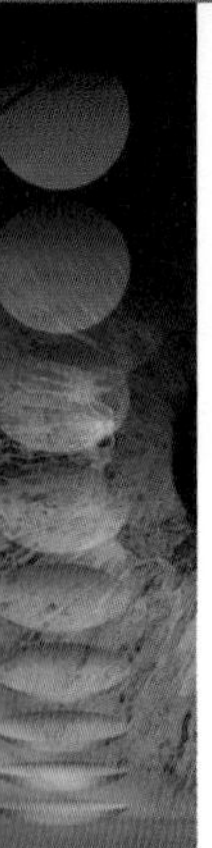

- Cosmetically, the large optic zone of full corneal clearance was ugly.
- As the steep optic had to remain filled with fluid for the wearer to see, a glove-like seal was required on the scleral zone. Any air seeping under the scleral portion resulted in an air bubble trapped in the steep apex of the lens in front of the pupil.
- Sattler's veil developed after some 2 hours of wear, visible to the wearer more readily indoors as a faint blue haze resembling tobacco smoke. Shortly after onset, the classic rainbow rings, resembling glaucoma haloes, would be seen. Few patients were able to pursue lens wear for more than about 30 minutes after the onset of these symptoms because the developing corneal oedema produced photophobia, blepharospasm and an unpleasant sensation of heat.

1933: Professor Hans Hartinger suggested blending the sharp junction between optic and scleral zones of the Zeiss lens. Zeiss trade literature offered the option of totally blended transition lenses (Dallos 1936). This removed the 'sharp edge' which touched the eye close to the limbal area. Using this same reasoning, Forknall (1948) later introduced the 'offset scleral lens'.

1935/36: Zeiss records show a number of companies and institutions to whom 20 mm glass 'corneal-type' contact lenses were supplied. Professor H. J. M. Weve used glass corneal lenses to maintain corneal clarity while performing detachment surgery (Mann 1938, Obrig & Salvatori 1957b).

Circa 1933, Kenneth Dunscombe was probably the first optometrist (ophthalmic optician) in the UK to fit contact lenses, followed by Frank Dickinson, Keith Clifford Hall and Geoff McKellen. Up until then, ophthalmologists and optical dispensers were predominantly the developers of the contact lens as a result of their working closely together in practice.

1936: Joseph Dallos in Budapest had accumulated so many glass shells from his earlier impressions that he was eventually able to fit from his stock of 'type shells'. He demonstrated that the secret of fitting scleral lenses was not just the initial selection or the initial impression but the careful tailoring of this first lens to the precise requirements of the individual eye. To this modification procedure Dallos gave the title 'haptics', which he described in 1936 as 'a new branch of prosthetics'. Because of his success, he continued to fit glass scleral lenses by this method until his death in 1979 (Dallos 1936).

1937: Ida Mann was the first woman to become a consultant ophthalmologist at Moorfields Eye Hospital, London (1927) and the first female professor at Oxford (1945). Together with **Andrew Rugg-Gunn**, an ophthalmologist from Western Eye Hospital, London, and Frederick Williamson-Nobel, a consulting surgeon to St Mary's, Paddington and Moorfields Eye Hospital, and later Consultant to the Royal Navy, visited Dallos in Budapest to 'learn the skills of making scleral lenses'. They soon realized that the skills required in scleral lens fitting were too complex to learn on a short trip and tried to persuade Dallos to move to the UK, but he refused.

The following year, Ida Mann returned to Hungary. Preparations for war had caused conditions to deteriorate and it was obvious that Dallos' work in Budapest could be destroyed. As a Hungarian of Jewish extraction he was at great risk. Ida Mann was able to persuade him to go to England where Theodore Hamblin, who owned the Hamblin Dispensing outlets, had agreed to set up a contact lens clinic for him in Cavendish Square attached to their London Wigmore Street premises.

- **1938: Joseph Dallos** and **George Nissel**, Dallos' brother-in-law and contact lens technician, arrived in London and commenced contact lens production and improvements in design.
- **1939+: Dallos** was able to successfully fit 84 late onset mustard gas keratitis casualties, their injuries dating from World War I, with scleral lenses (Mann 1973).

1942: Adolf Mueller-Welt and his wife Ruth travelled throughout Germany and occupied Europe during World War II fitting fluid-less glass scleral lenses to German officers who, in those years, were not allowed to wear spectacles while in uniform. They took with them cases of lens sets with five to six thousand lenses in each, and were thus able to fit almost all corrections (Schiller 1969). Deteriorating conditions of war stopped such travel by 1944.

1945: William Feinbloom in New York decided that minimal tangential touch would not only evoke less sensation but would enable a better balanced fit on the toroidally shaped sclera. He introduced the 'Feincone lens' with an optic radius of 8.5 mm and cone angles of 43°, 46° and 49°. Unfortunately, it was a full clearance lens and therefore did nothing to reduce the effects of Sattler's veil (Feinbloom 1945).

In the 1940s, further improvements of Dallos' minimum clearance lenses transformed patients' wearing times to all-day wear.

1945+: Norman Bier and **Phillip Cole,** both optometrists in the UK, introduced a small set of preformed fitting shells that supplemented the fitting sets of the Dixey lenses then in use. This was the 'transcurve lens' and its originators claimed cosmetic superiority by virtue of a total diameter larger than that of the Dixey-type preformed lens. The most significant contribution associated with the transcurve lens was the introduction of the separate corneal measuring caps, later referred to as fenestrated lenses for optic measurement (FLOM) (see Chapter 15) (Bier & Cole 1948).

1946+: Joseph Dallos and **Norman Bier,** working independently, formulated the fenestrated or 'ventilated' scleral lens (Bier 1945, 1948, Dallos 1946). Dallos happened upon the idea by accident when he was forced to cut a 4 mm hole in a glass scleral lens to relieve the pressure on a 'filtration scar' (trabeculectomy) (Fig. 1.14). Immediately the comfortable wearing time of the lens doubled. He experimented with slots and holes and found the most successful position for a small hole fenestration was on the temporal part of the lens close to the limbus, which had the effect of sucking in an air bubble on nasal gaze.

Independently, Norman Bier took out a patent (Fig. 1.15) for a series of slotted and fenestrated lenses in order to 'permit lachrymal fluid and air to flow' through the lens.

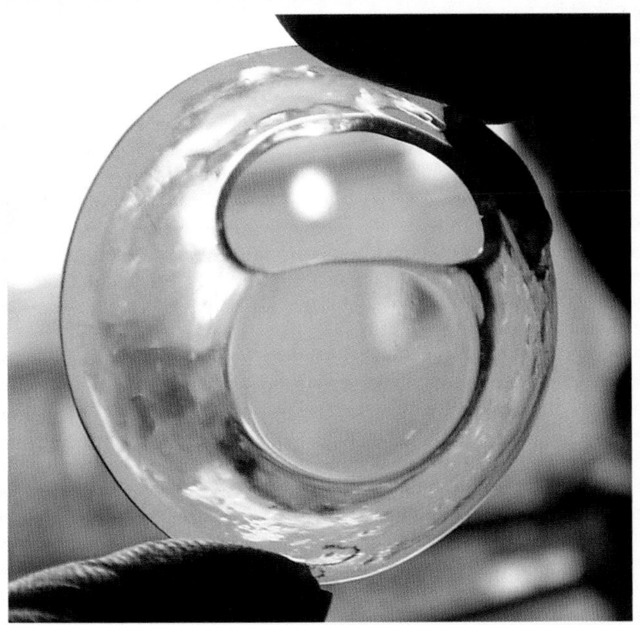

Figure 1.14 Dallos' original glass lens with a hole for the fenestrated filtration scar, lens engraved '... *3703*' with repair at the upper temporal edge

SCLERAL TO CORNEAL

1946: Kevin Tuohy, an optical dispenser and partner in the firm of Solex in California with Solon Braff and Xavier Villagram, was making a scleral lens of high negative power. He was finishing the optic zone when the corneal portion cracked away producing a perfect disc. He and his wife were both myopes and the corneal portion was about his wife's prescription. Tuohy polished the edges of the lens

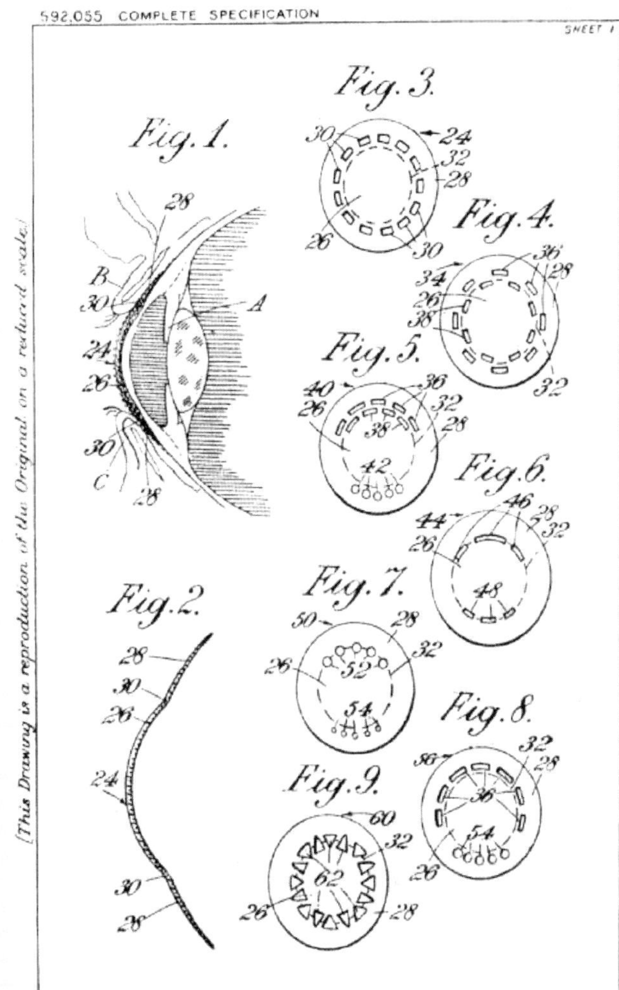

Figure 1.15 Norman Bier's patent for fenestrated lenses

and took it home to try on his wife. He then designed, manufactured and patented the corneal lens (patent granted in 1950).

The first Tuohy lens was 11 mm in diameter and 0.4 mm thick. It was a monocurve lens and fitted flatter than flattest *K* (www.nova.edu); 2 D of corneal astigmatism was considered to be the limit of its corneal astigmatic correction (Bier 1957).

1946: Heinrich Wöhlk, an engineer in Kiel, North Germany, designed his first PMMA lens, the 'Parabolar', after his 8 D of hypermetropia was corrected by Professor Leopold Heine with a Zeiss lens. Wöhlk's lens was similar in size to modern corneal lenses (Bier 1957).

1947: Raymond Kelvin Watson, an optometrist in Manchester, introduced his 'Kelvin Conic Lens' (Watson 1947), a scleral

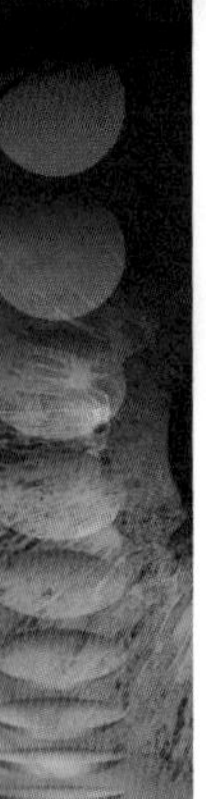

lens with a spherical optic zone and a conical sclera. It had an extra curve at the temporal side in an attempt to give a closer scleral fit (Sabell 1980b).

Watson started the Kelvin Contact Lens company and developed methods of moulding both scleral and corneal lenses (McKellen 1949).

1947: George Nissel had set up his own lens manufacturing laboratory in Siddons Lane, London, and produced the 'wide angle lens' based on the Feincone design. This was a scleral lens with spherical optic and scleral zones linked with a conical section. This, together with the Feincone and Kelvin Conic lenses, aimed to reduce the vast numbers of permutations introduced by the Dixey system by standardizing the diameter of the optic zone.

Numerous lens designs, searching for the ultimate in comfort and wearability, were becoming available:

1948: Arthur Forknall, an optometrist from Wollaton in Nottingham, designed the 'offset lens' – again a scleral lens with a spherical optic and an aspherical scleral zone attempting to give even pressure on the sclera. It simplified fitting by eliminating the need to adjust the scleral zone radius when the total diameter was changed. As McKellen (1963) pointed out, this design was neglected by most contact lens practitioners until it was later reintroduced by Montague Ruben as an offset corneal lens in 1966.

1950: George Butterfield, an optical dispenser in the USA, improved on Tuohy's design to produce a better fitting corneal lens. It was 9.50 mm diameter and approximately 0.2 mm thick with a bicurve design.

The performance and comfort of a corneal lens depends upon the ability of the upper lid to raise the lens on the cornea after each blink. PMMA, which was very light compared to glass, led to the success of corneal lenses.

1952: Frank Dickinson (UK), **Wilhelm Sohnges** (Germany) and **John C. Neil** (USA) made their own modifications to the corneal lens and introduced it into all three countries. It was lathe-cut in the UK and both lathe-cut and moulded in Germany. The lenses were fitted approximately 0.65 mm flatter than flattest corneal radius and manufactured as a single curve with a total diameter of 9.5 mm. They were much better than the larger Tuohy lenses (Dickinson 1954). Frank Dickinson's wife, Muriel, coined the name 'Microlens' and, due to its small diameter, it could correct up to 4 D of corneal toricity.

Both the Microlens and the Tuohy lens produced heavy apical touch, which caused corneal erosions. The smaller, thinner Microlens had obvious advantages and its designers specified that centre thickness should be calculated on the basis of an afocal lens of centre thickness 0.2 mm with no edge bevel.

Problems caused by long periods of flat lens wear led to further developments in corneal lenses:

1955: Norman Bier introduced his 'Contour Principle' lens. This was a corneal lens with multiple back surface curves. Of similar size and thickness to the Microlens, Bier's 'contour lens' was fitted nearly in alignment with the central corneal zone, thereby reducing the problem of corneal erosions.

Edge clearance was maintained by a peripheral curve some 1.25 mm wide. Bier postulated that flatter corneas were likely to require greater peripheral curve flattening, relative to the back optic zone radius (BOZR), than steeper corneas. He therefore recommended fitting sets in which the degree of peripheral flattening ranged from 0.3 mm for a BOZR of 7.3 mm to 0.7 mm for a BOZR of 8.5 mm. This system was complicated and, from about 1960, fitting sets with standard peripheral flattening were employed. It is interesting that 40 years later, fitting sets commonly use Bier's principle and have a constant edge lift (see Chapter 9).

Bier also laid down the principles of apical clearance fitting but this was not popular and did not gain acceptance until later design changes allowed its full exploitation (Bier 1956a,b).

1955: John de Carle, an optometrist in London, developed a bifocal corneal lens of concentric design with a centre portion focused for distance correction surrounded by the reading portion. It was based on an idea of ophthalmologist Frederick Williamson-Noble, who had adapted one of Dallos' scleral lenses (de Carle, J., personal communication; 2004) (Fig. 1.16). The lens was of limited success as the size of the optic was too small to be effective.

1960+: George Jessen and **Newton K. Wesley** in Chicago observed that when rigid contact lenses were fitted flat in relation to the cornea, the patient stopped becoming more myopic and could actually reverse their prescription over time. Many improved to the point where they no longer needed any corrective lenses and could see 6/6 (20/20) for short periods (see Chapter 19).

Between 1960 and 1970 corneal lenses continued to develop. Narrower intermediate and peripheral zones in multicurve lenses led to numerous variations of back surface designs: aspheric corneal lenses with tangential conic peripheries (Thomas 1968, Stek 1969), continuous offset bicurve lenses

(a)

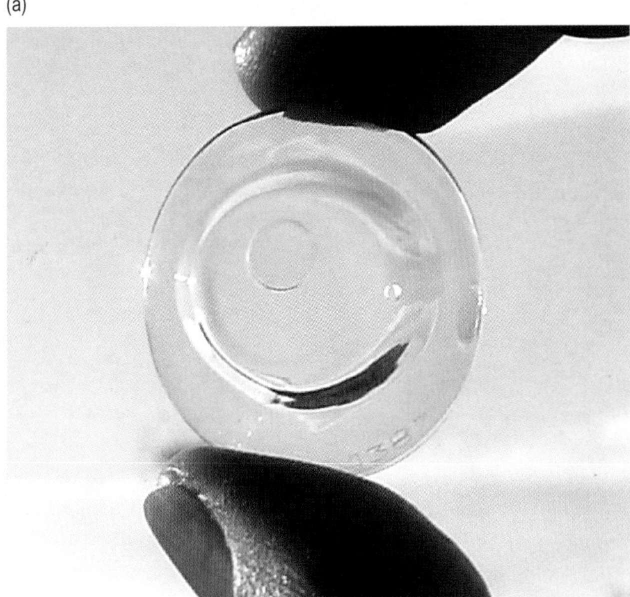

(b)

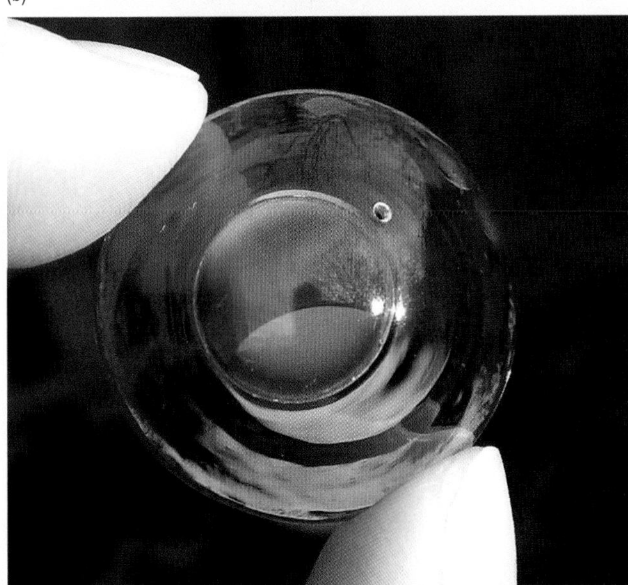

Figure 1.16 Two of Dallos' glass lenses adapted as bifocals: (a) engraved '7104387' with a circular reading zone close to the centre; (b) with a central bifocal lens fused onto the scleral carrier. Note the slight yellowing of the central fused lens

(Ruben 1966, Nissel 1967), lathe-cut continuous aspheric lenses (Nissel 1968) and the 'Kelvin Continuous Curve' corneal lens designed by Raymond Kelvin Watson.

Lenses could be fenestrated to minimize central corneal oedema (though this could cause 'dimple veil' in a steep fitting lens) or truncated in weighted prism ballasted cases. There were numerous variations.

1967: Fraser and Gordon designed the 'Apex lens' specifically for the hospital service. The name 'Apex' is derived from 'aphakic experiment'. The large semi-scleral design is quite thick and heavy in aphakic prescriptions but it provides stability of vision from its limbal locating characteristics (Ruben 1967). However, its long-term use in PMMA material led to corneal neovascularization in many cases (Fraser & Gordon 1967). The design is still used in high Dk materials for high prescriptions (see Chapter 21).

The time line now splits to describe the development of soft, rigid gas-permeable (RGP) and silicone rubber lenses. Developments are described separately although they occurred in parallel.

THE SOFT LENS

1961: Otto Wichterle was a Professor of Chemistry in Prague and director of the newly established Institute of Macromolecular Chemistry of the Czechoslovak Academy of Sciences. His second doctorate was in organic chemistry. From 1952, he worked with Dr Maximillian Dreifus, an ophthalmologist of the Second Eye Hospital in Prague. Wichterle, together with his assistant, Drahoslav Lim, had devoted themselves to studying the synthesis of cross-linking hydrophilic gels which expanded their volume in water with the aim of finding a material suitable for eye implants.

They succeeded in preparing a cross-linking gel, 2-hydroxyethylmethacrylate (pHEMA). It was transparent, absorbed up to 40% of water and exhibited good mechanical properties (Dreifus 1978). In December of 1961 Wichterle, continuing his experiments at home to transform hydrogels into a suitable shape for a contact lens, used his son's construction set to assemble the first prototype of a centrifugal casting device. It was driven by a bicycle dynamo and connected to a bell transformer and its glasswork was blown by Otto. With this he cast his first four lenses.

An announcement in the *New Scientist* on 18 January 1962 stated that Otto Wichterle had developed contact lenses made of a new 'hydrocolloid' material (Wichterle et al. 1961, ASCR Office Press Department 1962) (Figs 1.17, 1.18).

1964: Geltakt lens and **SPOFA-Lens** were the first soft lenses manufactured by Protetika in Prague, Czechoslovakia. Dr Dreifus produced the guidelines for their fitting and prescribing. The SPOFA lens was made with a single back surface curve steeper than the human cornea in the hope that it would conform to the corneal contours as the material was so flexible. The original lenses were spun cast and had an aspherical back surface derived from their mode of manufacture. The lenses were 10 mm and 12–13 mm in diameter, respectively.

Many difficulties were faced: the optical quality varied, as did the power and thickness. The resultant corneal oedema limited the wearing time to below 8 hours. There were also

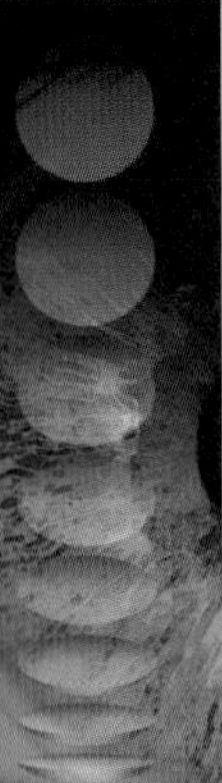

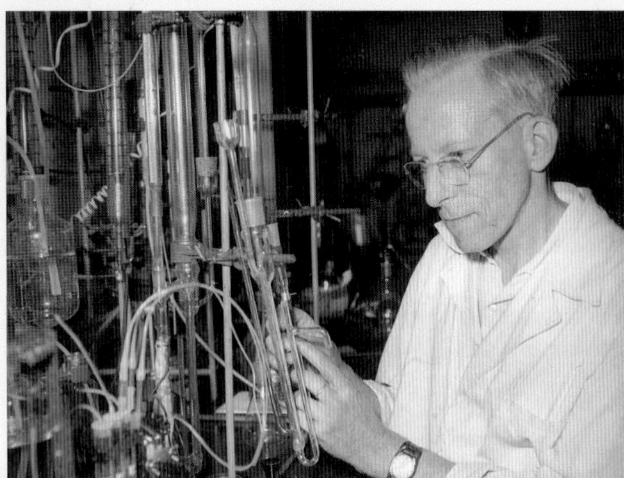

Figure 1.17 Portrait of Otto Wichterle made in his Institute of Macromolecular Chemistry of the Academy of Sciences, July 12 1962 (Courtesy of the Archives of the Academy of Sciences of the Czech Republic, from the personal papers of Otto Wichterle)

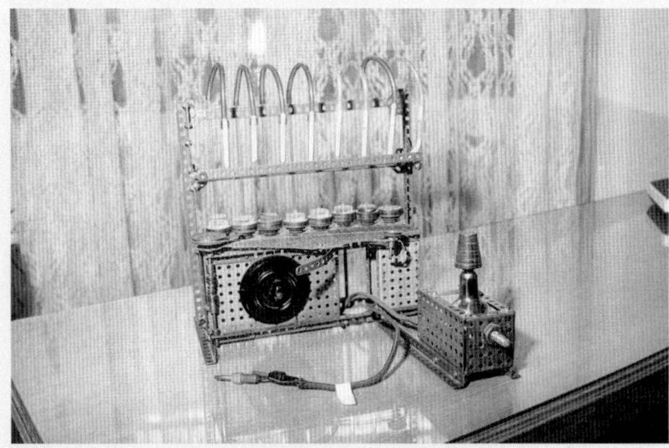

Figure 1.18 Apparatus devised by Otto Wichterle using a child's building kit, and the motor and moving parts of a gramophone to produce a 13-spindle device on which he produced spun-cast gel contact lenses (Courtesy of the Archives of the Academy of Sciences of the Czech Republic, from the personal papers of Otto Wichterle)

doubts at that time concerning bacterial contamination of soft lenses (Larke & Sabell 1971).

Although Otto Wichterle had taken out a patent on the lenses, in 1964 the Czech Academy of Sciences and Arts (CSAS) sold the patents to Robert J. Morrison, an enterprising optometrist from Harrisburg, USA. Two American investment capitalists – Martin Pollak and Jerome Feldman (who were also patent lawyers) – owned and operated the National Patent Development Corporation (NPDC) and saw the potential of the product. They were involved in the purchase of Morrison's rights by Bausch & Lomb.

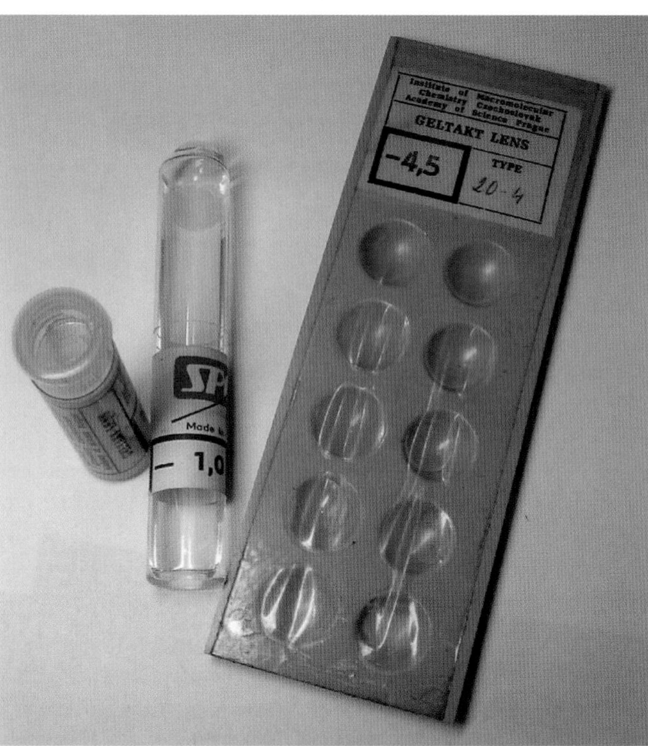

Figure 1.19 Geltakt and SPOFA lenses in original posting packets. Forty years on and the lenses are still visible, though the blister packets have dehydrated. Those in solution in the sealed glass test tubes are slightly opaque

1965 saw the availability of buttons of dehydrated HEMA material which allowed development of lathe-cutting techniques and the application of conventional back surface design (Turner 1964a,b). The Czechoslovakian lenses were used all over the world by institutes and hospitals experimenting with the new material (Fig. 1.19).

1967: Hydron Ltd was formed jointly by the NPDC and Smith & Nephew Associated Co. Ltd, to investigate other products made from Hydron (the registered name for polyHEMA).

1968: The United States Government decided that a soft lens should be regarded as a drug and needed Food and Drug Administration (FDA) approval before its general clinical use. This required extensive pre-market testing, toxicological and clinical trials, regulatory procedures and extensive documentation, slowing down the introduction of new designs and materials onto the American market. The long, safe use of PMMA lenses allowed them to be exempt from these regulations.

1970s: Allan Isen, an optometrist in New York, owned his own hard contact lens laboratories – Frontier Contact Lenses in the USA and Griffin Laboratory in Canada. He worked with Ken O'Driscoll, a local polymer chemist, to produce a new hydrogel material. The resultant Griffin lens material was a copolymer combining HEMA hydrogel with a pyrrolidone ring, producing a material called Bionite. It had a higher water content than HEMA but a lower tensile strength. Initial lenses had problems of tearing, variable fit and unreliable optics.

The FDA approved the Griffin lens as a therapeutic or bandage lens. It was 15.5 mm in diameter and had a 60% water content. As a therapeutic lens it was only available to ophthalmologists but it was most widely used for correction of refractive errors, when it was marketed as the Griffin Naturalens. The suggested cleaning regime consisted of soaking in 3% hydrogen peroxide followed by neutralization with saline (Isen 1972). This copolymer of HEMA/PV is currently still available in some medium water content lenses.

The Griffin lens later became the Softcon lens, which was sold to Warner-Lambert Pharmaceutical and assigned to their subsidiary, American Optical. Later still the Softcon lens was sold to CIBA Vision and became the basis for their Focus and NewVues lenses.

During this period, work was being carried out, both in America and the UK, on another type of soft lens. Instead of HEMA, it contained a copolymer of methylmethacrylate (MMA) and had a pyrrolidone ring as the hydrophilic unit – MMA/PV (Morris 1980). The concentrations of the monomers could be altered, producing a wide range of properties such as differing water contents, rigidity, swell rates, etc. Thus high-water-content lenses could be designed for extended wear.

1970: John de Carle began experiments developing a high-water-content soft lens material containing the pyrrolidone ring for extended wear (HEMA/VP). He designed the Permalens, later produced by Global Vision and then CooperVision. The water content was more than 70% and it was used as an extended-wear lens on healthy eyes (de Carle 1983). Initially the lenses were 11.5 mm in diameter, although 13.5 mm lenses were available. They were originally fitted in alignment or slightly steeper than the cornea.

1970: Contact Lens Manufacturing Group Ltd (CLM), a UK company, brought out a high-water-content soft lens made from MMA/PV. This was the Sauflon lens, a lathe-cut lens with 79% water when fully hydrated. Together with its sister material, the ultra high water content Sauflon 85, it was available in the UK for extended wear and therapeutic use (www.eyetech.me.uk).

David Clulow, an optometrist, fitted lenses made by his partner Philip Cordrey, a science graduate, in Earls Court in London. Together they formed CLM and subsequently opened a chain of practices specializing in contact lens fitting.

1971: Bausch & Lomb, a major American optical group who had bought the original patent to use pHEMA to manufacture contact lenses, were granted FDA approval for its clinical use. They began producing SOFLENS using a spin-casting technique.

Many of the initial problems faced by the Czech spun-cast lenses had been overcome and a more efficient fitting guide had been produced. Lenses were made in series C, F, N, J and B, which varied in posterior apical radius and diameter. Series C was 13.5 mm in diameter, the others were 12.5 mm. As the lenses were spun-cast, their inner surface was parabolic in shape. Initial lenses were chosen based on the *K* reading. If, after 20 minutes, the lenses proved unsuitable, the practitioner was guided to the next series. Recommended cleaning was to rub with saline after use, place in glass vials and heat in an Aseptor Patient Unit (Gruber 1970).

1972: Hydron Lenses Ltd (a subsidiary of Hydron Ltd in the UK) manufactured Hydron soft lenses, lathe-cut from solid buttons of dehydrated pHEMA. The lenses were of lenticular design, the optic zone decreasing as the power of the lens increased. The fitting guide suggested the initial lens should be fitted 1 mm flatter than flattest *K* and 2 mm larger in diameter than the corneal diameter. The edge geometry was constant for all powers: a 0.6 mm wide peripheral curve of 12.25 mm radius cut onto the posterior surface with constant 0.18 mm edge thickness. Total diameters ranged from 13.5 to 15.0 mm, although 14.0 and 14.5 mm were most common. Lenses were fitted from a trial set of around 30 hydrated lenses in glass bottles with screw tops. It was recommended that lenses were cleaned with 0.9% saline, replaced in their glass vials in fresh saline, and heated to 90°C in a lens hygiene unit for at least 15 minutes after use (Hydron Fitting & Service Manual 1973). In time the number of trial lenses reduced. Hydron's Z6 soft lenses had three standard BOZR (8.4, 8.7 and 9.00) and one standard diameter (14 mm).

1972: Titmus Eurocon, a subsidiary of the family business Schwind in Germany, began production of the Weicon pHEMA lens. It was lathe-cut with a spherical front surface and characteristic elliptical back surface and was produced in two back central optic radii: F (flat) and S (steep). In 1983, Titmus Eurocon was sold to CIBA Vision.

1975: Duragel MMA/PV material was developed by IH Laboratories in the UK. It was a 75% water content material and was used to manufacture lenses by lathe-cutting the dehydrated buttons. The material was marketed to many contact lens companies who produced their own branded lenses such as Scanlens 75 (CIBA Vision).

Over the next few years, as soft contact lenses became increasingly successful, many more companies started producing lenses. Soft lenses were of low (38%), medium (50–65%) or high (68–80%) water content, and were produced either by spin-casting or lathe-cutting. Spin-cast lenses were limited in design by means

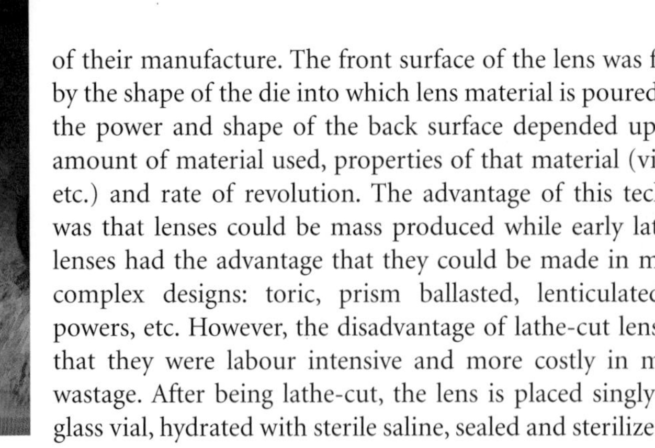

of their manufacture. The front surface of the lens was formed by the shape of the die into which lens material is poured, while the power and shape of the back surface depended upon the amount of material used, properties of that material (viscosity etc.) and rate of revolution. The advantage of this technique was that lenses could be mass produced while early lathe-cut lenses had the advantage that they could be made in multiple complex designs: toric, prism ballasted, lenticulated high powers, etc. However, the disadvantage of lathe-cut lenses was that they were labour intensive and more costly in material wastage. After being lathe-cut, the lens is placed singly into a glass vial, hydrated with sterile saline, sealed and sterilized.

Another method of manufacture soon emerged, that of injection or cast-moulding, where a measured amount of lens material was injected into the space between two dies, with polymerization taking place when the mould was full. Although costly to set up, no lens material was wasted and lens production could be significantly speeded up. This method of manufacture eventually led to the production of disposable lenses.

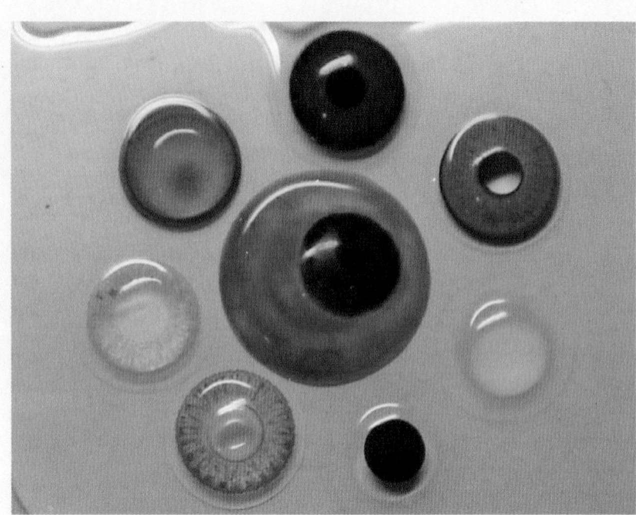

Figure 1.20 Selection of soft coloured lenses, from hand-painted prosthetic to visible handling tint

1974: Coloured Soft Lenses. Titmus Eurocon brought out the first cosmetic coloured soft lenses, the Weicon Iris print and the Weicon Iris hand-painted soft lenses. The original painted lenses used opaque colours which gave a false look to the eye. As more paint was used, the lens became thicker, changing its fitting characteristics and producing a stiff uneven lens. Later 'tinted' lenses evolved, the tint initially being bonded to the front surface of the lens. This caused problems with lens curling and surface deposits on the tint, so the bonding was transferred to the back surface.

John de Carle was one of the first to experiment with tinted lenses, having had the idea from a fluorescein contaminated soft lens (de Carle, J., personal communication; 2004). Experimenting with his wife's lenses, vegetable dye was dropped into her eye while wearing a corneal-sized high-water-content lens. The lens absorbed the dye, producing a desirable colour, which changed during the day as the dye leeched out. Subsequently, many of de Carle's patients, and others, adopted this technique.

Around 1987 Hydron produced its solid, opaque coloured lens, which produced an unnatural look. More successful coloured lenses were introduced with the dot matrix design, originally from Wesley–Jessen. These allowed the eye's natural colour to show, providing a natural depth of colour. Many modern lenses are of dot matrix design, using both opaque and tinted dots and mixtures of collaret patterns, although solid tints are still available (Fig. 1.20).

1976: Soft toric contact lenses were approved by the FDA. These had been evolving for several years. In 1972 Peter Fanti, who later worked for CIBA Vision, patented the thin zone stabilization lens (later manufactured as the Weicon toric lens). This was dynamically stabilized using the blinking action to keep the lens orientated correctly (see Chapter 12).

Other manufacturers were working on alternative toric designs. Hydron produced a truncated prism ballasted toric lens called the 'Rx toric lens' made in 38% water content HEMA. It was a stable lens that could correct high degrees of oblique astigmatism. Modern lenses are generally now a combination of prism ballast and thin-zone technology.

1977: Barnes-Hind produced one of the first aspheric soft bifocal lenses called the Alges. This was a centre-near lens of 14 mm in total diameter and 45% water content (Alges 1985).

Since then several companies have produced a variety of bifocal lenses (see Chapter 14).

1981: FDA approval was given for the use of extended-wear soft contact lenses to correct refractive errors. Therapeutic lenses were approved for extended wear in 1971.

1982: Disposable lenses. The first lens manufactured and marketed as a disposable lens was the Danalens invented by Michael Bay, a Danish ophthalmologist. It was made by MIA, who sold it to Johnson & Johnson.

1988: Vistakon (the optical subsidiary of Johnson & Johnson) launched the 'Acuvue' disposable lens. Johnson & Johnson used their vast knowledge and resources from the pharmaceutical industry to gear up production, improve quality and streamline packaging. The Danalens and the original Acuvue lenses were weekly extended wear lenses, worn constantly for 1 week and then discarded.

1995: Vistakon launched '1 Day Acuvue', their daily disposable lens. Technology patented by Ron Hamilton and sold to Vistakon, together with enormous investment in equipment and advertising, popularized the daily disposable contact lens. The logistics of 1-day disposable lenses are phenomenal, with each patient requiring 730 lenses a year.

RIGID GAS-PERMEABLE (RGP) AND SILICONE RUBBER

In 1970, corneal PMMA lenses were available in numerous designs and soft lenses were in their infancy. The quality of vision from hard (PMMA) lenses generally surpassed that of soft, but comfort was limited and the material impermeable, resulting in corneal hypoxia.

1971: Dr Leonard Seidner, an optometrist with Polymer Optics laboratories, together with his brother Joe, an engineer, commissioned Norman Gaylord, a polymer chemist, to produce a new material. The 'Gaylord patent' was awarded in 1974 for the first silicone/acrylate (S/A) rigid gas-permeable material. It was made into a corneal lens called Polycon, though it was some time before these lenses were available to the public.

1972: Dow Corning bought a silicone elastomer material from Breger Muller-Welt of Chicago and produced a flexible lens called SILCON. Silicone rubber was so highly oxygen permeable that it allowed normal levels of atmospheric oxygen to reach the cornea. Unfortunately, it was hydrophobic with poor wetting properties. The lens surface had been treated to improve its wettability but was prone to breaking down and it suffered badly from surface deposits. In 1984 they sold the silicone elastomer licence to Bausch & Lomb who still manufacture their Silsoft lenses (see Chapter 24).

1979: Cellulose acetate butyrate (CAB) was the first rigid gas-permeable contact lens material to be approved by the FDA in the United States. CAB was a grade of the polymer containing 2% water when fully hydrated. The lens had better in-eye wetting properties than PMMA and was comfortable. However, CAB was dimensionally unstable, could not be tinted, was difficult to manufacture and its oxygen permeability was poor. CAB was first available as Titmus Eurocon's elliptical Persecon E lens.

Silicone acrylate materials are more gas-permeable than PMMA and CAB but silicone is hydrophobic. Methylmethacrylic acid was therefore added to improve hydrophilic qualities, but this makes the surface more prone to cracking, so fluorine, another hydrophilic component, was incorporated (Morris 1980) to allow a reduction in the content of methacrylic acid. Gas permeability and hydrophilic properties could thereby be maintained, while reducing surface problems. The addition of fluorine also allowed other manufacturers to produce RGP materials without being restricted by the Gaylord patent.

1982: Boston II Material was granted FDA approval. Dr Perry Rosenthal, an ophthalmologist from Harvard Medical School, Boston, together with Louis Mager, a physicist, and Joseph Salamone, Professor of Chemistry at Lowell, Massachusetts, set up 'Polymer Technology' in 1974 to investigate oxygen permeable materials for contact lenses. In 1975 they began producing Boston RGP materials from a silicone/acrylate combination. Boston I was sold to a Canadian company, Boston II was developed and widely used, Boston III was researched but never released and Boston IV is still widely used today. Each development produced higher oxygen permeability. Polymer Technology was sold to Bausch & Lomb in 1983 where they continue to develop new materials.

The transition from PMMA to RGP materials was gradual. At first, standard PMMA lens designs were ordered in RGP material. However, these generally had smaller, steeper optic zones with very flat edge bevels. Materials with a high Dk can be fitted with larger optic zones in alignment with the central cornea and reduced edge clearance. This produces a more comfortable, optically stable lens, to which it is easier for new patients to adapt. RGP lenses are available in spherical, toric, bitoric, bifocal, keratoconic and scleral designs.

1982: The Diffrax bifocal lens by Pilkington was a simultaneous vision bifocal using the concept of a diffraction grating to create two foci: one for distance and one for near. The angled gratings produced interferometry patterns with good resolution (Ruben 1989), technology similar to that used in the production of holograms. The design worked well but had the disadvantage of needing to be fitted steep, otherwise the diffraction grating moulded the stepped shape into its surface. It was also expensive to make and the gratings tended to become clogged up with deposits.

1985: A combination or hybrid lens was first manufactured by Precision-Cosmet as the 'Saturn Lens' in 1977. It had an RGP centre of 8 mm diameter bonded to a hydrogel soft skirt, giving a total diameter of 14.3 mm. The lens was more comfortable than a corneal lens and gave better vision than a soft lens for keratoconic eyes; however, it was prone to splitting at the RGP–soft junction, especially as it dehydrated, and its oxygen transmissibility was low. Saturn II was an improvement on the initial design and later Pilkington Barnes Hind's 'Softperm' was brought out as a further improvement. More recently, a hybrid lens has been introduced by SynergEyes, Quarter Lambda Technologies, California, USA, with much higher oxygen permeability.

In 1998 the timelines of soft and RGP/silicone lenses join again and indeed the materials themselves are beginning to converge.

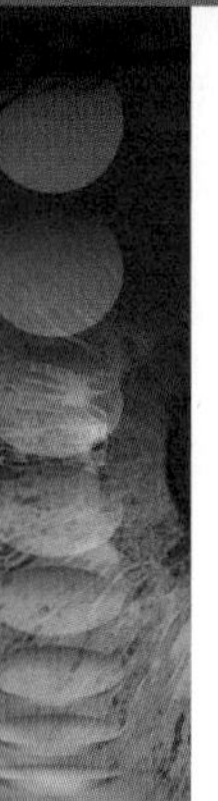

1998: CIBA's Night & Day was launched closely followed by **Bausch & Lomb's PureVision.** A combination of silicone and hydrogel, many of the previous problems of silicone have been overcome by developments in moulding and surface technology, combined with the disposable wearing modality. Unlike the old silicone elastomer lenses, which were impervious to fluid and sucked onto the eye, silicone hydrogel lenses contain water (Night & Day 24%; PureVision 36%), which allows fluid to pass through the material (see Chapter 10).

1998: CE marking compliance to the European Medical Device Directive 93/42/EEC (MDD) became mandatory. Contact lenses were regarded as a Class 2a medical device. CE marking had the advantage of quality assurance for the patients and, for the manufacturers, unrestricted access to export to more than 20 European countries. However, it had the disadvantage of being time consuming and costly, resulting in several small manufacturers going out of business.

1999: vCJD. Variant Creutzfeldt–Jakob disease was recognized and guidelines published by the Department of Health and the General Optical Council in the UK suggesting that: 'As a general rule a contact lens should not be re-used on another patient ... except in special circumstances in which complex diagnostic lenses may need to be used in the management of patients.' (www.official-documents.co.uk). This restricted the re-use of trial fitting sets in the UK.

2003: Vistakon Advance was introduced. Another silicone hydrogel lens, with a higher water content and lower Dk than the original silicone hydrogels, it is designed for improving physiology in daily wear.

2004: CIBA introduced their lower Dk silicone hydrogel lens **O_2Optix** for daily wear to compete with Johnson & Johnson.

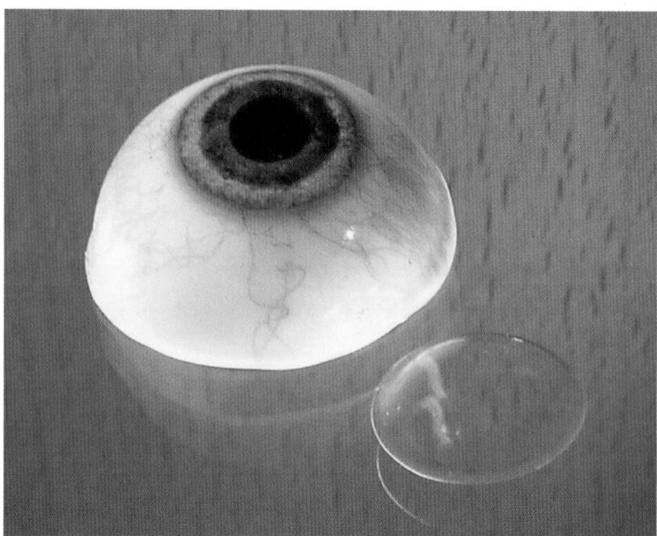

Figure 1.21 From hand-blown artificial glass eye to daily disposable hydrogel lens in 120 years

2006 and beyond: Improved optics in soft bifocal and toric lenses; second generation silicone-hydrogel lenses with Dks of 200 and more and improved surface properties; flexible RGP materials with good wettability, improving comfort while combining the optics of rigid lenses with the improved physiology of silicone; hybrid lenses with significant gains in oxygen transmissibility; and much more.

SUMMARY

This chapter shows how ideas from history can be reapplied with modern technology and materials to produce successful modern lenses (Fig. 1.21). Many items described are displayed in the Contact Lens Collection at the British Optical Association (BOA) Museum in London. The BOA museum would welcome any collections of contact lens-related items (www.college-optometrists.org/college/museum/clc.htm).

References

Airy, G. B. (1827) On a peculiar defect in the eye, and a mode of correcting it. Trans. Camb. Phil. Soc., 2, 267–271

ALGES™ Bifocal Contact Lenses Fitting Guide (1985) Trade catalogue

Anderson, J. M. (1952) Contact Lenses, Clinical and Other Observations, p. 11. Brighton: Courteney Press

ASCR Office Press Department (1962) Online. Available: http://press.avcr.cz/en/dpr.php

Bier, N. (1945) Application for British Patent No. 592055, 25th January 1945. Published in Contact Lens Theory and Practice, 2nd edn. London: Butterworths

Bier, N. (1948) The practice of ventilated contact lenses. Optician, 116, 497–501

Bier, N. (1956a) A study of the cornea. Am. J. Optom., 33, 291–304

Bier, N. (1956b) The contour lens – a new form of corneal lens. Optician, 132(3422), 397–399

Bier, N. (1957) Contact Lens Routine and Practice, 2nd edn. London: Butterworths, pp. 141–145

Bier, N. and Cole, P. J. (1948) The 'transcurve' contact lens fitting shell. Optician, 115(2987), 605–606

Dallos, J. (1936) Contact glasses, the 'invisible' spectacles. Arch. Ophthalmol., 15, 617–623

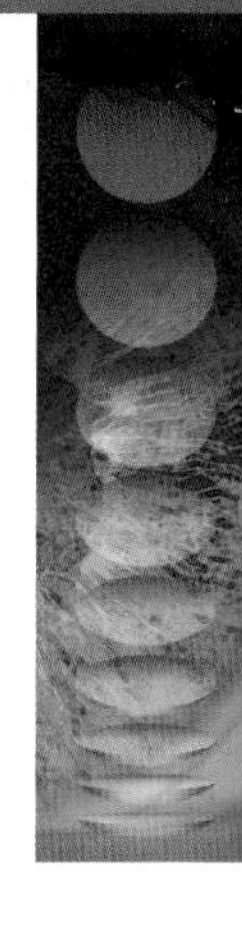

Dallos, J. (1946) Sattler's veil. Br. J. Ophthalmol., 30, 607–613
de Carle, J. (1983) Extended wear lenses – past, present and future. J. Br. Contact Lens Assoc., 6(4), 134–136
Descartes, R. (1637) Discours de la Methode, Discours No. 7, La Dioptrique, p. 79
Dickinson, F. (1954) Report on a new corneal lens. Optician, 128(3303), 3–6
Dickinson, F. and Hall, K. G. C. (1946) An Introduction to the Prescribing and Fitting of Contact Lenses. London: Hammond and Hammond
Dixey, C. W. & Son Ltd (1943) Dixey flexible contact lenses. Trade catalogue
Dor, H. (1892) Sur les verres de contact. Rev. Gén. Ophtalmol, 11, 493–497
Dreifus, M. (1978) The development of PHEMA for contact lens wear. In Soft Contact Lenses, pp. 7–16, ed. M. Ruben. London: Baillière Tindall
Duke-Elder, S. (1970) Ophthalmic Optics and Refraction, System of Ophthamology, Vol. 5, p. 713. London: Kimpton
Enoch, J. M. (1956) Descartes' contact lens. Am. J. Optom., 33, 77–85
Feinbloom, W. (1936) A plastic contact lens. Trans. Am. Acad. Optom., 10, 37–44
Feinbloom, W. (1945) The tangent cone contact lens series. Optom. Weekly, 36, 1159–1161
Ferrero, N. (1952) Leonardo da Vinci: of the eye. Am. J. Ophthalmol., 35, 507–521
Fick, A. E. (1888) A contact lens (trans. C. H. May). Arch. Ophthalmol., 19, 215–226
Forknall, A. J. (1948) Offset contact lenses. Optician, 116(3006), 419–421
Fraser, J. P. and Gordon, S. P. (1967) The 'apex' lens for uniocular aphakia. Ophthal. Opt., 7, 1190–1194, 1247–1253
Gasson, W. (1976) Leonardo da Vinci – ophthalmic scientist. Ophthal. Opt., 16, 393–541
Graham, R. (1959) The evolution of corneal contact lenses. Am. J. Optom., 36, 55–72
Gruber, E. (1970) Clinical experience with the hydrophilic contact lens. Am. J. Ophthalmol., 70(5), 833–842
Györffy, I. (1940) Kontaktschalen aus Kunststoffen. Klin. Mbl. Augenheilk., 104, 81–87
Györffy, I. (1950) Therapeutic contact lenses from plastic. Br. J. Ophthalmol., 34, 115–118
Györffy, I. (1964) The history of the moulded all-plastic lens. Br. J. Physiol. Opt., 21(4), 291–292
Györffy, I. (1968) The manufacture of haptic and corneal lenses in Budapest. Contact Lens, 2(1), 9–15
Györffy, I. (1980) Geschichte der Sklerallinsen aus PMMA. Contactologia, 2, 143–149
Györffy, I. (1981) Zur Geschichte der Korneallinsen aus PMMA. Contactologia, 3, 106–109
Heine, L. (1929) Die korrektur saemtlichr ametropien durch geschliffene kontaktschalen. Ber. 13' Congr. Ophthal. Amst., 1, 232–234
Heinz, R. (2003) The History of Contact Lenses, Vol 1: Early neutralization of corneal dioptric power. Ostend, Belgium: J. P. Wayenborgh
Herschel, J. F. W. (1845) 'Light' Section XII: 'Of the structure of the eye, and of vision'. Encyclopaedia Metropolitana, 4, 396–404
Hofstetter, H. W. and Graham, R. (1953) Leonardo and contact lenses. Am. J. Optom., 30, 41–44
Hydron Lenses Ltd (1973) Fitting and Service Manual, 2nd edn. Shanghai: Hydron Contact Lens Co. Ltd.
Isen, A. (1972) The Griffin lens. Am. J. Optom., 43, 275–286
Jessen, G. N. and Wesley, N. K. (1949) Concentric molding. Optom. Weekly, 40, 753
Koeppe, L. (1918) Die mikroskopie des lebenden augenhintergrundes mit starken vergrösserungen im fokalen lichte der Gullstrandschen Nernstspaltlampe. Graefes Arch. Ophthalmol., 95, 282–306
Larke, J. R. and Sabell, A. G. (1971) Some basic design concepts of hydrophilic gel contact lenses. Br. J. Physiol. Opt., 26, 49–60
Maisler, S. (1939) Casts of the human eye for contact lenses. Arch. Ophthalmol., 21, 359–361
Mann, I. (1938) The history of contact lenses. Trans. Ophthalmol. Soc. UK, 58, 129
Mann, I. (1973) Contact lenses and Dr Josef Dallos. The Contact Lens, 4(4), 16
McKellen, C. D. (1949) Conical contact lenses. Br. J. Ophthalmol., 33, 120–127
McKellen, G. D. (1963) The 'offset' haptic lens. Optician, 14, 105–107
Morris, J. (1980) Contact lenses in the eighties. Contact Lens J., 9(2), 3–5
Mueller-Welt, A. (1950) The Mueller-Welt fluidless contact lens. Optom. Weekly, 41, 831–834
Müller, A. (1889) Brillengläser und hornhautlinsen. Inaugural Dissertation p. 20. University of Kiel
Müller, F. A. and Müller, A. C. (1910) Das Kunstliche auge, pp. 68–75. Wiesbaden: J. F. Bergmann
Müller, F. E. (1920) Ueber die korrektion des keratokonus und anderer brechungsanomalien des auges mit mÜllers-chen kontaktschalen. Inaugural Dissertation. University of Marburg
Nissel. G. (1965) The Müllers of Wiesbaden. Optician, 150(3897), 591–594
Nissel, G. (1967) Offset corneal contact lenses. Ophthal. Opt., 6, 857–860
Nissel, G. (1968) Aspheric contact lenses. Ophthal. Opt., 7, 1007–1010
Obrig, T. E. (1938a) A cobalt blue filter for observation of the fit of contact lenses. Arch. Ophthalmol., 20, 657–658
Obrig, T. E. (1938b) Molded contact lenses. Arch. Ophthalmol., 19, 735–758
Obrig, T. E. (1943) A new ophthalmic impression material. Arch. Ophthalmol., 30, 626–630
Obrig, T. E. and Salvatori, P. L. (1957a) Contact Lenses, 3rd edn, pp. 340–345. New York: Obrig Laboratories
Obrig, T. E. and Salvatori, P. L. (1957b) Contact Lenses, 3rd edn, pp. 376, 378. New York: Obrig Laboratories
Pearson, R. M. (1978) August Müller's inaugural dissertation. J. Br. Contact Lens Assoc., 1(2), 33–36
Ridley, F. (1946) Recent developments in the manufacture, fitting and prescription of contact lenses of regular shape. Proc. R. Soc. Med., 39, 842–848
Ruben, M. (1966) The use of conoidal curves in corneal contact lenses. Br. J. Ophthalmol., 50, 642–645
Ruben, M. (1967) The apex lens. Contact Lens, 1(4), 14–28
Ruben, M. (1989) A Colour Atlas of Contact Lenses and Prosthetics, 2nd edn, p. 83. London: Wolfe Medical
Sabell, A. G. (1980a) An ophthalmic museum. Contact Lens J., 9(2), 15–19; 9(3), 16–22
Sabell, A. G. (1980b) An ophthalmic museum. Contact Lens J., 9(6), 3–18
Sabell, A. G. (1980c) An ophthalmic museum. Contact Lens J., 9(4), 10–18
Sattler, C. H. (1938) Erfahrungen mit haftgläsern. Klin. Mbl. Augenheilk., 100, 172–177

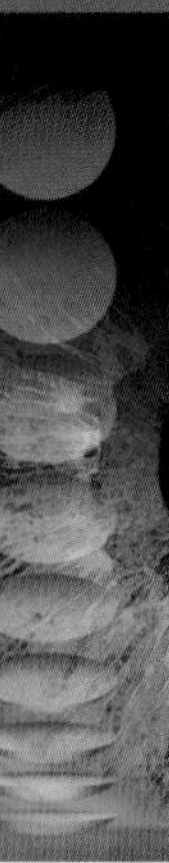

Schiller, F (1969) Testimonial to Dr Adolf Wilhelm Mueller-Welt, D.O.S. Online. Available: www.mueller-welt.com

Steele, E. (1948) American modifications of the contact lens moulding technique. Optician, 115(2968), 87

Stek, A. W. (1969) The Percon contact lens – design and fitting techniques. Contact Lens, 2(2), 12–14

Stevens, C. L. (1936) A method for making casts of the human cornea. Am. J. Ophthalmol., 19, 593–595

Stock, W. (1920) Über Korrektion des keratokonus durch verbesserte gechliffene kontaktgläser. Brichte der Deutschen Ophthalmologischen Gesellschaft Heidelberg, 352–354

Storey, J. K. (1972) The possible use of polysulphide rubber impression material in contact lens work. Ophthal. Opt., 12, 1017–1018

Straub (1888) Paper published in Centralblatt f. Augenheilk. (Title, vol. and page unknown) cited in Benson, A. H. (1902) A note on the value of the fluorescein test. Ophthalmol. Rev., 21, 121–130

Tallet, K. (1998) Mustard gas poisoning. Online. Available: http://ourworld.compuserve.com/homepages/kylet1/gas.htm

Thomas, P. (1968) The prescribing and fitting of conoid contact lenses. Contacto, 12(1), 66–69

Turner, R. (1964a) Hydrophilic contact lenses. Ophthal. Opt., 4(7,8), 343–346, 404–406

Turner, R. (1964b) An appraisal of the problems of hydrophilic contact lenses. Ophthal. Opt., 4(22), 1151–1159

von Csapody, I. (1929) Abgusse der lebenden augapfeloberfläche für verordnung von kontaktgläsern. Klin. Mbl. Augenheilk., 82, 818–822

von Rohr, M. and Stock, W. (1912) Über eine methode zur subjektiven prüfung von brillenwirkungen. Graefes Arch. Ophthalmol., 83, 189–205

Watson, R. K. (1947) The 'Kelvin' contact lens. Optician, 114, 228–230

Wichterle, O., Lim, D. and Dreifus, M. (1961) A contribution to the problem of contact lenses. Cesk. Oftal., 17, 70–75

www.dh.gov.uk/PublicationsAndStatistics/fs/en – Treatment of poisoning by selected chemical compounds. London: Department of Health, 2003

www.eyetech.me.uk – Eyetech (CLM) Ltd

www.nova.edu – A Brief History of the Contact Lens. Fort Lauderdale, FL: Nova Southeastern University

www.official-documents.co.uk – Transmissible spongiform encephalopathy agents: safe working and the prevention of infection. London: The Stationery Office

www.plastiquarian.com – London: Plastics Historical Society

www.rsm.ac.uk – London: The Royal Society of Medicine

www.zeiss.com – Germany: Carl Zeiss International

Young, T. (1801) On the mechanism of the eye. Phil. Trans. R. Soc., 16, 23–88

Chapter 2

Anatomy and physiology of the cornea and related structures

Gordon L. Ruskell and Jan P. G. Bergmanson

CHAPTER CONTENTS

When the first version of this chapter was written the task of selecting items for inclusion was quite simple. The few pages allocated were sufficient to cover most relevant information. Since then the growth of knowledge imposes a requirement for stricter selectivity but the criterion remains the same. Contact lens practitioners should be familiar with the structure and function of those tissues bearing the unnatural burden of a contact lens.

One important change is the adoption of the terminology recommended by the International Anatomical Nomenclature Committee (1989). More than 100 years ago it was recognized that eponyms are not descriptive and that more uniform anatomical terms should be developed. The first *Nomina Anatomica* was thus published in Latin in Basel in 1895 and has since been updated. Sections on embryology and histology have been added and the sixth and latest edition was published in 1985. Therefore, the terminology in this chapter has been determined internationally and agreed upon by acknowledged experts in the field.

Unfortunately, some of the eponymous ocular terms have resisted change. In the interest of progress towards the use of accepted and improved anatomical terms, the authors have elected not to refer to anatomical structures using an eponymous nomenclature.

THE CORNEA

The cornea occupies about 7% of the area of the outer coat of the eye and has a very regular layered structure composed of:

- Epithelium.
- Anterior limiting layer or Bowman's layer.
- Substantia propria or stroma.
- Internal limiting layer or Descemet's layer.
- Endothelium.

Corneal thickness is a factor that influences the intraocular pressure reading. A thicker cornea leads to an artificially higher reading and vice versa. The average human cornea is 535 μm thick with a range for normal between 445 and 600 μm (Doughty & Zaman 2000). It thickens by 23% from the centre to its periphery (Doughty & Zaman 2000) and it is steeper centrally and flatter peripherally, and has the shape of a minus meniscus lens (see also 'Pachometry/Pachymetry', Chapter 7).

The epithelium (epithelium anterius corneae)

- The outermost layer of the cornea is squamous stratified epithelium, from five to eight cells thick, and is probably the most regular of its type in the body (Fig. 2.1a).

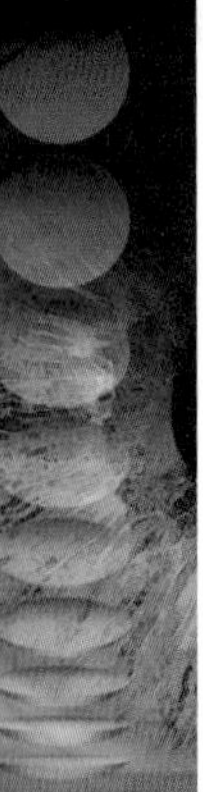

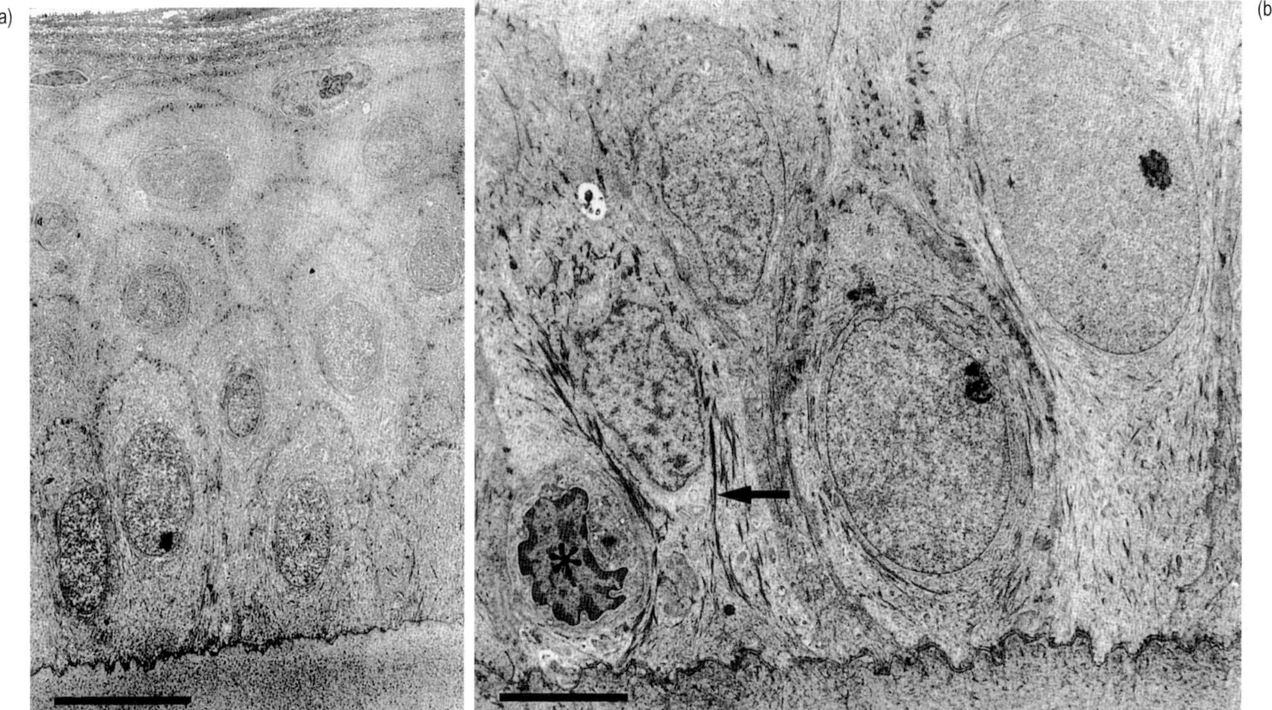

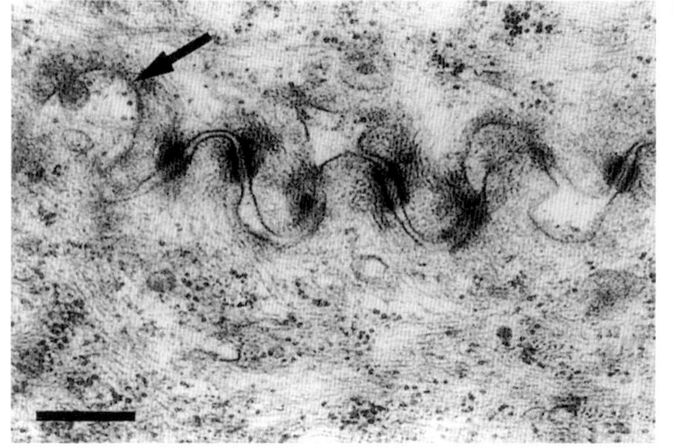

Figure 2.1 Electron micrographs of corneal epithelium. (a) Section close to the limbus. The squamous cell layers contain many vesicles (unstained) and the surface microvilli can be seen. Bar = 20 μm. (b) Detail of the basal region. Desmosomes give the cell perimeters a speckled appearance. Note the slightly undulating basement membrane and the dense intermediate filaments or tonofibrils (arrow). A Langerhans cell is marked with an arrow. Bar = 10 μm. (c) Reciprocal ridges of apposed cell membranes, desmosomes and a gap junction (arrow) are shown. The cytoplasm contains intermediate filaments mainly radiating from the desmosomes, and many free ribosomes. Bar = 0.5 μm

- It is thinnest centrally, between 48 and 51 μm thick (Holden et al. 1982, Li et al. 1997, Patel et al. 2001, Perez et al. 2003), increasing from about 50–60 μm, 3 mm from the centre (Reinstein et al. 1994) and about 70 μm near the limbus.
- It continues on to the conjunctiva where in most positions it thickens (see 'Conjunctiva') and shortly loses its smooth, regular surface.

The basal cells are columnar with a spherical or slightly oval nucleus containing dispersed chromatin (euchromatic). The cytoplasm contains many intermediate filaments, mostly grouped into bundles (tonofilaments), free ribosomes, sparse mitochondria, a little granular endoplasmic reticulum, glycogen granules and occasional Golgi complexes. They are covered by several layers of cells that become smaller, flatter and broader with distance from the base; the nuclei become more ovoid and finally disciform in the squamous superficial cells. The first two or three rows of suprabasal cells often overlap the apices of more than one underlying cell and are called umbrella or wing cells (Fig. 2.1). The organelles are similar throughout the epithelium except that filament aggregation is not observed in the squamous cells and they often contain numerous small vesicles.

Hemidesmosomes attach the basal cells to the epithelial basement membrane. They are so numerous they occupy at least one-third of the area of the membrane (Fig. 2.2). Hemidesmosomes are macula junctions continuous with basal cell tonofilaments and consist of local thickenings with increased density of the plasma membrane (the lamina densa) opposite a thickened zone of the basement membrane. The lighter interval between the two thickened membranes (lamina lucida) contains numerous fine connecting filaments. On the opposite side of the junction, the basement membrane is attached to the underlying stroma with anchoring filaments which in turn are attached to fine branched collagen structures called attachment plaques (Gipson et al. 1989) (Figs 2.3 and 2.4).

Cell borders are characterized by shallow interlocking ridges covering most of their surfaces, with little space between cells. The ridges are least frequent in the apposed membranes of basal

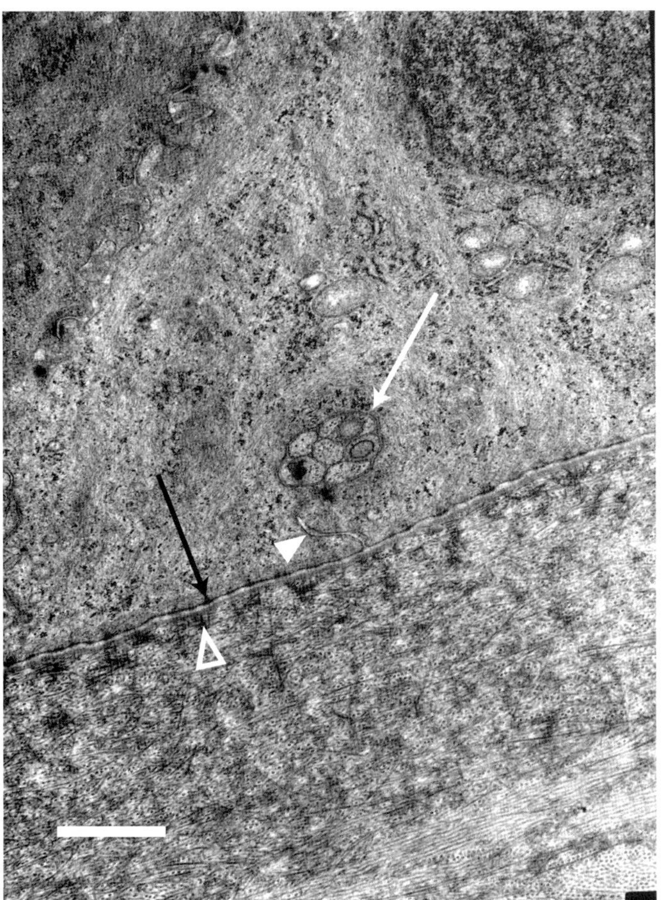

Figure 2.2 Electron micrograph of six epithelial axons (white arrow) in transverse section. They travel in an infolding of the cell membrane of the basal cell internal side (arrowhead), along which are numerous hemidesmosomes (black arrow). Fine filament, Type VII collagen and electron dense plaques (open arrowhead) are present. Bar = 3 μm. Monkey (*Macaque mulatta*)

cells. Cells are joined by many desmosomes, which, together with the interlocking ridges, provide the exceptional strength of the epithelium against shearing forces such as eye rubbing.

Gap junctions (Fig. 2.1c) are noted infrequently between the cells and at the epithelial surface, adjacent cells are joined by tight junctions (zonulae occludentes). Unlike the other junctions, they girdle the cells forming close contact but do not completely fuse. This limits permeability, allowing access to the intercellular space from the tear film, or vice-versa, only through discrete ion selective pores (Gumbiner 1993). Desmosomes are attached to the cytoplasmic tonofibrils, forming a girder-like desmosomal–cytoskeletal network supporting the epithelium layer. Gap junctions contribute to intercellular adhesion and are probably communicating junctions permitting ionic exchange.

CORNEAL SURFACE

Unlike surface skin cells, corneal cells are normally unkeratinized and retain their organelles, which suggests that metabolic processes are still functioning. Superficially the cells look smooth when examined at medium magnification through a

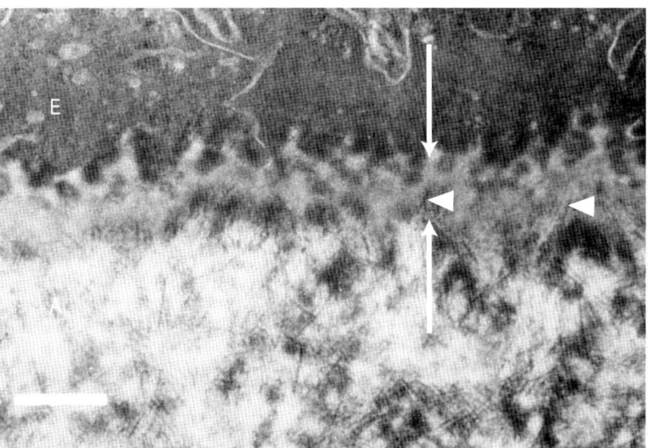

Figure 2.3 Electron micrograph of oblique or almost tangential section through the epithelial basement membrane. The extent of the basement membrane is indicated by arrows. Type VII collagen fibres (triangles) are deeply embedded in the basement membrane. E, epithelium; A, anterior limiting lamina/stroma. Bar = 1 μm. Rabbit

light microscope but with electron microscopy they resemble the pile of a carpet. The superficial squamous cells form tightly packed microvilli and/or microplicae (Figs 2.1 and 2.5) up to 0.75 μm long in humans.

As cells slough from the surface, desmosomes split to achieve detachment, and cytoplasmic extrusion at these points may be responsible for the microvilli development (Fig. 2.6) (Pedler 1962). Differences in the appearance of surface cells can be observed by specular (McFarland et al. 1983) or scanning microscopy (Pfister & Burstein 1977). The latter technique reveals light, intermediate and dark cells, depending on the surface form and size, which may change with age (Lemp & Gold 1986, Doughty 1990, 1991). The degree of overlap between the flat surface cells may account for this variation, although cells with a light electron reflex are generally smaller while dark reflex cells tend to be larger and have a greater number of sides (Doughty 1990).

A similar or slightly modified surface pattern is found in most wet epithelia, where the resultant increase in surface area provides the benefit of enhanced molecular adherence. The immediate molecular attachment to the surface of the corneal epithelium, as in other cases, is the glycocalyx, a thin glycoprotein layer (termed MUC1) produced by the surface epithelium. Watanabe et al. (1993) demonstrated that the corneal and conjunctival glycocalyx was absent until the eyes were opened after birth.

CELL PRODUCTION AND CORNEAL TROPHISM (NUTRITION)

Generation of new cells occurs mainly in the basal cell layer (Machemer 1966). Epithelial mitosis displays a circadian rhythm in rats, being most common at 2–7 a.m. and least common at 2–7 p.m. (Cardoso et al. 1968, Fogle et al. 1980, Lavker et al. 1991). Basal cells make room for new ones by migrating to the next layer and subsequently to the surface, becoming squamosed and

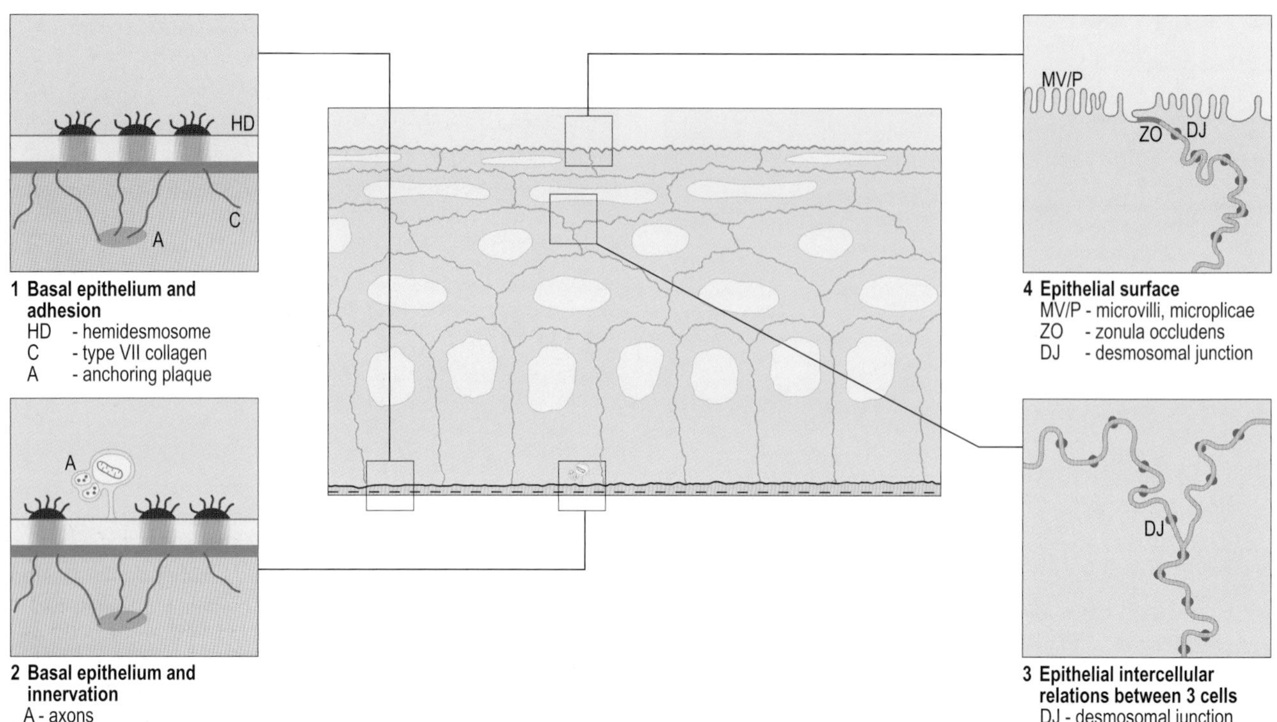

Figure 2.4 Corneal epithelial features. This diagram highlights the position of epithelial cell junctions, microvilli/plicae, basement membrane adhesion apparatus and the location of most nerve fibres (Published with permission from Jan Bergmanson; Clinical Ocular Anatomy and Physiology, 12th edition, 2005)

sloughed away by the action of the eyelids. These cells constitute the greater part of proteinaceous material found in tears.

Autoradiographic studies of epithelial cell nuclei, labelled with tritiated thymidine, indicate that the life cycle of cells is 3.5–7 days in a variety of young animals (Hanna & O'Brien 1960, Süchting et al. 1966). By arresting the division of cells at metaphase with colchicine, Bertanlanffy and Lau (1962) determined that 14.5% of epithelial cells are renewed daily in rats. Assuming surface cells desquamate at the same rate, and all cells are resident for a similar period, then the epithelium could be fully regenerated in 7 days. Hanna and O'Brien (1961) used results of isotope studies of enucleated eyes to estimate the life cycle of human corneal epithelial cells to be 7 days, but Cenedella and Fleschner (1990) suggested that complete turnover of the corneal epithelium took 14 days.

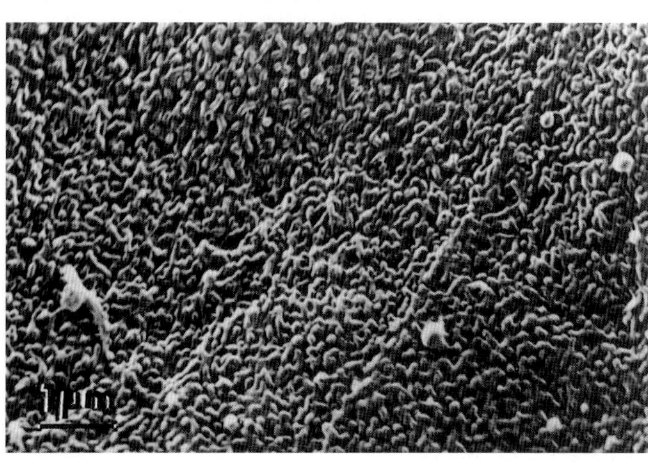

Figure 2.5 Scanning electron micrograph of the surface of the cornea showing microvilli and microplicae with a line marking the borders of adjacent epithelial cells

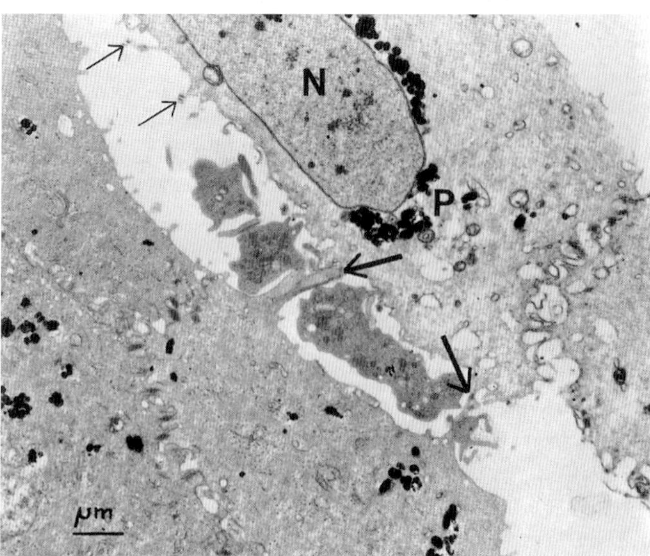

Figure 2.6 Electron micrograph showing partial detachment of surface cells from the perilimbal epithelium prior to sloughing. Cytoplasmic extrusions opposite desmosomes (thick arrows) mark the persisting attachment zones. Desmosomes have broken away from the attached cells and are suspended from microvilli of the detaching cell (thin arrows). N, nucleus; P, pigment granules

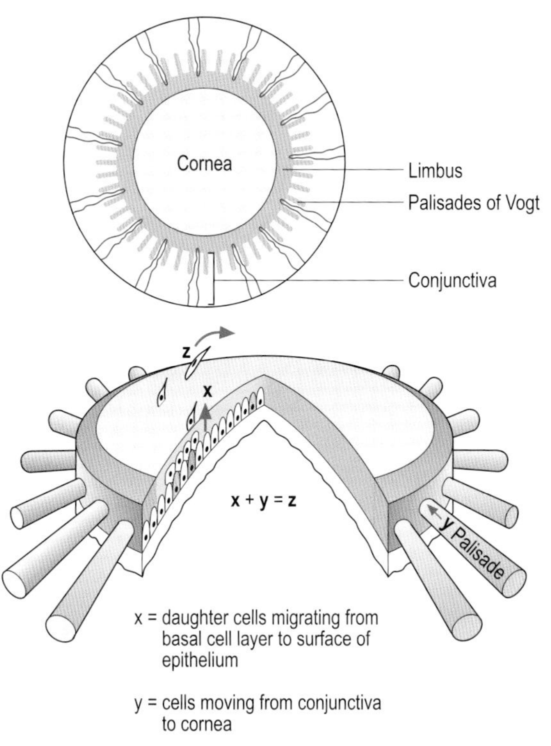

Figure 2.7 Epithelial stem cells and the X,Y,Z theory. Summary diagram of the Thoft and Friend (1983) X,Y,Z theory for epithelial regeneration. Darker blue represents the proposed location of epithelial stem cells (Published with permission from Jan Bergmanson; Clinical Ocular Anatomy and Physiology, 12th edition, 2005)

Cell renewal, a feature of all epithelia, is dependent upon stem cells and the cornea is no exception. The stem cell is a slowly cycling basal cell that divides to produce a replica of itself and a transient amplifying cell with the capacity to proliferate before differentiation. The self-renewed stem cell remains basal and the transient amplifying cell is responsible, by relatively rapid division, for cell turnover.

The cornea is exceptional in lacking stem cells, and the cell cycling described above is dependent on transient amplifying cells migrated from the limbal conjunctiva, the product of stem cells located in large numbers on the limbal basement membrane (Schermer et al. 1986, Cotsarelis et al. 1989, Kruse 1994, Zieske 1994). Stem cells may have a lifelong ability to slowly regenerate whereas the faster dividing transient amplifying cells can only divide a limited number of times (Lehrer et al. 1998).

Thoft and Friend (1983) proposed the X,Y,Z theory which suggests an orderly and continuous death and controlled regeneration of epithelial cells of the corneal surface.

- Cells move centripetally from limbus to cornea (Y).
- At the same time, basal cells move vertically towards the surface (X).
- X plus Y equals the cells desquamating from the corneal surface (Z) (Fig. 2.7).

Intrinsically orchestrated apoptosis is necessary for the development and healthy maintenance of human tissue. Ren and Wilson (1996) found that during normal homeostatic conditions approximately 1% of cells along the epithelial surface are undergoing apoptosis. This cell shedding is genetically controlled and regulated by a complex signal transduction cascade, which causes alterations in mitochondrial permeability and the execution of downstream death effectors. Apoptotic cell death occurs, unlike necrotic cell death, without concurrent inflammation and is characterized by cell shrinkage, chromatin condensation, cytoplasmic blebbing and nuclear degradation. Receptors in the cell membrane finish the process through phagocytosis.

Studies on rabbits have suggested that the highest incidence of apoptotic cell death occurs at the centre of the cornea (Yamamoto et al. 2002). This increased desquamation observed in the central cornea may be due to the overall centripetal movement of cells.

In the contact lens wearer, fewer cells are being shed from the ocular surface (O'Leary et al. 1998, Ren et al. 1999a, Yamamoto et al. 2002). Nitrogen goggle experiments and eyelid suturing suggest that hypoxia is an important factor in inhibiting epithelial shedding (Ren et al. 1999b). This stagnation in epithelial shedding among contact lens wearers may help explain the increased incidence of microbial corneal infections in these patients. Cells inhibited from programmed desquamation remain longer on the corneal surface, allowing more time for bacterial adhesion or indeed plasmalemmal (cell membrane) changes promoting bacterial adhesion.

Epithelial renewal slows during contact lens wear depending on the oxygen permeability of the lens (Ren et al. 1999b, Ladage et al. 2001, 2002). In particular:

- Basal cells divide more slowly.
- Epithelial cells migrate more slowly.
- Apoptotic epithelial cell surface death is inhibited.

This implies that there is a constant centripetal flow of epithelial cells in the cornea; this is suggested in dark irides where short, linear strands of pigment encroach into the cornea, especially at the lower limbus (Davanger & Eversen 1971).

Adrenaline (epinephrine) and sensory denervation by sympathectomy decrease the mitotic rate in rats (Friedenwald & Buschke 1944a), presumably as a result of denervation and adrenaline not circulating. In humans, the balance of evidence favours the presence of adrenergic innervation (Toivanen et al. 1987, Marfurt & Ellis 1993).

Appropriate regulation of mitosis is important in maintaining corneal epithelial trophism and of the cornea as a whole. Sensory denervation also decreases the mitotic rate (Sigelman & Friedenwald 1954), delays wound healing and increases epithelial permeability (Beuerman & Schimmelpfennig 1980), and may result in neurotrophic keratitis. Abelli et al. (1993) showed that corneal lesions induced by neonatal sensory denervation were limited by sympathectomy. This surprising result suggests that a balance in neuronal activity between sympathetic neurones and trigeminal sensory neurones may be critical for maintaining the normal physiology of the cornea.

LANGERHANS CELLS

Derived from bone marrow with a lifespan of weeks, Langerhans cells migrate from the bloodstream via the conjunctival

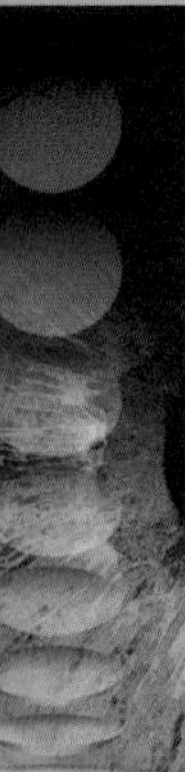

epithelium to the corneal epithelium, where they are much less common than in skin (Sugiura 1965).

Langerhans cells:

- Are smaller than epithelial cells.
- Have a limited perikaryon.
- Have numerous long thin processes.
- Are generally found on or close to the basement membrane (Fig. 2.1b).
- Are present at birth throughout the layer and reduce in number away from the limbus so that none is normally present in the centre of the adult cornea (Chandler et al. 1985).

Langerhans cells are an integral component of the local immune response to microbial and possibly other antigens. In response to various corneal insults their number increases substantially (Lewkowicz-Moss et al. 1987). For instance, overnight wear of contact lenses elevates their density (Hazlett et al. 1999) but exposure to ultraviolet B radiation leads to a loss (Hill et al. 1994). They bear HLA-DR antigens and may provide the first signal in host sensitization leading to corneal graft rejection (Braude & Chandler 1983, Treseler et al. 1984, Rodrigues et al. 1987).

EPITHELIAL DAMAGE

Corneal wounds

If these are smaller than a pin head, they are covered in about 3 hours by the neighbouring basal cells sending pseudopodia to cover the excavated area (Friedenwald & Buschke 1944b). Normal mitosis is inhibited and plays no part in healing. A series of animal studies showed that physical damage caused by contact lenses does not appear to extend beyond the epithelium, thus sparing the epithelial basement membrane and underlying anterior limiting lamina (Bergmanson & Chu 1982a, Bergmanson et al. 1985, Bergmanson 1987).

If a larger area of the cornea is denuded, cells from all layers of the surrounding epithelium migrate and flatten to cover the wound; mitosis is at first inhibited but recommences after a few hours and takes an active part in repair. Mann (1944) found that, in rabbits, an area 2–3 mm in diameter will become covered within 24 hours, and in 3 days the area will have a normal appearance as determined by fluorescein staining. The time course of repair is independent of the cause except in the case of burns, when it is delayed. Other experiments on rabbits have shown that the establishment of a tight adhesion of newly regenerated epithelium takes only a few days if the basement membrane is largely intact, but initially the new epithelium is not firmly attached and is susceptible to damage (Khodadoust et al. 1968).

Tight junction reformation is swift (McCartney & Cantu-Crouch 1992) and may re-establish the epithelial barrier well before the layer is firmly attached to the stroma. It is prudent, therefore, to discontinue contact lenses wear for a few days after incurring significant epithelial damage and for re-establishment of tight junctions following deep epithelial trauma.

If the lesion lies close to the limbus, conjunctival cells take part in the migration, as ascertained by the movement into the cornea of pigment cells from the limbus in rabbits and noted by Mann (1944) in African patients. Such migration may represent an acceleration of a normal slow centripetal movement of epithelial cells (Buck 1985). After total denudation of rabbit corneas, 50% coverage occurs after 24 hours, 75% after 48 hours (Langham 1960) and total coverage takes from 4 to 12 days (Mann 1944, Heydenreich 1958, Khodadoust et al. 1968).

Once the cornea is completely covered, the epithelium is one or two cells thick (Khodadoust et al. 1968), after 2 weeks it is two to three cells thick (Heydenreich 1958) but it takes several weeks before the epithelium is of normal thickness and adhesion structures are adequately reformed (Gipson et al. 1989). Langham (1954) found that normal thickness might be attained in one region of a previously denuded cornea while another area remains uncovered.

In rabbits, polymorphonuclear leucocytes appear in the basal lamina and at the edge of an abrasion possibly as soon as 3 hours following epithelial abrasions. These white blood cells reach the cornea via the tears following full thickness epithelial injuries from trauma or postrefractive surgery (Anderson et al. 1989, Snyder et al. 1998). Epithelial cells bordering the abrasion are flattened and develop surface ruffles and long, fine filopodia at their free edges (Pfister 1975). These extend to form attachments to the basal lamina, giving the impression of drawing the cells forward into the area of the defect. Epithelial cells bordering a defect appear to increase their water content and surface area, facilitating the production of cell extensions (Cintron et al. 1982). Marr (1967) found that epithelial repair in rabbits slows with age, although only slightly.

Weimar (1960) found evidence to suggest that chemotactic substances liberated from the epithelium are responsible for initiating the early stages of healing, both in the epithelium and the stroma. Immediately after deep corneal wounding in rats, proteolytic enzymes in the epithelium give rise to the invasion of polymorphonuclear leucocytes and to phagocytic activity by the stromal cells.

Epithelial thinning

Bergmanson and Chu (1982b) showed that wearing low Dk rigid or thick low water content HEMA lenses can, over an extended period, lead to a whittling away of epithelial cells layer by layer until only the basement membrane remains. A blunt shearing injury, such as a thumb in the eye, will cause the basal cells to be torn apart just beneath their nuclei, leaving the overlying epithelium intact but detached from the underlying cornea. This demonstrates the strength of the epithelium, allowing it to withstand shearing forces such as vigorous eye rubbing.

The ability of the epithelial cells to remain intact is best explained by the extensive interdigitations between cells and the vast number of desmosomal cell junctions. The tall columnar basal cells are the weakest. Excessive force causes them to rupture between the basal cell membrane and the nucleus, leaving the basal cell membrane with some internal cytoplasmic fragments attached by hemidesmosomes to the basement membrane. Because the untraumatized basement membrane remains intact, rapid and complete epithelial regeneration can take place. Repair after photorefractive keratectomy is significantly different.

Anaesthetics

Anaesthetics are protoplasmic poisons which alter cellular metabolism. Friedenwald and Buschke (1944a) showed that, if these or other agents such as adrenergic drugs were applied locally in experimental animals, mitosis and migration were inhibited, and epithelial healing in guinea-pigs was delayed by anaesthetics (Gunderson & Liebman 1944). This effect varied with concentration and tonicity but not with pH.

Excessive use of local anaesthetics causes:

- Epithelial and possibly stromal opacification.
- Eruption of cells.
- Bleb formation.
- Complete corneal staining.

Antibiotics and antimicrobials

Wound healing may also be slowed by some antibiotics and antimicrobials (Nakamura et al. 1993). High concentrations of fluoroquinolones and peptides slowed cultured corneal epithelial migration but aminoglycosides had little effect and penicillins none.

Microcysts

The epithelium in contact lens wearers is subject to the development of microcysts at basal cell level (Zantos & Holden 1978). This is an asymptomatic clinical manifestation of altered epithelial metabolism (see Chapter 13). Although the exact morphological composition of microcysts is unknown, Zantos (1983) proposed that they represent interepithelial pockets of cellular breakdown products. In clinical practice, microcysts indicate the level of epithelial stress but are not a serious threat to epithelial health.

Corneal wrinkling

If the eye has been bandaged, or if pressure is exerted through the eyelids, the epithelium wrinkles (Bron 1968) giving rise to a quickly fading mosaic visible with fluorescein staining.

Orthokeratology (OK)

The rapid refractive changes achieved in orthokeratology (see Chapter 19) are believed to occur primarily due to central thinning of the epithelium, together with an approximately equal thickening of peripheral epithelial regions (Swarbrick et al. 1998, Alharbi & Swarbrick 2003, Soni et al. 2003).

Corneal epithelium thinning can be achieved by:

- Pushing cells aside.
- Shedding cells.
- Flattening cells (Bergmanson et al. 1985, Bergmanson & Wilson 1989).

The tension exerted by closed eyelids on a flat fitting, rigid contact lens worn overnight has the ability to alter epithelial thickness. This can be observed on a fresh cadaver eye, where the mouldable, jelly-like properties of the epithelium can be demonstrated together with the plasticity of the structure.

Contact lens wear

Generally, contact lenses do not interfere with the smooth topography of the corneal surface but subtle refractive irregularities can be observed with computerized analysis (Ruiz-Montenegro et al. 1993). Cochet (in Guilbert 1963) argued that the softness or fragility of the epithelium varies, and observed a marked fragility in 5% of patients seeking to wear contact lenses. Millodot and O'Leary (1980a) demonstrated that the epithelial fragility threshold was lower than its touch threshold, i.e. superficial epithelial trauma could be induced without evoking an awareness of the insult.

Imprinting of the cornea can result from contact lens wear and takes the form of a raised crescent of tissue. Greenberg and Hill (1973) found that this was accompanied by the loss of a wing cell layer and increased mitosis in rabbit corneas, indicating a faster turnover of cells. This was questioned by Hamano et al. (1983) who found a reduced cell turnover.

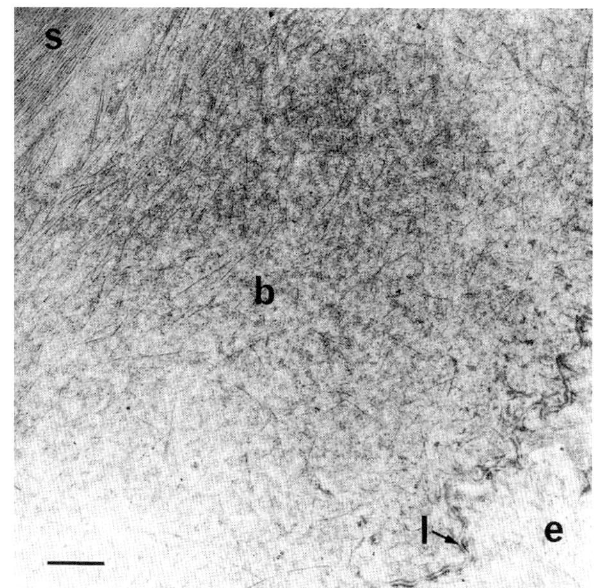

Figure 2.8 Electron micrograph of Bowman's layer (b). Note the random orientation of the collagen fibres. Bowman's layer merges with the stroma (s) in which the fibrils are regularly orientated. The basement membrane of the epithelium (e) is not smooth; the densities opposite the membrane are hemidesmosomes (the arrow indicates one). Bar = 1 μm

The anterior limiting lamina (lamina limitans anterior)

(eponym: Bowman's layer)

The anterior limiting lamina is:

- A cell-free layer of uniform thickness of about 8–9 μm in transverse section (Horne et al. 2003, Bergmanson 2006).
- A fine randomly orientated mesh of Type I collagen fibrils (Fig. 2.8), seen with electron microscopy, terminating at the peripheral extreme of corneal limbus (Fig. 2.9).
- Modified anteriorly where the anchoring filaments, collagen Type VII, bridge the basement membrane and the electron-dense anchoring plaques. This structural arrangement is believed to explain the firm attachment of the epithelial basement membrane to the underlying stromal tissue.

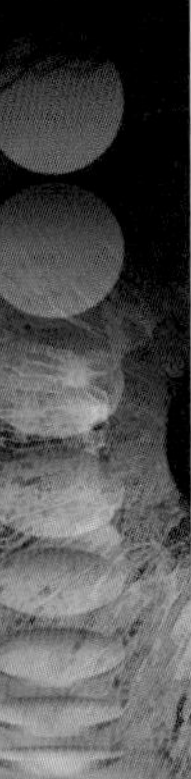

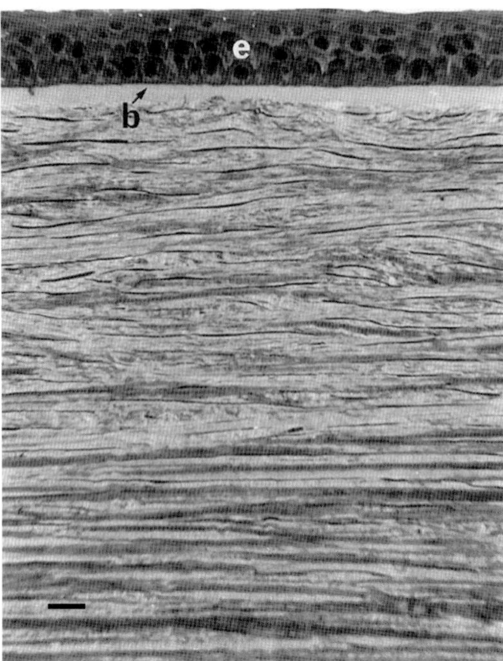

Figure 2.9 Light micrograph of the anterior half of the cornea in transverse section. The difference in density of the lamellae of the stroma is partly attributable to a difference in fibril orientation. The slight irregularity of the lamellae underlying Bowman's layer (b) is a normal feature. e, epithelium. Bar = 20 μm

- Penetrated, over its whole area, by fine unmyelinated sensory nerve fibres, which pass from the stroma to the epithelium, losing their Schwann cell sheaths as they leave the stroma. These are more frequent peripherally (see Corneal innervation, p. 38).
- Relatively tough, as evidenced by frequent epithelial damage without involvement of this layer. If it does become damaged, fibrous scar tissue is laid down, resulting in a permanent opacity – although some reduction of the initial scar area usually occurs.

The outcome of photorefractive keratectomy (PRK) is a more or less pronounced corneal haze depending on individual corneal wound healing characteristics. Visual function in individuals who have undergone this procedure is usually close to normal except for at night or in low contrast conditions.

The stroma (substantia propria)

The stroma:

- Constitutes 90% of the corneal thickness.
- Gives the cornea its strength.
- Is transparent because of its regular structure and absence of blood vessels.

STROMAL LAMELLAE

The basic component of the stroma is the lamella, consisting of parallel collagen fibres, separated by matrix. The lamellae cross each other at various angles while maintaining an overall orientation parallel to the corneal surface. A transverse section of the central human cornea has an average of 242 lamellae (Bergmanson et al. 2005).

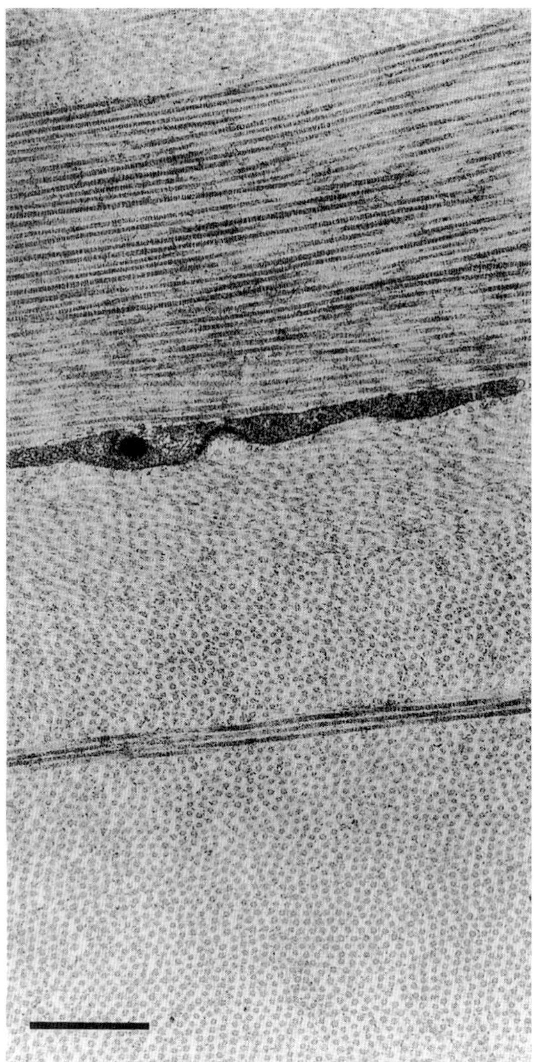

Figure 2.10 Electron micrograph of stromal lamellae showing different fibril orientation and lamellar thicknesses. A keratocyte process is interposed between two of the lamellae. Bar = 0.5 μm

The fibrils are buried in a matrix of proteoglycans and have a periodicity characteristic of collagen (Fig. 2.10). There are no elastic fibres in the adult human cornea (Alexander & Garner 1983). Collagen fibrils are of a regular size at any given depth in the stroma but vary in size from an average of 19 nm in the anterior layers to 34 nm in the posterior layers in humans (Jakus 1961).

Lamellae have an average thickness of 1.2 μm (Bergmanson et al. 2005). In the anterior third of the cornea, they run obliquely and become interwoven with each other, while posteriorly they are laid down more plainly with one over the other (Fig. 2.10). Schute (1974) discovered a diagonal upward and outward bias of the lamellae using polarized light, whereas Meek et al. (1987), using X-ray diffraction, revealed vertical and horizontal orientations. Towards the periphery, some lamellae

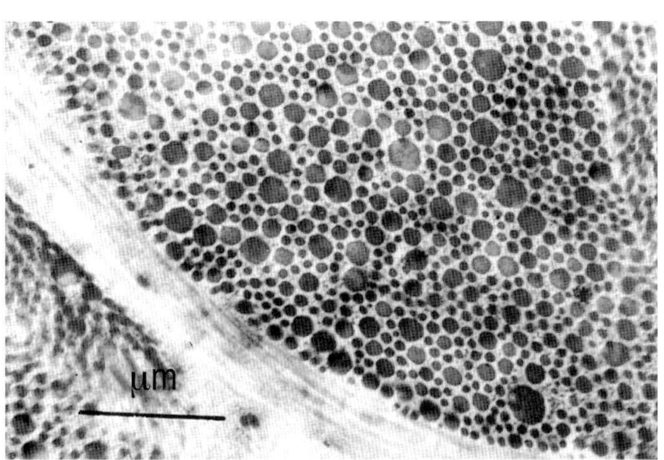

Figure 2.11 Electron micrograph of a transverse section through collagen fibrils of the scleral spur. The difference between adjacent collagen fibril diameters is dramatic

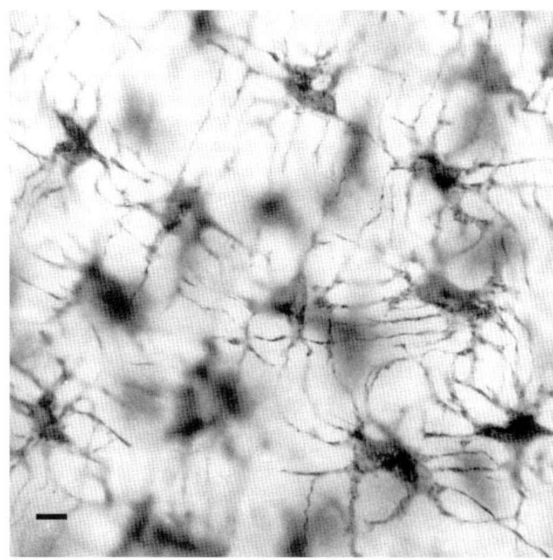

Figure 2.12 Stromal keratocytes. The full thickness of the cornea is viewed from the front and focused at a superficial stromal level. The keratocytes in focus probably all lie at a single lamella interface. Bar = 20 μm

lie approximately concentric with the limbus (Kokott 1938, Polack 1961).

The issue whether lamellae bridge the cornea from limbus to limbus and how much they extend into the sclera has yet to be determined. Most sources claim that stromal lamellae span the full width of the cornea (Duke-Elder & Wybar 1961, Hogan et al. 1971, Arffa 1997, Klyce & Beuerman 1998, Edelhauser & Ubels 2003) but Bron et al. (1997) proposed that this may not be the case. Bergmanson et al. (2005) explored the stromal anterior limiting lamina interface and provided evidence that at least some anterior lamellae appear to terminate halfway and that the dominant feature of the terminating lamellae was electron dense formations. These appeared to be a proteinaceous material anchoring the terminating collagen fibres in the stroma. Little or no overlapping was apparent at the stromal–anterior limiting lamina interface.

Lamellar widths are difficult to measure; most are up to 250 μm but some appear to be in excess of 1 mm. Adjacent lamellae appear to be discrete but there are occasional slightly oblique branches in the posterior two-thirds of the cornea, connecting one lamella with another. This arrangement explains the ease with which the deep stroma may be split parallel to the surface, as in preparation for corneal lamellar grafts.

At the corneoscleral margin, the stromal lamellae undulate, branch and probably interweave. The fibrils of single lamellae remain parallel to each other, which has a profound effect on how much the cornea swells (Doughty & Bergmanson 2004a). Fibril diameters vary 10-fold or more (Fig. 2.11) and there is some variation in diameter throughout the sclera. The sclera acts as a clamp to limit corneal swelling; with the sclera removed a cornea will swell several times more. The canal of Schlemm and the corneoscleral meshwork are located more posteriorly; a description of their structure and relationships is beyond the scope of this chapter.

STROMAL MATRIX

This is composed largely of glycosaminoglycans (GAGs) covalently bound to protein, constituting proteoglycans. The two major types are keratin sulphate and chondroitin sulphate. Hirsch et al. (1989) demonstrated their filamentous structure with filaments attaching through their core proteins to collagen fibrils, bridging the spaces between. Details of this 'bottle brush' organization are uncertain but Scott (1992) proposed a model explaining the manner in which the matrix influences the regular separation of collagen fibrils. During oedema resulting from a compromised endothelium, GAGs are lost from the cornea (Anseth 1969, Kangas et al. 1990).

KERATOCYTES

- The main cellular element of the stroma is the keratocyte (corneal fibrocyte, corpuscle or fixed cell), which is a flattened, dendritic cell predominantly disposed in the interface between adjacent lamellae (Fig. 2.10).
- In a single interface, the cell bodies are well spaced across the cornea but their thin, lengthy processes are so extensive that many come into contact with processes from neighbouring cells, giving the appearance of a delicate wide-mesh network (Fig. 2.12). This is repeated at each lamellar interface.
- They form a network (first noted by Clareus in 1857).
- Contacts between neighbouring cells are gap junctions (they allow intercellular communication) (Müller et al. 1995, Watsky 1995, Doughty et al. 2001). Thus keratocytes facilitate intercorneal communication, which may explain parts of the corneal response to injury.
- At intervals, keratocytes project long, attenuated, translamellar processes in an anterior or posterior direction (Doughty et al. 2001), which may allow different stromal levels to communicate with each other. These can project 30–50 μm from the cell body. Thus, an individual cell can bridge a corneal distance of about 100 μm, which is unusual for a non-neural cell but useful to maintain a transcorneal communicating network.

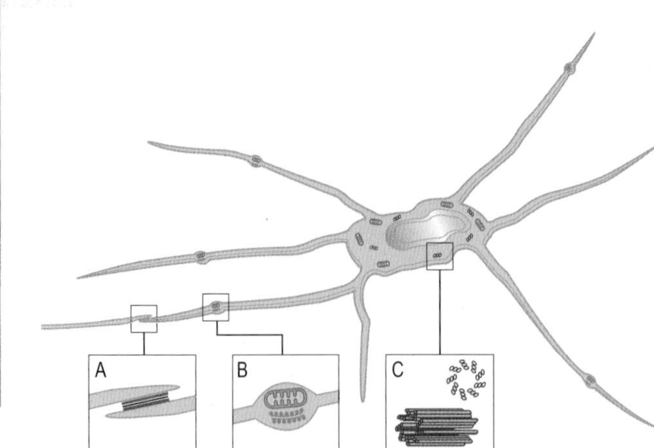

Figure 2.13 3-D reconstruction of a keratocyte. The keratocyte is of paper-thin proportions and through its long processes it may cover corneal distances of 100 μm. In achieving this impressive feat, processes may become too thin to harbour organelles, which may be located in local swellings along the process extending from the cell body (Published with permission from Jan Bergmanson; Clinical Ocular Anatomy and Physiology, 12th edition, 2005)

- There are approximately 2.4 million keratocytes in the human cornea.
- They are denser anteriorly than posteriorly. At the posterior limiting lamina, the cell density is 30% less than anteriorly (Moller-Pedersen & Niels 1995).
- They serve to maintain corneal health and facilitate repair following corneal injury, disease or surgery.
- They are flat and approximately 31 μm wide and 1.34 ± 0.46 μm thick in transverse section (Doughty et al. 2001) (Fig. 2.13).

Much of the cell body is occupied by the oval nucleus, which in transverse section occupies 75% of the perikaryon, leaving little room for other organelles. In coronal section, the nucleus-to-cytoplasm ratio is 44% (Doughty et al. 2001). Away from the perikaryon, a much higher number of organelles is noted (Snyder et al. 1998); these include mitochondria, rough endoplasmic reticulum and centrioles. Keratocytes associate closely and even interact with neighbouring collagen. This intimate association between cells and lamellae suggests that keratocytes are active not only in fibre synthesis but that they also have a tethering function (Müller et al. 1995, Doughty et al. 2001).

Functions of keratocytes

- Matrix turnover.
- Intracorneal communications.
- Reservoir for glycogen (energy source).
- Interlamellar tethering.
- Phagocytosis.
- Wound healing.

There is good evidence that corneal fibrocytes display a phagocytic function (Klintworth 1969, Fujita et al. 1987). Polymorphonuclear leucocytes and mast cells are present in the periphery of the stroma. Early autoradiographic studies of thymidine-labelled nuclei revealed little or no evidence of DNA synthesis among keratocytes, suggesting that they seldom divide (Hanna & O'Brien 1961, Machemer 1966). However, more recent work using different staining methods (BrdU-labelling) showed that keratocytes rarely divide in the normal cornea but can do so under stress, as in contact lens wear (Ladage et al. 2001). Contact lens wear diminishes the density of keratocytes (Jalbert & Stapleton 1999, Efron et al. 2002, Kallinikos & Efron 2004).

Keratocytic regeneration may use a different response pathway from that following post-excimer laser exposure or in traumatic scar formation, where activated stromal cells invade the lesion. The primary location of mitotic keratocytes is in the periphery of the contact lens-wearing cornea (Ladage et al. 2001).

The posterior limiting lamina (lamina limitans posterior)

(eponym: Descemet's layer)

- The posterior limiting lamina is a product of the endothelium and also the basement membrane of the endothelium.
- It is composed of collagen Type IV, as in all basement membranes.
- It is thinner than the anterior limiting lamina in the young – approximately 3 μm at birth, thickening to 5 μm by the age of 1 year then more slowly, approximately 1–1.3 μm each decade (Johnson et al. 1982, Murphy et al. 1984), reaching up to 17–20 μm in some older people. The stroma, by comparison, remains unchanged.
- The fetal posterior limiting lamina is recognizable as the banded portion in the adult membrane, while the non-banded portion is secreted after birth.

In tangential sections, the posterior limiting lamina has a two-dimensional lace network appearance of repeating hexagonal units with seven dense nodes marking each angle. These are connected by fine filaments of equal length. The networks are stacked in depth as revealed by transverse sections. Dark bands are discernible perpendicular to the plane of the cornea, consisting of columns of dark granules, which are the nodes of the tangential section network (Jakus 1964).

The posterior part of this layer has the same fine granular appearance in whichever plane it is sectioned and it shows no signs of a patterned organization. This layer becomes thicker than the fibrillar layer with age.

The posterior limiting lamina is uniformly thick in the centre. Local thickenings – Hassell-Henle warts – may occur in the periphery of healthy corneas. If these occur in the central cornea, they are known as corneal guttae and, if too numerous, the endothelial cells can no longer function normally. This can lead to uncontrolled corneal oedema and in a condition known as Fuchs' endothelial dystrophy. (Often, due to a misuse of the Latin language, these features are termed guttatae.)

The endothelium (epithelium posterius)

- The endothelium consists of a single thin layer of squamous cells, approximately 18 μm wide and 5 μm thick (Fig. 2.14).

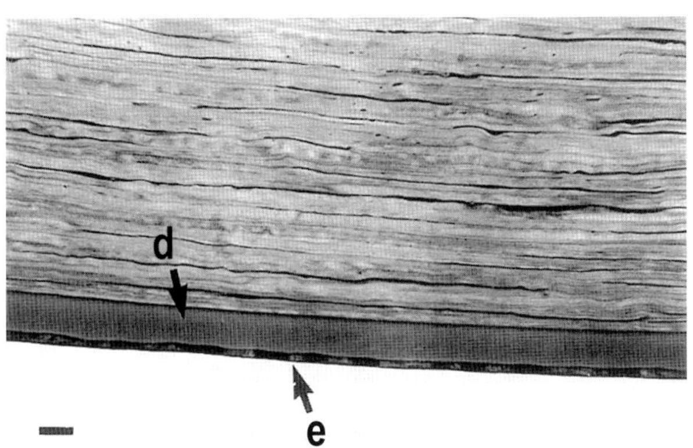

Figure 2.14 Structures of the cornea bordering the anterior chamber. d, Descemet's membrane; e, endothelium. Bar = 10 μm

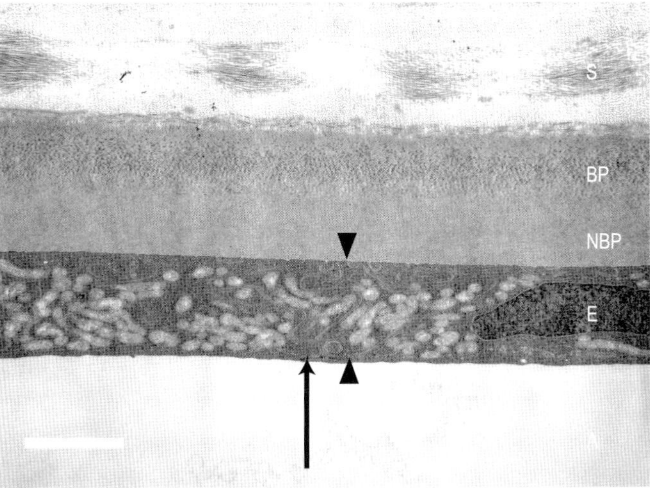

Figure 2.15 Electron micrograph of posterior cornea in transverse section. This field of view shows stroma (S), banded portion of posterior limiting lamina (BP), non-banded portion of posterior limiting lamina (NBP) and endothelium (E). An endothelial zonula occludens (arrow) is present and the anterior limit of the interdigitated lateral side (triangles) demonstrates that the lateral side of the non-polymegethous endothelial cell is approximately perpendicular to the plane of the cornea. Bar = 5 μm. Four-year-old human. A, anterior chamber

- The basal and apical sides are parallel to each other and to the corneal surface. They are smooth except for infrequent microvilli along the apical side.
- The lateral sides have extensive, deep invaginations which interdigitate with each neighbouring cell (Fig. 2.15).
- In transverse sections the cells are rectangular.
- Cells in the coronal plane are predominantly hexagonal but a normal cornea may contain many cells of different shapes.
- Tangential sections, viewed with a light microscope, show an oval or a kidney-shaped nucleus and granular cytoplasm.
- The cells are well stocked with organelles, especially mitochondria, and the endoplasmic reticulum is prominent.

On the lateral side of the cells, near the apex, the intercellular space is reduced to form a 10 nm wide tight junction (zonula occludens) which presumably restricts the movement of substances in and out of the cornea between the endothelial cells (Iwamoto & Smelser 1965). Unlike most other tissues with zonulae occludentes, the endothelial tight junction does not form a complete circle around the perimeter of the cell (Hirsch et al. 1977). Instead, there are discontinuities along this cell junction, which allows fluid to leak from the aqueous into the stroma. This explains the physiological description of the endothelium as a leaky membrane.

Gap junctions and intermediate junctions are also present. The gap junctions promote intercellular communications, while the intermediate cells are weaker variants of desmosomes or macula adherentes. The latter are junctions which support cell adhesion but do not need to be as strong as the desmosomes found in the epithelium along the ocular surface where shearing and other forces may challenge structural integrity. Endothelial junctions occur along the lateral sides, mostly in junctional complexes located near the apex of the cell.

In humans, most cell division ceases before birth (Murphy et al. 1984), although some mitosis may occur in very young (Speedwell et al. 1988). Cells increase in size during growth of the eye and spread to cover damaged areas when injured.

Clinically, the endothelium is visualized using specular reflection with a biomicroscope or an endothelial specular microscope. The view is:

- A two-dimensional image; three-dimensional assumptions cannot be made from it.
- Of the posterior face of the cells – the interface between the endothelium and the aqueous. All that is seen is the apical plasmalemma of the endothelial cell, and cellular size and volume cannot be assumed.

Inferences in the literature based on specular microscopy may therefore be flawed or should be accompanied by a clarification that observations concern only one of the multiple, mostly 8, sides forming these cells.

Polymegethism – the presence of large and small cells in the endothelial mosaic – was first described by Schoessler and Woloschak (1981) in polymethylmethacrylate (PMMA) contact lens wearers. The mosaic is uniform, especially in the young, and becomes less so with age and disease. Cell density also decreases with age (see Bergmanson 2000, 2006) and, where cells are lost, the lateral borders of adjacent cells expand to fill the space. Thus, the endothelium becomes more polymegethous with age.

Contact lens wear does not accelerate cell loss (Doughty 1989, Bergmanson & Weissman 1992). Studies assessing the functionality of the endothelium in contact lens wearers with polymegethism and comparing these with control groups failed to uncover any functional deficits in the polymegethous corneas (Bourne et al. 1999, Patel et al. 2002). Rao et al. (1979) suggested that contact lens-induced polymegethism would increase the chance of developing pseudophakic bullous keratopathy following cataract surgery, but Bates and Cheng (1988) refuted this.

Bergmanson (1992) proposed a three-dimensional explanation to polymegethism in contact lens wear. He observed that the

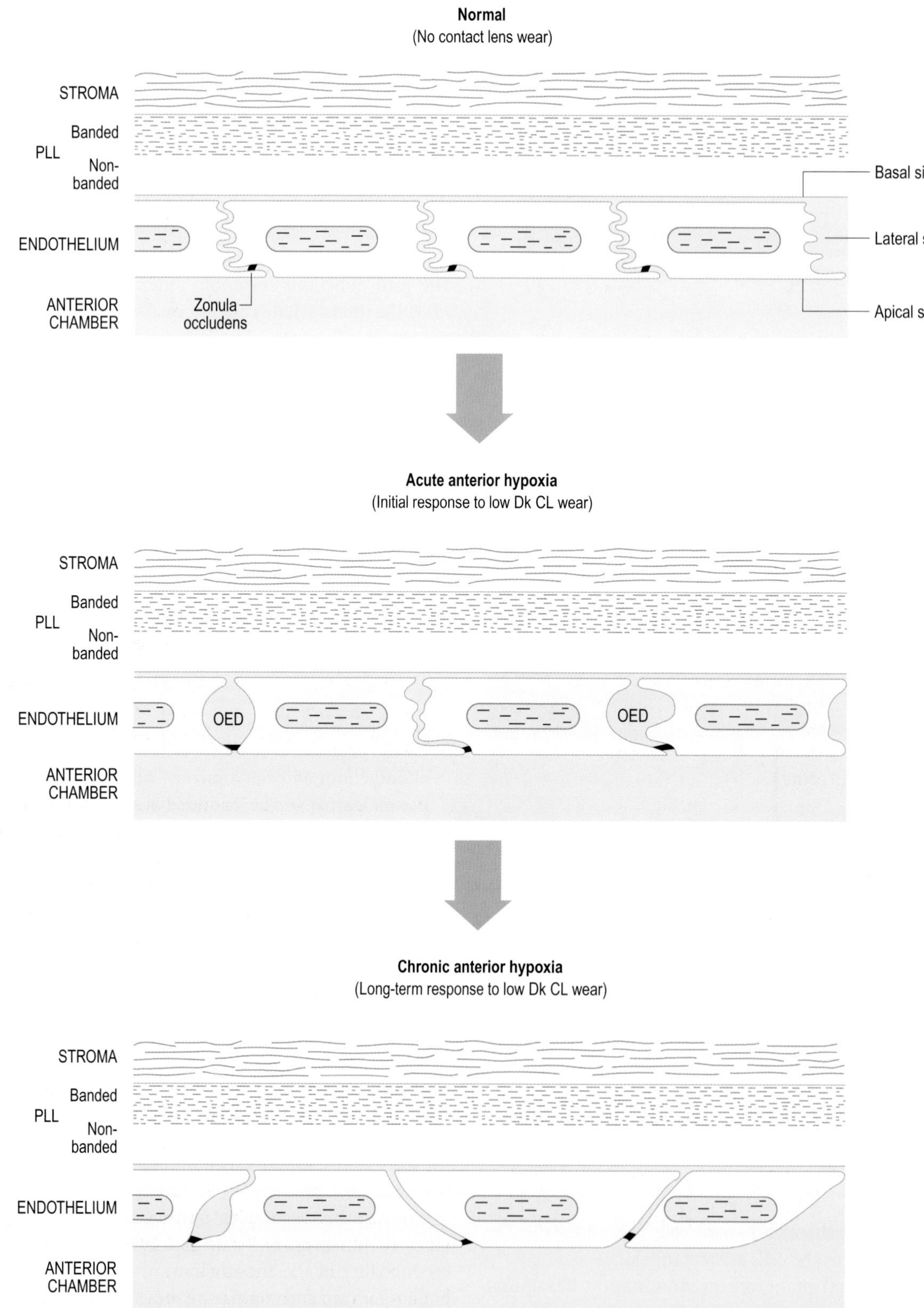

Figure 2.16 Polymegethism. Diagram after Bergmanson (1992) summarizing the events leading to endothelial polymegethism in contact lens wearers where the lateral sides straightened and reoriented to become oblique rather than perpendicular to the corneal plane. This theory suggests that cells with a large apical side may have a compensatory small basal side and vice versa. This three-dimensional imaging proposes that the endothelial cells only changed shape and did not become randomly bloated or shrivelled. PLL, posterior limiting lamina (Published with permission from Jan Bergmanson; Clinical Ocular Anatomy and Physiology, 12th edition, 2005)

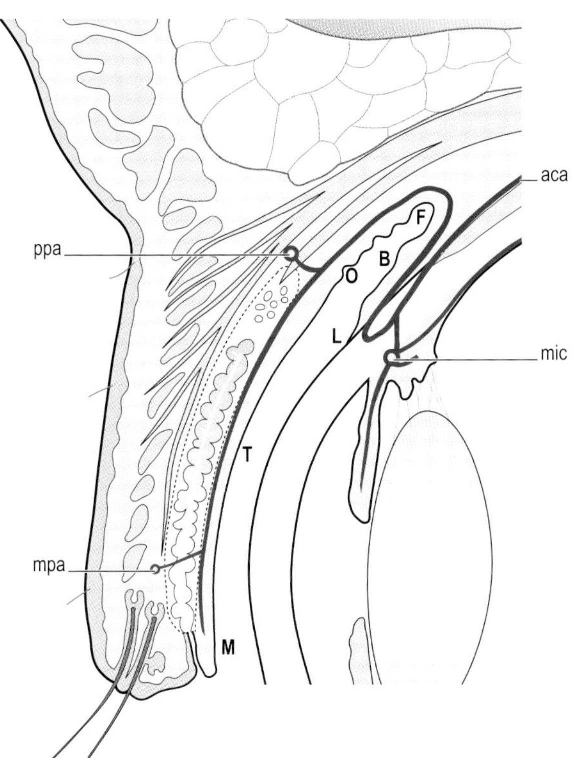

Figure 2.17 The subdivisions of the conjunctiva and the principal sources of blood. B, bulbar; F, forniceal; L, limbal; M, marginal; O, orbital; T, tarsal. The marginal, tarsal and orbital parts constitute the palpebral conjunctiva: aca, anterior ciliary artery; mic, major iridic circle; mpa, marginal palpebral arcade; ppa, peripheral palpebral arcade

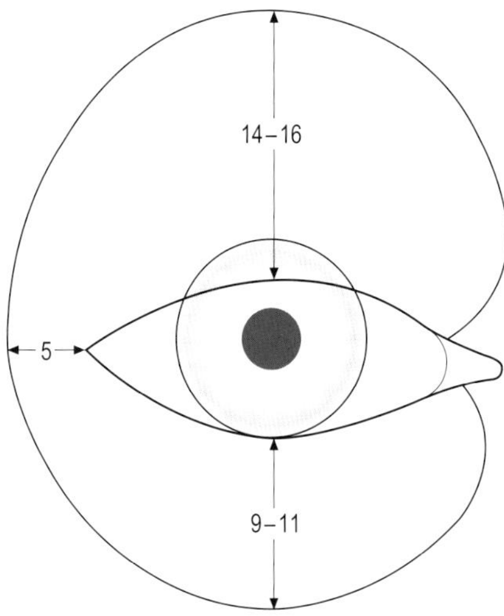

Figure 2.18 Approximate contours of the fornix and the dimensions of the unextended conjunctival sac in millimetres when the eye is open. [Based on the data of Whitnall (after Baker) and Ehlers (1965b)]

lateral sides, instead of being extensively perpendicularly interdigitated with the plane of the cornea, had in the polymegethous cornea become stretched out and reoriented in an oblique manner (Fig. 2.16). Cells with a small anterior surface area could therefore have a compensatory larger anterior surface and vice-versa and could rearrange their sides but maintain their volume. This may explain why polymegethism in contact lens wearers does not appear to cause any functional deficit.

Polymegethism persists at least as long as the contact lenses are worn (Stocker & Schoessler 1985) and does not resolve after 6 months without wear (Holden et al. 1986). However, two separate studies showed that, when patients are followed over 5 years, partial recovery occurs (Sibug et al. 1991, Odenthal et al. 2005).

THE CONJUNCTIVAL SAC AND THE EPITHELIAL SURFACE

The subdivisions of the conjunctiva are shown in Figure 2.17. It:

- Is a seromucous membrane.
- Provides mucus secretion.
- Contains the outlets for the ocular serous-producing glands.
- Lines the posterior surface of each eyelid, reflecting sharply at the fornix to line the anterior eyeball where it becomes continuous with the corneal epithelium.

The opposite faces of the conjunctiva are separated by a very thin liquid film. Estimates of the depth of the sac vary, and the measurements of the sac superiorly and inferiorly are presented in Figure 2.18.

- The sac circumference has a mean value of about 9.5 cm, and Ehlers (1965b) showed that the circumference varies with the width of the palpebral fissure.
- The conjunctiva covering the eyeball (bulbar), and especially that of the fornix, is thrown into numerous horizontal folds and consequently the sac is potentially larger than is shown in Figure 2.18.
- Ehlers (1965b) found that the sac may be distended inferiorly to 14–16 mm and superiorly to 25–30 mm, which is more than enough to lodge a displaced contact lens.

The wet, unkeratinized conjunctival epithelium presents a smooth surface of fine packed microvilli or microplicae approximately 0.75 μm in height. The tightly packed marginal and limbal epithelia are stratified and up to 12 cells thicker than elsewhere. The tarsal surface is also smooth but a subtarsal fold is often present, marking the marginal termination of the tarsal plate in the upper eyelid where small foreign bodies can lodge. Intercellular attachments are predominantly by desmosomes, and hemidesmosomes attach cells to the basement membrane with a similar anchoring mechanism as described in the cornea. A few gap junctions are present, and tight junctions girdle the apical walls.

In the tarsal area, the marginal stratified epithelium quickly gives way to a layer of mainly cuboidal cells three or four deep (Fig. 2.19). Beyond the tarsal plate, the orbital conjunctival epithelium thickens as the cells become columnar and the intercellular gaps increase, the stability of the layer being aided by reciprocal thin digital processes joined at or near their tips by

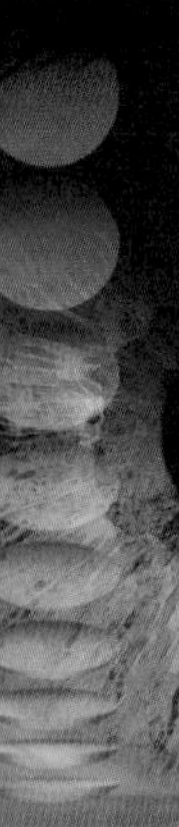

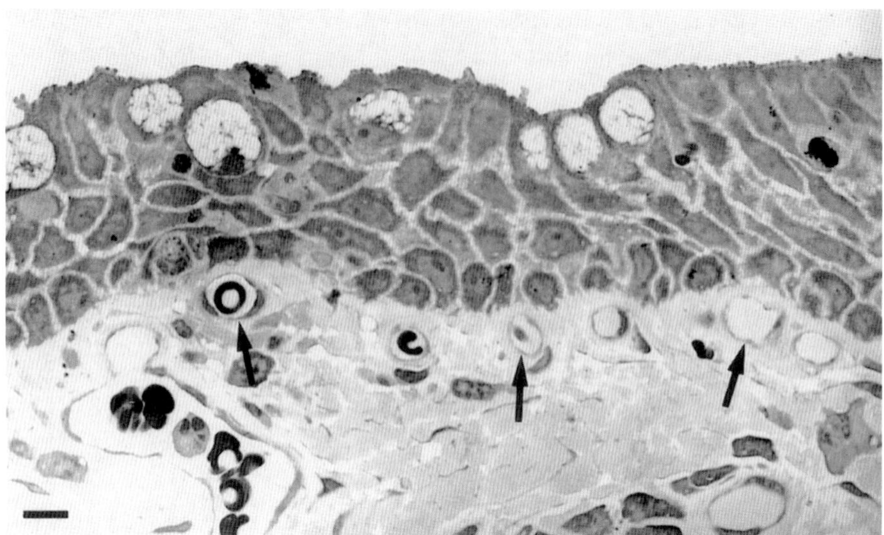

Figure 2.19 Conjunctiva from opposite the margin of the upper eyelid tarsal plate. The epithelium is four or five cells thick and contains a few goblet cells. Numerous capillaries (arrows) lie adjacent to the basement membrane. Further from the margin the epithelium thins slightly. Bar = 10 μm

desmosomes. Spaces between cells facilitate folding of the layer without jeopardizing cell integrity.

Little change in thickness occurs at the fornix or, at first, in the bulbar conjunctiva, but then it gradually thickens, the spacing between cells reducing as they become less columnar and more stratified on approaching the limbal region. Here the layer varies from three to 12 cells thick according to position in relation to the limbal palisades of Vogt. These are linear ridges of fibrous connective tissue in the conjunctival stroma, arranged radially at the limbus and terminating very close (0.5 mm or less) to the cornea. There are 5–10 per mm and they are up to 1 mm in length.

The conjunctival surface is smoothed by epithelium, ridged in complementary fashion, to fill the troughs between palisades. These troughs are 10–20 cells thick, reducing to three or four cells at the crests. Palisades of Vogt regularly occur sagittally, most clearly at 6 o'clock, but are often barely discernible or absent horizontally. They are most visible in pigmented conjunctivae where the pigment, located in the stroma between the epithelial ridges, highlights the palisades.

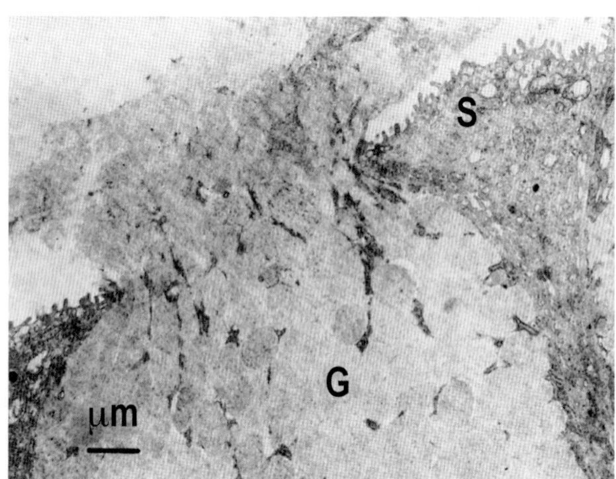

Figure 2.20 Electron micrograph of the apex of a conjunctival goblet cell. Nearly all the cytoplasm consists of secretion granules (G). The conjunctival surface is indicated by the microvilli of adjacent supporting cells (S). The material extruding from the apex of the cell includes secretion granules and other organelles of which granular endoplasmic reticulum can be recognized. Bar = 1 μm

GOBLET CELLS

Goblet cells are present in large numbers (Figs 2.19, 2.20) although their frequency varies:

- Low frequency in marginal epithelium.
- Slight increase in the tarsal area.
- High density in the orbital conjunctiva, fornix and neighbouring bulbar conjunctiva. This is greatest in children, falling to 50% of maximum in young adults, a level largely maintained in the following decades.
- Exposed areas of the bulbar conjunctiva have no goblet cells (Kessing 1968).
- Highest density in the lower nasal conjunctiva reaching a maximum at the plica semilunaris and caruncle.

Mature goblet cells measure 11 μm in diameter and are packed with secretory granules with an average diameter of 1 μm (Doughty & Bergmanson 2004b).

CONJUNCTIVAL EPITHELIUM

Epithelial cells along the ocular surface contain secretory granules which make an important contribution to the tear film. The discharged, long-branched mucoprotein chains remain attached to the epithelial cell membrane on the surface and provide an anchor for the mucus layer secreted by the goblet cells (Dilly 1985). They represent the glycocalyx of the surface cells and the vesicle-bearing surface cells of the cornea, those of the whole conjunctival surface producing their own glycocalyx. This thin layer appears in the newborn animal on first opening the eyes (Watanabe et al. 1993). Vesicles in the bulbar conjunctiva increase in number in contact lens wearers (Greiner et al. 1980).

Some cells appear to have the capacity to remove substances from the surface of the conjunctiva by ingestion through pinocytotic vesicles, which discharge into the intercellular spaces and subsequently to the subepithelium for removal by the vascular system (Steuhl & Rohen 1983).

The mucous products secreted by the epithelial cells are known as MUC 1 and MUC 4. They prevent adhesion of microorganisms and inflammatory cells and also act as wetting agents. MUC 1 and MUC 4, together with the mucins MUC 5AC and MUC 2 secreted from the goblet cells, form the deeper aspect of the tear film (see 'Precorneal film', below). This is essentially interposed between the watery phase of tears and the hydrophobic cell membrane (Phlugfelder et al. 2000, Argueso & Gipson 2001) and is vital for spreading the film over this hydrophobic surface. The gel-forming MUC 5AC also projects into the overlying water phase and probably helps stabilize the tears.

The conjunctival epithelium normally receives migratory cells including Langerhans cells, melanocytes and leucocytes, mainly T-lymphocytes of both suppressor and helper types, and neutrophils. The number of leucocytes is low in healthy conjunctival epithelium. Langerhans cells are largely concentrated at the limbus and lie on or close to the basement membrane as in the cornea (see above).

Melanocytes are small, dendritic and mainly basal, and are often confused with Langerhans cells if they lack melanosomes. Melanosomes are commonly absent in young Caucasians, although pigmentation may increase with age, but often occur in other races. Epithelial cells are derived from the neural crest. They cannot generate pigment but receive it from melanocytes.

CONJUNCTIVAL CIRCULATION

The blood vessels of the bulbar conjunctiva tend towards a radial arrangement. Arterioles pass from the anterior ciliary arteries before they penetrate the sclera while others pass round the fornix from arterioles of the palpebral conjunctiva (see Fig. 2.17). At the limbus, capillaries are again radially disposed, mainly within the palisades and form fine vascular loops at the margin of the cornea. Venules pass back, converge and anastomose frequently and many of the larger venules lie adjacent to the arterioles. The sclera overlaps the cornea anteriorly about the vertical meridian and gradually loses transparency across the transition, giving the impression that the limbal vessels penetrate the cornea. Conjunctival capillaries are commonly closed in the normal eye but irritation increases the number and size of blood-bearing vessels.

Small lymphatic vessels are present in the conjunctiva including fine lymphatic capillaries that extend to the corneoscleral border, often within palisades. They drain into larger subconjunctival vessels.

LYMPHOCYTES

These reside in the conjunctival stroma, especially in the palpebral region, where there are also discrete, dense accumulations accommodated in lymph follicles or nodules. Most of these lie in the orbital and peripheral tarsal conjunctiva, immediately underlying the epithelium, which is modified opposite the follicle. They appear topographically as translucent, white or yellowish elevations up to 1 mm in diameter. They enlarge and become more numerous in certain maladies.

Papillae are another form of inflammatory cell accumulation, with lymphocytes predominant (Kessing 1966). The distinction between papillae and follicles is unclear but, respectively, papillae are usually stated to have centrally and peripherally located blood vessels. Enlarged papillae occasionally infiltrate much of the tarsal area in contact lens wear or in the presence of other foreign bodies such as a prosthetic eye resulting in giant papillary conjunctivitis (see Chapter 17).

CONJUNCTIVAL INNERVATION

The upper conjunctiva receives a limited sensory innervation from the ophthalmic nerve. The lower conjunctiva is partly innervated by the infraorbital branch of the maxillary nerve in monkeys (Oduntan & Ruskell 1992) although the ophthalmic nerve is the major provider of sensory fibres. A few sensory terminals enter the epithelial layer where they lie on the basement membrane or between basal cells (Macintosh 1974) but most appear to be associated with blood vessels (Stone & McGlinn 1988). Infrequent complex encapsulated terminal forms are present in the stroma of the bulbar conjunctiva in humans, and these are presumed to be sensory (Lawrenson & Ruskell 1993). They occur more frequently in the upper temporal quadrant, and especially at the limbus in association with the palisades.

Sympathetic nerves from the superior cervical ganglion and parasympathetic nerves from the pterygopalatine ganglion are also found in the bulbar conjunctiva in primates (Macintosh 1974, Ruskell 1975) and subprimates (ten Tusscher et al. 1988, Elsas et al. 1994), both being substantially vasomotor.

THE EYELIDS

- The skin of the eyelids is very thin.
- The epidermis consists of only six or seven layers of epithelial cells beneath the keratinized surface layer.
- At the lid margin, the epithelium thickens and becomes moist and the keratinized layer terminates at and around the orifices of the tarsal glands. In fact, keratinization can be seen to project a few microns into these openings.
- The epithelium is continuous with that of the marginal conjunctiva where the epithelium is the thickest in the eyelid.
- The dermis contains small sweat glands.
- The hairs of the skin are extremely fine and short and, where the skin is regularly folded upon itself in the palpebral furrows, the hairs barely extend beyond their follicles.
- There are small sebaceous glands associated with the hairs.
- Nearly a third of the thickness of the eyelid is made up of the striated orbicularis oculi muscle, which is bordered anteriorly and posteriorly by loose non-adipose connective tissue (Fig. 2.21).

The orbicularis is a thin muscle surrounding the palpebral aperture and extending well beyond the orbital margin on to the face. Structurally and functionally, the muscle is divisible into orbital and palpebral portions. The orbital portion approximates a horizontal ellipse lying beyond the orbital

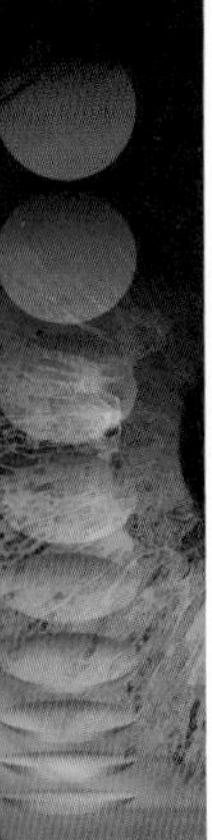

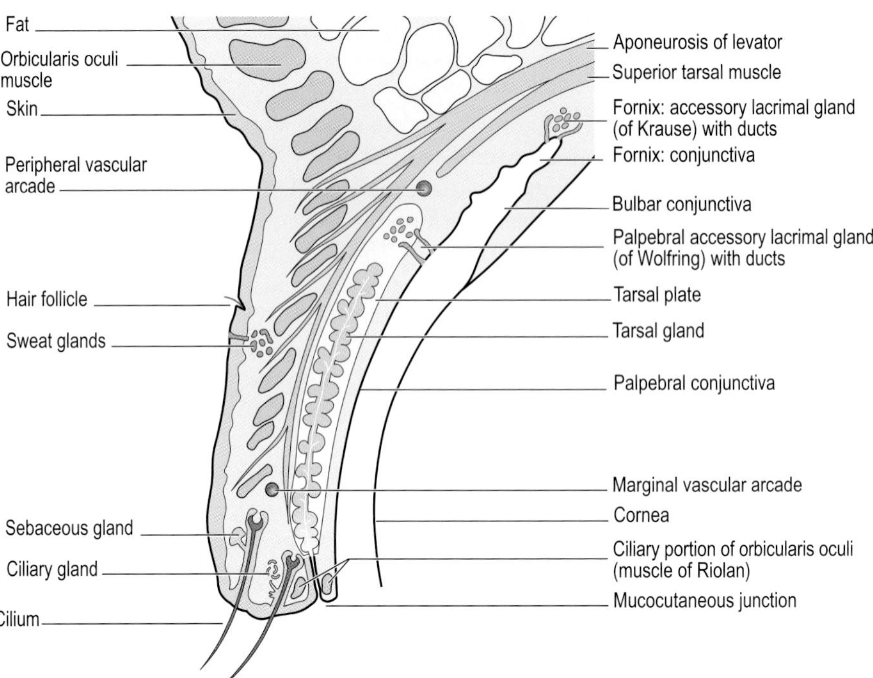

Figure 2.21 Transverse section through the upper lid showing pertinent lid structures and their relations (Published with permission from Jan Bergmanson; Clinical Ocular Anatomy and Physiology, 12th edition, 2005)

margin. It is continuous with the palpebral portion, which itself is clearly divisible into preseptal (lying in front of the orbital septum) and pretarsal parts, the latter terminating near the palpebral margins.

The muscle bundles along the lid margin, posterior to the follicles of the eyelashes, are sometimes referred to as the ciliary portion of the orbicularis oculi (muscle of Riolan) (see below).

Behind the orbicularis oculi lies the dense, fibrous tarsal plate, regarded as the skeleton of the eyelid. Its base is close to the lid margin. In the upper lid, it extends to the level of the superior palpebral furrow and its upper boundary describes an arc from the medial to the lateral canthus. In the lower lid the plate is only a third as deep.

TARSAL GLANDS

Lid eversion reveals the tarsal (meibomian) glands, which are buried within the tarsal plate.

- The glands run nearly the full length of the tarsus and beyond the tarsus at the lid margin.
- They are approximately parallel.
- There are about 25 in the upper eyelid and about 20 in the lower eyelid.
- The openings of the gland ducts are disposed in a single row along the lid margin, behind the lashes.
- The sebaceous and holocrine glands and ruptured pyknotic cells secrete the oily superficial layer of the tear film (see Chapter 5).

Tarsal glands commonly become infected, forming a chalazion or internal stye, a small, hard, discrete elevation of the inner surface of the eyelid, which may irritate the cornea. Chalazia may require surgical removal through an incision in the palpebral conjunctiva.

Embedded in the tarsal plate is the tarsal accessory lacrimal gland (of Wolfring), which has numerous openings, measuring from 10 to 100 μm in diameter. It secretes directly onto the cornea by a ductal system that traverses the palpebral conjuctiva (Bergmanson et al. 1999). This makes the conjunctiva a seromucous membrane and not simply a mucous membrane (Doughty 1997, Bergmanson et al. 1999, Doughty & Bergmanson 2003). In the rabbit, the ducts leading from the acini (small sacs) to the palpebral surface follow a tortuous and complex route to reach the surface (Fig. 2.22).

The palpebral conjunctiva lines the posterior face of the eyelids. It is firmly attached to the tarsal plate by a thin fibrous subepithelial layer that is rich in capillaries and venules. There is good evidence that the vessels nourish the cornea when the lids are closed. Some small lymphatic vessels are also present in this layer, which communicate with other lymphatics of the eyelids at the upper and lower margins of the tarsal plate. The epithelium is described above.

The levator palpebrae superioris is a striated muscle which elevates the upper eyelid. It therefore opposes the action of the orbicularis oculi. The levator passes above the superior rectus muscle within the orbit and has a broad tendinous insertion in the lid. Part of the insertion terminates at the upper border of the tarsus and the remainder passes in front of the tarsus between the fascicles of the orbicularis to the skin. The levator is innervated by the oculomotor nerve. Other eyelid musculature is beyond the scope of this chapter.

Structure of the eyelid margin

The line of tarsal gland orifices at the margins of the lids marks the sharp transition from the unkeratinized epithelium of the conjunctiva posteriorly to the keratinized epithelium of the skin. Two or three irregular rows of cilia, or eyelashes,

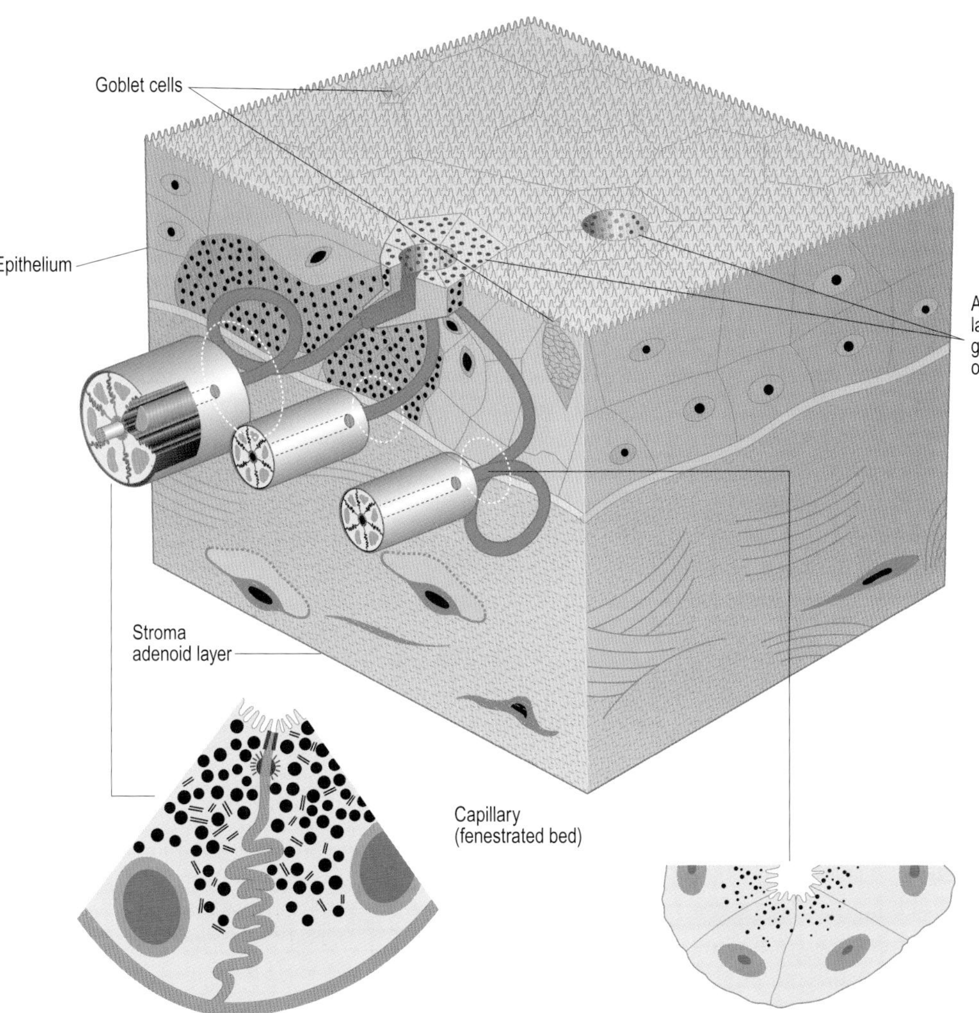

Figure 2.22 Palpebral accessory lacrimal gland (of Wolfring) and its relationship to palpebral conjunctiva. The ducts leading from the acini follow a tortuous and complex route to the palpebral surface. The ducts are lined by epithelial cells containing secretory granules (Published with permission from Jan Bergmanson; Clinical Ocular Anatomy and Physiology, 12th edition, 2005)

emerge from the skin in front of the tarsal gland orifices. The lashes are thick and strong, and those of the upper eyelid are longer and more numerous. The lash follicles are disposed between the terminations of the pretarsal portion of the orbicularis muscle and the lid margin; they lack arrectores pilorum. Lashes are replaced two or three times a year and regrow quickly after epilation. They are normally curved outwards and cause problems if they grow inwards (trichiasis) and touch the cornea.

Paired sebaceous glands (of Zeis) open into the lash follicles and their oily secretion moistens the lashes. Ciliary glands (of Moll) are also present in small numbers in the lid margins. Unlike sweat glands elsewhere, they are uncoiled and possess a wide lumen. Although they sometimes open into lash follicles, they usually exhibit the common feature of sweat glands of opening directly onto the skin.

Small bundles of striped muscle fibres (of orbicularis oculi – Riolan) are present immediately beneath the skin of the lid margins, mostly anterior to the tarsal gland ducts. In general, they run approximately parallel to the lid margins but some fibres pass obliquely between the ducts. It has been postulated that these fibres control the lumina of the ducts. This appears unlikely other than incidental to their function of maintaining the lid margins in apposition to the eye during lid closure.

The palpebral conjunctiva adjacent to the lid margin of the upper lid acts as a 'lid wiper' in sweeping the ocular surface. If this area stains with fluorescein or Rose Bengal, Korb et al. (2002, 2005) termed it 'lid wiper epitheliopathy' which can help in the diagnosis of patients with dry eyes.

The conjunctival face of the eyelid margins receives the richest innervation (Munger & Hulata 1984, Baljet et al. 1989) via the ophthalmic division of the fifth nerve.

Lid movements

A basic rhythm of blinking occurs at an approximate frequency of 12 blinks per minute (King & Michels 1957, Carney & Hill 1982), with considerable variation between individuals and circumstances. Alterations in blink rate result from many factors such as anxiety, noise or a stuffy atmosphere but, interestingly, not by a dry atmosphere.

A blink is completed in less than one-third of a second. During this period, the eye moves rapidly upwards between 40 and 70 minutes of arc and between 20 and 100 nasally (Ginsborg 1952) and then returns. In secondary positions of gaze, there is a tendency for the eye to move towards the primary position during blinking (Ginsborg & Maurice 1959). This small displacement is insufficient to account for the movement of a contact lens relative

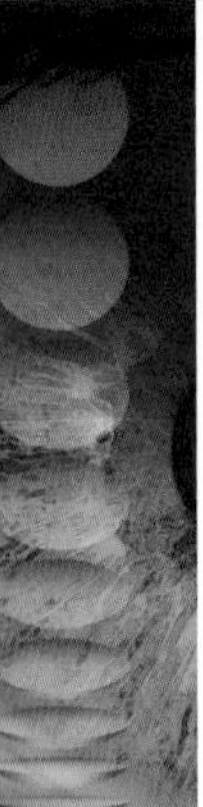

to the eye during a blink; clearly it is the traction of the eyelid that causes the lens movement. The blink rate is initially reduced when rigid contact lenses are worn (Brown et al. 1973).

If one eye is prevented from closing by holding the lid when a person attempts to shut both eyes, a movement upwards and outwards is usually seen. This displacement is known as Bell's phenomenon and is strikingly displayed in Bell's palsy. The movement is greater than that induced by blinking.

Closure on blinking is produced by relaxation of the levator followed by contraction of the palpebral portion of the orbicularis oculi. The whole orbicularis and frequently the accessory muscles contract when the eyes are squeezed shut. This may occur reflexly (optical blinking or menace reflex) together with a backward movement of the head when, for example, a tonometer or contact lens approaches the eye.

In downward gaze, as in reading, the orbicularis muscle plays no active part and relaxation of the levator alone is responsible for the partial closure of the palpebral aperture (Gordon 1951). In upward gaze, contraction of both the levator and the frontalis muscle occurs.

Corneal lens wear, especially extended wear, leads to a narrowing of the palpebral fissure or a slight ptosis (Fonn & Holden 1986, Fonn et al. 1996) (see also Chapter 9). Soft contact lenses do not have the same effect.

CORNEAL INNERVATION

The cornea is served by 70–80 small sensory nerves. These issue from ciliary nerves which branch from the ophthalmic division of the trigeminal nerve. They enter the sclera from the uvea at the level of the ciliary body and pass anteriorly to enter the cornea radially, predominantly in the middle layers. Other nerves from the same source enter the cornea superficially. They enter the conjunctival epithelium from the subepithelial tissue at the limbus and pass directly into the corneal epithelium at basal cell level (Lim & Ruskell 1978).

A minority of corneal nerve fibres possess a myelin sheath which is lost at the limbus or within 0.5 mm of entering the cornea. Occasionally, myelin persists further, even to the centre of the cornea, and appears opaque with a biomicroscope. The perineurium and the fibres and cells of the endoneurium also terminate at the limbus. Only the nerve fibre bundles advance into the cornea. Each bundle consists of several axons enclosed by a Schwann cell sheath (Matsuda 1968).

Initially, the fibre bundles of each nerve are grouped together. These separate and spread, overlapping and running together with branches from neighbouring nerves producing the plexiform arrangement seen in full thickness preparations of the cornea under low magnification with methylene blue stain (Zander & Wedell 1951, Oppenheimer et al. 1958) or with a stain for acetylcholinesterase (Fig. 2.23). The plexus is particularly dense beneath the anterior limiting lamina.

Axons separate and some divide at intervals and form fine terminal branches, some of which may lose their Schwann cell investment; the terminal axons follow a lengthy and tortuous course between the stromal fibrils (Fig. 2.24). They bear numerous small bead-like varicosities, with a final, often larger one marking the end of the axon.

Fibres from single nerve bundles at the limbus may be distributed to as much as two-thirds of the area of the cornea. Consequently, there is a considerable overlapping of nerve fibres from different nerve bundles. Measurements of receptive fields of the cornea of the cat recorded from ciliary nerves are consistent with the anatomical arrangement of nerve fibre bundles; indeed, overlapping of receptive fields of single nerve fibres has been demonstrated (Belmonte & Giraldez 1981). This arrangement explains why sensitivity persists in all areas of the cornea subsequent to large incisions and explains the inability to localize cornea stimuli.

The epithelium receives a prolific supply of terminal nerve fibres which pass perpendicularly from the plexus of the anterior stroma and penetrate the anterior limiting lamina (Bowman's layer). The small nerve fibre bundles lose their Schwann cell investment before entering the epithelium whereupon the fine naked axons disperse and turn sharply to lie nearly parallel to the anterior limiting lamina. They probably arborize (Ueda et al. 1989) as they pass between the basal cells. Varicosities similar to those present in the stroma occur in the epithelium. Such axons may run a course, often with little weaving, up to a length of 2 mm with fine beaded branches directed through successive layers of epithelial cells nearly to the surface of the cornea (Schimmelpfennig 1982, Tervo et al. 1985) (Figs 2.24, 2.25, 2.26). Matsuda (1968) observed epithelial nerve terminal beads of two types in rabbits and humans: one containing mitochondria and the other both mitochondria and vesicles. He suggested that beads without vesicles probably serve a sensory function, and those with vesicles are probably motor.

This leads to the question of whether the human cornea has an autonomic innervation. There is no reliable evidence of parasympathetic fibres in the cornea of any species and, in studies demonstrating the parasympathetic neurotransmitter – vasoactive intestinal polypeptide (VIP) – in various tissues of the eye, none is found in the cornea (Miller et al. 1983, Stone et al. 1986a). Various authors favour sympathetic innervation (Toivanen et al. 1987, Ueda et al. 1989, Marfurt & Ellis 1993) but doubt persists (Stone et al. 1986b, ten Tusscher et al. 1989) (see 'Cell production and corneal trophism' above).

Variety in their chemistry suggests that sensory fibres may consist of functionally distinct subgroups; some contain the neuropeptide substance P (Tervo et al. 1981, Stone et al. 1982), which is recognized as a neurotransmitter in the central nervous system, and others, of unknown chemical identity, do not (Lehtosalo 1984). Calcitonin gene-related protein (CGRP), another neuropeptide identified in the cornea, may coexist with substance P in the same terminal (Stone et al. 1986b).

Sensitivity of the cornea and conjunctiva

The sensitivity of the cornea is probably unsurpassed by that of any other part of the body. The stimulus employed in aesthesiometry was classically a fine hair or a series of hairs of different lengths and weights applied to the surface of the cornea but this was replaced by an unsupported nylon

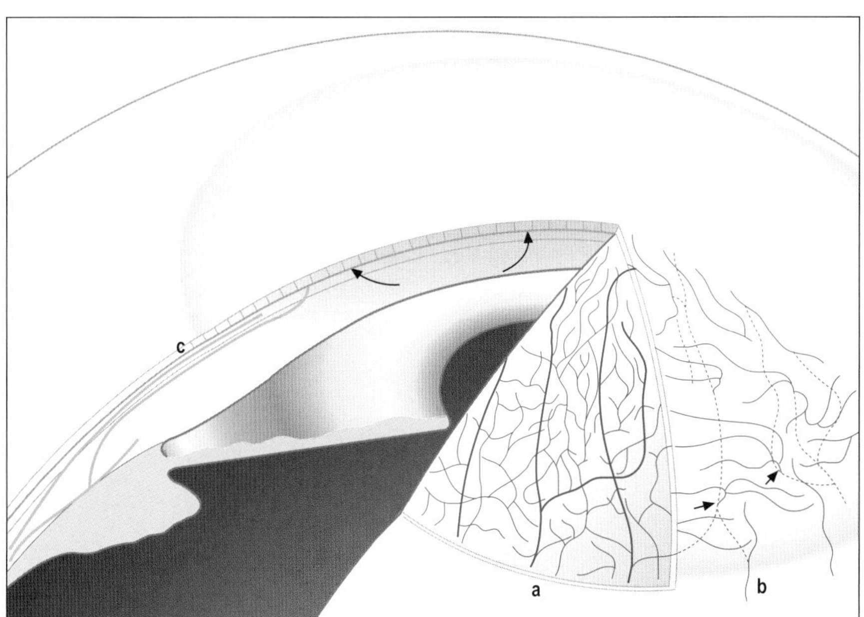

Figure 2.23 Anterior structures of the eye with a segment removed to reveal a meridional section; the topographical appearance of the stromal nerves of the cornea is presented at 'a' (the epithelium is removed), and the epithelial nerves at 'b'. The small arrows opposite 'b' indicate examples of stromal nerve (dotted) penetration to the epithelium. The longer arrows similarly show the penetration from the subepithelial plexus of nerves. The branch at 'c' enters the conjunctival epithelium very close to the cornea and crosses into the epithelium directly

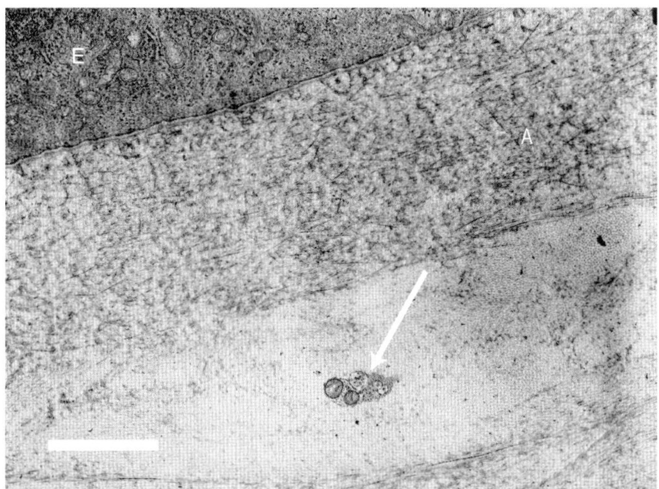

Figure 2.24 Electron micrograph of a stromal nerve terminal. Immediately adjacent to the anterior limiting lamina (A) is a single unmyelinated stromal nerve fibre bundle with varicose axons (arrow). It is within 15 microns of the epithelium (E) and its Schwann cell has opened up its mesaxons to promote transmission of stimulus. Bar = 4 μm. Monkey (*Macaque mulatta*)

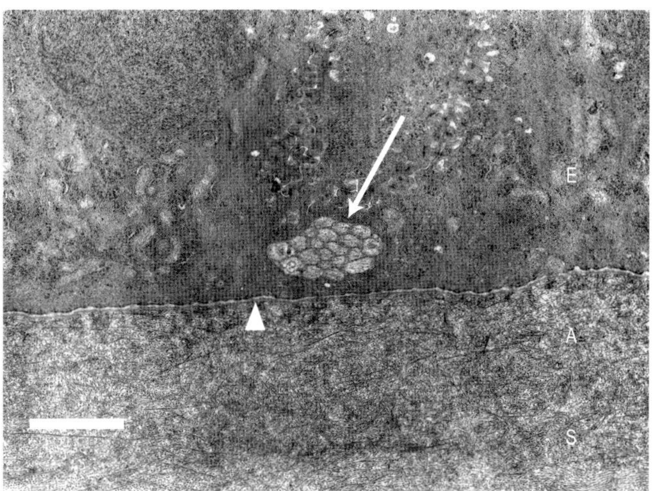

Figure 2.25 Electron micrograph of transverse section through the corneal epithelium (E). A group of naked axons (arrow) at terminal level travel deep in the basal cell layer and parallel to the basement membrane (triangle). Anterior limiting lamina (A) and stroma (S) are present in this view. Bar = 4 μm. Monkey (*Macaque mulatta*)

monofilament. The force exerted is measured in weight per unit area of contact. This remains constant and the weight or pressure is varied. Pressure on the instrument is increased until the monofilament bends and the force required to achieve this endpoint for any length of monofilament is precalibrated. The length of monofilament is decreased until a threshold response is elicited. The shorter the length of monofilament, the greater the pressure required to bend it.

An electronic aesthesiometer with an induction coil producing preset forces was developed by Draeger (1984). This has been superseded by the pneumatic aethesiometer, which uses controlled air flow as the stimulus (Vega et al. 1999). Threshold and differential responses can be measured electrophysiologically in experimental animals.

The sensitivity varies (Fig. 2.27):

- Maximum at the corneal apex – approximately 15 mg/mm^2 measured with a nylon filament
- Minimum at the periphery, but the highest peripheral corneal threshold is at the 12 o'clock position where it is

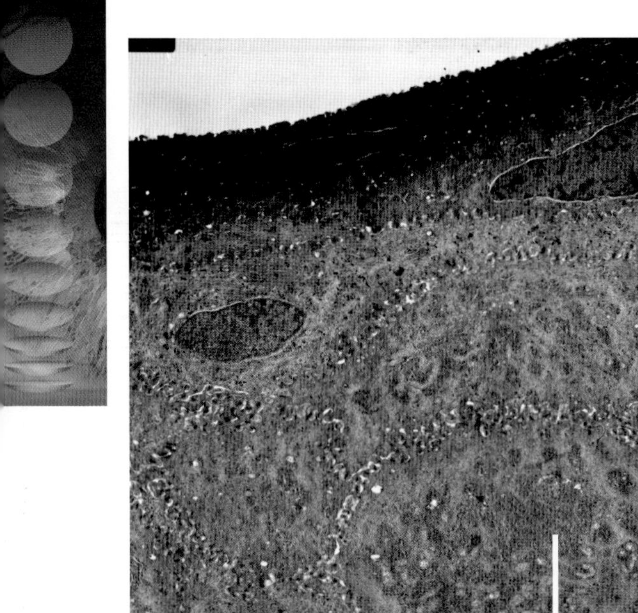

Figure 2.26 An electron micrograph of a group of epithelial nerve fibres. The naked axons travel close to the cell membrane of the basal cell internal side and parallel to the basement membrane. Consecutive varicosities (arrows) are present in some axons. E, epithelium. Bar = 8 μm

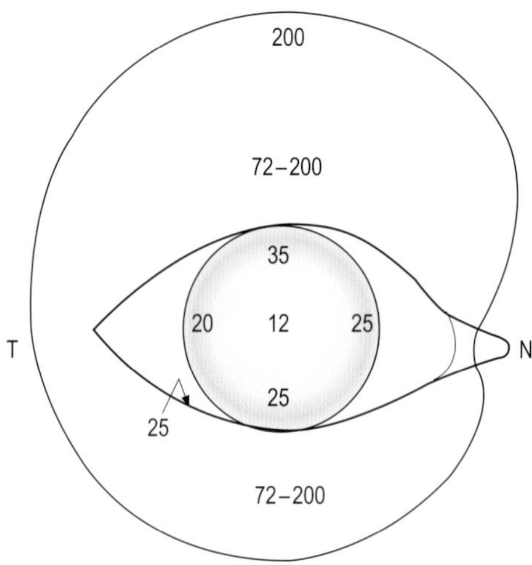

Figure 2.27 Touch thresholds (in mg/mm²) representing a synthesis of published results. Absolute values vary according to the technique used and those shown are considered the most likely to be obtained with careful use of a hand-held 0.12 mm nylon suture Cochet–Bonnet aesthesiometer. Lower thresholds would be obtained using a 0.08 mm instrument with mechanical control of application and microscopic viewing. The arrow indicates the marginal conjunctiva normally in contact with the eye

normally partially covered by the eyelid (Draeger 1984, Millodot 1984).

- Drops rapidly at the limbal conjunctiva.
- Reduces further to a minimum at the fornix.
- Increases at the lid margins.
- Continues to increase sharply from tarsal to marginal conjunctiva.
- Then reduces slightly at the narrow strip of conjunctiva contributing to the occlusal surface of the eyelid (Boberg-Ans 1955, Cochet & Bonnet 1960, Schirmer & Mellor 1961, McGowan et al. 1994).

When assessing sensitivity, the following should be considered:

- Age – in a study of 150 patients aged between 10 and 90 years, Boberg-Ans (1956) found a peak sensitivity in young patients three times that of his oldest patients. Millodot (1977) found a slightly greater difference. Most of the sensitivity reduction occurs between the ages of 50 and 65 years (Jalavisto et al. 1951) or later (Sédan et al. 1958).
- Inter-eye sensitivity is usually similar.
- Gender shows no reliable difference although Millodot and Lamont (1974) observed that the average sensitivity in nine women was approximately halved during the premenstruum and at the onset of menstruation (Fig. 2.28). Moreover, women may exhibit a transient reduction of sensitivity in the later weeks of pregnancy (Millodot 1977, Riss & Riss 1981).
- Diurnal variation – sensitivity increases by about one-third greater in the evening than in the morning (Millodot 1972).
- Iris colour – Millodot (1975b) found that blue-eyed people have a greater sensitivity than those with dark-brown irides (Fig. 2.29). Non-white people with dark-brown irides have less sensitive corneas than Caucasians with similar iris colour. On average, non-white people have four times less sensitive corneas than blue-eyed people and half as sensitive corneas as brown-eyed Caucasians. However, using a Belmonte pneumatic aesthesiometer, Henderson et al. (2005) were unable to demonstrate any relationship between sensitivity and eye colour but they did find that subjects with the palest irises appeared to show a linear association between eye colour and sensitivity to cooling stimuli.

Epithelial reinnervation of corneal transplants in humans may reach normal levels, whereas stromal reinnervation is sparse (Tervo et al. 1985). Recovery of sensitivity in the transplant area after several years is practically nil in some cases and slow and fractional in others (Ruben & Colebrook 1979, Lyne 1982, Draeger 1984, Macalister et al. 1993). Likewise, the recovery following excimer laser (LASIK, PRK) surgery is also incomplete. Trigeminal fibres to the cornea have some regenerative power but are unable to completely return to pre-trauma functionality.

Millodot (1984) studied the effect of various diseases on corneal sensitivity and found most reduced sensitivity. In particular:

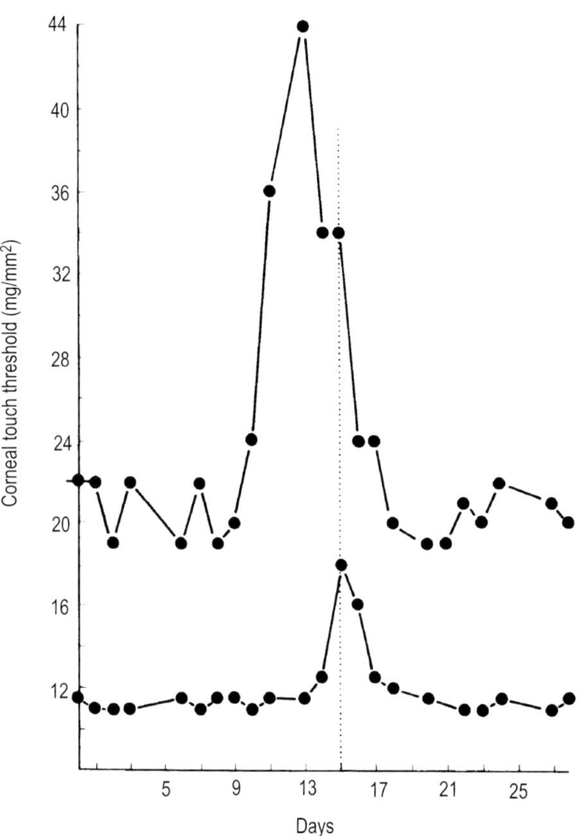

Figure 2.28 Relationship between corneal touch threshold and number of days of the menstrual cycle of two women. Days are numbered from the assumed occurrence of ovulation and the dotted line represents onset of menstruation (From Millodot and Lamont 1974, reproduced with permission from the BMJ Publishing Group)

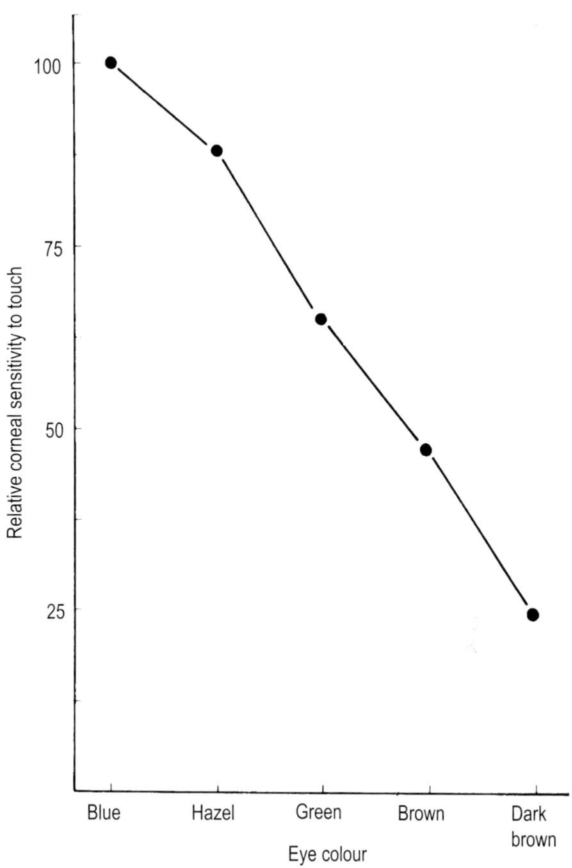

Figure 2.29 Relative corneal sensitivity to touch as a function of the colour of the iris (112 subjects). The dark brown group consists of non-white subjects. The sensitivity is the reciprocal of the touch threshold measured in mg/mm^2 and the group with greatest sensitivity has been assigned 100 (From Millodot, 1975b, by kind permission of the author and publishers)

- Keratoconus (Millodot & Owens 1983, Bleshoy 1986) – this does not correlate with the steepness of the cone and the reduction is largely confined to the central cornea.
- Diabetes (O'Leary & Millodot 1981).
- Albinism (Millodot 1978).

The effects of contact lenses on corneal sensitivity

Sensitivity reduction is chronic and slowly progressive, and after some years of daily PMMA lens wear, corneal sensitivity no longer returns to normal upon removal of the lenses (Fig. 2.30). Corneal sensitivity of long-term PMMA lens wearers improved substantially when transferred to rigid gas-permeable lenses (Bergenske & Polse 1987). Most of the improvement occurred within 7 days and was maintained for the remainder of the 6-month period of the study.

Thick soft lenses also depress corneal sensitivity but the amount is relatively small (Knoll & Williams 1970). Extended wear of conventional lenses appears to hasten the process, as sensitivity was less than half after 20 weeks (Larke & Hirji 1979). The rate of sensitivity loss also depends upon the lens material (Fig. 2.31) and well-controlled studies with silicone hydrogel lenses are awaited.

Oxygen deprivation is the major cause of corneal sensitivity loss and, presumably, mechanical assault is responsible for eyelid margin effects. Sensitivity reduces after sleep (see above) and when deprivation is extended by taping the lids, sensitivity reduction is much increased (Millodot & O'Leary 1980b). When atmospheric gases are controlled with goggles, sensitivity reduction is highly correlated with time of exposure to reduced oxygen levels.

Sensibility of the cornea and conjunctiva

One associates the sensations of pain and irritation with the cornea, possibly to the exclusion of any others. Lele and Weddell (1956) claimed that the sensibilities of touch, cold, warmth and pain may be experienced if the cornea is suitably stimulated.

Temperature-responsive corneal neurones have been identified in animals. Electrical recordings from rabbit anterior segments studied in vitro revealed cold-, mechano-, mechano/heat- and chemosensitive units (MacIver & Tanelian 1993) with different conduction rates (delta and C fibres) and related to different fibre orientations in the epithelium. For example, fibres running perpendicular to the corneal surface gave C fibre cold or chemosensitive responses. Gallar et al. (1993) found cold receptors, preferentially located at the periphery of the

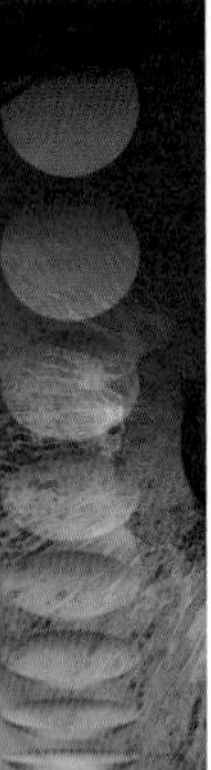

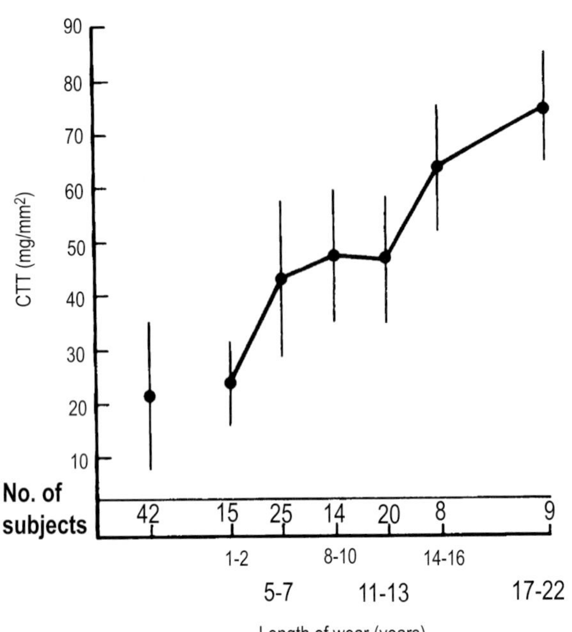

Figure 2.30 Chronic sensitivity reduction in PMMA contact lens wearers using a daily wear routine. The corneal touch threshold (CTT) was measured early on the day before insertion of the lenses. Vertical lines represent ± SD (From Millodot 1976, by kind permission of Blackwell Publishing)

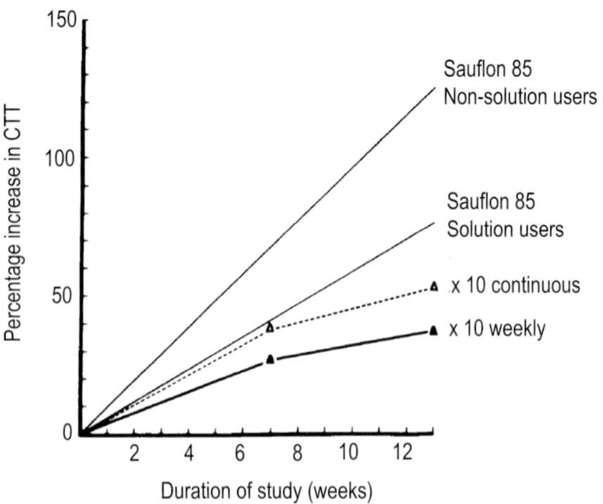

Figure 2.31 Variation in corneal touch threshold (CTT) with two types of high-water-content soft lenses worn differently. The Sauflon data were taken from the 20-week study of Larke and Hirji (1979) referred to in the text. ×10 is assumed to be an abbreviation for another type of extended-wear lens. (From Millodot 1984, by kind permission of Blackwell Publishing)

cornea in cats, which were distinguished from polymodal (mechanical, heat, chemical) receptors.

CORNEAL TRANSPARENCY

The most obvious and simple explanation for the transparency of the cornea is that its components all have the same refractive index, but a number of easily observed factors discount this. The structure of the cornea in unstained sections is discernible using phase contrast microscopy which is dependent on refractive index differences. Similarly, cellular detail is discernible in the living eye with a biomicroscope. The birefringence of the cornea is evident from the interference figures it displays when examined with polarized light, and this property has been examined in detail (Naylor 1953, Stanworth & Naylor 1953).

No satisfactory hypothesis explaining the transparency of the cornea as a whole has appeared but Maurice (1957, 1962a) offered an explanation of the transparency of the stroma. His hypothesis is precisely stated and does not invoke extravagant assumptions. It embraces light of all incidences and satisfactorily explains how transparency is lost in various circumstances. Maurice proposed that the stromal fibrils, which were found to have a refractive index of approximately 1.55 in the dry state, are so arranged as to behave as a series of diffraction gratings permitting transmission through the liquid ground substance (refractive index 1.34). We have already seen that the fibrils in adjacent regions of the stroma are of remarkably regular diameter and that they are probably regularly spaced so that, neglecting the curvature of the cornea, in any plane a reasonable facsimile of a diffraction grating exists. It is of interest to note that the fibrils of the opaque sclera do not show these properties.

A diffraction grating eliminates scattered light by destructive interference and permits the transmission of light energy maxima at angles θ to a normally incident beam, the angles depending on the physical characteristics of the grating and the light. Accordingly:

$$\sin \theta = m\lambda/d$$

where m is any integer, λ is the wavelength of light and d is the space between grating elements. The fibrils are the grating elements which, it is suggested, are disposed in a hexagonal lattice as shown in Figure 2.32. Only the first of the energy maxima applies because the grating or fibril interval is shorter than the wavelength of light, i.e. $\lambda/d > 1$, and the equation is only satisfied when m is zero and consequently θ is 0°. Thus, the transmission of normally incident light through the stroma, without deviation or significant scattering, is explained.

A light beam of other than normal incidence is covered by the hypothesis by considering an oblique lattice plane as shown in Figure 2.32. Other planes can be drawn, and together they explain the transmission of light through the cornea at different incidences.

The theory has gained wide acceptance as a reasonable explanation of transparency of the stroma, although Smith (1969) argued that Maurice's calculations of refractive index differences were incorrect.

The slight irregularities of collagen fibril separation as seen with the electron microscope were regarded by Maurice as preparation artefacts. Others, such as Hart and Farrell (1969), who computed the probability distribution function for the relative position of fibrils from electron micrographs, have taken them into account. They found that the mathematical summation of the phases of light waves scattered by the partially ordered array gave

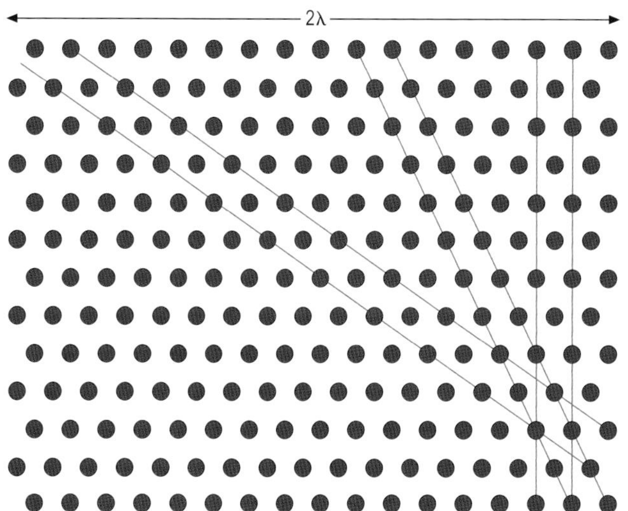

Figure 2.32 Lattice arrangement of the fibrils of the corneal stroma. If lines were drawn joining the adjacent fibrils, they would describe a lattice. The parallel lines pass through rows of fibrils and represent light wave fronts. The rows of fibrils may act as diffraction gratings (Maurice 1957) and hence, wave fronts of widely differing orientations may traverse the stroma

magnitude and wavelength dependence of the scattered light in good agreement with that found experimentally. Goldman and Benedek (1967) and Benedek (1971) presented proof that the scattering of light is produced only by fluctuations in the index of refraction (n) of wavelengths larger than one-half the wavelength of light in the medium (λ/2n). Since the index fluctuations are far shorter than this value, transparency of the stroma is explained without the need for a perfect lattice of collagen fibrils. It has the added advantage of explaining the transparency of the anterior limiting lamina. In practical terms, the cornea remains transparent as long as fibrils are not spaced further apart than λ/2n.

When the cornea is oedematous, its transparency is reduced. This can be explained in terms of the lattice theory in that the regularity of the fibrillar spacing is disturbed by the excess liquid and the efficiency of fibrils as grating elements is reduced. Local pressure on the cornea reduces transparency in the compressed region, again as a result of fibril disarray, but normal transparency returns immediately the pressure is withdrawn. The haze and haloes around bright lights which may become noticeable when contact lenses are worn are the result of corneal swelling, again explained in terms of the lattice theory. Alternatively, transparency loss with oedema may be explained by the formation of spaces within the stroma, free of collagen fibrils and larger than the critical size of half the wavelength of light.

Maintenance of corneal transparency is dependent on the forces which limit its hydration. These are susceptible to disturbances such as that produced on inserting a contact lens. In cases of severe corneal metabolic challenge, the overall corneal swelling is limited by the clamping effect of the sclera (Doughty & Bergmanson 2004a). The dehydrating forces are discussed in the following section.

Maintenance of corneal transparency

The cornea functions in a liquid environment and yet it has the capacity to maintain a steady solid/liquid ratio of about 1:4. If this ratio is increased by liquid uptake, the cornea loses its transparency. Removal of the epithelium in vivo leads to some hydration of the cornea but to a lesser extent than when the endothelium is removed (Maurice & Giardini 1951). Corneal swelling in rabbits caused by removing the epithelium is reversed from the periphery as cells from the conjunctiva slowly migrate across the cornea, while the remaining denuded area stays swollen. This situation is maintained even after 72 hours when 90% of the cornea is covered (Langham 1960).

The excised or damaged cornea can be remarkably hygroscopic and has a substantial swelling pressure. An excised cornea placed in water can increase to about four times its normal thickness (Müller et al. 2001) while an excised stroma might increase 10-fold in thickness (Doughty 2004). The cornea must therefore keep water out to maintain its transparency and this underlies the idea of a pump to remove water.

The integrity of the surface layers is essential for maintenance of corneal transparency and the pump must operate through them. The endothelium carries the major burden in this active process and could explain the high oxygen consumption per unit volume of the endothelium compared with that of the epithelium (Freeman 1972).

Maurice (1972) showed that the endothelium in rabbits can pump out water up to 12 times its own thickness in an hour. Both epithelium and endothelium act as inert partial barriers to ion and liquid influx under experimental conditions such as hypothermia or anoxia when the pump cannot be working; therefore, the pump must complement the structural barriers in effecting deturgescence of the cornea.

The barrier characteristics of the limiting layers are different, the epithelium being more impermeable to organic ions than the endothelium, while the endothelium is more resistant to diffusion of water (Maurice 1951, Donn et al. 1963). Current thinking is that the endothelium functions as a leaky membrane. The zonulae occludentes of the corneal endothelium do not encircle the entire cell, which is the case elsewhere in the body; thus there is a steady imbibing of water by the cornea, which must steadily be removed. This is commonly referred to as the pump leak theory. The cornea imbibes fluid and swells; in cases of corneal damage, there is a resultant increase in thickness and reduction in transparency. If significant leakage of fluid into the cornea occurs, whether caused by metabolic inhibition or damage, the 'pump' counters it.

The pump probably operates by expelling ions from the stroma to the fluids bathing the cornea, setting up an osmotic flow of water from the cornea. It is an active process and if corneal metabolism is inhibited the pump cannot operate and the cornea swells and loses transparency due to the uptake of water. A 'metabolic pump' therefore actively transports substances across the surface layers. Active transport describes the movement of a substance across a biological membrane against an electrochemical gradient, which requires energy. The potential gradient results from the inequality of distribution of electrolytes on the two sides of the membrane.

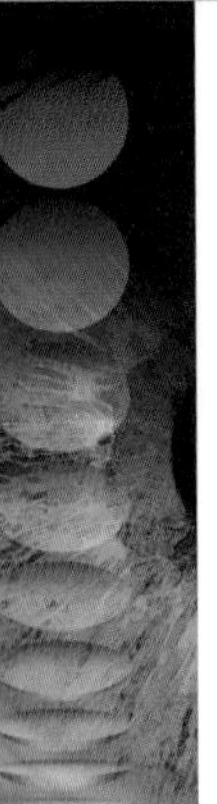

Sufficient reduction in temperature (Davson 1955, Harris & Nordquist 1955, Mishima 1968), deprivation of oxygen or the application of metabolic inhibitors such as ouabain (Trenberth & Mishima 1968), produces reversible swelling and opacification of the cornea, which demonstrates the importance of metabolism in maintaining corneal clarity.

Recovery of normal corneal thickness at body temperature after cooling of excised cornea, whether or not the epithelium is present, demonstrates that deturgescence is substantially the responsibility of the endothelium (Harris & Nordquist 1955). A punctate lesion of the corneal endothelium causes a well-circumscribed region of stromal opacification opposite it, suggesting that liquid intake is confined to the traumatized zone by the vigorous activity of the adjacent endothelium (Langham 1960).

The precise nature of the pump is not known but more than one type of ion is involved. Hodson and Miller (1976) demonstrated active transport of bicarbonate ions from endothelium to aqueous, activated by the enzyme carbonic anhydrase located adjacent to the posterior membrane of the endothelium.

The enzyme catalyses the conversion of carbon dioxide and water into bicarbonate and hydrogen ions. Bicarbonate is then actively transported to the aqueous humor. The endothelial pump is partly inhibited when carbon dioxide and bicarbonate are removed from the cornea. Sodium and bicarbonate ions are necessary for the pump to be fully active in maintaining the dehydrated cornea (Hodson 1977), indicating that the transport of bicarbonate is linked to that of sodium, most likely as indicated in Figure 2.33.

Sodium–potassium–adenosine triphosphate enzyme is present in the lateral walls of endothelial cells and probably contributes to the endothelial pump by promoting active transport of sodium from cell to aqueous. Ouabain, a specific inhibitor of this enzyme, causes corneal swelling (Geroski & Edelhauser 1984) and prevents reversal of oedema induced by cooling (Brown & Hedbys 1965). Other ions have also been implicated in the pump. The contribution of the epithelium to corneal deturgescence is unlikely to be attributable to its inert barrier characteristics alone, and a chloride pump acting through the epithelium to move water from the corneal stroma to the tear film has been identified in rabbits (van der Heyden et al. 1975, Klyce & Wong 1977, Beekhuis & McCarey 1986). Whether or not the chloride pump (see Klyce & Bonanno 1988) is generally applicable is uncertain as there is evidence of a chloride pump working in the opposite direction in humans (Fischer et al. 1978).

The picture becomes more uncertain if one considers the possible effects of various ions on the corneal stroma as well as on these pumps. For example, while corneal deturgescence can be remarkably sensitive to bicarbonate concentrations (Doughty 1985, 1987), the relative effect on the actual transendothelial fluid pump appears to be far less (Doughty & Maurice 1988). Doughty (1999) found that the hydroscopic properties of the corneal stroma can also be bicarbonate and pH sensitive, and that chloride ions might also play an important role (Guggenheim et al. 1995). From such a perspective, the leaky membrane of the corneal endothelium could play a role in regulating the anion composition of the corneal stroma in addition to transporting water out (Doughty 2003).

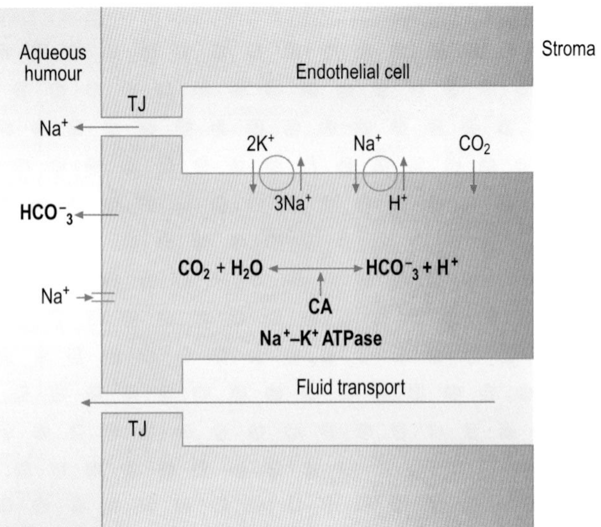

Figure 2.33 Scheme to show the principal components of the endothelial pump. The major factor is the combination of exogenous and endogenous CO_2 to form bicarbonate ions which act as a substrate for the endothelial transport mechanism resulting in translocation of bicarbonate ions to the aqueous. This mechanism is catalysed by carbonic anhydrase (CA) with hydrogen ions as a by-product. The carrier protein Na^+-K^+ ATPase, located in the lateral membranes, is responsible for transport of Na^+ to the intercellular space and presumably past the tight junctions (TJ) to the aqueous. It may also be indirectly coupled to the Na^+-H^+ exchange shown. The osmotic gradient generated by the active transport of these ions draws water out of the stroma into the aqueous. Opposing this outward pump is an inward 'leak' from the aqueous humour into the hygroscopic corneal stroma – the 'pump–leak' hypothesis. At steady-state stromal thickness, the fluid gain of the leak is offset by the fluid loss due to the pump

At the corneoscleral junction there is a potential liquid leak into the cornea, but Maurice (1962b) calculated that the endothelium has more than sufficient pumping power to deal with the influx of water from this region. The surrounding sclera, however, appears to play an important mechanical role in reducing the swelling of the corneal stroma (Doughty & Bergmanson 2004a).

GLUCOSE METABOLISM

De Roetth (1950) showed that carbohydrate metabolism predominates in the cornea as indicated by a respiratory quotient of 1, and glucose is the principal monosaccharide of this process. Much of the energy released in the metabolism of glucose is used in the phosphorylation of adenosine diphosphate (ADP) to adenosine triphosphate (ATP) and energy is stored in this form. The efficiency of a metabolic pathway may therefore be measured in terms of the number of ATP molecules produced. The processes of greatest importance in the metabolism of glucose

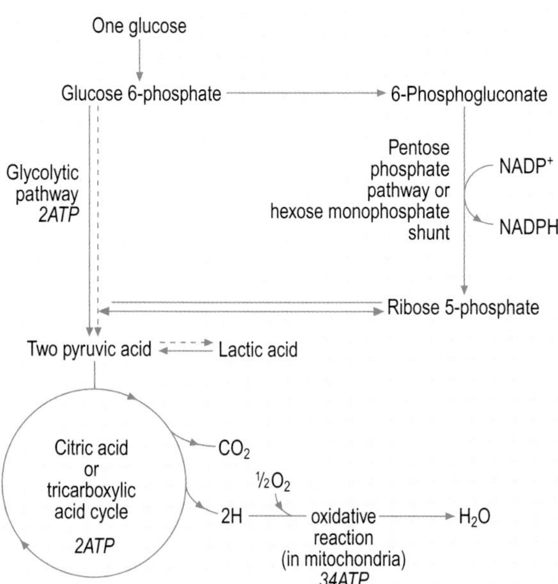

Figure 2.34 Outline of glucose metabolism in the cornea. Free oxygen does not take a direct part in the citric acid cycle, but its presence is essential and the cycle cannot operate in anaerobic conditions. Note the reversible connections between the pentose phosphate and glycolytic pathways

are, first, the glycolytic pathway followed by the tricarboxylic or citric acid cycle and, second, the oxidation of glucose directly by the pentose phosphate pathway or hexose monophosphate shunt. These will be considered in turn and then related specifically to corneal metabolism.

GLYCOLYSIS

In this complex glycolytic process, dehydrogenase enzymes act as catalysts for each stage in the process and finally split the glucose molecule into two molecules of pyruvic acid. In the third of the four stages of the glycolytic process, liberated energy is used to form two molecules of ATP from ADP and inorganic phosphate.

Under anaerobic conditions, pyruvic acid is converted to lactic acid without significant liberation or uptake of energy. Under aerobic conditions, glucose metabolism does not stop at this point but continues until the final products are carbon dioxide and water. This further breakdown is brought about by the citric acid cycle. During the cycle, carbon dioxide and hydrogen atoms are released. The hydrogen atoms eventually become oxidized to form water and the combined cycle and oxidative processes synthesize a further 36 ATP molecules (Fig. 2.34).

HEXOSE MONOPHOSPHATE SHUNT

Although the glycolytic pathway just described is the principal pathway for the oxidation of glucose, others are available. The hexose monophosphate shunt is the most important, in which glucose-6-phosphate takes part in a cyclic mechanism. Rather than producing ATP for general metabolic functions, this has the main purposes of providing reducing power in the form of reduced nicotinamide adenine dinucleotide phosphate (NADPH) which can be used for biosynthesis and to produce the ribose-5-phosphate necessary for the synthesis of nucleotides and nucleic acids. Due to the rapid production of epithelial cells, the cornea has a substantial requirement for these molecules.

CARBOHYDRATE METABOLISM IN THE CORNEA

Glycolysis is predominantly exhibited in the epithelium. The high level of enzyme and pyridine nucleotide concentration and the rate of oxygen consumption indicate that the endothelium also has a high glycolytic activity, but the relative inaccessibility of this layer has limited studies. In contrast, the stroma shows very little metabolic activity. Tissues exhibiting aerobic glycolysis accumulate lactate because the glycolytic pathway is more efficient than the aerobic mechanisms, which cause the combustion of pyruvate to carbon dioxide and water (Langham 1954).

Anaerobic glycolysis alone, with its low energy yield, is evidently inadequate to maintain the cornea in its normal state as, in the absence of oxygen, the cornea swells and loses its transparency (Heald & Langham 1956, and many others).

Kinoshita and his colleagues demonstrated that the hexose monophosphate shunt is unusually active in the cornea (Kinoshita & Masurat 1959, Kinoshita 1962). They estimated that, in the bovine corneal epithelium, about 65% of the glucose is metabolized by way of the glycolytic pathway followed by the citric acid cycle, and 35% by means of the hexose monophosphate shunt. Kuhlman and Resnick (1959) estimated that, in rabbit corneas, up to 70% of glucose is oxidized to carbon dioxide via the shunt mechanism.

The metabolism of the corneal layers is interrelated; for example, lactic acid is produced in all layers of the cornea but cannot be utilized in the absence of the epithelium (Hermann & Hickman 1948). Chen and Chen (1990) found about 95% of total corneal lactate in the stroma in rabbits but only 32% was produced there. The epithelium was the source of 47% and the endothelium 21%.

Sources of metabolites

There are three possible routes of metabolite supply into the cornea:

- Perilimbal blood vessels.
- Aqueous humor.
- Tear liquid.

The perilimbal blood vessels provide metabolites for the peripheral cornea but this route is of limited importance. Gunderson (1939) noted that corneal transparency was unaltered following complete peritomy of the cornea. Scarification of the conjunctiva in cases of perilimbal melanomas and experimental thermocoagulation of the perilimbal tissues in rabbits fails to interfere with corneal transparency. Diffusion of radioactive substances from the limbus into the cornea following subconjunctival or systemic injection is found in greater concentration peripherally than centrally (Maurice 1951, Pratt-Johnson 1959). Maurice (1962b) found that large molecules are the most likely to diffuse to the central cornea.

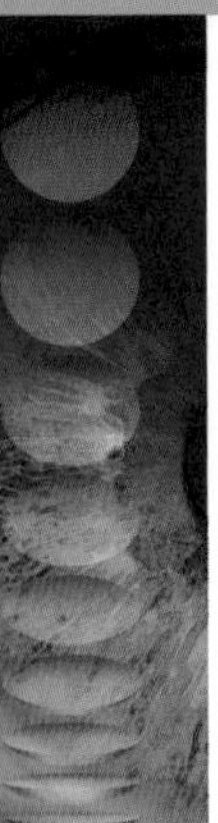

Bock and Maumenee (1953) inserted thin polythene sheets between stromal lamellae in rabbits and observed a thickening of the overlying stroma with complete degeneration of the epithelium in the central zone after 2 days. The deep underlying stroma and the endothelium were normal during this period and the epithelium maintained its integrity when the polythene sheet was trephined with several 2 mm holes. The authors concluded that the epithelium and stroma depend on the aqueous humor for metabolites. However, Pollack (1962) used water-impermeable polypropylene sheets inserted between stromal lamellae in cats and found they were tolerated for more than a year without pathological changes, deep or superficial to the sheet.

Clearly, the deeper layers flourish when isolated from the anterior layers and hence the aqueous must be a source of metabolites for the cornea. It is unlikely that much glucose moves in the other direction, from the tears to the cornea, as the concentration of 2.6 mg/100 ml in tears in humans (Giardini & Roberts 1950) is too little to be of much significance in the nourishment of the cornea (Maurice 1962b). Glucose concentration is more than ten times as great in the aqueous (Reim et al. 1967). A reduction in epithelial glycogen and ATP as well as glucose was demonstrated following the insertion of intralamellar membrane barriers (Turss et al. 1970) and these changes could not be prevented by tarsorrhaphy or the topical application of glucose.

Tears are an important source of atmospheric oxygen and vitamins in the form of ions such as calcium, potassium, magnesium and zinc (Bergmanson & Wilson 1989). A number of current dry eye tear formulations are formulated with these essential ions (e.g. Theratears) to better mimic the natural tears and provide necessary nutrition.

Thoft and Friend (1972) observed passive diffusion of labelled amino acid through the endothelium. The rapid turnover of epithelial cells demands a considerable utilization of amino acids in the synthesis of protein and, as expected, the concentration was high. It was actively accumulated by the epithelium only after it had appeared in the stroma, suggesting that none was taken up from the tears despite their rich amino acid content (Balik 1958). It appears, therefore, that epithelium has a very low permeability to amino acids and glucose.

The utilization of atmospheric oxygen by the cornea through the tear film has been demonstrated in a number of ways. In man, symptoms of corneal irritation, together with the haze and haloes known as Sattler's veil (Finkelstein 1952), were experienced when the cornea was deprived of atmospheric oxygen (Smelser 1952, Smelser & Ozanics 1952). These symptoms were induced 2.5 hours after pumping nitrogen saturated with water vapour into tight-fitting goggles. The introduction of oxygen relieved the symptoms. Langham (1952) exposed the eyes of rabbits to a pure oxygen atmosphere for 3–3.5 hours and found that the lactic acid concentration in the cornea was reduced by a third, indicating an increase in aerobic glycolysis. Using a nitrogen atmosphere for the same period of time, lactic acid concentration was increased by a third, a decrease in aerobic glycolysis.

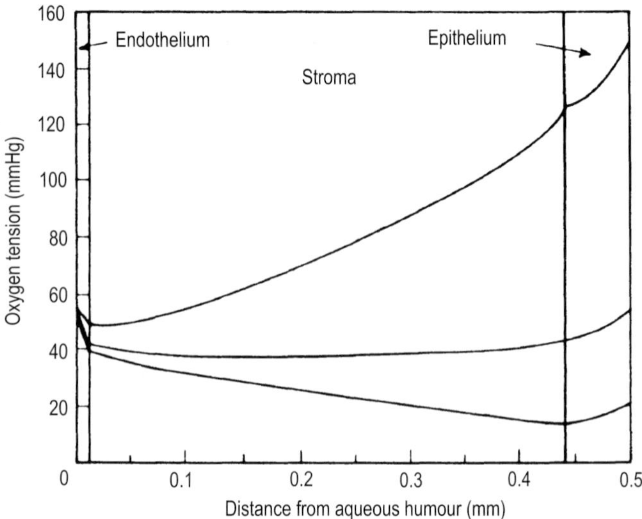

Figure 2.35 Summary of oxygen tension profiles for various conditions based on measurements made under each condition at the epithelial surface in rabbits. The curves joining the surface points were calculated. The upper and middle curves represent the eye in open and closed conditions, respectively. The lowest curve represents the profile with a soft contact lens of low permeability on the eye (Modified from Fatt et al. 1974)

Hill and Fatt (1964) measured the rate of oxygen uptake by the corneal epithelium in humans using oxygen electrodes embedded in a tight-fitting scleral lens with an oxygen-filled reservoir between the lens and cornea. They observed a rapid reduction in the oxygen tension in the reservoir as a result of oxygen uptake by the cornea. A rate of oxygen uptake of 4.8 μl/cm^2 per hour was calculated from their results. However, Farris et al. (1967), using the same technique, interpreted their data differently to arrive at a figure of 1.4 μl/cm^2 per hour.

Langham (1952) concluded that the rabbit cornea also utilizes aqueous oxygen. The lactic acid concentration decreased from a value of unity to 0.7, 3–3.5 hours after introducing an oxygen bubble into the anterior chamber. Barr and his co-workers found an oxygen gradient reducing from the front surface of the cornea to the anterior chamber in rabbits and concluded that atmospheric oxygen normally diffuses through the full thickness of the cornea to the anterior chamber (Barr & Roetman 1974, Barr et al. 1977). On the other hand, Fatt and Bieber (1968) and Fatt et al. (1974) concurred with Langham on the basis of calculated oxygen distribution profiles through the cornea, knowing the partial oxygen pressures at the two surfaces, stromal consumption, diffusion coefficients and solubility. The profile (Fig. 2.35) displays a trough at the stromal aspect of the endothelium, indicating that the endothelial layer receives oxygen from the aqueous. However, the crucial datum at the deep surface is difficult to determine and is supported by a single measurement.

Fatt and Bieber believed that the oxygen distribution profiles in rabbits represent, at least qualitatively, the situation in the human cornea. When the lids were closed long enough for equilibrium levels to be reached, the partial oxygen pressure at the epithelium reduced from 155 mmHg to the same level

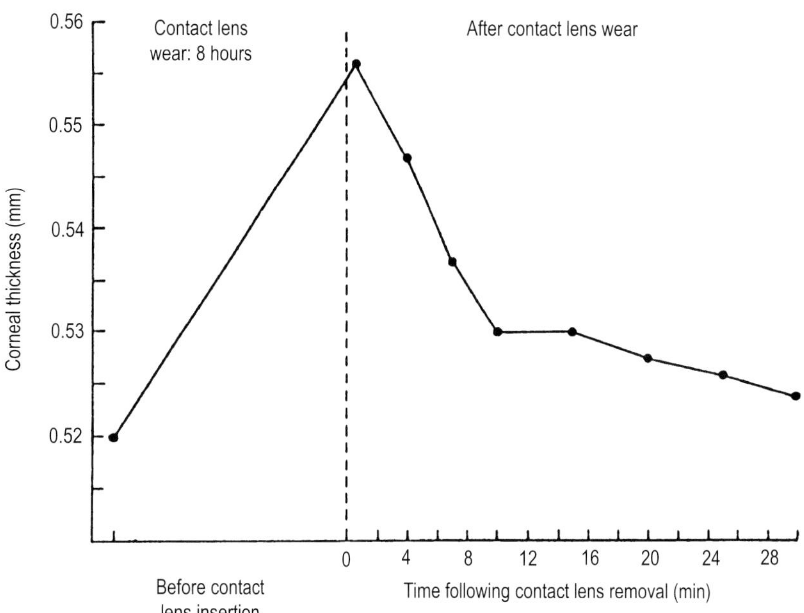

Figure 2.36 Relationship between central corneal thickness and the wearing of PMMA contact lenses for 8 hours. Each point represents the mean of 11 subjects. (After Millodot 1975a)

(55 mmHg) obtained at the endothelial surface (Fig. 2.35), with a trough within the stroma. Under these circumstances, it appears that the vessels of the palpebral conjunctiva must provide the epithelium with oxygen because if contact between these surfaces is prevented the partial oxygen pressure falls to zero. Earlier, Langham (1952) reached the same conclusion.

The altered profile suggests that aqueous oxygen is being used by deeper structures of the cornea. This interpretation is based on the assumption that aqueous oxygen levels are maintained whereas Barr and Silver (1973) claimed that it reduces as oxygen levels at the anterior surface of the cornea are reduced. Similar studies of the carbon dioxide partial pressures indicated that corneal and aqueous carbon dioxide passed out to the tears when the lids were open, but when they were closed some passed to the aqueous from the cornea.

The effects of contact lenses on corneal metabolism

A contact lens presents a barrier between the cornea and the atmosphere, which is likely to cause deprivation of oxygen with a consequent reduction in aerobic glycolysis. Oxygen uptake by the tears in front of the lens would continue but transference of oxygen through the lens is substantially impeded, especially with low Dk lenses. Lens movement will facilitate tears exchange at the lens perimeter which is the principal route for oxygen and carbon dioxide exchange with PMMA lenses.

The cornea can tolerate a reduction of the partial oxygen pressure at the epithelial surface from 155 mmHg (or a concentration of 21%) to 55 mmHg (7.5%), as when the lids are closed for some length of time as shown in Figure 2.35. Corneal metabolism is altered during sleep (which the middle profile of Fig. 2.35 may represent) as expressed by a slight oedema, thickening by about 4% (Mandell & Fatt 1965) and sensitivity reduction (Millodot 1972). Raised corneal temperature, lowered pH and hypotonicity of tears may contribute to these responses. Evidence shows that about 10% oxygen (70–75 mmHg) is necessary (Holden & Mertz 1984).

As discussed above, interference with normal corneal metabolism produces thickening and reduction of transparency of the cornea. The thickening observed with lens use varies between individuals and depends on the type and material of the lens. Numerous early studies of the effect of PMMA lens wear produced figures of corneal thickness increase of 4–8%, usually measured after 8 hours wear. Figure 2.36 shows a typical result and adds a temporal profile of recovery following lens removal. Epithelial swelling contributes to thickening (Farris et al. 1971).

Corneal thickening with early soft contact lenses was, at most, little more than the 4% or so incurred normally during sleep (Mandell & Fatt 1965). Corneal swelling with early rigid gas-permeable lenses was similar in amount to that induced with soft lenses when the two types were matched for oxygen transmissibility (O'Neale et al. 1984). The results of more recent materials are discussed in Chapter 13.

TEARS

The basic secretion of tears is largely derived from the lacrimal gland, with additional contributions from the accessory lacrimal glands: the mucous conjunctival glands and the sebaceous tarsal (meibomian) glands. A conjunctival gland or goblet cell is shown in Figure 2.20 in the process of releasing mucin granules into the tear film. The lacrimal gland is classified as a serous gland, but its cytology and histochemistry suggests some variety of output (Ruskell 1969, Allen et al. 1972). In the palpebral accessory lacrimal glands, the epithelial cells lining the ducts leading to the openings along the palpebral conjunctiva contained secretory granules. These granules have a

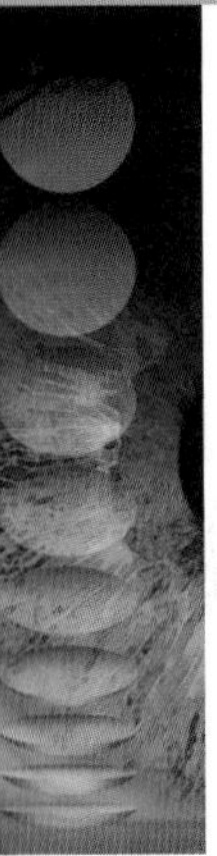

different electron density from those found within the acinar secretory cells (Bergmanson et al. 1999). It is possible that the ductal epithelial cells produce the mucoid secretion from this and the other lacrimal glands.

The eye remains moist if the lacrimal gland is congenitally absent, when the gland is removed or its motor nerve supply is interrupted, but this radically reduces basic tear secretion (Golding-Wood 1964, Ruskell 1969).

Superimposed on the basic secretion are the phasic increments in secretion induced reflexly by mechanical or chemical irritation and by psychogenic factors. To distinguish between the two, the words 'lacrimation' (to describe reflex tears) and 'weeping' (for psychogenic tears) have been suggested.

The precorneal film

Wolff (1948) considered the precorneal film to consist of a triple-layered structure with a central watery phase made up of the serous secretion of the lacrimal gland and constituting the bulk of the film. A thin superficial oily layer was thought to issue from the tarsal glands and a deep layer of mucoproteins from the conjunctival glands.

This postulated structure is still widely accepted. Using a variety of techniques, there was reasonable agreement that the precorneal tear film measured from 6 to 9 μm in thickness (Ehlers 1965a, Mishima 1965), reducing by about 20%, 5 seconds after a blink and by 50% after 30 seconds. Prydal et al. (1992) confounded the established view by claiming a thickness of 34–45 μm, figures that are close to the thickness of the epithelium, using laser interferometry and confirmed by confocal microscopy. Moreover, they considered the film to be composed substantially of mucin rather than an aqueous layer with some dispersed mucin (Holly & Lemp 1971). Petroll et al. (2003) argued that the confocal microscope is probably not the instrument of choice for tear thickness measurements because of the constant horizontal eye movements together with the anterior–posterior movements of the eyeball due to pulsation of orbital blood vessels.

The presence of a thin superficial lipid layer is suggested by the coloured interference fringes, which may be observed with a biomicroscope or Tearscope (see Chapter 5). Mishima and Maurice (1961) demonstrated that, in rabbits, tear film evaporation increases at least 10-fold in the absence of tarsal gland secretion. This amount of increased evaporation is approximately that expected of water in the absence of a surface lipid film. Despite this apparently straightforward evidence for tarsal gland function, when secretion, expressed from human tarsal glands, was spread over a saline solution, no significant reduction in evaporation was observed (Brown & Dervichian 1969). Although the experimental conditions of this study are not beyond criticism, the results serve at least to stimulate discussion of the matter.

The lipid layer extends from its sources at the openings of the tarsal glands at the lid margins to cover the tear film, and provides a stable interface between the aqueous layer and air. It is approximately 0.1 μm thick (Norn 1969), varying substantially with the size of the palpebral aperture and time of exposure. It compresses and thickens as the eyelids close, thinning gradually following a blink. In contrast to the remainder of the tear film, the lipid layer does not take part in the flow of tears from lateral to medial canthi and is essentially an independent part of the film. Lipid does not normally enter the conjuctival sac.

Mucins (MUC 5AC) from the conjunctival goblet cells form the deepest layer of the precorneal tear film and are absorbed by the epithelium producing a wettable hydrophilic surface essential for tear film stability (Holly & Lemp 1971, Holly 1973). The deep, glycoprotein part of the layer (or glycocalyx – MUC 1 – see above) is surface active and hydrophobic, and is responsible for attachment to the surface epithelial cell membrane. The strongly hydrophilic mucous portion is exposed to the aqueous layer. The figure of 0.8–1.0 μm obtained by direct measurement of the preserved mucous layer in histological preparations of the guinea-pig cornea (Nichols et al. 1984) suggests that the mucous layer might constitute a large fraction of the total tear film thickness in humans. A more complex picture of the tear film is emerging, where the gel forming MUC 5AC plays an important role in the aqueous part of the tear film (Pflugfelder et al. 2000, Argueso & Gipson 2001).

The precorneal tear film increases in thickness at the lid margins where a meniscus of tear fluid, the marginal tear strip, is formed; however, a thinning may occur along the line joining the film with the meniscus. Tear fluid flows medially within the marginal tear strips, hence the alternative name of lacrimal river or rivus lacrimus.

There is little tear flow across the cornea between blinks. The limited flow and the uniform thickness are the consequences of the 'framing' function of the eyelids which is eliminated if the eyelids are withdrawn from the eyeball, causing a spotty drying of the precorneal film.

Apposition of the eyelid margins during blinking permits replenishment of lipid from the tarsal glands, which is then spread across the surface of the reconstructed film as the eyelids part. Similarly, mucus is spread over the corneal and conjunctival epithelium by the massaging action of the eyelids. Spreading of the tear film is facilitated by the movement of the eyelids across the cornea. In the presence of a contact lens, the interfacial tension at three surfaces has to be considered. The desirable establishment of low interfacial tension at the two surfaces of the contact lens is partly related to the lens material and condition.

Function of tears

Tear liquid is essential for the maintenance of the normal optical properties of the cornea. Without it, corneal metabolic processes are impaired, as noted earlier, with consequent loss of transparency. The tears transport atmospheric oxygen and ions to the cornea and provide an excellent refracting surface. Tear liquid is the lubricant for eyelid movement over the cornea and the medium for flushing away foreign matter, which potentially endangers the optical integrity of the cornea.

Tears have antibacterial properties. Lysozyme, the enzyme originally described by Fleming (1922) in tear liquid, provides a degree of protection against certain Gram-positive bacteria lodged in the conjunctival sac. Claims for the presence of a non-lysozyme antibacterial factor (NLAF) in tears with far greater activity than lysozyme are broadly agreed. Lactoferrin is present in abundance in tears (Kijlstra et al. 1983) and may have an anti-inflammatory function (Veerhuis & Kijlstra 1982). Sack et al. (2001) suggested that lactoferrin is effective in disrupting the cell membrane of Gram-negative bacteria (*Pseudomonas aeruginosa*, *Escherichia coli* and *Proteus*).

Among the antibody proteins, IgA and IgG are prominent in tears but other immunoglobulins are also present (see also Chapter 4). Qu and Lehrer (1998) reported that the tear film concentration of secretory phospholipase A2 is sufficiently high to kill Gram-positive bacteria (*Listeria monocytogenes* and *Staphylococcus aureus*) but was not bactericidal against Gram-negative bacteria (*E. coli*, *Salmonella typhimurium* and *P. aeruginosa*).

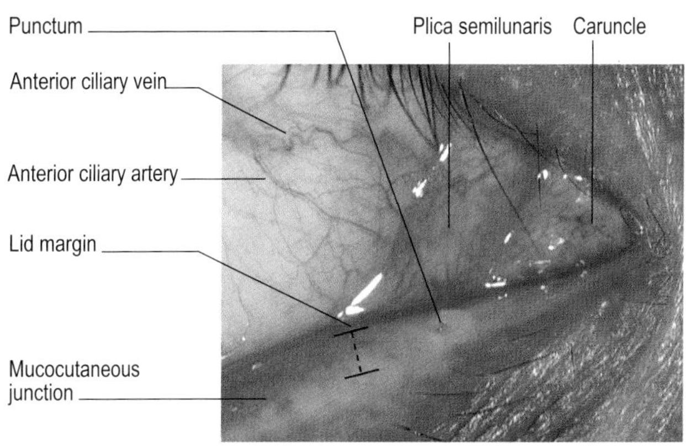

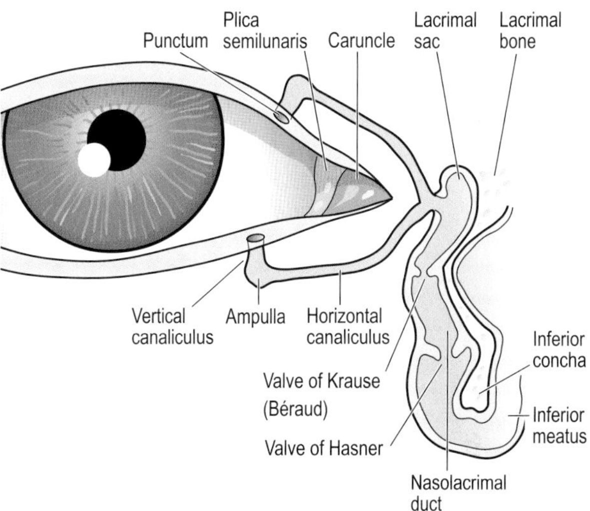

Figure 2.37 The tear drainage apparatus: its components and relation to the nose (Published with permission from Jan Bergmanson; Clinical Ocular Anatomy and Physiology, 12th edition, 2005)

Tear drainage

Much of the tear liquid lies in the marginal tear strips presenting a concave surface. Medially, the strips terminate in the so-called lacrimal lake, which is described as a reservoir of tear liquid bathing the caruncle and bounded by the inner canthus and the free edge of the plica semilunaris. Although this delimitation obviously changes as the eye moves from the primary position, under normal circumstances the inner canthus is moist but does not contain a pool of fluid. The punctum lacrimale of each papilla is turned in towards the cornea and interrupts the marginal tear strip.

Drainage of tears is initiated by the movement of tear liquid from the marginal tear strips through the punctum and into the canaliculus by:

- Capillary attraction.
- Negative pressure.
- Gravity.

This is facilitated by the continuous movement of liquid nasally which is effected by lid closure. Closure occurs first at the outer canthus and then, progressively, to the inner canthus. If a small spot of dye is applied to a marginal tear strip, blinking will cause the dye to spread towards the punctum; it will move neither to the fornix nor to the outer canthus (Ehlers 1965b).

The punctum leads to the canaliculus, which consists of a vertical and horizontal portion joined together by the ampulla (Fig. 2.37), a local dilatation of the drainage duct, which becomes compressed during the act of blinking. Compression of the ampulla creates a negative pressure that helps drive fluid into the drainage apparatus. In addition, the canaliculi, which are embedded in the orbicularis muscle, become shortened during the muscle contraction and this too assists to move the fluid in the direction of the lacrimal sac. Regurgitation is prevented by the simultaneous closure of the ampulla of each canaliculus. The muscular activity amounts to a milking action rather than a peristalsis. The preseptal portion of the orbicularis muscle is thought to have a deep insertion from each lid to the lacrimal diaphragm, which is the lateral fascial wall of the lacrimal sac, with the consequence that contraction causes a lateral movement of the lacrimal diaphragm. However, pressure measurements within the sac reveal little change during eyelid movement (Maurice 1973). It appears that gravity alone may account for the movement of the tears out of the lacrimal sac.

Tear output

Schirmer (1903) found the daily output of tears to be less than 1 g. This has been questioned because of the probable inaccuracy of his measuring technique. Nover and Jaeger (1952) calculated an average rate of 14 g of tear secretion daily, but Kirchner's (1964) results were similar to those of Schirmer. Norn (1965) subsequently reported a daily tear output of 15–30 g measured after instilling dye. The instillation of a stain (rose Bengal and/or fluorescein) will elevate the recorded figure for basic tear secretion, both by its own bulk and by its irritant

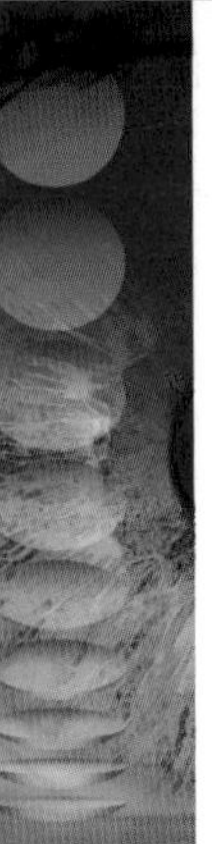

effect. Toker et al. (2002) found that full-term infants produced a mean basal tear production of 7.3 (± 3.2) mm as measured with the Schirmer test. Hence, it may be concluded that the lacrimal secretion normally produced is well in excess of 1 g as suggested by Schirmer but rather less than the 15–30 g measured by Norn.

In a study of full-term infants, Penbharkkul and Karelitz (1962) encountered shedding of tears as early as 5.5 hours of age and as late as 84 days. The onset of lacrimation occurred during the first 4 weeks in a majority of infants and in most it occurred first with crying associated with hunger and pain. Sjögren (1955) used nasal irritants to determine the onset of reflex lacrimation in infants and found that it occurred in all but 13% during the first few weeks of life.

With advancing years, basic tear secretion decreases gradually: the difference between the sexes is negligible (Norn 1965) except in early adult life, when females have a higher rate of secretion (Henderson & Prough 1950, de Roetth 1953). Sex differences concerning psychogenic tears or weeping are clearly a separate matter.

Schirmer's tear secretion test is unsatisfactory as a precise quantitative test for tear secretion but is of considerable value in comparing the production of tears between eyes of a pair and between eyes of different persons (see Chapters 5 and 8).

Neural control of tears

Irritation of the cornea, conjunctiva, nasal mucosa and any area served by the trigeminal nerve causes reflex lacrimation. The trigeminal nerve is responsible for the sensory input of the reflex pathway and, if it is blocked, or surface anaesthesia applied, reflex lacrimation is abolished. The paths of the central nervous system associated with psychogenic weeping are unknown, and a knowledge of the link between the trigeminal nerve and the facial nerve in the reflex lacrimation pathway is lacking.

Both parasympathetic nerve fibres (from the pterygopalatine or sphenopalatine ganglion) and sympathetic nerve fibres (from the superior cervical ganglion) have been thought to be responsible for motor control of lacrimal gland secretion but in experiments on cats and monkeys, only parasympathetic fibres could be shown to exercise this control (Botelho et al. 1966, Ruskell 1969, 1975). The gland has a limited sensory innervation (Matsumoto et al. 1992). There is no clear evidence of motor control of the tarsal and conjunctival glands although control of the former has been suggested (Chung et al. 1996).

Acknowledgements

Sadly my inspirational mentor, Gordon Ruskell, passed away during the spring of 2004. I am honoured to be able to add my name to his. Given that Professor Ruskell was a superb writer and exceptionally well versed in the subject matter of this chapter, there is little that needs to be upgraded or changed to keep this part of the text current. Consequently, I have attempted to add important new knowledge to the text rather than rewrite the entire chapter and have changed the text where recent findings have corrected previously held notions or in cases where accuracy of measurements has been improved.

I also wish to acknowledge Professor Michael Doughty, who has been my valued collaborator for many years and has helped with many of the research findings on the anatomy and physiology of the cornea and ocular adnexa. In preparing my part of the manuscript I was very ably supported by Dr Robin Bynum.

References

Abelli, L., Geppetti, P. and Maggi, C. A. (1993) Relative contribution of sympathetic and sensory nerves to thermal nociception and tissue trophism in rats. Neuroscience, 57, 739–745

Alexander, R. A. and Garner, A. (1983) Elastic and precursor fibres in the normal human eye. Exp. Eye Res., 36, 305–315

Alharbi, A. and Swarbrick, H. A. (2003) The effects of overnight orthokeratology lens wear on corneal thickness. Invest. Ophthalmol. Vis. Sci., 44, 2518–2523

Allen, M., Wright, P. and Reid, L. (1972) The human lacrimal gland. A histochemical and organ culture study of the secretory cells. Arch. Ophthalmol., 88, 493–497

Anderson, J. A., Murphy, J. A. and Gaster, R. N. (1989) Inflammatory cell responses to radial keratotomy. Arch. Ophthalmol., 101, 1113–1116

Anseth, A. (1969) Studies on corneal glycosaminoglycans in transient corneal edema. Exp. Eye Res., 8, 297–311

Arffa, R.C. (1997) Grayson's Diseases of the Cornea, pp. 446–454. St Louis: Mosby

Argueso, P. and Gipson, I. K. (2001) Epithelial mucins of the ocular surface: structure, biosynthesis and function. Exp. Eye Res., 73, 281–289

Balik, J. (1958) [The amino acid content of tears.] Sb. Lek. 60, 332–336, as cited in Ophthalmol. Lit., 12, No. 4847 (1958)

Baljet, B., van der Werf, F. and Otto, A. J. (1989) Autonomic pathways in the orbit of the human fetus and the rhesus monkey. Doc. Ophthalmol., 72, 247–264

Barr, R. E. and Roetman, E. L. (1974) Oxygen gradients in the anterior chamber of anesthetized rabbits. Invest. Ophthalmol., 13, 386–389

Barr, R. E. and Silver, I. A. (1973) Effects of corneal environment on oxygen tension in the anterior chambers of rabbits. Invest. Ophthalmol., 12, 140–144

Barr, R. E., Hennessey, M. and Murphy, V. G. (1977) Diffusion of oxygen at the endothelial surface of the rabbit cornea. J. Physiol., 270, 1–8

Bates, A. K. and Cheng, H. (1988) Bullous keratopathy: a study of endothelial cell morphology in patients undergoing cataract surgery. Br. J. Ophthalmol., 72, 409–412.

Beekhuis, W. H. and McCarey, B. E. (1986) Corneal epithelial Cl-dependent pump quantified. Exp. Eye Res., 43, 707–711

Belmonte, C. and Giraldez, F. (1981) Responses of cat corneal sensory receptors to mechanical and thermal stimulation. J. Physiol., 321, 355–368

Benedek, G. B. (1971) Theory of transparency of the eye. Appl. Optics, 10, 459–472

Bergenske, P. D. and Polse, K. A. (1987) The effect of rigid gas permeable lenses on corneal sensitivity. J. Am. Optom. Assoc., 58, 212–215

Bergmanson, J. P. G. (1987) Histopathological analysis of the corneal epithelium after contact lens wear. J. Am. Optom. Assoc., 58, 812–818

Bergmanson, J. P. G. (1992) Histopathological analysis of corneal endothelial polymegethism. Cornea, 11, 133–142

Bergmanson, J. P. G. (2000) Endothelial Complications: Anterior Segment Complications of Contact Lens Wear. Boston: Butterworth-Heinemann, pp. 37–66

Bergmanson, J. P. G. (2006) Clinical Ocular Anatomy and Physiology, 13th edn. Houston: Texas Eye Research and Technology Center, University of Houston College of Optometry

Bergmanson, J. P. G. and Chu, L. W. F. (1982a) Contact lens-induced corneal epithelial injury. Am. J. Optom. Physiol. Opt., 59, 500–506

Bergmanson, J. P. G. and Chu, L. W. F. (1982b) Corneal response to rigid contact lens wear. Br. J. Ophthalmol., 66, 667–675

Bergmanson, J. P. G. and Weissman, B. A. (1992) Hypoxic Changes in Corneal Endothelium: Complications of Contact Lens Wear. St Louis: Mosby, pp. 37–67

Bergmanson, J. P. G. and Wilson, G. S. (1989) Ultrastructural effects of sodium chloride on the corneal epithelium. Invest. Ophthalmol. Vis. Sci., 30, 116–121

Bergmanson, J. P. G., Ruben, C. M., and Chu, L. W. F. (1985) Epithelial morphological response to soft hydrogel contact lenses. Br. J. Ophthalmol., 69, 373–379

Bergmanson, J. P. G., Doughty, M. J. and Blocker, Y. (1999) The acinar and ductal organisation of the tarsal accessory lacrimal gland of Wolfring in rabbit eyelid. Exp. Eye Res., 68, 411–421

Bergmanson, J. P. G., Horne, J., Doughty, M. J., Garcia, M. and Gondo, M. (2005) Assessment of the number of lamellae in the central region of the normal human corneal stroma, at the resolution of the transmission electron microscope. Eye Contact Lens, 31, 281–287

Bertanlanffy, F. D. and Lau, C. (1962) Mitotic rate and renewal time of the corneal epithelium in the rat. Arch. Ophthalmol., 68, 546–551

Beuerman, R. W. and Schimmelpfenning, B. (1980) Sensory denervation of the rabbit cornea affects epithelial properties. Exp. Neurol., 69, 196–201

Bleshoy, H. (1986) Corneal sensitivity in keratoconus. Trans. Br. Contact Lens Assoc., 9, 9–12

Boberg-Ans, J. (1955) Experience in clinical examination of corneal sensitivity. Br. J. Ophthalmol., 39, 705–726

Boberg-Ans, J. (1956) On the corneal sensitivity. Acta Ophthalmol., 35, 149–162

Bock, R. H. and Maumenee, A. E. (1953) Corneal fluid metabolism: experiments and observations. Arch. Ophthalmol., 50, 282–285

Botelho, S. Y., Hisada, M. and Fuenmayer, N. (1966) Functional innervation of the lacrimal gland in the cat. Arch. Ophthalmol., 76, 581–588

Bourne, W. M., Hodge, D. O. and McLaren, J. W. (1999) Estimation of corneal endothelial pump function in long-term contact lens wearers. Invest. Ophthalmol. Vis. Sci., 40, 603–611

Braude, L. S. and Chandler, J. W. (1983) Corneal allograft rejection. The role of the major histocompatibility complex. Surv. Ophthalmol., 27, 290–305

Bron, A. J. (1968) Anterior corneal mosaic. Br. J. Ophthalmol., 52, 659–669

Bron, A. J., Tripathi, R. C. and Tripathi, B. J. (1997) The cornea and sclera. In Wolff's Anatomy of the Eye and Orbit, 8th edn, p. 247. London: Chapman & Hall Medical

Brown, S. I. and Dervichian, D. G. (1969) The oils of the meibomian glands. Arch. Ophthalmol., 82, 537–540

Brown, S. and Hedbys, B. (1965) The effect of ouabain on the hydration of the cornea. Invest. Ophthalmol., 4, 216–223

Brown, M., Chinn, S., Fatt, I. and Harris, M. G. (1973) The effect of soft and hard contact lenses on blink rate, amplitude and length. J. Am. Optom. Assoc., 44, 254–257

Buck, R. C. (1985) Measurement of centripetal migration of normal corneal epithelial cells in the mouse. Invest. Ophthalmol. Vis. Sci., 26, 1296–1298

Cardoso, S. S., Ferreria, A. L., Camargo, A. C. M. and Bohn, G. (1968) The effect of partial hepatectomy upon circadian distribution of mitosis in the cornea of rats. Experientia, 24, 569–570

Carney, L. G. and Hill, R. M. (1982) The nature of normal blinking patterns. Acta Ophthalmol., 60, 427–433

Cenedella, R. J. and Fleschner, C. R. (1990) Kinetics of corneal epithelium turnover in vivo: studies of lovastatin. Invest. Ophthalmol. Vis. Sci., 31, 1957–1962

Chandler, J. W., Cummings, M. and Gillette, T. E. (1985) Presence of Langerhans cells in the central corneas of normal human infants. Invest. Ophthalmol. Vis. Sci., 26, 113–115

Chen, C-H. and Chen, S. C. (1990) Lactate transport and glycolytic activity in the freshly isolated rabbit cornea. Arch. Biochem. Biophys., 276, 70–76

Chung, C. W., Tigges, M. and Stone, R. A. (1996) Peptidergic innervation of the primate meibomian gland. Invest. Ophthalmol. Vis. Sci., 37, 238–245

Cintron, C., Kublin, C. L. and Covington, H. (1982) Quantitative studies of corneal epithelial wound healing in rabbits. Curr. Eye Res., 1, 507–516

Cochet, P. and Bonnet, R. (1960) L'esthésia cornéenne. Sa measure clinique ses variations physiologiques et pathologiques. Clin. Ophthalmol., 4, 1–27

Cotsarelis, G., Cheng, S-Z., Dong, G., Sun, T-T. and Lavker, M. (1989) Existence of slow-cycling limbal epithelial basal cells that can be preferentially stimulated to proliferate: implications on epithelial stem cells. Cell, 57, 201–209

Davanger, M. and Eversen, A. (1971) Role of the pericorneal papillary structure in renewal of corneal epithelium. Nature, 229, 560–561

Davson, H. (1955) The hydration of the cornea. Biochem. J., 59, 24–28

de Roetth, A., Jr. (1950) Respiration of the cornea. Arch. Ophthalmol., 44, 666–676

de Roetth, A., Sr. (1953) Lacrimation in normal eyes. Arch. Ophthalmol., 49, 185–189

Dilly, P. N. (1985) Contribution of the epithelium to the stability of the tear film. Trans. Ophthalmol. Soc. UK, 104, 381–389

Donn, A., Miller, S. and Mallett, N. (1963) Water permeability of the living cornea. Arch. Ophthalmol., 70, 515–521

Doughty, M. J. (1985) New observations on bicarbonate–pH effects on thickness changes of rabbit corneas under silicone oil in vitro. Am. J. Optom. Physiol. Opt., 62, 879–888

Doughty, M. J. (1987) Sided effects of bicarbonate on rabbit corneal endothelium in vitro. Clin. Exp. Optom. 70, 168–177

Doughty, M. J. (1989) Toward a quantitative analysis of corneal endothelial cell morphology: a review of techniques and their application. Optom. Vis. Sci., 66, 626–642

Doughty, M. J. (1990) Morphometric analysis of the surface cells of rabbit corneal epithelium by scanning electron microscopy. Am. J. Anam., 189, 316–328

Doughty, M. J. (1991) Scanning electron microscopy study of cell dimensions of rabbit corneal epithelium surface. Cornea, 10, 149–155

Doughty, M. J. (1997) Scanning electron microscopy study of the tarsal and orbital conjunctival surfaces compared to peripheral

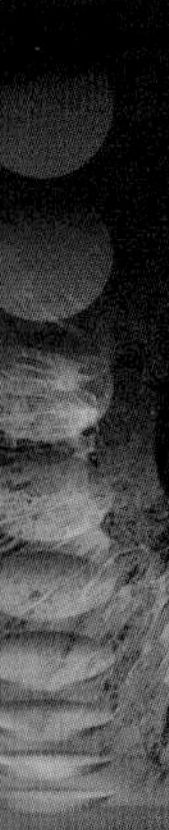

corneal epithelium in pigmented rabbits. Doc. Ophthalmol., 93, 345–371

Doughty, M. J. (1999) Re-assessment of the potential impact of physiologically-relevant pH changes on the hydration properties of the isolated mammalian corneal stroma. Biochim. Biophys. Acta, 1472, 99–106

Doughty, M. J. (2003) A physiological perspective on the swelling properties of the mammalian corneal stroma. Contact Lens Anterior Eye, 26, 117–129

Doughty, M. J. (2004) Impact of hypotonic solutions on the stromal swelling, lactate dehydrogenase and aldehyde dehydrogenase activity of the keratocytes of the bovine cornea. Cell Biol. Int., 28, 593–607

Doughty, M. J. and Bergmanson, J. P. G. (2003) New insights into the surface cells and glands of the conjunctiva and their relevance to the tear film. Optometry, 74, 485–500

Doughty, M. J. and Bergmanson, J. P. G. (2004a) Collagen fibril characteristics at the cornea–scleral boundary and rabbit corneal stromal swelling. Clin. Exp. Optom., 87, 81–92

Doughty, M. J. and Bergmanson, J. P. G. (2004b) Heterogeneity in the ultrastructure of the mucous (goblet) cells of the rabbit palpebral conjunctiva. Clin. Exp. Optom., 87, 377–385

Doughty, M. J. and Maurice, D. M. (1988) Bicarbonate sensitivity of rabbit corneal endothelium fluid pump in vitro. Invest. Ophthalmol. Vis. Sci., 29, 216–223

Doughty, M. J. and Zaman, M. L. (2000) Human corneal thickness and its impact on intraocular pressure measures: a review and meta-analysis approach. Surv. Ophthalmol., 44, 367–408

Doughty, M. J., Seabert, W., Bergmanson, J. P. J. and Blocker, Y. (2001) A descriptive and quantitative study of the keratocytes of the corneal stroma of albino rabbits using transmission electron microscopy. Tissue Cell, 33, 408–422

Draeger, J. (1984) Corneal Sensitivity: Measurement and Clinical Importance. Vienna: Springer-Verlag

Duke-Elder, S. and Wybar, K. C. (1961) The eye. In System of Ophthalmology, vol. II, p. 103. The Anatomy of the Visual System. London: Henry Kimpton

Efron, N., Perez-Gomez, I. and Morgan, P. B. (2002) Confocal microscopic observations of stromal keratocytes during extended contact lens wear. Clin. Exp. Optom., 85, 156–160

Ehlers, N. (1965a) The precorneal film. Biomicroscopical, histological and chemical investigations. Acta Ophthalmol., 18 (Suppl. 81), 19–34

Ehlers, N. (1965b) On the size of the conjunctival sac. Acta Ophthalmol., 43, 205–210

Edelhauser, H. F. and Ubels, J. L. (2003) The cornea. In Adler's Physiology of the Eye, p. 56, eds. P. L. Kaufman and A. Alm. St Louis: Mosby

Elsas, T., Edvinsson, L., Sundler, F. and Uddman, R. (1994) Neuronal pathways to the rat conjunctiva revealed by retrograde tracing and immunocytochemistry. Exp. Eye Res., 58, 117–126

Farris, R. L., Takahashi, G. H. and Donn, A. (1967) Corneal oxygen flux in contact lens wearers. In Corneal and Scleral Contact Lenses, pp. 413–425, ed. L. J. Girard. St Louis: Mosby

Farris, R. L., Kubota, Z. and Mishima, S. (1971) Epithelial decompensation with corneal contact lens wear. Arch. Ophthalmol., 85, 651–660

Fatt, I. and Bieber, M. T. (1968) The steady-state distribution of oxygen and carbon dioxide in the in vivo cornea. l: The open eye in air and the closed eye. Exp. Eye Res., 7, 103–112

Fatt, I., Freeman, R. D. and Lin, D. (1974) Oxygen tension distributions in the cornea: a re-examination. Exp. Eye Res., 18, 357–365

Finkelstein, I. S. (1952) The biophysics of corneal scatter and diffraction of light induced by contact lenses. Am. J. Optom., 29, 231–259

Fischer, F. H., Schmitz, L., Hoff, W. et al. (1978) Sodium and chloride transport in the isolated human cornea. Pflugers Arch., 373, 179–188

Fleming, A. (1922) On a remarkable bacteriolytic element found in tissues and secretions. Proc. R. Soc. Lond. B, 93, 306–317

Fogle, J. A., Yoza, B. K. and Neufeld, A. H. (1980) Diurnal rhythm of mitosis in rabbit corneal epithelium. Graefes Arch. Klin. Exp. Ophthalmol., 213, 143–148

Fonn, D. and Holden, B. A. (1986) Extended wear of hard gas permeable contact lenses can induce ptosis. CLAO J., 12, 93–94

Fonn, D., Pritchard, N., Garnett, B. and Davids, L. (1996) Palpebral aperture sizes of rigid and soft contact lens wearers compared with nonwearers. Optom. Vis. Sci., 73, 211–214

Freeman, R. D. (1972) Oxygen consumption by the component layers of the cornea. J. Physiol., 225, 15–32

Friedenwald, J. S. and Buschke, W. (1944a) Mitotic and wound-healing activities of the corneal epithelium. Arch. Ophthalmol., 32, 410–413

Friedenwald, J. S. and Buschke, W. (1944b) The effect of excitement of epinephrine and of sympathectomy on the mitotic activity of corneal epithelium in rats. Am. J. Physiol., 141, 689–694

Fujita, H., Ueda, A., Nishida, T. and Otori, T. (1987) Uptake of India ink particles and latex beads by corneal fibroblasts. Cell Tissue Res., 250, 251–255

Gallar, I., Pozo, M. A., Tuckett, R. P. and Belmonte, C. (1993) Responses of sensory units with unmyelinated fibres to mechanical, thermal and chemical stimulation of the cat's cornea. J. Physiol., 468, 609–622

Geroski, D. and Edelhauser, H. F. (1984) The effects of ouabain on endothelial function in human and rabbit corneas. Curr. Eye Res., 3, 331–338

Giardini, A. and Roberts, J. R. E. (1950) Concentration of glucose and total chloride in tears. Br. J. Ophthalmol., 34, 737–743

Ginsborg, B. L. (1952) Rotation of the eyes during involuntary blinking. Nature, 169, 412–413

Ginsborg, B. L. and Maurice, D. M. (1959) Involuntary movements of the eye during fixation and blinking. Br. J. Ophthalmol., 43, 435–437

Gipson, I. K., Spurr-Michaud, S., Tisdale, A. and Keough, M. (1989) Reassembly of the anchoring structures of the corneal epithelium during wound repair in the rabbit. Invest. Ophthalmol. Vis. Sci., 30, 425–434

Golding-Wood, P. H. (1964) The ocular effects of autonomic surgery. Proc. R. Soc. Med., 57, 494–497

Goldman, J. N. and Benedek, G. B. (1967) The relationship between morphology and transparency in the nonswelling corneal stroma of the shark. Invest. Ophthalmol., 6, 574–600

Gordon, G. (1951) Observations upon the movement of the eyelids. Br. J. Ophthalmol., 35, 339–351

Greenberg, M. H. and Hill, R. M. (1973) The physiology of contact lens imprints. Am. J. Optom., 50, 699–702

Greiner, J. V., Kenyon, K. R., Henriquez, A. S., Korb, D. R., Weidman, T. A. and Allansmith, M. R. (1980) Mucus secretory vesicles in conjunctival epithelial cells of wearers of contact lenses. Arch. Ophthalmol., 98, 1843–1846

Guggenheim, J. A., Armitage, W. J., Evans, A. D., Davies, H., Rebello, G. and Hodson, S. A. (1995) Chloride binding in the stroma of cultured human corneas. Exp. Eye Res., 61, 109–113

Guilbert, J. (1963) Contact lens fitting in France. J. Am. Optom. Assoc., 34, 1403–1405

Gumbiner, B. M. (1993) Breaking through the tight junction barrier. J. Biol., 123, 1631–1633

Gunderson, T. (1939) Vascular obliteration for various types of keratitis. Its significance regarding nutrition of corneal epithelium. Arch. Ophthalmol., 21, 76–107

Gunderson, T. and Liebman, S. D. (1944) Effect of local anaesthetics on regeneration of corneal epithelium. Arch. Ophthalmol., 31, 29–33

Hamano, H., Hori, M., Hamano, T. et al. (1983) Effects of contact lens wear on mitosis of corneal epithelium and lactate content in aqueous humor of rabbit. Jpn J. Ophthalmol., 27, 451–458

Hanna, C. and O'Brien, J. E. (1960) Cell production and migration in the epithelial layer of the cornea. Arch. Ophthalmol., 64, 536–539

Hanna, C. and O'Brien, J. E. (1961) Thymidine-tritium labelling of the cellular elements of the corneal stroma. Arch. Ophthalmol., 66, 362–365

Harris, J. E. and Nordquist, L. T. (1955) The hydration of the cornea. l: The transport of water from the cornea. Am. J. Ophthalmol., 40, 100–110

Hart, R. W. and Farrell, R. A. (1969) Light scattering in the cornea. J. Opt. Soc. Am., 59, 766–774

Hazlett, L. D., McClellan, S. M., Hume, E. B., Dajcs, J. J., O'Callaghan, R. J. and Willcox, M. D. (1999) Extended wear contact lens usage induces Langerhans cell migration into cornea. Exp. Eye Res., 69, 575–577

Heald, K. and Langham, M. E. (1956) Permeability of the cornea and blood–aqueous barrier to oxygen. Br. J. Ophthalmol., 40, 705–720

Henderson, J. W. and Prough, W. L. (1950) Influence of age and sex on flow of tears. Arch. Ophthalmol., 43, 224–231

Henderson, L., Bond, D. and Simpson, T. (2005) The association between eye color and corneal sensitivity measured using a Belmonte esthesiometer. Optom. Vis. Sci., 82(7), 629–632

Hermann, H. and Hickman, F. H. (1948) The adhesion of epithelium to stroma in the cornea. Bull. Johns Hopkins Hosp., 82, 182–207

Heydenreich, A. (1958) Die Hornhautregeneration. Marhold: Halle

Hill, J. C., Sarvan, J., Maske, R. and Les, W. G. (1994) Evidence that UV-B irradiation decreases corneal Langerhans cells and improves graft survival in rabbit. Transplantation, 57, 1281–1284

Hill, R. M. and Fatt, I. (1964) Oxygen measurements under a contact lens. Am. J. Optom., 41, 382–387

Hirsch, M., Renard, G., Faure, J. P. and Pouliquen, Y. (1977) Study of the ultrastructure of the rabbit corneal endothelium by freeze-fracture technique. Apical and lateral junctions. Exp. Eye Res., 25, 277–288

Hirsch, M., Nicolas, G. and Pouliquen, Y. (1989) Interfibrillary structures in fast-frozen, deep-etched and rotary-shadowed extracellular matrix of the rabbit corneal stroma. Exp. Eye Res., 49, 311–315

Hodson, S. (1977) Endothelial pump of cornea [editorial]. Invest. Ophthalmol. Vis. Sci., 16, 589–591

Hodson, S. and Miller, F. (1976) The bicarbonate ion pump in the endothelium which regulates the hydration of rabbit cornea. J. Physiol., 263, 563–577

Hogan, M. J., Alvarado, J. A. and Weddell, J. E. (1971) Histology of the Human Eye, p. 89. Philadelphia, PA: W. B. Saunders

Holden, B. A. and Mertz, G. W. (1984) Critical oxygen levels to avoid corneal edema for daily and extended wear contact lenses. Invest. Ophthalmol. Vis. Sci., 25, 1161–1167

Holden, B. A., Sweeney, D. F., Efron, N., Vannas, A. and Nilsson, K. T. (1985) Effects of long-term extended contact lens wear on the human cornea. Invest. Ophthalmol. Vis. Sci., 26, 1489–1501

Holden, B. A., Williams, L. and Sweeney, D. F. (1986) The endothelial response to contact lens wear. CLAO J., 12, 150–152

Holly, F. J. (1973) Formation and rupture of the tear film. Exp. Eye Res., 15, 515–525

Holly, F. J. and Lemp, M. A. (1971) Wettability and wetting of corneal epithelium. Exp. Eye Res., 11, 239–250

Horne, J., Fulton, J., Gondo, M. and Bergmanson. J. (2003) Anatomical evidence for the structural reinforcement of the stromal-anterior limiting lamina interface in the human cornea. Invest. Ophthalmol. Vis. Sci., 44, ARVO E-Abstract 885

Iwamoto, T. and Smelser, G. K. (1965) Electron microscopy of the human corneal endothelium with reference to transport mechanisms. Invest. Ophthalmol., 4, 270–284

Jakus, M. A. (1961) The fine structure of the human cornea. In The Structure of the Eye, pp. 343–366, ed. G. K. Smelser. New York: Academic Press

Jakus, M. A. (1964) Ocular Fine Structure. Selected Electron Micrographs. Retina Foundation, Inst. Biol. Med. Sci. Monographs & Conferences, Vol. 1. London: Churchill

Jalavisto, E., Orma, E. and Tawast, M. (1951) Ageing and relation between stimulus intensity and duration in corneal sensibility. Acta Physiol. Scand., 23, 224–233

Jalbert, I. and Stapleton, F. (1999) Effect of lens wear on corneal stroma: preliminary findings. Aust. N. Z. J. Ophthalmol., 27, 211–213

Johnson, D. H., Bourne, W. M. and Campbell, R. J. (1982) The ultrastructure of Descemet's membrane. I. Changes with age in normal corneas. Arch. Ophthalmol., 100, 1942–1947

Kallinikos, P. and Efron, N. (2004) On the etiology of keratocyte loss during contact lens wear. Invest. Ophthalmol. Vis. Sci., 45, 3011–3020

Kangas, T. A., Edelhauser, H. F., Twining, S. S. and O'Brien, W. J. (1990) Loss of stromal glycosaminoglycans during corneal edema. Invest. Ophthalmol. Vis. Sci., 31, 1994–2002

Kessing, S. V. (1966) On the conjunctival papillae and follicles. Acta Ophthalmol., 44, 846–852

Kessing, S. V. (1968) Mucous gland system of the conjunctiva. Acta Ophthalmol., Suppl. 85, 36–59

Khodadoust, A. A., Silverstein, A. M., Kenyon, K. R. and Dowling, J. E. (1968) Adhesions of regenerating corneal epithelium: the role of basement membrane. Am. J. Ophthalmol., 65, 339–348

Kijlstra, H., Jeurissen, S. H. M. and Koning, K. M. (1983) Lactoferrin levels in normal human tears. Br. J. Ophthalmol., 67, 199–202

King, D. C. and Michels, K. M. (1957) Muscular tension and the human blink rate. J. Exp. Psychol., 53, 113–116

Kinoshita, J. H. (1962) Some aspects of the carbohydrate metabolism of the cornea. Invest. Ophthalmol., 1, 178–186

Kinoshita, J. H. and Masurat, T. (1959) Aerobic pathways of glucose metabolism in bovine corneal epithelium. Am. J. Ophthalmol., 48, 47–52

Kirchner, C. (1964) Untersuchungen uber das Ausmass der Tränensekretion beim Menschen. Klin. Mbl. Augenheilk., 144, 412–417

Klintworth, G. K. (1969) Experimental studies on the phagocytic capability of the corneal fibroblast. Am. J. Pathol., 55, 283–294

Klyce, S. D. and Beuerman, R. W. (1998) Structure and function of the cornea. In The Cornea, p. 14, eds. H. E. Kaufmann, B. A. Barron and M. R. McDonald. Boston: Butterworth-Heinemann

Klyce, S. D. and Bonanno, J. A. (1988) Role of the epithelium in corneal hydration. In The Cornea: Transactions of the World Congress on the Cornea III, pp. 159–164, ed. H. D. Cavanagh. New York: Raven Press

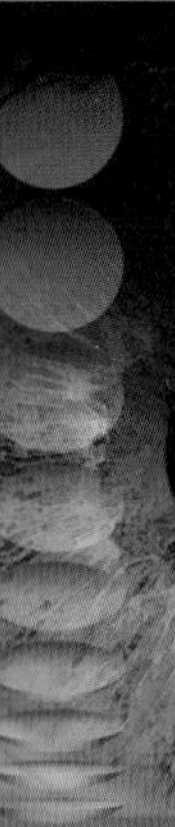

Klyce, S. D. and Wong, R. K. S. (1977) Site and adrenaline action on chloride transport across the rabbit corneal epithelium. J. Physiol., 266, 777–799

Knoll, H. A. and Williams, J. (1970) Effects of hydrophilic contact lenses on corneal sensitivity. Am. J. Optom., 47, 561–563

Kokott, W. (1938) Uber mechanisch funktionelle Strukturen des Auges. Graefes Arch. Klin. Exp. Ophthalmol., 138, 424–485

Korb, D. R., Greiner, J. V., Herman, J. P. et al. (2002) Lid-wiper epitheliopathy and dry-eye symptoms in contact lens wearers. CLAO J., 28, 211–216

Korb, D. R., Herman, J. P., Greiner, J. V. et al. (2005) Lid wiper epitheliopathy and dry eye symptoms. Eye Contact Lens, 31, 2–8

Kruse, K. (1994) Stem cells and corneal epithelial regeneration. Eye, 8, 170–183

Kuhlman, R. E. and Resnick, R. A. (1959) The oxidation C-14-labelled glucose and lactate by the rabbit cornea. Arch. Biochem. Biophys., 8, 29–36

Ladage, P. M., Yamamoto, K. and Ren, D. H. et al. (2001) Proliferation rate of rabbit corneal epithelium during overnight rigid contact lens wear. Invest. Ophthalmol. Vis. Sci., 42, 2804–2812

Ladage, P. M., Yamamoto, K., Li, L. et al. (2002) Corneal epithelial homeostasis following daily and overnight contact lens wear. Contact Lens Anterior Eye, 25, 11–21

Langham, M. E. (1952) Utilization of oxygen by the component layers of the living cornea. J. Physiol., 117, 461–470

Langham, M. E. (1954) Glycolysis in the cornea of the rabbit. J. Physiol., 126, 396–403

Langham, M. E. (1960) Corneal metabolism and its influence on corneal hydration in the excised eye and in the living animal. In The Transparency of the Cornea, pp. 87–109, eds S. Duke-Elder and E. S. Perkins. Oxford: Blackwell

Larke, J. R. and Hirji, N. K. (1979) Some clinically observed phenomena in extended contact lens wear. Br. J. Ophthalmol., 63, 475–477

Lavker, R. M., Dong, G., Cheng, S. Z. et al. (1991) Relative proliferation rates of limbal and corneal epithelia. Invest. Ophthalmol. Vis. Sci., 32, 1864–1875

Lawrenson, J. G. and Ruskell, G. L. (1993) Investigation of limbal touch sensitivity using a Cochet–Bonnet aesthesiometer. Br. J. Ophthalmol., 77, 339–343

Lehrer, M. S., Sun, T. T. and Lavker, R. M. (1998) Strategies of epithelial repair: modulation of stem cell and transit amplifying cell proliferation. J. Cell Sci., 111, 2867–2875

Lehtosalo, J. I. (1984) Substance P-like immunoreactive trigeminal ganglion cells supplying the cornea. Histochemistry, 80, 273–276

Lele, P. P. and Weddell, G. (1956) The relationship between neurohistology and corneal sensibility. Brain, 79, 119–154

Lemp, M. A. and Gold, J. B. (1986) The effects of extended-wear hydrophilic contact lenses on the human corneal epithelium. Am. J. Ophthalmol., 101, 274–277

Lewkowicz-Moss, S. J., Shimeld, C., Lipworth, K. et al. (1987) Quantitative studies on Langerhans cells in mouse corneal epithelium following injection with herpes simplex virus. Exp. Eye Res., 45, 127–140

Li, H. F., Petroll, W. M., Moller-Pederson, T., Maurer, J. K., Cavanagh, H. D. and Jester, J. V. (1997) Epithelial and corneal thickness measurements by in vivo confocal microscopy through focusing (CMTF). Curr. Eye Res., 16, 214–221

Lim, C. H. and Ruskell, G. L. (1978) Corneal nerve access in monkeys. Graefes Klin. Exp. Arch. Ophthalmol., 208, 15–23

Lyne, A. (1982) Corneal sensitivity after surgery. Trans. Ophthalmol. Soc. UK, 102, 302–305

Macalister, G., Woodward, E. G. and Buckley, R. J. (1993) The return of corneal sensitivity following transplantation. J. Br. Contact Lens Assoc., 16, 99–104

Machemer, R. (1966) Autoradiographische Untersuchungen des Regenerationzonen der Hornhaut. Graefes Arch. Klin. Exp. Ophthalmol., 170, 286–297

Macintosh, S. R. (1974) The innervation of the conjunctiva in monkeys. An electron microscopic and nerve degeneration study. Graefes Arch. Klin. Exp. Ophthalmol., 192, 105–116

MacIver, M. B. and Tanelian, D. L. (1993) Structural and functional specialization of Aδ- and C-fiber free nerve endings innervating rabbit corneal epithelium. J. Neurosci., 13, 4511–4524

Mandell, R. B. and Fatt, I. (1965) Thinning of the human cornea on awakening. Nature, 208, 292–293

Mann, I. (1944) A study of epithelial regeneration in the living eye. Br. J. Ophthalmol., 28, 26–40

Marfurt, C. L. and Ellis, L. C. (1993) Immunohistochemical localization of tyrosine hydroxylase in corneal nerves. J. Comp. Neurol., 336, 517–531

Marr, M. (1967) Zur Altersabhängigkeit der Heilung von Hornhautepitheldefekten. Graefes Arch. Klin. Exp. Ophthalmol., 173, 250–255

Matsuda, H. (1968) Electron microscopic study of the corneal nerve with special reference to its endings. Jpn J. Ophthalmol., 12, 163–173

Matsumoto, Y., Tanabe, T., Ueda, S. and Kawata, M. (1992) Immunohistochemical and enzyme-histochemical studies of peptidergic, aminergic and cholinergic innervation of the lacrimal gland of the monkey (Macaca fuscata). J. Auton. Nerv. System, 37, 207–214

Maurice, D. M. (1951) The permeability to sodium ions of the living rabbit's cornea. J. Physiol., 122, 367–391

Maurice, D. M. (1957) The structure and transparency of the cornea. J. Physiol., 136, 263–286

Maurice, D. M. (1962a) Clinical physiology of the cornea. Int. Ophthalmol. Clin., 2, 561–572

Maurice, D. M. (1962b) The cornea and sclera. In The Eye, Vol. 1, pp. 289–368, ed. H. Davson. New York: Academic Press

Maurice, D. M. (1972) The location of the fluid pump in the cornea. J. Physiol., 221, 43–54

Maurice, D. M. (1973) The dynamics and drainage of tears. Int. Ophthalmol. Clin., 13, 103–116

Maurice, D. M. and Giardini, A. (1951) Swelling of the cornea in vivo after the destruction of its limiting layers. Br. J. Ophthalmol., 35, 791–797

McCartney, M. D. and Cantu-Crouch, D. (1992) Rabbit corneal epithelial wound repair: tight junction reformation. Curr. Eye Res., 11, 15–24

McFarland, J. L., Laing, R. A. and Oak, S. S. (1983) Specular microscopy of corneal epithelium. Arch. Ophthalmol., 101, 451–454

McGowan, D. P., Lawrenson, J. G. and Ruskell, G. L. (1994) Touch sensitivity of the eyelid margin and palpebral conjunctiva. Acta Ophthalmol., 72, 57–60

Meek, K. M., Blamires, T., Elliot, G. F., Gyi, T. J. and Nave, C. (1987) The organisation of collagen fibrils in the human corneal stroma – a synchroton X-ray diffraction study. Curr. Eye Res., 6, 841–846

Miller, A. S., Coster, D. J., Costa, M. and Furness, J. B. (1983) Vasoactive intestinal polypeptide immunoreactive nerve fibres in the human eye. Aust. J. Ophthalmol., 11, 185–193

Millodot, M. (1972) Diurnal variation of corneal sensitivity. Br. J. Ophthalmol., 56, 844–847
Millodot, M. (1975a) Effect of hard contact lenses on corneal sensitivity and thickness. Acta Ophthalmol., 53, 576–584
Millodot, M. (1975b) Do blue-eyed people have more sensitive corneas than brown-eyed people? Nature, 255, 151–152
Millodot, M. (1976) Effect of the length of wear of contact lenses on corneal sensitivity. Acta Ophthalmol., 54, 721–730
Millodot, M. (1977) The influence of pregnancy on the sensitivity of the cornea. Br. J. Ophthalmol., 61, 646–649
Millodot, M. (1978) Corneal sensitivity in albinos. Arch. Ophthalmol., 96, 1225–1227
Millodot, M. (1984) A review of research on the sensitivity of the cornea. Ophthalmic Physiol. Opt., 4, 305–318
Millodot, M. and Lamont, A. (1974) Influence of menstruation on corneal sensitivity. Br. J. Ophthalmol., 58, 752–756
Millodot, M. and O'Leary, D. J. (1980a) Corneal fragility and its relationship to sensitivity. Acta Ophthalmol., 59, 820–826
Millodot, M. and O'Leary, D. J. (1980b) Effect of oxygen deprivation on corneal sensitivity. Acta Ophthalmol., 58, 434–439
Millodot, M. and Owens, H. (1983) Sensitivity and fragility in keratoconus. Acta Ophthalmol., 61, 908–917
Mishima, S. (1965) Some physiological aspects of the precorneal tear film. Arch. Ophthalmol., 73, 233–241
Mishima, S. (1968) Corneal thickness. Surv. Ophthalmol., 13, 57–96
Mishima, S. and Maurice, D. M. (1961) The oily layer of the tear film and evaporation from the corneal surface. Exp. Eye Res., 1, 39–45
Moller-Pedersen, T. and Niels, E. (1995) A three-dimensional study of the human corneal keratocyte density. Curr. Eye Res., 14, 459–464
Müller, L. J., Pels, L. and Vrensen, G. F. J. M. (1995) Novel aspects of ultrastructural organization of human corneal keratocytes. Invest. Ophthalmol. Vis. Sci., 36, 2557–2567
Müller, L., Pels, E. and Vrensen, G. F. J. M. (2001) The specific architecture of the anterior stroma accounts for maintenance of corneal curvature. Br. J. Ophthalmol., 85, 437–443
Munger, B. L. and Hulata, Z. (1984) The sensorineural apparatus of the human eyelid. Am. J. Anat., 170, 181–204
Murphy, C., Alvarado, J. and Juster, R. (1984) Prenatal and postnatal growth of the human Descemet's membrane. Invest. Ophthalmol. Vis. Sci., 25, 1402–1415
Nakamura, N., Nishida, T., Mishimo, H. and Otori, T. (1993) Effects of antimicrobials on corneal epithelial migration. Curr. Eye Res., 12, 733–740
Naylor, E. J. (1953) Polarised light studies of corneal structure. Br. J. Ophthalmol., 38, 77–84
Nichols, B. A., Chiappino, M. L. and Dawson, C. R. (1984) Demonstration of the mucous layer of the tear film by electron microscopy. Invest. Ophthalmol. Vis. Sci., 26, 464–473
Nomina Anatomica (1989) 6th edn. Authorised by the Twelfth International Congress of Anatomists in London. Edinburgh: Churchill Livingstone
Norn, M. S. (1965) Tear secretion in normal eyes estimated by a new method. The lacrimal streak dilution test. Acta Ophthalmol., 43, 567–573
Norn, M. S. (1969) Mucus flow in the conjunctiva. Acta Ophthalmol., 47, 129–146
Nover, A. and Jaeger, W. (1952) Kolorimetrische Methode zur Messung der Tränensekretion (Fluoreszein-Verdünnungstest). Klin. Mbl. Augenheilk., 121, 419–425
Odenthal, M. T., Gan, I. M., Oosting, J., Kijlstra, A. and Beekhuis, W. H. (2005) Long-term changes in corneal endothelial morphology after discontinuation of low gas-permeable contact lens wear. Cornea, 24, 32–48
Oduntan, O. and Ruskell, G. L. (1992) The source of sensory fibres of the inferior conjunctiva of monkeys. Graefes Arch. Klin. Exp. Ophthalmol., 230, 258–263
O'Leary, D. J. and Millodot, M. (1981) Abnormal epithelial fragility in diabetes and contact lens wear. Acta Ophthalmol., 59, 827–833
O'Leary, D. J., Madgewick, R., Wallace, J. and Ang, J. (1998) Size and number of epithelial cells washed from the cornea after contact lens wear. Optom. Vis. Sci., 75(9), 692–696
O'Neale, M. R., Polse, K. A. and Sarver, M. D. (1984) Corneal response to rigid and hydrogel lenses during eye closure. Invest. Ophthalmol. Vis. Sci., 25, 837–842
Oppenheimer, D. R., Palmer, E. and Weddell, G. (1958) Nerve endings in the conjunctiva. J. Anat., 92, 321–352
Patel, S., McLaren, J., Hodge, D. and Bourne, W. (2001) Normal human keratocyte density and corneal thickness measurements by using confocal microscopy in vivo. Invest. Ophthalmol. Vis. Sci., 42, 333–339
Patel, S., McLaren, J., Hodge, D. and Bourne, W. (2002) Confocal microscopy in vivo in cornea of long-term contact lens wearers. Invest. Ophthalmol. Vis. Sci., 43, 995–1003
Pedler, C. (1962) The fine structure of the corneal epithelium. Exp. Eye Res., 1, 286–289
Penbharkkul, S. and Karelitz, S. (1962) Lacrimation in the neonatal and early infancy period of premature and full-term infants. J. Pediatr., 61, 859–863
Perez, J. G., Meijome, J. M., Jalbert, I., Sweeney, D. F. and Erickson, P. (2003) Corneal epithelial thinning profile induced by long-term wear of hydrogel lenses. Cornea, 22, 304–307
Petroll, W. M., Kovoor, T., Ladage, P. M., Cavanagh, H. D., Jester, J. V. and Robertson, D. M. (2003) Can postlens tear thickness be measured using three-dimensional in vivo confocal microscopy? Eye Contact Lens, 29, S110–114
Pfister, R. R. (1975) The healing of corneal epithelial abrasions in the rabbit: a scanning electron microscope study. Invest. Ophthalmol., 14, 648–661
Pfister, R. R. and Bursetin, N. L. (1977) The normal and abnormal human corneal epithelial surface: a scanning electron microscopic study. Invest. Ophthalmol. Vis. Sci., 16, 614–622
Pflugfelder, S. C., Liu, Z., Monroy, D. et al. (2000) Detection of sialo mucin complex (Muc 4) in luman ocular surface epithelium and tear fluid. Invest. Ophthalmol. Vis. Sci., 41, 1316–1326
Polack, F. M. (1961) Morphology of the cornea. 1: Study with silver stains. Am. J. Ophthalmol., 51, 179–184
Pollack, I. P. (1962) Corneal hydration studied in stromal segments separated by intralamellar discs. Invest. Ophthalmol., 1, 661–665
Pratt-Johnson, J. A. (1959) Studies on the anatomy and pathology of the peripheral cornea. Am. J. Ophthalmol., 47, 478–488
Prydal, J. I., Artal, P., Woon, H. and Campbell, F. W. (1992) Study of human precorneal tear film thickness and structure using laser interferometry. Invest. Ophthalmol. Vis Sci., 33, 2006–2011
Qu, X. D. and Lehrer, R. I. (1998) Secretory phospholipase A2 is the principal bactericide for staphylococci and other gram-positive bacteria in human tears. Infect. Immun., 66, 2791–2797
Rao, G. N., Shaw, E. L., Arthur, E. J. and Aquavella, J. V. (1979) Endothelial cell morphology and corneal deturgescence. Ann. Ophthalmol., 11, 885–899
Reim, M., Lax, F., Lichte, H. and Turss, R. (1967) Steady state levels of glucose in the different layers of the cornea, aqueous humor, blood and tears in vivo. Ophthalmologica, 154, 39–50

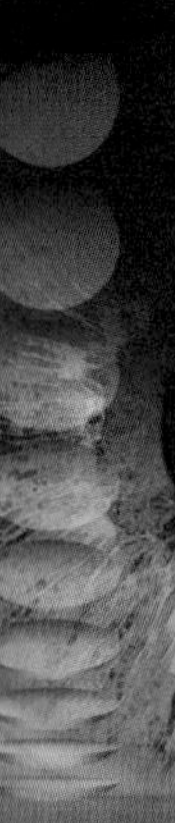

Reinstein, D. Z., Silverman, R. H., Rondeau, M. J. and Coleman, D. J. (1994) Epithelial and corneal thickness measurements by high frequency ultrasound digital signal processing. Ophthalmology, 101, 140–146

Ren, H. and Wilson, G. (1996) Apoptosis in the corneal epithelium. Invest. Ophthalmol. Vis. Sci., 37(6), 1017–1025

Ren, D. H., Petroll, W. M., Jester, J. V. and Cavanagh, H. D. (1999a) The effect of rigid gas permeable contact lens wear on proliferation of rabbit corneal and conjunctival epithelial cells. CLAO J., 25(3), 136–141

Ren, D. H., Petroll, W. M., Jester, J. V., Ho-Fan, J. and Cavanagh, H. D. (1999b) Short-term hypoxia downregulates epithelial cell desquamation in vivo, but does not increase Pseudomonas aeruginosa adherence to exfoliated corneal epithelial cells. CLAO J., 25(2), 73–79

Riss, B. and Riss, P. (1981) Corneal sensitivity in pregnancy. Ophthalmologica, 183, 57–62

Rodrigues, M. M., Rowden, G., Hackett, J. and Bakas, J. (1987) Langerhans cells in the normal conjunctiva and peripheral cornea of selected species. Invest. Ophthalmol. Vis. Sci., 21, 759–765

Ruben, M. and Colebrook, E. (1979) Keratoplasty sensitivity. Br. J. Ophthalmol., 63, 265–267

Ruiz-Montenegro, J., Mafra, C. H., Wilson, S. E. et al. (1993) Corneal topographic alterations in normal contact lens wearers. Ophthalmology, 100, 128–134

Ruskell, G. L. (1969) Changes in nerve terminals and acini of the lacrimal gland and changes in secretion induced by autonomic denervation. Z. Zellforsch. Mikroscop. Anat., 94, 261–281

Ruskell, G. L. (1975) Nerve terminals and epithelial cell variety in the human lacrimal gland. Cell Tissue Res., 158, 121–136

Sack, R. A., Nunes, I., Beaton, A. and Carol, M. (2001) Host-defense mechanism of the ocular surfaces. Biosci. Rep., 21, 463–479

Schermer, A., Galvin, S. and Sun, T-T. (1986) Differentiation-related expression of a major 64K corneal keratin in vivo and in culture suggests limbal location of corneal epithelial stem cells. J. Cell Biol., 103, 49–62

Schimmelpfennig, B. (1982) Nerve structures in human central corneal epithelium. Graefes Arch. Klin. Exp. Ophthalmol., 218, 14–20

Schirmer, K. E. and Mellor, L. D. (1961) Corneal sensitivity after cataract extraction. Arch. Ophthalmol., 65, 433–436

Schirmer, O. (1903) Studien zur Physiologie und Pathologie der Träanenabsonderung und Thränenabfur. Graefes Arch. Klin. Exp. Ophthalmol., 56, 197–291

Schoessler, J. P. and Woloschak, M. J. (1981) Corneal endothelium in veteran PMMA contact lens wearers. Int. Contact Lens Clin., 8, 19–25

Schute, C. C. D. (1974) Haidinger's brushes and predominant orientation of collagen in corneal stroma. Nature, 250, 163–164

Scott, J. E. (1992) Morphometry of cupromeronic blue-stained proteoglycan in animal corneas, versus that of purified proteoglycans stained in vitro, implies that tertiary structures contribute to corneal ultrastructure. J. Anat., 180, 155–164

Sédan, J., Farnarier, G. and Ferrand, G. (1958) Contribution … l'etude de la keraesthesie. Ann. Oculist, 191, 736–751

Sibug, M. E., Datiles, M. B. and Kashima, K. (1991) Specular microscopy studies on the corneal endothelium after cessation of contact lens wear. Cornea, 10, 395–401

Sigelman, S. and Friedenwald, J. S. (1954) Mitotic and wound-healing activities of the corneal epithelium. Effect of sensory denervation. Arch. Ophthalmol., 52, 46–57

Sjögren, H. (1955) The lacrimal secretion in newborn, premature and fully developed children. Acta Ophthalmol., 33, 557–560

Smelser, G. K. (1952) Relation of factors involved in maintenance of optical properties of cornea to contact-lens wear. Arch. Ophthalmol., 47, 328–343

Smelser, G. K. and Ozanics, O. (1952) Importance of atmospheric oxygen for maintenance of the optical properties of the human cornea. Science, 115, 140

Smith, J. W. (1969) The transparency of the corneal stroma. Vision Res., 9, 393–396

Snyder, M. C., Bergmanson, J. and Doughty, M. J. (1998) Keratocytes: no more the quiet cells. J. Am. Optom. Assoc., 69, 180–187

Soni, P. S., Nguyen, T. T. and Bonanno, J. A. (2003) Overnight orthokeratology: visual and corneal changes. Eye Contact Lens, 29, 137–145

Speedwell, L., Novakovic, P., Sherrard, E. and Taylor D. (1988) The infant corneal endothelium. Arch. Ophthalmol., 106(6), 771–775

Stanworth, A. and Naylor, E. S. (1953) Polarised light studies of the cornea. I. The isolated cornea. J. Exp. Biol., 30, 160–163

Steuhl, P. and Rohen, J. W. (1983) Absorption of horse-radish peroxide by the conjunctival epithelium of monkeys and rabbits. Graefes Arch. Klin. Exp. Ophthalmol., 220, 13–18

Stocker, E. G. and Schoessler, J. P. (1985) Corneal endothelial polymegethism induced by PMMA contact lens wear. Invest. Ophthalmol. Vis. Sci., 26, 857–863

Stone, R. A. and McGlinn, A. M. (1988) Calcitonin gene-related peptide immunoreactive nerves in human and rhesus monkey eyes. Invest. Ophthalmol. Vis. Sci., 29, 305–310

Stone, R. A., Laties, A. M. and Brecha, N. C. (1982) Substance P-like immunoreactive nerves in the anterior segment of the rabbit, cat and monkey eye. Neuroscience, 7, 2459–2468

Stone, R. A., Kuwayama, X., Terenghi, G. and Polak, J. M. (1986a) Calcitonin gene-related peptide: occurrence in corneal sensory nerves. Exp. Eye Res., 43, 279–284

Stone, R. A., Tervo, T., Tervo, K. and Tarkkarnen, A. (1986b) Vasoactive intestinal polypeptide-like immunoreactive nerves to the human eye. Acta Ophthalmol., 64, 12–18

Süchting, P., Machnemer, R. and Welz, S. (1966) Die Lebenszeit der Epithelzelle der Rattencornea und conjunctiva. Graefes Arch. Klin. Exp. Ophthalmol., 170, 297–310

Sugiura, B. (1965) The polygonal cell system of the corneal epithelium. In Die Struktur des Auges. II. Symposium, pp. 463–479, ed. J. Rohen. Eighth International Congress of Anatomists, Wiesbaden. Stuttgart: Schatauer

Swarbrick, H. A., Wong, G. and O'Leary D. J. (1998) Corneal response to orthokeratology. Optom. Vis. Sci., 75, 791–799

ten Tusscher, M. P. M., Klooster, J. and Vrensen, G. F. J. M. (1988) The innervation of the rabbit's anterior eye segment: a retrograde tracing study. Exp. Eye Res., 46, 717–730

ten Tusscher, M. P. M., Klooster, J., van der Want, J. J. L., Lamers, W. P. M. A. and Vrensen, G. F. J. M. (1989) The allocation of nerve fibres to the anterior eye segment and peripheral ganglia of rats. 1. The sensory innervation. Brain Res., 494, 95–104

Tervo, K., Tervo, T., Eränkä, L., Eränkä, O. and Cuello, C. (1981) Immunoreactivity for substance P in the Gasserian ganglion, ophthalmic nerve and anterior segment of the rabbit eye. Histochem. J., 13, 435–443

Tervo, T., Vannas, A., Tervo, K. and Holden, B. A. (1985) Histochemical demonstration of adrenergic nerves in the stroma of human cornea. Invest. Ophthalmol. Vis. Sci., 28, 398–400

Thoft, R. A. and Friend, J. (1972) Corneal amino acid supply and distribution. Invest. Ophthalmol., 11, 723–727

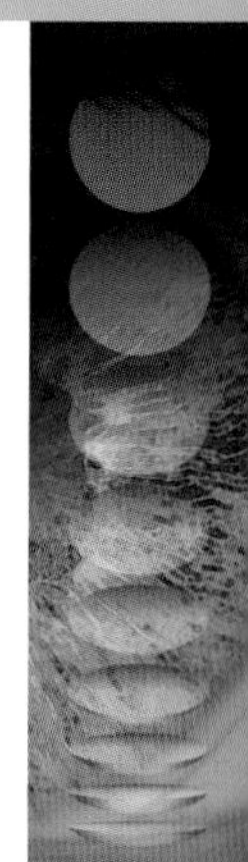

Thoft, R. A. and Friend, J. (1983) The X,Y,Z hypothesis of corneal epithelial maintenance. Invest. Ophthalmol. Vis. Sci., 24, 1442–1443

Toivanen, M., Tervo, T., Partanen, M., Vannas, A. and Hervonen, A. (1987) Histochemical demonstration of adrenergic nerves in the stroma of human cornea. Invest. Ophthalmol. Vis. Sci., 28, 298–400

Toker, E., Yenice, O., Ogüt, M. S., Akman, I. and Ozek, E. (2002) Tear production during the neonatal period. Am. J. Ophthalmol., 133(6), 746–749

Trenberth, S. M. and Mishima, S. (1968) The effect of ouabain on the rabbit corneal endothelium. Invest. Ophthalmol., 7, 44–52

Treseler, P. S., Foulks, G. N. and Sanfilippo, F. (1984) The expression of HLA antigens by cells in the human cornea. Am. J. Ophthalmol., 98, 763–772

Turss, R., Friend, J. and Dohlman, C. H. (1970) Effect of a corneal barrier on the nutrition of the epithelium. Exp. Eye Res., 9, 254–259

Ueda, S., del Cerro, M., Lo Cascio, J. A. and Aquavella, J. V. (1989) Peptidergic and catecholaminergic fibres in the human corneal epithelium: an immunohistochemical and electron microscopic study. Acta Ophthalmol., 67 (Suppl.), 80–90

van der Heyden, C., Weekers, J. F. and Schoffeniels, E. (1975) Sodium and chloride transport across the isolated rabbit cornea. Exp. Eye Res., 20, 89–96

Veerhuis, R. and Kijlstra, A. (1982) Inhibition of hemolytic complement activity by lactoferrin in tears. Exp. Eye. Res., 34, 257–265

Vega, J. A., Simpson, T. L. and Fonn, D. (1999) A noncontact pneumatic esthesiometer for measurement of ocular sensitivity: a preliminary report. Cornea, 18, 675–681

Watanabe, H., Tisdale, A. S. and Gipson, I. K. (1993) Eyelid opening induces expression of a glycocalyx glycoprotein of rat ocular surface epithelium. Invest. Ophthalmol. Vis. Sci., 34, 327–338

Watsky, M. A. (1995) Keratocyte gap junctional communication in normal and wounded rabbit cornea and human corneas. Invest. Ophthalmol. Vis. Sci., 36, 2568–2576

Weimar, V. (1960) Healing processes in the cornea. In The Transparency of the Cornea, pp. 111–124, eds. S. Duke-Elder and E. S. Perkins. Oxford: Blackwell

Wolff, E. (1948) The Anatomy of the Eye and Orbit, 3rd edn, p. 166. London: Lewis

Yamamoto, K., Ladage, P. M., Ren, D. H. et al. (2002) Effect of eyelid closure and overnight contact lens wear on viability of surface epithelial cells in rabbit cornea. Cornea, 21(1), 85–90

Zander, E. and Weddell, G. (1951) Observations on the innervation of the cornea. J. Anat., 85, 68–99

Zantos, S. G. (1983) Cystic formations in the corneal epithelium during extended wear of contact lenses. Int. Contact Lens Clin., 10, 128–146

Zantos, S. G. and Holden, B. A. (1978) Ocular changes associated with continuous wear of contact lenses. Aust. J. Ophthalmol., 61, 418–426

Zieske, J. D. (1994) Perpetuation of stem cells in the eye. Eye, 8, 163–169

Chapter 3

Contact lens materials

Brian J. Tighe

CHAPTER CONTENTS

INTRODUCTION

From silica to silicone hydrogels: the rebirth of silicone-based ophthalmic biomaterials

The years that have elapsed since the previous edition of this book was published have been significant for the development of contact lens materials. The most important feature of this period has been the commercial appearance of silicone hydrogels, which differ from conventional hydrogels in their enhanced oxygen permeabilities – a direct consequence of the inclusion of a significant proportion of siloxy groups. These groups contain the element silicon linked directly to both oxygen and carbon atoms. Thus the terms siloxy and silicone refer to organic compounds of silicon, whereas silica and silicates are inorganic glasses containing oxygen but no organic carbon.

Since their first commercial appearance in 1998, silicone hydrogel lenses have shown significant market growth. Because of their enhanced oxygen permeability, they were developed primarily with extended wear in mind, but they are now available for both overnight and daily wear use. This versatility is reflected in the growing range of commercial silicone hydrogels, some of which are specifically designed for daily wear only. At the outset, two commercial lenses were launched, bearing the USAN (United States Adopted Name) balafilcon A and lotrafilcon A, manufactured by Bausch & Lomb and CIBA Vision, respectively (see below). Once silicone hydrogels had become clinically established, the regulatory route for new materials became easier. This, in turn, makes it easier to track the development and progress to the launch of new products.

The patent literature provides initial information on new materials developments, but this is effectively supplemented by the application that companies make to the US Food and Drug Administration (FDA) for approval to market new, or modified, lenses. Once silicone hydrogel wear without significant adverse response became an established fact, new lens materials could be submitted for so-called 510(k) approval – the central point of this being a demonstration of 'substantial equivalence' to existing materials. Information relating to the submission is summarized on the FDA website and usually indicates the intention of the manufacturer to take the new material to market.

In this way, the appearance of three more silicone hydrogel lenses – galyfilcon A (Acuvue Advance, Vistakon), senofilcon A (Acuvue Oasys, Vistakon), and lotrafilcon B (AIR OPTIX, CIBA Vision) – was predictable before the event. Similarly, consultation of the FDA website showed the availability of

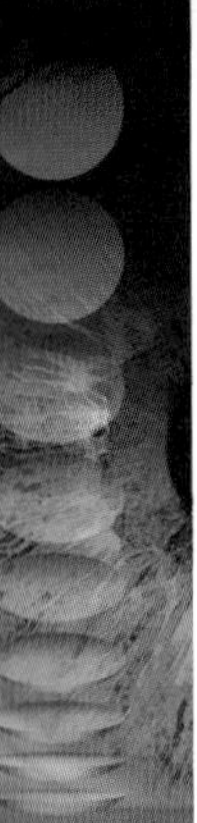

CooperVision material – comfilcon A. This has increased the number of commercial silicone hydrogel lenses to six, covering equilibrium water contents from 24 to 48% and oxygen permeabilities (Dk) from 60 to 140 barrers. Further details of these materials are contained in Table 3.3 and the associated text.

Silicon has re-emerged as a vitally important element in ophthalmic biomaterials. Glass, which is predominantly silicon dioxide, was the first material to be utilized clinically (see Chapter 1) but it was displaced by optically clear synthetic carbon-based polymers, notably polymethylmethacrylate (PMMA). Despite attempts to harness the outstanding oxygen permeability and resilience of silicone rubber, it was not until the development of the silicon-containing 'Tris' monomer, and its use to convert PMMA into gas permeable rigid lenses, that silicon made any real commercial impact in ophthalmic polymers. Now that economically viable solutions to the problem of incorporating essentially the same Tris monomer into hydrogels has been found, silicon is, once again, playing a unique and important role in the field of ophthalmic biomaterials. That is in essence the core message of this chapter.

The aim of this chapter is to provide systematic information on which the nature and behaviour of both existing and emerging materials can be understood. The subsequent sections are presented under four headings:

- The nature and behaviour of contact lens materials.
- Hard and rigid lens materials.
- Soft conventional hydrogel lens materials.
- Silicone hydrogel materials.

THE NATURE AND BEHAVIOUR OF CONTACT LENS MATERIALS

Silicon and glass

Although over 100 elements are known, and more than 80 exist in a stable form in the world around us, just four of these (carbon, nitrogen, oxygen and hydrogen) make up 95% (by weight) of all living matter on Earth. They are not, however, the four most abundant elements on Earth (which are oxygen, iron, silicon and magnesium). Historically, materials science was primarily dependent upon inorganic raw materials derived from the Earth itself, for example metals and ceramics. More recently the field of biomaterials has developed and here nature, particularly the structure and function of the human body, has provided inspiration. In this respect silicon is something of an anomaly. Its role in the formation of glass gave it an important position in civilization because of its unique clarity and rigidity. These properties made it an obvious choice for ophthalmic applications, examples of which stretch back more than 2000 years. For example, ancient civilizations used glass to represent the eye in statues of birds and animals, many of which still exist. Pellier de Quency, an 18th century French ophthalmologist, suggested the use of a glass shell, surrounded by a silver ring to accommodate sutures, as an artificial cornea. It was not until the 20th century, however, that successful glass tissue-contacting devices were made, in the form of scleral contact lenses.

The word 'glass' is used quite broadly in materials science to describe a solid material which is hardened and becomes rigid without crystallizing. Glass as we know it is more accurately described as silicate glass. It is formed by solidifying individual silicon dioxide (silica) clusters into a solid but non-crystalline (i.e. amorphous) framework. Commercial glasses are based on this silica framework, together with additives to break down any crystalline structure and reduce the melting point. The older forms of glass had only three basic ingredients: sand (silica), soda ash (Na_2O) and lime (CaO). Types of glass were then developed for more demanding applications which required chemical resistance or thermal stability by adding small amounts of other components. In all of these, however, silica is the predominant component, usually comprising 70–80% by weight of the total composition.

The fact that the element silicon is once more growing in importance in ophthalmic biomaterials is substantially unrelated to its place in materials history. Its new role is, on the face of it, unconnected to either its ability to form silicate glasses or its natural abundance. Nor is its use inspired by the way in which it performs in the human body – where it is largely absent. It might be argued that the abundance of the element stimulated research into its transformation into other useful forms of material, for it was in this way that the very useful properties brought by silicon to the field of organic materials (as distinct from inorganic or mineral-based materials) were discovered. To understand this difference, and the whole question of the interaction of modern contact lenses with the eye, it is necessary to build a picture of the nature and structure of the class of materials known as polymers.

The nature of polymers

The unique properties that polymers possess arise from the ability of certain atoms to link together to form stable bonds. This is quite different from the nature of glasses, in which the solid is held together by electrostatic forces. Foremost among the atoms that can form linking bonds with each other is carbon (C), which can link together with four other atoms, either of its own kind or alternatively atoms of, for example, hydrogen (H), oxygen (O), nitrogen (N), sulphur (S) or chlorine (Cl). It is this property of carbon that forms the basis of organic chemistry or the chemistry of carbon compounds. Most of the polymers that we encounter fall within the realm of organic chemistry, defined in this way. These polymers may be purely natural (such as cellulose), modified natural polymers (such as cellulose acetate) or completely synthetic (such as PMMA).

To some extent, silicon (Si) resembles carbon in this way, especially in its ability to link to carbon, hydrogen and oxygen. A much smaller family of polymers thus exists, based on silicon, rather than carbon. Their properties differ somewhat from those of the carbon-based polymers and they are best known in the form of siloxane polymers in which silicon and oxygen alternate in the backbone. Although both the number and structural versatility of silicon-based polymers is relatively small, they have some properties that are not achievable in carbon-based compounds. In the context of contact lenses, one of these

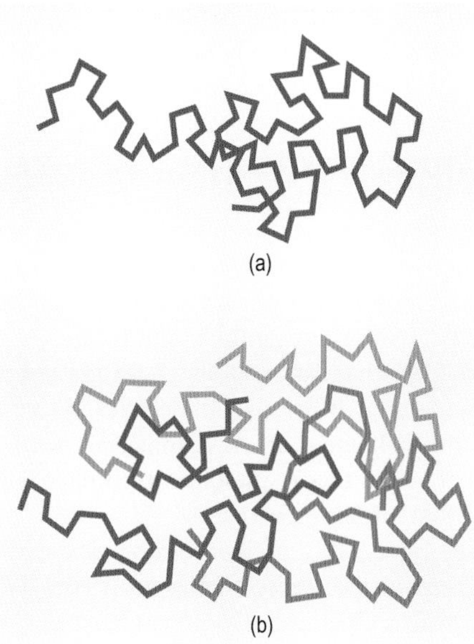

Figure 3.1 (a) Single polymer chain; (b) entangled polymer chains

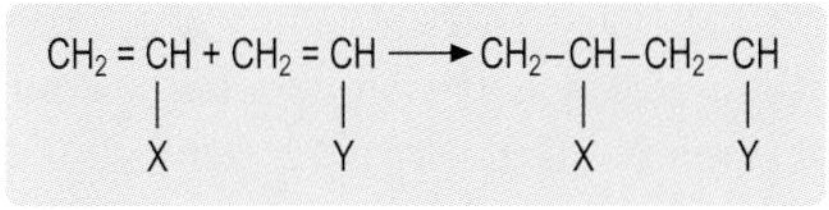

$$CH_2{=}\underset{\displaystyle X}{\underset{|}{CH}} + CH_2{=}\underset{\displaystyle Y}{\underset{|}{CH}} \longrightarrow CH_2{-}\underset{\displaystyle X}{\underset{|}{CH}}{-}CH_2{-}\underset{\displaystyle Y}{\underset{|}{CH}}$$

Figure 3.2 Monomer conversion to polymer

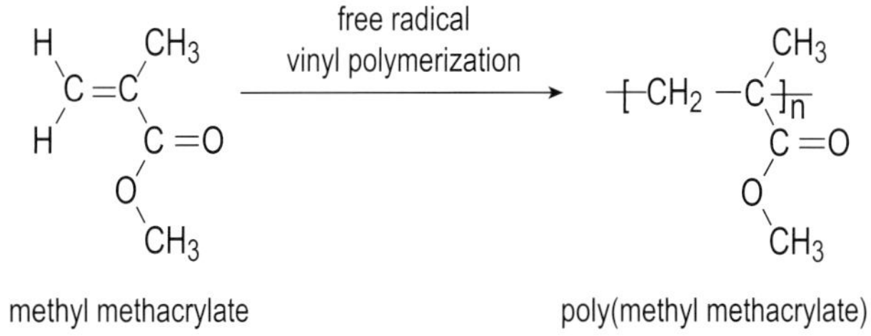

$$H_2C{=}C(CH_3){-}C({=}O){-}O{-}CH_3 \xrightarrow{\text{free radical vinyl polymerization}} {+}CH_2{-}C(CH_3)(C({=}O){-}O{-}CH_3){+}_n$$

methyl methacrylate → poly(methyl methacrylate)

Figure 3.3 Free radical polymerization of methyl methacrylate monomer (MMA)

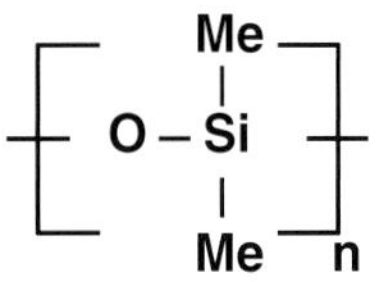

$$\left[O{-}\underset{\displaystyle Me}{\overset{\displaystyle Me}{Si}} \right]_n$$

Figure 3.4 Structure of silicone rubber

properties (oxygen permeability) is advantageous, whereas another (water repellency) is a disadvantage. The major advances in their use in contact lens materials have been based around the formation of hybrid structures which enable the versatility of carbon–carbon chemistry to be enhanced by the unique properties of the siloxane groups.

The single characteristic that unites both silicon- and carbon-based polymers is the fact that, as the name (poly-mer) suggests, they are composed of many units linked together in long chains. Thus, if we can imagine a molecule of oxygen and a molecule of water enlarged to the size of a tennis ball (the molecular size of water is very similar to that of oxygen), a molecule of polyethylene or poly(methyl methacrylate) on the same scale would be of similar cross-sectional diameter but something like 200 feet in length. It is the gigantic length of polymers (sometimes called macromolecules) in relation to their cross-sectional diameter that gives them their unique properties, such as toughness and elasticity. The links between individual atoms are inclined to each other at an angle (the bond angle) which means that chains are not straight and rod-like but 'kinked' as shown in Figure 3.1. One major difference between the siloxane (Si – O – Si) backbone and the carbon (C – C) backbone is in the ease of rotation (rather like a crankshaft in a car engine) resulting from differences in size and bond angles of the individual atoms.

The individual building blocks from which polymers are formed are termed 'monomers'. To indicate that a polymer contains more than one type of repeating monomer unit – for example when two different monomers are polymerized together – the description 'copolymer' is used. Copolymer is a general term and can be used to describe polymers obtained from mixtures of more than two monomers. Because most contact lens polymers are formed from monomers that are characterized by the presence of a carbon–carbon double bond that opens to form a linked chain, the resultant structures can be generalized as shown in Figure 3.2. It is the way in which the structural and functional groups represented in Figure 3.2 by X and Y interact with each other, and with their surrounding environment, that governs the interaction of polymer chains and the resultant properties of the polymer itself. The siloxane polymers are structurally different and, as a consequence, the methods of polymer synthesis are not interchangeable with those used for carbon backbone polymers. It is this simple fact that has made the preparation of hybrids of silicon- and carbon-based polymers very difficult to achieve.

Perhaps the best way of visualizing the way in which polymer chains arrange themselves is by taking several pieces of string to represent individual molecules. The usual arrangement is random, with the pieces of string loosely entangled rather than being extended. The interaction and entanglement of the individual molecules in this way gives polymers their characteristic physical properties. By changing the chemical nature of the polymer chain and their arrangement together we can change the physical properties and thus obtain either hard glassy behaviour or, at the other extreme, flexible, elastomeric behaviour. The best example of a hard glassy material is poly(methyl methacrylate) which is formed from methyl methacrylate monomer units (Fig. 3.3). This figure represents the assembly of '*n*' methyl methacrylate units to form a PMMA chain '*n*' units long. The best example of a biomaterial based on the flexible silicon–oxygen backbone is silicone rubber (Fig. 3.4) which is both elastomeric and highly permeable to oxygen.

One important way in which a hard glassy polymer can be converted into a flexible material is by the incorporation of a 'plasticizer'. This is a mobile component, often an organic liquid with a high boiling point, that will act as an 'internal lubricant'. Its presence separates the polymer chains, allowing them to move more freely. A good example is poly(vinyl chloride) or

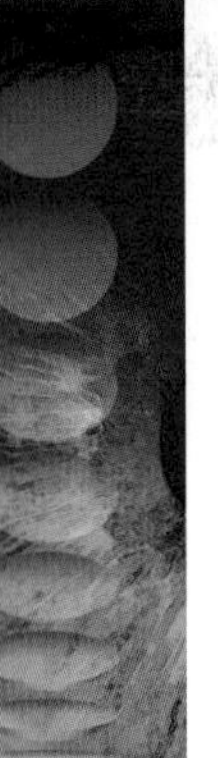

PVC (Fig. 3.2, X = Y = Cl) which in its unmodified state is a rigid glassy material and will be familiar as the clear corrugated roofing material used on car ports and similar domestic extensions. When a plasticizer is incorporated, the material is converted into the flexible material used, for example, as 'vinyl' seat coverings in cars and general domestic applications. In these cases, pigments and various processing aids will also have been added in order to enable the polymer to be produced in a variety of colours and textures.

When glass began to be replaced by PMMA, it signalled a new range of plastics which had various advantages:

- Easier to process.
- Better structural versatility.
- Lower price.

PMMA was an ideal candidate for a rigid contact lens material. It has:

- A similar appearance and ease of fabrication to glass.
- Acceptable surface wettability.
- Excellent durability.

The lenses compared favourably with scleral lenses as they were thin and lightweight, could be worn more comfortably and gave excellent visual correction. They were also relatively easy to clean and suffered little from tear deposition problems. Unfortunately, the material has one very significant drawback for use as a corneal lens – it is virtually impermeable to oxygen.

HARD AND RIGID LENS MATERIALS

Attractions and disadvantages of polymethyl methacrylate

To appreciate the way in which rigid, as distinct from soft, materials have developed it is necessary to go back to the period following World War II. The new availability of plastics materials, specifically PMMA, led to the design and development of the first corneal lens as a replacement for glass corneoscleral lenses. The PMMA lenses were prepared by adopting the polymerization of methyl methacrylate with a free radical initiation system shown in Figure 3.3 to form rods or buttons from which a lens was obtained by lathing and polishing.

By the 1960s a greater appreciation of the effects of contact lens wear on the anterior eye was developing and the fact that PMMA is essentially a barrier to oxygen transport became widely recognized. Corneal physiologists at that time were able to carry out theoretical calculations on the effect of contact lenses on corneal respiration and also well-differentiated experiments using PMMA and a different material with a much higher oxygen permeability – silicone rubber (see Fig. 3.4). It is instructive to examine why these two materials have such different oxygen permeabilities.

The oxygen permeability (P) of a material is determined by the product of two factors: D and K – diffusion and solubility. It is for this reason that the term DK, or more commonly Dk, is used to describe oxygen permeability (see also p. 73). The magnitude of the diffusion term, D, is determined by the rate at which oxygen molecules can pass through the polymer chains. The solubility term, K, is governed by the number of oxygen molecules within the polymer, i.e. the amount of oxygen that can be dissolved. Values of Dk are conveniently quoted in barrers (see p. 66):

$$\text{Dk (barrers)} = 10^{-11}\text{cm}^3\ \text{O}_2\ \text{(STP).cm/s.cm}^2\text{.mmHg}$$

Thus Dk (or P) is the permeability coefficient for a given material, whereas Dk/t or P/t refers specifically to the permeability (transmissibility) of a sample (such as a contact lens) of that material of a given thickness, t.

The paradox that has hindered the development of the ideal contact lens material over several decades is crystallized in Figures 3.3 and 3.4. Here are two materials with aspects of behaviour that make them suitable for contact lens use, but other aspects that inhibit their success.

PMMA (see Fig. 3.3) is a glassy thermoplastic material which has advantageous optical clarity, surface properties, processibility and ease of sterilization, but the disadvantage of being virtually impermeable to oxygen.

Silicone rubber (see Fig. 3.4) is the most significant member of a group of materials known as synthetic elastomers. It has oxygen permeability more than a thousand times greater than PMMA but is hydrophobic, making it difficult to use for contact lens materials.

Synthetic elastomers are flexible and show rubber-like behaviour, i.e. they are capable of being compressed or stretched and instantaneously return to their original shape when the deforming force is removed. They consist of polymer chains that possess high mobility, allowing oxygen to diffuse rapidly through the structure, and they are cross-linked at intervals along the polymer backbones. The extremely high oxygen permeability of silicone rubber arises from the backbone of alternate silicone and oxygen atoms which confers not only great freedom of rotation but also a much higher solubility for oxygen than rubbery polymers with simple carbon backbones.

Much effort has been expended to make hydrophobic materials adequately wettable for contact lens use. Silicone rubber lenses, surface-treated to give acceptable wettability, were developed in the mid-1960s (McVannel et al. 1967) and found clinically to have little deleterious effect on corneal respiration (Hill & Schoessler 1967) but the problems of maintaining adequate surface properties during routine clinical use have never been fully overcome. Silicone rubber lenses are still used only in specialized applications (see Chapter 24).

Elastomers, such as silicone rubber, are in many ways intermediate between thermoplastics such as PMMA and hydrogels, such as poly-2-hydroxyethyl methacrylate (polyHEMA). They possess some of the toughness associated with the former group and the softness of the latter, and in this sense are ideal candidates for contact lens usage. Unfortunately, the molecular features required for true elastic behaviour invariably produce polymers with hydrophobic surfaces. This problem is made worse by the virtually instantaneous elastic recovery of the materials, which causes them to 'grab' the cornea after being deformed by the blink, which in turn displaces the posterior tear film and leads to lens binding. Despite attempts to harness almost every available elastomeric material, as

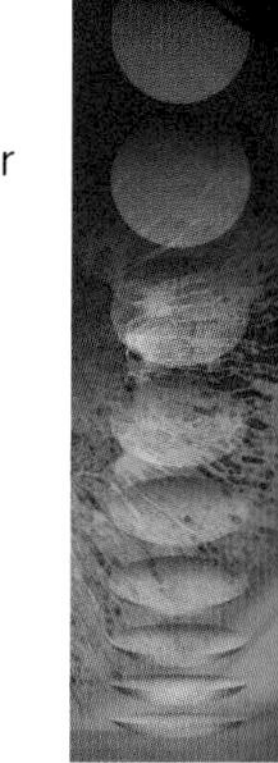

witnessed by the patent literature, no true elastomer has been successfully used as a commercial contact lens material.

It was not until the uniquely high oxygen permeability of the silicon–oxygen backbone could be copolymerized with the monomers used in contact lens manufacture that any real progress was made in this area. Once the breakthrough was made, it paved the way for two distinct types of contact lens material: silicone hydrogels and rigid gas-permeable (RGP) materials.

At first, the task of finding a material better than PMMA did not seem too difficult, since almost all thermoplastics are less rigid and more oxygen permeable. Several flexible thermoplastic materials were suggested in the patent literature, but none achieved clinical significance. The most promising results were obtained with cellulose esters such as cellulose acetate butyrate (CAB). The oxygen permeability is approximately 20 times greater than that of PMMA (Refojo et al. 1977) and the material could be moulded, which was cheaper than lathe cutting, the most widely used method of contact lens fabrication in the 1970s. Cellulose esters lack the dimensional stability of PMMA but this would not have affected their success, had it not been for the appearance, and almost instant success, of the silicone acrylates.

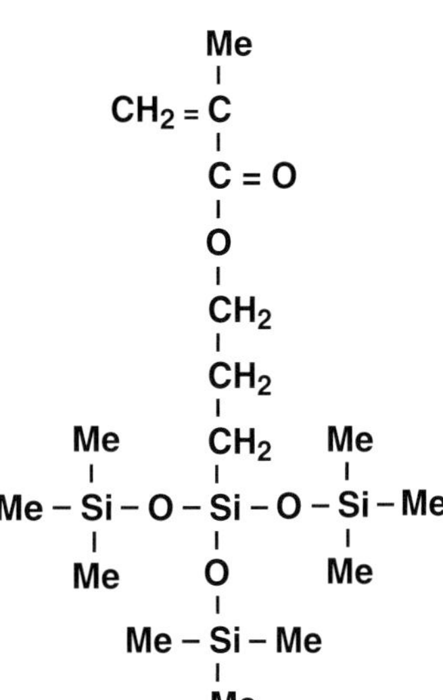

Figure 3.5 Tris (trimethyl-siloxy)-γ-methacryloxy-propylsilane (TRIS) monomer

Me
|
$CH_2 = C$
|
$C = O$
|
O
|
$CH_2 -(CF_2)_8 - H$

Figure 3.6 1,1,9-Trihydroperfluoro-nonyl methacrylate monomer

The hybrid rigid gas-permeable materials

Silicone acrylate materials combine, to a degree, the ease of preparation of PMMA and the oxygen permeability of silicone rubber. The problem lay in combining the polymers to achieve a balance of properties because different types of reaction are used in the formation of the two materials. This is illustrated by using the picture of polymers, such as PMMA and hydrogels, as 'washing line' polymers which are formed from precursors containing carbon–carbon double bonds (e.g. Fig. 3.3). The principle is that polymers of this type have a long backbone (i.e. the string or 'washing line') from which a variety of chemical groups may be suspended (the 'washing').

Silicone rubber is an example of what can be regarded as 'poppet bead' polymers. The individual units are joined just like the individual beads on a 'poppet bead' necklace. There is no 'washing' hanging from the chain and the properties of the polymer are controlled by the structure of the poppet beads themselves. The fundamental problem that prevented simple PMMA–silicone rubber combinations from being prepared is that the 'washing line' and 'poppet bead' chemistries are incompatible and beads cannot be inserted into the washing line. For an individual 'monomer' unit to be inserted into an acrylate or methacrylate polymer such as PMMA, it is necessary that the monomer should have a carbon–carbon double bond (see Fig. 3.3). Without the double bond, the washing cannot be 'pegged onto the washing line'.

Current siloxy-methacrylates get round this problem in a well-recognized, but nevertheless quite ingenious, way. Short segments of the poppet bead chain are turned into 'washing' by attaching them to a chemical intermediate that contains the necessary double bond. This can be seen in the structure of the siloxy-methacrylate monomer (Fig. 3.5) which in essence consists of the individual units of silicone rubber structure pasted onto a modified methyl methacrylate molecule – the silicone rubber units have been turned into washing and can now be pegged onto a PMMA washing line.

Much of the relevant information regarding gas-permeable lenses is contained in the patent literature, which is analysed in detail elsewhere (Kishi & Tighe 1988, Künzler and McGee 1995, Tighe 1997).

The Gaylord patents – harnessing silicone

The major advance that enabled the development of RGP contact lens materials is found in the work of Norman Gaylord at Polycon Laboratories, described in a series of patents (Gaylord 1974, 1978). Two aspects of this work are of note:

- The development of what has become the industry standard siloxy-methacrylate monomer, tris (trimethyl-siloxy)-γ-methacryloxy-propylsilane (see Fig. 3.5), commonly referred to as TRIS.
- The recognition of the value of incorporating fluoroalkyl methacrylates (e.g. 1,1,9-trihydroperfluoro-nonyl methacrylate, Fig. 3.6) principally to further enhance oxygen permeability.

Both these aspects have been subsequently developed and together, form the basis of most existing commercial gas-permeable contact lens materials. Although TRIS is still the most widely used siloxy-methacrylate monomer in RGP

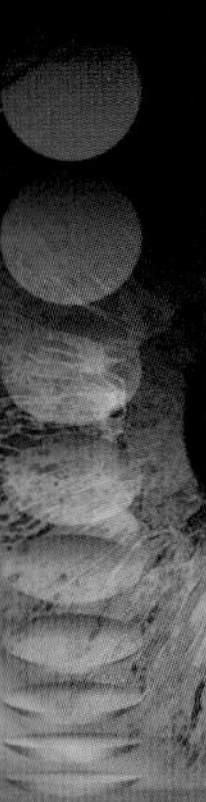

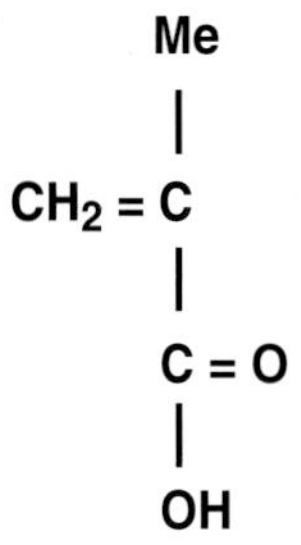

Figure 3.7 Methacrylic acid monomer

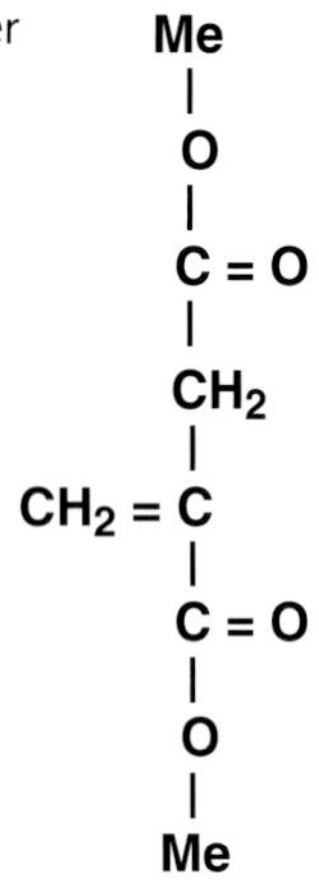

Figure 3.8 Dimethyl itaconate monomer

manufacture, the fluoromethacrylate monomers employed in current commercial materials are much simpler than that initially used by Gaylord.

A fluorine-containing contact lens was not new. Fluorocarbons dissolve more oxygen than hydrocarbons and give rise to polymers with higher oxygen permeabilities than their hydrocarbon equivalents. A series of Du Pont's patents described the advantages of contact lenses prepared from polymers derived from perfluoroalkylethyl methacrylates, but it took a further 10 years before significant commercial use was made of fluorocarbon-based contact lenses (Tighe 1997). This was because siloxy-methacrylates have a much greater oxygen permeability than fluorocarbon methacrylates, which on their own show little improvement over PMMA. Their advantages become evident when they are used to partially replace methyl methacrylate in copolymers with TRIS. The balance of the three components (fluoromethacrylate, methyl methacrylate and TRIS) is adjusted to optimize oxygen permeability, hardness (which influences processability) and wettability.

In 1978 and 1979, at about the time of the appearance of Gaylord's third patent, three workers began to file their separate patents related to siloxy-methacrylate-based contact lens materials. These were Kyoichi Tanaka (Toyo Contact Lens Co. Ltd), Edward Ellis (Polymer Technology Corporation) and Nick Novicky whose later patents (and presumably rights to the earlier) were assigned to Syntex (USA) Inc. The Ellis and Novicky patents form a clear line of continuation from Gaylord's early work and, because of this, are best considered together (Ellis & Salamone 1979, Novicky 1980).

The most important of the Ellis and Salamone patents used Gaylord's basic composition based on TRIS, but claimed novelty in the additional use of methacrylic acid (Fig. 3.7, a hydrophilic monomer referred to but not exemplified by Gaylord) to improve surface wettability, and by the incorporation of an itaconate ester (e.g. dimethyl itaconate; Fig. 3.8). This composition formed the basis of the influential Boston range of early gas permeable materials.

Tanaka's work has parallel filings in Japan and the USA and it has some slight and significant differences. One of these (Fig. 3.9) is the inclusion of a hydroxyl group into the siloxy monomer to improve wettability (Tanaka et al. 1979a,b). This was also a significant early step in overcoming the technical obstacles to the development of silicone hydrogels.

Tanaka's early Japanese patent marked the beginning of a rapid growth in Japanese patents, principally as a result of work assigned to Hoya Lens K. K. and Toyo Contact Lens Co. Ltd. Subsequent clinical interest in using RGPs for extended wear in Japan stimulated a series of patents, which provide valuable information on the use of fluoroalkyl methacrylates in conjunction with siloxy-methacrylates, and the properties of fluoroalkyl methacrylates themselves. For example, the relative permeability along the series of homopolymers of methyl methacrylate, trifluoroethyl methacrylate (Fig. 3.10) and hexafluoroisopropyl methacrylate (Fig. 3.11) is disclosed (1:60:100), which indicates the relative advantage, in terms of permeability, of replacing methyl methacrylate by either of these two fluoro monomers. These opened the way to the development of fluorine-containing siloxy-methacrylate gas-permeable materials (e.g. Equalens, FluoroPerm, Menicon SP).

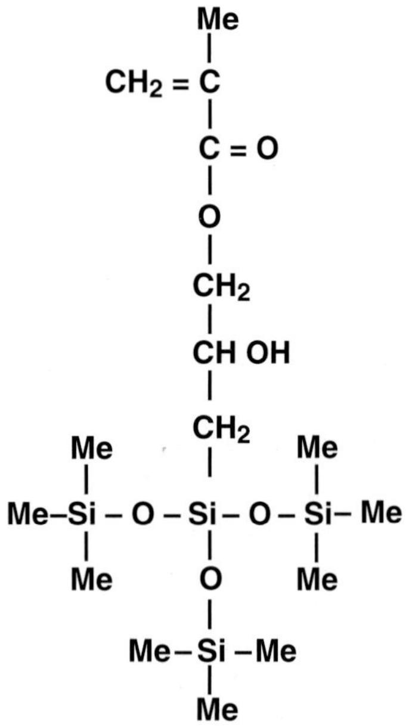

Figure 3.9 (3-methacryloxy-2-hydroxypropyloxy) propylbis(trimethylsiloxy) methylsilane monomer

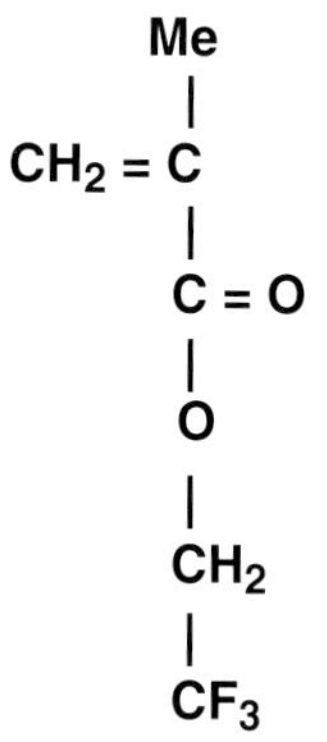

Me
|
$CH_2 = C$
|
C = O
|
O
|
CH_2
|
CF_3

Figure 3.10 Trifluoroethyl methacrylate monomer

Me
|
$CH_2 = C$
|
C = O
|
O
|
$CF_3 — CH — CF_3$

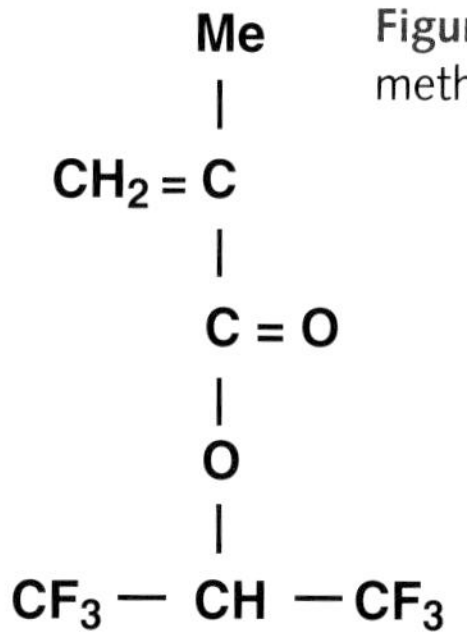

Figure 3.11 Hexafluoroisopropyl methacrylate monomer

Increasing oxygen permeability is balanced against the retention of acceptable dimensional stability and ocular compatibility (characterized by wettability and deposit resistance). The essential structural developments have centred around the following:

- The TRIS component, characterized by attempts to incorporate higher proportions of more highly branched siloxy derivatives.
- Fluorocarbon co-monomers in the place of hydrocarbon-based components such as methyl methacrylate.
- Improvement of wettability by incorporation of hydrophilic co-monomers, or subsequent surface modification of the formed lens.
- The development of cross-linking technology – RGPs contain much higher levels of cross-linking agents than soft lenses.

Despite much discussion in the patent literature, little that is truly new has appeared since Gaylord's 1974 work. The process since then has been of refinement and improvement.

Commercial RGP materials and their properties

Some commercially available RGP materials are shown in Table 3.1, together with information on chemical type, oxygen permeability, wettability, mechanical properties, density and refractive index. Values for PMMA, cellulose acetate butyrate and a silicone rubber lens are included for comparison. This information has been compiled from various sources and some comments on the methodologies used are included.

Oxygen permeability

Several experimental procedures for determining oxygen permeability may be distinguished. In each, oxygen at a known effective concentration passes from the donor side of the cell through the membrane (of known thickness and cross-sectional area) to a receiver side, also of known volume, where it is sensed. In the case of rigid polymers it is possible to use both gas-to-gas and liquid-to-liquid systems.

This has the advantage that reference values for standard materials can be obtained in the gas-to-gas system which does not suffer from some of the shortcomings of the liquid-to-liquid cell, in which the liquid is ideally stirred on both sides of the membrane.

The polarographic electrode technique, which is usually used for lens measurement, has several shortcomings.

- The cell is unstirred, giving rise to boundary layer problems.
- The thickness of the contact lens normally shows a centre-to-edge variation, producing uncertainties in the calculation.
- Because the lenses vary in curvature, the volume of the receiver side is not accurately fixed.

The last point is less important, because the technique is not usually operated in the manner that measures rate of increase in oxygen concentration of the receiver side of the cell, but rather the resultant equilibrium oxygen consumption by the electrode.

The measurement of oxygen consumption assumes that oxygen transported to the receiver side is efficiently consumed by the electrode sensor and therefore, as a result, the partial pressure of oxygen on the receiver side is always effectively zero. With very permeable samples, these assumptions are not justified.

In all cell configurations, the membrane separating donor and receiver chambers must be oxygen tight but this again is difficult to achieve with contact lens measurements, and edge effect corrections must be made. Much effort has gone into standardization of procedures and cross-correlation of results (Holden et al. 1990, Weissman & Fatt 1991).

Mechanical properties

Developments that produce higher oxygen permeabilities lead to problems with mechanical properties. In particular, when siloxy-methacrylate content is increased to achieve high oxygen permeabilities:

- Incompatibility, phase separation and deterioration in mechanical properties, particularly dimensional stability, limit the proportion of such monomers that can be incorporated.
- To improve wettability, they require the incorporation of hydrophilic monomers containing hydroxyl, carboxyl, amide or lactam groups, which tend to reduce oxygen permeability and produce low levels of water uptake that in turn reduce dimensional stability.

Current mechanical property measurements, such as hardness, do not indicate any clear distinction between materials (see Table 3.1) and poor mechanical behaviour cannot be correlated

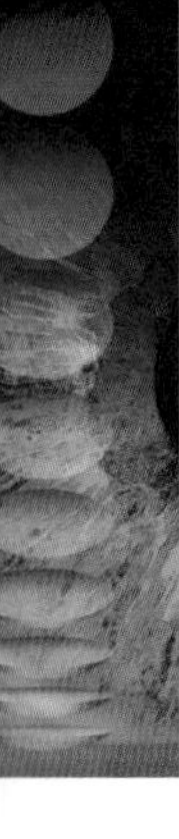

Table 3.1: Properties of typical commercial rigid lens materials

Product (Manufacturer/supplier)	Material type	Dk (34°C, barrers)	Contact angle (soaked)	Hardness	Refractive index	Specific gravity
Alberta S (Progressive Optical)	Polysulphone copolymer	28(a), 45(c)	28°(a), 9°(c)	85SD	1.475	1.140
Boston II (B&L/Polymer Tech)	Siloxy-methac. itaconate copolymer (Itafocon A)	12–14(a,b,c)	25°(b), 20°(c)	85SD, 119R(c)	1.471	1.130
Boston IV (B&L/Polymer Tech)	Siloxy-methac. itaconate copolymer (Itafocon B)	21(a), 28(b), 22(c)	25°(b), 17°(c)	80SD, 117R(c)	1.469	1.110
Boston 7 (B&L/Polymer Tech)	Siloxy-fluoromethac. copolymer (Satafocon A)	73(b), 49(c)	33°(b), 54°(c)	85SD, 117R(c)	1.428	1.220
Boston RXD (B&L/Polymer Tech)	Siloxy-fluoromethac. copolymer (Itabisflufocon A)	27,45(b), 24(c)	39°(b), 39°(c)	85SD, 121R(c)	1.435	1.270
Boston ES (B&L/Polymer Tech)	Siloxy-fluoromethac. copolymer (Enflufocon A)	31(b), 18(c)	52°(b), 52°(c)	118R(c)	1.443	1.220
Boston EO (B&L/Polymer Tech)	Siloxy-fluoromethac. copolymer (Enflufocon B)	82(b), 58(c)	49°(c)	83SD, 114R(c)	1.429	1.230
Boston XO (B&L/Polymer Tech)	Siloxy-fluoromethac. copolymer (Hexafocon A)	100(b),(c)	49°(c)	81SD, 112R(c)	1.415	1.270
Equalens (B&L/Polymer Tech)	Siloxy-fluoromethac. copolymer (Itafluorofocon A)	47,72(b) 47(c)	30°(c)	81SD, 115R(c)	1.439	1.196
Equalens II (B&L/Polymer Tech)	Siloxy-fluoromethac. copolymer (Oprifocon A)	125(b), 85(c)	40°(b), 30°(c)	114R(c)	1.423	1.240
Fluorocon 30,60,92,151 (WJ/PBH)	Siloxy-fluoromethac. copolymer (Paflufocon)	30,60,92, 151(c)	As FluoroPerm range	As FluoroPerm range	As FluoroPerm range	–
FluoroPerm 30 (Paragon Vision Sci)	Siloxy-fluoromethac. copolymer (Paflufocon A)	24(b), 30(c)	13°(c)	84SD	1.466	1.140
FluoroPerm 60 (Paragon Vision Sci)	Siloxy-fluoromethac. copolymer (Paflufocon B)	47(b), 60(c)	15°(c)	83SD	1.453	1.150
FluoroPerm 92 (Paragon Vision Sci)	Siloxy-fluoromethac. copolymer (Paflufocon C)	50(b), 92(c)	16°(c)	81SD	1.453	1.100
FluoroPerm 151 (Paragon Vision Sci)	Siloxy-fluoromethac. copolymer (Paflufocon D)	151(c)	42°(c)	79SD	1.442	1.100
Menicon SFP (Menicon Co)	Siloxy-fluoromethac. copolymer	102(c)	18°(c)	80SD(b), 7.6V(c)	N/A	1.120
Optacryl 60 (Paragon Vision Sci)	Siloxy-methac. copolymer	12, 14(b), 18(c)	25°(c)	83SD(b), 88SD	1.467	1.126
Optacryl K (Paragon Vision Sci)	Siloxy-methac. copolymer	21(b), 32(c)	25°(c)	81SD(b), 84SD	1.467	1.110
Paragon HDS (Paragon Optical Inc.)	Siloxy-methac. copolymer	58(c)	13°(c)	84SD	1.449	1.160
Paragon Thin (Paragon Optical Inc.)	Siloxy-methac. copolymer	29(c)	15°(c)	85SD	1.463	1.145
Paraperm O2 (Paragon Optical Inc.)	Siloxy-methac. copolymer	12(b), 15(c)	30°(b), 25°(c)	86SD	1.473	1.127
Paraperm EW (Paragon Optical Inc.)	Siloxy-methac. copolymer	40(b), 56(c)	26°(c)	10.6V(b), 82SD	1.467	1.070

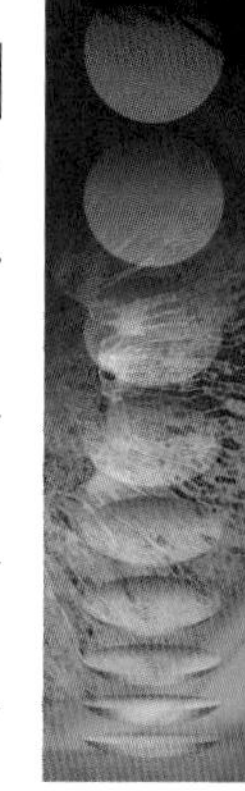

Table 3.1: Properties of typical commercial rigid lens materials (*cont'd*)

Product (Manufacturer/supplier)	Material type	Dk (34°C, barrers)	Contact angle (soaked)	Hardness	Refractive index	Specific gravity
Persecon 92E (CIBA Vision)	Siloxy-fluoromethac. copolymer (Paflufocon C)	50(b), 92(c)	16°(c)	81SD	1.453	1.100
Polycon II (WJ/PBH)	Siloxy-methac. copolymer (Silafocon A)	10(a), 12(c)	12°(c)	84.5SD	1.467	1.130
Polycon HDK (WJ/PBH)	Siloxy-methac. copolymer	30(b), 40(c)	40°(c)	85SD	1.469	1.148
Silicone rubber (e.g. Silsoft, B&L)	Silicone rubber	340–450(a,c)	–	–	1.44	1.13
PMMA (Various)	Poly methyl methacrylate	0.1(a)	15–35°(a,b)	>90SD(b)	1.49	1.195
CAB (e.g. Persecon E, CIBA)	Cellulose acetate-butyrate	7–9(a,c)	15–30°(a,c)	77.5SD	1.478	1.20

(a) Independent laboratories; (b) competitor laboratories; (c) manufacturers' information. Hardness: R, Rockwell; SD, Shore; V, Vickers.
Contact angles: captive air bubble in soaking solution (not identified).
Material type: siloxy-methac = copolymer includes siloxy compound (usually TRIS) and conventional methacrylate; siloxy-fluoromethac = copolymer includes siloxy compound (usually TRIS) and fluorinated methacrylate; other components include wetting agents (e.g. NVP, methacrylic acid), cross-linking agents, itaconate esters (Boston materials).
A variety of names are used for lenses made from equivalent materials, including original name (e.g. Boston), own name (e.g. AL 01, 02…, Eureka, Novagas, etc.) or rebranded materials name (e.g. Optacryl range also made as Vistacryl; FluoroPerm becomes Fluorocon, Oxyflow, Persecon).

with current test measurements (Kerr & Dilly 1988, Jones et al. 1996). Hardness tests do not reflect the type of mechanical failure that normally arises. These are usually associated with fracture, chipping or splitting, or distortion. In the absence of agreed standards for suitable methods, manufacturers' data are usually quoted, using one of the standard hardness test methods.

Hardness can be defined as resistance to penetration. In a hardness test an indicator is pressed on the surface of the material under test, and the extent to which it sinks in for a given pressure and time is an inverse measure of the hardness. Hardness testers available for plastics and rubbers include the Vickers indenter, the Rockwell hardness tester and the Shore durometers. These measure:

- Resistance of a material to indentation by an indenting probe (e.g. Brinell, Vickers and Shore durometers)
  - indentation with the load applied.
  - residual indentation after the load is removed.
- Resistance of a material to scratching by another material (e.g. the Bierbaum scratch test, the Moh hardness test). Similar techniques are commonly used in paint testing and involve pulling the sample beneath a loaded indenter.
- Recovery efficiency or resilience (e.g. the various Rockwell testers).
- Rockwell tests where the amount of rebound or recoverable deformation is important.

There is no common method of measurement in these tests and each uses an arbitrary scale. Although the scales can be approximately compared, precise correlation is not possible. For example, the Rockwell A scale hardness test measures the depth of penetration with the load applied, whereas the Rockwell R, L, M and E scale tests measure depth caused by a spherical indenter after most of the load has been removed. In the Vickers Microhardness test, a microscope measures the diagonals of the pits left by a diamond-shaped indenter on a square base. There is a linear relationship between the depth of impression and the hardness number.

Surface properties

Wide variations occur when measuring wettability by contact angle techniques because of:

- The effect of soaking on water uptake and thus the wettability of materials.
- The inverted or captive air bubble technique in solutions other than water.

The water wettability of materials provides a good primary indication of the ability of tears to form a coherent and stable layer on the surface of the material; it tells nothing of the compatibility of the material with tears.

Unfortunately, the inverted (captive) air bubble technique, which has been identified as a standard in contact lens work, is not an easy and reproducible method to use. The measurement is made after an air bubble is allowed to impinge, from underneath, onto the surface of the sample, which is suspended in an aqueous liquid. This is the most difficult type of contact angle to measure correctly, since it involves

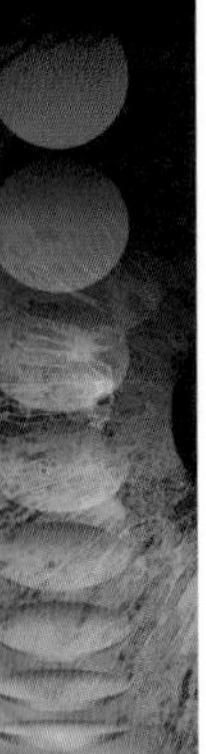

Figure 3.12 2-Hydroxyethyl methacrylate monomer (HEMA)

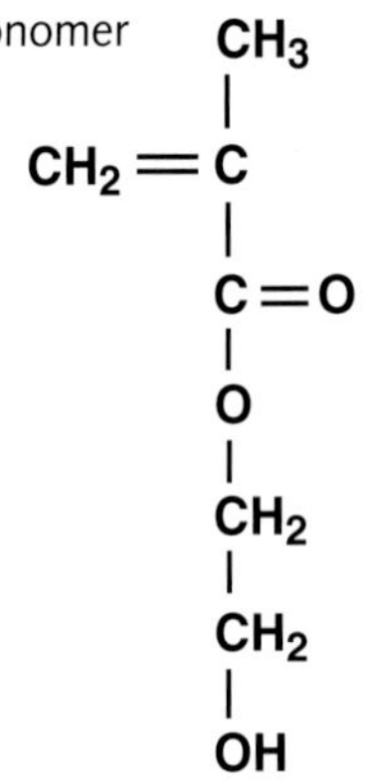

$$CH_2{=}C(CH_3){-}C(=O){-}O{-}CH_2{-}CH_2{-}OH$$

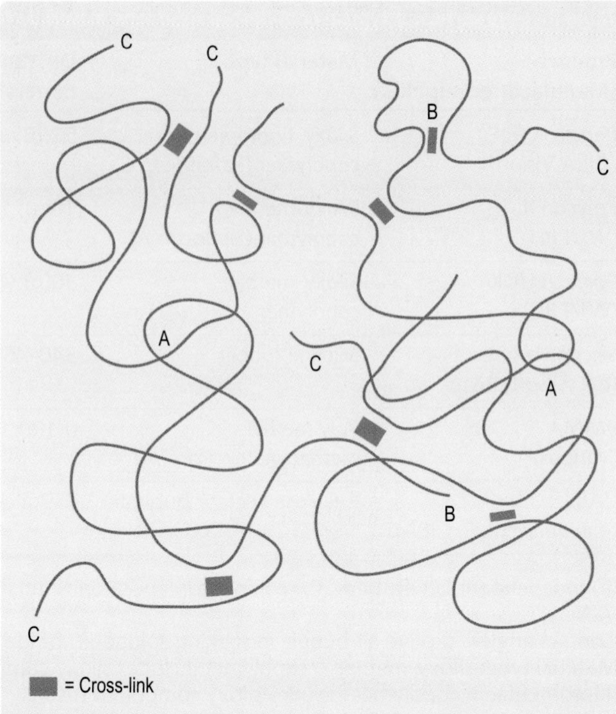

Figure 3.13 Cross-linked polymer network, showing (A) chain entanglements, (B) chain loops and (C) chain ends

judging where the base of a distorted sphere just impinges on a surface. More importantly, the air bubble has to displace water from the surface of the sample, which is frequently pre-soaked. Since all the siloxy-methacrylate gas-permeable materials contain appreciable amounts of hydrophilic monomer to improve surface wettability, they all retain a strongly adsorbed water layer at the surface under these conditions. Not surprisingly, therefore, with this method, similar low so-called 'wetting angles' are often obtained with current RGP materials. What is measured is the value for a diffuse layer of water on a polymer surface and is similar to values obtained by this technique with hydrogels. However, the biological and biochemical effects on the surfaces occur at a molecular level. Measurement methods do not recognize the diffuse water layer 'barrier' that is sensed by macroscopic 'droplet' techniques. This is the underlying reason for the lack of relevance, as presently measured, to clinically measured 'wetting angle'.

SOFT CONVENTIONAL HYDROGEL LENS MATERIALS

The principles discussed in the preceding section are similarly involved in the formation of hydrogel polymers. The structure of poly(methyl methacrylate) can be made more hydrophilic by the incorporation of hydroxyl groups, because groups of this type have an affinity for water. The simplest methacrylate structure that can be made in this way is 2-hydroxyethyl methacrylate, or HEMA (Fig. 3.12). PolyHEMA is obtained by polymerizing a 2-hydroxyethyl methacrylate (HEMA) monomer. In the absence of water, polyHEMA is a hard glassy material which can be lathe-cut. Upon hydration, the rigid glassy dehydrated polymer is transformed into the familiar contact lens material.

It is simplest to describe hydrogel polymers using the 'washing line' analogy previously described and the following points apply:

- The function of the chemical groups (the 'washing') in hydrogels is primarily to attract and bind water within the structure.
- Greater physical stability is achieved by fastening the washing lines together at intervals by the use of cross-links, shown schematically in Figure 3.13.
- Cross-links are introduced by cross-linking agents which are monomers with two active carbon–carbon double bonds.

Figure 3.14 *N*-vinyl pyrrolidone monomer (NVP)

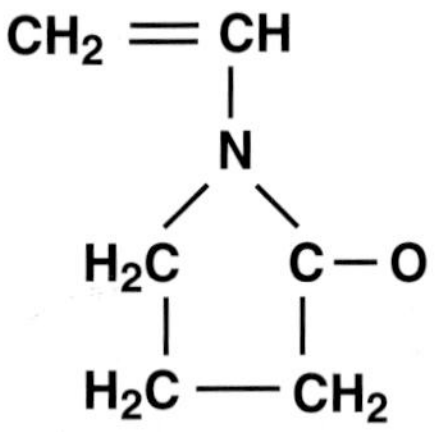

$$CH_2{=}CH{-}N<\begin{matrix} H_2C - CH_2 \\ | \quad\quad | \\ H_2C - C{=}O \end{matrix}$$

- Networks are never perfect and contain entanglements (A), chain loops (B) and wasted chain ends (C) (see Fig. 3.13).
- In addition to HEMA, other important monomers used to achieve an attraction for water include *N*-vinyl pyrrolidone (Fig. 3.14, widely used, particularly in FDA Group II materials) and methacrylic acid (see Fig. 3.7, used in all FDA Group IV materials).
- In silicone-hydrogels, groups that contain siloxy or silicone units are attached in order to increase oxygen permeability. This is achieved with the monomer commonly referred to as TRIS (see Fig. 3.5) which is a component of both RGP and silicone hydrogel materials.

Hydrogels are, both historically and potentially, the largest group of contact lens materials in terms of structural variety. The first hydrogel to achieve commercial significance, polyHEMA, was developed by Otto Wichterle and his co-workers in Czechoslovakia. They developed both HEMA monomer and a method for the fabrication of soft contact lenses (Wichterle & Lim 1960, 1961). PolyHEMA is in many ways typical of other hydrogels and is still undoubtedly the most important single

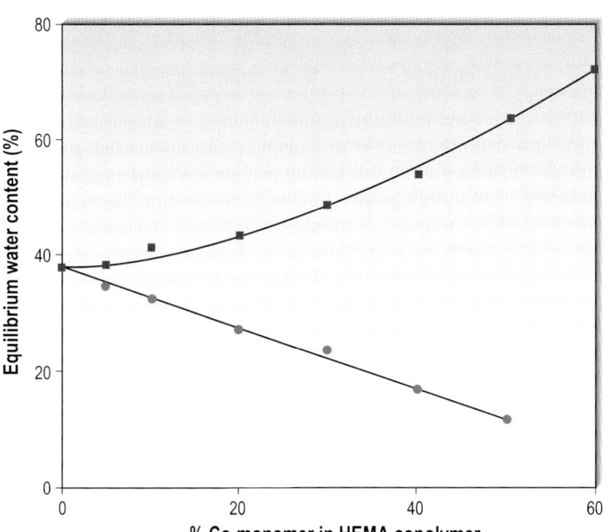

Figure 3.15 Equilibrium water contents of: HEMA-MMA copolymers (circles) and HEMA-NVP copolymers (squares)

material of its class across a wide range of biomedical applications.

The function of the chemical groups (the 'washing') in hydrogel polymers is primarily to attract and bind water within the structure. The extent of this ability controls the equilibrium water content, the most important property of a hydrogel. The equilibrium water content (EWC) is defined in the following way:

$$\text{EWC (\%)} = \text{weight of water/weight of hydrated gel} \times 100\%$$

It is important to define the temperature at which the measurement was made and the nature of the hydrating medium (e.g. pure water or saline solution). The EWC of a gel measured in water at 20°C can be different from its value at eye temperature and in isotonic saline.

PolyHEMA hydrogel has an EWC of approximately 38% (depending upon the degree of cross-linking and the conditions of measurement). This can be reduced by copolymerizing with a hydrophobic monomer such as methyl methacrylate, or increased by copolymerizing with more hydrophilic monomers such as *N*-vinyl pyrrolidone (NVP, see Fig. 3.14) or methacrylic acid (see Fig. 3.7). By using a range of monomers in various combinations, it is possible to 'purpose-design' or 'tailor-make' polymers for contact lens use. For example, Figure 3.15 shows how the equilibrium water content of HEMA is affected by copolymerization with methyl methacrylate and with *N*-vinyl pyrrolidone.

The first basic principle of hydrogel design is fairly simple. To achieve a particular water content, a mixture of monomers is chosen such that the balance of more hydrophilic and less hydrophilic gives the required water content. A cross-linking agent (usually about 1% of the total monomer mix) is added to produce a network that will give elastic stability.

A particular combination of monomers and cross-linking agent is classified in the United States in two ways. It is given a USAN identity (e.g. etafilcon A) which is unique to that specific composition. It will also fall into one of the four groups of the FDA classification scheme, which offers a simple but effective subdivision of lens materials, on the basis of water content and ionic character:

I Low water content non-ionic.
II High water content non-ionic.
III Low water content ionic.
IV High water content ionic.

The division between low and high water content is set at 50% and an ionic hydrogel is defined as containing more than 0.2% ionic material. There are anomalies:

- High-water-content polymers with levels of methacrylic acid only marginally above 0.2% (e.g. perfilcon) are placed in Group IV; however, they do not behave like typical Group IV materials (e.g. etafilcon and vifilcon) in the way that they interact with tear components. This topic is outside the scope of this chapter but is dealt with extensively elsewhere (Tighe & Franklin 1997).
- Some years ago, the same USAN was given to two or more different ratios of the same ingredients, hence the same USAN is given to materials of different water content which appear in more than one FDA Group (e.g. bufilcon and phemfilcon) (see also Chapter 10).

Commercial lens materials and their properties

The way in which different hydrogels have emerged to form the wide range of commercially successful contact lenses is best understood from the patent literature (Tighe 1997) and the situation is constantly changing. It is instructive, however, to collect together a representative range of materials. Table 3.2 shows principal components and water contents of various conventional hydrogel materials, including significant historical materials and also examples of materials that are marketed in several lens forms which may differ in, for example, design and centre thickness or different replacement frequencies (daily, monthly, etc.).

Hydrogel behaviour is controlled predominantly by the amount of water in the gel. It is convenient, therefore, to describe the generic properties of hydrogels relevant to contact lens applications and discuss their dependence upon water content (Tighe 1976, Peppas & Yang 1981).

Swell factor and dimensional stability

Linear and volume swell occurring on hydration of hydrogel materials are a direct consequence of the volume of water absorbed. Therefore, any phenomenon that causes a change in water content will cause a change in lens dimensions.

PolyHEMA is an extremely stable hydrogel and variations in temperature, pH and tonicity (osmolality or salt concentration) have relatively little effect on its water content. However, the use of more hydrophilic monomers can have a marked effect on the stability of the material, whether the monomer is more

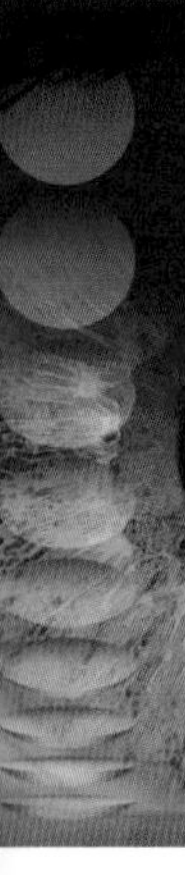

Table 3.2: Conventional soft lenses

Name	Manufacturer/supplier	Principal components	Water content (%)	USAN nomenclature
FDA Group I (<50% EWC <0.2% ionic content)				
Biomedics 38	Ocular Sciences	HEMA	38	Polymacon
Cibasoft	CIBA Vision	HEMA	38	Tefilcon A
Classic	PBH/WJ	HEMA, VP, MMA	43	Tetrafilcon A
CSI	PBH/WJ	GMA, MMA	38	Crofilcon A
Durasoft	PBH/WJ	HEMA, EEMA, MA	30	Phemfilcon A
Frequency 38	CooperVision	HEMA	38	Polymacon
Ultra Vision 38	Ultra Vision	HEMA	38	Polymacon
Medalist 38	Bausch & Lomb	HEMA	38	Polymacon
Menicon Soft	Toyo contact Lens	HEMA, VA, PMA	30	Mafilcon A
Omega 38	Ultra Vision	HEMA	38	Polymacon
Optima 38	Bausch & Lomb	HEMA	38	Polymacon
SeeQuence	Bausch & Lomb	HEMA	38	Polymacon
Soflens 38	Bausch & Lomb	HEMA	38	Polymacon
Softspin	Bausch & Lomb	HEMA	38	Polymacon
Zero 6	CooperVision	HEMA	38	Polymacon
FDA Group II (>50% EWC <0.2 ionic content)				
Actifresh 400	CooperVision	MMA, VP	73	Lidofilcon
Actisoft 60	CooperVision	GlyMA	60	Hioxifilcon A
Dailies	CIBA Vision	Polyvinyl alcohol	69	Nelfilcon A
ES 70 (Lunelle)	Ocular Sciences	AMA, VP	70	–
Gentle Touch	WJ/PBH	MMA, DMA	65	Netrafilcon A
Igel 67	Ultra Vision Optics	MMA, VP, CMA	67	Xylofilcon A
Omniflex	CooperVision	MMA, VP	70	Lidofilcon A
Medalist 66	Bausch & Lomb	HEMA, VP	66	Alphafilcon A
Permaflex	WJ/PBH	MMA, VP	74	Surfilcon A
Precision UV	WJ/PBH	MMA, VP	74	Vasurfilcon A
Proclear	CooperVision	HEMA, PC-HEMA	62	Omafilcon A
Rythmic	Lunelle	MMA, VP	73	Lidofilcon
Soflens Oneday	Bausch & Lomb	HEMA, VP	65	Hilfilcon A
Softlens 66	Bausch & Lomb	HEMA, VP	66	Alphafilcon A
FDA Group III (<50% EWC >0.2 ionic content)				
Comfort Flex	Capital Contact Lens	HEMA, BMA, MA	43	Deltafilcon A
Durasoft 2	WJ/PBH	HEMA, EEMA, MA	38	Phemefilcon A
Soft Mate II	WJ/PBH	HEMA, DAA, MA	45	Bufilcon A
FDA Group IV (>50% EWC >0.2 ionic content)				
Acuvue	Vistakon	HEMA, MA	58	Etafilcon A
Biomedics 55	CIBA Vision	HEMA, PVP, MA	55	Vifilcon A
Durasoft 3	WJ/PBH	HEMA, EEMA, MA	55	Phemefilcon A
Focus Monthly	CIBA Vision	HEMA, PVP, MA	55	Vifilcon A

Table 3.2: Conventional soft lenses (*cont'd*)

Name	Manufacturer/supplier	Principal components	Water content (%)	USAN nomenclature
Frequency 55	CooperVision	HEMA, MA	55	Methafilcon A
Hydrocurve II/3	WJ/PBH	HEMA, DAA, MA	55	Bufilcon A
Permalens	WJ/PBH	HEMA, VP, MA	71	Perfilcon A
Surevue	Vistakon	HEMA, MA	58	Etafilcon A
Ultraflex 55	Ocular Sciences	HEMA, MA	55	Ocufilcon D

AMA, alkyl methacrylate; BMA, butyl (probably isobutyl) methacrylate; CMA, cyclohexyl methacrylate; DAA, diacetone, acrylamide; DMA, *N*,*N*-dimethyl acrylamide; EEMA, ethoxyethyl methacrylate; GlyMA, glyceryl, methacrylate; GMA, glycidyl, methacrylate; HEMA, 2-hydroxyethyl methacrylate; MA, methacrylic acid; MMA, methyl methacrylate; PVP, polyvinyl pyrrolidone (i.e. graft copolymer); VA, vinyl acetate; VP, *N*-vinyl pyrrolidone.
USAN, United States Adopted Name Council: Many USAN equivalents exist, e.g. Hefilcon (Unilens, Miracon); Deltafilcon (Amsoft, Aquasoft, Aquasight, Metrosoft, Soft Form, Softics, Softflow, Softact); Lidofilcon (CV 70, Genesis 4, Hydrosight 70, Q&E 70, Lubrisof. PDC 70, N&N 70); Tefilcon (Cibathin, Torisoft, Softint, Bisoft); Metafilcon (Kontur, Metro 55, Biomedics 55, Mediflex 55, Omniflex 55); Polymacon (CustomEyes 38, Vesoft, Versaflex, Synsoft, Cellusoft). Polymacon has become used as a generic term for polyHEMA, and Lidofilcon for NVP-MMA copolymers. The SoftLens 2000 database (adp Consultancy, Bristol, UK) provides clinically relevant information and brand equivalents on soft lenses in various modalities.

hydrophilic because of a basic nitrogen atom (as in *N*-vinyl pyrrolidone) or an acidic hydrogen atom (as in methacrylic acid).

If the temperature of a hydrogel increases from 4 to 90°C, the thermal energy increases causing greater mobility of the chains and enabling water to interact more freely with each functional group. This causes a rise in water content and an increase in swell factor. Up to around 40°C, however, there is less thermally induced disorder, but as the chains gain a little more rotational freedom, the functional side groups rearrange and more effectively 'match' the interaction of their polar elements. As a result, during this 'optimization' process, water is less able to hydrate the individual groups and a decrease in water content occurs. There is frequently a minimum in the water content, therefore, at around 40°C, particularly for copolymers (i.e. polymers with more than one type of functional group). A secondary consequence is that the water content of hydrogels frequently drops significantly between room temperature and eye temperature.

Materials in Group I, particularly polyHEMA, show little temperature dependence, whereas Group IV materials show a significant drop in water content between 20 and 40°C. This change occurs rapidly and the lens quickly reaches its new equilibrium water content on insertion into the eye. All lenses dehydrate over time in the eye but that process is separate from thermal re-equilibration and is no better or worse for any particular class of hydrogel.

The sensitivity of water content to tonicity is similarly affected by monomer structure. In general, hydrogels show some small decrease in water content when the equilibration solution is changed from pure water to isotonic saline. However, such a change, and others induced by changing the nature of the storage solution, is much greater than those brought about by tonicity variations in the eye.

Variations in water content with respect to pH are more marked and are monomer dependent. The pH ranges required to bring about such changes are, however, greater than those found diurnally or on a patient-to-patient basis in the eye, which lie well within one pH unit. Anionic monomers, such as methacrylic acid, are too sensitive to changes greater than this and used to be the major reason for their lack of success in soft contact lenses.

The advent of disposability has meant that high water content anionic hydrogels (FDA Group IV materials) could be used as disposable lenses. Their highly ionic nature produces dramatic parameter changes in solutions of different pH and these were the solutions that were available in the 1970s (i.e. just before solution regulation). As a result, Group IV materials were prone to instability problems and were never a serious option. To maintain the stability of disposable lenses during storage, and to minimize dimensional changes between storage container and eye, lenses are packed in buffered saline solution which ensures that both pH and tonicity are controlled.

Mechanical properties

In its dehydrated state, polyHEMA (and indeed most other hydrogel-forming polymers) is hard and brittle. In this it resembles PMMA. When swollen in water, however, it becomes soft and rubber-like with a very low tear and tensile strength. As well as water content, the chemical structure of a polymer also plays a large part in mechanical strength within a given family of materials. This is illustrated by comparing the strength of synthetic hydrogels such as polyHEMA with that of natural composite hydrophilic gels, such as articular cartilage, intervertebral disc and the cornea. Cartilage has a tensile strength more than 10 times greater than that of polyHEMA despite having double the water content (around 80%).

In summary, the elastic behaviour and rigidity of hydrogels are closely governed by monomer structure and effective cross-link density, including covalent cross-link and also ionic, polar and steric interchain forces. Modified monomer combinations and cross-linking agents allow high-water-content polymers

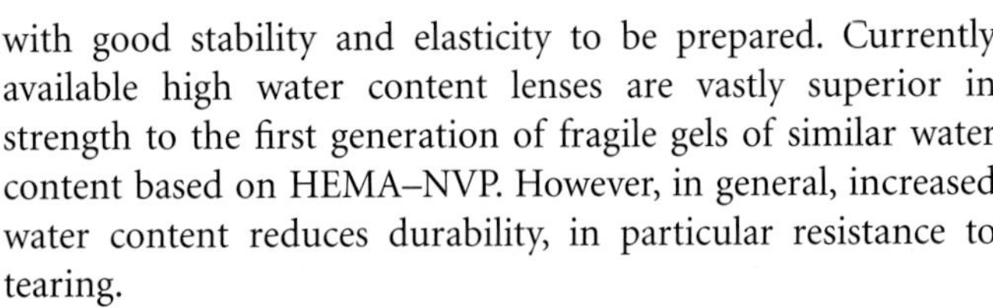

with good stability and elasticity to be prepared. Currently available high water content lenses are vastly superior in strength to the first generation of fragile gels of similar water content based on HEMA–NVP. However, in general, increased water content reduces durability, in particular resistance to tearing.

Surface properties

Two contributing factors influence the behaviour of hydrogels in the eye:

- The anterior surface of the lens will progressively lose water, especially in adverse environmental conditions.
- Polymer chains are able to rotate rapidly in response to a changed interface. In contact with aqueous fluids, the hydrophilic groups rotate to the surface whereas in contact with more hydrophobic interfaces, such as air or lipids, the hydrophilic groups 'bury' themselves within the gel and a more hydrophobic surface is exposed.

Chain rotation is a dynamic process whereas evaporative water loss is progressive. Molecular processes such as protein deposition and denaturation are able to respond to the dynamic processes, which is why the eye presents such a challenging environment. The progressive dehydration has a more influential effect on the gross surface properties of the hydrogel and is part of the complex process that produces end of day discomfort for many wearers.

Surface properties that can be used to characterize hydrogels are:

- Surface energy (which manifests itself as wettability).
- Coefficient of friction (which underlies the biotribological behaviour of the lens).

These properties are linked to the water-binding ability of the lens. Frictional studies show that both synthetic hydrogels and natural hydrogels (e.g. the cornea) are normally lubricated by a hydrodynamic (water) boundary layer. This dominates the dynamic coefficient of friction to the extent that when an intact lubricating layer separates the hydrogel and substrate, it is the properties of the solution rather than those of the material or substrate that govern the value of sliding friction. The simplest analogy is that of a car aquaplaning – the ease of sliding is independent of the rubber from which the tyres have been fabricated. When this water layer breaks down there is an increase in the resistance to sliding. The surface energy of a hydrogel is a more progressive property. It rises rapidly up to a water content of around 30% and much more slowly thereafter. As previously stated, however, at a hydrophobic interface the surface energy drops dramatically because of chain rotation.

The clinical consequence of these facts is relatively simple to state but complex to relate to direct measurement. All conventional hydrogels have adequate wettability and frictional behaviour when fully hydrated, no matter what the initial water content. Problems only arise because of progressive dehydration and the dynamic responsiveness of the lens material to air and lipids (caused primarily by tear break-up). These processes in turn influence the irreversible deposition of tear components and the onset of symptoms such as end of day dryness, which are linked to biotribological phenomena.

Density

The density of hydrogel polymers depends upon both the water content and the monomer composition. Low-water-content (and fairly rigid) gels containing hydrophobic monomers have the greatest densities of the common hydrogels. These are around 1.22 g/ml at 10% water content and 20°C. These materials are currently used as flat sheets or membranes, rather than contact lenses, and even the emerging generation of low water content, high-Dk hydrogels are unlikely to rise to this value. Typical contact lens copolymers containing HEMA and the more hydrophilic monomers decrease progressively from around 1.16 at 38% water content to around 1.05 at 75% water content (all at 20°C).

Refractive index

Refractive index also decreases progressively with increasing water content in an almost linear fashion. The results for hydrogels used in contact lenses lie within a fairly narrow, almost rectilinear band, decreasing from 1.46–1.48 at 20% water content to 1.37–1.38 at 75% water content. Refractive index can be used, therefore, as a rapid method of determining the approximate water content of an unknown gel although the method suffers from inherent inaccuracies, including the assumption that dehydrated hydrogels all have the same refractive index. Despite this, the procedure is convenient and enables the approximate water content of a lens to be determined quickly (see also Chapters 10 and 16).

Optical transmittance

Not all hydrogels are optically transparent. Translucence and opacity in hydrogels are associated with microphase separation of water which produces regions of differing refractive index within the gel. Hydrogels that show this type of behaviour (typically synthesized by making copolymers with large blocks or segments of hydrophobic and hydrophilic monomers rather than randomly dispersing them) do have advantages in terms of enhanced strength and permeability performance. Phase-separated hydrogels in which the domain sizes are small enough to retain optical transparency are of interest where strength and/or permeability are particularly important (e.g. extended wear contact lenses and synthetic cornea). The lack of optical clarity in simple copolymers of hydrophilic monomers such as HEMA (see Fig. 3.12) and TRIS (see Fig. 3.5) has led to considerable ingenuity in developing monomers and polymerization methodologies to overcome this problem.

Oxygen permeability: principles and definitions

The earlier comments relating to oxygen permeability need to be expanded here in order to appreciate the greater complexity

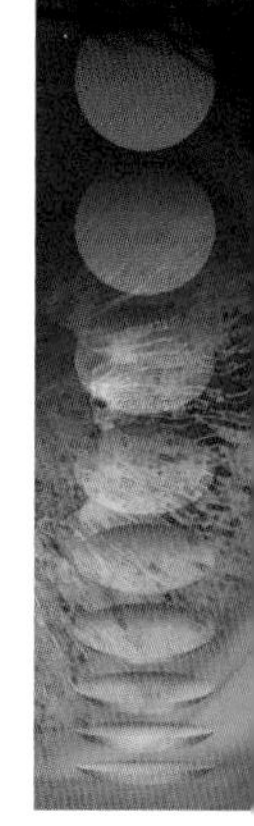

of hydrogel polymers, where there are two (polymer and water) phases able to promote or impede transport. The simple fundamental definition:

$$P = DS$$

applies equally to hydrogel membranes where P is the permeability coefficient for the combination of polymer and water in conjunction with a given permeant (i.e. gas), D is the diffusion coefficient of the gas, and S is the solubility of the gas in the water-swollen polymer.

Much of the work on oxygen permeability of contact lens materials was carried out by Irving Fatt, who chose to use the alternative term K to represent gas solubility (e.g. Weissman & Fatt 1991) (see also p. 62). For this reason, the contact lens literature favours the term Dk, whereas in membrane science DS or, more commonly, P is used. Thus Dk (or P) is the permeability coefficient for a given material, whereas Dk/t or P/t refers specifically to the permeability (transmissibility) of a sample (such as a contact lens) of that material of a given thickness, t. The symbol L was also used to represent lens thickness, hence Dk/L. To determine the permeability coefficient (P or Dk) of a material at a given temperature, it is necessary to measure the rate (volume per unit time) at which the chosen gas passes through a sample of membrane of given dimensions (area and thickness) for a given gas pressure. Dk units which take these variables into account are quite complex. The still often quoted traditional units based on Fatt are $cm^2/s.ml\ O_2/(ml.mmHg)$ but membrane scientists usually quote values using the pressure difference expressed in cmHg, rather than mmHg, and so quote the value in barrers:

$$Dk\ (barrers) = 10^{-11} cm^3\ O_2\ (STP).cm/s.cm^2.mmHg$$

However, for ISO nomenclature, when the international standard unit of pressure, the hectopascal, is used instead of mmHg, the units of Dk are: $cm^2/s.ml\ O_2/(ml.hPa)$. As a result, the equivalence often quoted is 1 barrer = $10^{-10}\ cm^2.s^{-1}.cmHg^{-1}$ or, to convert from traditional units to ISO units, multiply by the constant 0.75006.

Since the oxygen passing through the contact lens is consumed by the cornea, it is apparent that, in principle, it should be possible to balance this consumption requirement with the oxygen flux through a contact lens of given dimensions and given conditions, and to define the required lens behaviour in terms of a permeability (Dk value). There are however, two problems:

- The measurement of a true permeability (Dk) value for the material (Refojo & Leong 1979, Fatt & Weissman 1992, Compan et al. 1999).
- The use of the specific permeability value of the material in the prediction of the effective transmissibility of a lens of given design and prescription on the eye (Harvitt & Bonanno 1999, and references therein).

The measured and quoted Dk values for lenses are a good guide to their relative ability to deliver oxygen to the cornea, which is much more critical in the case of extended (overnight) wear. It is important, therefore, to identify between the factors that affect the oxygen permeability of conventional hydrogels and to examine the principles involved in the development of so-called silicone hydrogels.

Oxygen permeability: conventional and silicone-containing hydrogels

While diffusion (D) is related to the mobility of the polymer chains and the ease with which the oxygen molecule can meander through them, solubility (K) is governed by the amount of oxygen that the material can dissolve. Incorporating water into a glassy polymer which resembles PMMA not only increases the ease of diffusion but also provides a medium that effectively dissolves oxygen. Therefore, the more water a polymer contains, the more oxygen it will dissolve and the higher the resultant permeability. Additionally, the water acts as a plasticizer (see above) and progressively increases the ease of diffusion. Because of this combined effect, the product of diffusion and solubility (i.e. permeability or Dk) in a conventional hydrogel is always significantly below the value for water itself, which at 34°C is around 100.

The relationship between oxygen permeability and water content is empirical: permeability (Dk) increases exponentially with the equilibrium water content (W%). That is:

$$Dk = A\ e^{-BW*}$$

where A and B are experimentally determined constants for a given temperature. Therefore, if water content and the constants A and B are known at a given temperature (say 34°C), a reasonably exact value of the oxygen permeability can be calculated.

However, because the water content of different materials varies with temperature, comparative predictions of the permeabilities at 34°C cannot be made from their water contents at room temperature. Unlike other polymers, polyHEMA is atypically well-behaved in this respect (see above). If water content of hydrogels were to remain unchanged between 20 and 34°C, oxygen permeability would almost double over that temperature range; however, since water contents usually fall with this temperature rise, the gain in oxygen permeability between room temperature and eye temperature is significantly less for most contact lens materials.

The methodology for measuring Dk values is well established but the factors identified above produce variability in quoted permeabilities, even of ostensibly identical materials. Figure 3.16 shows the quoted Dk values for a series of commercial lenses as a function of water content, and contains reference data for Dk and water contents of hydrogel membranes at both 25 and 34°C. Quoted water contents and Dk values, taken together, should be used only as a guide to on-eye transmissibility, but no more than that.

* e is a mathematical symbol like 'pi'. It signifies the base of the natural system of logarithms and has a value of approximately 2.718. It signifies that Dk on one hand, and the water content, W, on the other are related by an exponential (or logarithmic) relationship.

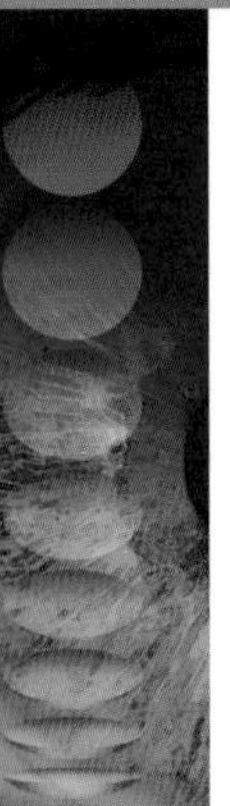

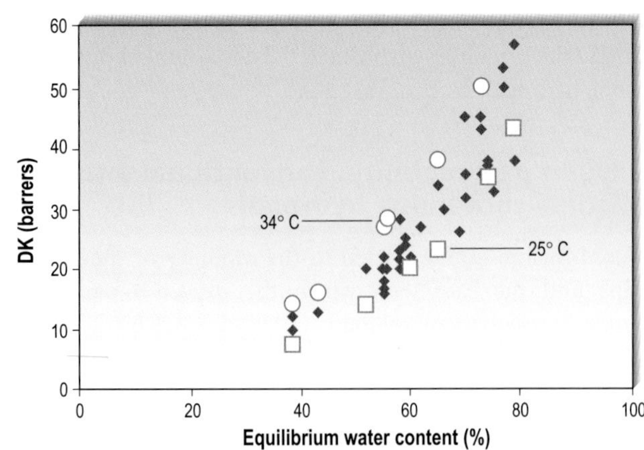

Figure 3.16 Variation of Dk with water content for conventional hydrogels: quoted manufacturers' data (solid diamonds); reference materials at 25°C (open squares); reference materials at 34°C (open circles)

SILICONE HYDROGEL MATERIALS

As discussed above, poly(dimethyl siloxane), in the form of silicone rubber (see Fig. 3.4), has both oxygen solubility and oxygen permeability (Dk = diffusion × solubility) several times greater than that of water and over 100 times greater than either PMMA or dehydrated polyHEMA. Its incorporation into a hydrogel, therefore, produces a marked gain in oxygen permeability, and comparative permeability values for conventional hydrogels and a family of silicone hydrogels are shown as a function of water content in Figure 3.17. As the proportion of silicone-based polymer increases, and water content consequently decreases, the Dk rises to values in excess of 100 barrers.

Commercial realization

The elements of silicone rubber (see Fig. 3.4) must be combined with those of a typical hydrogel-forming monomer such as HEMA (see Fig. 3.12) to form a copolymer that combines the properties of both. The logical answer is to combine HEMA with the monomer that has been so successfully used in the preparation of RGP lens materials, commonly referred to as TRIS (see Fig. 3.5). However, to combine hydrophobic TRIS with hydrophilic HEMA and then hydrate the product presents the same fundamental difficulty as trying to combine oil and water to form an optically clear product. Phase separation occurs and the optical clarity is impaired. Although true molecular compatibility of the two species may not be possible, it is necessary to improve the compatibility to a level where optical clarity is not disturbed – the submicron region.

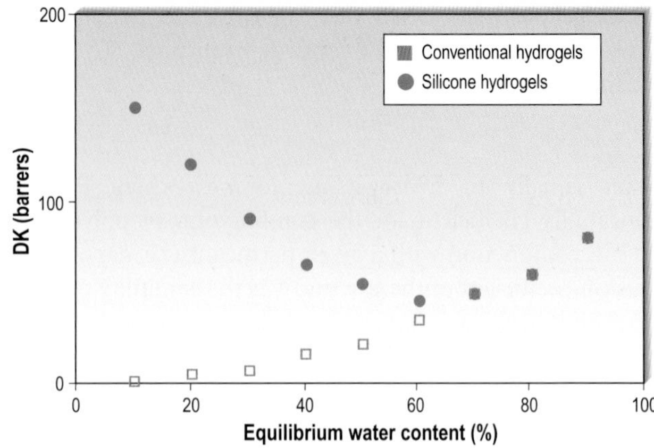

Figure 3.17 Variation of Dk with water content for TRIS-based silicone hydrogels

There are two approaches to this problem (Tighe 2000, 2004):

1. The insertion of more polar groups into the TRIS molecule (see Fig. 3.9) (Tanaka et al. 1979a,b, Künzler & Ozark 1994, 1995).
2. The development of macromer technology. Macromers are large monomers formed by preassembly of structural units that are designed to bestow particular properties on the final polymer (Fig. 3.18).

At the time of writing there are six distinct products in commercial production (Table 3.3). These fit into three distinct categories in terms of their bulk chemistry and surface properties. (One further material [Biofinity, CooperVision] is being launched. It is claimed to combine high [48%] equilibrium water content with a Dk of 128 barrers and a surface that needs no separate treatment process.)

- Tanaka's monomer (3-methacryloxy-2hydroxypropyloxy) propylbis(trimethylsiloxy)methylsilane (see Fig. 3.9), was the first of this type to be exemplified in the patent literature in 1979 but was not converted into a commercial silicone hydrogel in the lifetime of the patent. It eventually formed the basis of the third commercial silicone hydrogel lens made by Vistakon. They improved the synthesis for the Tanaka monomer to produce the Acuvue Advance (galyfilcon A) lens, which was launched in 2004 upon the expiry of the original patent (McCabe et al. 2003).

Both Bausch & Lomb and CIBA Vision developed extensive patent portfolios in the field of silicone hydrogels and launched the first two commercial silicone hydrogels in 1998.

- Bausch & Lomb's PureVision (balafilcon A), based on (1) above, developed a range of novel monomers, one of which forms the basis of PureVision (Fig. 3.19) (Bambury & Seelye 1991, 1997).

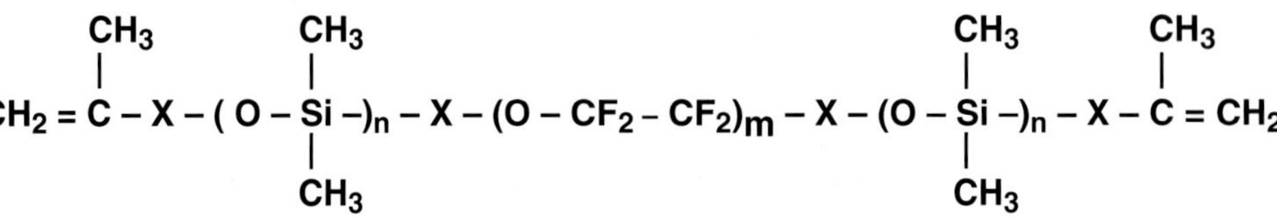

Figure 3.18 Siloxy fluoroether macromer

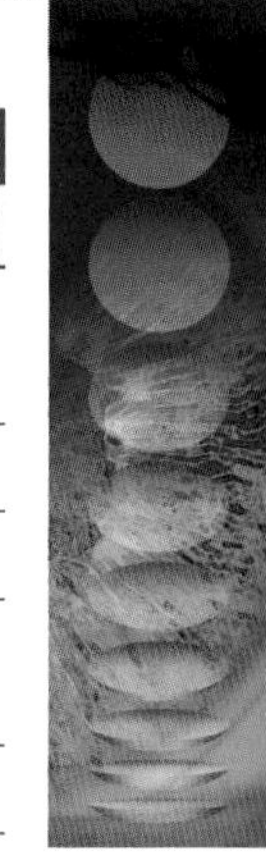

Table 3.3: Silicone-hydrogel lens materials

Proprietary name	Focus Night & Day	AIR OPTIX	PureVision	Acuvue Oasys	Acuvue Advance	Biofinity
United States Adopted Name	lotrafilcon A	lotrafilcon B	balafilcon A	senofilcon A	galyfilcon A	comfilcon A
Manufacturer	CIBA Vision	CIBA Vision	Bausch & Lomb	Vistakon	Vistakon	CooperVision
Water content	24%	33%	36%	38%	47%	48%
Oxygen permeability Dk × 10^{-11}	140	110	99	103	60	128
Tensile modulus (psi)	238	190	148	68	65	105
Initial modulus (MPa)	1.4	1.2	1.1	0.6	0.4	0.8
Elast mod @ 5 kHz (kP)	58	43	44	36	28	40
Initial advancing contact angle (°)	80	78	95	68	65	n/a
Relative initial dehydration rate	1	1.5	1.9	1.8	2.4	2.3
Surface treatment	Plasma coating	Plasma coating	Plasma oxidation	Internal wetting agent (PVP)	Internal wetting agent (PVP)	None

See also Table 10.2.

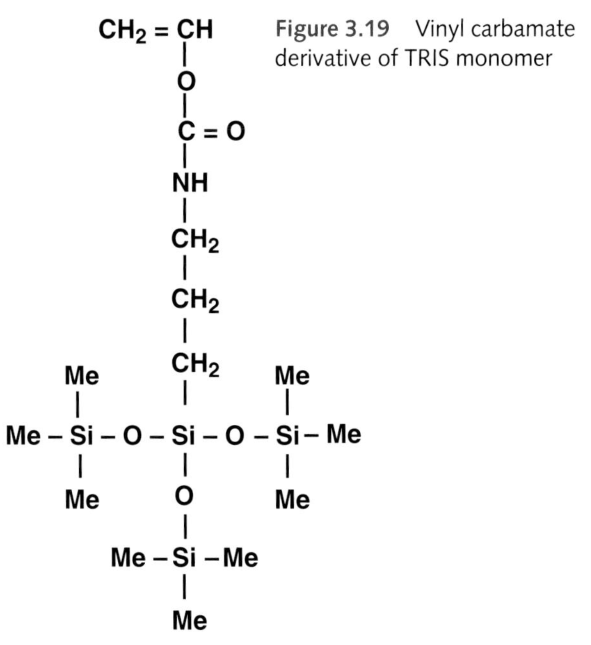

Figure 3.19 Vinyl carbamate derivative of TRIS monomer

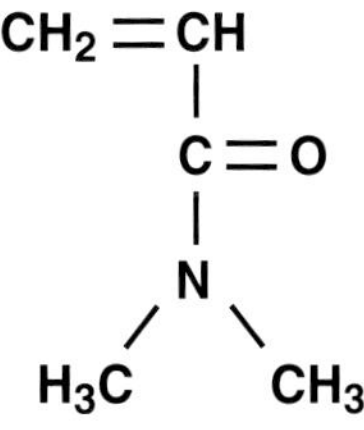

Figure 3.20 *N,N*-dimethyl acrylamide monomer (NNDMA)

- CIBA Vision's Focus Night & Day (lotrafilcon A) was based on (2). CIBA's patent contains poly(fluoroethylene oxide) segments and oxygen-permeable polysiloxane units. This focused on macromers and polymerization methodologies, and culminated in the appearance of a group of patents (e.g. Greisser et al. 1996, Nicolson et al. 1998) with two broad features:
  - the preparation of biphasic materials with channels enabling both high oxygen permeability and high ion (e.g. sodium) permeability to be achieved.
  - minimum levels of ion or water permeation that are required to enable the lens to move adequately on the eye.

The CIBA Vision materials – lotrafilcon A and lotrafilcon B (see Table 3.3) – both employ a co-continuous biphasic or two-channel molecular structure, in which the phases persist from the front to the back surface of the lens. The siloxy phase facilitates the solubility and transmission of oxygen and the hydrogel phase transmits water and sodium ions, allowing good lens movement. The two phases work concurrently, to allow the co-continuous transmission of oxygen and aqueous salts. The lotrafilcon platform comprises a fluoroether macromer of the type shown in Figure 3.18, copolymerized with TRIS monomer (see Fig. 3.5) and *N,N*-dimethyl acrylamide (Fig. 3.20), in the presence of an inert diluent, such as ethanol, which is removed on hydration.

The Bausch & Lomb PureVision material, balafilcon A, is based on the combination of the vinyl carbamate derivative of TRIS (see Fig. 3.19) copolymerized with the hydrophilic monomer *N*-vinyl pyrrolidone (see Fig. 3.14). There is no deliberate attempt in the polymerization process described to

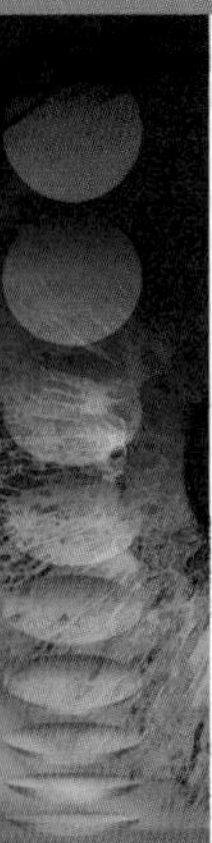

induce phase separation or channels, but some biphasic character may be an inevitable consequence of the nature of the monomer combination used.

Both Bausch & Lomb and CIBA employ surface treatment techniques to improve lens wettability. Both are treated using gas plasma techniques but whereas Bausch & Lomb have opted for plasma oxidation, CIBA have chosen to apply a plasma coating. In the former case (PureVision) oxidation of TRIS produces hydrophilic glassy silicate 'islands' on the surface (Salamone et al. 1999), whereas the surface of Night & Day is coated with a 25 nm thick, dense, high refractive index coating.

Vistakon's materials – galyfilcon A and senofilcon A – are a more recent family of silicone hydrogel materials and again, share a common chemical framework. The silicone hydrogel matrix is based on a combination of the 'Tanaka' monomer (3-methacryloxy-2hydroxypropyloxy) propylbis(trimethylsiloxy) methylsilane (see Fig. 3.9) copolymerized with HEMA (see Fig. 3.12) and *N,N*-dimethyl acrylamide (see Fig. 3.20), together with a simple siloxy macromer. The siloxy macromer is effectively a silicone rubber (see Fig. 3.4) chain approximately 11 units long with a polymerizable methacrylate unit at the end of the chain. The additional feature is the incorporation of polyvinyl pyrrolidone to enable an adequate degree of lens wettability to be achieved without subsequent surface treatment. The polyvinyl pyrrolidone is referred to as HydraClear™ technology and is sometimes described as functioning as an internal wetting agent.

Relatively little is known about CooperVision's (USAN comfilcon A) material which is only just becoming available at the time of writing. Although comments in the optical press raised expectation of a silicone hydrogel incorporating CooperVision's PC technology (inherited from Biocompatibles), the comfilcon material has emerged from a different stable. It is interesting for two reasons:

- The absence of either surface treatment or an internal wetting agent.
- The oxygen permeability is unexpectedly high for its water content compared to other materials (see Table 3.3). This is not completely unexpected. The oxygen permeabilities of gas-permeable materials vary over a wide range, indicating that the structure of the non-aqueous part of a silicone hydrogel will, equally, be capable of influencing the achievable oxygen permeability at a given water content.

The technology underpinning the comfilcon material originates in a Japanese patent filed in December 2000 by the Asahikasei Aime Co. Ltd, which formed a research and development agreement with Ocular Sciences in 2001. This allowed Ocular Sciences to apply its cast moulding manufacturing process to the newly developed silicon-based material created by Asahikasei Aime to produce a 'state of the art, high performance contact lens'. Following the merger of Ocular Sciences and CooperVision, a further patent was filed naming Arthur Back as co-inventor (Iwata et al. 2006).

There are two possible reasons for the departure of comfilcon from previous silicone hydrogel developments.

- Conventional 'TRIS' monomer and its derivatives are not used. Instead the patent claims that two siloxy macromers of different sizes, one of which is only monofunctionalized (contains only one polymerizable double bond), when used together produce advantageously high oxygen permeabilities.
- The use of vinyl amides as hydrophilic monomers. Whereas these monomers are well-known (indeed *N*-vinyl pyrrolidone is a vinyl amide), the specific advantages of *N*-methyl-*N*-vinyl acetamide, which is a central component in the Iwata patent, have not been previously harnessed in silicone hydrogels.

The patent contains other subtleties which, taken together, appear to have enhanced the compatibility of silicone moieties with hydrophilic domains.

Physical properties of soft lenses

Until the mid-1990s, contact lens materials were judged on:

- Wettability.
- Mechanical behaviour.
- Oxygen permeability.

Other properties – such as optical clarity, cost, processibility, toxicity and deposit resistance – were also important.

COMPARING SILICONE HYDROGELS WITH CONVENTIONAL HYDROGELS

The properties of silicone hydrogels are broadly similar to those of conventional hydrogels.

Water content, permeability and mechanical properties

As a general rule of thumb, the most significant effect of increasing water content in silicone hydrogels is a decrease in both oxygen permeability and stiffness.

The extensive CIBA patent (Greisser et al. 1996) proposed another type of property measurement, which is linked to lens movement on the eye: hydraulic and ionic permeability. The patent, which underpins CIBA's Night & Day material, describes the preparation of biphasic materials with high oxygen permeability. It also defines minimum levels of ion or water permeation to enable silicone hydrogel lenses to move adequately on the eye. These correspond approximately to those measured for polyHEMA. Because of this, the relevance of this property increases as water contents of silicone hydrogels fall markedly below that of polyHEMA, especially since the elastomeric 'grab' of the materials also increases with decreasing water content. CIBA's Focus Night & Day has a water content far below that of polyHEMA such that this property becomes significant.

The other materials in Table 3.3 (CIBA's AIR OPTIX may be a borderline case) have sufficient water to enable them to show ion transport at a level typified by polyHEMA. The benefits of the CIBA biphasic approach are primarily in the achievement of higher oxygen permeabilities while maintaining ion transport at the level achieved by, for example, polyHEMA. With the range of silicone hydrogels increasing, the relative perceived importance of higher oxygen permeability, at a cost of compromise in other properties, will be demonstrated by success in the marketplace.

The relative oxygen permeability of all but one (comfilcon) of the six materials shown in Table 3.3 falls with increasing

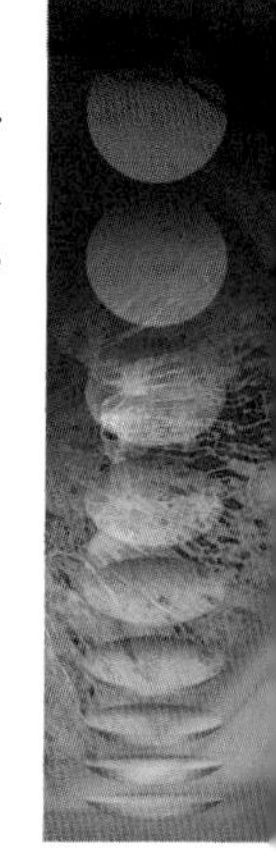

water content. The reason for the apparently anomalous behaviour of confilcon is discussed above. Materials with higher water contents are less stiff but the silicone content produces elements of elastomeric behaviour. One aspect of this is that the stiffness changes as the rate of deformation increases – the faster the deformation, the stiffer the material appears to be. The deformational movement of the eyelid is rapid, whereas the deformation produced by handling a material is slow. There has been no need with conventional materials to employ sophisticated testing techniques but with the increasing range of silicone hydrogels becoming available, there is a need for standardization using a relevant method.

The manufacturers' initial information for PureVision and Focus Night & Day indicated that the two materials were appreciably stiffer than conventional hydrogels but quite similar to each other. Comparative tests, using the same method, proved that Night & Day is appreciably stiffer than PureVision, as the difference in water contents would suggest. Results from two laboratories using different methods (and units) are shown in Table 3.3. For comparison, Acuvue (etafilcon A) would have a modulus of around 37 psi or 0.24 MPa.

The newer silicone hydrogels have moved to higher water contents for two reasons:

- Clinical research suggests that less stiff materials produce better clinical outcomes.
- Laboratory evaluation showed that the high frequency elastomeric behaviour described above is easier to eliminate as percentage water contents rise above the mid 30s.

Wettability and dehydration

Hydrogels show both hydrophilic and hydrophobic behaviour at their surface, depending upon the environment. The polymer chains orient themselves to present their hydrophobic aspect when introduced to an air interface and their hydrophilic aspect in an aqueous environment. This is useful as it reflects the break and reformation of the tear film. Polymers, particularly hydrogels, undergo relatively rapid rotation around the atoms that link to form the backbone.

Using the analogy of the washing line, if the washing line, with washing in place, is immersed in water, the washing will be randomly arranged around the washing line and it will be quite difficult to see the continuous line. If the line and washing are removed from water the washing will be drawn down by gravity, leaving the line much more exposed. This happens in hydrogels, not because of gravity, but because of the affinity for an aqueous environment by the functional groups on the hydrogel (the washing).

When covered by the tear film, the polar water-loving groups surround the hydrophobic polymer backbone. When the tear film breaks, leaving the surface of the hydrogel exposed to air or to a deposited lipid layer (both of which are relatively hydrophobic), the polar groups turn away from the surface into the aqueous environment of the gel. This leaves a polymer surface with a relatively hydrophobic polymer backbone and, consequently, the intrinsic wettability of the surface structure of the polymer changes. This is reflected in the change in contact angle as an aqueous layer advances and recedes from the surface, which is represented by the equation:

$$\theta_H = \theta_A - \theta_R$$

where

θ_H is the change in contact angle (contact angle hysteresis).

θ_A is the advancing angle, which reflects the wettability of the material after it has been exposed to air for a predetermined time period.

θ_R is the receding angle, which reflects the wettability of the material after it has been immersed in water or saline.

The dipping technique should be short to reflect break up and reformation of the tear film and the contact angle hysteresis should be as small as possible. Both conventional and silicone hydrogels have receding contact angles between 25° and 45° with silicone hydrogels at the upper end of the range. However, the advancing angle for silicone hydrogels is higher than for conventional hydrogels, often above 100°, depending upon the time of exposure to air, while for conventional hydrogels measured under the same conditions, it would be around 70°.

The wettabilities of current silicone hydrogels are therefore inferior to the best conventional hydrogels, especially when exposed to air, when the advancing contact angle rises sharply with the length of exposure. The clinical consequence is that, as the front surface of the lens begins to dehydrate, it becomes hydrophobic and can consequently accumulate lipid deposits. These depend on tear break-up time and interblink period as well as tear lipid profile.

The data in Table 3.3 include information on wettability and relative initial dehydration. Under the same test conditions, Acuvue (etafilcon A) shows a relative dehydration rate of 3 and an initial advancing contact angle of 65°. Although Acuvue has a more marked rate of dehydration, its less hydrophobic polymer structure means that the wettability does not deteriorate as fast as that of the silicone hydrogels.

Of the silicone hydrogel lenses:

- Acuvue Advance shows the best wettability at the beginning of the dipping cycle but the greatest deterioration in wettability with dehydration.
- Focus Night & Day has the lowest water content and less good initial wettability characteristics but shows the lowest rate of dehydration and deterioration in wettability.

There are no industry standard methods for characterizing wetting and dehydration behaviour, and an agreed basis for comparative in vitro characterization of silicone hydrogels is needed.

There is still some way to go in the perfection of the surface properties of silicone hydrogel contact lenses, although tremendous strides have already been made with this exciting group of materials. The wettability of all the silicone hydrogel lenses is clinically acceptable and perceived differences are likely to be as much patient-driven as by material variations.

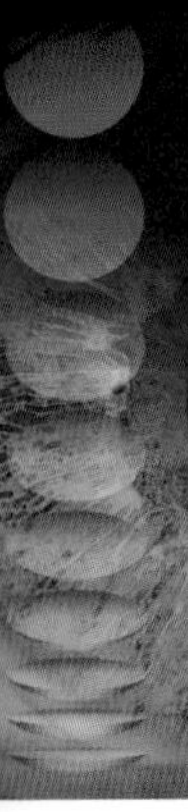

References

Bambury, R. E. and Seelye, D. (1991) Vinyl carbonate and vinyl carbamate contact lens material monomers. US Patent 5070215

Bambury, R. E. and Seelye, D. (1997) Vinyl carbonate and vinyl carbamate contact lens materials. US Patent 5610252

Compan, V., Lopez, M. L., Andrio, A., Lopez-Alemany, A. and Refojo, M. F. (1999) Determination of the oxygen transmissibility and permeability of hydrogel contact lenses. J. Appl. Polym. Sci., 72(3), 321–327

Ellis, E. J. and Salamone, J. C. (1979) (to Polymer Technology Corp) Silicone-containing hard contact lens material. US Patent 4152508

Fatt, I. and Weissman, B. A. (1992) Influence of polarographic cathode diameter on measured oxygen transmissibility of hydrogel contact-lenses with power. Optom. Vis. Sci., 69(12), 931–935

Gaylord, N. G. (1974) (to Polycon Lab Inc.) Oxygen-permeable contact lens composition: methods and article of manufacture. US Patent 3808178

Gaylord, N. G. (1978) (to Syntex USA Inc.) Methods of correcting visual defects: compositions and articles of manufacture useful therein. US Patent 4120570

Greisser, H. J., Laycock, B. G., Papaspiliotopoulos, E. et al. (1996) Extended wear ophthalmic lens. WO 96/31792

Harvitt, D. M. and Bonanno, J. A. (1999) Re-evaluation of the oxygen diffusion model for predicting minimum contact lens Dk/t values needed to avoid corneal anoxia. Optom. Vis. Sci., 76(10), 712–719

Hill, R. M. and Schloessler, J. (1967) Optical membranes of silicone rubber. J. Am. Optom. Assoc., 38, 480–483

Holden, B. A., Newton-Howes, J., Winterton, L. et al. (1990) The DK project – an interlaboratory comparison of DK/L measurements. Optom. Vis. Sci., 67(6), 476–481

Iwata, J., Haki, T., Ikawa, S. and Black, A. (2006) Silicone hydrogel contact lens, US Patent application 2006 006 3852, March 23, 2006

Jones, L., Woods, C. A., and Efron, N. (1996) Life expectancy of rigid gas permeable and high water content contact lenses. CLAO J 22(4), 258–260

Kerr, C. and Dilly, P. N. (1988) Problems of dimensional stability in RGPs. Optician, 195(5134), 21–23

Kishi, M. and Tighe, B. J. (1988) RGP materials: a review of the patent literature. Optician, 196(5160), 21–28

Künzler, J. and Ozark, R. (1994) Fluorosilicone hydrogels. US Patent 5321108

Künzler, J. and Ozark, R. (1995) Hydrogels based on hydrophilic side-chain siloxanes. J. Appl. Polym. Sci., 55(4), 611–619

Künzler, J. F. and McGee, J. A. (1995) Contact lens materials. Chem. Ind., 21, 651–653

McCabe, K. P., Molock, F. F., Hill, G. A. et al. (2003) (to Johnson & Johnson) Biomedical devices containing internal wetting agents. US Patent 6822016

McVannel, D. E., Mishler, J. L. and Polmanteer, K. E. (1967) (to Dow Corning Corp.) Hydrophilic contact lens and method of making same. US Patent 3350216

Nicolson, P., Baron, R., Chabrecek, P. et al. (1998) (to CIBA Vision) Extended wear ophthalmic lens. US Patent 5760100

Novicky, N. N. (1980) Oxygen permeable hard and semi-hard contact lens compositions, methods and articles of manufacture. US Patent 4242483

Peppas, N. A. and Yang, W. H. M. (1981) Properties-based optimisation of the structure of polymers for contact lens application. Cont. Intraoc. Lens Med. J., 7, 300–314

Refojo, M. F., Holly, F. J. and Leong, F. L. (1977) Permeability of dissolved oxygen through contact lenses I. Cellulose acetate butyrate. Cont. Intraoc. Lens Med. J., 3(4), 27–33

Refojo, M. F. and Leong, F. L. (1979) Water-dissolved oxygen permeability coefficients of hydrogel contact lenses and boundary layer effects. J. Memb. Sci., 4, 415–426

Salamone, J. C., Grobe, G. L., Seelye, D. and Künzler, J. (1999) Silicone hydrogels for contact lens application. Proc. ACS-PMSE, 80, 108–109

Tanaka, K., Takahashi, K., Kanada, M. et al. (1979a) Copolymer for soft contact lens, its preparation and soft contact lens made therefrom. US Patent 4139513

Tanaka, K., Takahashi, K., Kanada, M. and Toshikawa, T. (1979b) (to Toyo Contact Lens Co. Ltd, Japan) Methyl di(trimethylsiloxy)silylpropyl glycerol methacrylate. US Patent 4139548

Tighe, B. J. (1976) The design of polymers for contact lens applications. Br. Polym. J., 8, 71–77

Tighe, B. J. (1997) Contact lens materials. In Contact Lenses, 4th edn, Ch. 3, eds. A. J. Phillips and L. Speedwell. London: Butterworth-Heinemann

Tighe, B. J. (2000) Silicone hydrogel materials – how do they work? In Silicone Hydrogels: The Rebirth of Continuous Wear, Ch. 1, ed. D. Sweeney. London: Butterworth-Heinemann

Tighe, B. J. (2004). Silicone hydrogel materials – structure, properties and behaviour. In Silicone Hydrogels, 2nd edn, Ch. 1, ed. D. Sweeney. London: Butterworth-Heinemann

Tighe, B. J. and Franklin, V. J. (1997) Lens deposition and spoilation. In The Eye in Contact Lens Wear, 2nd edn, Ch. 4, ed. J. R. Larke. London: Butterworth-Heinemann

Weissman, B. A. and Fatt, I. (1991) Contact-lens wear and oxygen permeability measurements. Curr. Opin. Ophthalmol., 2(1), 88–94

Wichterle, O. and Lim, D. (1960) Hydrophilic gels for biological use. Nature, 185, 117–118

Wichterle, O. and Lim, D. (1961) Method for producing shaped articles from three-dimensional hydrophilic polymers. US Patent 2976576

Chapter 4

Microbiology, lens care and maintenance

Lewis Williams and Fiona Stapleton

CHAPTER CONTENTS

Contact lens care and maintenance are central to the safety and efficacy of lens wear and one of many reasons for lens wear cessation (McMonnies 1988, Young 2004). However, in recent years there has been a decline in the perceived importance of lens maintenance due to the following:

- The advent of frequent replacement and disposable lenses with a lower complication rate (Freeman 1997).
- Convenience lens care products (e.g. one-step disinfectants) and the advent of one-bottle lens care systems (OBSs).
- No-rub products.

This is unfortunate because:

- Although daily disposable lenses require no conventional lens care, they do not dominate the market.
- It is unlikely that *all* future lenses will be disposable, or worn on an extended-wear or continuous-wear basis.
- High ametropes are unlikely to be catered for by disposable lenses in the near future.

Hind (1979) first became involved with lens solutions and their problems in the 1940s (glass, polymethylmethacrylate [PMMA] or hybrid scleral lenses), although the early solutions were intended to overcome physiological problems (e.g. Sattler's veil), not care issues. The earliest attempts at altering the physical condition of contact lenses were intended to improve lens wetting and employed polyvinyl alcohol. Subsequently, it was realized that if the lens surface was unclean (Fig. 4.1), the wetting solution was less effective and so work began on an effective lens 'cleaner'. Eventually, a suite of products that cleaned, disinfected and wetted lenses was produced (Hind 1979) and lens care had 'arrived'.

The roles of lens care

Lens care will ideally:

- Disable and remove all viable and necrotic microorganisms from contact lenses to eliminate the possibility of lens-borne eye infections or other untoward effects.
- Remove all other biological and non-biological lens contaminants.
- Restore and maintain the lens in as-new condition.

Subsequently to:

- Maintain the lens in as-new condition.

Unfortunately, these ideals are not realizable in practice but, by striving for the ideal, an acceptable lens condition can usually be achieved, i.e. a lens that can be worn safely.

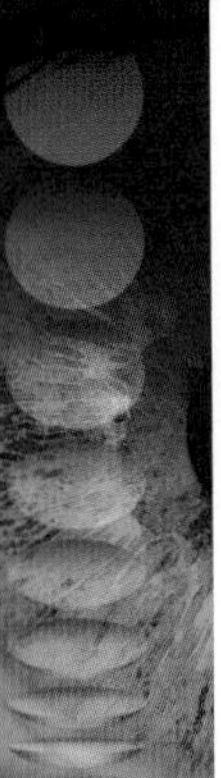

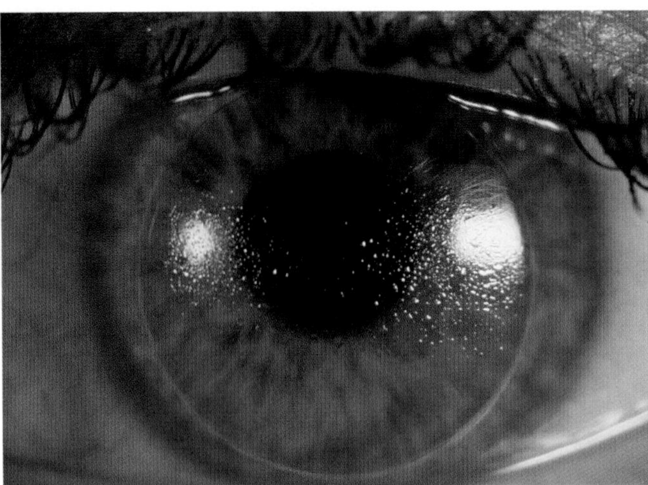

Figure 4.1 PMMA lens showing anterior surface lipid and mucus deposition along with numerous surface scratches (shown in specular reflection) (Courtesy of D. Goldsbury)

The foregoing could be restated simply as:

- To *attain* a ready-to-wear state after each lens use.
- To *maintain* this ready-to-wear state until the next use.

In general, a lens care system should:

- Clean.
- Rinse.
- Disinfect.
- Maintain/store.
- Rewet/rehydrate.
- Lubricate.
- Remove tear proteins and other lens contaminants.

Other considerations when formulating or prescribing care regimens include:

- Efficacy.
- Safety.
- Convenience.

Maintaining good vision and comfort, and keeping the lens storage case clean are other important factors.

Lens contaminants

Lenses should arrive in sterile, sealed packaging. Once this is opened, 'contaminants' can reach the lens from:

- The atmosphere.
- The wearer's (or carer's) hands during handling/insertion/ removal.
- Lens care products.

Contaminants can include:

- Viable and necrotic microorganisms.
- Viruses.
- Prions.
- Cellular debris.
- Tear components:
  - proteins.
  - mucus.
  - lipids.
  - other tear film constituents.
- Skin lipids.
- Finger-borne debris.
- Eye and other cosmetics.
- Air-borne contaminants.
- Care products and/or their derivatives.
- By-products of any interactions between lens, care products, and contaminants.

In this chapter, challengers (microorganisms and other biological entities) and challenges (everything else) are treated separately.

GENERAL MICROBIOLOGY

Microorganisms consist of nucleic acids, proteins, lipids and carbohydrates (sugars). The nucleic acids may be either deoxyribonucleic acid (DNA) or ribonucleic acid (RNA). DNA codes genetic information that determines the phenotype (physical manifestation) of the microorganism and RNA molecules participate in protein synthesis. Each microorganism also contains enzymes which determine its metabolic activity. These enzymes regulate cellular reactions and the biosynthesis of macromolecules from nutrients derived from the environment.

The structural unit of fungi, algae and mammalian cells is a *eukaryotic* cell, and is more complex than the *prokaryotic* cell of bacteria. Table 4.1 summarizes the differences between these types of cell.

Bacterial cells have an average diameter of approximately 1–2 μm, viral cells <0.5 μm, fungal cells 3–5 μm and protozoa 15–30 μm.

Microorganisms are commonly unicellular or acellular and include most bacteria, algae, viruses, protozoa and some fungi. All except algae can produce systemic and ocular disease. Most of these cells are enclosed by a cytoplasmic membrane, a double-layered structure of lipid and protein that encloses all structures and molecules for the maintenance of biological function. It acts as a semi-permeable membrane and controls the passage of solutes between the cell and external environment. Many of the antimicrobials and preservatives in lens care products target the cytoplasmic membrane.

Table 4.1: Characteristics of eukaryotic and prokaryotic cells

Eukaryotic cells	Prokaryotic cells
Nuclear membrane present	No nuclear membrane
Multiple chromosomes	Single chromosome
Membrane-bound organelles present (mitochondria, lysosomes)	Membrane-bound organelles absent
Intracellular digestive vacuoles present	Intracellular digestive vacuoles absent
Cells divide by mitosis	Cells divide by binary fission

(a)

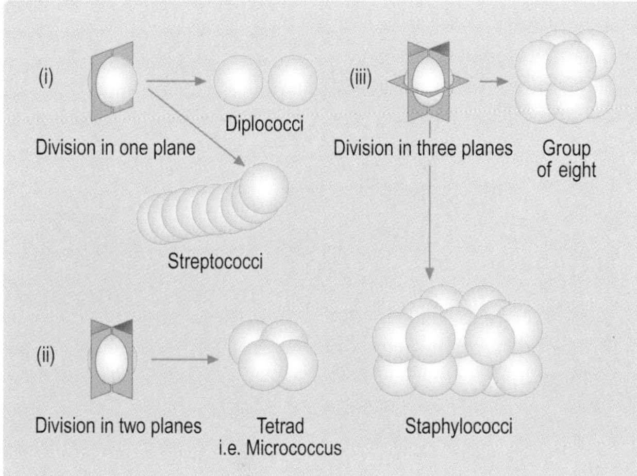

(b)

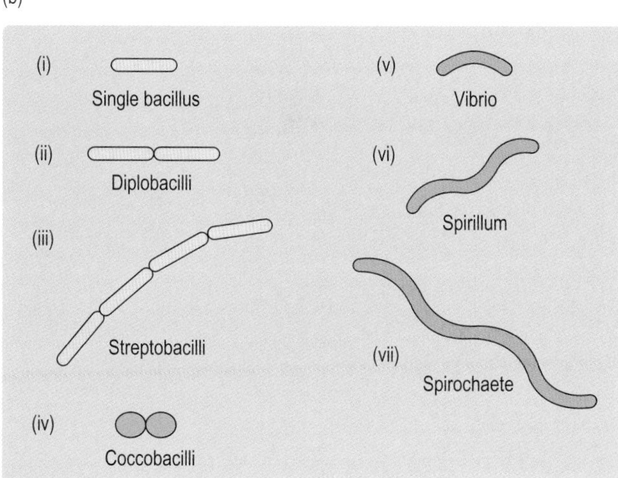

Figure 4.2 Morphology of (a) bacterial cocci and (b) rods

While multicellular microorganisms may originate from a single cell, single cells may also attach to one another to form threads or filaments while still functioning as a single cell. Some bacteria and algae exist in this form. *Coenocytic* structures describe those not composed of discrete cellular subunits, but which have a continuous cytoplasm. Such microorganisms, including some fungi and algae, grow in size without undergoing cellular division.

Bacteria

Bacteria are classified according to their morphology, staining characteristics, growth requirements, biochemical type or antigenic structure as follows (Sleigh & Timbury 1990).

MORPHOLOGY

- Spherical (*cocci*). The morphology of cells depends on how single cells divide. Possible options include:
  - if cocci divide in a single plane, they form pairs (*diplococci*, e.g. *Neisseria* spp.) or chains (e.g. *Streptococcus* spp.).
  - if cocci divide in two planes, they form a group of four (*tetrads*, e.g. *Micrococcus* spp.).
  - if cocci divide in three planes, they form a cluster of eight either as a cube (*sarcinae*) or as a cluster (e.g. *Staphylococcus* spp.).
- Cylindrical (*bacilli* or *rods*, e.g. *Pseudomonas* spp.). Again these may take several forms:
  - *Coccobacilli* are short rods with a more rounded appearance (e.g. *Acinetobacter* spp.).
  - *Filamentous* rods which grow as elongated forms.
  - *Vibrios* which look like commas (e.g. *Vibrio cholerae*).
- Helical, known as *spirochaetes*.

These different morphologies are illustrated in Figure 4.2.[†]

Bacteria may also be differentiated by their carbohydrate metabolism, protein metabolism, enzyme production, or other specific biochemical reactions (biotyping). For microorganisms that are biochemically similar, other methods of typing include:

- *Antibiogram typing.* This method is based on the microorganism's susceptibility to different antibiotics.
- *Bacteriophage typing.* Differentiation on the basis of the microorganism's susceptibility to various bacterial viruses and is used commonly to differentiate between strains of *Staphylococcus aureus*.
- *Bacteriocin typing.* Differentiation on the basis of inhibitory protein (bacteriocin or pyocin) production. Certain microorganisms, including *Pseudomonas aeruginosa*, produce proteins that inhibit the growth of other members of the same species.
- *Serotyping.* Differentiation on the basis of antigenic structure. This method is used to differentiate between strains of, for example, *P. aeruginosa* and *Legionella pneumophila*.
- *Molecular typing.* These techniques involve differentiation between microorganisms at the DNA level and have been used for a wide range of species. Such molecular biology methods include random amplified polymorphic DNA and restriction fragment polymorphism techniques. Both methods have been used in differentiating species of organisms derived from the ocular surface. The polymerase chain reaction (PCR) provides a means for amplification of DNA sequences of microorganisms.

CELL WALL

Bacteria are grouped by their Gram staining reaction[*] which reflects the structure of the cell wall. The cell wall of Gram-positive microorganisms comprises a cytoplasmic membrane surrounded by a thick peptidoglycan layer (a mucopeptide) cross-

---

[†] For further information see: http://www.cdc.gov/od/ohs/biosfty/bmb14/bmb14s7d.htm

[*] The Gram staining procedure involves sequentially staining a heat-fixed smear of bacterial cells with crystal violet, iodine, decolorizing with an organic solvent and counterstaining. Gram-positive bacteria resist decolorization and remain stained purple. Gram-negative bacteria decolorize and take up a red/pink counterstain. Figure 4.3 illustrates Gram-positive and Gram-negative bacilli and cocci.

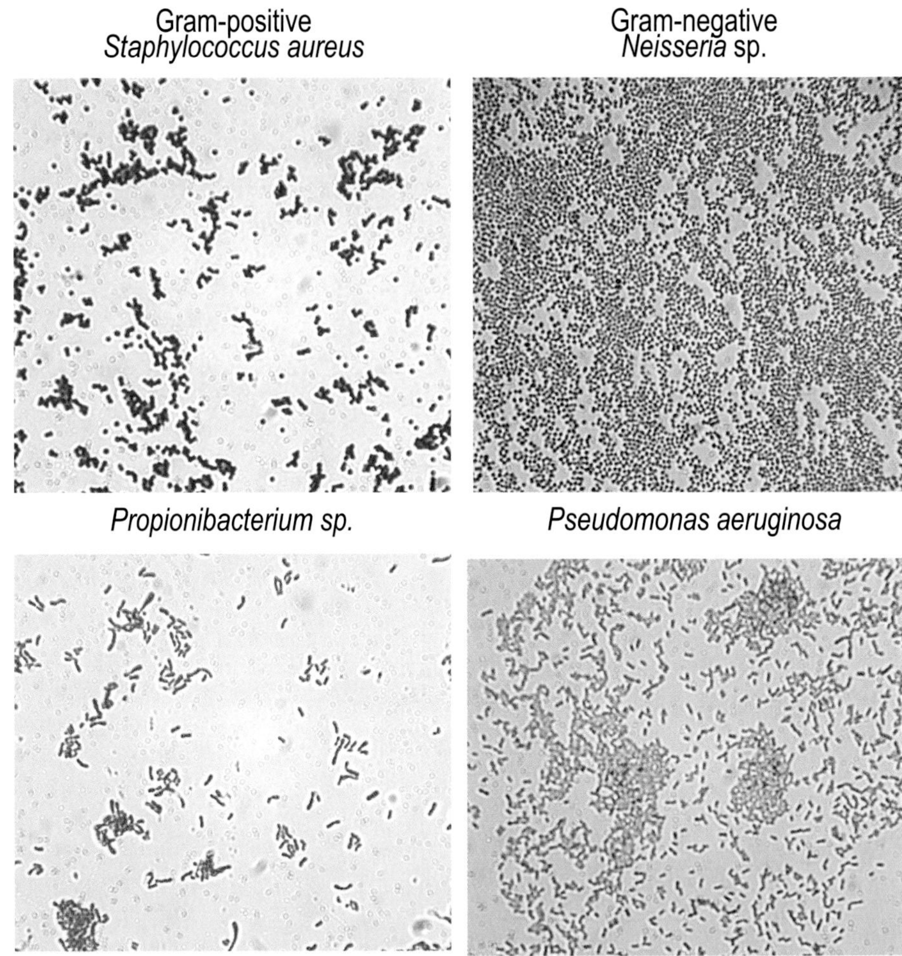

Figure 4.3 Gram stain of Gram-positive and Gram-negative rods and cocci

linked with peptide subunits (these give rigidity to the structure) and interspersed with (lipo-) teichoic or teichuronic acid.

In contrast, Gram-negative microorganisms have a cytoplasmic membrane with a smaller peptidoglycan layer, surrounded by an outer protein membrane and lipopolysaccharide (LPS) enclosing the periplasmic space. In the eye, this difference is important in defence, since the tear protein lysozyme cleaves peptidoglycan and causes bacterial death, either by allowing other bactericidal proteins to penetrate the cell or by causing osmotic death. Peptidoglycan damage is more of a problem for Gram-positive microorganisms and lysozyme is much less effective against Gram-negative bacteria that are protected by their outer wall (which is impermeable to enzymes).

Outside the cell wall, there may be other external structures present such as flagella, pili and capsules. Flagella are filaments of the protein flagellin, responsible for bacterial motility. Pili are shorter filaments of the protein pilin that emerge from the cytoplasmic membrane. Pili are responsible for bacterial adhesion and the transfer of non-chromosomal genetic material, such as plasmids, between bacteria. These are general gene-carrying, mobile DNA elements found in the cell cytoplasm that are not essential for bacterial survival but which provide some selective advantage (e.g. antimicrobial resistance).

Capsules are frequently a polysaccharide matrix comprising the outermost layer of certain bacteria. Capsules are a major determinant in the virulence of a microorganism, which act by protecting the bacteria from phagocytosis and from other antimicrobial agents. Capsules also play a role in the binding to host tissue.

GROWTH REQUIREMENTS

Bacteria can be further classified according to their environmental requirements for growth. These could include oxygen requirements, growth temperature, pH, salinity and micronutrients.

Atmospheric requirements can be classified as follows:

- Aerobic microorganisms that require oxygen for growth.
- Facultative anaerobic microorganisms that grow in the presence or absence of oxygen.
- Anaerobic microorganisms that grow only in the absence of oxygen.
- Microaerophilic microorganisms that grow in the presence of trace oxygen and carbon dioxide.

The temperature ranges for optimal growth are as follows:

- Thermophilic microorganisms – 55–80°C.
- Mesophilic microorganisms – 25–40°C.
- Psychrophilic microorganisms – below 20°C.

External ocular infections tend to be caused by mesophilic microorganisms that may be aerobes, facultative aerobes or microaerophilic microorganisms.

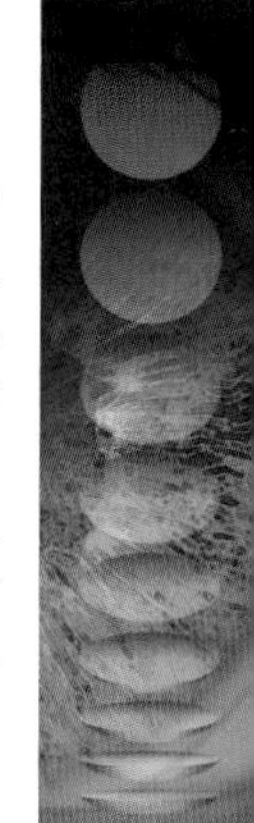

BACTERIA AND DISEASE

Bacteria may cause disease either by:

- Direct invasion of tissue and subsequent replication of microorganisms.
- Toxin or enzyme production that may in turn activate the immune system causing an inflammatory tissue response. Dead or dying bacteria also release toxins.

In diseases associated with Gram-negative microorganisms, endotoxin has been implicated as a cause of major tissue damage. Endotoxin is an outer membrane component of Gram-negative microorganisms comprised of lipopolysaccharide that is known to cause antibody and cytokine production, neutrophil migration and complement activation.

Chlamydiae

Chlamydiae are intracellular parasites, originally believed to be viruses because of their small size and difficulty in culturing by traditional bacteriological techniques. This group is now recognized as a bacterial species.

Chlamydia are between 0.2 and 1 μm in size with an outer membrane similar to Gram-negative bacteria but without peptidoglycan in the cell wall. On Gram stain they look like tiny Gram-negative bacteria. Unlike viruses, chlamydiae can make their own DNA, RNA and protein, but rely on host cells for energy sources such as adenosine triphosphate.

In the eye, *Chlamydia trachomatis* is the species that causes both trachoma and inclusion keratoconjunctivitis. Diagnosis is often difficult as chlamydiae are intracellular organisms that will not grow using conventional laboratory media. Cell culture techniques are laborious and expensive and diagnosis is based on the presence of inclusion bodies and laboratory testing of swabs using monoclonal antibodies to detect chlamydial antigens. Antibodies may be conjugated with a fluorescent tag to make the antigens visible under fluorescence microscopy. PCR is frequently used to amplify small amounts of nucleic acids and to identify chlamydial serotypes.

Fungi

Most fungi are found in soil, where they degrade organic matter. They rarely cause disease in healthy humans, but are a major cause of eye infections in immunocompromised individuals or in association with ocular trauma in rural areas.

All fungi are either aerobes (moulds) or facultative anaerobes (yeasts). Structurally, fungi are larger than bacteria, contain multiple chromosomes, and the cytoplasm contains mitochondria and endoplasmic reticulum. Their cell walls are quite different from bacteria, are very thick, and contain no peptidoglycan making them resistant to host defences and difficult to eliminate once infection is established. They lack structures for movement and have fewer mechanisms for adherence to host cells, making it more difficult for fungi to invade the host initially.

FUNGI AND DISEASE

Fungi release spores into the environment that are carried by air or water. Spores are highly resistant to environmental factors and can survive extremes of temperature and pH. This resistance is due partly to surface components, such as hydrophobic glycoproteins or lipoglycoproteins, which also help dissemination. They are ubiquitous in the environment and are found on skin, and are ingested or inhaled frequently. Despite their frequency in the environment, fungal disease is rare and requires the spores to penetrate the host tissue and germinate.

Species pathogenic in the eye include filamentous fungi, *Aspergillus* spp., *Fusarium* spp. and the yeast *Candida* spp.

Actinomycetes

Actinomycetes are a group of bacteria that share some common characteristics with fungi and in the eye can cause similar disease to fungi. They are able to form hyphae, usually considered a trait of fungi only. Structurally, in all other ways, they are prokaryotic cells that resemble bacteria and are susceptible to penicillin, which fungi are not.

Examples of Actinomycetes include *Streptomyces* spp. These are an important group of soil bacteria used in the synthesis of antibiotics such as streptomycin. Species that are pathogenic in the eye include *Corynebacterium* spp. and *Mycobacterium* spp.

Viruses

Viruses are responsible for many human, animal and plant diseases, including disease at all ocular sites. Viruses are small (20–250 nm), acellular obligate parasites that are different structurally from cellular microorganisms such as bacteria with different chemical composition and mode of growth.

One useful definition of a virus is 'a subcellular agent, consisting of a core of nucleic acid surrounded by a protein coat (and sometimes an outer protein and lipid envelope) that must use the metabolic machinery of a living host to replicate'.

Viruses can exist in either an extracellular or intracellular form. The extracellular form, or virion, comprises either single- or double-stranded DNA or RNA molecule(s) (nucleocapsid) within a protein coat or capsid. Viruses can be differentiated by how their nucleic acid is packaged, i.e. rod shaped, helical, spherical or isometric. The virion contains no structures for growth or multiplication and, therefore, requires a host cell to undergo replication (Stainer et al. 1981) and must be released subsequently from the host cell after replication.

Ocular infections may be caused by the herpes virus (cytomegalovirus, varicella-zoster virus, Epstein–Barr virus [MSV] and human virus-6) and adenoviruses, although infections may be caused by other groups.

VIRUSES AND DISEASE

Viruses can produce disease in several ways:

- Directly by inhibiting cell metabolism and synthesis. Cells infected by viruses lyse and this can lead to temporary or permanent loss of function.

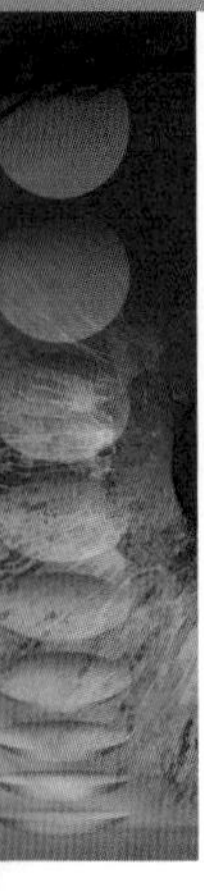

Table 4.2: Comparison of biochemical characteristics of eukaryotes, prokaryotes, viruses, and prions

Biochemical trait	Eukaryotic cells	Prokaryotic cells	Viruses	Prions
Protein	✓	✓	✓	✓
Nucleic acids	✓	✓	✓(DNA or RNA not both)	✗
Carbohydrates	✓	✓	✓/✗	✗
Lipids	✓	✓	✓/✗	✗
Ribosomes	✓	✗	✗	✗
Chloroplasts/ mitochondria	✓	✗	✗	✗
Nuclear membrane	✓	✗	✗	✗
Multicellular	✓	✗	✗	✗
Intracellular growth	✓/✗	✓/✗	✓	✗

- Indirectly by compromising host defences so that opportunistic microorganisms such as bacteria can colonize. One example of this is the influenza virus that damages the respiratory epithelium and cilia so that the surface cannot be cleared of bacteria. Bacteria such as *Haemophilus influenzae* are then able to adhere to the damaged tissue and to colonize and produce disease.
- By inducing tumour formation (*oncogenic* viruses). This is controversial but both DNA and RNA viruses carry genes closely related to host cell genes that are able to transform cells and alter their physiological properties.

Protozoa

Protozoa comprise a number of diverse groups of unicellular microorganisms that range from 5 μm to 1 mm in diameter. Most are aquatic, and may live as parasites in a range of species, or may be free living. Under certain environmental conditions many protozoa become encysted as a means of protection. This allows the cell to survive adverse environments and to survive outside the host until they can enter a new host. From the perspective of the contact lens environment, this enables them to resist lens care products and wait until conditions are more suitable.

There are approximately 40,000 species of protozoa, but only a few cause disease in humans.

Ocular infections may be caused by *Toxoplasma* spp. and by *Acanthamoeba* spp.

Prions

Prions are unconventional infectious agents that cause transmissible fatal brain disease in humans and animals. They are not living microorganisms in the conventional sense (Table 4.2). Prions are an aberrant isoform of a normal cellular protein (PrP^c) that exists in normal human and animal neuronal tissue. Prions enter brain tissue and, through mechanisms that are not yet fully understood, cause the conversion of the normal PrP^c into copies of the aberrant prion protein PrP^{sc} in a self-propagating process. Conversion to the prion protein PrP^{sc} appears to be associated with abnormal protein folding, rendering the protein insoluble, resistant to protease degradation, resistant to many biocides, and transmissible.

PRIONS AND DISEASE

Prions cause cross-species neurodegenerative diseases known as transmissible spongiform encephalopathies in humans and animals. The most common acquired human prion diseases include Creutzfeldt–Jakob disease (CJD) and new variant Creutzfeldt–Jakob disease acquired through eating infected cattle meat and kuru (ritual cannibalism in New Guinea). Iatrogenic CJD has been reported following administration of prion-containing growth hormone and transplantation of prion-containing nervous system grafts. There have been one proven case (Duffy et al. 1974) and three possible cases following corneal transplantation (Uchijama et al. 1994, Heckmann et al. 1997, Rabinstein et al. 2002).*

MICROBIOLOGY OF THE EYE

NORMAL OCULAR BIOTA

It is generally accepted that the external ocular surface is sparsely colonized and microorganisms are removed by the normal ocular defence mechanisms rather than leading to persistent and increased colonization over time.

The most common microorganisms isolated from the eyelids and conjunctiva are Gram-positive bacteria, specifically coagulase-negative staphylococci, *Corynebacterium* spp. and *Propionibacterium* spp. Other bacterial species include *Staphylococcus aureus*, *Micrococcus* spp., *Bacillus* spp. and *Bacteroides* spp. (Perkins et al. 1975, Fleiszig & Efron 1992b, Seal et al. 1998). The conjunctival fornices may harbour small numbers of anaerobic organisms, with *Propionibacterium* and *Peptostreptococcus* being the most common genera (Perkins et al. 1975, Fleiszig & Efron 1992b). The cornea and anterior chamber are considered to be sterile. Gram-negative micro-organisms are isolated in less than 5% of cases and tend to be present as transient microorganisms rather than persistent colonizers in normal healthy eyes.

In adults, fungi are more rarely isolated, although regional variations have been reported, with fungal recovery from the eyelids occurring in 2–52% of samples and in 2–28% of conjunctival samples (Ainley & Smith 1965, Wilson et al. 1969). An increased recovery rate of fungi from the ocular surface has been reported using PCR for the detection of fungal DNA (Wu et al. 2003).

* For further information see: http://www.cdc.gov/ncidod/diseases/cjd/cjd_fact_sheet.htm

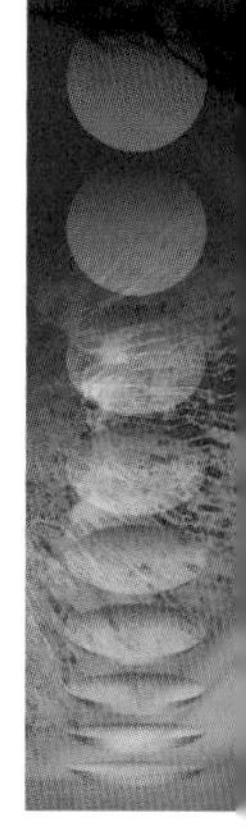

Ocular biota is also influenced by sleep, the number and frequency of recovery of Gram-positive microorganisms increasing with sleep (Ramachandran et al. 1995) such that patching of the eye overnight following foreign body removal should be accompanied by prophylactic antibiosis.

MICROORGANISMS AND EYE DISEASE

Table 4.3 summarizes the common causative microorganisms for different ocular diseases and Figure 4.4 shows the classification of organisms associated with ocular infections.

The effect of lens wear on ocular biota

Alterations to the normal ocular biota during lens wear may, theoretically, suppress the ocular defence mechanism and enable colonization by pathogenic organisms. There is considerable controversy in the literature as to the effect of contact lens wear. Much of this confusion is likely to reflect differences in methodology, sampling techniques, subject groups, lens types, wear modality, and type and duration of wear. Increased conjunctival biota has been reported in daily hydrogel lens wearers (Morgan 1979, Callender et al. 1986, Larkin & Leeming 1991, Stapleton et al. 1995b) although the spectrum of organisms was not found to differ. This increase in conjunctival biota may be secondary to quantitative changes in lid margin biota (Larkin & Leeming 1991). In one study, the conjunctival biota could be related to the contaminants of the lens storage case (Morgan 1979) although no such association was confirmed in a later study (Fleiszig & Efron 1992b). An alteration in the spectrum of organisms was found to occur in a mixed group of rigid and soft lens wearers (Høvding 1981) and in extended wear hydrogel wearers (Stapleton et al. 1995b) where increased numbers of both sterile cultures and Gram-negative organisms were isolated. However, other studies have reported no differences in conjunctival biota between lens wearers and non-lens wearers (Tragakis et al. 1973, Rauschl & Rogers 1978, Higaki et al. 1998).

Increased conjunctival colonization by pathogenic non-resident organisms has been demonstrated during extended wear of rigid gas-permeable (RGP) lenses (Fleiszig & Efron 1992a). Adherence and colonization of lenses by pathogenic organisms has been reported in association with lens-related keratitis (Stapleton & Dart 1995) and high numbers of pathogenic organisms have been recovered from lenses during episodes of acute adverse responses (Baleriola-Lucas et al. 1991, Holden et al. 1996). One possibility is that pathogenic organisms adhere and easily colonize lenses and are not removed as easily as normal biota. Inhibition of the clearing of pathogenic organisms from the eye during lens wear may be one of several factors modulating this alteration in biota with lens wear. This alteration in biota has been reported as persisting subsequent to cessation of lens wear (Fleiszig & Efron 1992a). It is not clear, however, whether this effect is limited to wearers discontinuing wear due to adverse responses.

THE INTERACTION BETWEEN LENSES AND MICROORGANISMS

In asymptomatic lens wear, a contact lens is infrequently colonized by small numbers of microorganisms (Hart et al. 1993) derived from the hands (Mowrey-McKee et al. 1992), lids (Willcox et al. 1997), lens care solutions (Sweeney et al. 1999), storage cases (Clark et al. 1994, Donzis et al. 1987, Gray et al. 1995, Larkin et al. 1990, Kanpolat et al. 1992), the domestic water environment (Willcox et al. 1997) or from environmental sources (Stapleton et al. 1995).

Storage cases have also been implicated as a source of lens contamination by fungi and amoebae. Fungal contamination of storage cases appears to be widespread (Donzis et al. 1987, Gray et al. 1995), with 24% of cases in asymptomatic wearers showing contamination by filamentous fungi and yeasts (Gray et al. 1995). Species isolated most commonly included *Cladosporidium* spp., *Candida* spp., *Fusarium solarni*, *Aspergillus* spp., *Exophiala* spp. and *Phoma* sp. Contamination of storage cases by *Acanthamoeba* has been shown in 4–10% of wearers (Devonshire et al. 1993, Larkin et al. 1990). However, where tap water rinsing of cases was avoided and cases were replaced monthly, no amoebic contamination was reported (Seal et al. 1999). Amoebic contamination of lenses in asymptomatic wearers appears rare (Saddiq et al. 1998).

Under certain circumstances, a contact lens may act as a vector by presenting organisms to the cornea, either by prolonging retention of organisms on the ocular surface or by organisms colonizing the lens surface in-eye or during storage. Large numbers of bacteria have been recovered from lenses during corneal inflammation and infection.

Colonization of lenses by large numbers of Gram-negative bacteria (*P. aeruginosa*, *Serratia marcescens* and *H. influenzae*) (Holden et al. 1996, Sankaridurg et al. 1996) or *Streptococcus pneumoniae* (Sankaridurg et al. 1999) has been reported in contact lens-induced acute red eye (CLARE). Contact lens-induced peripheral ulcer (CLPU) has been associated with Gram-positive contamination of lenses, particularly *S. aureus* (Jalbert et al. 2000) and *Strep. pneumoniae* (Sankaridurg et al. 1999). In microbial keratitis, concordance between the corneal isolate and contact lens isolate is frequently reported (Martins et al. 2002, Stapleton et al 1995).

Bacteria can adhere to both unworn and worn lenses (Dart & Badenoch 1986, Duran et al. 1987, John et al. 1989, Miller & Ahearn 1987, Willcox et al. 2001). There is a large literature on the effect of adsorbed tear components, lens material and surface properties, bacterial species, strain, phenotypic characteristic and growth requirements on adhesion, which is a necessary step in retaining organisms on a lens surface sufficiently for colonization to occur. The predominant mode of growth for bacteria within natural ecosystems is within glycocalyx-enclosed microcolonies, forming a biofilm on inert surfaces (Costerton et al. 1981), mucosal surfaces (Gristina & Costerton 1984), in osteomyelitis (Gristina & Costerton 1985), and on the surfaces of prostheses (Jacques et al. 1992). Motile bacterial cells lacking this protective mechanism (swarmer or

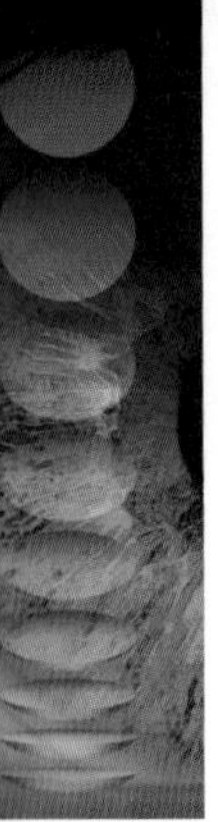

Table 4.3: Common causative organisms in ocular infections

Ocular site	Disease	Microorganisms
Lacrimal drainage	Canaliculitis	*Propionibacterium* sp.
Lid margin	Blepharitis, blepharoconjunctivitis, blepharokeratoconjunctivitis	*S. aureus*
Conjunctiva	Acute bacterial conjunctivitis (adult)	*S. aureus* *Strep. pneumoniae* *H. influenzae* *Strep. pyogenes* *Proteus* spp. *Moraxella* spp. Enteric Gram-negative bacteria Less commonly anaerobic species
Conjunctiva	Acute bacterial conjunctivitis (childhood)	*H. influenzae* *Neisseria gonorrhoeae* *Neisseria meningitidis* *S. aureus* *Strep. pneumoniae*
Conjunctiva	Phlyctenular conjunctivitis	*Mycobacterium tuberculosis* *S. aureus* *C. albicans*
Conjunctiva	Membranous conjunctivitis	*Strep. pyogenes* *Neisseria* spp. *Corynebacterium* spp.
Conjunctiva	Follicular conjunctivitis	*Chlamydia trachomatis* Adenovirus 1, 2, 4–6, 19
Conjunctiva	Viral conjunctivitis	*Herpes simplex* Adenovirus (pharyngoconjunctival fever) 3, 7 Herpes zoster Epstein–Barr virus Measles, mumps, hepatitis A virus
Conjunctiva	Acute haemorrhagic conjunctivitis	Adenovirus 11 Coxsackie virus 24 Enterovirus 70
Cornea	Microbial keratitis	*S. aureus* Coagulase-negative staphylococci *Strep. pneumoniae* *Strep. pyogenes* *Strep. viridans* *P. aeruginosa* *Moraxella* sp. *Proteus* sp. *Klebsiella* sp. *Serratia* sp. Other Gram-negative bacteria *Chlamydia trachomatis* Herpes simplex Herpes zoster Adenovirus *Aspergillus* sp. *Fusarium* sp. *C. albicans*

(cont'd)

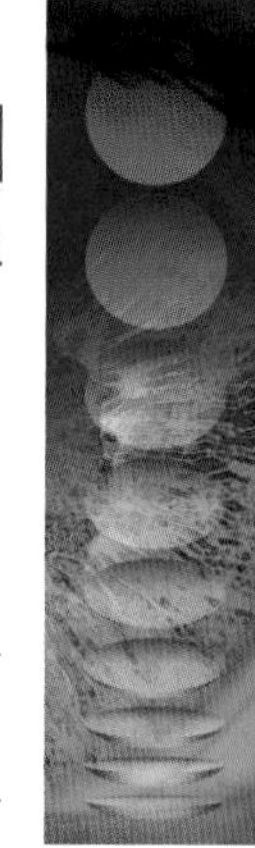

Table 4.3: Common causative organisms in ocular infections (*cont'd*)

Ocular site	Disease	Microorganisms
Cornea	Contact lens-related microbial keratitis	*P. aeruginosa* *S. marcescens* Other Gram-negative bacteria *S. aureus* *Strep. pneumoniae* *Acanthamoeba* spp. (Group 2)
Sclera	Scleritis	*Strep. pneumoniae* *Acanthamoeba* spp. (Group 2)
Anterior chamber	Acute endophthalmitis	*S. aureus* *Strep. pyogenes* *Strep. pneumoniae* Enteric microorganisms
Anterior chamber	Chronic endophthalmitis	Coagulase-negative staphylococci *Propionibacterium* sp. *Corynebacterium* sp. *Haemophilus* spp. *Pseudomonas* spp. *C. albicans* *Fusarium* spp. *Aspergillus* sp. Herpes simplex Herpes zoster

Sources: Alfonso et al. 1986, Brazier & Hall 1993, Galentine et al. 1984, Hyndiuk et al. 1988, Lass et al. 1981, Limberg 1991, Perkins et al. 1975, Piccolo 1989, Schein et al. 1989, Seal et al. 1981, 1982, 1998, Stehr-Green et al. 1989, Wilhelmus et al. 1988, Wilson 1979, Wilson et al. 1981.

planktonic cells) are released from the body of the biofilm to invade surrounding tissues or to colonize further surfaces (Fig. 4.5). Within this favourable adherent environment, propagation of organisms is enhanced and enclosed organisms are protected from host defences (Gristina & Costerton 1984) and antibiotics (Anwar et al. 1990). Formation of such a bacterial biofilm on lenses will result in increased numbers of organisms and prolonged exposure to the cornea. This has been demonstrated in an animal model (Dart et al. 1988) on lenses incubated with bacteria in vitro (Stapleton et al. 1993), on worn lenses in vivo (Slusher et al. 1987), and on lenses from wearers with culture-proven microbial keratitis (Holland et al. 1988, McLaughlin-Borlace et al. 1998, Stapleton & Dart 1995). The role of biofilm formation in lens-related disease is unclear. However, a bacterial biofilm on a contact lens or within a storage case (Fig. 4.6) renders organisms more resistant to the antimicrobial effects of lens care systems (Evans & Dart 1995, McCulloch et al. 1988, Wilson et al. 1991) and enables the organisms to persist on a lens surface with the potential for tissue damage, either directly or via toxin production (Figs 4.5 and 4.6).

Sterilization, disinfection and decontamination

Disinfection is the most important safety issue in lens care. Lens and storage case contamination is associated with both corneal infection (Mayo et al. 1986, Stapleton et al. 1995a, McLaughlin-Borlace et al. 1998) and inflammation (Bates et al. 1989). Disinfection describes the process by which vegetative microorganisms are killed or their growth is inhibited on surface, object or in liquid. Antiseptics remove or kill vegetative microorganisms on tissue while sterilization refers to killing of all living microorganisms, including bacterial endospores and cysts. Sterilization of soft lenses by manufacturers may take place via autoclaving (a process involving pressure to achieve a temperature of 121°C for 10–15 minutes) that destroys critical enzymes and disrupts DNA; via gamma irradiation that ionizes and denatures proteins; or ethylene oxide gas that alkylates, i.e. it attaches C_2H_5 to biochemical molecules. Rigid lenses are not supplied sterile following manufacture and cleaning and disinfection are required prior to their use.

Table 4.4 describes the mode of action of commonly used systems (McDonnell & Russell 1999).

GENERAL CONCEPTS IN DISINFECTION EFFICACY

The efficacy of many chemical systems is related to the concentration of the active agent, its contact time, and the form of delivery. There is invariably a trade-off between antimicrobial activity and ocular toxicity, and comfort and convenience.

Many disinfectants, including contact lens solutions, are neutralized by organic materials (Schunk & Schweisfurth

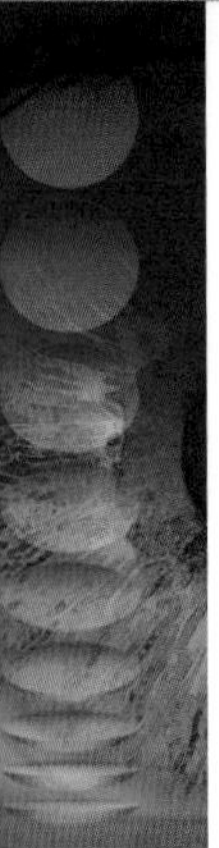

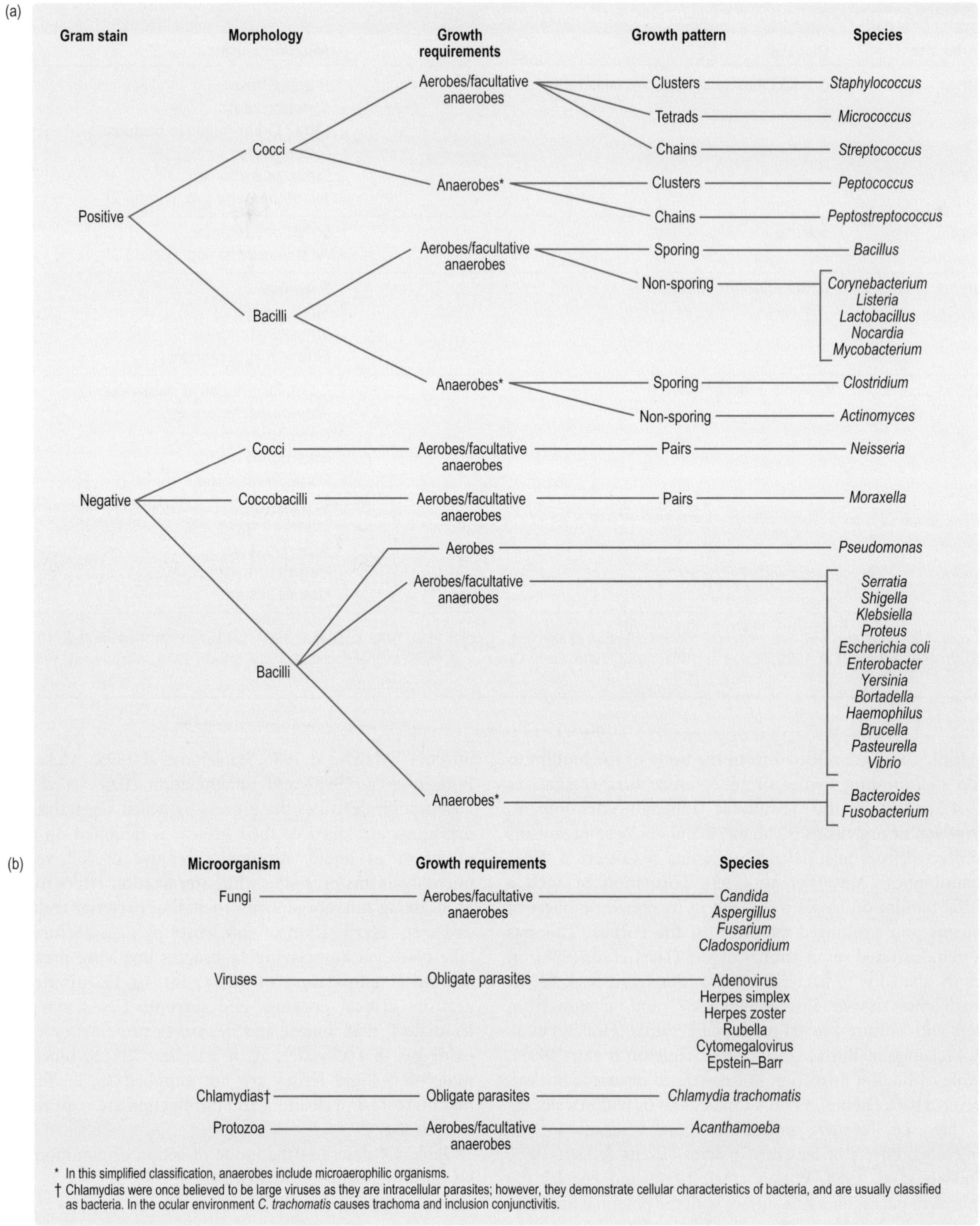

(a)

Gram stain	Morphology	Growth requirements	Growth pattern	Species
Positive	Cocci	Aerobes/facultative anaerobes	Clusters	*Staphylococcus*
			Tetrads	*Micrococcus*
			Chains	*Streptococcus*
		Anaerobes*	Clusters	*Peptococcus*
			Chains	*Peptostreptococcus*
	Bacilli	Aerobes/facultative anaerobes	Sporing	*Bacillus*
			Non-sporing	*Corynebacterium* *Listeria* *Lactobacillus* *Nocardia* *Mycobacterium*
		Anaerobes*	Sporing	*Clostridium*
			Non-sporing	*Actinomyces*
Negative	Cocci	Aerobes/facultative anaerobes	Pairs	*Neisseria*
	Coccobacilli	Aerobes/facultative anaerobes	Pairs	*Moraxella*
	Bacilli	Aerobes		*Pseudomonas*
		Aerobes/facultative anaerobes		*Serratia* *Shigella* *Klebsiella* *Proteus* *Escherichia coli* *Enterobacter* *Yersinia* *Bortadella* *Haemophilus* *Brucella* *Pasteurella* *Vibrio*
		Anaerobes*		*Bacteroides* *Fusobacterium*

(b)

Microorganism	Growth requirements	Species
Fungi	Aerobes/facultative anaerobes	*Candida* *Aspergillus* *Fusarium* *Cladosporidium*
Viruses	Obligate parasites	Adenovirus Herpes simplex Herpes zoster Rubella Cytomegalovirus Epstein–Barr
Chlamydias†	Obligate parasites	*Chlamydia trachomatis*
Protozoa	Aerobes/facultative anaerobes	*Acanthamoeba*

* In this simplified classification, anaerobes include microaerophilic organisms.

† Chlamydias were once believed to be large viruses as they are intracellular parasites; however, they demonstrate cellular characteristics of bacteria, and are usually classified as bacteria. In the ocular environment *C. trachomatis* causes trachoma and inclusion conjunctivitis.

Figure 4.4 (a) Classification of common bacteria associated with external ocular infections. (b) Classification of common organisms associated with external ocular infections

1989), so that binding to organic material effectively reduces the concentration of the antimicrobial agent. Bacterial endospores are more resistant to disinfectants than are vegetative organisms due to their lower water content and slower metabolism. Not all microorganisms are equally susceptible to disinfection. Generally, viruses with lipid membranes are the most susceptible > vegetative bacteria > fungi > non-lipid viruses > mycobacteria > bacterial spores > cysts > prions.

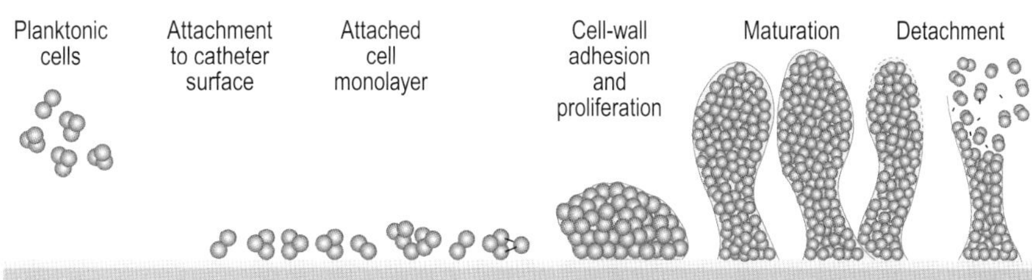

Figure 4.5 Diagrammatic representation of biofilm development on a surface

Microorganisms can acquire resistance to disinfectants:

- Through transfer of non-chromosomal genetic material on plasmids.
- Altering the binding sites for antimicrobials such as through phosphorylation.
- Altering the drug enzymatically.
- Developing effective pumps for removal of the drug.

Organisms with a complex cell wall composition tend to be more resistant than those with a simple cell wall structure. Certain bacteria (e.g. staphylococci) and fungi produce the enzyme catalase, which neutralizes hydrogen peroxide. This may account for higher contamination rates with Gram-positive organisms in one-step peroxide systems (Gray et al. 1995). Acquired resistance of *Serratia marcescens* to solutions containing chlorhexidine and benzalkonium chloride in rigid lens solutions has been documented (Wilson et al. 1991, Gandhi et al. 1993), and Lakkis and Fleiszig (2001) reported resistance of cytotoxic strains of *Pseudomonas aeruginosa* to hydrogel lens solutions containing polyaminopropyl biguanide (PAPB) and polymeric quaternary ammonium compounds (QAC).

Solution licensing requirements

Lens care systems are mainly designed to reduce microbial contamination introduced during wear and handling. The safety and efficacy requirements for marketing approval of care products are described by the Food and Drug Administration (FDA 510[k]; Services 1997) and the International Organization for Standardization (ISO-14729; Standardization 2001).

IN-OFFICE DISINFECTION OF TRIAL LENSES*

To limit the transfer of microorganisms between patients, trial lenses ideally should be used once and discarded. Where this is not possible, in-office disinfection needs to be effective against bacteria, fungi, viruses and *Acanthamoeba*. A recent concern is the theoretical risk of the transmission of vCJD via trial lens fitting or through other ophthalmic procedures.

The Health and Safety Executive of the Department of Health in the UK have advised the following procedure for removal of prions:

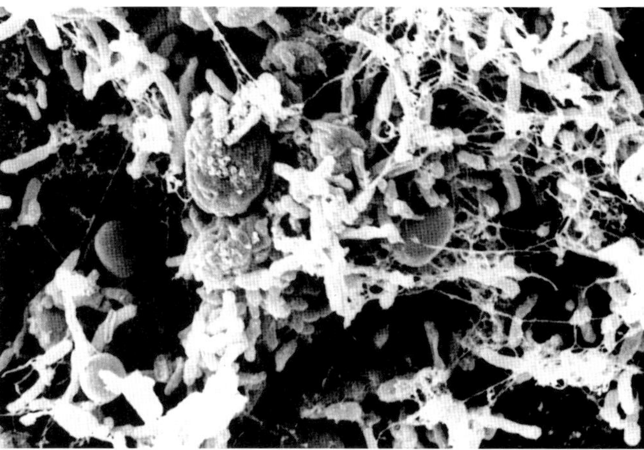

Figure 4.6 Scanning electron micrograph showing polymicrobial biofilm on a lens storage case (Courtesy of L. McLaughlin-Borlace)

- Soak in sodium hypochlorite at 20,000 ppm (2%) for 1 hour.
- Rinse thoroughly.
- Store in disinfecting solution prior to reuse or store dry in the case of rigid lenses.

It is not clear whether soft lens parameters are stable with this process although RGP lenses appear stable. For patients in a high-risk category for vCJD, disposal of the device or lens following use is recommended. An ISO standard is currently being developed although it does appear that the risk of transmission of prion infections by contaminated lenses is negligible (Hogan 2003).

Removal of agents other than prions can be achieved with heat disinfection using sterile saline. This provides:

- A rapid, cheap and effective method for lens and vial disinfection.
- An effective method against bacteria, fungi, viruses and *Acanthamoeba*, including cysts, utilizing temperatures of 78–90°C for 20 minutes to 1 hour (Busschaert et al. 1978, Statement 1988).

Drawbacks of heat disinfection of trial lenses include:

- Regrowth of organisms over time.
- The stability of lens parameters, particularly high-water-content lenses.
- Reduced lens life.
- The periodic requirement to ensure that the disinfection cycle for in-office heating units maintains the required temperature for an appropriate period (i.e. procedure validation).

* See ISO/TS 1997:2004 (E) Ophthalmic optics – contact lenses – Hygiene management of multi-patient use trial contact lenses.

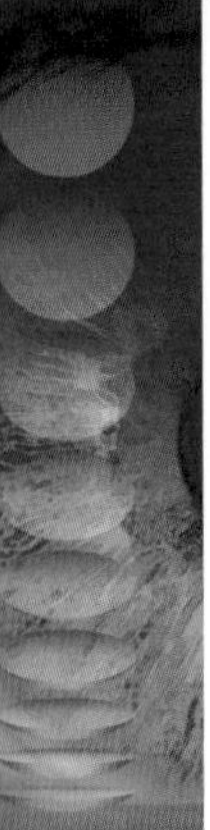

Table 4.4: Mode of action of common disinfection agents

Agent	Mode of action	Antimicrobial effect
Alcohol (ethanol or isopropyl alcohol)	Lipid solvent causing membrane damage and protein denaturation	Broad spectrum – vegetative bacteria, viruses, fungi. Not sporicidal
Quaternary ammonium compounds (QACs)	Interact with lipids in cell wall, surface active predominantly at the cytoplasmic membrane. Damage the outer membrane of Gram-negative bacteria	Broad spectrum – bactericidal, sporostatic, lipid viruses, enveloped viruses but not non-enveloped viruses, limited effect on fungi and *Acanthamoeba*
Biguanides:		
Chlorhexidine (CHX)	Damage to outer membrane, diffusion across the cell wall and cytoplasmic and inner membrane damage	Broad spectrum – vegetative bacteria (e.g.: *S. marcescens*), viruses, fungi, *Acanthamoeba* trophozoites and some effect against cysts. Not sporicidal
Polymeric biguanides (PHX)	Initially binds to phospholipids of the outer membrane and subsequently cytoplasmic membrane causing altered cell permeability and loss of membrane function	Broad spectrum. Variable resistance against fungi, yeasts, *Acanthamoeba*
Chlorine release compounds	Free chlorine acts as an oxidizing agent which destroys the cellular activity of proteins, lipids and bacterial DNA	Bactericidal activity, some effect on spores, limited effect on *Acanthamoeba* and fungi
Hydrogen peroxide	Hydroxyl (OH) radical acts as an oxidizing agent which destroys the cellular activity of proteins, lipids and bacterial DNA	Broad spectrum. Depending on the available concentration and duration of exposure, activity against bacteria, spores, viruses, fungi and *Acanthamoeba*
Heat	Disruption of tertiary structures of DNA, proteins and cell membrane	Non-specific. Activity dependent on duration and temperature. Sterilization results in removal of all organisms including spores

A 3% concentration of hydrogen peroxide is an effective method for the removal of bacteria, fungi, viruses and *Acanthamoeba* including cysts (Anger et al. 1990). Exposure periods ranging from 10 minutes to 4 hours have been recommended, depending on the organism type. Non-neutralized peroxide has activity against organisms within a biofilm (Wilson et al. 1991, Evans & Dart 1995).

Drawbacks of hydrogen peroxide in trial lens disinfection include:

- The requirement for a neutralization step after 24 hours.
- Leakage of fluid from one-step cases (Seal et al. 1999).
- Regrowth of organisms in neutralized peroxide (Penley et al. 1981, Rosenthal et al. 1995).
- The need for a vented case (see later).

The USA Centers for Disease Control recommends disinfection of trial lenses with hydrogen peroxide or heat to prevent transmission of HIV (Report 1985). For hydrogel lenses, there are no recommended decontamination procedures for removal of prions, and the consensus appears to be to discard the lenses wherever possible. If this is not possible, patients should be informed of the risks associated with multiple-use lenses and this should be documented.

The recommended procedure for hydrogel trial lenses is as follows:

- Clean and rinse on removal. Digitally clean for at least 20 seconds on each side of the lens with an alcohol-based or mildly abrasive cleaner followed by a sterile-saline rinse. This is associated with at least a 2 log unit reduction in viable organisms (Shih et al. 1985, Liedel & Begley 1996) and also removes HIV from lens surfaces (Vogt et al. 1986).
- Soak in 3% hydrogen peroxide for 2–3 hours and then neutralize for 10–60 minutes.
- Store in a cold chemical system with redisinfection every 30 days (Callender et al. 1992). To prevent contamination while handling, use the same storage container and refill with the chemical system (Standardization 2000).
- Replace lenses annually or as specified by the manufacturer.

For rigid trial lenses (Lakkis 2002):

- Digitally clean for at least 20 seconds on each side of the lens with an alcohol-based or mildly abrasive cleaner, followed by a sterile-saline rinse.

Either then:

- Soak in 2% hypochlorite for 1 hour followed by rinsing with sterile saline, or
- Soak in 3% hydrogen peroxide for 5–10 minutes. Remove and rinse with sterile saline.

Store dry and, prior to reuse, clean and rinse lenses as above.

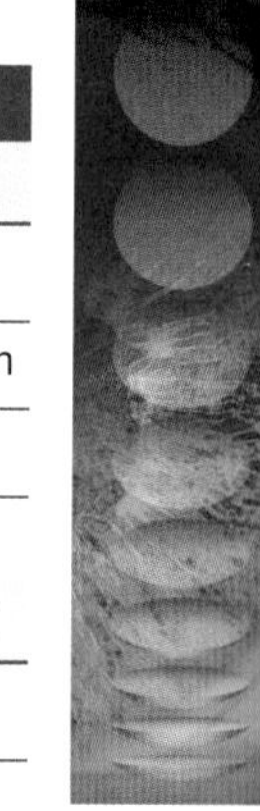

REDUCING STORAGE CASE CONTAMINATION

The frequency of storage case contamination in asymptomatic wearers suggests that the lens disinfection process alone, at least in the home environment, is not sufficient to maintain contamination-free cases. However, it is not clear how wearers should perform this task and there has been controversy in the literature in recommendations for case hygiene and the frequency of case disposal. Nonetheless, storage case contamination is reduced:

- With monthly storage case replacement.
- By the avoidance of contact with tap water.
- With the use of multipurpose or two-step peroxide care systems.

Daily lens storage case hygiene should include:

- Discarding the used solution.
- Rinsing with boiled, cooled water and air drying.

Weekly case hygiene should include:

- Scrubbing the case with lens care solution then disinfecting with either hydrogen peroxide or sodium hypochlorite for a minimum of 20 minutes followed by rinsing with sterile saline prior to reuse.

The manufacture of disposable storage cases may also reduce the frequency and level of microbial contamination (Larkin et al. 1990, Kanpolat et al. 1992).

Further information on disinfection procedures can be found at the websites listed in the footnote below.*

LENS DEPOSITS

Lens deposits may be adsorbed onto or absorbed into lens materials, regardless of type, although daily disposable lenses are discarded before any deposition can cause problems. However, acute deposit problems (e.g. an industrial issue such as embedded metallic particles) apply as much to daily disposable lenses as to conventional lenses. Table 4.5 shows the clinical classification of deposits.

Variables affecting lens deposition (after Franklin et al. 2001) include:

- Material water content and ionicity (especially protein deposition).
- Differences between wearers:
  - differences in protein adhesion (Keith et al. 2003).

Table 4.5: Lens deposit classification system (modified Rudko)

Class	Degree of deposit
I	Clean
II	Visible under oblique light when wet using 7× magnification
III	Visible when dry without special lighting, unaided eye
IV	Visible wet or dry with the unaided eye
Class	**Type of deposit**
C	Crystalline
G	Granular
F	Filmy
P	Plaque
D	Debris
Co	Coating
Class	**Extent of deposit**
a	0–25% of lens
b	26–50% of lens
c	51–75% of lens
d	76–100% of lens

Data from Hathaway & Lowther (1978).

- Differences within wearers:
  - differences of up to 30% in lipid levels between eyes (Franklin et al. 1991, 2001).
  - differences in protein adhesion (Keith et al. 2003).

Some of the more common lens deposits include the following.

CHALLENGES: ORGANIC

- Tear proteins.
- Lipids. Although having only limited solubility in water, some have greater solubility in the lens polymers themselves (Franklin et al. 2001). This means that the deposit may be both on and in the lens matrix. Lipid deposition is greatest with material containing vinyl pyrrolidone (Jones et al. 1997a, Franklin et al. 2001).
- Mucin.
- Other tear components.
- Discolorations.
- Finger-borne contaminants (skin lipids, dirt, microorganisms, other).
- Air-borne contaminants.

CHALLENGES: INORGANIC

- Metallic:
  - colours are often characteristic of the metal.
  - metal may corrode in situ (e.g. iron), leading to rust spots, pitting and deposit protrusion.
  - occupational/industrial.

* Relevant websites include the following:
(i) British College of Optometry: http://www.college-optometrists.org/membersarea/extranet/infection.pdf
(ii) Decontamination protocols for prions: http://www.who.int/topics/spongiform_encephalopathies_transmissible/en/
(iii) Procedures for hydrogel lenses: http://www.moh.gov.sg/cmaweb/attachments/publication/Contact_Lens_Care_Guidelines.pdf
(iv) Instrument disinfection: http://www. moh. gov.sg/cmaweb/attachments/publication/Contact_Lens_Care_Guidelines.pdf

- Non-metallic:
  - may be inactive (e.g. asbestos dust).
  - non-asbestos brake linings, disc-brake pad dust.
  - occupational/industrial.
- Clothing residues (lint).
- Discolorations (non-metallic).
- Accumulation of care products or their derivatives.
- Finger-borne contaminants.
- Air-borne contaminants.

Environmental issues include:

- Workplace location and activities.
- Residential location and environmental factors (e.g. proximity of residence to roadways, railways, factories, smoke-stacks, etc.).
- Commuting/travelling environment.

Time course of deposit formation

Spoilage of lenses by tear components, particularly lipids and proteins, is rapid (Franklin 1997). Largely because of its exposure to a 'resurfacing–evaporation–resurfacing' cycle, the lens front surface is more prone to deposits.

Leahy et al. (1990) reported that several proteins including lysozyme could be detected on some lenses after as little as 1 minute of wear. The complexities of the tear film and the eye's environment, as well as the nature of lens materials, probably make lens deposits unavoidable (Ilhan et al. 1998). Fowler and Allansmith (1980) observed that within 30 minutes of wear, approximately 50% of contact lens front surfaces were coated with ocular debris and mucus-like material. Eight hours of wear showed 90% coverage of a more complex nature that professional cleaning failed to remove completely. They concluded that, with further wear, coatings become more complex.

Not surprisingly, protein deposition increases with lens wear but the rate is more dependent on water content and ionicity than on intersubject differences.

Protein deposition: hydrogel lenses

Franklin et al. (1992) described protein deposits as discrete, elevated, film-like coatings that are thin, semi-opaque, white, and layered superficially. Their coverage varies in extent and ranges from small patches to complete coverage. Over time they grow increasingly hazy which reduces visual acuity progressively and increases rugosity. Hathaway and Lowther (1976) measured shorter tear film break-up time when deposition was greater and reported that albumin, in addition to lysozyme, was involved in protein deposits.

Heiler et al. (1991) found the distribution of protein on worn hydrogel lenses was FDA group-dependent, with ionic materials having significantly more protein deposited in the periphery than the central 'core', whereas non-ionic lenses had similar protein deposition all over. Tomlinson and Caroline (1990) recommended high-water-content, non-ionic lenses for heavy depositors.

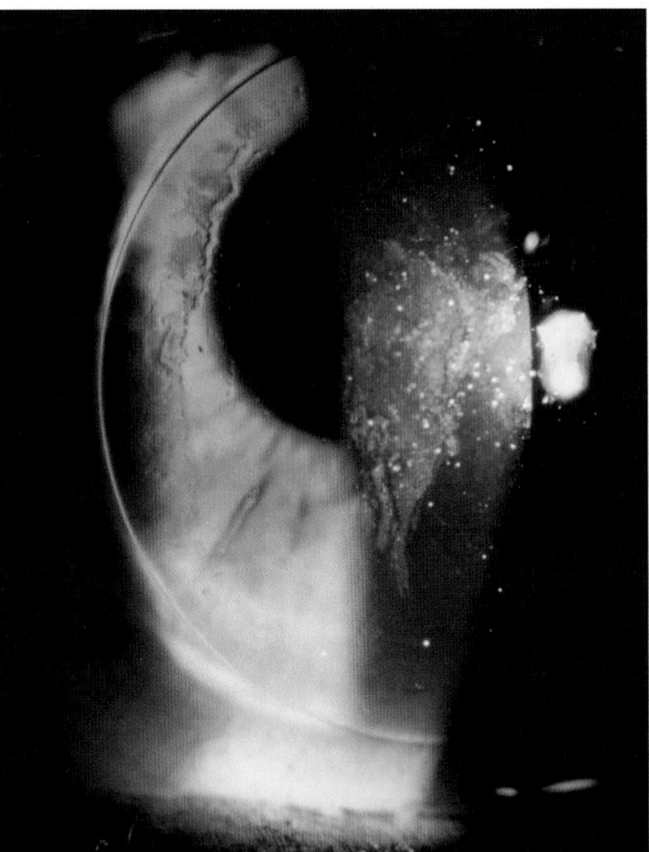

Figure 4.7 Lipid deposits on a rigid gas-permeable lens (Courtesy of D. Fonn)

Protein deposition: RGP lenses – material characteristics

RGP lens polymers are quite different despite having much chemistry and some formulation steps in common with hydrogels. Principally, they differ by having fewer charged sites and low matrix porosity. Their relatively neutral nature limits their water-binding potential and reduces the potential for some types of deposit, but they are not exempt from deposition/contamination.

RGP deposits take longer to appear and progress more slowly than on hydrogels. Generally, white spots do not appear because, although lipid deposits may occur on and in a lens matrix, an absence of calcium ions within the matrix precludes the formation of calcium–lipid complexes (alluded to by Hart 1984) necessary for white spot formation (Franklin et al. 2001) (Fig. 4.7).

Walker (1988) implicated a material's methacrylic acid content (greater in higher-Dk siloxane acrylates) in its deposit susceptibility.

Lenses, deposits, and microorganisms

Microorganisms that attach to lenses are not usually derived from the anterior eye, with most biological contaminants sourced from the fingers and inappropriate lens care regimens (Hart & Shih 1987) or from the lid margins (Hart et al. 1996).

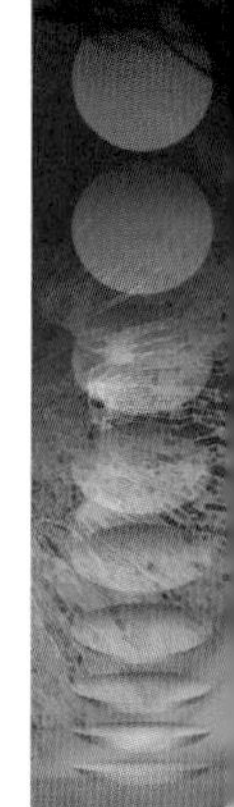

DEPOSITS AND MICROORGANISMS: BACTERIA

The frequency of corneal inflammation or infection increases for wearers of protein-deposited lenses (Keith et al. 2003), possibly because of increased adherence of microorganisms (e.g. *S. aureus*) to lenses with bound lysozyme deposits (Thakur et al. 1999), even after enzymatic protein treatment (Baines et al. 1990, and others).

DEPOSITS AND MICROORGANISMS: FUNGI

Fungal colonization of contact lenses is relatively uncommon (Wilhelmus et al. 1988). While not all wearers of contaminated lenses show signs of mycotic disease they reported ocular irritation traceable to their lenses (Berger & Streeten 1981).

Aspergillus sp., *Candida albicans, Fusarium* sp. and *Penicillium* sp. are the most common fungal lens contaminants, although *Candida* sp. is responsible for the majority of fungal infections (Wilhelmus et al. 1988).

DEPOSITS AND OCULAR REACTIONS

Patients' symptoms are not always related to lens deposition (Gellatly et al. 1988). Even with weekly replacement, hydrogel lenses can still trigger a contact lens-related papillary conjunctivitis (CLPC) response in some wearers, whereas RGP lenses, even in extended wear (EW), have a low incidence of CLPC (Grant et al. 1989). Minno et al. (1991) suggested that visual rating/classification scales need cautious application because of the poor correlation between the appearance of protein deposition and a subsequent assay of the total protein on a lens.

DEPOSITS: TYPES

Franklin et al. (2001) divided deposits into broad classes:

- *Discrete elevated deposits,* e.g. white spots (Fig. 4.8), variously described as jelly bumps, mulberry deposits (Pennington 1979), calcium deposits, calcium–lipid deposits and mucoprotein–lipid deposits. These deposits vary from clusters of small discrete white spots that are barely visible to the naked eye, to single, large, semi-translucent, very conspicuous, multifaceted (and probably multilayered) 'lumps' up to 1 mm or more in diameter. There is still no universal agreement on their chemistry. Fonn (1999) reported small, white, circular deposits on balafilcon A (silicone hydrogel) lenses similar to the jelly bumps and 'calcium deposits' seen on hydrogel lenses.
- *Lens coatings, surface films and plaques.* This category includes films of tear protein which are thin and semi-opaque to white in appearance (possibly thickness and protein-conformation dependent). They are layered and may affect vision. The 'lens' surface is rougher and this can increase lens movement in situ because of enhanced lid–lens interaction. Fonn (1999) reported reduced protein deposits with lotrafilcon A silicone hydrogels (compared to etafilcon A hydrogels), even though they were worn four times longer.
- *Lens discoloration.* This is relatively uncommon in modern practice. Generally, the combination of materials research and shorter lens-life expectations has seen most issues resolved. Most colours have been reported – yellow, orange, amber, brown, grey and pink (Stone et al. 1984) as well as blue and green (Franklin et al. 2001). Some are attributable to the combination of lens material and care regimen; for example, high water materials and thermal disinfection (Franklin & Tighe 1991) producing a yellow discoloration from denatured protein in and on the lens. However, colours such as pink and yellow occur in lenses that attract little protein, which must be attributed to care products and/or tear components other than proteins (Stone et al. 1984).

  Aetiological factors include calcium deposition, nicotine from cigarettes, metallic foreign bodies, selective absorption of preservatives (care products and ocular medications), dyes (e.g. from cosmetics), pigments (paints, artists' supplies) or other ambient chemical entities, skin contaminants, mucus and cells, microorganisms and eye drops containing phenylephrine or adrenaline (epinephrine) (Phillips 1976).

  Franklin and Tighe (1991) noted that, in yellow–brown discolorations, the lens' physical properties were often altered (e.g. a marked reduction in elasticity often accompanies yellow–brown discoloration).
- *Coloured microorganisms and fungi* colonize in and on the lens proper (as distinct from microorganisms and fungi residing opportunistically on, or in, lens defects only) (Fig. 4.9).

Bacterial colonies can cause discoloration or be coloured themselves, and may thwart attempts at eradication by collective behaviour such as the production of a glycocalyx or biofilm (a protective slime) over themselves as protection from the antimicrobials in lens care products. The protected organisms can re-emerge once the threat has passed. Slusher et al. (1987) investigated biofilms and demonstrated polysaccharide-mediated adhesion of *P. aeruginosa* and *Staphylococcus epidermidis* to extended wear soft lenses. Adherence must be an active process because killed or altered bacteria adhere less (John et al. 1989).

Acanthamoebae can encyst rapidly under unfavourable circumstances. In trophozoite form, they are susceptible to most disinfectants but once encysted they are only susceptible to heat, strong alcohol-based solutions, and solutions containing special anti-amoebic components.

Coloured or opaque fungi – for example, *Aspergillus niger* (dark brown) (Fig. 4.9a) and *C. albicans* (white translucent/opaque) (Fig. 4.9b) – are easily visible because the hyphae of the fungi can cover a significant area of a lens and/or they are strongly coloured. Such infestations are seen most commonly after extended storage in unpreserved or weakly preserved storage solution.

Although fungal and acanthamoebic infections of the eye are relatively uncommon, their effects can be devastating and their treatment difficult with a poor prognosis.

DEPOSITS AND COMFORT

Lever et al. (1995) found no correlation between total lens protein and patient comfort. They concluded that total lens-bound protein was not the sole or primary determinant of lens comfort or tolerance. However, Wardlaw and Sarver (1986) found that deposits generally decreased comfort even when they were not conspicuous.

(a)

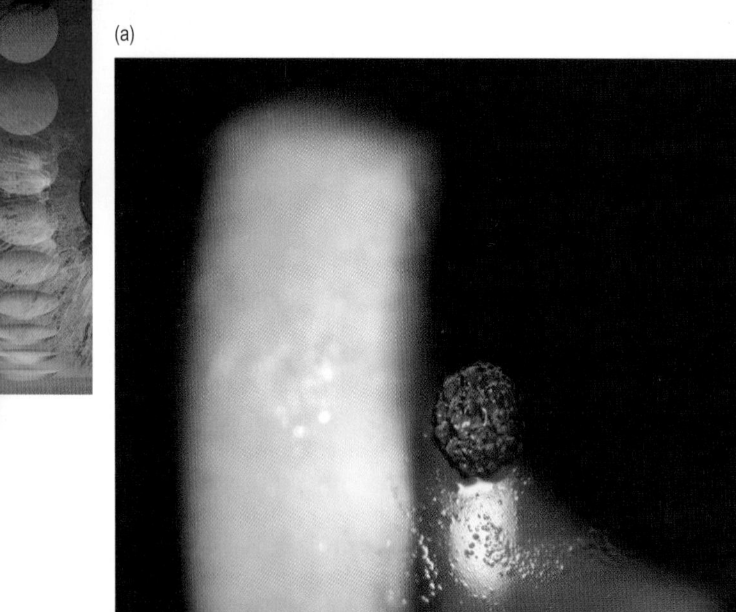

(b)

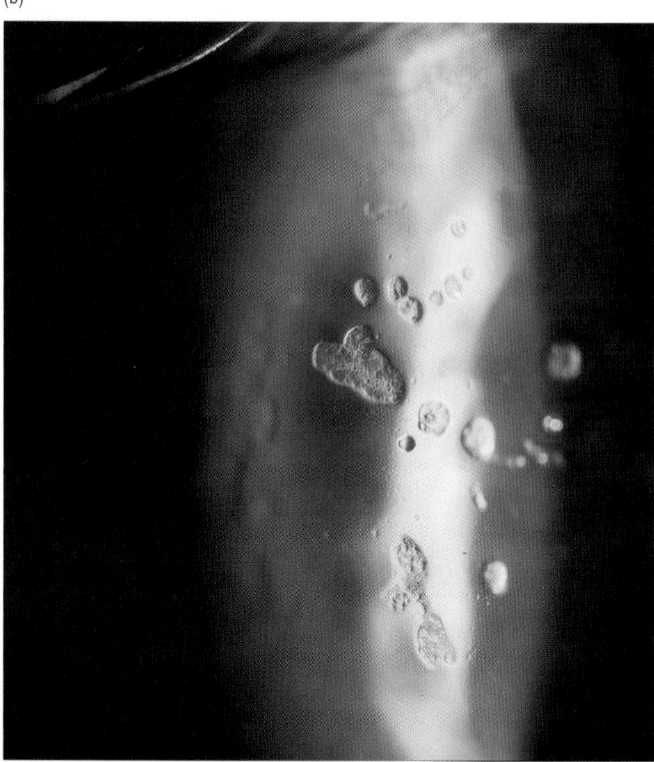

(c)

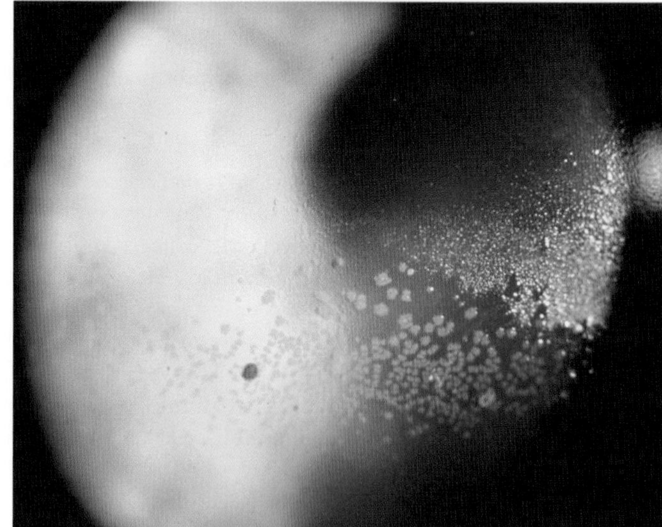

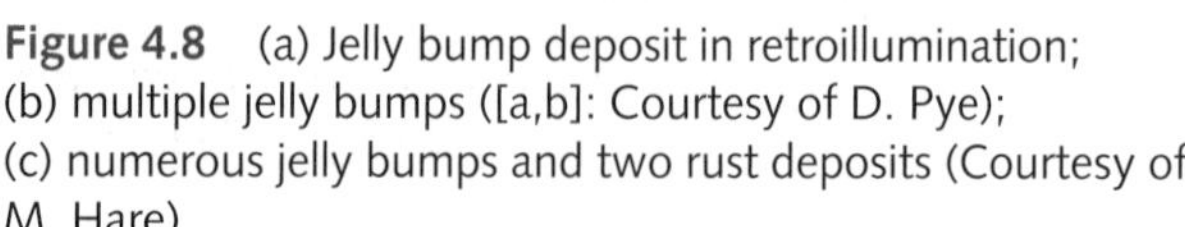

Figure 4.8 (a) Jelly bump deposit in retroillumination; (b) multiple jelly bumps ([a,b]: Courtesy of D. Pye); (c) numerous jelly bumps and two rust deposits (Courtesy of M. Hare)

THE HANDS

Barrier creams and cosmetics contain oils, fats, waxes, perfumes and colorants, and should be quarantined from lenses as completely as possible. A surfactant cleaner is the best method of cleaning lenses contaminated by cosmetics (Tighe et al. 1991).

Before touching their lenses, the wearer should wash their hands thoroughly with soap (liquid, gel or bar), paying particular attention to the fingernails, fingertips, the areas between the fingers, and the palms. To reduce the presence of lint and fluff, dry the hands with a towel that is as lint-free as possible (this excludes many paper products).

Where good hand hygiene is not possible due to ingrained contaminants (e.g. oil from car engines) or if the skin is rough, a no-rub solution is preferable. This can be a mechanical agitator (Fig. 4.10) and a no-rub solution or daily lens replacement.

PROTEIN DEPOSITS: REMOVAL – ENZYMATIC

Enzymatic protein removers are not completely effective in removing lens protein and even less effective against other types of lens deposits (Lowther 1977). Only about 75% of adherent tear protein is removed by enzymatic cleaners and that is replaced rapidly (Baines et al. 1990). Begley et al. (1990) found the three

(a)

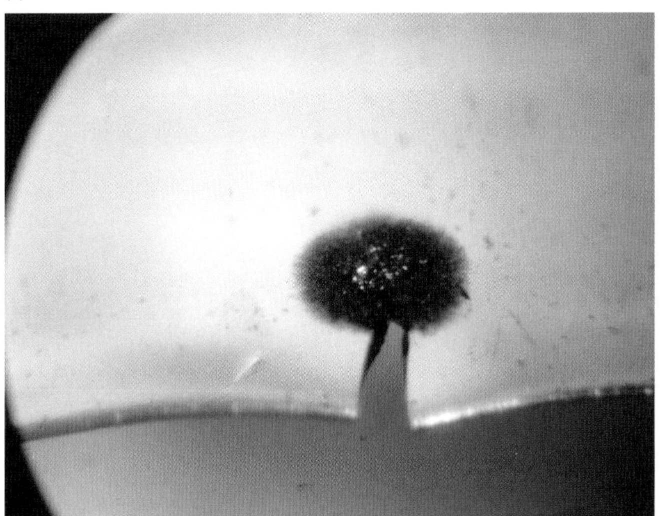

(b)

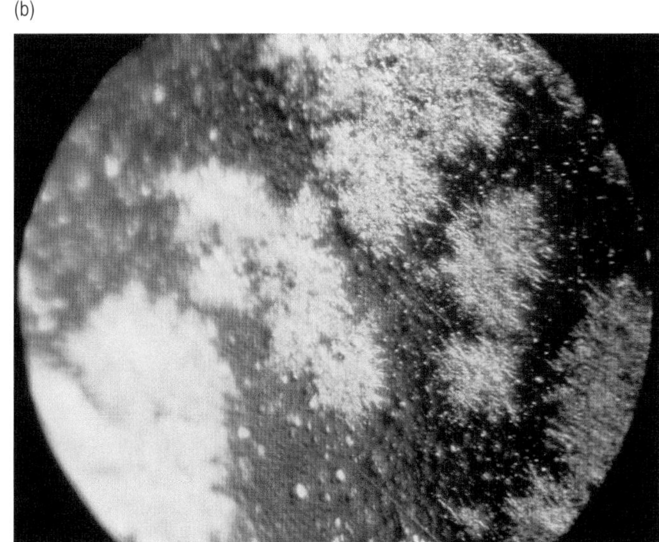

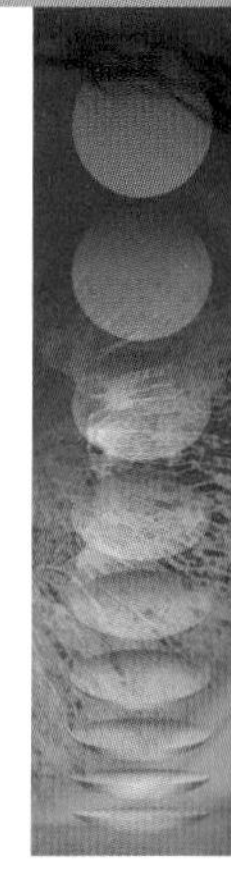

Figure 4.9 (a) Coloured fungus (*Aspergillus niger*) colonizing a soft contact lens edge defect. (b) White fungus (*Candida albicans*) colonizing the anterior surface of a soft lens (Courtesy of M. Hare)

enzymes, papain, pancreatin and subtilisin, to be statistically equally effective but the rate of protein deposit replacement was dependent on the enzyme used (pancreatin use appeared to result in a reduced deposit replacement rate).

Protein is usually removed with proteolytic enzymes (proteases), most notably papain (a cysteine protease from the papaya plant *Carica papaya,* Caricaceae) and subtilisin (a serine protease or carbonyl hydrolase from the bacterium *Bacillus subtilis* (or *Bacillus lichenformis*) (Begley et al. 1990).

Nowadays, lenses are usually discarded before deposits become clinically significant. Dave and Patel (1999) concluded that an enzymatic cleaner should be used with multipurpose solutions (MPSs) when lenses are used for more than 1 month.

Generally, in vivo, proteases catalyze the hydrolysis of certain proteins and peptide amines (Clarke 2004), thereby rendering them soluble or more soluble. Both cysteine and serine proteases do this by cleaving peptide bonds (actually the disulphide bonds) within their target proteins, transforming them into smaller molecular weight proteins making them more readily removable with rubbing and rinsing.

Partial removal of deposited proteins (exposure too short or product incapable of removing the full spectrum of proteins present) leaves an altered lens matrix and surface (Franklin et al. 2001) which could induce:

- Discomfort.
- Further deposition.
- Altered wettability.
- Tear film irregularity.

Other enzymes targeting proteins, lipids and mucins include:

- Pancreatin, a plant or animal pancreatic enzyme with properties of a lipase, protease and amylase. Note: pancreatin is often a porcine derivative and the use of such products is prohibited by some religions.
- Amylase, targeting carbohydrates.
- Lipases, targeting fats and lipids.
- Pronase, a mixture of endo- and exo-proteinases that are capable of cleaving almost any peptide bond.

RGP lens daily cleaners that contain a proteolytic enzyme (pancreatin) are also available (e.g. Optifree® Supra Clens™).

PROTEIN DEPOSITS: REMOVAL – NON-ENZYMATIC

Non-enzymatic products can assist in the removal of deposits. These include:

- Protein:
  - citrate (Lebow & Schachet 2003).
  - Hydranate® (Pederson 1999).
- Lipids:
  - surfactants (Pederson 1999).
  - alcohol-based cleaners.

For RGP lenses, Menicon Progent is a two-solution product that targets deposits and protein. Progent's solutions contain sodium hypochlorite (Part A – useful against bovine spongiform encephalopathy [BSE]) and potassium bromide (Part B).

LENS CARE PROCEDURES

Cleaning

Rubbing and rinsing a lens is important for successful wear (Sibley 1988) as it minimizes microbial load and long-term surface deposition, both of which can reduce disinfection efficacy (Tonge et al. 2001a) especially with heavy lipid deposition (Franklin et al. 2001) (see 'Cleaners: MPSs' below).

LENS CLEANING: PURPOSES

- To loosen (or solubilize) and subsequently assist in the

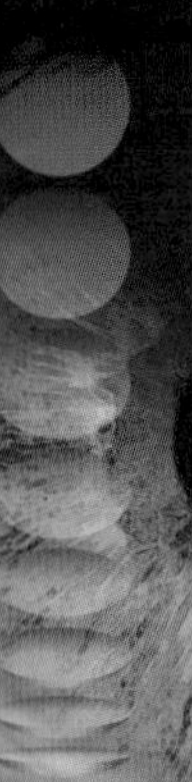

(a)

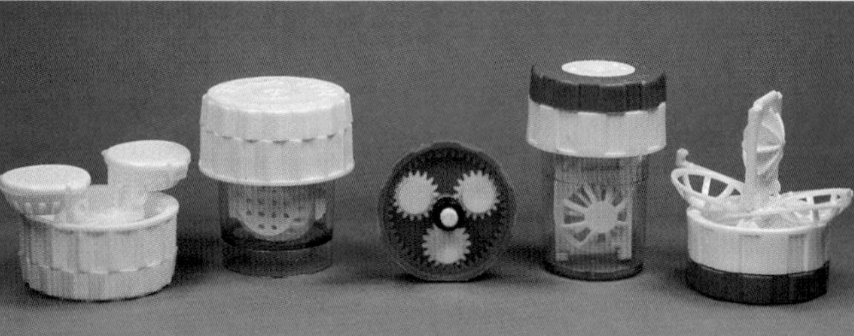

(b)

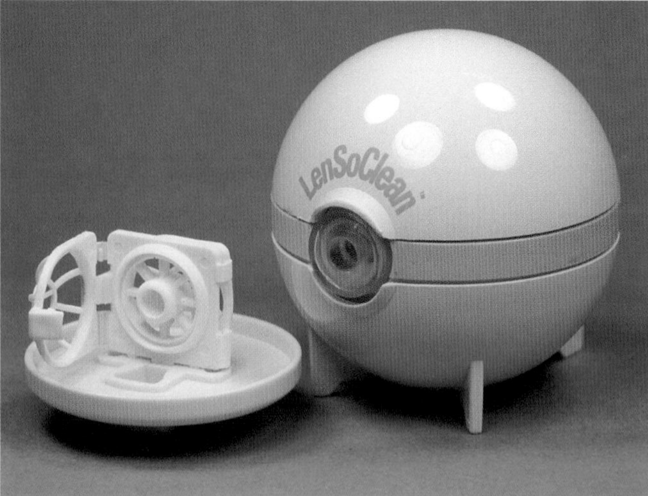

(c)

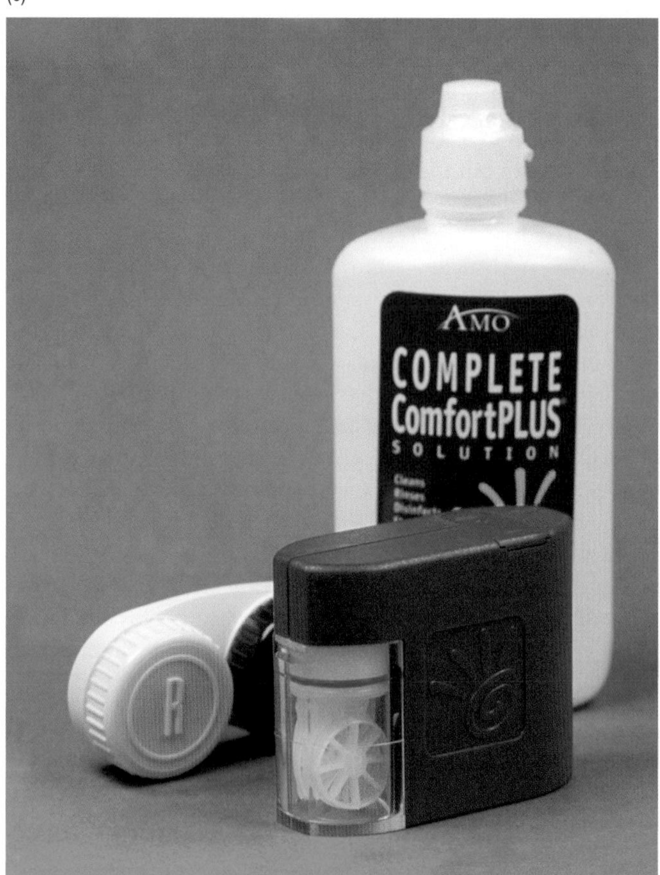

Figure 4.10 (a) Planetary-geared swishers; (b) LenSoClean™; (c) Complete® RapidCare™

removal of all lens contaminants (including deposits) bound to or located on the lens surface.

- To kill and remove the majority of microorganisms residing on a lens in preparation for disinfection, thereby increasing the disinfectant's 'margin of safety'.

Surfactant cleaners, single-purpose disinfectants, MPSs and enzymatic cleaners have at least some cleaning capability (Franklin et al. 2001).

For a solution to wet a lens, its surface tension must be lower than that of the lens. Traditionally, a surfactant is used to lower the solution surface tension by altering the interactions between its surface molecules (Fig. 4.11). Surfactants are compounds whose molecules have a longer, non-polar, hydrophobic, hydrocarbon tail and shorter, polar, hydrophilic head (Fig. 4.12).

For cleaners to be effective, they need to 'solubilize' rather than simply 'dissolve' lens contaminants. Taking oil as an example, oil tends to break up into small droplets and disperse. The hydrophobic tails of the surfactant's molecules attach to, and ultimately surround the oil, forming a 'micelle' (see Fig. 4.12), i.e. a sphere with the 'captive' oil at its centre. Once the critical micelle concentration (CMC) of the surfactant has been reached, micelles can form spontaneously as surfactant molecules start to associate with one another. Micelles and their surfactants are dynamic, and surfactant molecules join and leave constantly. The hydrophilic heads of the surfactant face the watery surround and, because they are polar, interact or disrupt the water's local network of hydrogen bonds, thereby reducing the water's cohesive forces. Because of their polar nature, they also repel one another and once an oil droplet is surrounded by a monolayer of surfactant, coalescence of oil is prevented by surfactant mutual repulsion. In this way, the oil is held in solution although *suspension* may be a more appropriate description.

Polymeric beads (e.g. polyamide in Alcon's Polyclens® [Opticlean®]) in a cleaner act as both a safe 'abrasive' (confirmed by Phillips & Czigler 1985) targeting protein deposits, and a normal cleaner, eliminating the need for regular protein removal (Stein & Harrison 1983). However, Reindel et al. (1989) reported no performance differences between alcohol-based, particulate-containing and 'conventional' cleaners, although the alcohol-based product removed protein less effectively from Group II lenses.

Simmons et al. (1996) found that cleaning lenses immediately after removal was more efficacious than cleaning after overnight disinfection. The authors attributed the differences to lens contaminants added during lens handling *after* disinfection.

CLEANERS: MPSs

MPSs are generally designed to clean, rinse, disinfect, rehydrate and store.

They usually contain (Franklin 1997):

- Antimicrobial agents, usually large-molecule, polymeric disinfectants not intended to enter the lens matrix.

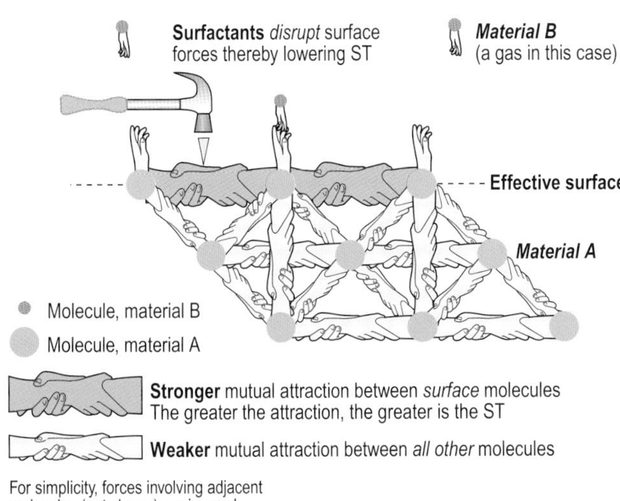

Figure 4.11 Surface tension (ST) and the effect of surfactant

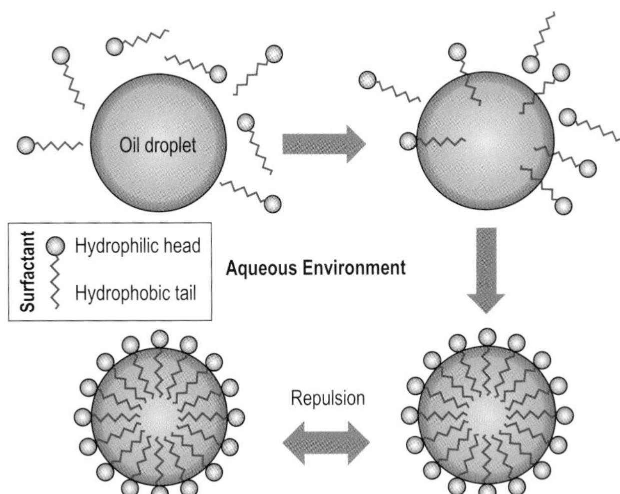

Figure 4.12 Surfactants and micelle formation

- Surfactant (especially if employed as a one-bottle solution [OBS]).
- Buffer system.

Products containing surfactants performed better at removing lipids if used in a soaking solution. Franklin (1997) concluded that the rub and rinse steps were still vital. Several MPSs now include more or different surfactants to enhance lens cleaning when the rub and rinse step is omitted (see below).

Rinsing

Normal saline (0.9%) for rinsing can be either preserved (for repeated use) or unpreserved (single-dose packaging or aerosol). The dangers of using multi-use unpreserved saline are highlighted periodically by reports of eyes or vision lost to microbial keratitis (especially *Acanthamoeba* keratitis) resulting from solution contamination.

Various authors investigated bulk saline (Jenkins & Phillips 1986, Phillips & Copley 1990, Sweeney et al. 1992, 1999) and reported the following:

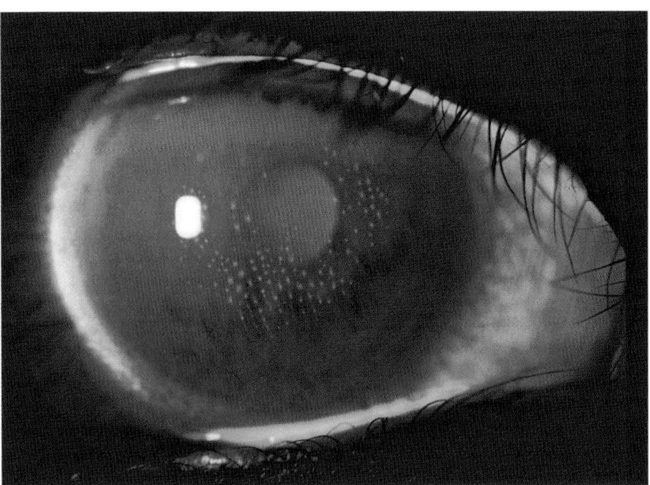

Figure 4.13 Dimple veiling caused by inserting an RGP lens using aerosol saline (nitrogen propellant)

- Unpreserved saline could become heavily contaminated (predominantly by Gram-negative bacteria) after 1 week.
- 35% of unpreserved saline was contaminated within 2 weeks of use (even when all sensible precautions were taken).
- 55–100% of unpreserved salines were contaminated by 4–6 weeks.
- Borate-buffered saline containing EDTA showed a lower incidence of contamination (6% over 1 month).
- Preserved salines also became contaminated with Gram-positive bacteria (Gram-negative in unpreserved salines).
- Bulk unpreserved saline should be removed from the market.
- Use aerosol saline as a preinsertion rinse with caution because bubbles of the propellant (usually nitrogen) can cause dimple veiling (Fig. 4.13).

Disinfection

Historically, PMMA lenses were disinfected with solutions containing benzalkonium chloride (BAK) introduced as far back as 1947 (Anger & Currie 1995). Early soft lens disinfection was with heat, a cold chemical system based on either chlorhexidine gluconate (CHX), povidone iodine or a quaternary ammonium compound (QAC) (Hind 1979), or selected varieties of pharmacy-grade hydrogen peroxide. The evolution of higher-water-content soft lenses necessitated the development of non-thermal disinfectants because repeated heating altered their materials and/or parameters, irreversibly.

There are different types of disinfecting system:

- Heat.
- Chemical:
  - hydrogen peroxide (H_2O_2).
  - other chemical.

DISINFECTION: HEAT

Heat is the most effective disinfection method (Thompson & Mansell 1976, Anger & Currie 1995). In 1988, CLAO recom-

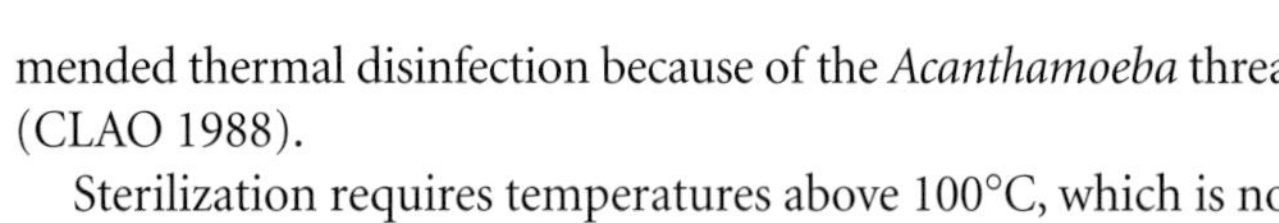

mended thermal disinfection because of the *Acanthamoeba* threat (CLAO 1988).

Sterilization requires temperatures above 100°C, which is not possible without special equipment. However, for disinfection, temperatures between 70° and 80°C for at least 5 minutes are adequate (Dallos & Hughes 1972, Luibinas et al. 1987, Sibley 1988). The combination of lower temperature and shorter duration also reduces protein denaturation.

Despite simplicity, speed, economy and lens disposability, thermal disinfection is rarely used now, as it is not convenient.

As most RGP materials (and PMMA) are thermoplastics, i.e. they soften at elevated temperatures, thermal disinfection is not used for rigid lens disinfection.

Microwave heating

Hiti et al. (2001) showed microwave ovens to be effective against *Acanthamoeba* (trophozoite and encysted forms) in as little as 3 minutes. At 10% output, they were effective against bacteria in 15 minutes (Kastl & Maehara 2001) with minimal effects except with high-water or tinted lenses (Harris et al. 1990, Crabbe & Thompson 2001a,b).

Using a no-rub MPS (ReNu® Multipurpose Solution), Crabbe and Thompson (2004) reported flocculation of solution components and foaming, leading to loss of solution, but concluded that lenses could be disinfected in 10–15 seconds, provided surfactants were avoided.

DISINFECTION: CHEMICAL – HYDROGEN PEROXIDE

Neutralization of peroxide produces safe by-products (water and oxygen). However, the need for neutralization and the unpleasant effects of unneutralized peroxide applied to the eye have reduced its popularity.

Peroxide concentrations vary from 0.6 to 3% but, with surfactant cleaning, only 1.5% is required for disinfection (Stokes & Morton 1987).

To enhance shelf-life, and to preclude the possibility of significant decomposition both before and after opening, a stabilizer is normally incorporated.

Hydrogen peroxide – neutralization

Hydrogen peroxide neutralization can be complex because of the pH of the neutralized solution and its osmolality. If the pH is outside the cornea's comfort range of 6.6–7.8 (Harris et al. 1988), abnormal lens fitting behaviour and/or significant discomfort can ensue. In multistep systems, solution parameters can be restored by including pH and osmolality-modifying agents in the neutralizer.

In one-step systems, either the peroxide must be supplied with the parameters preset (e.g. AOSept®) or the neutralizing system must restore the parameters of the peroxide (e.g. Omnicare or UltraCare®) (Fig. 4.14).

'Neutralization' can be achieved by any of the following:

- *Serial dilution*: The peroxide-soaked lens is rinsed repeatedly with saline and stored in saline for a minimum time to elute residual peroxide from the lens, although some traces remain.

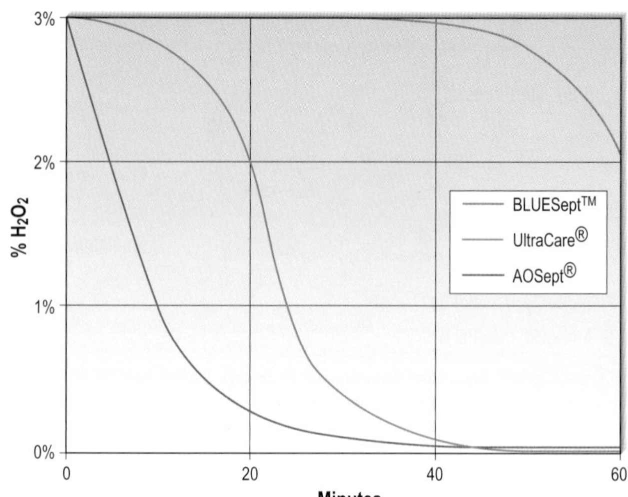

Figure 4.14 Hydrogen peroxide neutralization curves – one-step systems

- *pH shifting*: Sodium bicarbonate is used to raise the pH to 7.8–8.0. Peroxide is less stable and decomposes slowly (Thomas 1972): $2H_2O_2 \rightarrow 2H_2O + O_2\uparrow$.
- *Stoichiometric*: By a simple chemical reaction, hydrogen peroxide can be altered into compounds inherently non-threatening. For example:
  - *sodium pyruvate* ($NaC_3H_3O_3$) and peroxide produce water, carbon dioxide (dissolves in water), and sodium acetate: $NaC_3H_3O_3 + H_2O_2 \rightarrow NaC_2H_3O_2 + H_2O + CO_2$.
  - *sodium sulphite* (Na_2SO_3): $Na_2SO_3 + H_2O_2 \rightarrow Na_2SO_4 + H_2O$.
  - *sodium thiosulphate* ($Na_2S_2O_3$) (Ogunbiyi 1986): $2Na_2S_2O_3 + H_2O_2 \rightarrow Na_2H_2S_4O_6 + 2NaOH$ (i.e. sodium tetrathionate and sodium hydroxide; while the latter is known to be deleterious to the eye, the quantity produced is inconsequential. Hydrochloric acid and sodium hydroxide are both used in small quantities to adjust the pH of many ophthalmic products).
- *Catalytic decomposition*: In the presence of a suitable catalyst, hydrogen peroxide decomposes into water and oxygen, the latter given off as a gas, sometimes vigorously: $2H_2O_2 \rightarrow 2H_2O + O_2\uparrow$. Suitable catalysts are heavy metals (e.g. platinum or palladium) or biological catalysts such as catalase derived from a plant, animal or microorganism.
- *Indication of neutralization*: To avoid omitting the neutralizer tablet from their one-step system, AMO include vitamin B12 which turns pink when neutralization has been achieved. Similarly, BLUEvision™/BLUEsept™ use a blue solution. With two-step systems, Jones et al. (1993) recommended overnight neutralization rather than overnight disinfection.

Hydrogen peroxide disinfection – lens case considerations

Peroxide neutralization may release oxygen vigorously, so cases must be vented. Venting must be 'one-way', i.e. the oxygen must escape without lens contaminants, especially microorganisms, entering the case.

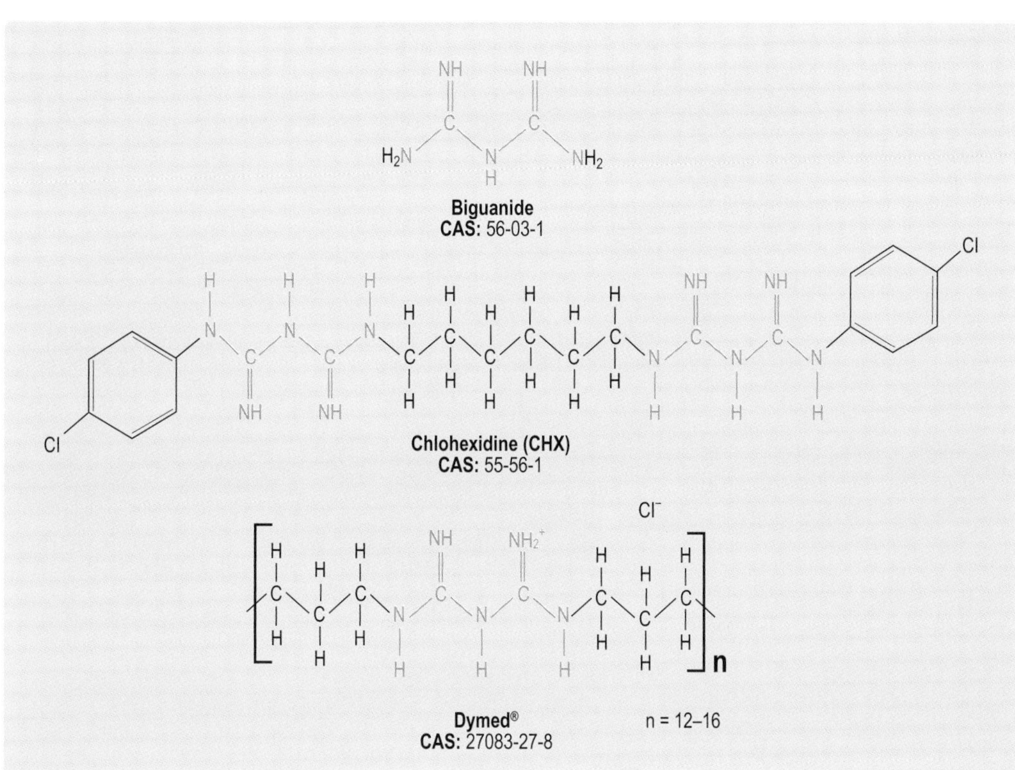

Figure 4.15 Structures of relevant biguanides including PHX (Dymed®)

Hydrogen peroxide disinfectants – effect on lens tints

Despite being a strong inorganic oxidizing agent, hydrogen peroxide, especially in one-step systems, has no significant effect on common lens tints (reactive or vat dyes) (Janoff 1988, Gentsch & Edrington 1990).

Hydrogen peroxide-like systems

Advanced Eyecare Research's Regard™ have produced a disinfection system using a combination of sodium chlorite ($NaClO_2$; used to disinfect mains water) and trace amounts (100 ppm) of hydrogen peroxide (Atkins 2004). The peroxide stabilizes the inherently unstable chlorine dioxide (ClO_2) generated and the combination is said to be effective against Gram-positive and Gram-negative bacteria, fungi and yeasts. Decomposition products are sodium chloride, water and oxygen.

When lenses are removed from solution, the residual sodium chlorite decomposes readily into sodium chloride and oxygen. No peroxide neutralization per se is needed and the residual peroxide (up to 100 ppm) is non-irritating to the anterior eye.

DISINFECTION: CHEMICAL – NON-PEROXIDE SYSTEMS

Biguanides

The first biguanide used was chlorhexidine (CHX) (Fig. 4.15) (Thomas 1972). Biguanides are available in several forms.

Polymeric biguanides – PHMB, PAPB, polyhexanide (PHX) (Fig. 4.15)

Trade names of various relevant polihexanides include:

- Cosmocil CQ (originally ICI Ltd. now Arch Chemicals Inc.).
- Arlagard E (Larkin et al. 1992).
- Vantocil IB or TG (Arch Chemicals Inc.).
- Baquacil (Arch Chemicals Inc.).
- Polyhexanide.
- Dymed® (Bausch & Lomb).
- Trischem™ (AMO's description of PHX combined with a tris buffer system (tris[hydroxymethyl] aminomethane) (Tonge et al. 2001a).

Polihexanide (PHX) properties include:

- Fast acting, broad spectrum antimicrobial.
- Good fungicide.
- Variable virucide.
- Good Gram-negative (e.g. *Pseudomonas* spp.) biocide.
- Broad range of pHs (4–10).
- Stable (>2 years).
- Heat stable to >140°C (autoclavable).
- Odourless, clear, colourless, non-foaming.
- Miscible with water in all proportions.
- Incompatible with chloride, calcium and magnesium ions.

Applications range from preservation of cosmetics and lens care products to swimming pool maintenance. PHX (0.02%) has been successful in the treatment of the encysted form of *Acanthamoeba* keratitis (Larkin et al. 1992).

PHXs share their hexamethylene-biguanide repeating molecular unit with CHX, have a molecular weight approximately four times that of CHX, and can be used in concentrations 20–25 times less than CHX (Meakin 1989).

The main differences in PHX-containing products are the concentrations of PHX (greater in RGP care products) and the combination with antimicrobial enhancers, buffers and surfactants (Tonge et al. 2001a).

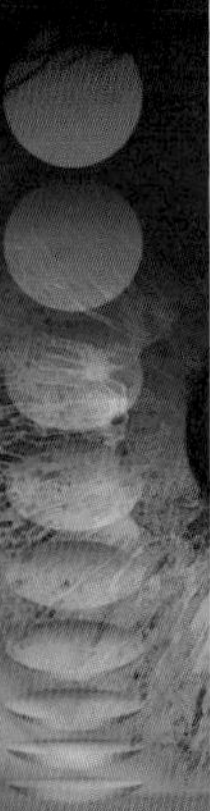

Figure 4.16 Structure of PQ-1 (Polyquad®)

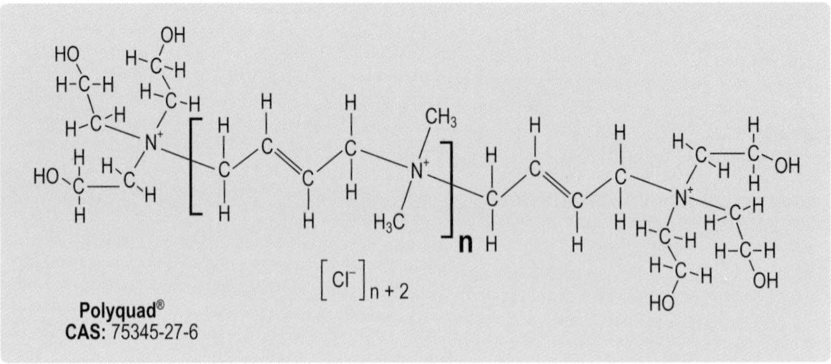

Polyquad®
CAS: 75345-27-6

Jones et al. (1997b) reported that higher concentrations of PHX reduced comfort and produced more corneal staining in users of Group II and IV (high-water) lenses.

Quaternary ammonium compounds (QACs)

QACs were first released commercially circa 1935 (Russell 2002). An early example of this class of antimicrobials is BAK, often employed for its antifungal properties. Anionic (–ve) detergents can interact with cationic (+ve) preservatives such as BAK (and other QACs, e.g. cetyl-pyridium chloride) and such a combination needs to be avoided if maximum efficacy is to be realized.

Wong et al. (1986, of Allergan) reported that siloxane acrylate lenses did not accumulate significant amounts of BAK from RGP care products. However, Iwamoto et al. (1993) reported BAK-caused surface deterioration in RGP lenses due to the formation of benzyl methacrylate, greater with higher Dk materials. Iwamoto et al. concluded that BAK should not be used with RGP lenses.

Polymeric QACs

Long-chain QACs have good antibacterial activity, the most common being polyquaternium-1 (PQ-1) (e.g. Polyquad®). Its molecule is larger than that of PHXs (molecular weight 1200–3100 versus 900–1600 with a chain length of 22.5 nm). However, it is a less potent antimicrobial than PHX and consequently is used in higher concentrations (Fig. 4.16) (Tonge et al. 2001a).

Polixetonium chloride

Polixetonium chloride is a water-soluble, cationic polymer used in RGP solutions (e.g. AMO's Total Care®). It is a copolymer of ethylene oxide (itself a disinfectant) and dimethyl ethylene amine, combined in a ratio of 1:2, respectively. Like PHX, it is used as a swimming pool disinfectant and algistat. Its molecular weight is 3500 with a small molecule size of 18.1 nm. It appears to be more effective against moulds than PQ-1 (Tonge et al. 2001a).

Chlorine

Chlorine-based disinfection systems, based on sodium dichloroisocyanurate (stabilized halane, Softab™) or *p*-(dichlorosulfamoyl) benzoic acid (stabilized halazone, Aerotab™), produced relatively high rates of infection, even when used according to manufacturers' instructions (Stapleton et al. 1993). They are not currently available.

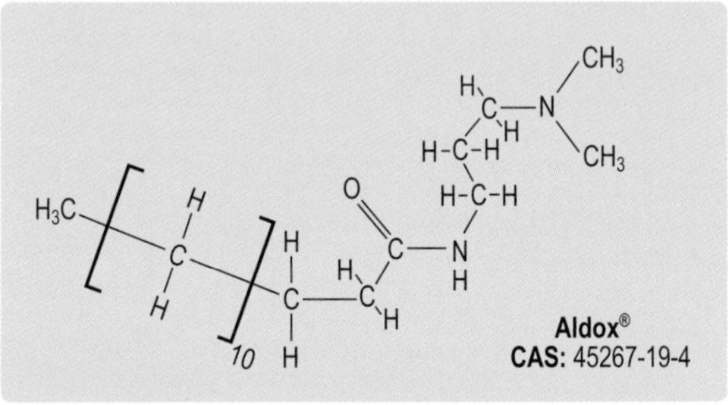

Aldox®
CAS: 45267-19-4

Figure 4.17 Structure of MAPD (Aldox®)

DISINFECTANTS: EXCIPIENTS THAT ENHANCE ANTIMICROBIAL ACTIONS

Because many polymeric antimicrobials have relatively weak actions against fungi (yeasts and moulds), they are used in combination with other solution excipients that enhance the solution's overall antimicrobial efficacy.

- *EDTA*: A sequestering and chelating agent and water softener. Although not regarded as a 'disinfectant' per se it is often described as a preservative enhancer (see below).
- *Boric acid* enhances the efficacy of polymeric antimicrobials, thereby reducing the necessary quantities of other antimicrobials (Tonge et al. 2001a).
- *Ethanol*: Promotes activity against cell walls in certain viral groups.
- *Isopropyl alcohol.*
- *Myristamidopropyl dimethyl amine* (MAPD) or Aldox®: An anti-acanthamoebal and antifungal additive in several of Alcon's MPSs used in combination with PQ-1 (Polyquad®) against *Acanthamoeba* sp. (see 'Disinfectant efficacy' below) (Fig. 4.17).
- *Hexetidine*: This propamidine-type agent (similar to that used in Brolene™ eye drops) is used in low concentrations (e.g. 0.000025%) in combination with EDTA (0.05–0.065%) in OSI's Concerto™ Soft Multi-Function. Its low molecular weight makes it accumulate within lenses over time (Tonge et al. 2001a).

MPS FORMULATIONS: SPECIAL CONSIDERATIONS

Both PHX and PQ-1 adhere to negatively charged (anionic) sites on hydrogel lens surfaces, leading potentially to lens

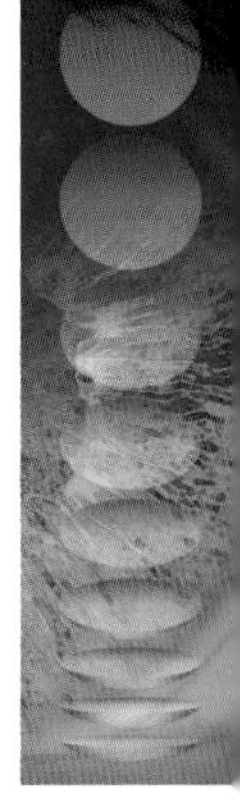

wettability issues. To address these, additional solution excipients are incorporated including the following:

- Chelating agents, buffers or surfactants that either compete for the charged lens surface sites (e.g. the Trischem™ system in AMO's Complete® MPS) or bind to the charged sites on the antimicrobial polymer, thereby preventing it from adhering to the lens (e.g. the citrate buffer system in Alcon's Optifree®).
- In Optifree® *EXPRESS*®, the highly negatively charged citrate buffer system interacts with the positively charged PQ-1 disinfectant to form a loose complex that prevents or reduces uptake by lenses. Similarly, the solution's poloxamine forms a loose complex with MAPD preventing the latter's uptake by the lens (Ewbank 2000). Furthermore, negatively charged groups on the citrate molecules may also bind to positively charged tear proteins such as lysozyme and lactoferrin, facilitating their removal.
- Bausch & Lomb's ReNu® MultiPlus® product incorporates Hydranate® to aid protein removal but does not affect lipid removal because their hydrophobic nature requires a surfactant to solubilize them (Tonge et al. 2001a).
- To address the problems of lipids, manufacturers of MPSs include high-molecular-weight (e.g. 12,600 or larger) non-ionic surfactants that are usually block copolymers of poly(ethylene oxide) and poly(propylene oxide) known as poloxamers (also a trade name – Poloxamer™), a family of products differentiated by a number (e.g. Poloxamer 407, average molecular weight: 12,500), or polyethylene-polypropylene glycol, or poloxamines. These high-molecular-weight surfactants are reputedly non-irritating because they cannot cross the corneal glycocalyx readily and stimulate corneal nerve endings (Tonge et al. 2001a).
- CIBA Vision uses the Tri-Klens™ combination (EDTA, a phosphate buffer system, and Poloxamer™ 407 that targets proteinaceous lens deposits) in their Solo-care® 10 Minute MPS. EDTA and the phosphate buffer work together to break the calcium bridges between protein deposit and lens (see Hydranate's description earlier) while Poloxamer™ 407 surfactant dislodges the now 'undocked' protein, thereby facilitating its dissolution and removal.
- Lubricating agents such as hydroxypropyl methylcellulose (HPMC) are used in Bausch & Lomb's and AMO's MPSs as an aid to on-eye comfort (Tonge et al. 2001a).
- To enhance the comfort of MPSs, artificial tear lubricants (e.g. methyl cellulose and related entities) can be added (Donshik et al. 2000).
- Generally, MPSs contain high molecular weight (MW) surfactants (e.g. poloxamers/poloxamines) because they have a lower potential to cause discomfort by crossing the corneal glycocalyx and stimulating the free nerve endings within the cornea. Complete® ComfortPLUS contains a high molecular weight surfactant (Christie 1999).

EXPERIMENTAL CARE PRODUCTS

Evans et al. (1993) demonstrated that experimental eyedrops containing bendazac lysine (a non-steroidal anti-inflammatory drug) inhibited protein deposition on conventional hydrogel lenses. A product incorporating bendazac lysine has been released (Bausch & Lomb Preservative Free Lubricating and Rewetting Drops).

OTHER FACTORS THAT AFFECT ANTIMICROBIAL EFFICACY

Anything that attracts, binds to, or alters an antimicrobial affects its function. Mucus binds readily to preservatives/disinfectants (Christie 1999), thereby decreasing overall efficacy. Ionic preservatives/disinfectants are unsuitable because of their potential to bind to ionic lenses. Moreover, bound antimicrobials also pose a threat to the lens-wearing eyes by their increased presence on lenses.

EDTA

EDTA's antibacterial activity is believed to be due to its ability to remove metal ions such as calcium and magnesium from bacterial cell surfaces (Pinney 1976).

ALCOHOL

Alcohol probably affects the lipids of cell membranes. Alcohols can also dehydrate cells along a concentration gradient. Both mechanisms can alter or kill living cells.

HYDROGEN PEROXIDE

The efficacy of hydrogen peroxide depends on its concentration, pH, presence of catalysts (intentional and unintentional), temperature and exposure times.

Penley et al. (1985) concluded that if cleaning were omitted, at least 45 minutes was needed in 3% hydrogen peroxide to kill several types of fungus (most bacteria required less than 5 minutes) and recommended 1 hour to cover the worst cases.

After comparing thermal and peroxide disinfection, Hara et al. (1989) found no positive cultures from either group but fewer adverse clinical signs in the peroxide group.

Közer-Bilgin et al. (1993) studied a disc-based, one-step peroxide system (AOSept) and found only a 55% kill rate of *P. aeruginosa*.

Tachikawa et al. (1991) and Hiti et al. (2004) showed that 3% one-step peroxide was ineffective against the encysted form of *Acanthamoeba* spp. but if a chitin or cellulose-decomposing enzyme, such as lysozyme, was added, peroxide killed all encysted forms of *Acanthamoeba* within 30 minutes (Izumi et al. 1991).

Unneutralized peroxide at 0.6% concentration (e.g. two-step Titmus H202, CIBA Vision) is more efficacious against encysted *Acanthamoeba* than either a 3% one-step system (Oxysept® Comfort) or a PHX containing RGP solution (Meni Care Plus) (Hiti et al. 2002). However, Beattie et al. (2002) expressed concern about low peroxide concentrations because of the ability of co-contaminating bacteria to produce catalases to reduce it to potentially unsafe levels. For better compliance, they recommended 3% peroxide or an MPS, and a 'no *Acanthamoeba*' approach to lens care, i.e. no tap water at any point in a regimen,

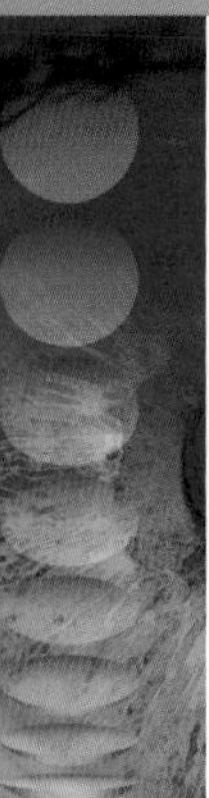

the use of only sterile solutions, and monthly lens case replacement.

Using a worst-case scenario, Grant (1988) rated overnight peroxide disinfection as having the greatest safety factors. Factors <1 were considered unsafe:

- Hydrogen peroxide 3%: overnight – 12.2, 20 minutes – 0.7, 10 minutes – 0.3.
- Hydrogen peroxide 0.6%: overnight – 3.1.
- CHX/EDTA/thiomersal: 0.2.

Disinfectant efficacy

PHX

Lambert et al. (1999) used the ISO/CD and FDA guidance documents to show that the stand-alone criteria were exceeded within 10 minutes of exposure with a PHX-based, 10-minute care system (Solo-care® 10 Minute). However, Noble et al. (2002) found that CHX was more effective against *Acanthamoeba* spp. than PHX.

POLYQUATERNIUM-1 WITH MAPD

Rosenthal et al. (1999, 2000) of Alcon challenged Optifree® *EXPRESS*® containing MAPD (Aldox®) with Gram-positive and -negative bacteria, yeasts, moulds and *Acanthamoeba* spp., and found it to be effective even when used non-compliantly.

Codling et al. (2003) and others studied the modes of action of PQ-1 and MAPD on encysted and trophozoite forms of *Acanthamoeba castellanii* and *Acanthamoeba fumigatus*, *C. albicans*, *P. aeruginosa*, *S. marcescens*, and *S. aureus* and found that PQ-1 behaved mainly as an antibacterial whereas MAPD was active against all of the test organisms, particularly fungi.

Wetting/conditioning solutions

The term 'conditioning' solution is used to describe a combined disinfecting, storing, wetting and hydrating solution for RGP lenses.

The roles of wetting solutions include:

- Enveloping the lens in a viscous liquid or gel to:
  - enhance its wettability by raising its surface tension.
  - assist the rapid spread of a uniform tear film over the lens.
  - 'cushion' the lens upon insertion.
  - reduce the foreign body sensation after lens insertion.
- Improving the optical quality of the lens front surface by helping sustain a regular pre-lens tear film:
  - increase tear break-up-time.
  - increase lens lubricity.
- Delaying onset of dryness and/or discomfort symptoms.

For tears to wet an RGP lens, the lens surface tension needs to be raised by a wetting agent. This may be the basis of a stand-alone (wetting) solution or a component added to an MPS. One of the earliest wetting agents was polyvinyl alcohol (PVA) (Hind 1979) while Rankin and Trager (1970) used hydroxy-ethyl cellulose as a 'cushioning' solution.

Modern 'wetting' solutions include the in-eye products detailed below. Like wetting solutions, these incorporate viscosity-increasing agents and wetting agents (e.g. PVA) to coat the lens (Parker 1988). Unfortunately, these remain effective for only a short time, the limiting factor being how long it takes the tears to take over the lens-wetting role.

Rewetting, lubricating, cleaning, rehydrating, moisturizing solutions (in-eye products)

In-eye products are intended to:

- Alleviate symptoms of dryness and/or discomfort.
- Flush contaminants, including irritants, from the lens.
- Soothe.
- Rehydrate and cushion the lens.
- Clean the lens and reduce deposition.
- Decrease tear protein denaturation.

Products intended for in-eye use confront several challenges (Tonge et al. 2001b):

- Short contact time.
- Narrow and stable range of tear pH.
- Low corneal permeability.
- Rapid tear drainage.

In-eye cleaners include non-irritating surfactants and appropriate buffers (Hom & Simmons 2002). Surfactants lower the surface tension of lens contaminants and surround them, forming micelles. These repel one another, facilitating contaminant removal by lid action and tear flushing.

Wearers should be cautioned not to use in-eye products just before lens removal because they make lenses slippery. In addition, some are hypertonic which tightens hydrogel lenses on the eye making removal difficult and lens damage more likely.

Multipurpose solutions (MPSs) – soft lenses

MPSs include a variety of functions:

- Disinfection.
- If no-rub, a surfactant cleaner must be included.
- Anti-*Acanthamoeba*.
- Comfort formula, depending on:
  - pH.
  - osmolality.
  - low toxicity.
  - viscosity.

  Of these, pH (in a buffer system) and viscosity are easiest to control.
- Moisture locking (the solution assists water retention by the lens and tears).

Bausch & Lomb ReNu® MPS with MoistureLoc™ contains polyquaternium 10 (CAS: 68610-92-4), a cellulosic material, with hydroxyethyl groups that bind water, which the manufacturers claim cushions, assists debris removal, inhibits deposit formation and resists protein denaturation.

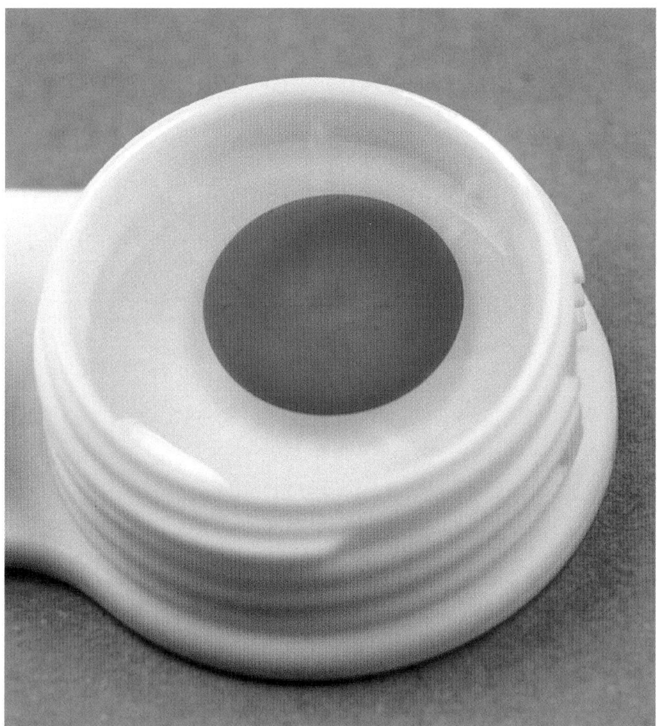

Figure 4.18 Originally, a clear soft lens until disinfected repeatedly (experimentally) in pharmacy-grade hydrogen peroxide

Multipurpose solutions – RGP lenses

One of the principal differences in RGP MPSs is their greater concentration of disinfectant. For example, the soft lens solution ReNu® MPS has 0.00005% PHX and EDTA and ReNu® MultiPlus® with Hydranate® has 0.0001% PHX and EDTA, whereas Boston Simplicity™ Multi-Action RGP solution contains 0.0005% PHX, 0.003% CHX and 0.05% EDTA. This is possible because of the lower adsorption and absorption of disinfectant by RGP materials because of their non-ionic nature, small 'pore' size and insignificant water content.

Care products – general

SOLUTION BUFFER SYSTEMS

Buffers are constituents of solutions that resist pH changes. Usually buffer systems are a combination of a weak acid or a weak base and one of its salts (e.g. boric acid and sodium borate).

The four common buffers are:

- Borate.
- Citrate.
- Bicarbonate – thermally unstable.
- Phosphate – can precipitate calcium phosphate, resulting in white spots and lens calculi.

Only borate and citrate systems are used in current care products.

For overall performance (antimicrobial and cleaning efficacies), synergies appear to exist between particular buffers and antimicrobials; for example, borate buffers and PHX (Lever & Miller 1999 of Bausch & Lomb), and citrate buffers and PQ-1 (Hong et al. 1994 of Alcon, Franklin 1997).

Hill et al. (1988) suggested that adverse reactions may be buffer-system related, necessitating a change to a care product with different buffer chemistry.

SOLUTION pH

While pH affects the properties of solutions, including the biocidal performance of any preservative or disinfectant therein (Parker 1988), pH can affect lens parameters (and fitting behaviour) by altering the lens water content and also a product's ability to remove protein, particularly from Group IV lenses (see Chapters 3 and 10). In negatively charged soft lenses, pH affects hydrogel expansion, facilitating the release of soluble proteins into the lens storage medium (Tonge et al. 2001a).

SOLUTION VISCOSITY

Viscosity is a measure of the resistance of a fluid to deformation in shear: in effect, resistance to flow or pouring. It is due to intermolecular friction, and molecular adhesion and cohesion within the fluid. Viscosity decreases with elevated temperatures (increased atomic/molecular activity decreases intermolecular cohesion and friction). The terms *thick* (high viscosity) and *thin* (low viscosity) are used as qualitative descriptions of a liquid.

Increased viscosity will enhance in-eye 'contact time' of a product and also provides demulcent properties, i.e. soothing, irritation-reducing and slippery. Solution demulcents include PVP, PVA, and polyethylene glycol (PEG).

Vigorous products for professional use only (RGP and soft lenses)

The advent of frequent replacement/disposable lenses has seen the almost total disappearance of this product category. Exceptions are Menicon's Progent, Paragon's Fluorosolve and Boston® Lab Lens Cleaner for RGP lenses.

Sodium hypochlorite (Milton™ Liquid Bleach – a dilute solution of sodium hypochlorite with up to 20% sodium chloride) can be used diluted, to bleach some soft lens discolorations or to remove reactive dye lens tints (vat tints are more bleach resistant).

Lens cases

Contamination of lens cases (Fig. 4.19) is often visible to the naked eye when the colonizing organism is a coloured fungus. Case replacement is important to avoid biofilm (see pp. 85, 87, 93 and Figs 4.5 and 4.6) formation and other debris from accumulating. Ideally, lens cases should withstand thermal disinfection but they are usually made of acrylic, PVC, or polypropylene which cannot be boiled without deforming.

The case lid must remain sealed during all reasonable circumstances (Fig. 4.20). Raised temperature and therefore pressure results from carrying a 'sealed' case close to the body, while reduced pressures and temperatures occur in aircraft. If the contents leak, there is:

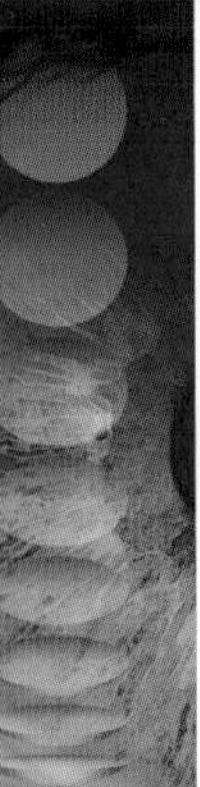

(a)

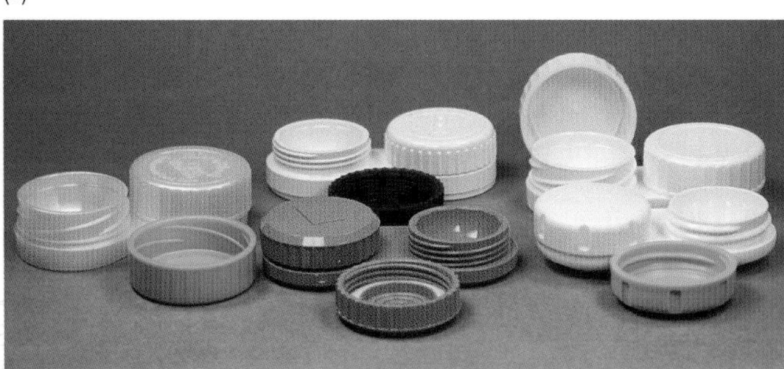

(b)

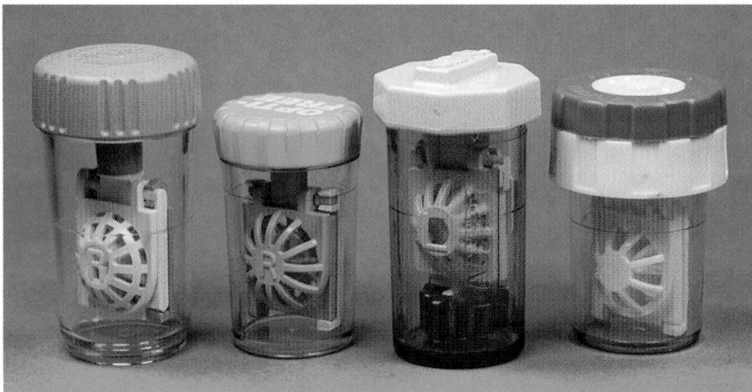

(c)

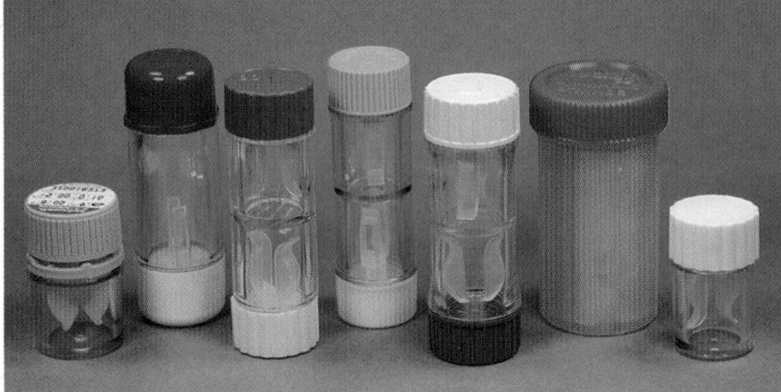

Figure 4.19 Lens cases: (a) flat packs; (b) barrels; (c) rigid gas-permeable containers

- Loss of solution.
- Loss of antimicrobial action as external contaminants are 'ingested'.
- Partial lens hydration.
- Mess.

RGP lenses: wet or dry storage?

Hind and Szekely (1959) found that with PMMA lenses, initial comfort was superior with wet storage even though dry storage was simpler. Siloxane acrylates and fluorosiloxane acrylates do not wet well but have a small but clinically significant water content, which can affect lens parameters, surface wetting, on-eye behaviour and initial comfort. Wet storage improves wettability and controls microbial contamination.

Care products and silicone hydrogel lenses

Higher levels of visible lens deposits have been associated with silicone hydrogel lenses (Brennan et al. 2002, and others).

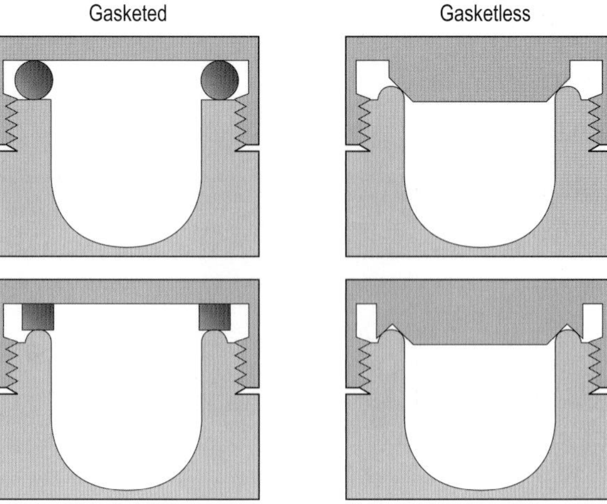

Figure 4.20 Lens case lid seals – diagrammatic.

Incompatibilities between silicone hydrogels and certain MPSs have become apparent, with signs of corneal staining. Although the signs of corneal staining were present, symptoms were usually absent. Jones et al. (2004) concluded that the corneal staining produced by silicone hydrogels differed from that produced by HEMA-based materials, and that new care regimens required careful performance evaluation with silicone hydrogels.

Although Beattie et al. (2003) reported significantly greater attachment of *A. castellanii* trophozoites to silicone hydrogels than to conventional hydrogels, risk of *Acanthamoeba* keratitis is no greater (Tomlinson 2002).

Miscellaneous effects of care products

LENS TINTS

Thermal and chemical disinfection has no significant effect on lens tints (Stanek & Yamane 1985), nor does ophthalmic-grade hydrogen peroxide (see also Fig. 4.18).

DRY EYE

Symptoms of end-of-day dryness are frequently reported by lens wearers. Smythe (2003) suggested that hydrogel-care solutions should be suspected if the wearer has no problems in spectacles or daily disposable lenses. If the solution was PHX-based, one with a lower concentration, a different antimicrobial system or, preferably, a hydrogen peroxide system should be tried instead.

Bishop (2004) recommended Complete® MoisturePLUS™ MPS and Blink-N-Clean™ Lens Drops for lens wearers who fly frequently.

Incompatibilities

Instances of solution incompatibilities are few, provided products are not misapplied (e.g. RGP lens products applied to soft lenses).

With catalytic disc-based systems, the catalyst must not be 'poisoned' by or coated with incompatible products (although if this does happen, the disc becomes less effective and disinfection efficacy increases). Eventually, residual peroxide becomes too uncomfortable to tolerate.

If frothing occurs with effervescent peroxide systems, contaminants – including viable microorganisms – can gain access to the inside roof of the case, beyond the reach of the disinfectant, and recontamination can occur. Wearers should be instructed to shake their lens case vertically immediately after filling with fresh peroxide to release these organisms.

Solutions used for thermal disinfection can alter their chemistry or induce reactions between the components and the lens material. Generally, unpreserved, unbuffered normal saline should be used at between 70 and 80°C.

Longer-term storage

For those lenses that are not disposable and require longer-term storage, one-step peroxide systems are unsuitable, as the residual solution has no antimicrobial action remaining. OBSs are not ideal because of their compromise between disinfection power and ocular cytotoxicity. Preferably, lenses should be disinfected thermally and then left unopened, or stored in hydrogen peroxide (in a vented case as some peroxide decomposition may raise the pressure inside the case). Lenses must be neutralized before wear. A peroxide – the pH and osmolality of which are near normal (e.g. AOSept®) – is the most suitable.

THE FUTURE

As lens costs decrease and lens replacement rates increase, the lens care market will diminish. OBSs are likely to increase their market share due to convenience, and fewer RGP-specific products will be available, being replaced by 'universal' products and specialized care products, particularly those that are more biocompatible.

Work is underway on antimicrobial or microbial contamination-resistant lenses, which ultimately may remove the need for lens care.

Epilogue

In writing a chapter such as this, it is disturbing to note that many papers are company sponsored and with predictable outcomes, particularly those relating to multipurpose solutions. Unfortunately, this is unlikely to change significantly and practitioners should ensure that information emanates from unbiased sources or that the sponsorship of the author(s) is known.

Acknowledgements

The significant help and attention to detail of Debbie McDonald in the preparation of the final manuscript is gratefully acknowledged as is the use of the extensive resources of the IER Library (UNSW). Images contributed to this chapter by others are identified with the photographer's name.

References

Ainley, R. and Smith, B. (1965) Fungal flora of the conjunctival sac in healthy and diseased eyes. Br. J. Ophthalmol., 49, 505–515

Alfonso, E., Mandelbaum, S., Fox, M. J. et al. (1986) Ulcerative keratitis associated with contact lens wear. Am. J. Ophthalmol., 101, 429–433

Anger, C. B. and Curie, J. P. (1995) Preservation and disinfection. In Contact Lenses. The CLAO Guide to Basic Science and Clinical Practice, Vol. II: Soft and Rigid Contact Lenses, p 197, ed. P. R. Kastl. Dubuque: Kendall/Hunt Publishing

Anger, C. B., Ambrus, K., Stoecker, J. et al. (1990) Antimicrobial efficacy of hydrogen peroxide for contact lens disinfection. Cont Lens Spectrum, 5, 46–51

Anwar, H., Dasgupta, M. K. and Costerton, J. W. (1990) Testing the susceptibility of bacteria in biofilms to antibacterial agents. Antimicrob. Agents Chemother., 34, 2043–2046

Atkins, N. (2004) Regard: a multipurpose solution. Optician, 228(5976), 14–16

Baines, M. G., Cai, F. and Backman, H. A. (1990) Adsorption and removal of protein bound to hydrogel contact lenses. Optom. Vis. Sci., 67(11), 807–810

Baleriola-Lucas, C., Grant, T., Newton-Howes, J. et al. (1991) Enumeration and identification of bacteria on hydrogel lenses from asymptomatic patients and those experiencing adverse responses with extended wear. Invest. Ophthalmol. Vis. Sci., 32, 739

Bates, A. K., Morris, R. J., Stapleton, F. et al. (1989) 'Sterile' corneal infiltrates in contact lens wearers. Eye, 3, 803–810

Bausch & Lomb (1998) ReNu MultiPlus: an everyday solution to an everyday problem. Optom. Today, 38, 28

Beattie, T. K., Tomlinson, A. and Seal, D. V. (2002) Anti-acanthamoeba efficacy in contact lens disinfecting systems. Br. J. Ophthalmol., 86, 1319–1320

Beattie, T. K., Tomlinson, A., McFadyen, A. K. et al. (2003) Enhanced attachment of acanthamoeba to extended-wear silicone hydrogel contact lenses: a new risk factor for infection? Ophthalmology, 110(4), 765–771

Begley, C. G., Paragina, S., Sporn, A. et al. (1990) An analysis of contact lens enzyme cleaners. J. Am. Optom. Assoc., 61, 190–194

Berger, R. O. and Streeten, B. W. (1981) Fungal growth in aphakic soft contact lenses. Am. J. Ophthalmol., 91, 630–633

Bishop, D. H. (2004) Fitting tip: dry eye care for frequent flyers. Cont. Lens Today, May 23. Online. Available: www.cltoday.com/archive.asp

Brazier, J. and Hall, V. (1993) Propionibacterium propionicum and infections of the lacrimal apparatus. Clin. Infect. Dis., 17, 892–893

Brennan, N. A., Coles, C., Comstock, T. L. et al. (2002) A 1-year prospective clinical trial of balafilcon A (PureVision) silicone-hydrogel contact lenses used on a 30-day continuous wear schedule. Ophthalmology, 109, 1172–1177

Busschaert, S. C., Good, R. C. and Szabocsik, J. (1978) Evaluation of thermal disinfection procedures for hydrophilic contact lenses. Appl. Environ. Microbiol., 35(3), 618–621

Callender, M. G., Tse, L. S. Y., Charles, A. M. et al. (1986) Bacterial flora of the eye and contact lens cases during hydrogel lens wear. Am. J. Optom. Physiol. Opt., 63, 177–180

Callender, M. G., Charles, A. M. and Chalmers, R. L. (1992) Effect of storage time with different lens care systems on in-office hydrogel trial lens disinfection efficacy: a multi-center study. Optom. Vis. Sci., 69, 678–684

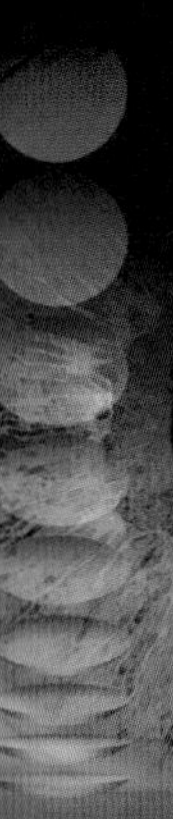

Christie, C. (1999) Solutions: same or different? Optician, 218(5717), 20–24

CLAO (1988) Contact lens care: new guidelines. CLAO Policy Statement, issued April 1987. CLAO J., 14(1), 55–56

Clark, B. J., Harkins, L. S., Munro, F. A. et al. (1994) Microbial contamination of cases used for storing contact lenses. J. Infect., 28, 293–304

Clarke, K. (2004) Bioinformatics project. Online. Available: http://homepages.uel.ac.uk/cla8045v/tsld011.htm

Codling, C. E., Maillard, J. Y. and Russell, A. D. (2003) Aspects of the antimicrobial mechanisms of action of a polyquaternium and an amidoamine. J. Antimicrob. Chemother., 51, 1153–1158

Costerton, J. W., Irvin, R. T. and Cheng, K. T. (1981) The bacterial glycocalyx in nature and disease. Ann. Rev. Microbiol., 35, 299–324

Crabbe, A. and Thompson, P. (2001a) Clinical trial of a patient-operated microwave care system for hydrogel contact lenses. Optom. Vis. Sci., 78, 605–609

Crabbe, A. and Thompson, P. (2001b) Effects of microwave irradiation on the parameters of hydrogel lenses. Optom. Vis. Sci., 78, 610–615

Crabbe, A. and Thompson, P. (2004) Testing of a dual-mode microwave care regimen for hydrogel lenses. Optom. Vis. Sci., 81, 471–477

Dallos, J. and Hughes, W. H. (1972) Sterilization of hydrophilic contact lenses. Br. J. Ophthalmol., 56(2), 114–119

Dart, J. K. and Badenoch, P. R. (1986) Bacterial adherence to contact lenses. CLAO J., 12, 220–224

Dart, J. K., Peacock, J., Grierson, I. et al. (1988) Ocular surface, contact lens and bacterial interactions in a rabbit model. Transaction of B.C.L.A. Conference, Birmingham, 95–96

Dave, J. and Patel, V. (1999) When is enzymatic protein cleaning necessary? Optician, 218(5713), 30–31

Devonshire, P., Munro, F. A., Abernethy, C. et al. (1993) Microbial contamination of contact lens cases in the west of Scotland. Br. J. Ophthalmol., 77, 1–25

Donshik, P., Madden, R. and Simmons, P. A. (2000) Pursuing comfort in a multi-purpose solution. Cont. Lens Spectrum, 15(12), 33–36

Donzis, P. B., Mondino, B. J., Weissman, B. A. et al. (1987) Microbial contamination of contact lens care systems. Am. J. Ophthalmol., 104, 325–333

Duffy, P., Wolf, J., Collins, G. et al. (1974) Possible person to person transmission of CJD. N. Engl. J. Med., 290, 692–693

Duran, J. A., Refojo, M. F., Gipson, I. K. et al. (1987) Pseudomonas attachment to new hydrogel contact lenses. Arch. Ophthalmol., 105, 106–109

Evans, E. and Dart, J. K. G. (1995) Efficacy of contact lens disinfecting solutions on Pseudomonas aeruginosa biofilms growing on contact lens storage case plastics. Invest. Ophthalmol. Vis. Sci., 36, 4714(4695)

Evans, T. C., Levy, B. and Szabocsik, J. (1993) Clinical study of bendazac lysine for in vivo contact lens cleaning. Optom. Vis. Sci., 70(3), 210–215

Ewbank, A. (2000) The product performance of a new generation multi-purpose CL solution. Optician, 219(5749), 32–38

Fleiszig, S. M. J. and Efron, N. (1992a) Conjunctival floral in extended wear of rigid gas permeable contact lenses. Optom. Vis. Sci., 69, 354–357

Fleiszig, S. M. J. and Efron, N. (1992b) Microbial flora in eyes of current and former contact lens wearers. J. Clin. Microbiol., 30, 1156–1161

Fonn, D. (1999) Factors affecting the success of silicone hydrogels. Optician, 218(5750), 12–14

Fowler, S. A. and Allansmith, M. R. (1980) Evolution of soft contact lens coatings. Arch. Ophthalmol., 98, 95–99

Franklin, V. J. (1997) Cleaning efficacy of single-purpose surfactant cleaners and multi-purpose solutions. Cont. Lens Ant. Eye, 20(2), 63–68

Franklin, V. J. and Tighe, B. J. (1991) Hydrogel lens spoilation. The structure and composition of white spot deposits. Optician, 202, 18–23

Franklin, V., Horne, A., Jones, L. et al. (1991) Early deposition trends on group I (polymacon and tetrafilcon A) and group III (bufilcon A) materials. CLAO J., 17(4), 244–248

Franklin, V. J., Bright, A., Pearce, E. and Tighe, B. (1992) Hydrogel lens spoilation. Part 5: Tear proteins and proteinaceous films. Optician, 204(5367), 16–26

Franklin, V., Tighe, B. and Tonge, S. (2001) Contact lens care: Part 4 – Contact lens deposition, discoloration and spoilation mechanisms. Optician, 222(5808), 16–20

Freeman, M. I. (1997) Guest editorial – Disposable contact lenses: where we have been – what we have learned. CLAO J., 23(1), 10–12

Galentine, P. G., Cohen, E. J., Laibson, P. R. et al. (1984) Corneal ulcers associated with contact lens wear. Arch. Ophthalmol., 102, 891–894

Gandhi, P. A., Sawant, A. D., Wilson, L. A. et al. (1993) Adaptation and growth of Serratia marcescens in contact lens disinfectant solutions containing chlorhexidine gluconate. Appl. Env. Microbiol., 59, 183–188

Gellatly, K. W., Brennan, N. A. and Efron, N. (1988) Visual decrement with deposit accumulation on HEMA contact lenses. Am. J. Optom. Physiol. Opt., 65(12), 937–941

Gentsch, T. F. and Edrington, T. B. (1990) The bleaching effect of hydrogen peroxide on DuraSoft 3 Colors. CL Spectrum, 5(7), 53–56

Grant, R. (1988) Comparative efficacy of three soft contact lens disinfection systems. J. B.C.L.A. (Transaction of B.C.L.A. Conference), 11(5), 106–109

Grant, T., Holden, B. A., Rechberger, J. et al. (1989) Contact lens related papillary conjunctivitis (CLPC): influence of protein accumulation and replacement frequency. Invest. Ophthalmol. Vis. Sci., 30(3)(Suppl), 166

Gray, T. B., Cursons, T. M., Sherwan, J. F. et al. (1995) Acanthamoeba, bacterial and fungal contamination of contact lens storage cases. Br. J. Ophthalmol., 79, 601–605

Hara, J., Araki, K., Ushio, K. et al. (1989) Clinical evaluation of SCL sterilization with hydrogen peroxide: comparison with boiling. J. Jpn Cont. Lens Soc., 31, 148–154

Harris, M. G., Torres, J. and Tracewell, L. (1988) pH and H_2O_2 concentration of hydrogen peroxide disinfection systems. Am. J. Optom. Physiol. Opt., 65, 527–535

Harris, M., Rechberger, J., Grant, T. et al. (1990) In-office microwave disinfection of soft contact lenses. Optom. Vis. Sci., 67(2), 129–132

Hart, D. E. (1984) Lipid deposits which form on extended wear lenses. I.C.L.C., 11(6), 348–360

Hart, D. E. and Shih, K. L. (1987) Surface interactions on hydrogel extended wear contact lenses: microflora and microfauna. Am. J. Optom. Physiol. Opt., 64(10), 739–748

Hart, D. E., Hosmer, M., Georgescu, M. et al. (1996) Bacterial assay of contact lens wearers. Optom. Vis. Sci., 73(3), 204–207

Hart, D. E., Reindel, W., Proskin, H. M. et al. (1993) Microbial contamination of hydrophilic contact lenses: quantitation and identification of micro-organisms associated with contact lenses while on the eye. Optom. Vision Sci., 70, 185–191

Hathaway, R. A. and Lowther, G. E. (1976) Appearance of hydrophilic lens deposits as related to chemical etiology. I.C.L.C., 3, 27–35

Hathaway, R. A. and Lowther, G. E. (1978) Factors influencing the rate of deposit formation on hydrophilic lenses. Aust. J. Optom., 61, 92–96

Heckmann, J., Lang, C. J., Petruch, F. et al. (1997) Transmission of Creutzfeldt–Jakob disease via a corneal transplant. J. Neurol. Neurosurg. Psychiatry, 63, 388–390

Heiler, D. J., Gambarcorta-Hoffman, S., Groemminger, S. F. et al. (1991) The concentric distribution of protein on patient-worn hydrogel lenses. CLAO J., 17(4), 249–251

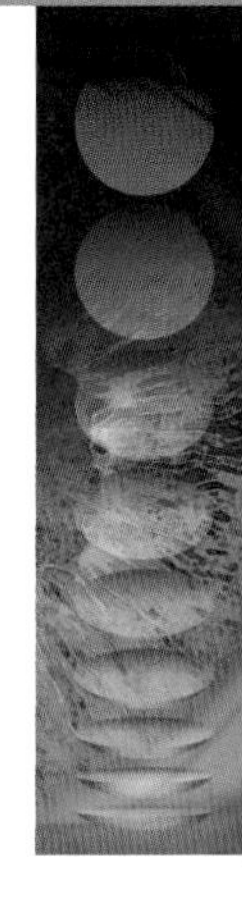

Higaki, S., Ohshima, T. and Shimomura, Y. (1998) Extended wear soft contact lenses don't change the ocular flora. Acta Ophthalmologica, 76, 639–640

Hill, R. M., Carney, L. G., Barr, J. T. et al. (1988) The boric acid buffer questions. Cont. Lens Spectrum, 3(12), 44–46

Hind, H. W. (1979) Contact lens solutions: yesterday, today, and tomorrow. Cont. Lens Forum, 4(11), 17–27

Hind, H. W. and Szekely, I. J. (1959) Wetting and hydration of contact lenses. Contacto, 3(3), 65–68

Hiti, K., Walochnik, J., Faschinger, C. et al. (2001) Microwave treatment of contact lens cases contaminated with Acanthamoeba. Cornea, 20(5), 467–470

Hiti, K., Walochnik, J., Haller-Schober, E. M. et al. (2002) Viability of Acanthamoeba after exposure to a multipurpose disinfecting contact lens solution and two hydrogen peroxide systems. Br. J. Ophthalmol., 86, 144–146

Hiti, K., Walochnik, J., Fashinger, C. et al. (2004) One- and two-step hydrogen peroxide contact lens disinfection solutions against Acanthamoeba: how effective are they? Eye (Advance Online Publication), 81(6), 442–454

Hogan, R. N. (2003) Potential for transmission of prion disease by contact lenses: an assessment of risk. Eye Cont. Lens, 29, S44–S48

Holden, B. A., La Hood, D., Grant, T. et al. (1996) Gram-negative bacteria can induce contact lens related acute red eye (CLARE) responses. CLAO J., 22, 47–52

Holland, S., Ruseska, I., Alfonso, E. et al. (1988). Pseudomonas and extended wear contact lenses. ARVO (Suppl. to Invest. Ophthalmol. Vis. Sci.), 11, 278

Hom, M. and Simmons, P. (2002) In-eye contact lens cleaners. Cont. Lens Spectrum, 17(7), 33–38

Hong, B.-S., Bilbault, T. J., Chowhan, M. A. et al. (1994) Cleaning capability of citrate-containing vs. non-citrate contact lens cleaning solutions: an in vitro comparative study. I.C.L.C., 21, 237–240

Høvding, G. (1981) The conjunctival and contact lens bacterial flora during lens wear. Acta Ophthalmologica, 59, 387–401

Hyndiuk, R. A., Skorah, D. N. and Burd, E. M. (1988) Bacterial Keratitis, pp 321–323. Boston: Little, Brown

Ilhan, B., Irkec, M., Orhan, M. et al. (1998) Surface deposits on frequent replacement and conventional daily wear soft contact lenses. A scanning electron microscopic study. CLAO J., 24(4), 232–235

Iwamoto, H., Yamada, M., Hagino, A. et al. (1993) Gas-permeable HCl surface deterioration by benzalkonium chloride. J. Jpn Cont. Lens Soc., 35, 219–225

Izumi, Y., Kamei, Y., Fujisawa, S. et al. (1991) The efficacy of disinfection system using hydrogen peroxide against Acanthamoeba. J. Jpn Cont. Lens Soc., 33, 282–286

Jacques, M., Marrie, T. J. and Costerton, J. W. (1992) Review: Microbial colonization of prosthetic devices. Microb. Ecol. Health Dis., 13, 173–191

Jalbert, I., Willcox, M. D. and Sweeney, D. F. (2000) Isolation of Staphylococcus aureus from a contact lens at the time of a contact lens-induced peripheral ulcer; case report. Cornea, 19, 116–120

Janoff, L. E. (1988) The effect of thirty cycles of hydrogen peroxide disinfection of CIBA Softcolor lenses. I.C.L.C., 15(5), 155–164

Jenkins, C. and Phillips, A. J. (1986) How sterile is unpreserved saline? Clin. Exp. Optom., 69(4), 131–136

John, T., Refojo, M. F., Hanninen, L. et al. (1989) Adherence of viable and non-viable bacteria to soft contact lenses. Cornea, 8(1), 21–33

Jones, L., Davies, I. and Jones, D. (1993) Effect of hydrogen peroxide neutralisation on the fitting characteristics of group IV disposable contact lenses. J. B.C.L.A., 16(4), 135–140

Jones, L., Evans, K., Sariri, R. et al. (1997a) Lipid and protein deposition of N-vinyl pyrrolidone-containing Group II and Group IV frequent replacement contact lenses. CLAO J., 23(2), 122–126

Jones, L., Jones, D. and Houlford, M. (1997b) Clinical comparison of three polyhexanide-preserved multi-purpose contact lens solutions. Cont. Lens Ant. Eye, 20(1), 23–30

Jones, L., Dumbleton, K., Bayer, S. et al. (2004) Corneal staining associated with silicone-hydrogel materials used on a daily-wear basis with ReNu and AOSept care regimens. Paper presented at Am. Acad. Optom. Meeting – Academy 2004 Global-Pacific Rim, Honolulu, 4 April 2004

Kanpolat, A., Kalayci, D., Arman, D. et al. (1992) Contamination in contact lens care systems. CLAO J., 18, 104–107

Kastl, P. R. and Maehara, J. R. (2001) Low-power microwave disinfection of soft contact lenses. CLAO J., 27(2), 81–83

Keith, D. J., Christensen, M. T., Barry, J. R. et al. (2003) Determination of the lysozyme deposit curve in soft contact lenses. Eye Cont. Lens, 29(2), 79–82

Közer-Bilgin, L., Manav, G., Tutkun, I. T. et al. (1993) Efficacy of a one-step hydrogen peroxide system for disinfection of soft contact lenses. CLAO J., 19(1), 50–52

Lakkis, C. (2002) Contact lens care: Part 12. Industrial contact lens sterilisation, in practice disinfection and daily disposables. Optician, 223(5840), 22–28

Lakkis, C. and Fleiszig, S. M. J. (2001) Resistance of Pseudomonas aeruginosa isolates to hydrogel contact lens disinfection correlates with cytotoxic activity. J. Clin. Microbiol., 39, 1477–1486

Lambert, S., Sevilla, C., Lindley, K. et al. (1999) Efficacy data on SOLOcare – a new 10 minute contact lens multi-purpose disinfection regimen. Optom. Vis. Sci., 76(12)(Suppl), 160

Larkin, D. F. P. and Leeming, J. P. (1991) Quantitative alterations of the commensal eye bacteria in contact lens wear. Eye, 5, 70–74

Larkin, D. F. P., Kilvington, S. and Dart, J. K. G. (1990) Contamination of contact lens storage cases by Acanthamoeba and bacteria. Br. J. Ophthalmol., 74, 133–135

Larkin, D. F. P., Kilvington, S., Dart, J. K. G. (1992) Treatment of Acanthamoeba keratitis with polyhexamethylene biguanide. Ophthalmology, 99, 185–191

Lass, J. H., Haaf, J., Foster, S. C. et al. (1981) Visual outcome in eight cases of Serratia marcescens keratitis. Am. J. Ophthalmol., 92, 384–390

Leahy, C. D., Mandell, R. B. and Lin S. T. (1990) Initial in vivo tear protein deposition on individual hydrogel contact lenses. Optom. Vis. Sci. 67(7), 504–511

Lebow, K. A. and Schachet, J. L. (2003) Evaluation of corneal staining and patient preferences with use of three multi-purpose solutions and two brands of soft contact lenses. Eye Cont. Lens, 29(4), 213–220

Lever, A. M. and Miller, M. J. (1999) Comparative antimicrobial efficacy of multi-purpose lens care solutions using the FDA's revised guidance document for industry: Stand–alone primary criteria. CLAO J., 25(1), 52–56

Lever, O. W., Groemminger, S. F., Allen, M. E. et al. (1995) Evaluation of the relationship between total lens protein deposition and patient-rated comfort of hydrophilic (soft) contact lenses. I.C.L.C., 22(1), 5–13

Liedel, K. K. and Begley, C. G. (1996) The effectiveness of soft contact lens disinfection systems against Acanthamoeba on the lens surface. J. Am. Optom. Assoc., 67, 135–141

Limberg, M. B. (1991) A review of bacterial keratitis and bacterial conjunctivitis. Am. J. Ophthalmol., 112, 2–9

Lowther, G. E. (1977) Effectiveness of an enzyme in removing deposits from hydrophilic lenses. Am. J. Optom. Physiol. Opt., 54(2), 76–84

Luibinas, J., Swenson, G. and Carney, L. G. (1987) Thermal disinfection of contact lenses. Clin. Exp. Optom., 70(1), 8–14

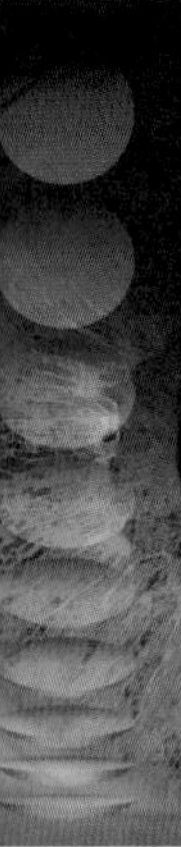

Martins, E. N., Farah, E. E., Alvarenga, L. S. et al. (2002) Infectious keratitis: correlation between corneal and contact lens cultures. CLAO J., 28, 146–148

Mayo, M. S., Cook, W. L., Schlitzer, R. L. et al. (1986) Antibiograms, serotypes, and plasmid profiles of Pseudomonas aeruginosa associated with corneal ulcers and contact lens wear. J. Clin. Microbiol., 24, 372–376

McCulloch, R. R., Torres, J. G., Wilhelmus, K. R. et al. (1988) Biofilm on contaminated hydrogel contact lenses protects adherent Pseudomonas aeruginosa from antibacterial therapy. ARVO (Suppl. to Invest. Ophthalmol. Vis. Sci.), 12, 228

McDonnell, G. and Russell, A. D. (1999) Antiseptics and disinfectants: activity, action and resistance. Clin. Microbiol. Rev., 12, 147–179

McLaughlin-Borlace, L., Stapleton, F., Matheson, M. et al. (1998) Bacterial biofilm on contact lenses and lens storage cases in wearers with microbial keratitis. J. Appl. Microbiol., 84, 827–838

McMonnies, C. W. (1988) Is there a way through the maintenance minefield? J. B.C.L.A. (Transaction of B.C.L.A. Conference), 11(5), 47–51

Meakin, B. J. (1989) Contact lens care systems: an update. J. B.C.L.A., 12 (Sci Meeting Suppl.), 26–31

Miller, M. J. and Ahearn, D. G. (1987) Adherence of Pseudomonas aeruginosa to hydrophilic contact lenses and other substrata. J. Clin. Microbiol., 25, 1392–1397

Minno, G. E., Eckel, L., Groemminger, S. et al. (1991) Quantitative analysis of protein deposits on hydrophilic soft contact lenses: I. Comparison to visual methods of analysis. II. Deposit variation among FDA lens material groups. Optom. Vis. Sci., 68(11), 865–872

Morgan, J. F. (1979) Complications associated with contact lens solutions. Ophthalmology, 86, 1107–1113

Mowrey-McKee, M. F., Sampson, H. J. and Proskin, H. M. (1992) Microbial contamination of hydrophilic contact lenses. Part II: quantitation of microbes after patient handling and after aseptic removal from the eye. CLAO J., 18, 240–245

Noble, J. A., Ahearn, D. G., Avery, S. A. et al. (2002) Phagocytosis affects biguanide sensitivity of Acanthamoeba spp. Antimicrob. Agents Chemother., 46(7), 2069–2076

Parker, J. (1988) Interaction of contact lens materials and available lens care products. J. B.C.L.A. (Transaction of B.C.L.A. Cont. Lens Seminar), 11, 45–48

Pederson, K. (1999) Exploring the differences in today's lens care options. Cont. Lens Spectrum, 14(5), 25–32

Penley, C. A., Schlitzer, R. L., Ahearn, D. G. et al. (1981) Laboratory evaluation of chemical disinfection of soft contact lenses. Cont. Intraocular Lens Med. J., 7, 101–110

Penley, C. A., Llabres, C., Wilson, L. A. et al. (1985) Efficacy of hydrogen peroxide disinfection systems for soft contact lenses contaminated with fungi. CLAO J., 11(1), 65–68

Pennington, R. N. (1979) Toric optic soft lenses. Optician, 178, 34–38

Perkins, R. E., Kundsin, R. B., Pratt, M. V. et al. (1975) Bacteriology of normal and infected conjunctiva. J. Clin. Microbiol., 1, 147–149

Phillips, A. J. (1976) Contact lens solutions. Ophthalmol. Optician, 16(22), 3–8

Phillips, A. J. and Copley, C. A. (1990) Bacteriostatic saline – does it work? Clin. Exp. Optom., 73(1), 1–2

Phillips, A. J. and Czigler, B. (1985) Polyclens (Opti-clean) – a further study. Aust. J. Optom., 68(1), 36–39

Piccolo, M. G. (1989) How to diagnose and treat bacterial conjunctivitis. Rev. Optom., 126, 55–57

Pinney, R. J. (1976) The disinfection of contact lenses. Ophthalmol. Optician, 16(22), 1–4

Rabinstein, A., Whiteman, M. and Shebert, R. (2002) Abnormal diffusion-weighted magnetic resonance imaging in Creutzfeldt–Jakob disease following corneal transplantations. Arch. Neurol., 59(4), 637–639

Ramachandran, L., Sharma, S., Sankaridurg, P. et al. (1995) Examination of the conjunctival microbiota after 8 hours of eye closure. CLAO J., 21, 195–199

Rankin, B. F. and Trager, S. F. (1970) Wetting of contact lenses. Am. J. Optom. Arch. Am. Acad. Optom., 47(9), 698–702

Rauschl, R. T. and Rogers, J. J. (1978) The effect of hydrophilic contact lens wear on the bacterial flora of the human conjunctiva. I.C.L.C., 5, 56–62

Reindel, W., Ploscowe, V., Minno, G. et al. (1989) Comparison study of hydrophilic contact lens surfactant cleaners: a clinical evaluation of residual deposits. I.C.L.C., 16(7–8), 232–236

Report: C.f.D.C.M.a.M.W. (1985) Atlanta, GA: Centers for Disease Control, pp 34, 533–534

Rosenthal, R. A., Stein, J. M., McAnally, C. L. et al. (1995) A comparative study of the microbiologic effectiveness of chemical disinfectants and peroxide neutraliser systems. CLAO J., 21, 99–110

Rosenthal, R. A., Buck, S., McAnally, C. et al. (1999) Antimicrobial comparison of a new multi-purpose disinfecting solution to 3% hydrogen peroxide system. CLAO J., 25(4), 213–217

Rosenthal, R. A., McAnally, C. L., McNamee, L. S. et al. (2000) Broad spectrum antimicrobial activity of a new multi-purpose disinfecting solution. CLAO J., 26(3), 120–126

Russell, A. D. (2002) Mechanisms of antimicrobial action of antiseptics and disinfectants: an increasingly important area of investigation. J. Antimicrob. Chemother., 49, 597–599

Saddiq, S. A., Azuara-Blanco, A., Bennett, D. et al. (1998) Evaluation of contamination of used disposable contact lenses by Acanthamoeba. CLAO J., 24, 155–158

Sankaridurg, P. R., Sharma, S., Willcox, M. D. et al. (1999) Colonization of hydrogel lenses with Streptococcus pneumoniae: risk of development of corneal infiltrates. Cornea, 18, 289–295

Sankaridurg, P. R., Sharma, S., Willcox, M. D. P. et al. (1996) Haemophilus influenzae adherent to contact lenses is associated with the production of ocular inflammation. J. Clin. Microbiol., 34, 2426–2431

Schein, O. D., Ormerod, L. D., Barraquer, E. et al. (1989) Microbiology of contact lens-related keratitis. Cornea, 8(4), 281–285

Schunk, T. and Schweisfurth, R. S. (1989) Disinfection performance of oxidising contact lens solutions: quantitative suspension tests with organic soil contaminants. Contactologia, 11, 84–89

Seal, D. V., McGill, J. L., Flanagan, D. et al. (1981) Lacrimal canaliculitis due to Arachnia (Acinetomyces) propionica. Br. J. Ophthalmol., 65, 10–13

Seal, D. V., Barrett, S. P. and McGill, J. I. (1982) Aetiology and treatment of acute bacterial infection of the external eye. Br. J. Ophthalmol., 66, 357–360

Seal, D., Bron, A. and Hay, J. (1998) Ocular Infection. Investigation and Treatment in Practice. London: Martin Dunitz

Seal, D., Dalton, A. and Doris, D. (1999) Disinfection of contact lenses without tap water rinsing: is it effective? Eye, 13, 226–230

Shih, K. L., Hu, J. and Sibley, M. J. (1985) The microbiological benefits of cleaning and rinsing contact lenses. I.C.L.C., 12(4), 235–242

Sibley, M. J. (1988) Soft contact lens hygiene: an overview. In Contact Lenses: The CLAO Guide to Basic Science and Clinical Practice, Update 3, Ch. 40, ed. O. H. Dabezies. Orlando: Grune and Stratton

Simmons, P. A., Edrington, T. B., Pfondevida, C. J. et al. (1996) Comparison between evening and morning surfactant cleaning of hydrogel lenses. I.C.L.C., 23(5), 172–175

Sleigh, J. D. and Timbury, M. C. (1990) Bacteria: organisation, structure, taxonomy. In Notes on Medical Bacteriology, 3rd edn, eds. J. D. Sleigh, M. C. Timbury. Edinburgh: Churchill Livingstone

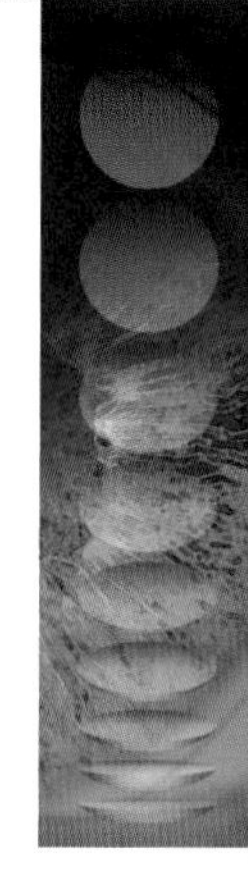

Slusher, M. M., Myrvik, Q. N., Lewis, J. C. et al. (1987) Extended-wear lenses, biofilm, and bacterial adhesion. Arch. Ophthalmol., 105, 110–115

Smythe, J. L. (2003) Managing solution-related dryness. Cont. Lens Spectrum, 18(3), 27

Stainer, R. Y., Adelberg, E. A. and Ingraham, L., eds. (1981) The viruses. In General Microbiology, 4th edn, pp 364–400. London: Macmillan

Standardization, I.O.o. (2000) Geneva: International Organization of Standardization

Stanek, S. R. and Yamane, S. J. (1985) Do thermal disinfection systems harm tinted soft lenses? Cont. Lens Forum, 10(3), 35–39

Stapleton, F. and Dart, J. K. G. (1995) Keratitis associated with bacterial biofilm formation in a disposable contact lens wearer. Br. J. Ophthalmol., 79, 864–865

Stapleton, F., Dart, J. K. and Minassian, D. (1993) Risk factors with contact lens related suppurative keratitis. CLAO J., 19(4), 204–210

Stapleton, F., Dart, J. K., Matheson, M. et al. (1993) Bacterial adherence and glycocalyx formation on unworn hydrogel lenses. J. Br. Contact Lens Assoc., 16(3), 113–117

Stapleton, F., Dart, J. K. G., Seal, D. V. et al. (1995a) Epidemiology of Pseudomonas aeruginosa keratitis in contact lens wearers. Epidemiol. Infect., 114, 395–402

Stapleton, F., Willcox, M., Fleming, C. et al. (1995b) Changes to the ocular biota with time in extended- and daily-wear disposable contact lens use. Infect. Immun., 63, 4501–4505

Statement, C. P. (1988) Contact lens care: new guidelines. CLAO J., 14, 55–56

Stehr-Green, J. K., Bailey, T. M. and Visvesvara, G. S. (1989) The epidemiology of Acanthamoeba keratitis in the United States. Am. J. Ophthalmol., 107, 331–336

Stein, H. and Harrison, K. (1983) The safety and effectiveness of Polyclens – an all purpose cleaner for hydrophilic soft contact lenses. CLAO J., 9(1), 39–42

Stokes, D. J. and Morton, D. J. (1987) Antimicrobial activity of hydrogen peroxide. I.C.L.C., 14(4), 146–149

Stone, R. P., Mowrey-McKee, M. F. and Kreutzer, P. (1984) Protein: a source of lens discoloration. Cont. Lens Forum, 9(9), 33–41

Sweeney, D. F., Taylor, P., Holden, B. A. et al. (1992) Contamination of 500ml bottles of unpreserved saline. Clin. Exp. Optom., 75(2), 67–75

Sweeney, D. F., Willcox, M. D., Sansey, N. et al. (1999) Incidence of contamination of preserved saline solutions during normal use. CLAO J., 25(3), 167–175

Tachikawa, T., Fuzisawa, S., Okuno, Y. et al. (1991) The efficacy of hydrogen peroxide against Acanthamoeba cysts using the modified Lowry's method. J. Jpn Cont. Lens Soc., 33, 179–184

Thakur, A., Chauhan, A. and Willcox, M. D. (1999) Effect of lysozyme on adhesion and toxin release by Staphylococcus aureus. Aust. N. Z. J. Ophthalmol., 27, 224–227

Thomas, P. F. (1972) The influence of environment on Bionite Naturalenses. Aust. J. Optom., 55(9), 354–357

Thompson, R. E. M. and Mansell, P. E. (1976) The cleansing and decontamination of hydrophilic contact lenses. Eye, Mar., 4–6

Tighe, B., Bright, A. and Franklin, V. (1991) Extrinsic factors in soft contact lens spoilation. J. B.C.L.A., 14(4), 195–200

Tomlinson, A. (2002) Silicone hydrogel risk analysed. Optician, 224(5880), 5

Tomlinson, A. and Caroline, P. J. (1990) Comparative evaluation of surface deposits on high water content hydrogel contact lens polymers. CLAO J., 16(2), 121–127

Tonge, S., Tighe, B. and Franklin, V. (2001a) Contact Lens Care: Part 5 – The design and development of wetting and multi-purpose solutions. Optician, 222(5812), 22–27

Tonge, S., Tighe, B. and Franklin, V. (2001b) Contact Lens Care: Part 6 – Comfort drops, artificial tears and dry-eye therapies. Optician, 222(5817), 27–33

Tragakis, M. P., Brown, S. I. and Pearce, D. B. (1973) Bacteriologic studies of contamination associated with soft contact lenses. Am. J. Ophthalmol., 75, 496–499

Uchijama, K., Ishido, C., Yago, S. et al. (1994) An autopsy case of CJD associated with corneal transplantation. Dementia, 8, 466–473

Ueda, K. (2000) A case of suspected corneal and conjunctival complications induced by polidronium chloride (Polyquad®). J. Jpn Cont. Lens Soc., 42, 164–166

Vogt, M. W., Ho, D. D., Bakar, S. R. et al. (1986) Safe disinfection of contact lenses after contamination with HTLV-III. Ophthalmology, 93, 771–774

Walker, J. (1988) A clinical and laboratory comparison of the deposition characteristics of both silicone/acrylate and fluoro-silicone acrylate lenses. J. B.C.L.A. (Transaction of B.C.L.A. Conference), 11(4)(Suppl), 83–86

Wardlaw, J. C. and Sarver, M. D. (1986) Discoloration of hydrogel contact lenses under standard care regimens. Am. J. Optom. Physiol. Opt., 63(6), 403–408

Wilhelmus, K. R., Robinson, N. M., Font, R. A. et al. (1988) Fungal keratitis in contact lens wearers. Am. J. Ophthalmol., 106, 708–714

Willcox, M., Power, K., Stapleton, F. et al. (1997) Potential sources of bacteria that are isolated from contact lenses during wear. Optom. Vision Sci., 74, 1030–1038

Wilson, L. (1979) External Diseases of the Eye, pp 31–46. Hagerstown, MD: Harper and Row

Wilson, L. A., Ahearn, D. G., Jones, D. B. et al. (1969) Fungi from the normal outer eye. Am. J. Ophthalmol., 67, 52–56

Wilson, L. A., Schlitzer, R. L. and Ahearn, D. G. (1981) Pseudomonas corneal ulcers associated with soft contact-lens wear. Am. J. Ophthalmol., 92, 546–554

Wilson, L. A., Sawant, A. D. and Ahearn, D. G. (1991) Comparative efficacies of soft contact lens disinfectant solutions against microbial films in lens cases. Arch. Ophthalmol., 109, 1155–1157

Wong, M. P., Dziabo, A. J. and Kiral, R. M. (1986) Adsorption of benzalkonium chloride by RGP lenses. Cont. Lens Forum, 11(5), 25–32

Young, G. (2004) Why one million contact lens wearers dropped out. Cont. Lens Ant. Eye, 27, 83–85

Chapter 5

Tears and contact lenses

Jean-Pierre Guillon and Andrew Godfrey

CHAPTER CONTENTS

The introduction of any contact lens into the eye will adversely affect the tear film and ocular environment. This will, in most cases, result in an unstable tear film, both over the contact lens and elsewhere in the eye. Our aim as contact lens practitioners is to manage this effect. Of those who stop using contact lenses, most do so because of decreased comfort, which is often caused by a poor tear film and its interaction with the lens.

Changes are most likely caused by one or more of the following:

- Nature of the contact lens surface.
- Nature of the contact lens design (lens edge and structure).
- Instillation of contact lens solutions with the lens (temporary).
- Instillation of eye drops during wear (artificial tears).
- Characteristics of the wearer's tear film.

The assessment of the tear film and its related ocular effects can indicate a patient's suitability as a contact lens wearer:

- Ideal.
- Normal.
- Problematic (symptomatic and asymptomatic).
- Not suitable.

As the tear film will be destabilized, we need to ensure that, before fitting, it is as good as possible.

TEAR FILM ASSESSMENT

History and symptoms

Many patients report that they suffer from dry eye or tear film problems, with scratchy, gritty, burning, watery or itchy eyes. Tired eyes late in the day may signify an inadequate tear film. A sharp stabbing eye pain lasting only a few seconds may also be a pointer towards a poor tear film. People doing concentrated near work or using computers in air-conditioned or heated buildings reduce their blink rate, resulting in dry eyes.

Some patients may be asymptomatic subjectively but have a poor tear film when examined objectively. Therefore, history and symptoms must be followed by more direct measurements.

Slit-lamp

CONJUNCTIVAL HYPERAEMIA

The location of the injection can indicate the cause of the dryness (Fig. 5.1).

- Between the lids – most often caused by exposure and resulting dryness.

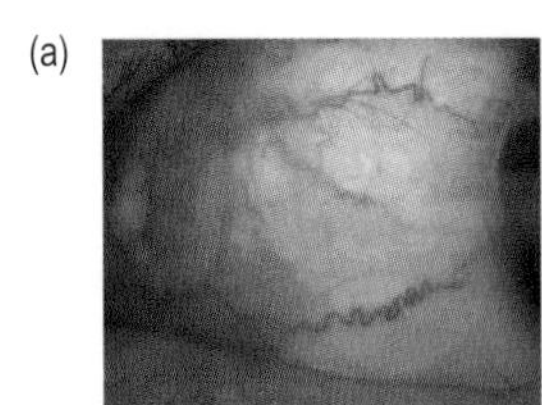
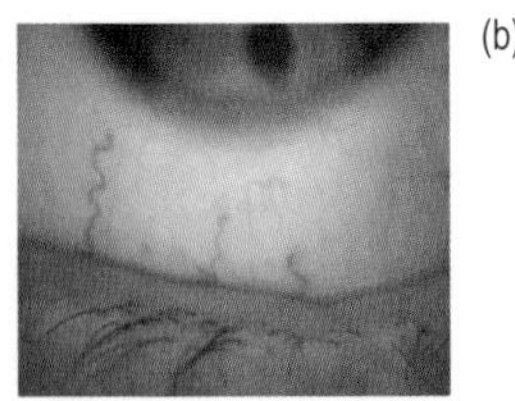

Figure 5.1 Conjunctival hyperaemia: (a) nasal conjunctiva; (b) inferior conjunctiva

- All over the eye – possibly results from an extreme dry eye or an infective/inflammatory reaction which may be worsened with dry eyes.
- Worse near the limbus – suggestive of poor lens fitting, inadequate oxygen permeability or lens-related drying effects.
- Below the lids – infective or severe dry eye.

CONJUNCTIVAL FOLDS

Conjunctival folds produce an abnormal apposition to the lid edge that prevents the formation of a normal tear reservoir. They are one of the main signs of conjunctival dryness and hyperaemia, and can easily be detected in white light (Fig. 5.2). They may also result from age-related changes.

Conjunctival folds can be graded according to their position and severity:

- Grade 1 – commonly seen in the temporal conjunctiva.
- Grade 2 – nasal conjunctiva.
- Grade 3 – centrally in the area adjacent to the inferior cornea (Fig. 5.2).

Conjunctival folds reduce the amount of fluid available, resulting in increased friction that may increase the severity of the folds. They can interfere both with the fitting of a contact lens as well as the distribution of the tears across the lens.

When folds are detected, ocular lubrication is needed by means of a gel rather than eye drops. The gel should be used at night (e.g. Viscotears [CIBA] or Genteal Gel [Novartis]) and slightly viscous liquid lubricants (e.g. Systane [Alcon] (only to be used before or after contact lens wear) or Refresh Plus [Allergan]) during the day.

CORNEA

With less lubrication, the mechanical effect of the lens upon the cornea will increase. Thus scattered punctate erosions can be a result of contact lens-related dry eyes. With thin, soft lenses, pervaporation may occur through the lens in areas of repeated dryness.

LID APPEARANCE

Any occurrence of meibomian gland dysfunction (MGD) or blepharitis should be treated before attempting contact lens fitting.

PAPILLARY CONJUNCTIVITIS

As one of the main causes of papillary conjunctivitis is a combination of mechanical and allergic response to lens surface deposition, a deposit-resistant material with good wetting properties is advisable, together with regular lens replacement.

Conjunctival and corneal staining

The main uses of biological stains are to detect areas of epithelial defects (punctuate staining) or dead/desiccated cells (Eliason & Maurice 1990) to make it easier to view the tear film and assess tear break-up time (TBUT), and in contact lens fitting.

SODIUM FLUORESCEIN

Sodium fluorescein is a water-soluble dye which takes up a yellow–green colouration. It can be excited with illumination by near UV light, such as that produced by the 'cobalt blue' light of a Burton lamp. In practice, the blue filter of the slit-lamp and a yellow barrier filter (Wratten 12) is the most effective combination.

Fluorescein is strictly a pH indicator rather than a dye, so the fluorescence is affected by the concentration and pH of the solution. Fluorescein does not usually stain intact cells. Where the damage is superficial, fluorescence is bright and well demarcated, but if corneal damage penetrates further than Bowman's layer, the fluorescence becomes less bright and the edges less well circumscribed.

Maximum fluorescence is obtained for a concentration of 0.08 g/l. For maximum effect, it is better to observe the staining a few minutes after instillation. The dye spreads in the aqueous phase of the tears and accumulates in intercellular spaces; it can, over time, even diffuse into the anterior chamber. Maximum fluorescence is obtained with a low concentration of fluorescein; by instilling more, the fluorescence may actually decrease.

The concentration usually instilled from a unit dose Minim is 1 or 2% fluorescein solution. For surface staining assessment this is usually too large to have any real value in assessing the tear film or tear reservoir. The best alternative is to use fluorescein-impregnated strips (e.g. Fluorets) wetted with saline to provide

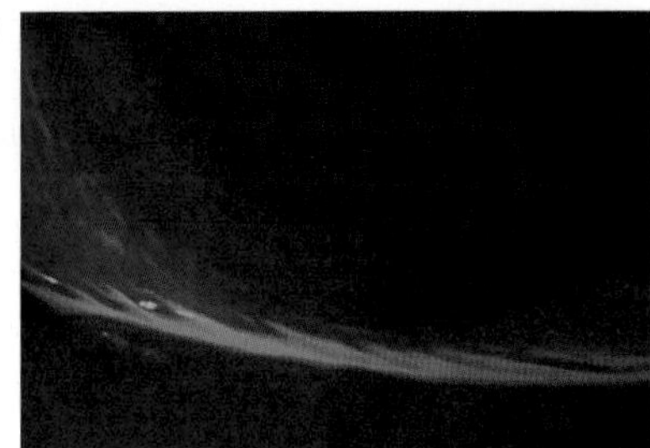
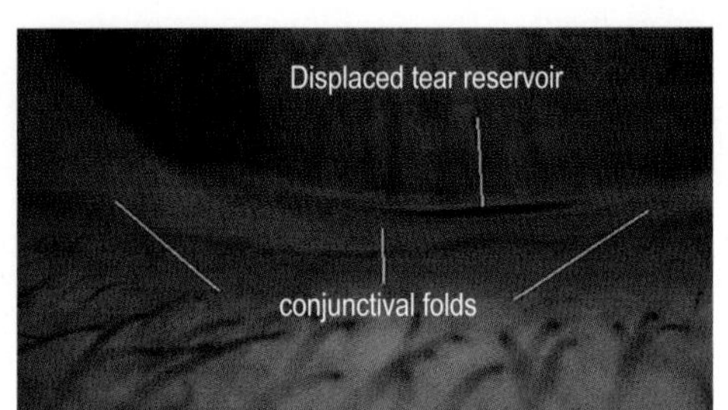

Figure 5.2 Conjunctival folds: (a) fluorescein view; (b) Tearscope view

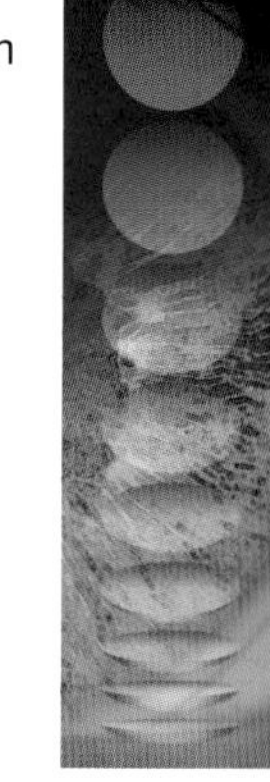

the minimal amount of stain to allow an adequate measurement of the fluorescein tear break-up time (TBUT), observation of the tear reservoir and ocular surface disruption. Thinning of the tear film becomes evident as a localized loss of fluorescence that is shortly followed by a break (Fig. 5.3).

A more measured rate of fluorescein instillation for TBUT is possible with the dry eye test (DET) method (Korb et al. 2001). This comprises 10 × 1 mm strips, which reduce the amount of fluorescein applied prior to measurement. By giving a fixed amount of fluorescein dye they appear to give improved repeatability compared to Fluorets.

The presence of staining may not necessarily be a definitive diagnosis, as normal eyes have been shown to exhibit corneal staining and, of course, staining may result from other causes.

HIGH-MOLECULAR-WEIGHT FLUORESCEIN

If fluorescein is used to assess the fit of a soft lens on the eye, then high-molecular-weight fluorescein is needed. The molecular weight is made sufficiently great to prevent immediate penetration into most soft lens materials (e.g. Fluoresoft and Fluorexon). However, care is still required with high water content lenses as there may be some uptake and discolouration. As the degree of fluorescence is less than with standard fluorescein, a yellow filter is recommended for observation. The picture seen is not always easy to assess.

SULPHORHODAMINE B

Sulphorhodamine B is an orange fluorescent dye that gives a greater contrast than fluorescein when observed by the appropriate excitation and barrier filters. The tear film is seen covering the surface of the conjunctiva as well as the usual concentration in its folds; transient tear film thinning at the limbus is also more obvious with this dye.

ROSE BENGAL

Rose Bengal is a water-soluble dye which stains devitalized cells, mucous fibrils (Norn 1972) and plaques. Staining occurs mostly in the interpalpebral conjunctiva, particularly in cases of aqueous tear deficiency. A faint punctuate line along the line of Marx may also be evident, which research has suggested is the site of frictional contact between the lid margin and bulbar conjunctiva/cornea (Donald et al. 2003, Hughes et al. 2003). Heavier punctuate staining can indicate a posterior blepharitis.

The dye is available at 1% concentration in Minim form but may cause intense stinging and should be used sparingly. It can also be used as impregnated strips as they sting significantly less. These are copiously wetted and applied to the lower conjunctiva.

LISSAMINE GREEN

Lissamine green has been recommended as an alternative to Rose Bengal as it causes insignificant stinging. It is mostly available in strips to be wetted with saline, which gives some control over the concentration used. It is a diagnostic dye for evaluating the cornea and conjunctiva but is not readily available worldwide.

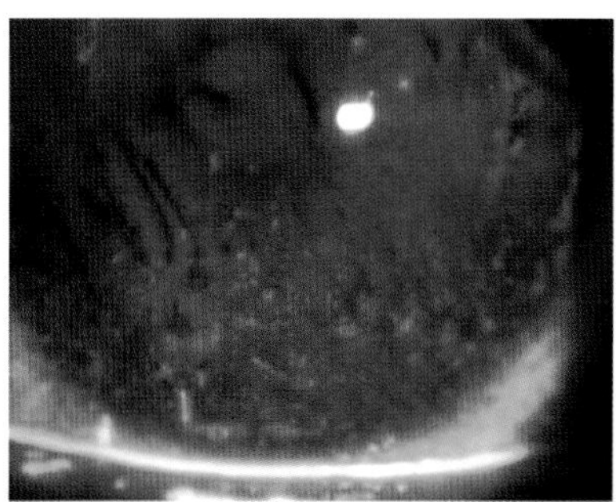

Figure 5.3 Fluorescein tear break-up

Tear break-up time (TBUT)

Norn (1969) proposed the tear film break-up time as 'corneal wetting time'. Fluorescein is instilled and, once spread evenly after a few blinks, the eye is viewed with cobalt blue illumination and yellow filter observation. When the uniform green film is interrupted with a dark area it represents the break-up of the tear film and the time since the last blink is recorded as the tear break-up time (TBUT) (Fig. 5.3). An average TBUT value of 30 seconds was found by Norn (1969) but with large variations. A TBUT less than 10 seconds is usually considered abnormal. If the tear film continually breaks at the same spot, then a superficial epithelial abnormality should be suspected (Lemp et al. 1970). In addition, an incomplete blinker will often show tear breaks in the inferior portion of the corneal surface.

Variations in measurement of TBUT may be caused by:

- Use of local anaesthetic.
- Use of lubricants.
- Forced blinking prior to measurement.
- Air movement during testing (air-conditioning/heating).
- Holding lids open during testing (forcibly).

The main problem is the invasive nature of fluorescein. Once fluorescein is instilled, the tear film is no longer 'normal' and may react in different ways to the presence of the dye, producing results that do not necessarily reflect the normal eye situation.

TEAR MEASUREMENT

Various tests are available for measuring tear output, the quality of the tears and precorneal film, and the rate of drying or thinning of the tears. Schirmer (1903) described a test for the measurement of tear output, whereby paper strips are bent at one end and inserted over the lower lid (Fig. 5.4). It is only adequate for the detection of gross abnormality as the test papers irritate the eye; however, it does reveal very dry eyes and can be useful before fitting any type of contact lens (Cho & Yap 1993). More accurate results can be obtained if a local anaesthetic is instilled first.

Norn's test (Norn 1965), although rarely used, is more accurate than Schirmer's. It involves judging the dilution of the tears in the lacrimal rivus over the central part of the lower lid, 5 minutes after 10 μl of a mixture of 1% Rose Bengal and 1% fluorescein is instilled into the lower fornix. Using the slit-lamp

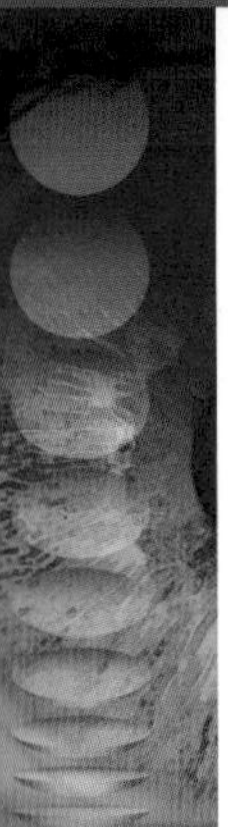

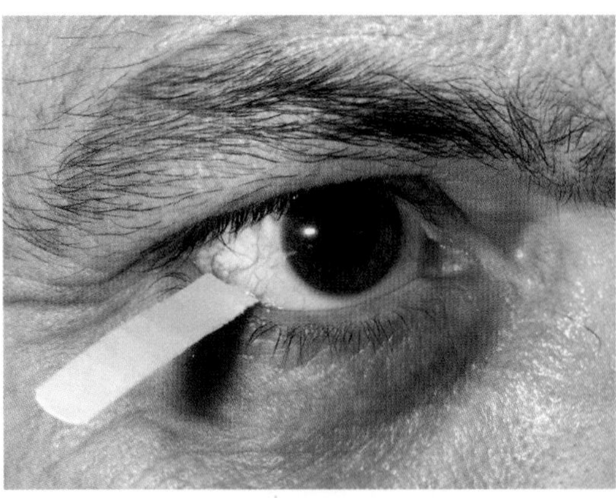

Figure 5.4 Schirmer's test showing how the tear fluid wets the paper strip

a comparison is made with known dilutions of the mixture in capillary tubes.

PHENOL RED THREAD

This method of assessing tear film quantity is less invasive than the Schirmer test as it produces less reflex secretion. It utilizes a two-ply cotton thread (0.2 mm) impregnated with the phenol red dye. Phenol red is pH sensitive and changes from yellow to red when wetted by the tears. The thread is 70 mm long with a small bend at one end, not unlike the Schirmer paper. This bent part is placed in the inferior conjunctival sac on the temporal side and left in position for 15 seconds only. On removal the amount of the thread that has undergone a colour change is measured. Little and Bruce (1994) showed it to be reliable and repeatable, and suggested that, for Caucasian subjects, tear secretion was low if, in 15 seconds, less than 11 mm of the thread is wetted, borderline if less than 16 mm, with 21 mm representing normal.

TEAR RESERVOIR

A normal pre-ocular (or pre-lens) tear film should be continuous over the cornea, conjunctiva and lid margin. The height of the tear reservoir at the lid margin represents the volume of tears available for resurfacing the eye (Fig. 5.5). Both can be observed non-invasively with the Tearscope (see below) or after instillation of a small amount of fluorescein.

Any discontinuity over the conjunctival surface is a sign of conjunctival dryness and is often seen in the presence of early conjunctival folds. The use of gels is recommended to limit their progression. Patients should be warned of the possibility of symptoms that may limit contact lens wear.

Reservoir height

The normal lacrimal rivus height is approximately 1.0 mm with a reduced height or scalloped edge indicating a potential dry eye. The use of artificial rewetting drops is strongly advised for adequate contact lens wear and acceptable comfort.

Marked aqueous and mucus deficiencies

- *Rose Bengal/lissamine green* (mucus deficiency): If the cornea itself stains with Rose Bengal or lissamine green, the patient should not be fitted with contact lenses unless indicated for medical purposes (see Chapter 26).
- *Schirmer's test* (aqueous deficiency): Less than 10 mm wetted in 3 minutes indicates a gross aqueous insufficiency.
- *Phenol red thread test* (aqueous deficiency): In the most popular test, Menicon's Zone-Quick, less than 10 mm wetted in 15 seconds indicates a significant aqueous deficiency.

LID AND BLINK ABNORMALITIES

Although less common, eyelid and blink abnormalities can contribute to an evaporative dry eye by increasing the ocular surface exposure. These include:

- Incomplete blink.
- Lagophthalmos from facial nerve palsies.
- Diseases that cause reduced blink (e.g. Parkinson's disease).
- Reduced blink rate associated with prolonged reading or computer use.
- Nocturnal lagophthalmos (check by taping one eyelid closed at bedtime).
- Proptosis (most commonly from thyroid eye disease).
- Positional eyelid abnormalities (e.g. ectropion or entropion).

DISEASES OF THE MUCOUS LAYER

Mucus deficiency

- Sjögren's syndrome.
- Late keratoconjunctivitis sicca (KCS).
- Thermal burns.
- Alkali burns.
- Vitamin A deficiency.
- Anaesthetic cornea.
- Stevens–Johnson syndrome.
- Cicatricial ocular pemphigoid.

Mucus overproduction

- Giant papillary conjunctivitis.
- Vernal conjunctivitis.
- Early KCS.
- Atopy.
- Mucus fishing syndrome.

COSMETICS

An abnormal appearance of the lipid layer and resulting dry eye is commonly caused by cosmetics. This can take several forms,

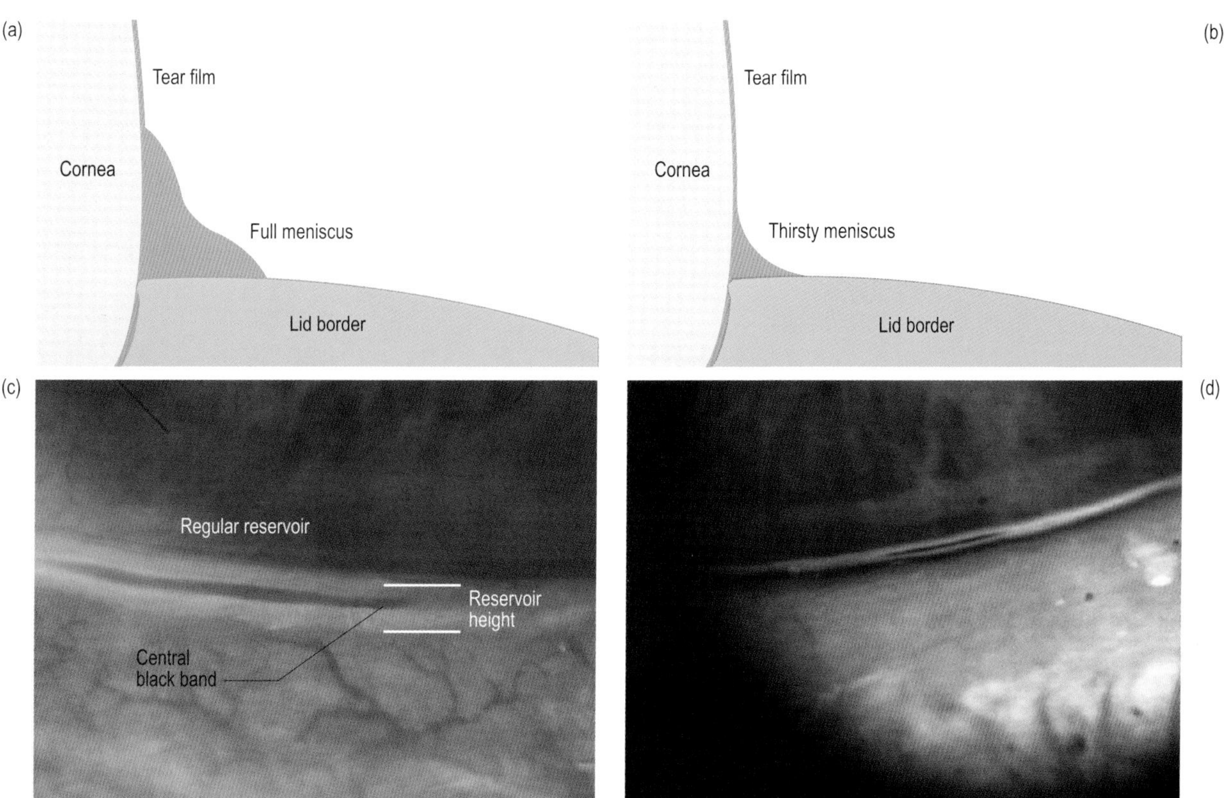

Figure 5.5 The tear reservoir showing a normal or regular meniscus (a, c) and a narrow or 'thirsty' meniscus (b, d) with a reduced reservoir height

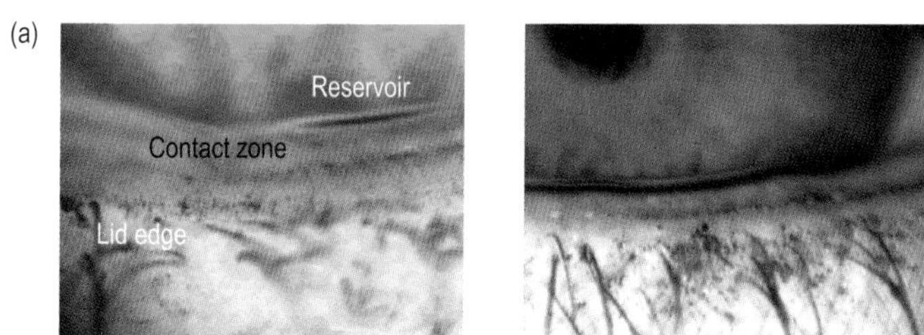

Figure 5.6 (a) Normal lid margin with make-up contamination shown in (b)

from specks in the tear film to a coating of the lid margin and blockage of the meibomian glands, preventing the normal lipid discharge into the tear film (Fig. 5.6).

Cosmetics are mostly surface-active products designed to stick to and penetrate the skin surface and alter its wetting properties. As their surface activity is greater than that of the meibomian secretion, they will break up the lipid layer and stick to the contact lens surface, producing an area of non-wetting.

The composition of the meibomian gland secretion and its physicochemical properties produce a barrier that normally prevents any skin secretion from invading the ocular surface. Similarly, the meibomian lipid secretion cannot spread further than the line of Marx (the line between the palpebral conjunctiva and the lid epithelium), allowing the formation of a normal tear reservoir.

The use of make-up and skin or medicated products has a detrimental effect on this fragile separation. It affects the tear film, resulting in rapid evaporation, which in turn causes dry eye symptoms and arcuate corneal epithelial desiccation and staining, similar to that found in blepharitis.

Make-up removers

Oily make-up removers cause most problems in the eye as they temporarily destroy the spreading capabilities of the tear lipid layer (Fig. 5.7). If this oil coats the lid margins, it affects the lipid layer at every blink, and the effect may even be visible more than 20 hours after their use. This results in dry eye symptoms.

One hypoallergenic make-up remover (Phas Respectissime by La Roche) has been designed to cause minimal effect to the ocular surface and lipid layer. It contains sodium hyalorunate as one of its ingredients, which appears to make the lipid layer more stable following its use.

- *Eyeliners* applied directly to the rim of the lid will interfere with the proper function of the meibomian glands by blocking their orifices and contaminating their secretion. When the eyeliner covers the line of Marx, it creates a bridge for any invading skin secretion or make-up products. Further, their removal will require contact with the lid margin and possible further disturbance to the tear film. Eyeliner should only be used on the outside of the lashes.
- *Waterproof mascara* can flake or break up and increase the debris level on the superficial lipid layer. It can only be

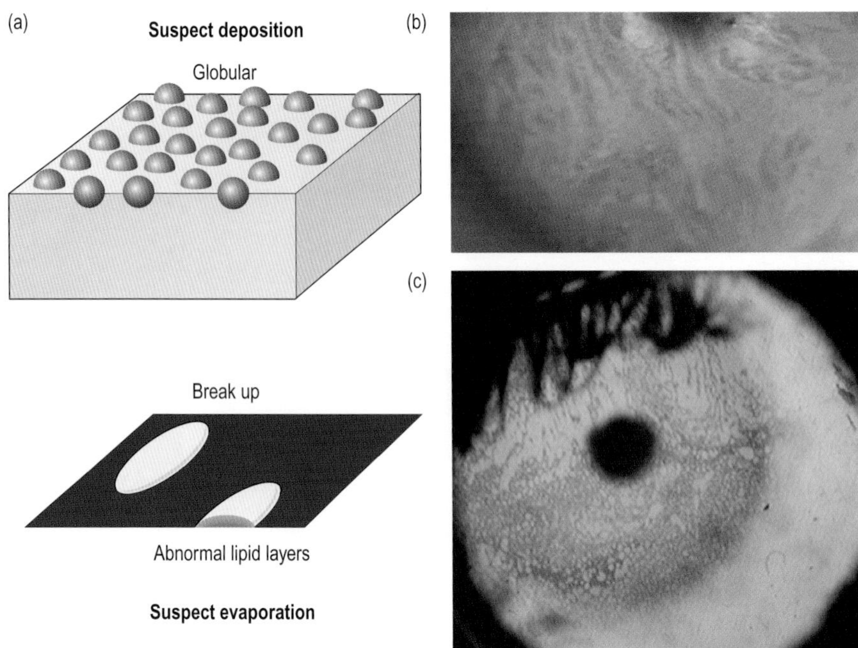

Figure 5.7 (a) Lipid layer broken up by make-up remover showing the abnormal globular layer at the top and the broken-up picture at the bottom. (b) Suspect deposition; (c) suspect evaporation

removed by an oily make-up remover which will disturb the tear film.

- *Water-based mascaras* are better but if heavily applied can deposit themselves on the lid margin and on the contact lens surface. This type of mascara should be applied in only moderate quantities and reapplied as necessary during the day. One mascara (Phas Respectissime mascara by La Roche) has been developed to avoid these problems.
- *Eye shadow* can release particles onto the tear film surface and increase debris formation.
- *Face powder* can spread very small particles over the lens surface and dry the pre-lens tear film.
- *Moisturizers* are designed to stay on the surface of the skin and limit evaporation. People suffering from marginal dry-eye symptoms commonly use moisturizers, as they often have a combination dry skin. Unfortunately, the best products for the skin are usually the worst for the tear film. When present in the tear film they appear as oily droplets or plaques. Their effect is worst when applied to the outer canthus as repeated contact with the superficial tear film increases the disturbance. Moisturizers cause non-wetting areas on the lens surface.
- *Rehydrating creams* are usually better as they are designed to penetrate the skin and rehydrate its inner layer.

The general advice should be to always apply the make-up after insertion of the contact lenses to avoid most of the mechanical contamination via the fingers.

With dry eyes, lens deposition increases as there is a less efficient tear film to remove make-up debris.

TEARSCOPE (KEELER)

Dry eye symptoms are present in about 25% of the contact lens-wearing population (more in less humid areas) and account for a large number of contact lens drop-outs. The Tearscope-plus is an effective diagnostic tool and allows accurate diagnosis and classification of dry-eye symptoms, together with the ability to monitor the effect of any treatment (Fig. 5.8). It allows non-invasive assessment of the tears under 'normal' eye conditions.

Use of fluorescein, while valuable, does not represent the normal in-eye situation. Fluorescein cannot be used with soft contact lenses without staining them (except for high molecular weight fluorescein such as Fluorosoft or Fluorexon). The Tearscope provides accurate information about the tear film behind and in front of the lens without the need for fluorescein.

Uses

Developed by one of the authors (JPG), the Tearscope is used to classify the various aspects of the tear film:

- Appearance.
- Volume.
- Stability (invasive and non-invasive).
- Morphology of the tear reservoir – regularity, height and curvature.
- The tear layers present both anterior and posterior to a contact lens.
- Effect on the ocular surface.
- Effect on the contact lens surface.

Measurements taken with the Tearscope are:

- NIBUT (non-invasive break-up time) – the first break of the tear film is recorded, as well as the type and location of the break (average 5 seconds).
- NIDUT (non-invasive drying-up time) – the point where there are no interference fringes visible and the lens is devoid of tears (average 20 seconds). This varies with the

(a)

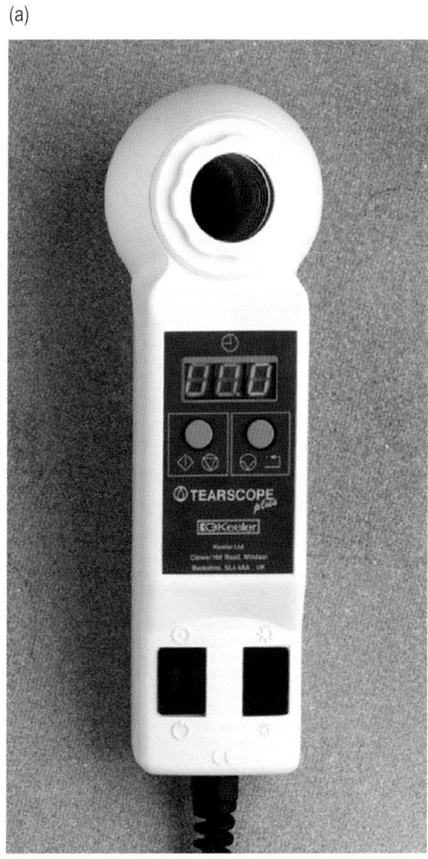

(b)

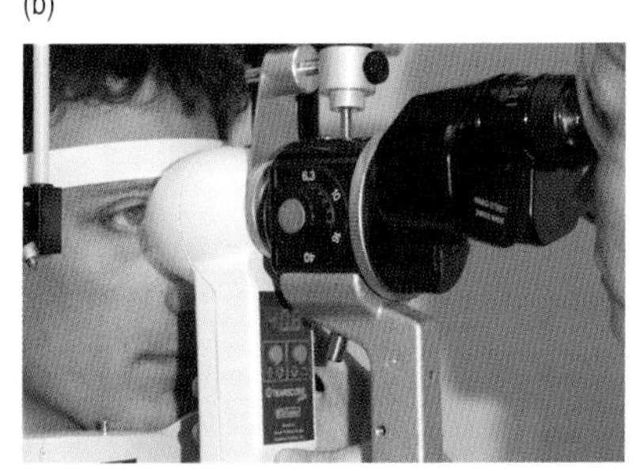

(c)

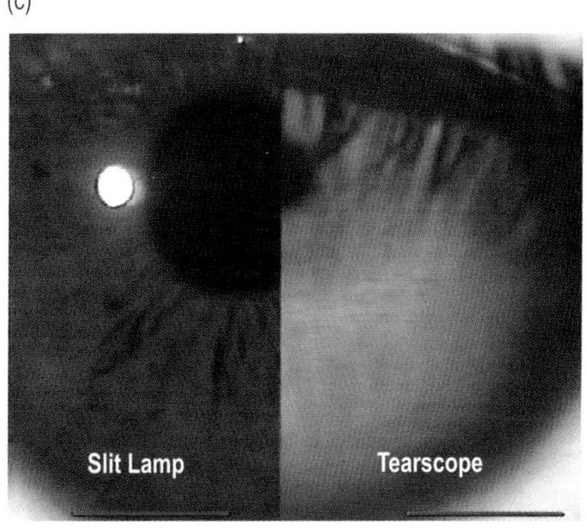

(d)

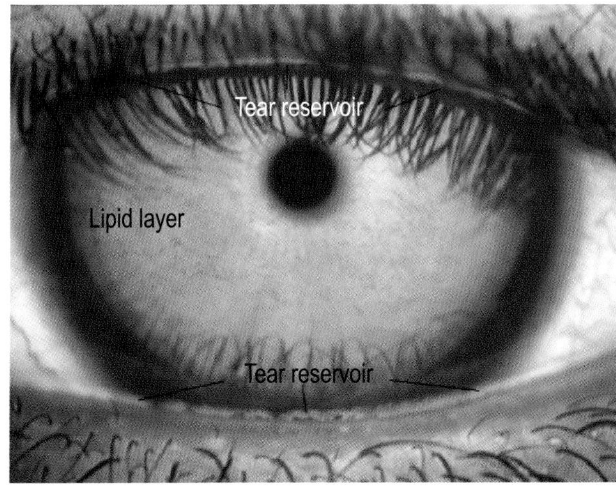

Figure 5.8 (a) Tearscope instrument, (b) being used mounted on a slit-lamp. Courtesy of staff at Great Ormond Street Hospital, London, (c) comparative view with and without Tearscope illumination, (d) superficial tear film structures imaged by the Tearscope

age of the lens and its surface condition (deposits and scratches).

The quality and quantity of each tear layer is important as well as their interaction with the eye and the pre- and post-contact lens surfaces. The tear film is not homogeneous; it relies on the separation of its layers for stability and protection of the surface it covers.

The design of the Tearscope

The Tearscope-plus has an internally illuminated tapered tubular design which permits proximity to the eye and eliminates obstruction from the nose, thereby allowing full corneal specular coverage (Fig. 5.9).

The two-level illumination system uses cold cathode light with reflectors to provide shadow-free viewing and reduced retroillumination. The light source is located at a maximal distance from the eye and a heat sink draws the heat away from the light via the handle and away from the patient's face. This reduces any heat-related drying effect which would interfere with accurate measurements. The instrument design allows for binocular examination with a slit-lamp using the 'R' tonometer mount so it can be swung in and out as needed. The Tearscope should be mounted at a 10° angle to ensure easy access to the switches and timer.

A hand-held magnifying lens provides 2× or 3× magnification when viewed from 30 to 50 cm.

A timer at the back of the instrument allows for accurate measurement of NIBUT/NIDUT to 1/10th of a second.

The following filters are available:

- A coarse grid.
- A fine grid (Fig. 5.9b).
- Concentric rings for corneal topography assessment (Fig. 5.9d).
- Filters for observing fluorescein in the tear film.

The coarse grid is used for NIBUT measurement when the Tearscope is hand-held to allow easier focusing than with the fine grid. It allows for detection of irregular and abnormal tear films to be observed without a slit-lamp. It can be used for both pre-ocular tear film (POTF) and pre-lens tear film (PLTF) observations along with NIBUT.

The fine grid insert is best used with slit-lamp magnification, allowing for a more sensitive measurement of the tear film. The

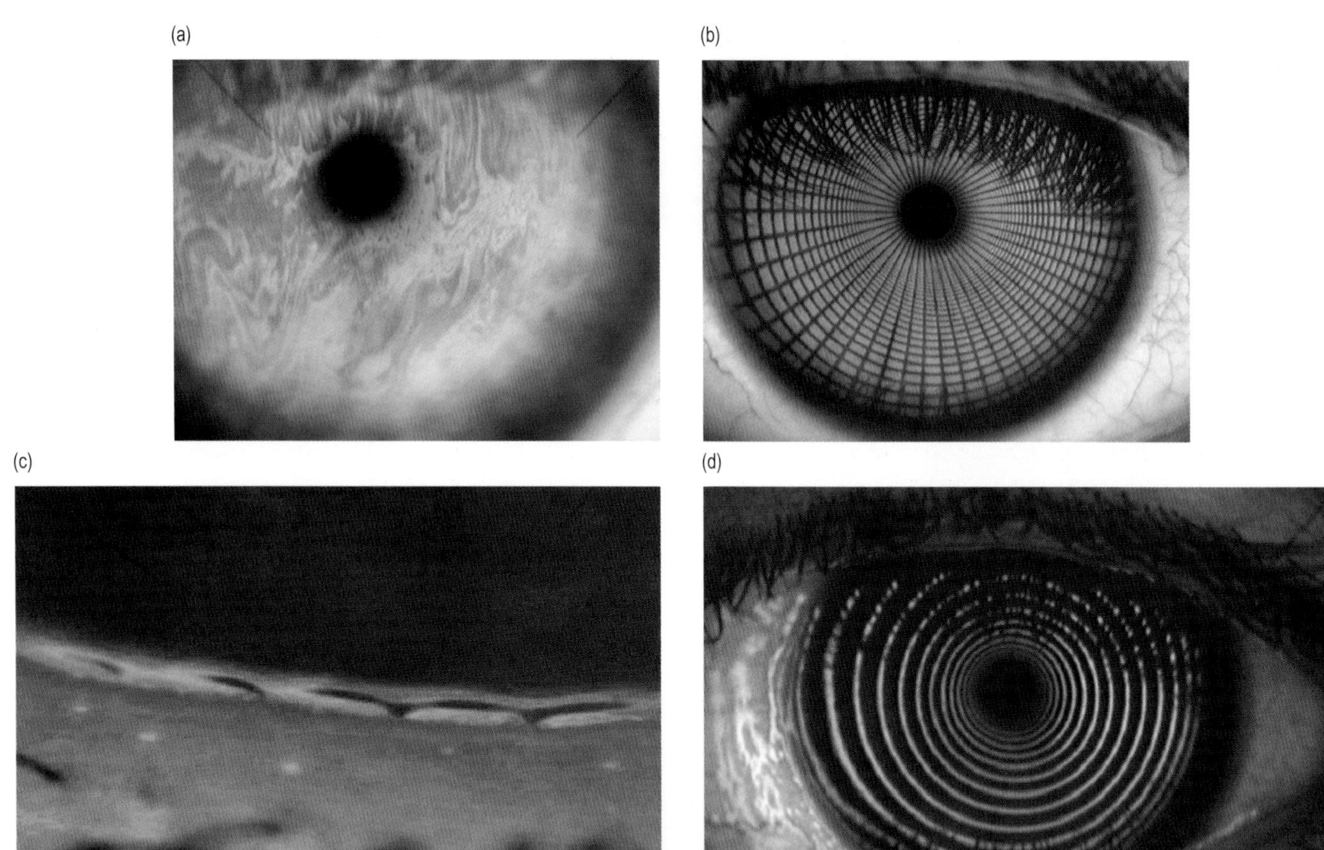

Figure 5.9 Observations with the Tearscope, (a) superficial lipid layer, (b) observation with fine grid insert, (c) irregular inferior reservoir observation, (d) observation with concentric ring insert

tear film is viewed against the white background to assess its structure, then the slit-lamp focused on the grid to measure the reflective quality of the tear film and the NIBUT.

The concentric rings act as an internally illuminated Placido disc, providing full corneal coverage. This is useful for rapid determination of:

- Keratoconus.
- Irregular or high astigmatism.
- Surface distortion of contact lenses.
- Distortion following corneal graft or refractive surgery.
- Effect of pterygia on the corneal shape.

The blue and yellow filter combination allows viewing of the fluorescein-stained tear film under low magnification and dynamic conditions. This has an advantage over UV lamps as the emission is mainly in the visible range, allowing easy fluorescein evaluation through lenses incorporating a UV filter.

The filter combination allows:

- Measurement of invasive break-up time with fluorescein (TBUT).
- Tear prism assessment for regularity.
- Rigid gas-permeable (RGP) lens fitting patterns.
- Corneal staining.

A dark field observation of contact lenses allows for a projection viewing system. A lens placed in the suitable holder can be illuminated and the image projected onto a dark background to show deposits and scratches as bright secondary light sources. This can be demonstrated to the patient to reinforce cleaning advice or the need for lens replacement.

Images seen with the Tearscope

LIPID LAYER

When present, the outermost layer of the tear film is highly reflective and can be seen moving at the surface.

AQUEOUS PHASE

This is visible as interference fringes and is seen when:

- The lipid layer is thin or absent.
- The lens surface is reflective.
- Reduced ocular surface mucous coverage is present.
- The pre-lens tear film is unstable.

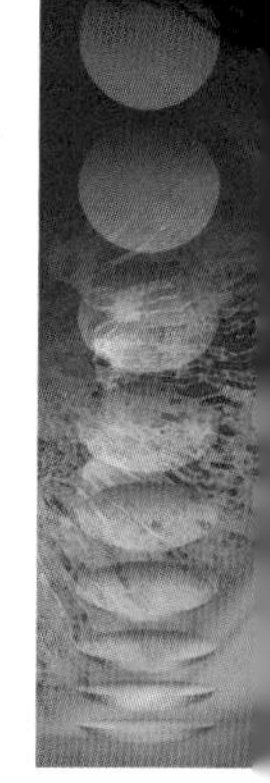

It is only visible over a large area during the interblink interval.

MUCOUS LAYER

This is visible when the aqueous phase has disappeared.

LENS SURFACE

In especially dry eyes, a blink does not resurface the lens with any tear film and the lens surface becomes visible.

INTERFERENCE FRINGES

Interference fringes depend on the thickness of the layer being observed and the reflectivity of bordering surfaces. This is greatest in very thin films of high refractive index such as soap bubbles and, conveniently, the lipid layer of the tear film. The Tearscope allows for bright interference colours to be seen in the lipid layer and some peak emission wavelengths allow for visualization of the thick aqueous layer over soft and RGP lenses.

Clinical usage

The following observations, grading and measurements can be made for both the POTF and PLTF on both prospective and current contact lens wearers:

- Lipid layer grading and observation.
- Tear reservoirs – regularity, height and curvature.
- Observation of the blink sequence.
- Measurement of the non-invasive break-up time.
- Grading of meibomian gland blockage.

Examining the PLTF

- Lipid layer grading and observation.
- Aqueous phase grading and observation.
- Tear reservoirs – regularity, height and curvature.
- Measurement of the NIBUT.

PRE-SOFT LENS TEAR FILM

The tear film that normally covers a soft contact lens is reduced and resembles the tear film seen in Sjögren's syndrome, with poor surface wettability and surface deterioration. The lipid, aqueous and mucous layers are thinner than the patient's normal pre-ocular tear film. Current hydrogel lenses also have reduced wetting properties compared with the normal cornea, which has epithelial anchorage for the mucous layer.

Observation of the pre-soft lens tear film can be used for the early detection of dry eye symptoms as these are always preceded by a decrease in tear film stability. The Tearscope can be used to provide information about the thickness and integrity of the various tear layers. It is possible to observe the aqueous phase which displays coloured interference fringes. The lipid layer is also visible when present. The interference fringes are visible due to interactions at the lipid/aqueous interface and the aqueous/mucus interface (Fig. 5.10).

The PLTF is important to reduce lens deposition and dehydration. It affects the cornea via the lens to the post-lens tear film through evaporation and pervaporation (where fluid is moved from the cornea through the post-lens tear film and lens to the pre-lens tear film where it subsequently evaporates). In advanced cases this can lead to severe drying of the corneal surface and damage.

The Tearscope can be used to assess:

- Presence or absence of the lipid layer.
- Thickness of the tear film.
- Presence of lens surface contaminants.
- Measurement of NIBUT.

The NIBUT rate and tear film thickness determine the optimum replacement frequency for disposable contact lenses. The lenses should be replaced when the NIBUT has decreased by 25% from the measurement taken with a new lens.

The Tearscope can also assess the effectiveness of any dry eye treatment such as changes in lens design, material, modality, lubricants, lens care solutions, more effective lens cleaning, artificial tears and lid care. It can be used to monitor both the quality and quantity of tears, allowing for a direct and easy comparison between after-care visits.

PLTF – RGP

The PLTF over an RGP lens is thin and less stable than that of a soft contact lens (Fig. 5.11). The lipid layer is often not present and quickly disappears, and the aqueous layer thins through evaporation and drainage due to the absence of the lipid layer. The aqueous phase can be assessed by counting the number of fringes visible in that area (Fig. 5.11).

The Tearscope can assess the PLTF time (when the first break occurs) and drying-up time (when full drainage has occurred). Following a blink, the break-up of the pre-lens tear film can be seen after 4–6 seconds and complete surface drainage within 20–25 seconds.

Repeated horizontal break-up of the pre-lens tear film, combined with break-up of the pre-ocular tear film along the lens edge, is an early sign that 3 and 9 o'clock desiccation staining is likely and modifying the lens edge lift should be considered (see Chapters 9 and 17).

Rapid or excessive lens movement will accelerate the destabilization of the PLTF.

PLTF – SILICONE HYDROGEL

Lenses that do not dehydrate retain a good PLTF. Clinical findings by the authors show that the PLTF of silicone hydrogel lenses is a hybrid between the pre-rigid and pre-soft lens tear films. A lipid layer is usually present which limits evaporation and the visibility of the aqueous fringes is enhanced compared to those found at the surface of hydrogel lenses. The effectiveness of silicone hydrogel lenses in dry-eye problems may be limited compared to alternative materials such as Proclear (CooperVision).

Observation of the pre-ocular tear film (POTF)

The lipid layer of the POTF

This is the outermost layer, and it is altered by blinking or reflex tearing. The thickness and the normal/abnormal appearance should be assessed (Figs 5.10 and 5.12).

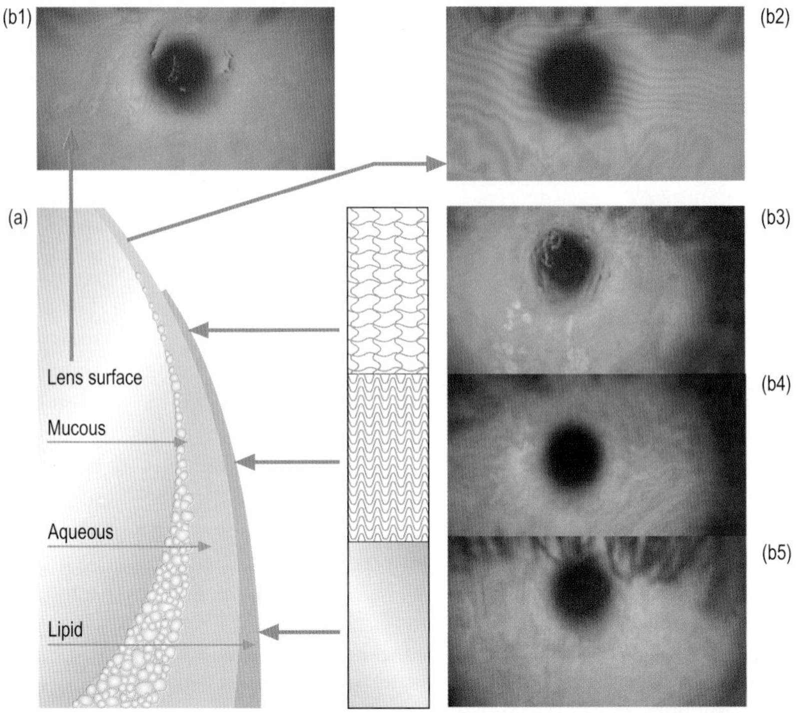

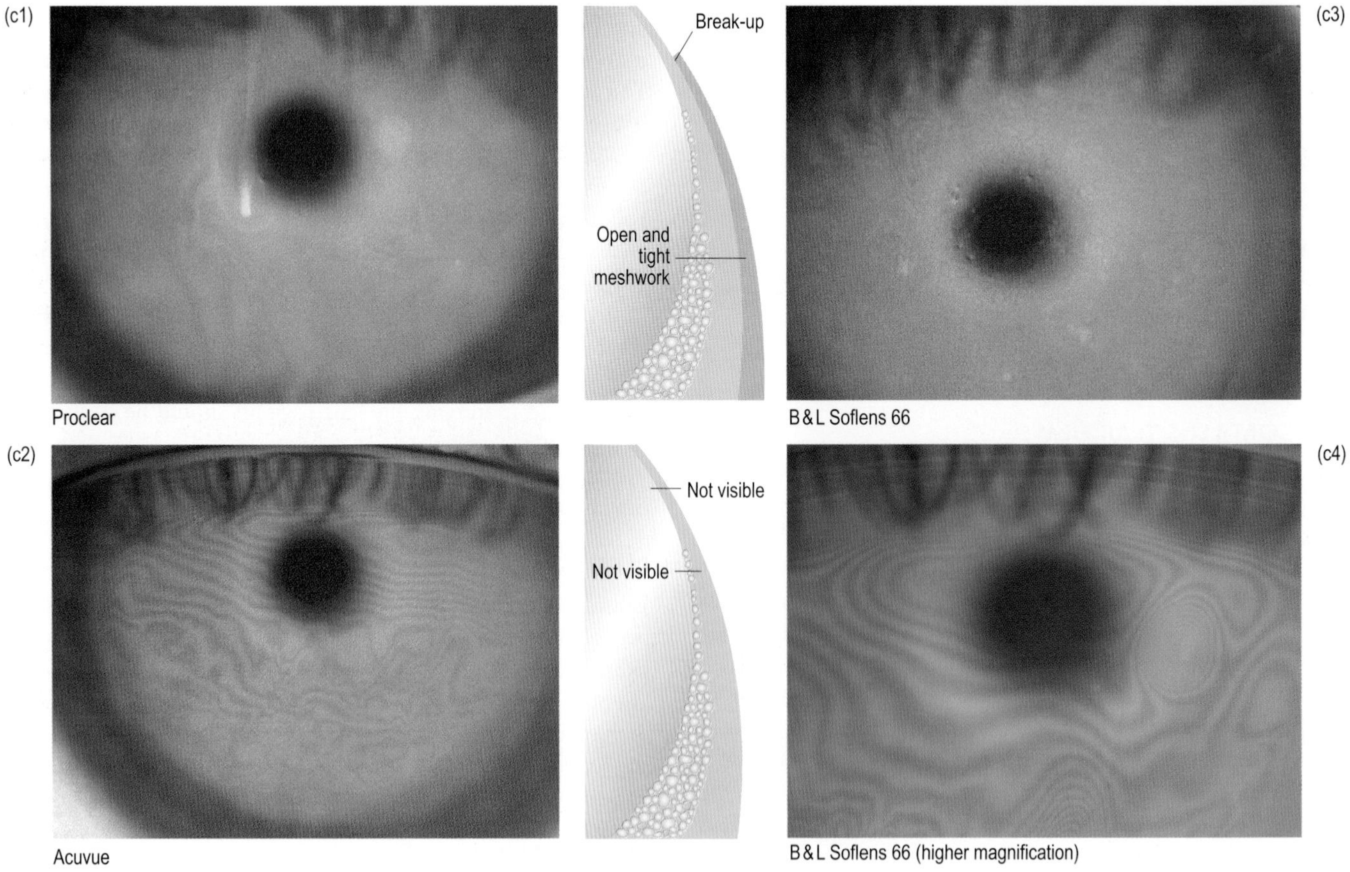

Figure 5.10 Tear film seen through Tearscope. (a) Pre-soft lens tear film grading: (b1) drying tear film; (b2) absent lipid layer, <1.0 μm aqueous; (b3) meshwork lipid layer, <1.0 μm aqueous; (b4) wave lipid layer, ~2.5 μm aqueous. (b5) amorphous lipid layer, >2.5 μm aqueous. (c) The lipid layer and aqueous fringes on three lens types after 6 hours of wear: (c1) Proclear; (c2) Acuvue; (c3) B&L Soflens 66; (c4) B & L Soflens 66 at higher magnification. The diagrammatic appearance of the tear film in this and later pictures is shown centrally

(b1) (b2)

(a) (b3)

Lens surface

Mucous (b4)

Aqueous (b5)

Lipid

(c1) Break-up (c3)

Open and tight meshwork

Proclear B&L Soflens 66

(c2) (c4)

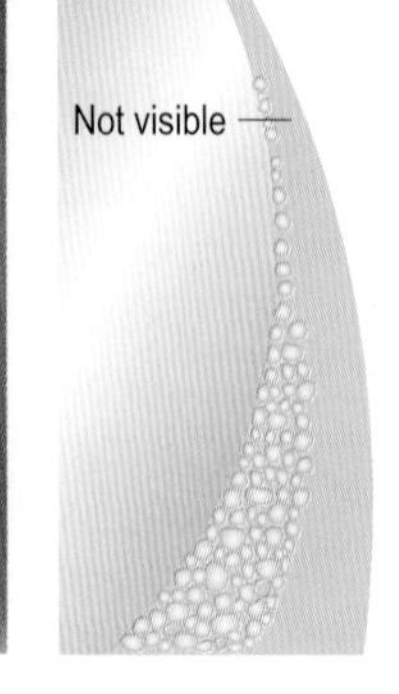

Acuvue B&L Soflens 66 (higher magnification)

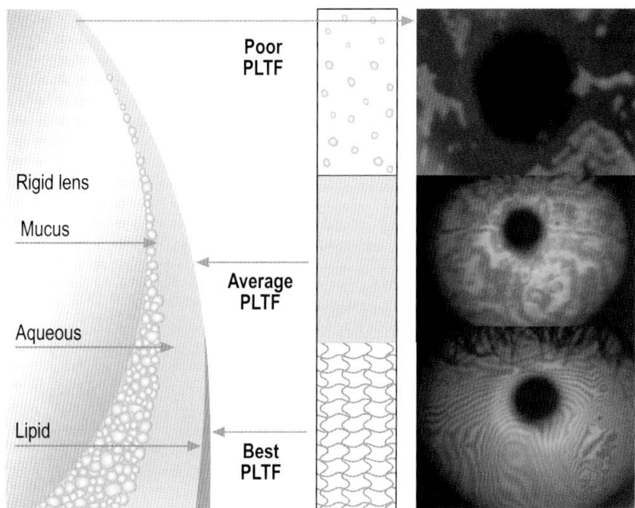

Figure 5.11 Pre-RGP lens tear film (PLTF) structure and grading images

The grading system developed by one of the authors (J-PG) is as follows:

Open meshwork (Fig. 5.12b1)

An open meshwork is very thin and may not be visible under normal magnification. It is seen only during a blink as it displaces upwards and becomes thickened for a few moments before disappearing. Such a thin lipid layer may not provide enough coverage over a soft contact lens and any cosmetics entering the eye from the lid margin are likely to attach to the lens.

Closed meshwork (Fig. 5.12b2)

When the lipid layer thickens it appears as a closed meshwork pattern, which is more visible and commonly seen. It takes a few seconds after the blink for the lipid layer to stabilize and is often thicker inferiorly.

Wave pattern (Fig. 5.12b3)

A thicker lipid layer shows as a flowing appearance with increased contrast. Both a vertical and a horizontal flow pattern (with increased lipid secretion) is possible and this is one of the most common appearances of the lipid layer.

Mixed pattern

The closed meshwork and the wave pattern can appear together on the same eye. The closed meshwork is often observed in the superior area where the lipid layer is thinner and the wave pattern seen inferiorly.

Amorphous pattern (Fig. 5.12b4)

This is the ideal lipid layer and provides excellent protection against evaporation. It shows high reflectivity and is thick and evenly distributed. These eyes usually do well with contact lenses.

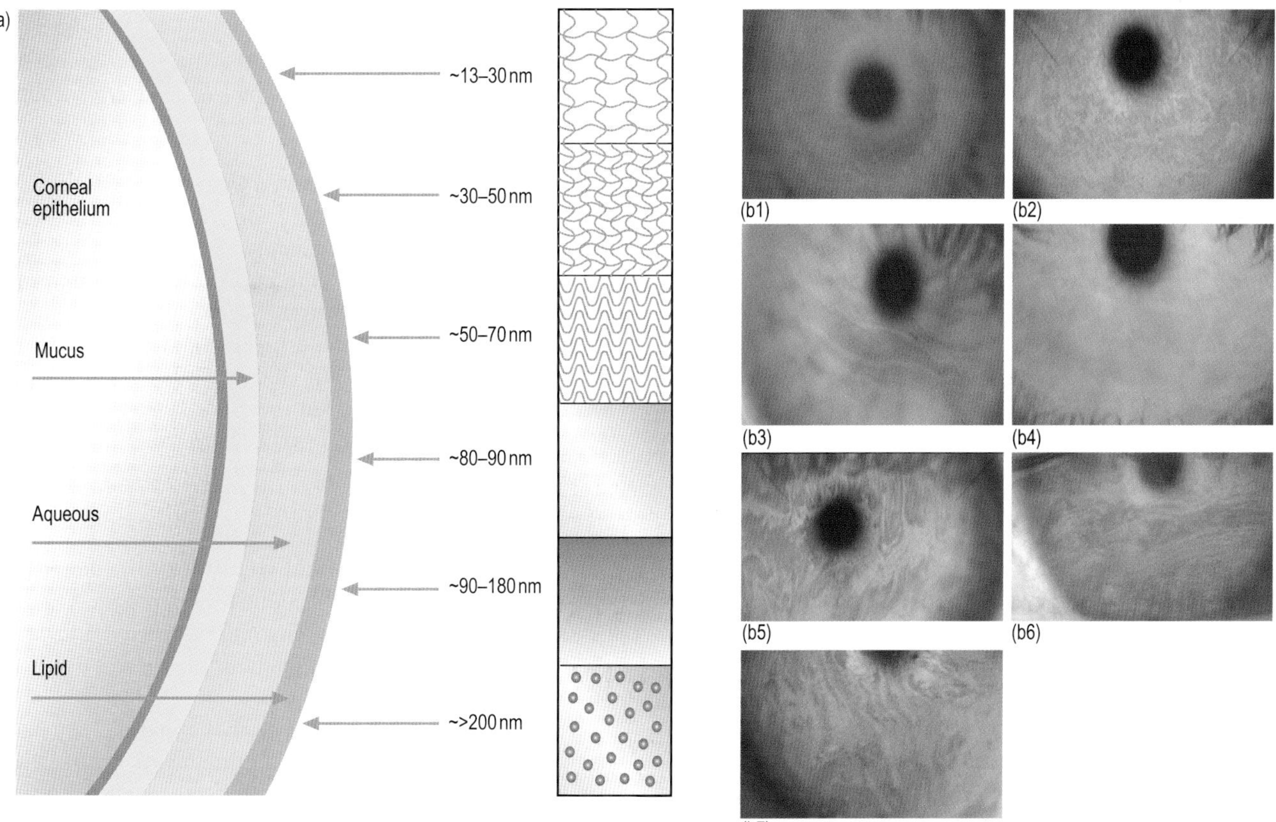

Figure 5.12 Pre-ocular tear film lipid grading: (a) diagrammatic representation of thickness and pattern; (b) Tearscope appearances: (b1) open meshwork, (b2) closed meshwork, (b3) wave, (b4) amorphous, (b5, b6) colour fringes, (b7) globular

(a)

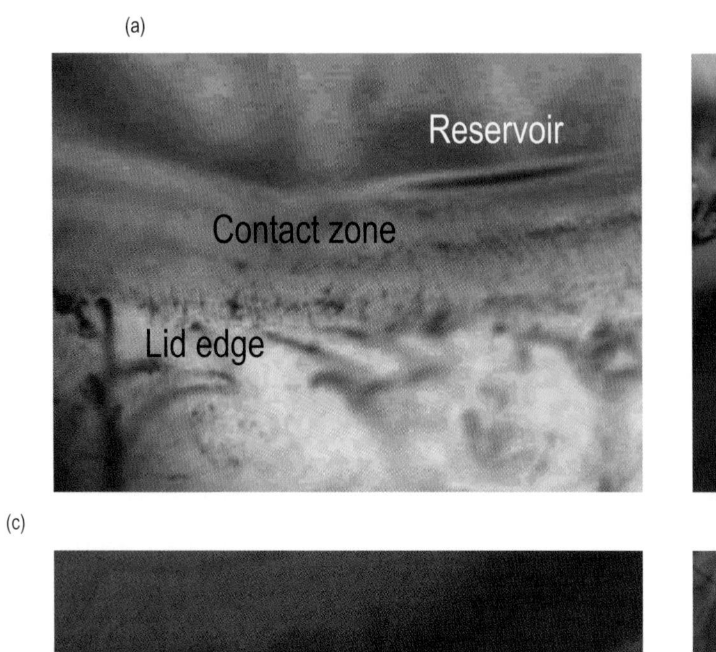

(b)

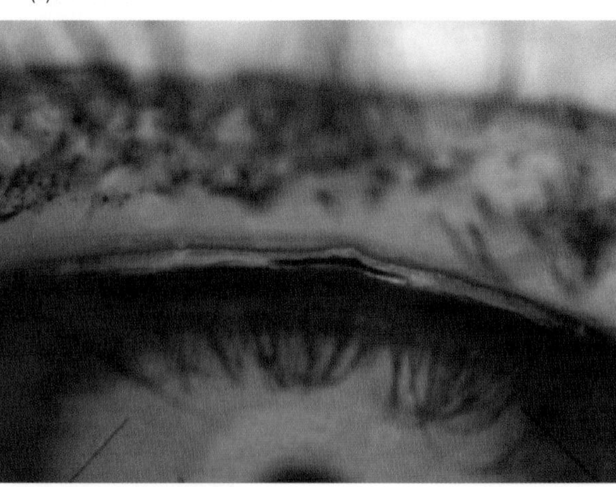

(c)

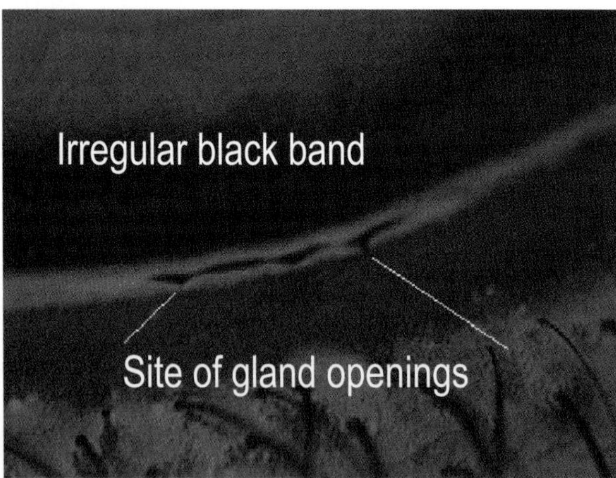

(d)

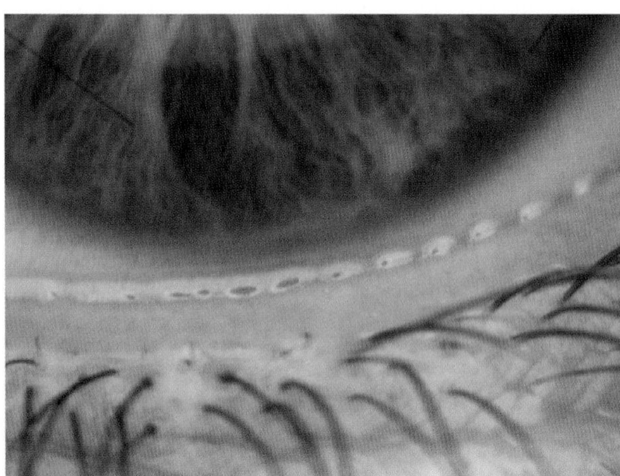

Figure 5.13 Irregular tear reservoirs: (a) make-up contaminated lid edge, (b) superior lid notch, (c) meibomian gland dysfunction, (d) non-continuous reservoir due to meibomian gland blockage

Coloured fringes (Fig. 5.12b5)
As the lipid layer thickens further, coloured fringes become visible. First-order fringes appear first as brown, blue and purple fringes. They are widely spread over the surface and in a homogeneous layer. This pattern is good for soft lenses.

Second- and third-order fringes (bright green and red) are present when there is oversecretion of the lipid layer, often seen following gland expression or from ocular irritation.

Globular appearance (Fig. 5.12b7)
A globular appearance is present in abnormally high secretions, which represent an unstable tear film so both thin and thick lipid layers are not satisfactory. It appears globular because the thick film cannot spread evenly and is often seen in blepharitis, meibomitis and ocular inflammation. Contact lens fitting should not be attempted in these patients until the underlying cause is resolved.

The lipid layer is produced by the meibomian glands and it is sometimes possible to visualize the secretion from a single gland. After lid manipulation, waves of lipid can be seen as interference fringes. If the secretion is globular it has been forced out before normal melting has occurred and does not flow freely. If the mixing is very poor, gland abnormality should be suspected and should be treated with hot compresses and lid massage morning and evening for 2 weeks before any lens fitting is attempted (see also Chapters 17 and 18).

The lipid layer may become invaded by cosmetic products and moisturizers that are surface active. These can cause the lipids to gather as a small oil droplet in an isolated area viewed against the dark zone of the aqueous phase. This will cause break-up of the tear film after every blink, resulting in dry eye symptoms in an otherwise normal eye/tear film.

Tear reservoir

The majority of the tear fluid secreted can be found in the upper and lower tear reservoir along the lid margin. This should be assessed for height, regularity and curvature, and provides excellent predictive information about the success or otherwise of new contact lens patients.

A full reservoir has a convex shape at the lid edge and concave centrally (Fig. 5.13). A thin meniscus forms when the aqueous is reduced and is characterized by a smaller height and increased curvature of the reservoirs. Tearscope appearance of the reservoir shows as a central black band inside two white bands. The central black band can be graded

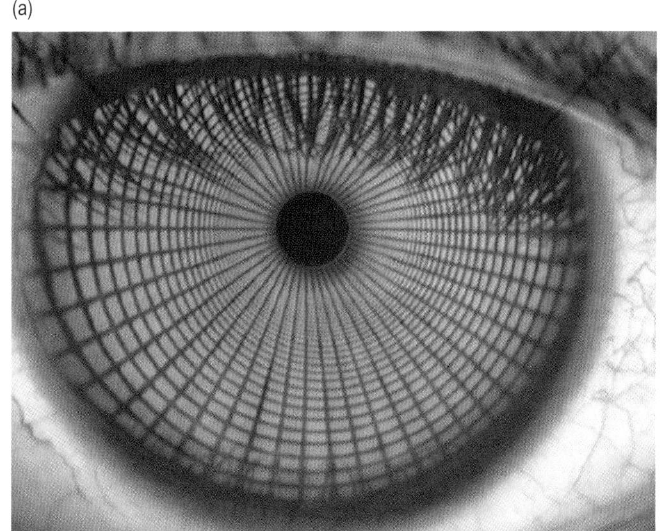

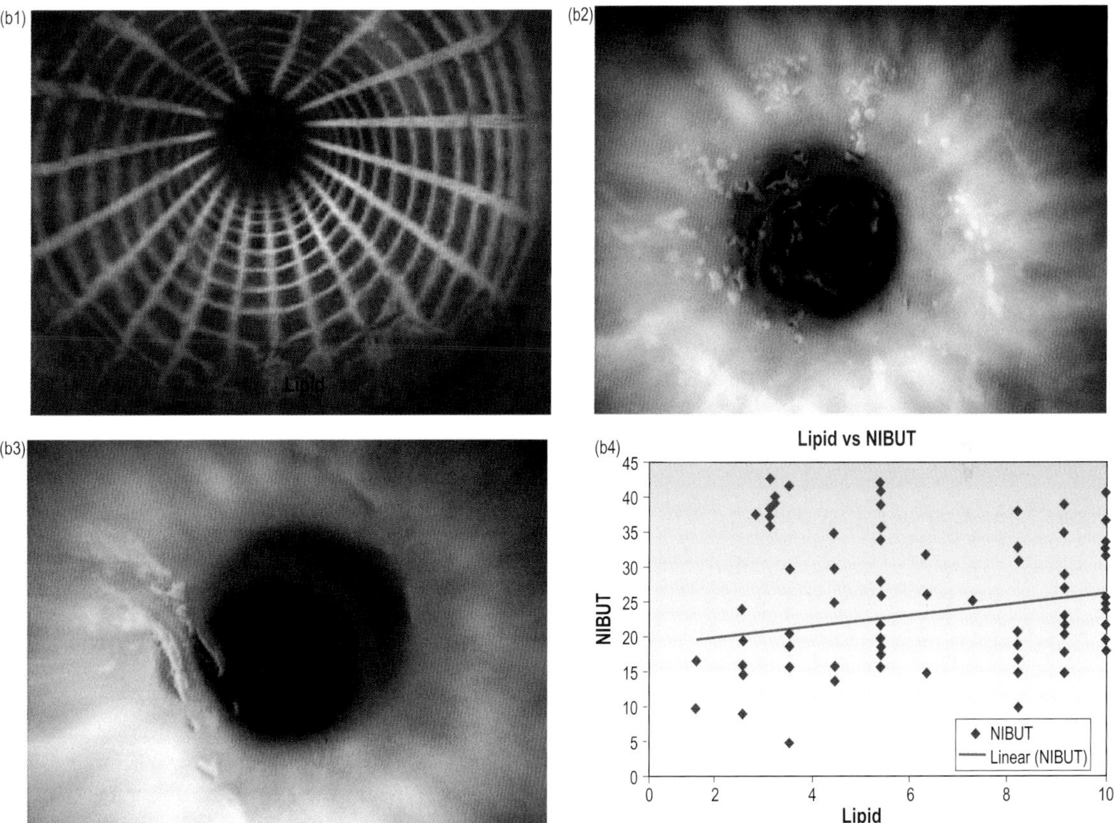

Figure 5.14 (a) Fine grid pattern prior to tear film break-up, (b1) grid pattern showing inferior break-up, (b2) example of spot break-up of tear film, (b3) example of streak break-up of tear film, (b4) relationship between the reduced lipid layer and decreasing non-invasive break-up time (NIBUT)

as thin, normal, full or overflowing. The reservoir may also be irregular, showing meibomian gland orifices and abnormal lid margins (chronic lid changes). Conjunctival folds can disturb the morphology and cause abnormal behaviour during the blink.

The tear reservoir should be measured when punctual occlusion is being considered. The measurement is taken before and after inserting temporary (collagen) plugs in order to determine their effectiveness.

Non-invasive break-up time

NIBUT can be measured either directly or indirectly. Direct measurement is recorded when a full thickness break in the tear film occurs. This is usually an elongated form or streak break, or a rounded/spot break. Indirect measurement is performed using the fine grid insert and by assessing disturbances to the regular grid pattern. This measurement is shorter because distortion appears prior to the full break (Fig. 5.14).

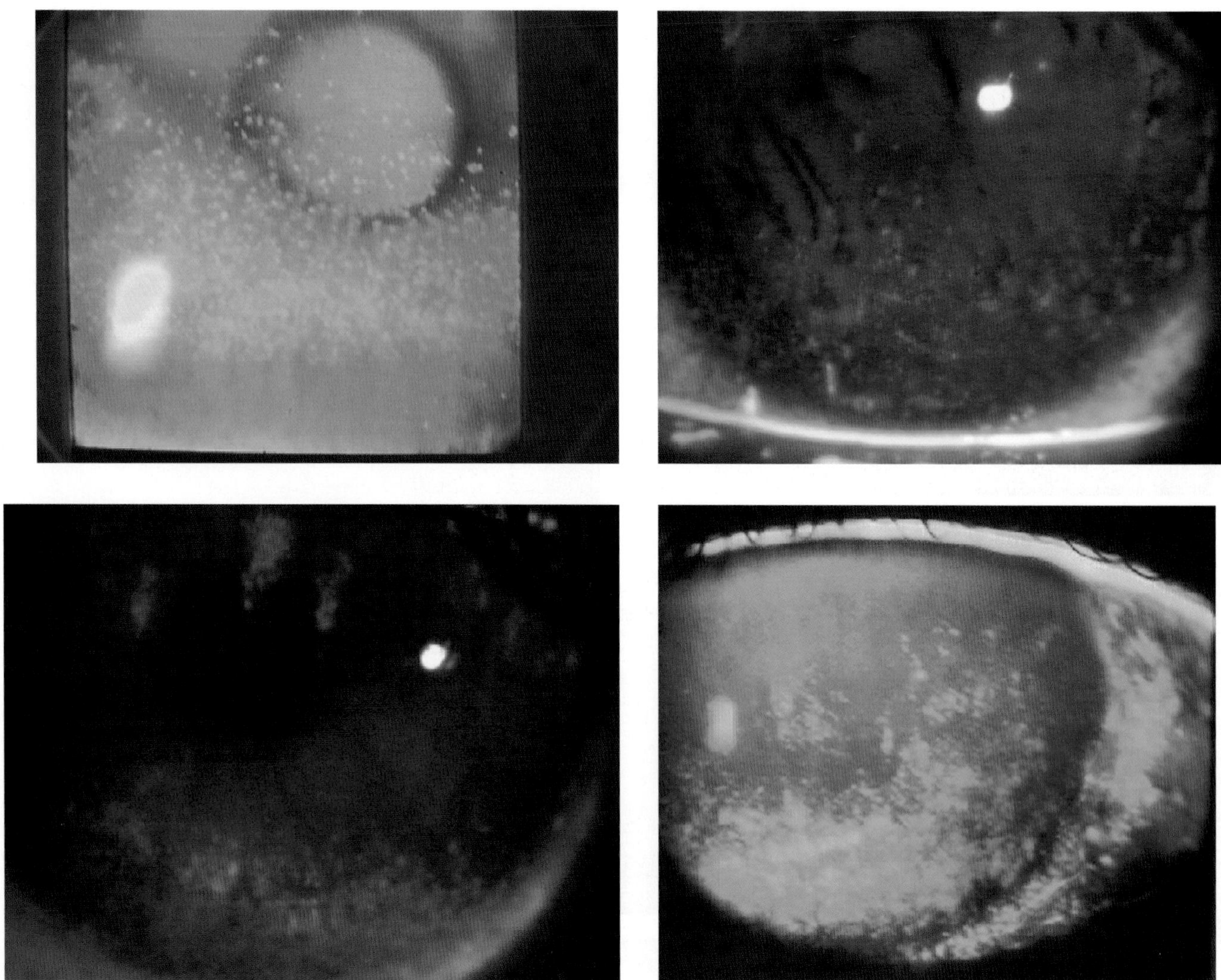

Figure 5.15 Corneal surface damage due to dessication seen through the Tearscope

Corneal damage

This can be assessed using the ring insert and gross distortion is often seen in abnormal lid coverage. The coarse and fine grids can be used to show distortion induced by 3 and 9 o'clock dryness or inferiorly when incomplete blinking or blepharitis has caused changes (Fig. 5.15).

MANAGEMENT

In the past, if a patient presented with dry/tired eyes they were simply advised to cease or reduce lens wear. We now have better control, not only of the contact lens type and design, but also better lens materials and treatment. The following gives some general advice for help.

Tip 1 – Separate the 'complainers' from the 'damagers'

- Complainers are symptomatic patients who have an adequate feedback mechanism producing reflex tearing which prevents epithelial surface damage. For complainers, artificial tears are used to decrease the occurrence or the severity of their symptoms.
- Damagers (asymptomatic) have a deficient feedback mechanism and a localized reduced sensitivity, which allows continual low-level damage that increases with time. For damagers, the use of artificial tears is to accelerate epithelial recovery over a very short period and to prevent further damage.
- Make sure a full explanation is given to the patient.

Tip 2 – Artificial tears use in damagers

- The surface epithelium continuously heals itself but can only do so in the presence of covering tear fluid. Epithelial damage occurs when tear coverage is deficient. In the dry-eye patient there is a continuing battle between damage and recovery of the epithelial cells.
- Long-term damage produces a decrease in subjective symptoms that allows a further increase in cellular damage.

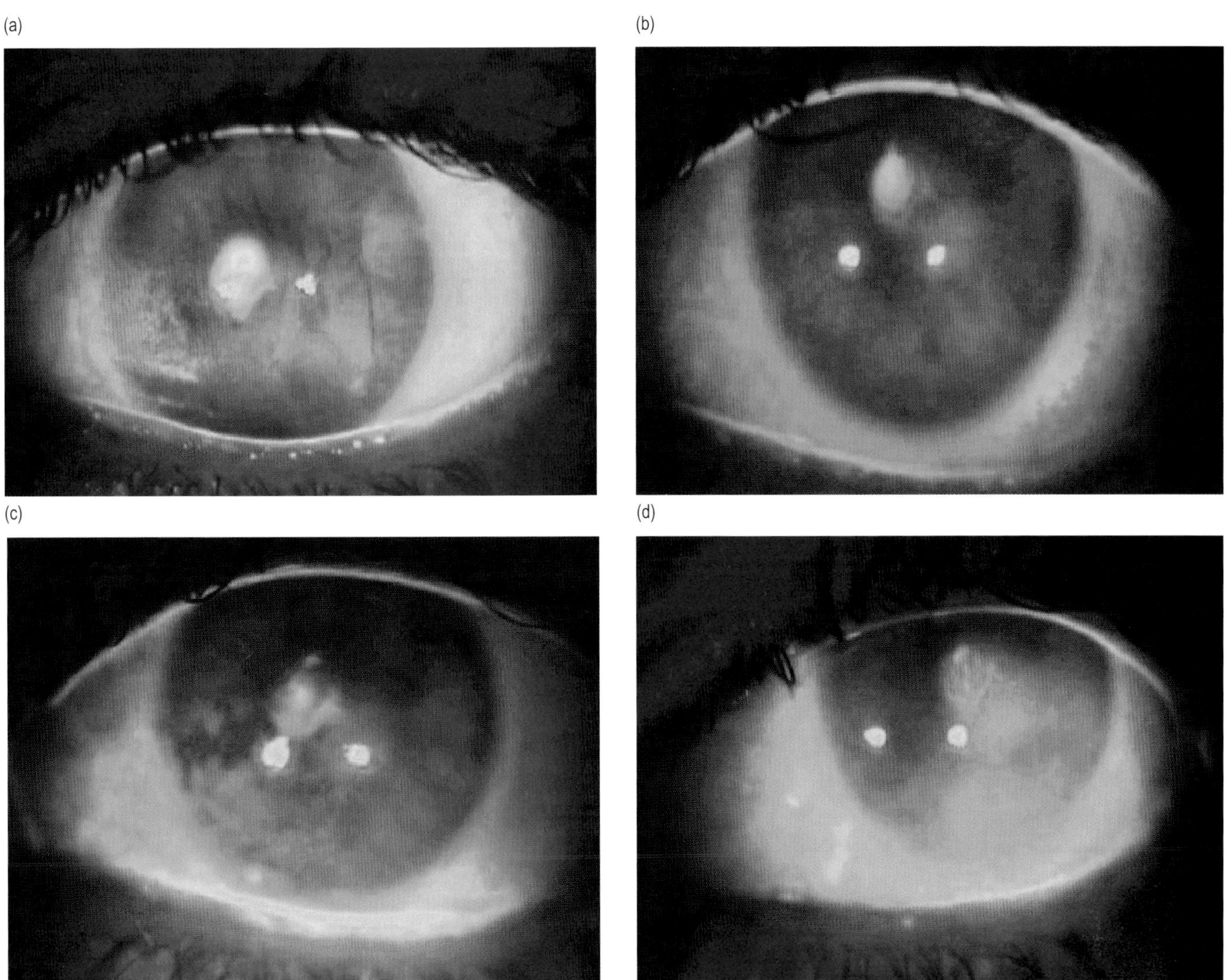

Figure 5.16 Corneal ulceration surface damage recovery following use of the 'flooding system' with Systane (Alcon): (a) Day 0; (b) Day 7; (c) Day 15; (d) Day 28

- In the presence of epithelial damage, recommend the use of a 'flooding system' lasting 3–4 days. This creates an artificial situation where the ocular surface is not allowed to dry:
  - Use lubricants hourly as a minimum and possibly as often as every 30 minutes (more frequently if necessary), especially during concentrated visual tasks such as computer work in air-conditioned offices.
  - This should be done for 3–4 days.
  - Following recovery of the epithelial surface, the use of the drops can be reduced to the minimum that prevents symptoms.
- Flooding the system with an artificial tear formulation achieves the following:
  - A quicker recovery of the epithelial surface.
  - Recovery of sensitivity of the ocular surface.
  - Feedback to the patient who will experience an irritation-free wet eye.
  - Enhancement of long-term patient compliance.
  - The system has been shown to be sufficiently effective that it has been successful in treating cases of corneal ulceration (Fig. 5.16).

Tip 3

- Advise the use of a thick gel at night for all cases of dry-eye symptoms on waking.

Tip 4

- Symptomatic patients not showing corneal damage may have conjunctival dryness.
- Increased daytime lubrication with gels is recommended.

Tip 5 – General points

- Consider punctum plugs when reduced tear secretion and a low tear reservoir are present (Fig. 5.17).

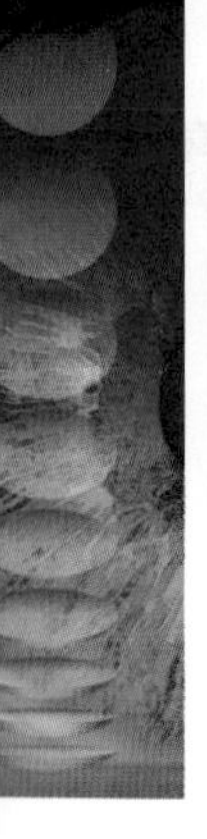

(a)

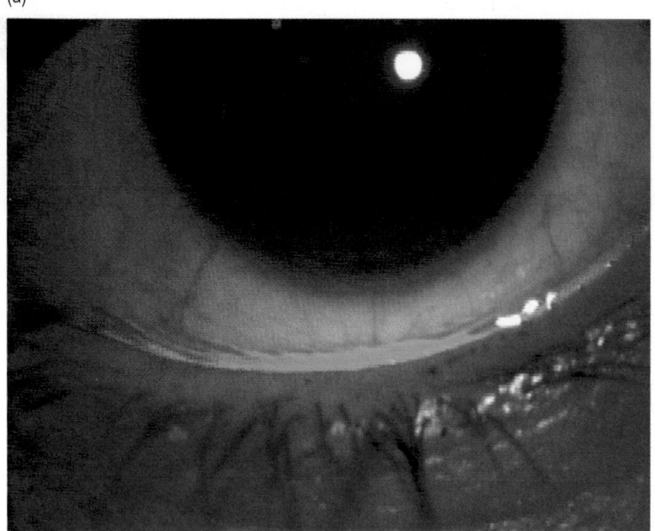

(b)

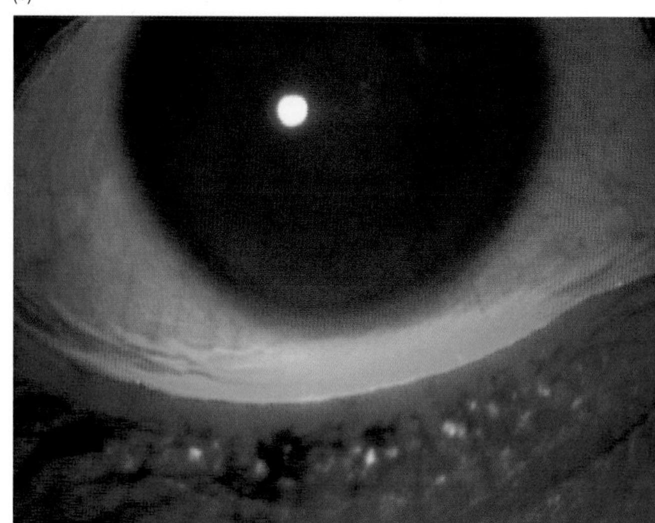

Figure 5.17 The benefit of punctum plugs showing the increased lacrimal rivus: (a) before; (b) after

- Lubricants – try hyaluronic acid-containing solutions; compare gels versus drops.
- Lens care solutions – try newer solutions with taurine or hyaluronic acid.
- Consider Lid-Care (CIBA Vision) for blepharitis if present.
- Try hot compresses and lid massage (see Chapters 17 and 18).

Tip 6 – The contact lens

- Try lens materials such as Proclear, Extreme H_2O, Complete Aquavision and silicone hydrogel lenses.
- Thicker, conventional soft lenses of low water content are more resistant to pervaporation. However, the effect on Dk/t should be noted.
- Refit soft lens wearers with RGPs.

Tip 7 – Living or working in a hot or dry environment

- Use a humidifier/pot-plants on gravel dishes.
- Drink plenty of water, not coffee.
- Wrap-around sunglasses outside.
- Blink exercises; close eyes occasionally.
- Keep heating as low as possible.
- Avoid being near air-conditioner vents.

SUMMARY

Poor detection and management of tear film abnormalities can make the difference between a happy or unhappy patient.

Initial detection of a problem can allow for:

- Treatment of any underlying cause.
- Monitoring of any treatment.
- Advice regarding potential symptoms and/or the effect on wearing time.
- Selection of the appropriate lens material or type to minimize potential problems.
- In severe cases, advice against the wearing of any type of lens.

Care and thoroughness in both the initial and follow-up examinations can save considerable chair-time and patient aggravation.

References

Cho, P. and Yap, M. (1993) Schirmer test II. A clinical study of its repeatability. Optom. Vis. Sci., 70, 157–159

Donald, C., Hamilton, L. and Doughty, M. J. (2003) A qualitative assessment of the location and width of Marx's line along the marginal zone of the human eyelid. Optom. Vis. Sci., 80(10), 564–572

Eliason, J. A. and Maurice, D. M. (1990) Staining of the conjunctiva and conjunctival tear film. Br. J. Ophthalmol., 74(9), 519–522

Hughes, C., Hamilton, L. and Doughty, M. (2003) A quantitative assessment of the location and width of Marx's line along the marginal zone of the human eyelid. Optom. Vis. Sci., 80(8), 564–572

Korb, D. R., Greiner, J. V. and Herman J. (2001) Comparison of fluorescein break-up time measurement reproducibility using standard fluorescein strips versus the Dry Eye Test (DET) method. Cornea, 20(8), 811–815

Lemp, M. A., Dohlman, C. H. and Holly, F. J. (1970) Corneal desiccation despite normal tear volume. Ann. Ophthalmol., 2, 258–261

Little, S. A. and Bruce, A. S. (1994) Repeatability of the phenol-red thread and tear thinning time tests for tear film function. Clin. Exp. Optom., 77, 64–68

Norn, M. S. (1965) Tear secretion in normal eyes estimated by a new method. The lacrimal streak dilution test. Acta Ophthalmol., 43, 567–573

Norn, M. S. (1969) Desiccation of the pre-corneal film. I. Corneal wetting time. Acta Ophthalmol., 47(4), 865–880

Norn, M. S. (1972) Vital staining of the cornea and conjunctiva. Acta Ophthalmol. (Kbh) Suppl., 113, 9–66

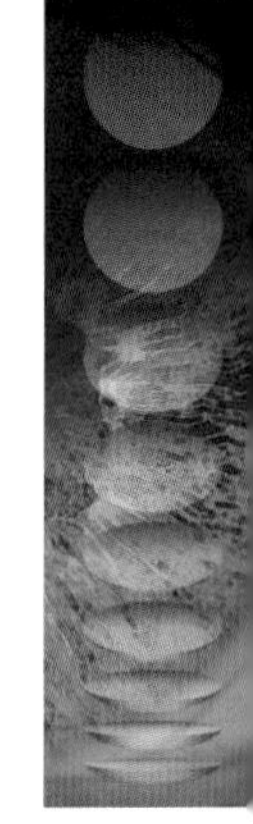

Schirmer, O. (1903) Studien zur Physiologie und Pathologie der Tränenabsonderung und Tränenabfuhr. Graefes Arch. Ophthalmol., 56, 197–291

Other references

A full list of references and recommended reading is available at: http://tearscope.eye5.com.au including a fully interactive CD-ROM for Tearscope and tear film evaluation. Tear film structure of the contact lens wearer. Based on: Guillon, J. P. (1990) PhD thesis dissertation. London: The City University.

Chapter 6

Optics and lens design

Morley Ford and Janet Stone, revised by Ronald Rabbetts

CHAPTER CONTENTS

Some aspects of contact lens design and optics are applied rarely nowadays as they are less relevant to modern practice but readers may still need to refer to them. They have therefore been moved onto the CD-ROM which accompanies this book while the more relevant topics are included here.

There are two main aspects to be considered when dealing with the optics of contact lenses: the effects on the wearer of the optical differences from spectacles, and the necessity for the practitioner to understand the components which affect the back vertex power of the contact-lens/liquid-lens system. There is some overlap of these two aspects, but for the sake of convenience they are discussed separately in the first two sections of the chapter. In the second section a set of approximate rules is included, the use of which should permit practitioners to make quick and reasonably accurate estimates of changes in power caused by altering certain lens parameters. The Cartesian sign convention is used throughout. For further understanding of the basic principles involved readers are referred to the works of Obstfeld (1982), Bennett (1985), Tunnacliffe (1993), Douthwaite (2006), Rabbetts (2007) and Freeman and Hull (2003).

Readers are particularly encouraged to consider the more realistic schematic eye data suggested by Bennett and Rabbetts (1988) and Rabbetts (1998), which take account of up-to-date research into the ocular components of the eye.

THE PRACTICAL EFFECTS OF OPTICAL DIFFERENCES BETWEEN CONTACT LENSES AND SPECTACLES

The various differences, and similarities, between contact lenses and spectacles will be considered.

Cosmetic appearance

Aside from the generally improved appearance achieved by doing away with spectacles, the magnification of the spectacle lenses is also eliminated. An observer therefore sees the eyes looking their normal size – smaller than with spectacles for a hypermetrope and larger for a myope. Disturbing appearances due to the prismatic effects and surface reflections of spectacle lenses are also removed.

Field of view or field of fixation, and field of vision

The field of view of someone wearing centred contact lenses equals the field of fixation and it is limited only by the extent to which the eyes can move. This normally gives a clear field of view of about 100°.

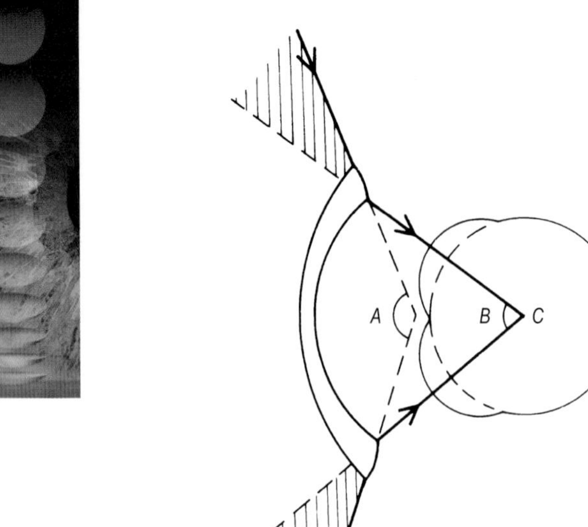

Figure 6.1 Field of view of a myope through a spectacle lens. A, actual macular field of view; B, apparent macular field of view; A > B; C, centre of rotation of eye. Hatched area is seen double due to prismatic effect (doubling is minimized by the spectacle frame, if present)

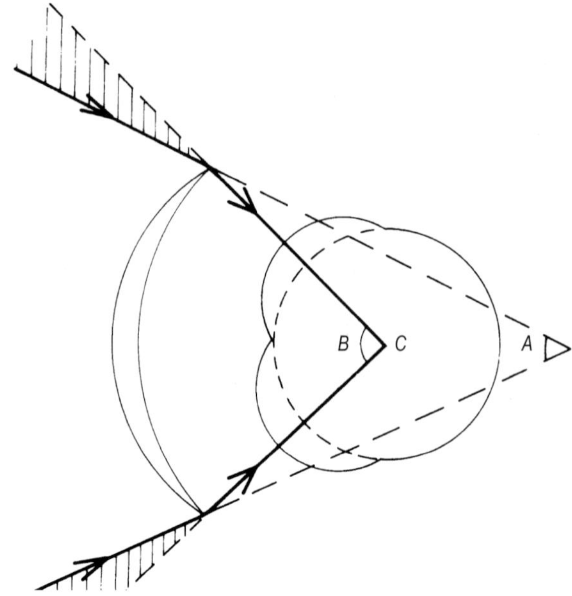

Figure 6.2 Field of view of a hypermetrope through a spectacle lens. A, actual macular field of view; B, apparent macular field of view; A < B; C, centre of rotation of eye. Blind area due to prismatic effect (and spectacle frame when present) is shown hatched

By comparison, the clear field of view of the spectacle wearer is limited by the size and vertex distance of the spectacle lens and is restricted to an apparent field of about 80° (although blurred vision is possible beyond the limits of the spectacle lens or frame as far as the eyes can rotate). Figure 6.1 shows that in fact the myopic spectacle wearer has a much larger real field of view than this, depending on the power of the spectacle lens. On the other hand, the hypermetropic spectacle wearer (Fig. 6.2) has a real field of view smaller than 80°. This means that, on transferring to contact lenses, the myope must move the eyes more to see the same area of the visual field as seen with spectacles. The reverse applies to the hypermetrope.

The sizes of the real and apparent fields of view through the spectacle lens are easily calculated. The angular subtense of the spectacle lens at the eye's centre of rotation, *C*, gives the apparent macular field of view, *B*.

For example, size of spectacle lens, 50 mm; thus, the semi-diameter is 25 mm.

Distance from spectacle lens to *C* is 25 mm.
Therefore $\frac{1}{2} B = \arctan^{*} (25/25) = 45°$ and thus $B = 90°$.

To obtain the size of the real macular field of view, *A*, requires that the position of the image of *C*, as formed by the spectacle lens, be found. *A* is then the angular subtense of the spectacle lens at that point. Using the same example as above and reversing the path of the light rays shown in Figure 6.1, if the lens has a power of –10.00 D and making use of the usual nomenclature for object and image distances then $l = -25$ mm and therefore $L = -40.00$ D; $F = -10.00$ D.

* Arctan = $\tan^{-1}$ or inverse tan

Thus, $L' = L + F = -50.00$ D
$l' = 1000/L' = -20$ mm
C is thus imaged 20 mm from the spectacle lens, on the same side as *C*.
Therefore, $\frac{1}{2} A = \arctan' (25/20) = 51.3°$. And thus $A = 102.7°$.

In addition, the prismatic effects of the spectacle lenses cause blind areas in the peripheral visual field of the hypermetrope and areas of doubled vision for the myope, as illustrated in Figures 6.2 and 6.1, respectively. The blind area experienced by a hypermetrope is enlarged due to the thickness of the spectacle frame. This prismatic effect and the blind area are particularly troublesome to aphakics owing to the high power of the spectacle lenses. Contact lenses afford great relief.

Oblique aberrations

Even best-form spectacle lenses allow objects viewed through their periphery to suffer from the effects of oblique aberrations:

- Oblique astigmatism.
- Coma.
- Distortion.
- Transverse chromatic aberration.
- Curvature of field.

Contact lenses remain almost centred in all directions of gaze, and distortions are therefore kept to a minimum.

The higher the spectacle prescription, the greater the aberration effects. The relief afforded by contact lenses is then considerable; conversely, however, returning to spectacles from contact lenses can give rise to disorientation and nausea and may require modification of the spectacle prescription to keep the power as low as possible consistent with adequate visual acuity. Any cylindrical correction needs to be kept to an absolute minimum and possibly removed altogether, provided visual acuity is not unduly compromised. The size of spectacle lenses should be kept as small as possible to avoid some of the peripheral distortion.

Prismatic effects

There are two types of prismatic effect caused by spectacles:

- Those of spectacle lenses during convergence.
- Those due to the anisometropic spectacle correction, when the eyes make version movements.

CONVERGENCE

Spectacles, optically centred for distance vision but which are used for all distances of gaze, differ from contact lenses, which move with the eyes remaining centred (or nearly so) for all distances and positions of gaze.

Thus, during near vision, a spectacle-wearing myope experiences a base-in prism effect and a spectacle-wearing hypermetrope a base-out effect, as shown in Figure 6.3. Provided that contact lenses remain optically centred, the contact lens wearer experiences no such prism effect. Therefore, for a given object distance, the contact-lens-wearing myope exerts more convergence and the hypermetrope less convergence than with spectacles.

Table 6.1 gives the amount of convergence in prism dioptres (Δ) exerted by both eyes in various degrees of ametropia, assuming spectacles centred for a distance CD of 60 mm and worn 27 mm in front of the eyes' centres of rotation; and contact lenses giving an equivalent power, remaining centred for all distances of gaze and worn 15 mm in front of the eyes' centres of rotation. The method of calculation of the convergence in Δ is as described for the calculation of prismatic effects in anisometropia (see pp. 131–133). Table 6.1 is used as a basis for the graph in Figure 6.4.

The significance of this difference in convergence must be considered in association with changes in accommodation (see 'Accommodation', p. 140, where it is shown that the ratio between accommodation and convergence remains the same with spectacles and contact lenses). The effect of the change in convergence alone, when transferring from spectacles to contact lenses, is only likely to prove difficult in a myope whose near point of convergence is abnormally remote, when the removal of the base-in prism may be sufficient to disrupt binocular vision at near.

The general effect of transferring from spectacles to contact lenses for near vision is as if the myope had brought the near task a little closer, since more convergence and accommodation are required, whereas for the hypermetrope the reverse applies and it is as if the working distance had been increased.

ANISOMETROPIA

Since contact lenses move with the eyes, the visual axes always pass through their optical centres or very close to them. Thus,

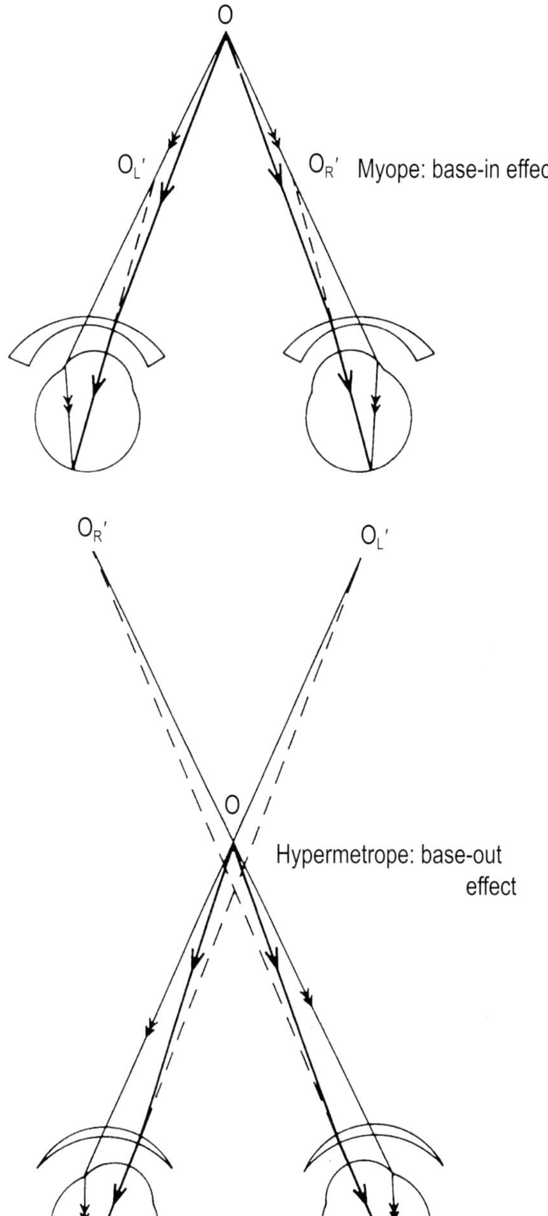

Figure 6.3 Spectacles centred for distance vision give prismatic effects when the eyes converge

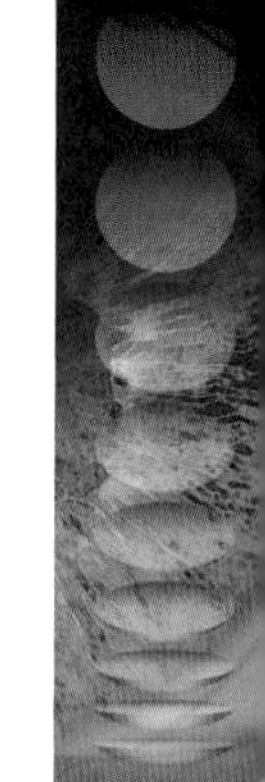

differential prismatic effects which can create difficulties for anisometropic spectacle wearers are virtually removed. (The effects of contact lens movement on the eyes are considered in 'Incorporation of prism', p. 133.)

An example will serve to illustrate this:

Spectacle correction: R – 4.00 DS
L + 1.00 DS

Prismatic effect when looking down at an object 10 cm below the horizontal and 25 cm in front of the spectacle plane (assumed to be 25 mm in front of the centres of rotation of the eyes):

Table 6.1: Comparison of convergence with spectacles and contact lenses

Spectacle refraction (D)	Convergence (Δ) at 0.33 metre from spectacle plane: Spectacles	Convergence (Δ) at 0.33 metre from spectacle plane: Contact lenses	Convergence (Δ) at 0.25 metre from spectacle plane: Spectacles	Convergence (Δ) at 0.25 metre from spectacle plane: Contact lenses
−20	11.11	16.66	14.56	21.66
−15	12.11	16.66	15.87	21.66
−10	13.33	16.66	17.56	21.66
−5	14.80	16.66	19.31	21.66
0	16.66	16.66	21.66	21.66
+5	19.03	16.66	24.67	21.66
+10	22.19	16.66	28.63	21.66
+15	26.64	16.66	34.14	21.66

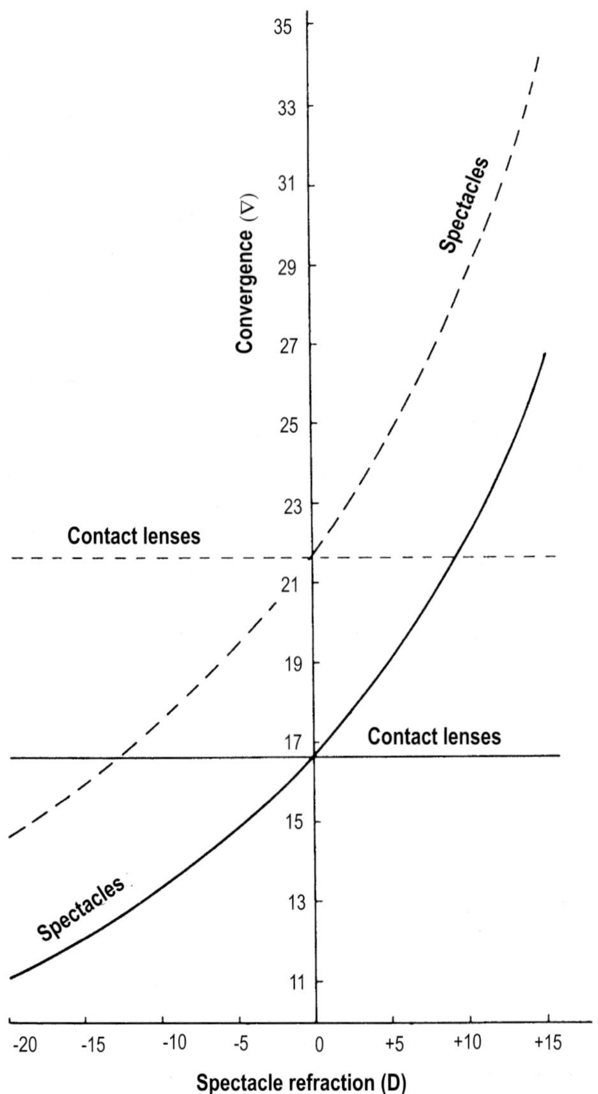

Figure 6.4 Convergence with spectacles and contact lenses. -- at 0.25 metre; — at 0.33 metre using figures from Table 6.1 (compare this with Fig. 6.16)

R 3.33Δ, base-down
L 1.00Δ, base-up

The difference between the two eyes in the vertical meridian is over 4 Δ, which is too great for the patient to obtain comfortable binocular single vision. This spectacle correction would therefore necessitate vertical head movements rather than eye movements. Figure 6.5 illustrates the difference in vertical eye rotation that would be required with this spectacle correction, as well as the difference in magnification (see 'Relative spectacle magnification', p. 138).

For calculation of the prismatic effect, the positions and sizes of the images O_R' and O_L' formed by the spectacle lenses are first found (Fig. 6.5).

Thus, for the right eye, $l = -25$ cm
Therefore, $L = -4$ D
Now $F = -4$ D, and since $L' = L + F$, $L' = -8$ D
Therefore $l' = -12.5$ cm
Since, $\frac{h'}{h} = \frac{L}{L'}$, $h'_R = \frac{-4}{-8} \times 10 \text{ cm} = 5 \text{ cm}$

For the left eye, l again $= -25$ cm. Therefore, $L = -4$ D

Now $F = +1$ D, and therefore $L' = -3$ D
Therefore, $l' = 33.33$ cm
and $h'_L = \frac{-4}{-3} \times 10 \text{ cm} = 13.33 \text{ cm}$

Points T, at which the two visual axes intersect the spectacle lenses, must then be found.

Using the similar triangles for each eye, that is with apex at C and bases at O′ and ST and assuming the distance s (SC) to be 25 mm.

For the right eye, $\frac{ST}{h'_R} = \frac{s}{s - l'}$

and ST $= 5 \times \frac{2.5}{15.0} = 0.833$ cm

For the left eye, $\frac{ST}{h'_L} = \frac{2.5}{35.83}$

and ST $= 13.33 \times \frac{2.5}{35.83} = 0.930$ cm

From Prentice's law (see p. 133), the prismatic effect of the right lens is $-4\,\Delta \times 0.833 = 3.33\,\Delta$ base-down and for the left lens it is $+1\,\Delta \times 0.930 = 0.93\,\Delta$ base-up. This gives over 4.26 Δ difference between the two eyes.

An alternative way of looking at this is to calculate the actual angles through which each eye rotates downwards, and then find the difference.

The right eye rotates downwards by an angle of θ_R given by:

$$\tan \theta_R = \frac{h'_R}{s - l'}$$

Since the angle θ in prism dioptres is given by the value 100 × tan,

$$\theta_R = 100 \times \frac{5}{2.5 - (-12.5)} = 100 \times \frac{5}{15} = 33.33\,\Delta$$

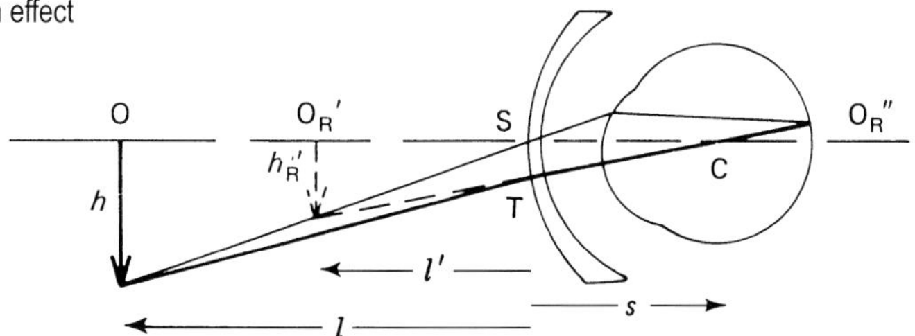

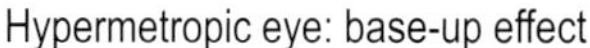

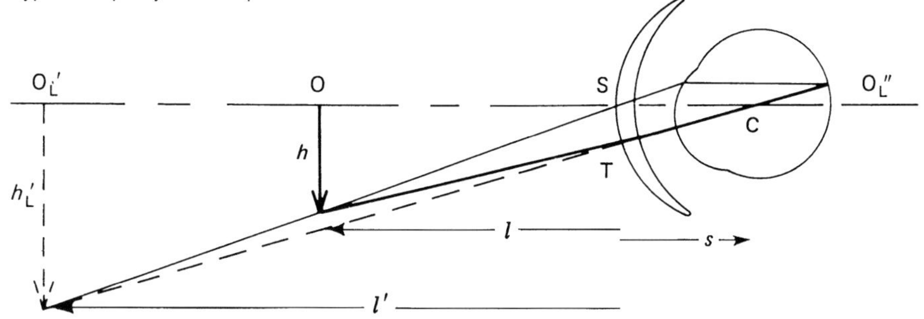

Figure 6.5 Anisometropia: during near vision when wearing spectacles the visual axis of the hypermetropic eye is depressed more than that of the myopic eye. The image seen by the hypermetropic eye is also larger than that seen by the myopic eye. O, object; O_R' and O_L', images of O formed by the spectacle lenses; O_R'' and O_L'', retinal images

The left eye rotates downwards by an angle of

$$\theta_L = 100 \times \frac{13.33}{2.5 - (-33.33)} = 100 \times \frac{13.33}{35.83} = 37.20\ \Delta$$

The difference between the rotation required of the two eyes is thus 3.87 Δ, which differs a little from the value measured in the spectacle plane, which was 4.26 Δ.

The latter method of determining the angles through which each eye rotates is the way in which angular values for convergence are also calculated. An object located on the midline between the two eyes (see Fig. 6.3) is then considered as an object of height (h) equal to half the interpupillary distance, because this is its distance from the optical axis of the spectacle lens.

Horizontal prism differences are more easily tolerated than vertical differences. During version movements of the eyes, the anisometropic spectacle wearer learns to make allowance for the increasing prismatic difference as the visual axes intersect points at increasing distances from the optical centres. This habit of allowing for the prismatic difference shows as a non-comitant heterophoria which may persist for some time after contact lenses are first worn, and this can at first cause difficulty on lateral rotation of the eyes. From habit, one eye moves more than the other, and objects tend to be seen double until a new extraocular muscle balance is achieved.

Incorporation of prism

Most manufacturers prefer not to incorporate more than 3 Δ into a contact lens as the thickness difference makes more than this amount impracticable (except in higher powers) with such steeply curved surfaces.

Because the prism base always rotates down and slightly in, it is impossible to prescribe a horizontal prism satisfactorily and a vertical prism is therefore also limited to 3 Δ as it can only be prescribed in one lens. Thus most prisms must be incorporated in spectacles to be worn in addition to contact lenses. It may be possible, at least in theory, to incorporate a low power horizontal prism in just the optic zone of a soft lens, relying on a different method of peripheral stabilization to give the required alignment (see Chapter 12), and scleral lenses can be made with a horizontal prism.

Sometimes contact lenses provide a better standard of binocular vision than spectacles and the expected prism proves to be either unnecessary or reduced. This is where tolerance trials in contact lenses are useful, as are tests for uncompensated heterophoria.

With contact lenses, some unwanted prismatic effect occurs due to movement of the lenses on the eyes. One of the aims of correct fitting is to ensure that this movement is similar for both lenses so that little prismatic difference between the two eyes is experienced.

The prism effect due to such movement is given by:

$$P = c \times F \qquad \text{(Prentice's law)}$$

where

P is prism effect in Δ
F is back vertex power, in dioptres, of the contact-lens/liquid-lens system
c is displacement in cm.

If the powers of the two lenses are the same and the movement is similar, then no prismatic difference occurs. If the two lens powers are not the same, the amount of movement enables the prismatic difference to be calculated. It is worth noting that, if a person wears a negative-powered contact lens in one eye and a positive-powered lens in the other, to counteract the prismatic effects due to vertical lens movement, the negative

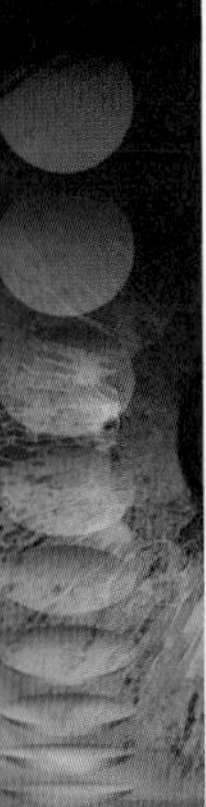

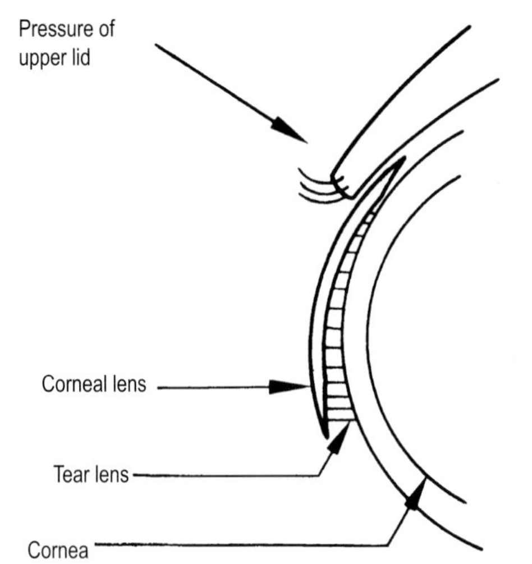

Figure 6.6 Prism base-down liquid lens: this effect is due to tilt of a corneal lens caused by pressure of the upper lid

lens should move up (prism base-down) as the positive lens moves down (also prism base-down). With corneal lenses, because of the position of the centre of gravity and the action of the lids during blinking (see Chapter 9), this desirable opposite movement of positive and negative lenses frequently occurs.

If a lens tilts due to pressure of the upper lid on a corneal lens or to downward lag of a scleral lens, then a certain amount of extra prism base-down is introduced due to the liquid lens, as shown in Figure 6.6. Bennett (1985) showed that this may be enough to counteract the prism base-up effect of a high negative scleral lens. Again, this tilt may be ignored as long as it is similar in the two eyes.

Where a contact lens has prism worked on it, then the power of the prism on the eye is the same as that in air. The liquid lens (unless it contains a prism element of its own due to tilt of the contact lens) has no effect on the prismatic element of the contact lens.

Cylinder effect introduced by prism, slip and tilt

It has been suggested that a prism in a contact lens introduces a significant cylindrical element; this is incorrect. Although the refracted pencil through the front surface is slightly oblique, the amount of cylinder introduced is negligible. For example, taking a lens of back vertex power (BVP) +10.00 D, back optic zone radius (BOZR) 7.80 mm and centre thickness 0.40 mm, calculation using the Coddington differential equations shows that the cylindrical element introduced is only 0.28 D for a prism of 3 Δ, and drops to 0.12 D for a 2 Δ prism. Expressed as a positive cylinder, the power is along the prism base–apex line and the axis perpendicular to it. Thus, in the example given, if the prism is base-down along 90, there will be +0.28 DC × 180. (In this calculation, it is assumed that the eye has rotated to view the object, so that the chief ray and visual axis still pass normally through the back surface, unlike with a spectacle lens incorporating a prism. The astigmatic effect is therefore solely caused by the tilt in the front surface; in this case the angle of incidence is just over 5° and the surface power nearly +71.5 D.)

Lenses can also tilt by slipping on the eye. If the slipping occurs as a rotation about the centre of curvature (C_2) of the back surface, then C_2 will not be displaced, but C_1, the centre of curvature of the front surface, is displaced. This introduces a small amount of prism, and hence, as shown in the previous example, astigmatism. The axis of the induced positive cylinder is perpendicular to the direction of slip.

In the case of negative lenses of similar numerical power, the astigmatism induced is less because of the flatter front surface. In the normal range, the BOZR has little influence on the result.

Note that in the above examples the effect of the back surface has been ignored as the refractive index (RI) change at this surface is small.

Clearly, the induced astigmatism may be increased if the lens actually tilts on the eye as well as slipping. When the whole lens tilts through a small angle, the resulting astigmatism can be found approximately by the equation:

$$\text{Cylinder} = F \tan^2 \theta$$

where θ is the angle of tilt and F is the back vertex power of the lens. The cylinder axis is perpendicular to the direction of tilt. Thus, if $F = +10.00$ D and $\theta = 5°$, the induced cylinder is +0.0765 D. If the direction of tilt is vertical, i.e. about a horizontal axis, then the cylinder axis is horizontal. Such a lens tilted in the vertical about a horizontal axis, due to upper lid pressure on the top of the lens, is shown in Figure 6.6. There is also a very small change in the spherical element given approximately by the equation:

$$\text{Sphere} = F\,(1 + \tfrac{1}{3} \sin^2 \theta)$$

Thus, in the same example, the sphere is increased to +10.025 D, which is of no significance.

Sarver (1963) studied the effect of contact lens tilt on residual astigmatism and his experimental observations confirmed the above theoretical findings.

Magnification

Any correction, be it a spectacle lens or a contact lens, alters the size of the basic retinal image. (The basic retinal image is taken to be the size in the uncorrected eye assuming blur circles of zero diameter, i.e. 'pinpoint' pupils.) This is known as 'spectacle' magnification, even when it is the magnification due to contact lenses. To compare spectacles and contact lenses, the differences in magnification for both spherical and toric correcting lenses must be considered. This is affected by the form and thickness of the lens.

SPHERICAL LENSES

Positive spectacle lenses magnify and negative lenses minify, and both effects increase with the vertex distance. Only if a corrective lens is worn in the plane of the eye's entrance pupil is

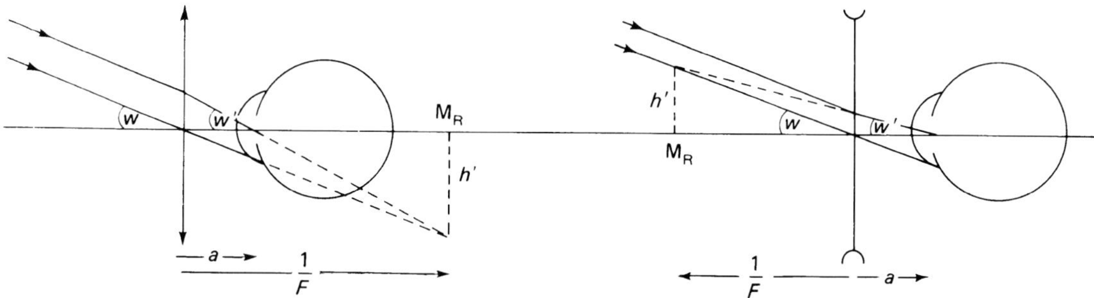

Figure 6.7 Spectacle magnification is w'/w. A distant off-axis object, subtending an angle w at the spectacle lens, is imaged by the lens of power F, in the far-point plane M_R. The image is of size h' and subtends an angle w' at the centre of the entrance pupil, which is situated at a distance of a metres from the spectacle lens. The left-hand diagram shows the situation in hypermetropia, and the right-hand diagram in myopia

unit magnification of the basic retinal image achieved. Thus, a contact lens worn on the cornea approaches unit magnification. (An intraocular implant is fitted closer to the entrance pupil plane.) Bennett (1985) showed that spectacle magnification can be expressed as:

$$\frac{1}{1 - aF}$$

where F is the power in dioptres of the correcting lens which is assumed to be infinitely thin, and a is the distance in metres from the correcting lens to the entrance pupil plane. Figure 6.7 shows how this expression is derived.

The size of the retinal image is proportional to the angular subtense of the object at the entrance pupil. The angular subtense is w' when the spectacle lens is present and w when it is not (a distant object is assumed).

Now, $w' = \dfrac{h'}{(1/F) - a}$ and $w = \dfrac{h'}{(1/F)}$

Thus, spectacle magnification $\dfrac{w}{w'} = \dfrac{(1/F)}{(1/F) - a} = \dfrac{1}{1 - aF} \approx 1 + aF$

Note that with a contact lens, a is about 3 mm (the approximate distance of the entrance pupil plane from the cornea); with a spectacle lens, a equals the vertex distance plus the approximate distance of the entrance pupil plane from the cornea, i.e. 3 mm. Therefore, a is approximately 15 mm and the approximate expression gives 1.5% per dioptre.

Thus, it can be seen that myopes who change from spectacles to contact lenses see objects larger than before, and hypermetropes see objects smaller than before. This is illustrated by the graph in Figure 6.8, which shows the percentage increase or decrease in retinal image size given by theoretically infinitely thin contact lenses as compared with infinitely thin spectacle lenses. This is based on a vertex distance of 12 mm and a distance of 3 mm between anterior cornea and entrance pupil plane. More realistic values are shown for typical aligning corneal lenses, soft lenses and scleral lenses, again compared with infinitely thin spectacle lenses. For positive lenses, the slope for soft lenses falls somewhere between the corneal and scleral lens slopes depending on thickness and RI, and for negative lenses approximates to that of corneal lenses, again

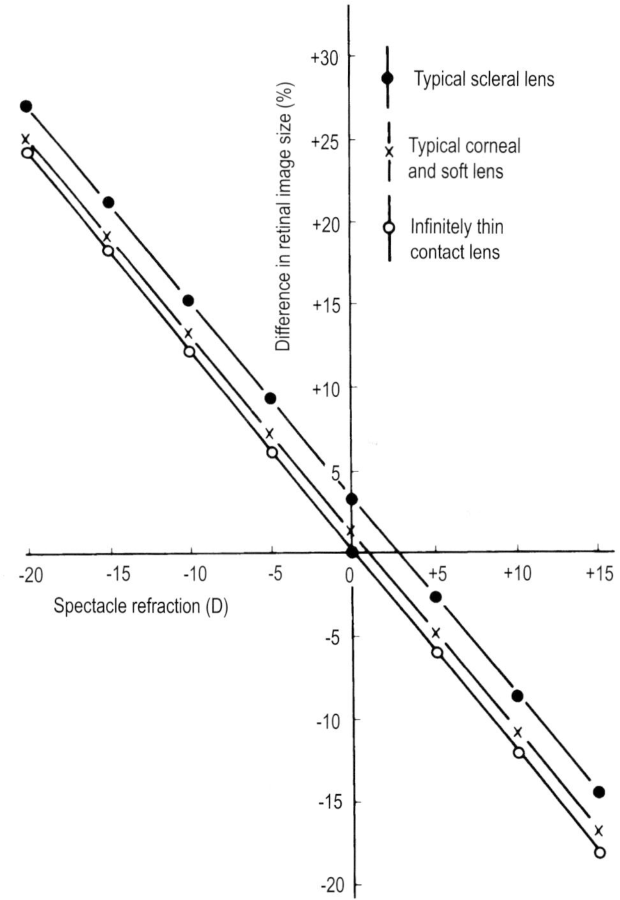

Figure 6.8 Percentage difference in retinal image size: comparison with a thin spectacle lens

depending on thickness and RI. (Lenses of low RI are normally thicker than their higher RI counterparts.)

Myopes might expect increased acuity in contact lenses but may experience some disorientation when they are first worn owing to the apparent increase in the size of objects.

Conversely, hypermetropes may have poorer acuity with contact lenses but, since the difference in image size is only of real significance in the higher powers (except for those with poor visual acuity), it is only the high hypermetropes and aphakes who

Figure 6.9 Variation of magnification with type and form of correcting lens: —•— typical scleral lens; —×— typical corneal and soft lens; —⊗— 'thin' contact lens; —○—'thin' spectacle lens

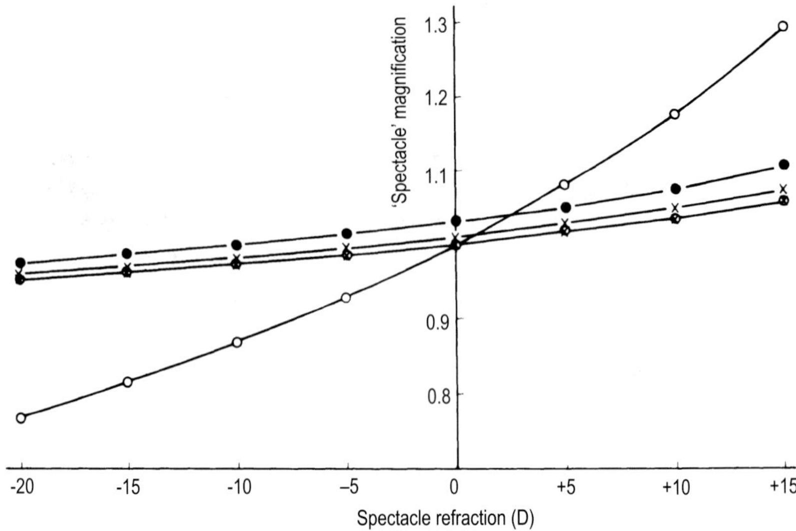

are affected (see Chapter 21). The latter are able to see objects reduced to only slightly larger than their normal size again.

The graph in Figure 6.9 shows the different values for spectacle magnification given by four types of lens. Theoretical values are drawn for spectacle lenses (assumed infinitely thin and worn 12 mm from the cornea) and contact lenses (also assumed infinitely thin and worn on the cornea, 3 mm in front of the entrance pupil) as well as more realistic values for typical rigid corneal, soft and scleral lenses, taking form and thickness into account. Soft lenses fall close to the values for corneal lenses but there are slight differences due to their lower RI, the absence of any tear lens, and small thickness differences (for the effects of thickness and RI, and the tear lens, see 'Shape factor', below). The spectacle magnification of an infinitely thin contact lens should be multiplied by this factor to obtain a truer idea of the retinal image size when making comparisons with spectacles. This is borne out in Figure 6.8.

TORIC LENSES

The graph in Figure 6.9 shows that contact lenses cause less change in size of the basic retinal image than do spectacle lenses.

A toric spectacle lens gives different magnification in different meridians, which produces distortion of the retinal image. This is particularly noticeable where the principal meridians are at oblique axes, as Bennett (1985) pointed out. A square object seen through a toric spectacle lens may look rectangular if the principal meridians are horizontal and vertical, or diagonal like a parallelogram if the principal meridians are oblique (Fig. 6.10). This distortion of shape is minimized with a contact lens because the meridional difference in magnification is reduced (see Fig. 6.9).

Difficulty may arise when a toric spectacle correction has been worn for many years and a perceptual allowance has been made for the distortion. On transferring to contact lenses which give a less distorted retinal image, the perceived image may again appear distorted until the processes of perception become readjusted to the new situation (see Fig. 6.10).

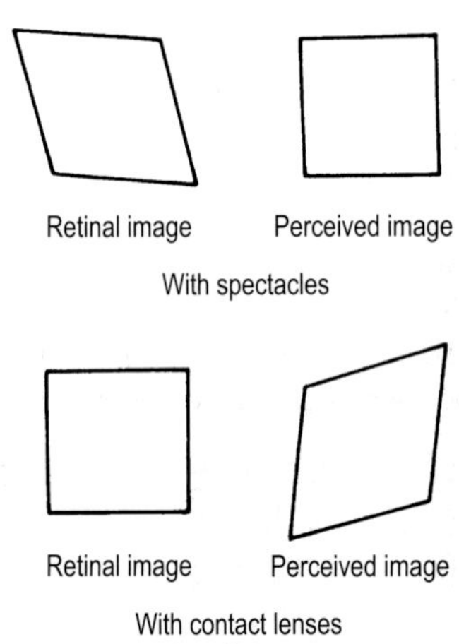

Figure 6.10 Perceptual compensation for retinal image distortion: this is acquired during spectacle wear and continues when contact lenses are first worn

SHAPE FACTOR

The magnification of two lenses having the same back vertex power is affected by their front surface power and thickness. Shape factor, a term which is unfortunately also applied to the asphericity $e^2 = (1 - p)$ of conic sections (see 'Corneal shape', Chapter 9), is the allowance which must be made for the increase in magnification due to the form and thickness of the lens and is given as:

$$\frac{1}{1 - (tF_1/n)}$$

which is the ratio between back vertex power and equivalent power, where

n = RI
t = central optic thickness in metres
F_1 = front surface power in dioptres.

The values for spectacle magnification for the 'thin' lenses in Figure 6.9 should therefore be amended to:

$$\frac{1}{1-aF} \times \frac{1}{1-(tF_1/n)}$$

if shape factor is to be taken into account. This expression is easily applied to spectacle lenses but a contact lens system comprises a plastic lens and a tear lens in combination. The expression for the shape factor is correspondingly more involved. Bennett (1985) derived an approximate simplified expression for shape factor of a contact lens system, based on values which are normally known. This is:

$$1 + t(K + C) - (t_1/n_1)F_2$$

where

t (total reduced thickness in metres of plastic lens and liquid lens) $= t_1/n_1 + t_2/n_2$
K = ocular refraction in dioptres
C* = keratometer reading in dioptres (assuming RI of calibration equals RI of tears, i.e. 1.336)
t_1 = thickness of plastic contact lens in metres
n_1 = RI of plastic material of contact lens
F_2 = interface power in dioptres at the back optic zone surface of the contact lens.

This expression was used in calculating values for the graphs in Figures 6.8, 6.9 and 6.11 which show that corneal and soft lenses give smaller retinal images than the corresponding scleral lens, because a scleral lens has a larger shape factor.

Figure 6.11 shows the shape factors for soft, corneal and scleral lenses. Soft lenses were assumed to be 0.1 mm thick, corneal lenses 0.2 mm and scleral lenses 0.75 mm, and the liquid lens was taken to be 0.01 mm and 0.1 mm thick in the latter two cases respectively, with zero thickness assumed behind a soft lens. Negative lenses, especially those of high power, are normally thinner than the values stated, while positive lenses may be considerably thicker. However, the values assumed permit sufficient illustration of the effect of thickness on shape factor. Had more accurate thickness values been used, the graphs shown would have sloped slightly more steeply.

Positive soft lenses are generally a little thicker than positive corneal lenses, whereas negative soft lenses are often thinner than negative corneal lenses, and as they generally have a lower RI than rigid corneal lenses, the shape factor is slightly less than for corneal lenses.

A keratometer reading (C*) of +42.00 D (8.00 mm) was assumed. The corneal lenses have the same BOZR as the corneal radius. For comparison, values are shown for scleral lenses having different back optic zone radii (BOZR) of 8.00 mm and 8.75 mm. (It is normal for the back optic zone of a scleral lens to be fitted about 0.50–0.75 mm flatter than the keratometer radius value.) It can be seen from the graph that this flattening has little effect on the shape factor as compared with the thickness difference between corneal and scleral lenses.

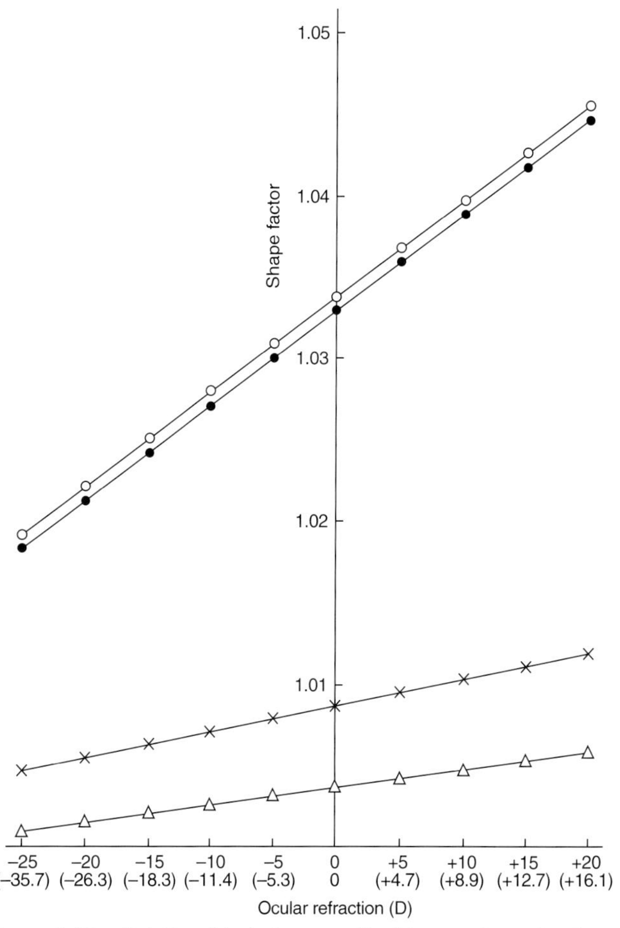

Figure 6.11 Relationship between retinal image sizes, due to shape factor differences, with scleral, corneal and soft lenses. The ocular refraction (D) = back vertex power of contact lens system. The values in parentheses are the spectacle refraction (D). —○— aligned PMMA scleral lens; —•— flat PMMA scleral lens; —×— aligned RGP corneal lens; —Δ— aligned soft lens (n = 1.4)

Values used for the graph in Figure 6.11 are:

	Soft lens	Aligned corneal lens	Aligned scleral lens	Flat scleral lens
n_1	1.40	1.47	1.49	1.49
n_2	1.336	1.336	1.336	1.336
t_1 (mm)	0.10	0.20	0.75	0.75
t_2 (mm)	0.00	0.01	0.1	0.1
BOZR (mm)	8.00	8.00	8.00	8.75
F_2 (interface) (dioptres)	−8.00	−16.75	−19.25	−17.60
Corneal radius (mm)	8.00	8.00	8.00	8.00
Keratometry reading (C) (dioptres)	+42.00	+42.00	+42.00	+42.00

* Although many contact lens practitioners refer to the corneal curvature as measured by keratometry as the 'K' reading, and indeed this applies elsewhere in this book, because in visual optics the letter K is reserved for ocular refraction, to avoid confusion this chapter adopts the use of 'C' to denote the power of the cornea as measured by a keratometer.

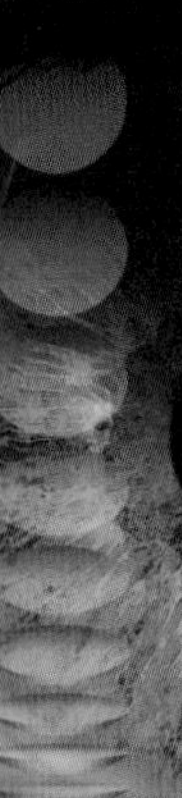

Relative spectacle magnification

This is defined as the ratio between the retinal image sizes in a corrected ametropic eye and a standard emmetropic eye. Various formulae have been given to calculate this, depending on whether the difference between the two eyes is axial or refractive (see below). Its main use is in determining whether a particular type of correction is likely to improve or disrupt binocular vision, by comparing the two retinal image sizes.

Bennett (1985) pointed out such formulae can be misleading because the human emmetropic eye does not always have the standard length and power; indeed the range of values found is quite large. A much simpler approach is used therefore in this chapter, based on 'reduced eye' data and values for 'spectacle' magnification to determine retinal image sizes.

Where a person has different ocular refractions in the two eyes, the different magnification given by the two spectacle lenses (or contact lenses) may result in poor binocular vision. This is usually due to fusion difficulties resulting from unequal retinal image sizes. (Similar distribution of the retinal receptors in the two eyes is assumed although this may be a false assumption.)

It is common to think of anisometropia as being either axial or refractive. Sorsby et al. (1962) showed that most naturally occurring anisometropia is predominantly *axial*, but this is often accompanied by a smaller *refractive* component.

By contrast, one obvious example of *refractive* anisometropia is unilateral aphakia. It is in such cases that contact lenses give greater similarity in retinal image sizes than do spectacle lenses. As can be seen in Figure 6.9, a soft or corneal lens for the aphakic eye renders the minimum amount of magnification of the basic retinal image, but in two eyes of the same length only an intraocular implant for the aphakic eye can achieve 'equality' of retinal image sizes.

The diagrams in Figure 6.12 illustrate how two eyes of the same length and corneal power, one aphakic and the other phakic, have similar basic retinal image sizes. Contact lenses give rise to a minimum change in this basic retinal image size, thereby permitting a good chance of binocular vision although difficulties may still occur. Retinal image size differences of as little as 1% may give rise to binocular problems in some patients.

Figure 6.13 shows how two eyes of unequal length have unequal basic retinal image sizes. In such cases, contact lenses – which scarcely affect this basic size – are theoretically unsatisfactory if fusion is to be achieved, assuming equally spaced retinal receptors in the two eyes. A spectacle lens worn by the ametropic eye, because it is positioned close to the eye's anterior focal plane, makes the retinal image in that eye closer in size to that of the other eye. Typical of such a case is unilateral myopia. However, the retinal receptor distribution may be different in the two eyes, being more widely spaced in the bigger myopic eye, thus reducing the enlargement caused by the longer axial length (Table 6.2). In practice it is found that axially anisometropic patients achieve better binocular fusion in contact lenses than in spectacles (Winn et al. 1986) (see Chapter 21). Thus, all types of anisometropia and antimetropia are better corrected by contact lenses than spectacles, if optimum binocular vision is to be achieved.

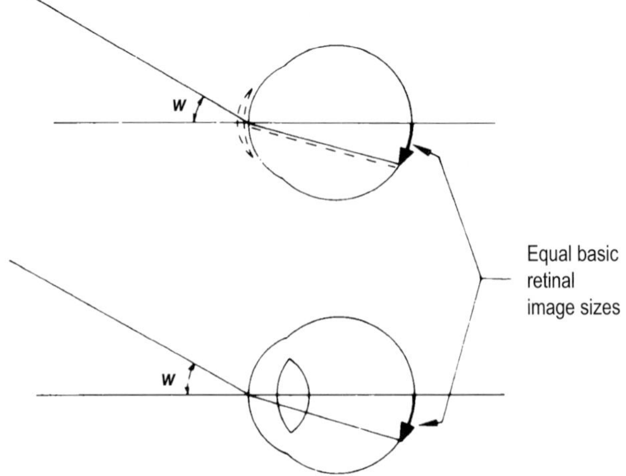

Figure 6.12 Refractive anisometropia: corneal and soft lenses cause minimum change in the basic retinal image size. *w*, angular subtense of distant object

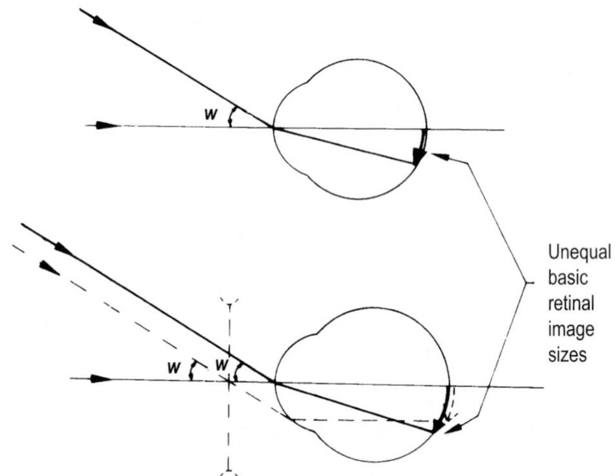

Figure 6.13 Axial anisometropia: a spectacle lens suitably placed before the ametropic eye can give equality of retinal image sizes, but this may not be desirable (see text). *w*, angular subtense of distant object

To compare or calculate retinal image sizes, it is simplest to assume a reduced eye as shown in Figure 6.13 with a RI of 1.336 and a single spherical refracting surface of radius 5.6 mm giving it a power of +60.00 D.

When the refractive error (K) is known to be *axial*, then the power of the reduced eye (F_e') is assumed as +60.00 D and its length is k'.

Now, $k' = \frac{n'}{K'}$, where $K' = K + F_e$

Thus, if the ocular refraction, $K = -10.00$ D then

$K' = +50$ D and $k' = \frac{1.336 \times 1000}{60} = 26.72$ mm

Table 6.2: Differences between axial and refractive anisometropia

	Spectacle correction (D)		Ratio of basic retinal image sizes in uncorrected eyes (R:L)	With spectacle correction			With contact lenses		
				Spectacle magnification		Difference in retinal damage sizes (%)	Spectacle magnification		Difference in retinal image sizes (%)
	R	L		R	L		R	L	
(1)	+2	+12	60.00:60.00	1.03	1.22	18.29	1.01	1.04	3.75
(2)	−1	−10	51.07:59.01	0.99	0.87	1.98	1.00	0.97	12.87

A standard emmetropic eye has an axial length

$$f'_e = \frac{n'}{F'_e} = \frac{1.336 \times 1000}{60} = 22.27 \text{ mm}$$

When the error is known to be *refractive* (as in aphakia) then the power of the eye (F_e') is determined from its length (k') and its ocular refraction (K). For example, $K = +12.00$ D, $k' = 22.27$ mm.

Thus, $K' = \dfrac{1.336 \times 1000}{22.27} = +60.00$ D

and $F_e' \;= K' - K = 60 - 12 = +48.00$ D

As can be seen from Figure 6.13, the principal ray determining the basic retinal image size undergoes refraction according to Snell's law at the principal point of the eye.

Considering this principal ray, prior to refraction the angle subtended at the eye's principal point is w, and after refraction the angle subtended by the basic retinal image is thus w/n'. (All angles are small, and the sine, tangent and angle in radians then all become equal.)

But $\dfrac{w}{n'} = \dfrac{\text{Basic retinal image size}}{k'}$

Thus, basic retinal image size $= k'(w/n') = w/K'$ (in metres).

Note that the principal ray may already have undergone refraction at a spectacle lens or contact lens, so that w is then equivalent to the w' of Figure 6.7. Thus, the spectacle magnification is taken into account in determining the angular subtense at the principal point prior to refraction by the eye. The final retinal image size then becomes

$$\frac{1}{1 - aF} \times \frac{w}{K'} \text{ (in metres)}$$

In the standard emmetropic eye the retinal image size is thus $w \times 60$ metres.

Table 6.2 illustrates the differences between axial and refractive anisometropia. The vertex distance is assumed as 12 mm and the distance from cornea to entrance pupil as 3 mm. Shape factor has not been taken into account.

- *Refractive* anisometropia is demonstrated by a unilateral aphakic with equal retinal image sizes because both eyes are similar in length. Thus, the spectacle magnification afforded by both spectacles and contact lenses has a direct effect on the retinal image sizes. With spectacles, the difference in magnification between the two eyes is large and so, therefore, is the percentage difference between retinal image sizes. With contact lenses, it is small, providing a greater chance of binocular vision.

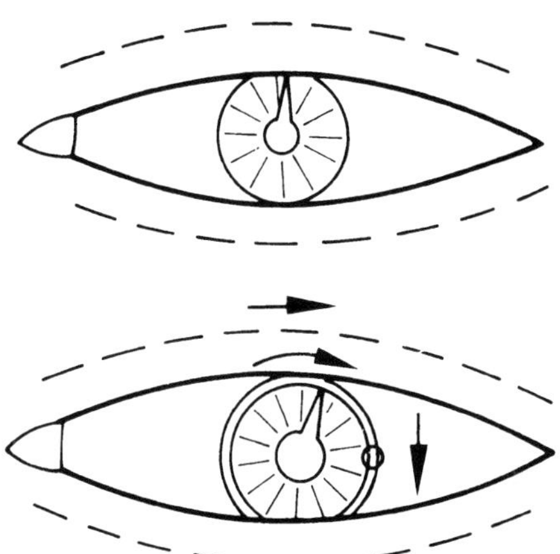

Figure 6.14 The effect of a high positive scleral lens: there is a wider lid aperture and the eye tends to rotate in the directions shown

- *Axial* anisometropia is demonstrated by unilateral axial myopia in which the power of both eyes is assumed to be 60.00 D. Thus, the basic retinal image sizes are proportional to the axial lengths (or inversely proportional to the dioptric lengths, $K'_L{:}K'_R$, as shown in Table 6.2, after remembering to calculate these on the basis of ocular refraction). These basic image sizes are then affected by the spectacle magnifications; so that, with spectacles, where the difference in magnification is large there is only a small difference in the retinal image sizes. With contact lenses, the spectacle magnifications are almost the same but the retinal images are very different in size. Theoretically, spectacles provide the better chance for binocular vision although this is often not the case in practice (see above).

The extremes of purely refractive or purely axial anisometropia, as shown in the examples in Table 6.2, are rare. In most anisometropes, contact lenses afford other advantages such as absence of differential prism. In the authors' experience (Ford & Stone), the perceptual process which allows fusion of different-sized images is more readily adaptable than is the extraocular musculature which has to cope with dissimilar prismatic effects (Ford & Stone 1997).

Soft lenses, being more stable than corneal lenses, are the better type of lens to use for anisometropia, unless large corneal lenses with very little movement can be satisfactorily fitted. In scleral lenses, the weight of the high positive lens may cause hypophoria and excyclophoria of the aphakic eye (Fig. 6.14). This is an extreme example.

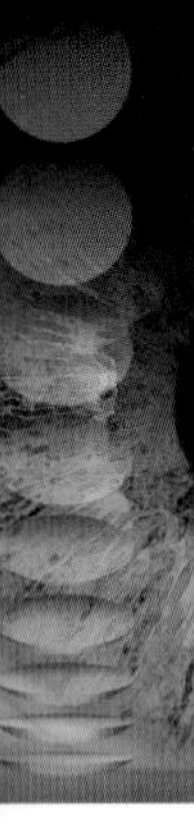

Table 6.3: Comparison of accommodation with spectacles and contact lenses

Spectacle refraction (D)	Ocular accommodation (D) at 0.33 metre from spectacle plane		Ocular accommodation (D) at 0.25 metre from spectacle plane	
	Spectacles	*Contact lenses*	*Spectacles*	*Contact lenses*
–20	1.89	2.90	2.50	3.82
–15	2.09	2.90	2.76	3.82
–10	2.32	2.90	3.06	3.82
–5	2.58	2.90	3.40	3.82
0	2.90	2.90	3.82	3.82
+5	3.27	2.90	4.31	3.82
+10	3.72	2.90	4.89	3.82
+15	4.25	2.90	5.61	3.82

Accommodation

The accommodation exerted for a given working distance varies, depending on whether spectacles or contact lenses are worn. More accommodation is required by myopes and less by hypermetropes when they transfer from spectacles to contact lenses (Table 6.3 and Fig. 6.16).

In order to calculate the ocular accommodation (A) (the actual amount of accommodation exerted by the eye), it is necessary to determine the ocular refraction (K) and the distance (b) at which the near object of regard is imaged by the spectacle lens of power F_s.

For example, Figure 6.15a shows a myope wearing a spectacle lens of –8.00 D, who reads at a distance (l) 25 cm from the spectacle plane. Thus, the demand on spectacle accommodation (A_{sp}) is 4 D. Now if the spectacle lens is worn 12 mm from the eye, the ocular refraction (K) is –7.30 D (see Appendix A and **Formula *I*** on the accompanying CD-ROM, where ocular refraction is denoted as F_O instead of K due to the use of the symbol K for keratometer readings). The CD-ROM also has a program that converts spectacle to ocular refraction.

(The method of calculating ocular refraction from spectacle refraction and vertex distance, d, should be apparent from Figure 6.17 if K is substituted for L and k for l.)

In Figure 6.15a the near object, O, is imaged by the spectacle lens at O′.

Now $l = -250$ mm
Therefore, $L = -4$ D
$F_s = -8$ D
Therefore $L' = -12$ D
Thus, $l' = -83.3$ mm
But $b = l' - d = -83.3 - 12 = -95.3$ mm

$$B = \frac{1}{b \text{ (in metres)}} = -10.5 \text{ D}$$

But –7.30 D of this corrects the ocular refraction. The remaining 3.20 D must be overcome by the use of the myope's accommodation, i.e. $A = K - B$.

This demonstrates the effectivity of the spectacle lens in permitting such a myope to use only 3.2 D of accommodation, whereas if a contact lens were worn, the same near object would be 262 mm from the eye, necessitating 3.82 D of accommodation.

Figure 6.15b shows a similar situation for a hypermetrope. $F_s = +8$ D, $l = -250$ mm and $d = 12$ mm. Thus, $K = +8.85$ D (see Appendix A and **Formula *I*** on the CD-ROM).

Now $L = -4$ D, $F_s = +8$ D
Therefore, $L' = +4$ D and $l' = +250$ mm
But $b = l' - d = +250 - 12 = +238$ mm
Therefore, $B = +4.2$ D
Since $A = K - B$, $A = +8.85 - 4.2 = +4.65$ D

This demonstrates how the ocular accommodation of a hypermetrope wearing spectacles is greater than that required when contact lenses are worn. In this example, 4.65 D of accommodation is required as compared to 3.82 D in contact lenses.

If a comparison is made of the graphs of convergence in Figure 6.4 and the graphs of accommodation in Figure 6.16, it will be noted that the slopes showing convergence and accommodation with spectacles are the same. They are also the same with contact lenses. As Westheimer (1962) stated, this implies that the accommodation/convergence ratio (A/C ratio)

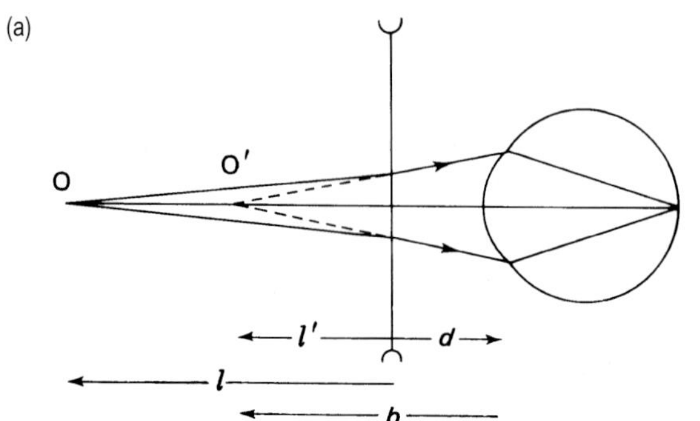

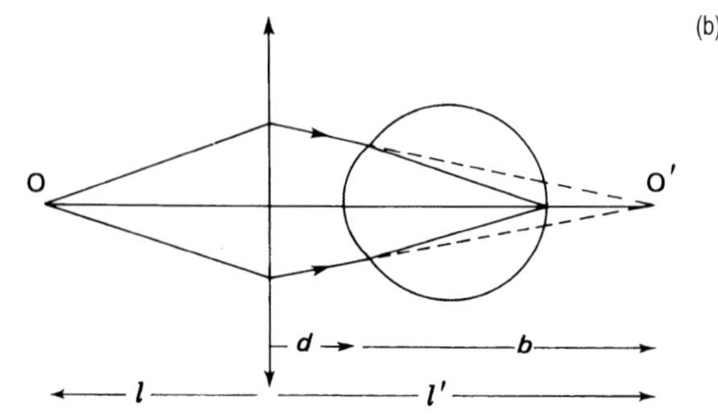

Figure 6.15 Near vision through spectacle lenses. The near object of regard, O, is imaged at O′, which is at a distance b from the eye. The object, image and vertex distances from the spectacle lens are l, l', and d respectively. (a) Myopia; (b) hypermetropia

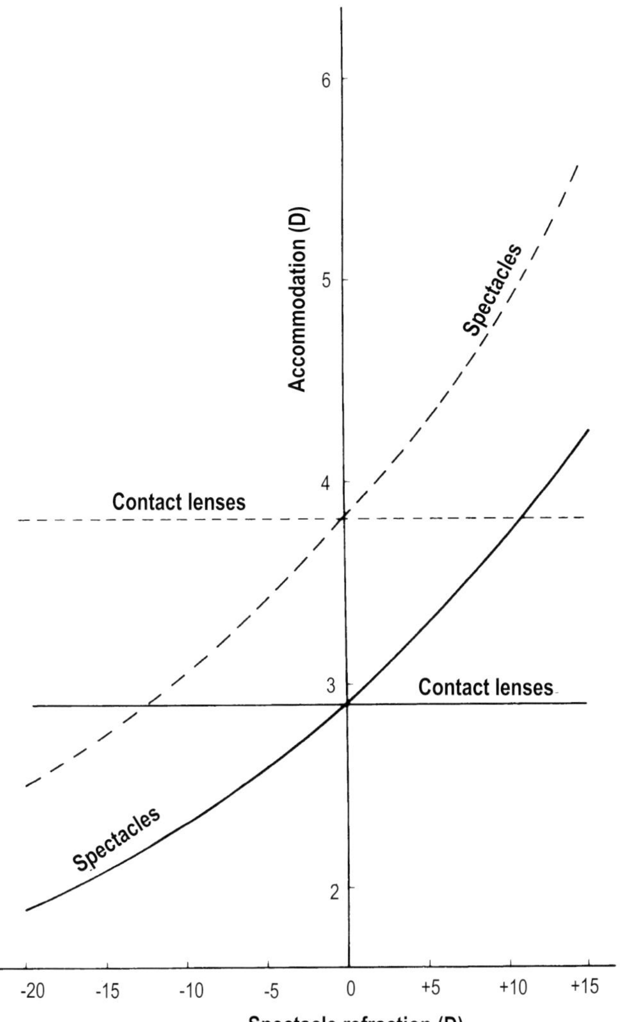

Figure 6.16 Accommodation with spectacles and contact lenses. -- at 0.25 metre; — at 0.33 metre (compare this with Fig. 6.4)

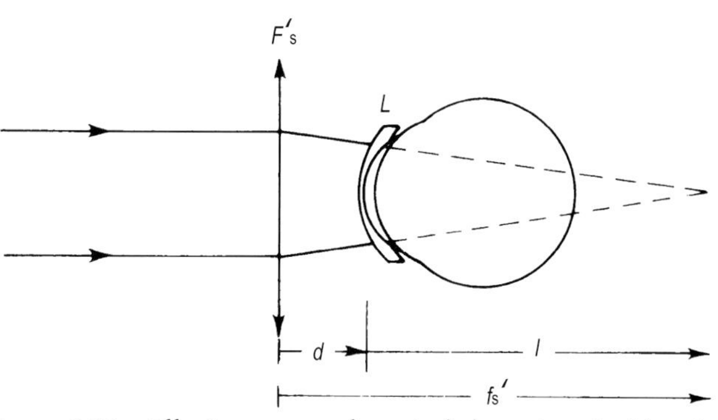

Figure 6.17 Effective power of spectacle lens at contact lens is: $L = 1/l = F_s'/(1 - dF_s')$ (see Appendix A and **Formula *I*** on the CD-ROM)

Table 6.4: Ratio between accommodation and convergence with spectacles and contact lenses

Spectacle refraction (D)	Ratio of accommodation (D) to convergence (Δ) at			
	0.33 metre from spectacle plane		0.25 metre from spectacle plane	
	Spectacles	*Contact lenses*	*Spectacles*	*Contact lenses*
−20	0.170	0.174	0.172	0.176
−15	0.173	0.174	0.174	0.176
−10	0.174	0.174	0.174	0.176
−5	0.174	0.174	0.176	0.176
0	0.174	0.174	0.176	0.176
+5	0.172	0.174	0.175	0.176
+10	0.168	0.174	0.171	0.176
+15	0.160	0.174	0.164	0.176

is the same with contact lenses as it is with spectacles. Stone (1967) also showed that if contact lenses remain centred for all working distances and a comparison is made with spectacles centred for distance vision, the accommodation/convergence ratio remains approximately the same with both forms of correction (Table 6.4).

The figures for the basis of this table are derived from Tables 6.1 and 6.3 and show that:

$$\frac{\text{A/C ratio with spectacles}}{\text{A/C ratio with contact lenses}} \approx 1 - F_{sp}(z - 2d)$$

where

F_{sp} = spectacle lens power in dioptres
z = distance from spectacle plane to centre of rotation of eye, in metres
d = back vertex distance of spectacle lens in metres

Now, if $d = z/2$ it can be seen that the A/C ratio is the same with both spectacles and contact lenses.

In Table 6.4, d was taken as 12 mm and z as 27 mm, which accounts for the slight discrepancies between the values found for the two forms of correction. But as d is always approximately $z/2$, the ratios are always approximately the same. The PD and spectacle centre distance was taken as 60 mm.

Changes in accommodation should therefore only cause difficulty in the presbyopic or pre-presbyopic myope, who may have trouble in exerting the extra accommodation and convergence when transferring to contact lenses from spectacles.

OPTICAL CONSIDERATIONS OF CONTACT LENSES ON THE EYE

To understand why a contact lens correction often differs considerably from a spectacle correction, the significance of the following points must be fully understood:

- Effectivity – the difference between spectacle and ocular refraction.
- The contribution made by the liquid (tears) lens.

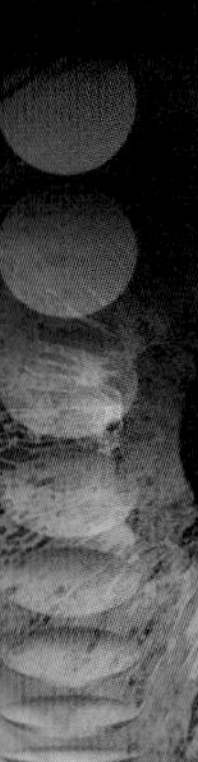

- The effects of radius changes on the back vertex power of the contact lens–liquid lens system.
- The differences between total and corneal astigmatism.

This section is intended as a practical guide in determining soft and rigid corneal lens powers, and it employs the method of specifying BOZR in millimetres rather than in terms of the keratometer reading in dioptres.

To correct fully an eye's refractive error, the back vertex power of the contact-lens/liquid-lens system must equal the ocular refraction (K) – not to be confused with the keratometer reading, also often denoted as 'K'.

The principle of effectivity is shown in Figure 6.17 which illustrates a hypermetropic eye corrected by a spectacle lens of power F'_s and hence of focal length f'_s giving the position of the far point plane M'_R. The distance from the corneal vertex to this plane is reduced by the vertex distance d, so the required power of the contact-lens/liquid-lens system of the ocular refraction K is given by:

$$k = f'_s - d$$

$$\text{hence } K = \frac{1}{f'_s - d} = \frac{F'_s}{1 - dF'_s}$$

$$\text{or approximately } F'_s(1 + dF'_s) = F'_s + dF'^2_s$$

Since dF'^2_s is always positive, the ocular refraction and hence the contact-lens/liquid-lens system power for a hypermetrope is always greater than the spectacle refraction, while it is numerically less for a myope.

Conversely, given K, the spectacle refraction is given by:

$$F'_s = \frac{K}{1 + dK}$$

In the following considerations, it will be assumed that surface powers are additive provided that their separations are small. This leads to some approximations. It will also be assumed that the back vertex power of a contact lens can be directly added to the vergence of the light reaching it – although this, again, is an approximation.

Approximate methods of calculation are useful to cross-check that formulae and computer programs have been used correctly. However, a contact lens having an entirely different back vertex power from that required should not be used for refraction.

In addition, a combination of positive spectacle lens and negative contact lens, which constitutes a Galilean telescope system, should be avoided wherever possible since it gives a higher magnification than that obtained with the final contact lens. Hence, a false assessment of visual acuity may be made, and disappointment will follow when the final contact lens gives poorer vision.

Different aspects of refraction with contact lenses will now be considered.

Ocular refraction

  BVP of final contact lens in air
\+ BVP of liquid lens in air (liquid lens assumed thin)

= Ocular refraction

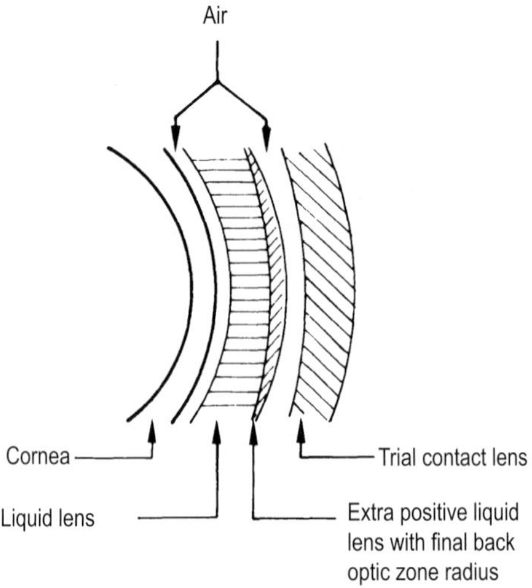

Figure 6.18 Refraction with a trial contact lens: the trial contact lens has too flat a back optic zone radius

REFRACTION WITH A CONTACT LENS OF INCORRECT BOZR

When a refraction is carried out using a lens of incorrect BOZR, for example if a rigid trial lens is fitted that is slightly different from the lens to be ordered, then:

  Liquid lens power in air
\+ trial contact lens BVP in air
\+ effective power at the contact lens of the additional spectacle lens

= Ocular refraction

If the BOZR is flatter than that to be ordered, the liquid lens is more negative than it will be with the final contact lens (Fig. 6.18). The vergence of the light reaching the front surface of the liquid lens must therefore be adjusted to allow for this. Negative power must be added to counteract the extra positive power of the final liquid lens.

When fitting soft lenses, this does not apply because they conform to the central corneal contour. However, if there are large differences in radius between lens and cornea, there may be an effect on the liquid lens. This effect is unpredictable:

- Thick soft lenses and relatively inelastic lenses such as silicone hydrogel will have more of an effect on the liquid lens than ultrathin soft lenses. This effect can be as much as 0.50 D.
- If the back surface of the lens closely parallels the entire cornea, then the liquid lens will have zero power, but if the lens touches the apex region of the cornea and clears the mid-peripheral region, there is likely to be a small negative-powered liquid lens.

APPROXIMATE RULE [1]

*If, when fitting rigid corneal lenses, the BOZR is flatter than that to be ordered, for each 0.20 mm that the BOZR is too **flat**, add **–1.00 D** to the BVP of the contact lens.*

When the BOZR is steeper than that to be ordered, for each 0.20 mm that the BOZR is too ***steep****, add* ***+1.00 D*** *to the BVP of the contact lens.*

This rule can be shown to be approximately correct by checking on a Heine's scale (see Bennett 1985) or by using radius/power tables for a RI of 1.336 (see **Formulae *III*** and ***V*** on the CD-ROM).

Examples

(i) A typical corneal lens problem
(ii) A typical scleral lens problem

		(i)	*(ii)*
BOZR used (mm)		8.10	8.25
BOZR ordered (mm)		8.00	8.50
Change in power (D) of liquid lens front surface in air	From:	+41.48	+40.73
	To:	+42.00	+39.53
	By:	+0.52	−1.20
Contact lens BVP change (D) to counteract this	Accurate method:	−0.52	+1.20
	Approximate method:	−0.50	+1.25
Error of approximate method (D)		+0.02	+0.05

These examples show that the error of the approximate method is sufficiently small to be ignored. (However, see also Chapter 20 where the lens BOZR fall out of the normal physiological range.)

Ocular astigmatism

Front surface corneal astigmatism
\+ back surface corneal astigmatism
\+ crystalline lens astigmatism (referred to the corneal plane)

= Total ocular astigmatism

Note that the front surface of the cornea usually has greater positive power in the near vertical meridian, i.e. 'with-the-rule' astigmatism, whereas the back surface of the cornea and the crystalline lens normally have 'against-the-rule' astigmatism. The total effect is usually with-the-rule, although this decreases and may reverse with age.

ASTIGMATISM OF THE FRONT SURFACE OF THE CORNEA AND THE EFFECT OF THE LIQUID LENS

RI of tears, n_t = 1.336
RI of cornea, n_c = 1.376

When a rigid contact lens with spherical back surface is placed on the eye, the front surface of the liquid lens is spherical because it is formed by the back surface of the contact lens. If the front surface of the cornea is toroidal, then the back surface of the liquid lens is also toroidal, with radii (r) in mm equal to that of the cornea, but having negative power.

The powers in air of the back surface of the liquid lens are given by:

$$F = \frac{(1 - 1.336)\ 1000}{r}$$

and the powers of the front surface of the cornea are given by:

$$F = \frac{(1.376 - 1)\ 1000}{r}$$

This means that the front surface astigmatism of the cornea is partly neutralized by the back surface astigmatism of the liquid lens. The amount neutralized thus is 336/376, which is almost 90%. This is of importance with toroidal corneas because it is likely that the back surface of the cornea itself will neutralize the remaining 10% of its front surface astigmatism.

Thus, with a rigid, non-flexing, spherical contact lens on the eye, any residual astigmatism found is almost entirely due to the crystalline lens since practically all the corneal astigmatism is corrected, i.e.

Back surface astigmatism of liquid lens
\+ front surface astigmatism of cornea
\+ back surface astigmatism of cornea

= Zero (approximately)

Keratometry and corneal astigmatism

Keratometers measure front surface corneal radii but give total corneal power on the assumption, given above, that the back surface of the cornea has −10% of the power of the front surface.

The true RI of the cornea (1.376) is therefore not used to calibrate keratometers. Instead, an index of 1.3375 is usually used (n_k). This allows the instrument to read total corneal power (or approximately 90% of the front surface power).

However, n_k and n_t are almost the same (1.3375 and 1.336). Indeed, some keratometers are calibrated for an index of 1.336 or even 1.332. Therefore, the astigmatism measured by the keratometer is almost the same as that corrected by the back surface of the liquid lens. In fact, the use of n_k instead of n_t gives a *power* value which is slightly too high:

For a radius of 8 mm:

n_k gives F_k = 42.19 D and
n_t gives F_t = 42.00 D.

Astigmatism is the *difference between the two principal powers*, therefore the error due to the slight difference in the refractive indices is reduced to an insignificant amount. This is illustrated in the following example of a highly astigmatic cornea.

Example

Keratometry (n_k = 1.3375)	8 mm (+42.19 D) along 180 7 mm (+48.21 D) along 90
Total corneal astigmatism	+ 6.02 DC × 180
Liquid lens back surface powers (n_t = 1.336)	8 mm (−42.00 D) along 180 7 mm (−48.00 D) along 90
Liquid lens back surface astigmatism	−6.00 DC × 180

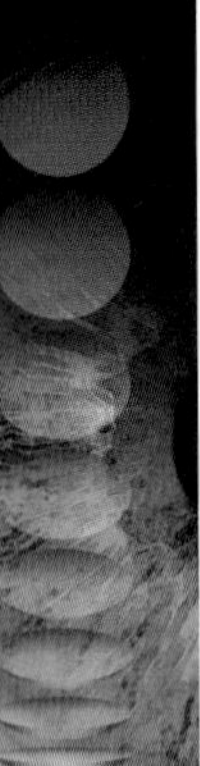

Even in such an extreme example it can be seen that the amount of total corneal astigmatism uncorrected by the liquid lens is an insignificant amount (+6.02 – 6.00 = +0.02 D). It is therefore valid to state that all the astigmatism measured by keratometry is corrected by the back surface of the liquid lens.

Although this large difference of 1 mm between the two meridians gave 6 D of corneal astigmatism, a difference of 0.2 mm at the average corneal radius of 7.8 mm results in approximately 1.00 D of corneal astigmatism, the same relation as for changes in BOZR of a rigid corneal lens.

Residual astigmatism

Residual astigmatism is defined as that remaining when a non-flexing rigid contact lens is placed on an eye.

Since the amount of astigmatism corrected by the back surface of the liquid lens can be measured by keratometry (as shown above), the amount of residual astigmatism with a spherical contact lens may be predicted in advance, although this assumes that the lens is reasonably thick and does not flex (see p. 152). If this is so:

  Total ocular astigmatism
– astigmatism measured by keratometry

= Residual astigmatism

When determining the total ocular astigmatism, the effective change in power of *both* the spherical and the cylindrical elements must be calculated from the spectacle refraction and the vertex distance as shown in the following example:

Spectacle refraction	–6.00/–1.00 × 180
Back vertex distance	12 mm
Spectacle refraction in crossed cylinder form	–6.00 × 90/–7.00 × 180
Ocular refraction in crossed cylinder form after allowing for vertex distance (see Appendix A and the CD-ROM)	–5.60 × 90/–6.46 × 180
Ocular refraction	–5.60/–0.86 × 180

This shows that the 1 D cylinder is reduced to 0.86 D due to the associated sphere power, whereas if the sphere power were ignored there would be no significant change in the power of the cylinder – which is demonstrably incorrect. The higher the powers of sphere and cylinder, the greater is the effect of vertex distance.

Prediction of residual astigmatism allows the effect of this amount of astigmatism to be simulated by the use of a trial cylinder in front of the patient's usual spectacle correction. The sphere power may then be adjusted to obtain the best visual acuity. If this is inadequate, it is obvious that the contact lens must incorporate a cylinder for the correction of the residual astigmatism in order to obtain satisfactory visual acuity. A suitable lens design may then be selected at the outset of the fitting.

With spherical soft lenses, owing to their replication of corneal astigmatism (see p. 150), the residual astigmatism is usually almost the same as the ocular astigmatism; if this is 1 D or more, a toric soft lens or a spherical rigid lens may be necessary to obtain adequate visual acuity.

Rigid gas permeable (RGP) materials vary in the amount of lens flexure that takes place on a toroidal cornea (see Chapter 9). In addition, a thin spherical RGP lens that corrects all the corneal astigmatism when first worn, may, after several weeks of wear, alter shape, thereby increasing the amount of residual astigmatism.

APPROXIMATE RULE [2]

When rigid non-flexing spherical lenses are to be fitted, if the corneal astigmatism and total ocular astigmatism are both with-the-rule or against-the-rule and ***the difference between them is less than 0.75 D****, this cylinder (which represents the expected residual astigmatism) may be ignored.*

When spherical soft or RGP lenses are to be fitted, ***ocular astigmatism of 0.75 D or less*** *may usually be ignored, though for RGP lenses this assumes that the corneal astigmatism is also low.*

In those rare cases where the ocular astigmatism is low but corneal astigmatism is significant, i.e. the corneal astigmatism is neutralized by the crystalline lens, a spherical soft lens is the lens of choice as the corneal astigmatism is transferred through the lens to the front surface.

TORIC CONTACT LENSES (see Chapter 12)

Both optical and fitting considerations of toric polymethyl-methacrylate (PMMA) corneal lenses have been dealt with in detail by Capelli (1964), Stone (1966) and Westerhout (1969). In summary, it may be said that if the back optic zone of a rigid contact lens is to be made toroidal, the BVP required should ideally be found by refraction over a lens having the correct toroidal BOZR and appropriate power. Many laboratories will manufacture a diagnostic lens if given the patient's spectacle prescription, vertex distance and keratometry readings. Rabbetts (1992) published a spreadsheet program, which enabled the appropriate powers to be ordered (see also CD-ROM). Alternatively, an over-refraction may be carried out with a spherical lens having a BOZR equal to the flatter meridian of the toric lens to be ordered. The calculation method will be taken first.

Calculation method – induced astigmatism and toric back optic zone rigid lenses

Induced astigmatism is that astigmatism generated when a rigid toric lens is placed on an eye. It is simplest to take an example.

K readings	8.00 along 180
	7.60 along 90
Refractive error	–3.25/–2.50 × 180 at 12 mm

Using a notional n_k of 1.336, the same as tears, the corneal astigmatism is 2.21 D with-the-rule, as shown in the following table:

	Flat meridian	Steep meridian	Astigmatism
Keratometry (mm)	8.00	7.60	
Corneal powers (D)	42.00	44.21	−2.21 × 180
Spectacle refraction	−3.25	−5.75	
Ocular refraction	−3.13	−5.38	−2.25 × 180
	Spherical lens – radius 7.90		
Liquid lens	+0.53	−1.68	−2.21 × 180
BVP of required lens	−3.66	−3.70	negligible
	Toric lens: 8.00 × 7.60		
Lens back surface power (n = 1.487)	−60.88	−64.08	−3.20
Liquid lens	0.00	0.00	0.00
BVP required = ocular refraction – liquid lens power	−3.13	−5.38	−2.25
But if the lens has power of −3.13 in the flat meridian, power in steep meridian =		−6.33 (−3.13 − 3.20)	
Hence induced astigmatism =			+0.95 {−5.38 −(−6.33)}

When a spherical lens is placed on the eye, for example one of BOZR 7.90 which lies between the two keratometry readings, the liquid lens in one meridian is positive since the lens is steeper than the cornea, while in the other it is negative since the lens is flatter. In this example, the residual astigmatism is negligible (about 0.05 D).

When a toric lens exactly matching the keratometry readings is placed on the eye, the liquid lens is of zero power in both meridians. The back surface of the toric lens has, however, −3.20 D of astigmatic power while the eye needs only −2.25 D. Hence the eye is now over-corrected by the difference, +0.95 D × 180.

APPROXIMATE RULE [3]

If the cornea has 2 D of astigmatism, then an aligning rigid contact lens will show approximately 3 D of astigmatism in air, while on the eye there is an overcorrection of approximately −1 D, the negative sign signifying that the sign of the induced refractive error is opposite to the original.

This is a simple 3:2:−1 rule.

Several points arise:

- It is often simplest to do the power calculation in the two meridians separately. It is only necessary at the end to consider astigmatic powers, i.e. the difference between the meridional powers needed on the lens and the astigmatic power of the back surface of the contact lens.
- If all the ocular astigmatism is in the cornea, then fitting a toric contact lens will always induce some astigmatic error, though a partial match will reduce the induced error: in the example above, a fit of 7.95 × 7.65 reduces the induced error to +0.70 D. The ideal patient for a toric fitting is the rare individual with greater ocular than corneal astigmatism.
- The rule comes from the relative refractive effect of tears or the cornea and of the contact lens. Since the RI of lens material is around 1.5, its refractive effect in air is proportional to (1.5 − 1.0 = 0.5); the refractive effect of tears on the cornea is proportional to (1.336 − 1.0 ≈ 1/3); whilst the refractive effect of the lens on the eye is proportional to (1.5 − 1.336 ≈ 1/6).

Toric power measurement from refracting through a spherical lens

In this case, which is not as straightforward as refracting through a lens with the correct toric back optic surface, some calculation is necessary in order to determine the BVP of the final toric lens to be ordered. Since the BOZR of one meridian is to be steepened by a known amount when ordering, the calculation is the same as that for a spherical lens where refraction has been carried out with a trial lens of incorrect BOZR, as outlined on page 142 and summarized in Approximate rule [1]. It is a simple matter of allowing for the fact that the liquid lens power in one meridian will be different, with the final lens in place, from the value with the spherical trial lens in place. An allowance for this difference must therefore be made on the contact lens itself.

Example

BOZR of lens to be ordered	8.10 along 180 7.50 along 90
BOZR of spherical trial lens for refraction	8.10 mm
BVP of spherical trial lens for refraction	−2.75 D
Over-refraction	−1.00/−0.75 × 90

which, when converted to crossed cylinder form, gives
−1.75 D × 90/−1.00 D × 180

BVP of final lens along 180 is −2.75 + (−1.75) = −4.50
BVP of final lens along 90 is approximately −2.75 + (−1.00) + allowance of −3.00 D for radius change (see Approximate rule [1]) = **−6.75 D** in total

When the radius change is as large as this, it is more accurate to work out the change in power of the liquid lens, remembering that this is a change of the front surface of the liquid lens in air (see p. 143 and **Formulae *III*** and ***V*** on the CD-ROM) for a RI difference of 1.336 − 1. In this example, this gives a change of −3.32 D, i.e. 0.32 D more than the value given by Approximate rule [1]. Thus, the BVP of the final contact lens along 90 should be **−7.07 D.**

It can now be established whether or not a front toroidal surface will also be necessary on the final toroidal back surface lens. This depends on whether or not the cylinder power of the back surface in air is the same as the required cylinder element of the BVP of the lens in air:

Required BVP of final lens (in air)	−4.50 along 180 −7.07 along 90 = −4.50/−2.57 × 180
For an RGP lens back surface powers (in air) (from **Formula *III*** for surface power (1.487 − 1))	−64.93 along 90 and −60.12 along 180
Back surface cylinder in air is thus	−4.81 × 180
Front surface cylinder required (ignoring thickness)	(−2.57− [−4.81]) × 180 = +2.24 × 180

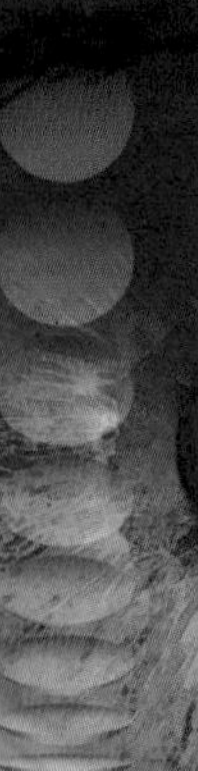

The induced astigmatism in this example is −1.49 D × 90, augmented for the final cylinder by the over-refraction at the same orientation.

Rabbetts (1992) gives a spreadsheet listing for calculating the required powers when refracting over a toric or spherical lens, as in this example.

The computer program on the accompanying CD-ROM may also be used to determine the back surface cylinder power in air and, if each meridian is treated separately, **Formula *III***, also on the CD-ROM, may be used. An alternative calculator is available at www.rgpli.org/mandell.htm.

The above example is an obvious case where a front surface cylinder is necessary to give good visual acuity. Frequently the front surface cylinder calculated in this way is quite small and the practitioner may prefer to order a lens with a spherical front surface and risk leaving the patient with a small amount of uncorrected (but usually overcorrected) astigmatism. The final lens may be ordered stating that it is to have a back toroidal surface only, and giving the back vertex power along the flattest meridian, i.e. the maximum positive or least negative power.

If the lens is ordered quoting the power along both meridians, then the cylinder element must be altered by the amount of front surface cylinder being ignored, i.e. the cylinder element of the BVP is then the same as the back surface cylinder in air.

Although, in theory, the contact lens powers can be obtained this way, the stability of a spherical lens on a toroidal cornea in the example given above would produce a poorly fitting lens and may cancel out the notional advantages. It may be preferable to calculate a trial toric lens specification as in the first example, or to send the refraction and keratometry details to the laboratory and let them do the calculations.

Compensated bitoric or spherical power equivalent bitoric lenses

These are rigid lenses in which the front toroidal surface in air has an equal and opposite cylindrical power to the back toroidal surface in tears. It thus acts like a spherical lens on the eye, both in terms of power and in that rotation of the lens on the eye does not induce any cylindrical effect (see Chapter 12). Such a lens may be required for reasons of comfort or fit, or if a spherical lens flexes on a toroidal cornea.

If, for example, a rigid spherical RGP lens corrects the astigmatism of an eye, but for physiological (and/or fitting) reasons the lens is likely to flex, thereby inducing unwanted astigmatism, it may be desirable to fit an RGP lens with a toroidal back surface to match the corneal radii. This prevents flexure but introduces astigmatism at the interface of the lens back surface with the liquid lens. The amount of this induced astigmatism is given by:

$$\frac{1000(n'-n)}{r_F} - \frac{1000(n'-n)}{r_S}$$

where n' = RI of contact lens
n = RI of tears = 1.336
r_F = BOZR along flattest meridian of lens back surface
r_S = BOZR along steepest meridian of lens back surface.

To compensate for this astigmatism introduced at the back surface of the lens in situ, a front toroidal surface with principal meridians parallel to those of the back surface must be made which, since it is in air, will not be as toroidal as the back surface. The ratio between front and back surface toricity depends on the RI of the lens material and is given by:

$$\frac{1/(n'-1)}{1/(n'-1.336)} = \frac{n'-1.336}{n'-1}$$

For PMMA this is

$$\frac{1.49-1.339}{1.49-1} = 0.314 \text{ or approximately } 1/3$$

For an RGP material of RI 1.45 it is

$$\frac{1.45-1.336}{1.45-1} = 0.253 \text{ or approximately } 1/4$$

Thus to provide a spherical effect on the eye, a compensated parallel bitoric lens has a front surface cylinder which counteracts in the region of a third to a quarter of the back surface cylinder in air, depending on the RI of the lens material. This information is useful when checking the lens on a focimeter. Its total cylindrical effect is thus two-thirds to three-quarters of the back surface cylinder in air, the latter being easily obtained from radiuscope readings (see Chapter 16) and then by radius/power conversion (see **Formulae *III–V*** on the CD-ROM).

If such lenses are not accurately manufactured with the principal meridians absolutely parallel on the front and back surfaces, then not only is the cylinder power of the lens in air different from that expected but the lens will also not provide the correct 'spherical equivalent' effect on the eye (Douthwaite 1988).

Similarly, if the power of the cylinder on the front surface does not have the correct ratio to that of the back surface then again it will not be the equivalent of a spherical lens on the eye. This may not be problematical unless the lens rotates when the effect of the swinging cylinder may give rise to a reduction and variation in visual acuity. These erroneous effects are compounded if the front surface cylinder is both incorrect in power and not parallel to that of the back surface – which may explain the reluctance of some manufacturers to supply such lenses, as they are extremely difficult to manufacture accurately.

Any resultant cylindrical effect from misalignment of the two astigmatic surfaces or of the lens on the eye can be found graphically by Stokes' construction, calculated by 'astigmatic decomposition' (Bennett 1984, Rabbetts 1998), Fourier decomposition (Thibos et al. 1997, Rabbetts 2007) or by using the CD-ROM program.

Stokes' construction

This is an excellent method of compounding two cylinders, F_1 and F_2, with an angle between their axes of α, into an equivalent sphere/cylinder power (Fig. 6.19) (Rabbetts 2007).

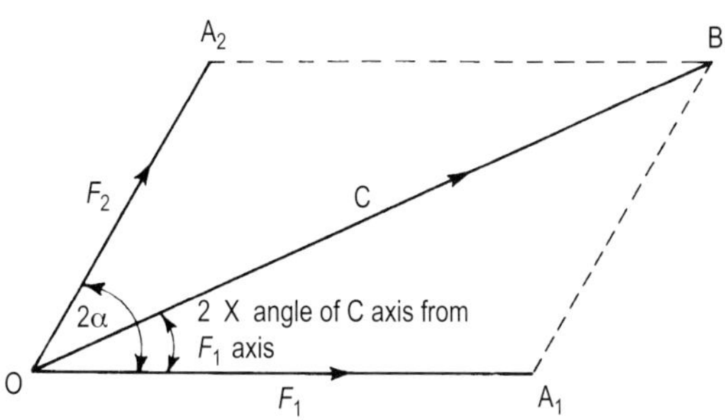

Figure 6.19 Stokes' construction

A parallelogram is constructed with the two sides OA_1 and OA_2 proportional to F_1 and F_2, with the angle between them equal to 2α, where α is the acute angle between the two cylinder axes.

The parallelogram is completed and the resultant OB drawn. This is proportional to the resultant cylinder C. The angle between OB and OA_1 is twice the angle between the axis of C and that of F_1.

The equivalent or mean sphere S resulting from *only* the combination of the two cylindrical components is given by:

$$S = \tfrac{1}{2}(F_1 + F_2 - C)$$

Astigmatic and Fourier decomposition

These methods are based on the principle that any astigmatic power C at any axis α may be regarded as the resultant of an astigmatic power with axis 180° and another power with axis 45°, or hence may be resolved or decomposed into two other astigmatic components. For methods of calculation, readers are referred to Rabbetts (2007).

POWER VARIATIONS AS A SEQUEL TO OTHER CHANGES

Back vertex power and thickness

This section applies particularly to high positive corneal and soft lenses and to scleral lenses.

With some lenses, particularly sclerals, it may not be possible to make an accurate measurement of the back vertex power with a focimeter. It may be easier to measure the front vertex power of the trial contact lens and provide the laboratory with the central optic thickness of the trial lens so that its BVP may be calculated. It is preferable, however, for practitioners to calculate this for themselves (see **Formula *XVIII*** on the CD-ROM).

Example

BVP of trial scleral lens	+5.62 D
t_c	0.50 mm
BOZR	8.00 mm
FVP	+5.40 D

If the lens were to be ordered on the basis of FVP without t_c being specified, it might be returned from the laboratory as:

FVP	+5.40 D
t_c	0.75 mm
BOZR	8.00 mm
BVP (instead of +5.62 D)	+5.75 D

This error increases with thickness and power (see **Formulae *VI*** and ***XVIII–XXV*** on the CD-ROM). Care is therefore needed when ordering high positive lenses, although corneal lenses are usually much thinner than sclerals, even in high positive powers, and the errors due to thickness differences are correspondingly much smaller.

Power changes of soft lenses

Before being placed on an eye, a soft contact lens is normally in a fully hydrated state in physiological saline solution and the RI is at its lowest value. The lens is also at room temperature and its curvature (i.e. its BOZR, or posterior apical radius, PAR, if the back surface is aspherical) and power should be as specified by the manufacturer.

After being placed on the eye, several changes occur, all of which affect the power of the lens.

FIRST CHANGE – FLEXURE

The centre of the back surface of the lens alters to take up the same curvature as the central cornea, or almost so. This change in curvature is commonly referred to as flexure or draping. The amount of the resultant power change due to flexure, be it spherical or toroidal, is small for thin lenses, but becomes significant for lenses of high positive power (Fatt & Chaston 1981).

Various empirical methods of predicting the power change due to this flexure have been suggested, such as assuming that the front optic zone radius (FOZR) changes by the same amount as the BOZR (Baron 1975), or alternatively that the two surfaces change in the same ratio. Strachan (1973) termed this ratio between the pre-wear and post-wear BOZR, the 'wrap-factor'. The most plausible explanation and theoretical exposition was given by Bennett (1976). He based his argument on the following:

- The volume of the lens remains constant even though its curvature changes.
- There was no redistribution of lens thickness.
- The centre thickness remains unchanged.
- The front surface of the lens remains spherical if the cornea is spherical.

Bearing these factors in mind he calculated that both positive and negative lenses change power with flexure by the same amount as concentric lenses (i.e. lenses which have a common centre of curvature for back and front surface radii) change power when they are bent. These changes are summarized in Table 6.5 which is reproduced by kind permission of A. G. Bennett. He not only calculated the values from exact equations, but also derived a simplified equation for the back vertex power of a lens with concentric surfaces:

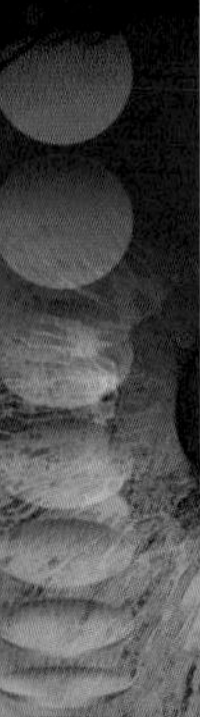

Table 6.5: Change in power when a soft lens is moulded by the cornea to a steeper back optic zone radius, refractive index (1.43–1.44) and volume remaining the same

Thickness	Change† in power (D) for change of back optic zone radius, r_0 (mm) (see note*)						
t (mm)	9.5–9.0	9.0–8.5	8.5–8.0	8.0–7.5	7.5–7.0	7.0–6.5	6.5–6.0
0.10	–0.03	–0.05	–0.05	–0.07	–0.08	–0.10	–0.12
0.15	–0.06	–0.07	–0.08	–0.09	–0.12	–0.15	–0.18
0.20	–0.07	–0.09	–0.11	–0.13	–0.15	–0.20	–0.24
0.25	–0.10	–0.11	–0.13	–0.16	–0.19	–0.24	–0.30
0.30	–0.12	–0.13	–0.16	–0.19	–0.23	–0.28	–0.36
0.35	–0.13	–0.15	–0.18	–0.22	–0.27	–0.33	–0.41
0.40	–0.14	–0.18	–0.21	–0.25	–0.30	–0.37	–0.47
0.45	–0.16	–0.19	–0.24	–0.28	–0.34	–0.41	–0.53
0.50	–0.19	–0.21	–0.26	–0.31	–0.37	–0.46	–0.58
0.55	–0.20	–0.24	–0.28	–0.33	–0.41	–0.51	–0.63
0.60	–0.21	–0.26	–0.30	–0.37	–0.44	–0.55	–0.68

†The change is invariably an addition of minus power and is virtually independent of the back vertex power of the original lens. For every 0.01 increase in refractive index over 1.44 the above figures should be increased by 1.5%.
* The following example shows the method of use of the table: if a lens of BOZR 9.00 mm and *t* 0.20 mm is fitted to a cornea of radius 8.00 mm, the power change expected, if *n* is 1.43, is –0.09 D + –0.11 D = –0.20 D. (The values in all columns between the two appropriate radii are added together to arrive at the power change.)

$$F'_v = -\frac{(n-1)}{n} \times \frac{t}{r_2^2} \quad *$$

where F'_v is back vertex power, n is RI, t is centre thickness, and r_2 is BOZR, where both of these are in millimetres.

For a value of n of 1.43, this gives:

$$F'_v = -\frac{-300t}{r_2^2}$$

Thus the change in power on flexing the lens is given by:

$$\Delta F'_v = -300t\left[\frac{1}{(r_2')^2} - \frac{1}{r_2^2}\right]$$

where r_2' is the radius to which r_2 changes after flexure. Now the RI of different soft lenses in their hydrated state varies between 1.36 and 1.46, but even if this variation is allowed for, the values in Table 6.5 would be altered by an insignificant amount and can safely be applied to all materials. (The greatest error introduced would be of the order of 0.10 D for a lens of centre thickness 0.60 mm and a change in r_2 from 6.5 mm to r_2' of 6.0 mm, the value for the change in power for n = 1.36 being –0.59 D and that for n = 1.46 being –0.71 D.) It is interesting that Wichterle (1967), by a completely different method, arrived at a value for $\Delta F'_v$ only 10% different from Bennett's, namely:

$$\Delta F'_v = -270t\left[\frac{1}{(r_2')^2} - \frac{1}{r_2^2}\right]$$

Had Bennett assumed a RI of 1.37 for soft lens materials instead of 1.43, he and Wichterle would have arrived at exactly the same expression.

Although it could be argued that Bennett's assumptions – that the centre thickness and volume of the lens remain unchanged and the front surface remains spherical if the cornea is spherical – are not absolutely correct, mathematical considerations show that errors introduced by their acceptance are of an insignificant order (Wichterle 1967, Bennett 1970, 1976).

The following example shows the effects of such flexure, as described by Bennett (1976). Figures 6.20 and 6.21 illustrate this flexure on a positive and a negative lens, respectively.

Example

In order to assist calculation, a positive lens of knife-edge form is illustrated, but the same arguments can be applied to a lens of any specified edge thickness. A lens has BOZR 9.50 mm, TD 14.50 mm, BVP +6.00 D, n = 1.44. This lens must have t_c 0.616 mm and FOZR 8.599 mm to give a knife edge (Jalie 1988) (Fig. 6.20).

The volume of this lens can be calculated, as explained by Bennett (1976), by subtracting the volume of the spherical cap bounded by the back surface from the volume of the spherical cap bounded by the front surface. The volume of a spherical cap = $(\pi/3)(3r - s)s^2$ where r = radius and s = sag.

* This system of calculation was used before the symbols used in the current International Standard were adopted. Formerly the subscript $_1$ was used to denote front surface parameters, for example r_1 and r_2 were used for back surface parameters. Now with BS EN ISO 8320-1:2003, r_1 has become r_{a0} and r_2 has become r_0. However, for optical calculations, subscripts 1 and 2 are still valid and have been retained here.

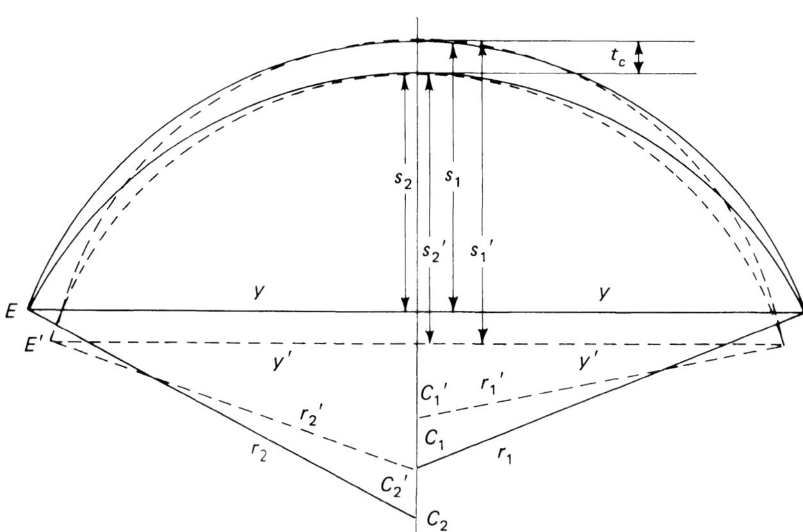

Figure 6.20 Steepening of a positive soft lens with knife edge: solid line before steepening and broken line after steepening. Before steepening: edge E, centres of curvature of front and back surfaces C_1 and C_2 with their radii of curvature r_1 and r_2 and sagitta s_1 and s_2 respectively, and semi-diameter y. After steepening these become: E', C_1', C_2', r_1', r_2', s_1', s_2' and y', respectively. Centre thickness t_c is the same before and after steepening

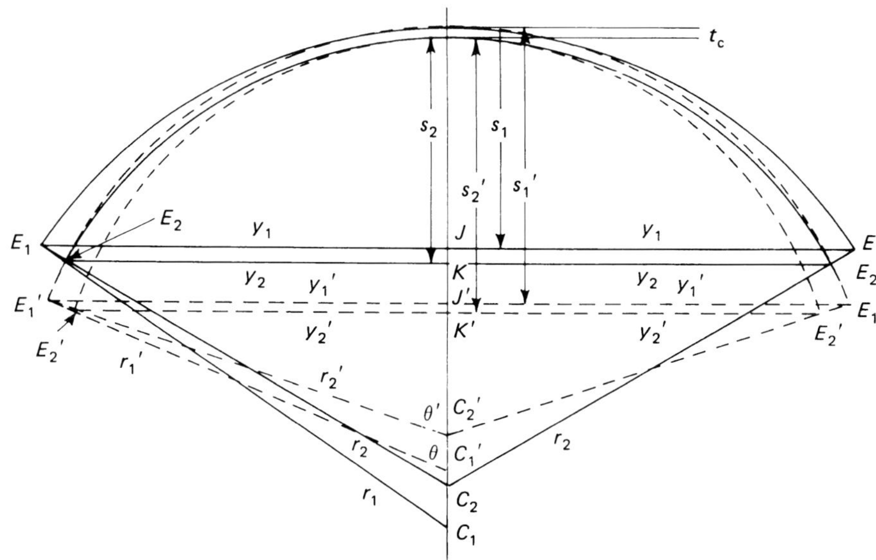

Figure 6.21 Steepening of a negative soft lens: solid line before steepening and broken line after steepening. Before steepening: front and back surface edges E_1 and E_2 with semi-diameters y_1 and y_2 intersecting the primary axis at J and K and subtending an angle θ at C_2. After steepening these become: E_1', E_2', y_1', y_2', J', K' and θ' at C_2', respectively. Other symbols are as in Figure 6.20

For the unstressed lens defined above, the volumes are thus:

Front spherical cap = 361.113 mm³
Back spherical cap = 297.379 mm³
Volume of lens, thus = 63.734 mm³

If this lens is applied to a spherical cornea of radius 8.00 mm, the semi-diameter y (7.25 mm) is reduced to some new value y', and since the BOZR is assumed to equal the corneal radius, the sag s_2' of the new back surface can be calculated, as therefore can the volume. Because (for a knife-edge lens), $s_1' = s_2' + t_c$ and the semi-diameter y' is common to both front and back surfaces (Fig. 6.20), the new front surface radius r_1' is obtainable from the expression relating radius to sag and semi-diameter, namely:

$$r = \frac{y^2 + s^2}{2s} \quad \text{(see **Formula XVII** on the CD-ROM)}$$

The volume of the new front surface spherical cap can also be calculated.

The value of y' must be found iteratively, the correct value being the one which gives the flexed lens the same volume as the unstressed lens. In this example:

$y' =$ 6.9 mm, $r_1' = 7.496$ mm, BVP = +5.21 D, showing a power change of –0.79 D.

After steepening, the volumes become:

Front spherical cap = 391.951 mm³
Back spherical cap = 328.217 mm³
Flexed lens (= that of unstressed lens) = 63.734 mm³

From the above it can be seen that whereas the BOZR has shortened by 1.5 mm (from 9.5 to 8.0 mm) the FOZR has shortened by only 1.103 mm. If both radii had shortened by 1.5 mm the volume of the lens would have increased to:

Front spherical cap = 460.939 mm³
Back spherical cap = 328.217 mm³
Volume of lens, thus = 132.722 mm³(!)

and the centre thickness would have increased to 1.479 mm!

If the front surface radius steepened more than the BOZR, both volume and centre thickness would increase to an even more ridiculous extent.

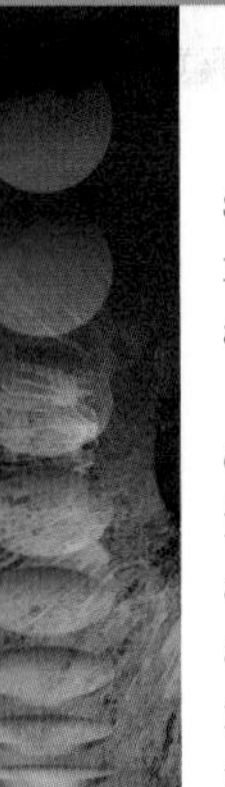

Because the front surface radius of a positive contact lens is shorter than that of the back surface, the front surface radius must alter by substantially less than the BOZR if the volume and thickness of the lens are to remain the same.

Negative lenses are treated in much the same way, except that edge thickness must be taken into account, and so it is necessary for the convenience of calculation to make one further assumption. It is assumed that the lens has a conical edge, with the apex of the cone at C_2 (see Fig. 6.21). The edge E_1E_2 is therefore normal to the back surface and it is assumed that E_1E_2 and its relationship to the back surface remain unchanged after flexure.

The volume of the lens is the volume of the front spherical cap plus the volume of the frustum of the cone bounded by E_1E_2, minus the volume of the back spherical cap. (Volume of frustum of cone = $(\pi/3)([y_1^2 \times JC_2] - [y_2^2 \times KC_2])$; Bennett 1976.)

Although highly unlikely to become flattened, hydrophilic lenses acquire additional positive power when in this state. The change of power due to flexure is given by:

$$\Delta F'_v = \frac{-(n-1)}{n} t \left[\frac{1}{(r_2')^2} - \frac{1}{r_2^2} \right]$$

(n = RI and other symbols are as in Fig. 6.20 and as given on p. 148).

It is evident from the above formula that the change of power due to flexure is dependent on RI, centre thickness and the amount of bending, and is independent of the original BVP (Bennett 1976), although the centre thickness of positive powered lenses is greater than that of negative powered lenses, and increases with increased power.

Plainis and Charman (1998) provided both a review paper of other formulae for predicting power changes when a soft lens is placed on an eye, and an experimental survey of various lenses fitted. Their results fitted both Bennett's analysis and an equation based on a constant sagittal change for the two surfaces. The effects for negative powered lenses of the thickness currently used are negligible.

Unfortunately, these theoretical power changes are not always those found in practice and some of the differences may be caused by temperature and evaporation changes (see below). It would appear from the work of Sarver et al. (1974, 1975) that aspherical back surface lenses may have a different power change from lathe-cut lenses, due to flexure. The change in power induced by the flexure of the lens and any liquid lens present was termed the 'supplemental power effect'. The BOZR of modern soft lenses is fitted considerably flatter than the central cornea (see Chapter 10) and so flexure induces an increase in negative power (see Table 6.5).

On toroidal corneas, the back surface of a flat spherical soft lens steepens differentially to conform to the eye in both meridians (Bennett 1976). This corrects the corneal astigmatism slightly, since there is a greater negative flexure effect along the steeper meridian. The amount of corneal astigmatism which can be corrected in this way is small – from 2 to 13% depending on centre thickness.

SECOND CHANGE – TEMPERATURE EFFECTS

As the temperature of the cornea is 37°C and room temperature is about 20°C, there is a change in temperature of the lens when it is put on the eye (Fatt & Chaston 1980a,b, 1981). This leads to steepening with an accompanying slight increase in the negative power of the lens (Table 6.6).

THIRD CHANGE – EVAPORATION EFFECTS

The increase in temperature and the exposure of the front surface of the soft lens to air leads to evaporation. This causes the water content of the lens to decrease slightly on the eye, which in turn leads to a small increase in RI and further steepening of the lens. The result is an increase of negative power (Table 6.7).

Ford (1976) termed this altered state of the lens on the eye as 'the equilibrated state', which takes into account changes due to:

- Flexure.
- Temperature.
- Evaporation.

Unfortunately, the amount of change in the lens due to evaporation depends on the tear output of the wearer (Ford 1974). Thus, greater changes occur in lenses worn in dry eyes than in those with normal or excessive tear output. According to Ford, variations in tear output alone can contribute to differences in power of over 1 D for high-powered lenses.

The determination of the required soft lens power for a given eye is imprecise, therefore. It depends on:

- The manufacturing process for the lens.
- Whether it has a spherical or aspheric back surface (although in general the effects of flexure are similar).
- The rate of peripheral corneal flattening.
- The tear output of the wearer.
- The temperature and evaporation from the lens. This is affected by:
  - external atmosphere
  - temperature
  - lens material
  - lens thickness.

It is important therefore to allow soft lenses adequate time to settle before over-refracting and to use diagnostic lenses of approximately the correct power, so that flexure on the eye will be similar. The discussion may explain why, however, the final power worn may not agree with the ocular refraction.

The effects on astigmatism of power changes due to soft lens flexure and equilibration

Spherical soft lenses flex to match the corneal contour (see pp. 147–150). They therefore replicate the front surface corneal toricity on their own front surface. The lens thickness may reduce the amount of toricity transferred, but as almost all soft lenses have a RI higher than that of the cornea, the amount of astigmatism transferred to the soft lens front surface is usually about the same as that of the corneal front surface.

Different soft materials have different RIs, most of which range from 1.36 to 1.46 when fully hydrated. RI also varies as the soft lens reaches equilibrium on the eye. Thus, the amount

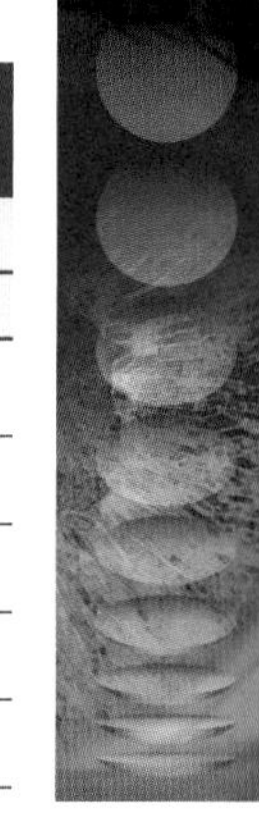

Table 6.6: Rate of change of surface power in air, in terms of D/0.10 mm change in radius *r*, for surfaces of various curvatures and various refractive indices

Refractive indices	d*F*/d*r* (D/0.10 mm change) at surface radius of curvature values (mm) of						
	6.50	7.00	7.50	8.00	8.50	9.00	9.50
1.33	0.781	0.673	0.587	0.516	0.457	0.407	0.366
1.34	0.805	0.694	0.604	0.531	0.471	0.420	0.377
1.35	0.828	0.714	0.622	0.547	0.484	0.432	0.388
1.36	0.852	0.735	0.640	0.562	0.498	0.444	0.399
1.37	0.876	0.755	0.658	0.578	0.512	0.457	0.410
1.38	0.899	0.776	0.676	0.594	0.526	0.469	0.421
1.39	0.923	0.796	0.693	0.609	0.540	0.481	0.432
1.40	0.947	0.816	0.711	0.625	0.554	0.494	0.443
1.41	0.970	0.837	0.729	0.641	0.567	0.506	0.454
1.42	0.994	0.857	0.747	0.656	0.581	0.519	0.465
1.43	1.018	0.878	0.764	0.672	0.595	0.531	0.476
1.44	1.041	0.898	0.782	0.688	0.609	0.543	0.488
1.45	1.065	0.918	0.800	0.703	0.623	0.556	0.499
1.46	1.089	0.939	0.818	0.719	0.637	0.568	0.510
1.47	1.112	0.959	0.836	0.734	0.651	0.580	0.521
1.48	1.136	0.980	0.853	0.750	0.664	0.593	0.532
1.49	1.160	1.000	0.871	0.766	0.678	0.605	0.543
1.50	1.185	1.022	0.890	0.782	0.693	0.618	0.554
1.51	1.209	1.042	0.908	0.798	0.706	0.630	0.565
1.52	1.233	1.063	0.925	0.813	0.720	0.642	0.577
1.53	1.256	1.083	0.943	0.829	0.734	0.655	0.588

of astigmatism transferred to the front surface of the soft lens depends on a number of factors:

- Type of material.
- Flexibility.
- Thickness.
- RI in the equilibrated state on the eye.

The astigmatism on the front surface of the soft lens is partly neutralized by:

- The back surface astigmatism of the cornea.
- The astigmatism at the cornea/soft lens interface.
- The crystalline lens astigmatism (possibly).

A soft lens fitted with its back surface flatter than the cornea corrects a small amount of corneal astigmatism (Bennett 1976) (see p. 150). As it flexes to match the steeper cornea, the power of the soft lens becomes more negative, more so along the steeper meridian, hence the slight correction of corneal astigmatism.

It may be helpful at times to be able to determine the astigmatism of the front surface of a soft lens and how it may alter while in situ on the eye. Table 6.6 shows the amount of astigmatism introduced by the toroidal surface of any lens (soft or hard), provided its radii of curvature and RI are known. It shows the change in surface power in air for a change of radius of 0.10 mm for refractive indices between 1.33 and 1.53 in steps of 0.01. (Interpolation permits power changes for even smaller gradations in RI than 0.01 to be obtained.)

As a change of radius of 0.10 mm induces different power changes, depending on whether the curvature of the surface is steep or flat, this is allowed for by taking surface radii in 0.50 mm steps between 6.50 and 9.50 mm.

Thus, for example, for a large change in radius, from 7.00 to 8.00 mm and RI 1.45, the figure in the intermediate (r = 7.50 mm) column should be used. So, for a lens of front surface radii 7.00 × 8.00 mm, the power difference (or astigmatism) is 10 × 0.800 = 8.00 D, which gives an error of only 0.036 D when compared with accurate calculations.

If there is only a moderate radius change, as for a surface of radii 7.00 × 7.50 mm, then (using the same RI of 1.45) it is best to average the figures in the two relevant columns to obtain the effect of a 0.10 mm change in radius, i.e. the average of 0.918 and 0.800 is 0.859 D, and for the 0.50 mm difference is 5 × 0.859 = 4.295 D of astigmatism. This gives an error of 0.009 D.

For small differences in radii, say 7.00 × 7.20 mm and RI 1.44, the value in the column applying to the nearest radius

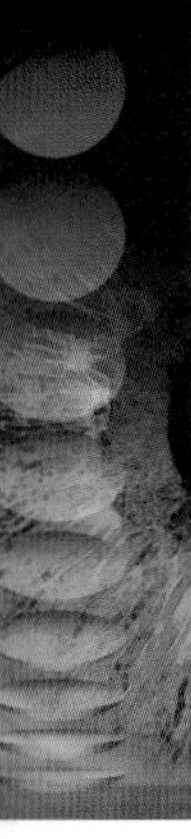

Table 6.7: Rate of change of surface power in air (*F*) for changes in refractive index (*n*) of 0.01 for various radii of curvature (*r*)

r (mm)	d*F*/d*n* (D)	*r* (mm)	d*F*/d*n* (D)
6.40	1.5625	8.00	1.2500
6.50	1.5385	8.10	1.2346
6.60	1.5152	8.20	1.2195
6.70	1.4925	8.30	1.2048
6.80	1.4706	8.40	1.1905
6.90	1.4493	8.50	1.1765
7.00	1.4286	8.60	1.1628
7.10	1.4084	8.70	1.1494
7.20	1.3699	8.80	1.1236
7.30	1.3889	8.90	1.1369
7.40	1.3514	9.00	1.1111
7.50	1.3333	9.10	1.0989
7.60	1.3158	9.20	1.0870
7.70	1.2987	9.30	1.0753
7.80	1.2821	9.40	1.0638
7.90	1.2658	9.50	1.0526

should be used – in this case 7.00 mm. Thus 0.898 D is found for a 0.10 mm radius change. So 0.20 mm difference in surface radii would give 2 × 0.898 = 1.796 D of astigmatism, an error of only 0.05 D.

If the front surface of a soft lens alters curvature while it is on the eye, as for example due to temperature changes or evaporation, then there is a surface power change which may also be obtained from Table 6.6. Suppose the front surface of a lens of RI 1.43 steepens from 9.50 to 9.40 mm, its power will change by 0.476 D. As this is a steepening of a convex surface, the power will become more positive. Changes in toricity of a surface lead to changes in astigmatism, which can be determined from Table 6.6 in the same way.

Such changes in radius of a soft lens occurring while it is on the eye are often accompanied by changes in RI. Table 6.7 shows how the surface power may alter if this occurs. For example, evaporation might lead to a rise in RI from 1.39 to 1.40 for a surface of radius 8.50 mm. There is then a resultant power change of 1.1765 D, while a change from 1.39 to 1.41 would lead to twice this amount, i.e. 2.353 D.

- A rise in RI leads to an increase in power of the surface.
- A drop in RI leads to a decrease in surface power.

Note that, in Table 6.7 as indicated in the above paragraph, the changes in power are linear at any one radius; thus for a radius of 7.50 mm, a change of RI of 0.06 would give a surface power change of 6 × 1.3333 = 7.9998 D, and a change of RI of 0.006 would give a power change of 0.79998 D.

The effects of flexure on rigid corneal lenses

In the same way that a soft lens flexes to conform to the corneal contour, there is a tendency for rigid lenses to flex on toroidal corneas, partially replicating the corneal astigmatism. Harris and Chu (1972) found that with PMMA lenses with centre thicknesses of less than 0.13 mm:

- The thinner the lens, the more it flexes.
- The more corneal astigmatism present, the greater is the lens flexure.

They found that thin lenses flexed in a predictable manner and induced astigmatism which affected the amount of residual astigmatism. Their results are summarized in Figure 6.22. As can be seen, this flexure-induced astigmatism can be used to benefit the patient.

As explained on page 144, if the lens does not flex, all corneal astigmatism is corrected by the liquid lens and any residual astigmatism is due to the crystalline lens. The latter is normally a small to moderate amount of against-the-rule astigmatism. If such is found on a with-the-rule cornea, then by fitting a thin lens, the induced with-the-rule astigmatism caused by lens flexure can be used to partially or completely neutralize the against-the-rule residual astigmatism. The standard of visual acuity and quality may thus be improved (see also Chapter 12).

Lens flexure can be minimized by fitting the BOZR as flat as possible (Pole 1983, Stone & Collins 1984) and by keeping the BOZD as small as possible (Brown et al. 1984) (see Chapter 9). Such flexure is rarely beneficial optically, and more often prevents the lens from adequately correcting the corneal astigmatism. Although the flexure is not as great with an RGP lens as with a soft lens, it may necessitate fitting a compensated bitoric lens (Douthwaite 1988).

As flexure affects both front and back surfaces of the contact lens, thereby altering the front surface of the liquid lens, the cumulative effect on astigmatism is complex. Provided the changes in radius are known, and the front surface of a lens can be measured on the eye by keratometry, the power effects can be obtained from Table 6.6 or from **Formulae *III–V*** on the CD-ROM.

Measurement of the BOZR with a radiuscope may also give a toric reading, since although initially the lens may recover its spherical form on removal from the eye, it may warp permanently with time. Since both front and back surfaces will have changed by similar amounts, there will be no significant astigmatic effect visible on the focimeter in air. Unfortunately, flexure may vary as the lens moves on the eye and is best assessed by refractive techniques (both objective and subjective) with the lens in situ.

Aberrations of contact lenses

Spherical aberration is an important consideration when dealing with steeply curved surfaces of contact lenses. The cornea's potential contribution to the overall spherical aberration of the eye is reduced by its peripheral flattening. When a rigid lens is placed on the eye, the overall aberration is likely to increase, particularly for positive powered lenses with their steeper

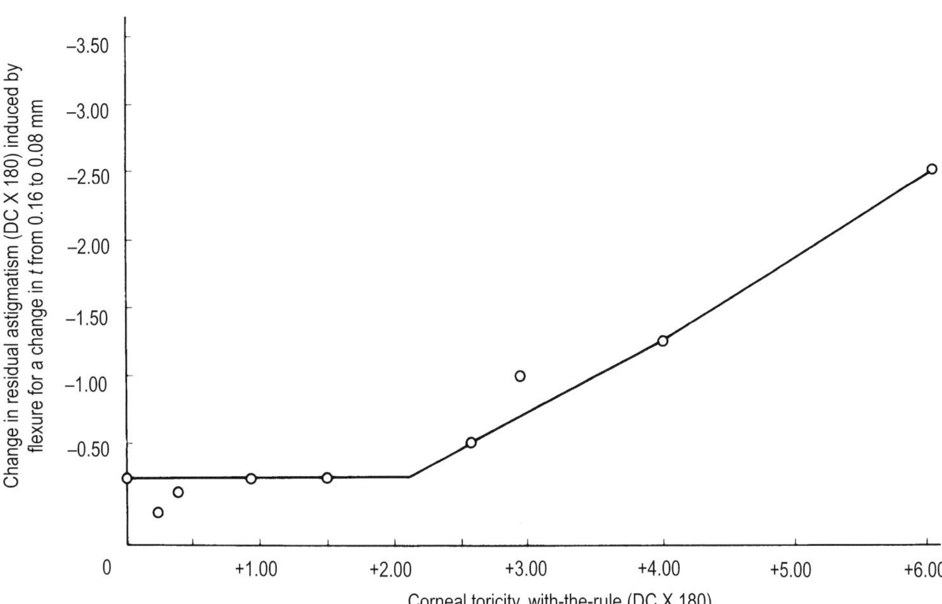

Figure 6.22 The difference in residual astigmatism between that induced by a thick PMMA lens (0.16 mm) and that induced by a thin lens (0.08 mm) for corneas of various toricities. For example, if a patient had −1.25 DC × 90 residual astigmatism with a 0.16 mm thick lens, on a 4.00 D with-the-rule toroidal cornea, then changing the lens to one of 0.08 mm thickness would induce −1.25 DC × 180 of astigmatism due to flexure, thereby eliminating the residual astigmatism. (Reproduced by kind permission of M. G. Harris and C. S. Chu)

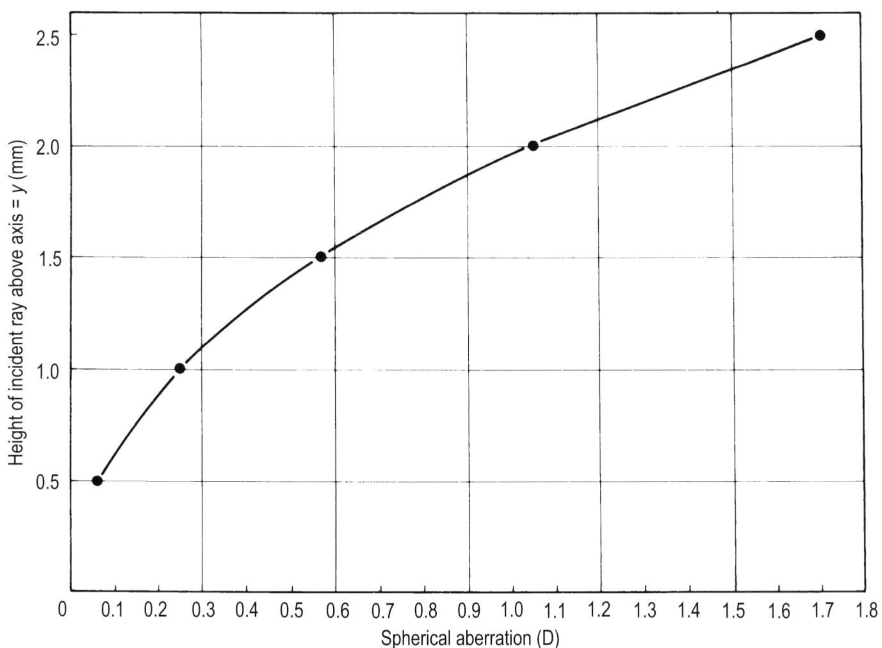

Figure 6.23 Variation of spherical aberration with aperture for a contact lens (n = 1.490) of +12.00 D BVP, BOZR of 7.80 mm and t_c of 0.35 mm. Parallel incident light is assumed

curves. Cox (1990) suggested that this was true for lenses of power more positive than −3.00 D.

The effects on vision may be greater when the lens moves on the eye. For example, an aphake fitted with a single vision distance lens may be able to do some close work. As the wearer looks down, the lens becomes displaced off-centre (usually upwards) relative to the pupil. Due to spherical aberration, the effective power of the lens is increased. Unfortunately, not all spherical aberration effects are so beneficial, and a high positive lens which does not centre well on the cornea may give poorer distance acuity than expected, as positive spherical aberration is introduced.

Figure 6.23 shows that a decentration of 2.5 mm on the eye leads to an addition of +1.7 D for a lens of BVP +12.00 D, centre thickness of 0.35 mm and BOZR of 7.80 mm.

With soft lenses, it is uncertain how much corneal asphericity is transferred to the front surface of the lens during flexing, and what effect the different anterior radius of curvature has on the p-value. Cox's (1990) calculations suggest that soft lenses would increase ocular aberrations for powers outside the range −6.00 to +3.00 D.

In an experimental study, Cox and Holden (1990) fitted subjects with both normal contact lenses and with trial lenses designed to provide known positive or negative spherical aberration. They found significant losses of contrast sensitivity with 6 mm pupils with the aberrated lenses, but these had little effect on high contrast acuity. There were no deleterious effects when the pupil diameter was 3 mm. de Brabander et al. (1998) tried experimental contact lenses which had been designed to

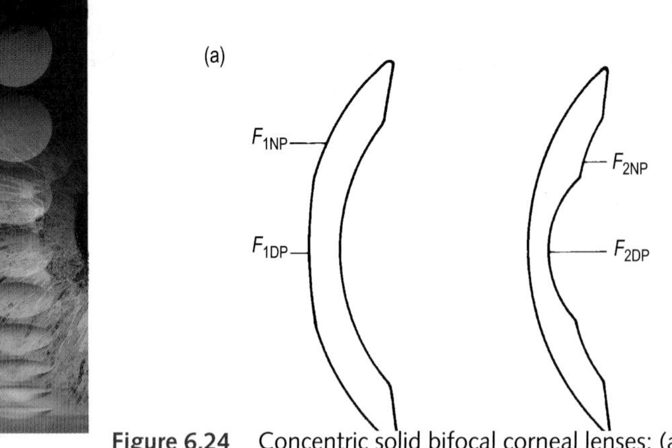

Figure 6.24 Concentric solid bifocal corneal lenses: (a) front surface addition; (b) back surface addition

correct their in-air rather than on-eye spherical aberration, only to find that standard lenses gave better contrast sensitivity.

Kerns (1974) showed that aspherical lenses improve acuity in patients with residual astigmatism. He suggested that both the astigmatism and spherical aberration result in a blurred image on the retina and removing either the astigmatic or the aberration element should improve acuity.

Aberrations are more complicated in rigid lenses with aspheric back surfaces, particularly as these move on the eye. The extra aberrations and astigmatism induced by this surface may require the front surface to be also aspheric in order to cancel them out (Hammer & Holden 1994, El-Nashar 1999, Hong et al. 2001). Aspheric front surfaces are also used to create an 'extended' focus or progressive power (see 'Progressive power contact lenses', below and Chapter 14).

BIFOCAL CONTACT LENSES

Chapter 14 deals with the various designs and methods of fitting of all types of bifocal contact lens. An appreciation of the optical principles of concentric solid bifocals with the distance portion in the centre and the fused bifocal with the near segment on the back surface permits a general understanding of all other designs of bifocal contact lens.

Concentric and flat-top solid bifocals

These are available with the addition worked on either the front or back optic surface (Fig. 6.24) (and, of course, a combination of back and front surface additions can be used). When the addition is on the front surface (a plastic/air interface), the front optic zone has two radii worked on it, the steeper corresponding to the near portion of the lens. Then, provided that the lens is assumed to be infinitely thin, the near addition is equal to the difference between the two front surface powers.

For example, if the near addition to be incorporated in an RGP lens is +3.00 D and where F_{1DP} and F_{1NP} are the front surface powers of the distance and near portions, respectively (see footnote, p. 148), then $F_{1NP} = F_{1DP} + 3.00$. Since this is a plastic/air interface, the appropriate front optic zone radii may be obtained from **Formulae *III–V*** on the CD-ROM using $n_2 = 1.47$ and $n_1 = 1.00$. If, in a particular case, F_{1DP} is calculated to be +58.00 D, this gives a radius, r_{1DP}, of

$$\frac{(1.470 - 1)1000}{58.00} = 8.10 \text{ mm}$$

For an addition of +3.00 D, F_{1NP} must therefore be +61.00 D, giving a radius of 7.70 mm.

If thickness is to be taken into account, reference to **Formula *VI*** on the CD-ROM should be made. In the example just given, if the centre thickness of the distance portion were 0.20 mm and that of the near portion 0.22 mm,

since L_1 = 0.00 D
and F_{1DP} = +58.00 D
L'_1 = +58.00 D for the distance portion.

It can be seen that 0.20 mm thickness adds 0.46 D to this power. The reduced vergence reaching the back surface is thus +58.46 D.

Similarly, for the near portion

since L_1 = 0.00 D
and F_{1NP} = +61.00 D
L'_1 = +61.00 D.

0.22 mm thickness adds 0.56 D to the reduced vergence reaching the back surface.

The difference between 0.46 D and 0.56 D is 0.10 D and is small enough to be ignored, but it indicates that F_{1NP} should be reduced by this amount, from +61.00 D to 60.90 D, giving r_{1NP} as 7.72 mm instead of 7.70 mm. In practice this small radius change is not worth making.

There is a tendency for a small negative-powered liquid lens to collect in front of the upper and lower portions of any corneal lens due to the tears prism along the eyelid margins. The configuration of the front surface of a solid bifocal with front surface addition (Fig. 6.24a) is such that this tear lens may slightly reduce the front surface positive power at the periphery. It is wise, therefore, to err on the positive side (by as much as +1.00 D) to allow for this negative tear lens although it varies depending on tear output and evaporation.

Executive-style segments are also available as solid front surface bifocals, with a junction ridge (see Chapter 14). The optical theory is the same as for concentric bifocals.

When the addition is on the back surface (Fig. 6.24b), no allowance for the effect of thickness need be considered; however, the major consideration here is that it is a plastic/tears interface, rather than a plastic/air interface.

In air the power of the RGP surface depends on

$$\frac{1.470 - 1}{r}$$

whereas in tears it depends on

$$\frac{1.470 - 1.336}{r}$$

This is a factor of 0.470/0.134 or approximately 3.51 for RGP lenses of this index. (For a RI of 1.45, this factor becomes 3.95,

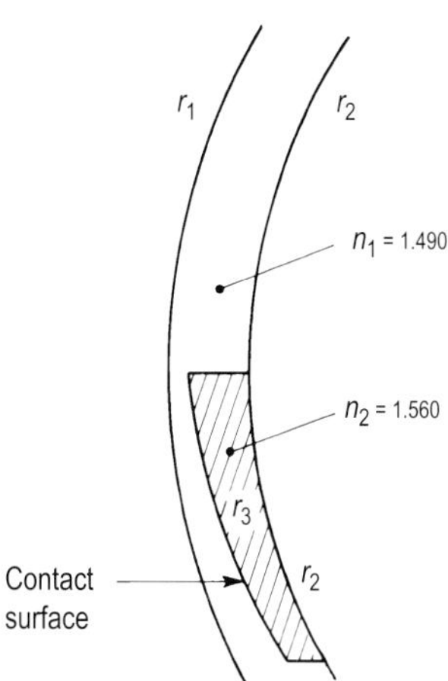

Figure 6.25 Fused bifocal corneal lens: r_1, r_2 and r_3 are the radii of the front, back and contact surfaces, respectively; n_1 and n_2 are the refractive indices of the main lens and the near segment

and for soft lenses of RI of 1.43 the factor becomes 4.57.) The back surface radii must therefore provide approximately three to four times the addition on the back surface (when measured in air) than is really required, due to the neutralizing effect of the tears (see Chapter 14).

Usually this type of bifocal is fitted with a steep BOZR (r_{2DP}) (see footnote, p. 148) and a small back optic zone diameter (BOZD), with the back peripheral optic zone radius (r_{2NP}) providing the near addition and fitted so as to align or be just flatter than the cornea. For example:

- If the BPOZR (r_{2NP}) is 8.50 mm, reference to **Formula *III*** on the CD-ROM for 1.336–1.470 shows F_{2NP} to be –15.764 D. (It is negative in power because the medium of higher RI has a concave surface.)
- To give a +3.00 D addition requires that F_{2DP} be –18.764 D; thus r_{2DP} (the BOZR) is 7.14 mm (from **Formula *IV*** on the CD-ROM).

If this lens is measured in air on a focimeter, the radii of 8.50 mm and 7.14 mm would have surface powers, for 1–1.470, of –55.2 9 D and –65.82 D, respectively (see **Formula *III*** on the CD-ROM).

Thus the near addition measured in air is +10.52 D, i.e. the near addition in tears × 3.51 (approximately) as stated above, depending on the RI of the material used.

Fused bifocals

These are very similar to fused bifocal spectacle lenses except that most corneal lenses have the segment on the back surface, and the RI of the fused segment is usually 1.56. The optical theory is easily understood if reference is made to Figure 6.25. **Formulae *VII–X*** on the CD-ROM should be consulted in connection with this section. In the formulae $r_{CS} \equiv r_{BCS}$ or r_{FCS} (depending on whether the fused segment is a back surface or front surface segment) while the alternative symbols, based on BS EN ISO 8320-1:2003, are used. Thus $r_1 \equiv r_{a0}$, $r_2 \equiv r_0$ and subscripts for powers F are similarly denoted. The contact surface F_{CS} must have a positive power (F_{BCS}) with a back surface fused segment (Fig. 6.25) and a negative power (F_{FCS}) when the segment is on the front surface.

Since the back surface is a negative surface and the segment has the higher RI, there is actually a gain in negative power at the back surface of

$$\frac{1.560 - 1.490}{r_2}$$

and where r_2 is in millimetres this expression becomes

$$\frac{-70}{r_2}\text{D}$$

For example, if the BOZR (r_2) is 8.00 mm, this gives a power of –70/8 = –8.75 D.

Alternatively, the back surface powers in tears are:

$$F_{2DP} = \frac{(1.336 - 1.490)1000}{8.00}\text{D} = -19.25\text{ D}$$

(see **Formula *III*** on the CD-ROM)

$$F_{2NP} = \frac{(1.336 - 1.560)1000}{8.00}\text{D} = -28.00\text{ D}$$

The difference is $F_{2NP} - F_{2DP} = -8.75$ D as before.

The power difference due to the segment is the same whether the power is determined in air or in tears, because the BOZR, (r_2), is the same throughout (as distinct from the back surface solid bifocal where $r_{2DP} < r_{2NP}$). This is easily shown using the same value for r_2 as above. The back surface powers in air are

$$F_{2DP} = \frac{(1 - 1.490)1000}{8.00}\text{ D} = -61.25\text{ D}$$

$$F_{2NP} = \frac{(1 - 1.560)1000}{8.00}\text{ D} = -70.00\text{ D}$$

The difference, $F_{2NP} - F_{2DP} = -8.75$ D.

This is exactly the same as when the back surface powers were determined in tears (see above). Because the back surface addition is the same measured in air as in tears, the addition read on a focimeter is the same as that on the eye.

Since the fused segment gives rise to a gain in negative power on the back surface, it must give rise to a gain in positive power at the contact surface, sufficient to overcome the negative gain as well as to provide the near addition, i.e. if the power of the contact surface is F_{CS} then for the refractive indices already given

$$F_{CS} = \text{Addition} - \left(-\frac{70}{r_2}\right) = \text{Addition} + \frac{70}{r_2}$$

Now F_{CS} (which is convex for the medium of higher RI)

$$= \frac{1.560 - 1.490}{r_{CS}}\text{D} = \frac{70}{r_{CS}}\text{D (where } r_{CS} \text{ is in mm)}$$

And since $F_{CS} = \text{Addition} + \dfrac{70}{r_2}$

(see **Formula *IX***)

$$r_{CS} = \frac{70}{\text{Add} + \dfrac{70}{r_2}}$$

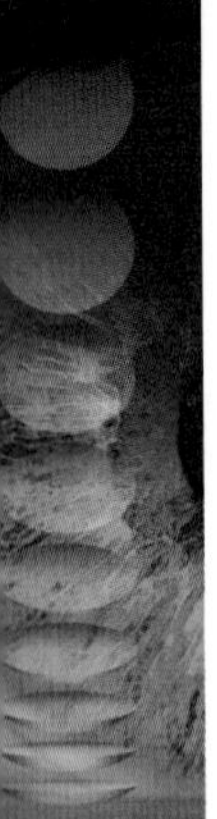

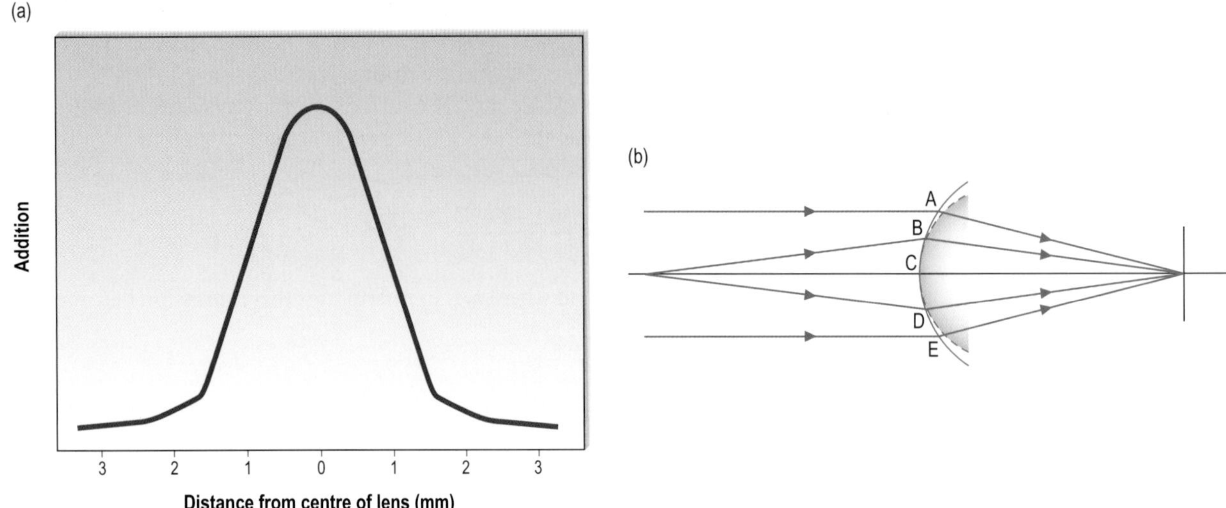

Figure 6.26 (a) Power profile of a centre-near, front surface, progressive power lens. (b) Schematic view (grossly out of scale) of the image formation by the front surface. The dotted line indicates a spherical surface having the same radius of curvature as the apical radius of the lens

(where the addition is in dioptres, and r_2 and r_{CS} are in millimetres).

Where the segment is fused on the front surface, **Formulae *VIII*** and ***X*** apply (see Example 13 on the CD-ROM).

The above example illustrates a PMMA fused bifocal but RGP bifocal lenses are available with similar straight-top segments (see Chapter 14).

Progressive power contact lenses

Rather like progressive power spectacle lenses, contact lenses may be made with a steadily flattening or steepening surface in order to give a continuous variation of power to provide a longer range of focus. In contact lens form, these lenses are made with radial symmetry. Soft lenses of this type will, like soft bifocal lenses, be of simultaneous vision design. A possible power profile for a centre near design is shown in Figure 6.26a, while a ray trace, grossly out of scale, is shown in Figure 6.26b. Provided the lens is reasonably well centred on the eye, rays from a distant object passing through A and E will be brought to a focus on the retina, while those from a nearer object passing through the more steeply curved central part at B and D will similarly be in focus. If the lens decentres, however, the behaviour will be more like that of the rigid lens described below.

Aspheric curves can also be used in rigid lenses. A centre distance design is used so that as the lens moves up on the cornea in down-gaze for near vision, the peripheral zone slides in front of the pupil, thus giving a partly alternating design. Simplistically, a single aspheric curve could be used, as with a soft lens. Figure 6.27 shows, again grossly exaggerated, the front surface of a steepening ellipse ($p > 1$), having decentred on the eye. In order to provide the near addition, the radius of curvature of the element TT of the lens surface in the plane of the diagram at point P, given by PC_T, has to be shorter than the apical radius of curvature AC_0. The sagittal radius of curvature, PC_S, corresponding to an element of the surface SS at right angles to the plane of the diagram, will differ again. If the wearer has a small pupil, the bundle of light forming the image is that from a small zone surrounding P. Light passing through this single peripheral zone may be significantly astigmatic, whereas, with the soft lens, the useful image is that provided by rays passing symmetrically either side of the apex of the lens. Just as in video-keratoscopy or keratometry, it is the sagittal or axial radius of curvature that is important with the soft lens.

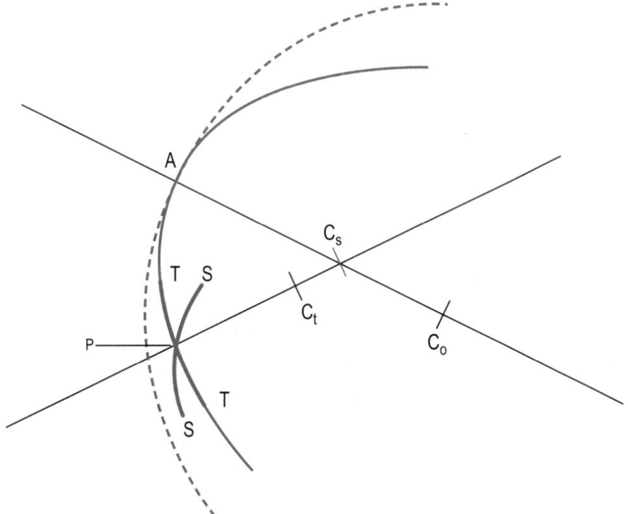

Figure 6.27 The astigmatic effect when viewing through a peripheral zone of an aspheric surface. The lens is assumed to have moved up on the wearer's cornea, while the visual axis of the wearer lies along the line PC_S. The dotted line indicates a spherical surface having the same radius of curvature as the apical radius of the lens

It is instructive to consider the astigmatism for a rigid lens. For example, a front surface progressive lens with an addition of +2.00 D at 3 mm from the apex in a material of RI 1.45 would have a p-value of 1.164 giving:

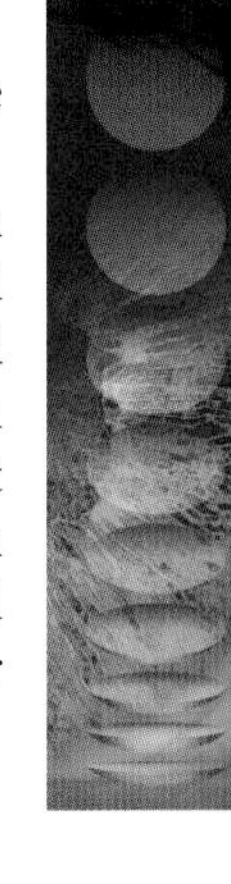

Height from apex (mm)	Addition (D)	Surface astigmatism (D)
1	0.22	0.14
2	0.87	0.58
3	2.00	1.34
4	3.64	2.45

where the astigmatism is calculated from the difference between the sagittal and tangential powers. However, in practice, oblique refraction at the surfaces will slightly alter the value entering the eye.

Not only is the induced astigmatism clinically significant, but the variation in power in the tangential plane across the pupil is large. The resulting beam pattern reaching the retina will be very irregular.

Charman and Saunders (1990) investigated the modulation transfer function for several types of multifocal and progressive power lens. They concluded that the reduced contrast in the image would make little difference to high contrast acuity. Woods et al. (1993) investigated, amongst other factors, the performance of bifocal lenses as a function of the relative sizes of central and peripheral optic zones, and decentration, but found their results too complicated for simple summary.

References

Baron, H. (1975) Some remarks on the correction of astigmatic eyes by means of soft contact lenses. Contacto, 19(6), 4–8

Bennett, A. G. (1970) Variable and progressive power lenses: 1. Optician, 160, 421–427

Bennett, A. G. (1976) Power changes in soft contact lenses due to bending. Ophthalmol. Opti., 16, 939–945

Bennett, A. G. (1984) A new approach to the statistical analysis of ocular astigmatism and astigmatic prescriptions. In Transactions of the First International Congress: The Frontiers of Optometry, Vol. 2, pp. 35–42, ed. W. N. Charman. London: British College of Ophthalmic Opticians (Optometrists)

Bennett, A. G. (1985) Optics of Contact Lenses, 5th edn. London: Association of Dispensing Opticians

Bennett, A. G. and Rabbetts, R. B. (1988) Schematic eyes – time for a change? Optician, 196(5169), 14–15

BS EN ISO 8320–1:2003 Contact lenses and contact lens care products – Vocabulary – Part 1: Contact lenses. London: British Standards Institution

Brown, S., Baldwin, M. and Pole, J. (1984) Effect of the optic zone diameter on lens flexure and residual astigmatism. Int. Contact Lens Clin., 11, 759–766

Capelli, Q. A. (1964) Determining final power of bitoric lenses. Br. J. Physiol. Opt., 21, 256–263

Charman, W.N. and Saunders, B. (1990) Theoretical and practical factors influencing the optical performance of contact lenses for the presbyopes. J. Br. Contact Lens Assoc., 13, 67–75

Cox, I. (1990) Theoretical calculations of the longitudinal spherical aberration of rigid and soft contact lenses. Optom. Vis. Sci., 67, 277–282

Cox, I. and Holden, B. A. (1990) Soft contact lens-induced longitudinal spherical aberration and its effect on contrast sensitivity. Optom. Vis. Sci., 67, 679–683

de Brabander, J., Chateau, N., Bouchard, F. and Guidollet, S. (1998) Contrast sensitivity with soft contact lenses compensated for spherical aberration in high ametropia. Optom. Vis. Sci., 75, 37–43

Douthwaite, W. A. (1988) Technical note: compensated toric rigid contact lenses. J. Br. Contact Lens Assoc., 11(2), 35–38

Douthwaite, W. A. (2006) Contact Lens Optics and Lens Design, 3rd edn. Oxford: Butterworth-Heinemann

El-Nashar, N. F. (1999) Spherical aberration and contact lenses. Ophthalmic Physiol. Opt., 19, 441–445

Fatt, I. and Chaston, J. (1980a) Temperature of contact lens on the eye. Int. Contact Lens Clin., 7, 195–198

Fatt, I. and Chaston, J. (1980b) The effect of temperature on refractive index, water content and central thickness of hydrogel lenses. Int. Contact Lens Clin., 7, 250–255

Fatt, I. and Chaston, J. (1981) The response of vertex power to changes in dimensions of hydrogel contact lenses. Int. Contact Lens Clin., 8(1), 22–28

Ford, M. W. (1974) Changes in hydrophilic lenses when placed on an eye. Paper read at the joint International Congress of The Contact Lens Society and The National Eye Research Foundation, Montreux, Switzerland

Ford, M. W. (1976) Computation of the back vertex powers of hydrophilic lenses. Paper read at the Interdisciplinary Conference on Contact Lenses, Department of Ophthalmic Optics and Visual Science, The City University, London

Ford, M. W. and Stone, J. (1997) Practical optics and computer design of contact lenses. In Contact Lenses, 4th edn, pp. 154–231, eds. A. J. Phillips and L. Speedwell. Oxford: Butterworth-Heinemann

Freeman M. H. and Hull, C. G. (2003) Optics, 11th edn. Oxford: Butterworth-Heinemann

Hammer, R. M. and Holden, B. A. (1994) Spherical aberration of aspheric contact lenses on eye. Optom. Vis. Sci., 71, 522–528

Harris, M. G. and Chu, C. S. (1972) The effect of contact lens thickness and corneal toricity on flexure and residual astigmatism. Am. J. Optom., 49, 304–307

Hong, X., Himebaugh, N. and Thibos, L. N. (2001) On-eye evaluation of optical performance of rigid and soft contact lenses. Optom. Vis. Sci., 78, 872–880

Jalie, M. (1988) The Principles of Ophthalmic Lenses, 4th edn, pp. 324–326. London: Association of British Dispensing Opticians

Kerns, R. L. (1974) Clinical evaluation of the merits of an aspheric front surface contact lens for patients manifesting residual astigmatism. Am. J. Optom., 51, 750–757

Obstfeld, H. (1982) Optics in Vision, 2nd edn. London: Butterworths

Plainis, S. and Charman, W. N. (1998) On-eye power characteristics of soft contact lenses. Optom. Vis. Sci., 75, 44–54

Pole, J. J. (1983) The effect of the base curve on the flexure of Polycon lenses. Int. Contact Lens Clin., 10(1), 49–52

Rabbetts, R. B. (1992) Spreadsheet power calculation for toric lenses. J. Brit. Contact Lens Assoc., 15, 75–76; (1993), 16, 41

Rabbetts, R. B. (1998) Bennett and Rabbetts' Clinical Visual Optics, 3rd edn. Oxford: Butterworths

Rabbetts, R. B. (2007) Bennett and Rabbetts' Clinical Visual Optics, 4th edn. Oxford: Elsevier

Sarver, M. D. (1963) The effect of contact lens tilt upon residual astigmatism. Am. J. Optom., 40, 730–744

Sarver, M. D., Ashley, D. and Van Every, J. (1974) Supplemental power effect of Bausch & Lomb Soflens contact lenses. Int. Contact Lens Clin., 1(1), 100–109

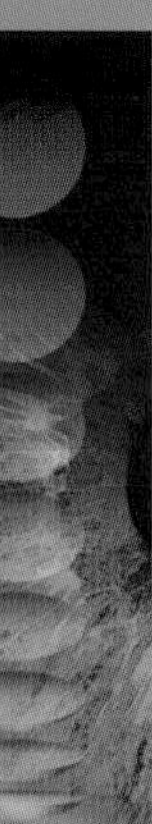

Sarver, M. D., Harris, M. G. and Polse, K. A. (1975) Corneal curvature and supplemental power effect of the Bausch & Lomb Soflens contact lenses. Am. J. Optom., 52, 470–473

Sorsby, A., Leary, G. A. and Richards, M. J. (1962) The optical components in anisometropia. Vision Res., 3, 43–51

Stone, J. (1966) The use of contact lenses in the correction of astigmatism. Optica Int., 3, 6–23

Stone, J. (1967) Near vision difficulties in non-presbyopic corneal lens wearers. Contact Lens 1(2), 14–25

Stone, J. and Collins, C. (1984) Flexure of gas permeable lenses on toroidal corneas. Optician, 188(4951), 8–10

Strachan, J. P. F. (1973) Some principles of the optics of hydrophilic lenses and geometrical optics applied to flexible lenses. Aust. J. Optom., 56, 25–33

Thibos, L. N., Wheeler, W. and Horner, D. (1997) Power vectors: an application of Fourier analysis to the description and statistical analysis of refractive error. Optom. Vis. Sci., 74, 367–375

Tunnacliffe, A. (1993) Introduction to Visual Optics, 4th edn. London: Association of British Dispensing Opticians

Westerhout, D. (1969) Clinical observations in fitting bitoric and toric forms of corneal lenses. Contact Lens, 2(3), 5–21, 36

Westheimer, G. (1962) The visual world of the new contact lens wearer. J. Am. Optom. Assoc., 34, 135–140

Wichterle, O. (1967) Changes of refracting power of a soft lens caused by its flattening. In Corneal and Scleral Contact Lenses, Proceedings of the International Congress, March 1966, Paper 29, pp. 247–256, ed. L. J. Girard. St Louis, MO: Mosby

Winn, B., Ackerley, R. G., Brown, C. A., Murray, F. K., Prais, J. and St John, M. F. (1986) The superiority of contact lenses in the correction of all anisometropia. Trans. BCLA Conference, 95–100

Woods, R. L., Saunders, J. E. and Port, M. J. A. (1993) Concentric-design rigid bifocal contact lenses, Part 1: Optical performance. J. Br. Contact Lens Assoc., 16, 25–36

Chapter 7

Clinical instrumentation in contact lens practice

Frank Eperjesi and James S. Wolffsohn

CHAPTER CONTENTS

The contact lens practitioner has a range of instrumentation available with which to assess the anterior eye for its suitability to wear or continue to wear lenses, and to determine the most appropriate lenses to be fitted. The most useful of these are the corneal topographer and the slit-lamp biomicroscope, although there are many others such as the Tearscope (see Chapter 5), which can further aid contact lens fitting and after-care.

CORNEAL TOPOGRAPHY

Keratometry

The determination of the corneal curvature is of prime importance with rigid contact lens fitting. Virtually all attempts to quantify corneal curvature have used the reflection of light off the convex cornea, which alters depending on the topography of the surface. Early methods were purely observational, with the first clinically applicable technique being the keratometer.

The keratometer provides a measurement of the radius of curvature of the 'corneal cap'. At a fixed viewing distance, an object of known size will be imaged so that the image size is a function of the radius of curvature of the reflecting surface (Fig. 7.1). The working distance of the keratometer is usually monitored through a Scheiner disc or similar system. This produces a doubled image of the object in the eyepiece unless the instrument is used at the exact working distance required by the instrument design (Fig. 7.2).

The eye is constantly moving, even during apparently steady fixation. It is therefore difficult to measure directly the size of an image reflected by the cornea. However, if the image is doubled by passing it through a prism or a doubly refractive crystal, when the base of one resultant image is aligned with the top of the other, the displacement will equal the exact height of the object (Fig. 7.3). This principle can be either:

- Fixed doubling where a predetermined amount of doubling is incorporated and the mire moved until the image produced is of the predetermined height (e.g. Javal–Schiötz mires – see Fig. 7.5).
- Variable doubling where the object is set to a predetermined size while the doubling system is varied until the image is displaced through its exact height (e.g. Bausch & Lomb mires; see Fig. 7.2).

The mires reflected from the corneal surface vary in appearance between manufacturers (Figs 7.2, 7.4, 7.5).

As the distance of the eye and change in image size resulting from its reflection from the cornea are now known, the radius of curvature can be calculated. It is read off an internal or external scale, in millimetres or in dioptres (the latter making the assumption that the refractive index of the cornea is on average 1.3375, including a compensation for the back surface of the cornea having a power of –10% of the power of the front surface).

As the cornea usually has two principal meridians at 90° to each other, the instrument is rotated until the horizontal limbs

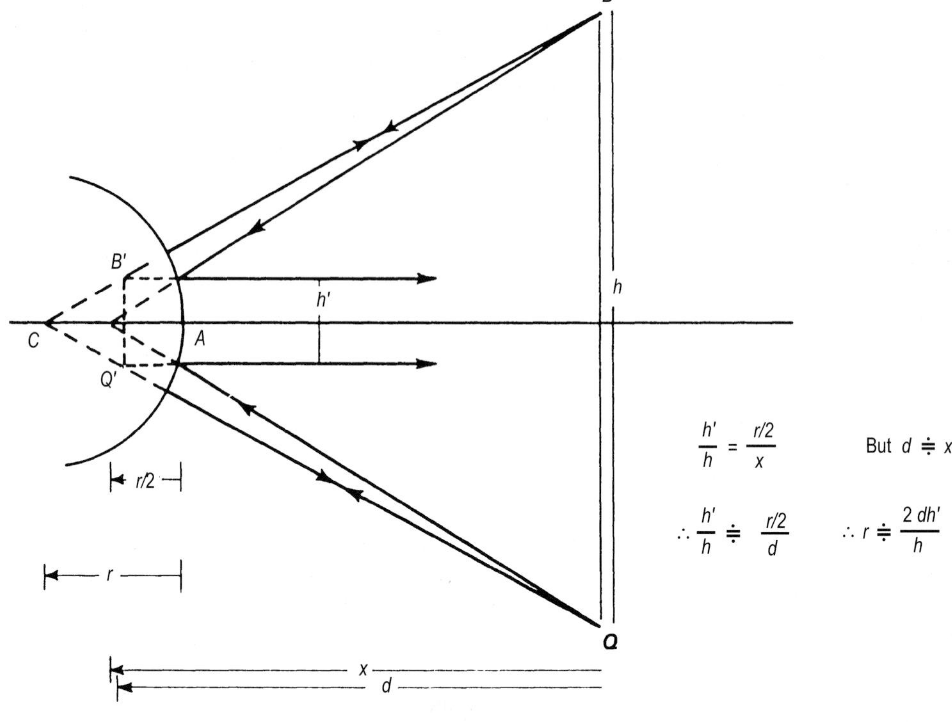

Figure 7.1 Optical principle of keratometry

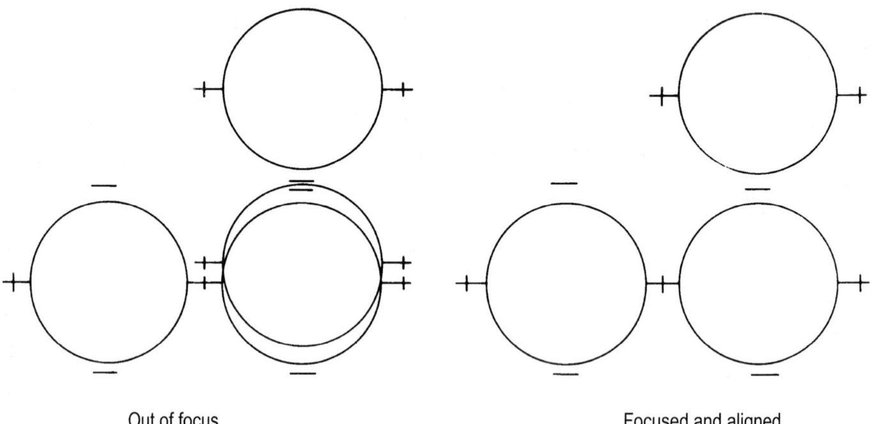

Figure 7.2 The Bausch & Lomb keratometer mires. When not set at the correct working distance a Scheiner disc creates a doubled image of the mires in the eyepiece

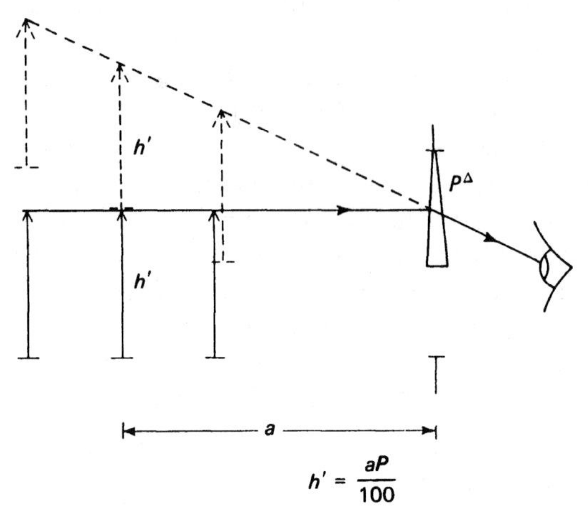

Figure 7.3 The principle of doubling used to measure image height

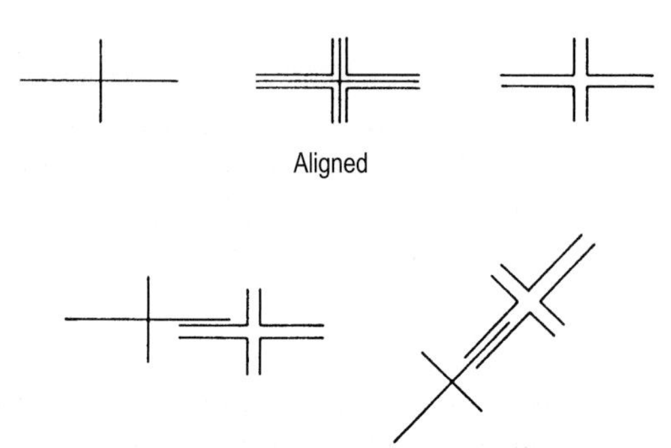

Figure 7.4 The Zeiss mire

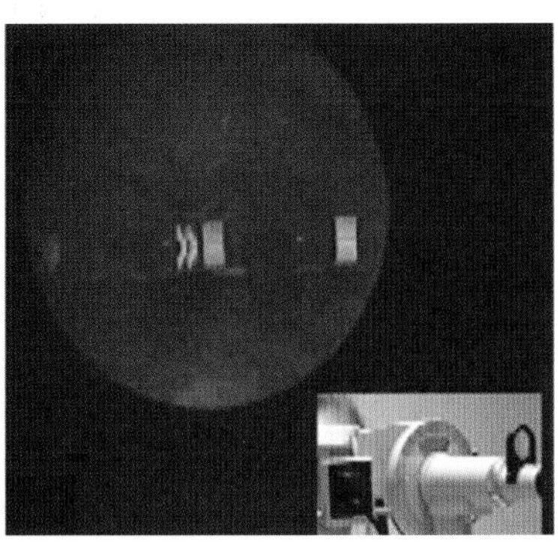

Figure 7.5 The Javal–Schiötz mire. The steps on the green mire represent 1 dioptre intervals of astigmatism

of the mires are coincident. If the keratometer is a one-position instrument (e.g. Bausch & Lomb), the image is doubled in two directions at right angles to each other which provides a means of measuring the two meridians simultaneously. The instrument is then adjusted until the two parts of the mire are superimposed. The circular mire readily demonstrates any corneal distortion, lens flexure and tear film instability (Hirji et al. 1989). Two-position instruments (e.g. those incorporating Zeiss or Javal–Schiötz mires) only assess the corneal curvature in one meridian and therefore need to be rotated by 90° to measure the second principal meridian. The two meridians may not be at 90° to each other if the astigmatism is irregular. Javal–Schiötz mires are usually of two different colours so that any overlapping of the mires produces a change in mire colour. With the mires aligned in the steeper meridian, rotation of the instrument head through 90° will result in one mire-step overlap for each dioptre of astigmatism (see Fig. 7.5).

Errors in the use of a keratometer involve:

- Features of the instrument design
  - inaccuracies in paraxial ray theory.
  - the assumption that the peripheral areas from which the mires are reflected have the same curvature as the corneal pole.
- Operator-induced errors
  - inaccurate alignment.
  - focusing errors.
  - proximal accommodation.
  - orientation of the instrument.
- Patient-induced errors, such as poor fixation and the presence of corneal distortions.

Although keratometry has traditionally been used for selection of the first trial contact lens, it is a poor guide to overall corneal shape as it assesses only a central area of 3.0–3.5 mm diameter. Comparing corneal astigmatism as measured by keratometry, with the spectacle astigmatism, can also assist lens selection. Such comparisons help predict whether rigid or soft lenses are likely to give a better visual result or whether a toric lens might be necessary (*see* Chapters 9, 10 and 12).

Topography

Corneal shape is generally considered more complex than that found by keratometry. It can be represented by a prolate ellipse (one that flattens in the periphery), although there is wide variation between individuals (Guillon et al. 1986).

Videotopographers have an illumination source to produce rings of light (mostly bowl or cone shaped). A camera, attached to an internal or external computer, images the rings as they are reflected off an area of approximately 10 mm diameter of the central cornea. Image capture can be manually triggered when the image is centred and in focus (often highlighted by indicator scales on the screen) or this can be activated automatically.

Image processing detects the location of the rings in multiple meridians. The data are displayed in the form of contour maps and simulated keratometry readings in the principal axes. These are generated from the innermost rings, the diameters of which most nearly equate with a conventional keratometer. The average eccentricity of the cornea can also be calculated.

The contour maps are generated from the point contour values, with similar values connected to form zones of equal curvature. The zones are coloured in spectral order, with the red end (warm colours) corresponding to steeper (shorter) corneal radii and the blue end (cooler colours) corresponding to flatter (longer) corneal curvatures.

Relative scales grade the image presentation to cover the entire difference in curvature across the image, highlighting any differences occurring regardless of their magnitude. Absolute scales are set by the user and attribute each scale increment to a set radius or power change. Careful note must be made of the type of scale used and the magnitude of the increments in order to correctly interpret contour maps (see also Chapter 19).

Contour maps are presented in four principal ways:

- *Sagittal maps* (also called axial presentation), based on a single refracting surface formula (paraxial ray theory), assume rotational symmetry of the surface and predict that all rays will be focused on the axis of symmetry (Fig. 7.6a). They are easy to verify, have the highest repeatability and are most widely used, but distort the position of the apex and features such as ablation areas.
- *Tangential maps*, or instantaneous representation, are based on a mathematical derivation of the radius of curvature with radii centres not restricted to a single axis. This gives a more accurate representation of the position of the apex and other corneal structures (Fig. 7.6b) and a better corneal shape when comparing the plot to the observed fluorescein pattern. The tangential plot is difficult to verify and has a lower repeatability than the sagittal plot.
- *Corneal height maps* (or X,Y,Z coordinates or Z values; Figure 7.6c) are based on the difference in height from a reference sphere (the reference sphere may be different on individual instruments). They are the most direct measure of corneal shape, but have the lowest repeatability.
- *Refractive power maps* (Fig. 7.6d) convert the detected curvature at any point into presumed refractive power based on assumptions of the refractive index of the cornea.

In addition to presentational distortions in accuracy, there are other sources of error.

- Difficulties caused by the virtual image not being accurately detected or being broken-up due to

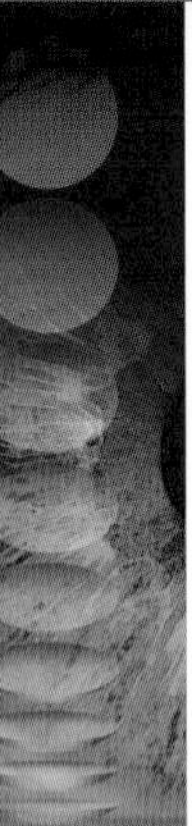

Figure 7.6 Contour maps: (a) axial curvature view; (b) tangential curvature view; (c) corneal height; (d) refractive power. (Reproduced with permission from Medmont International)

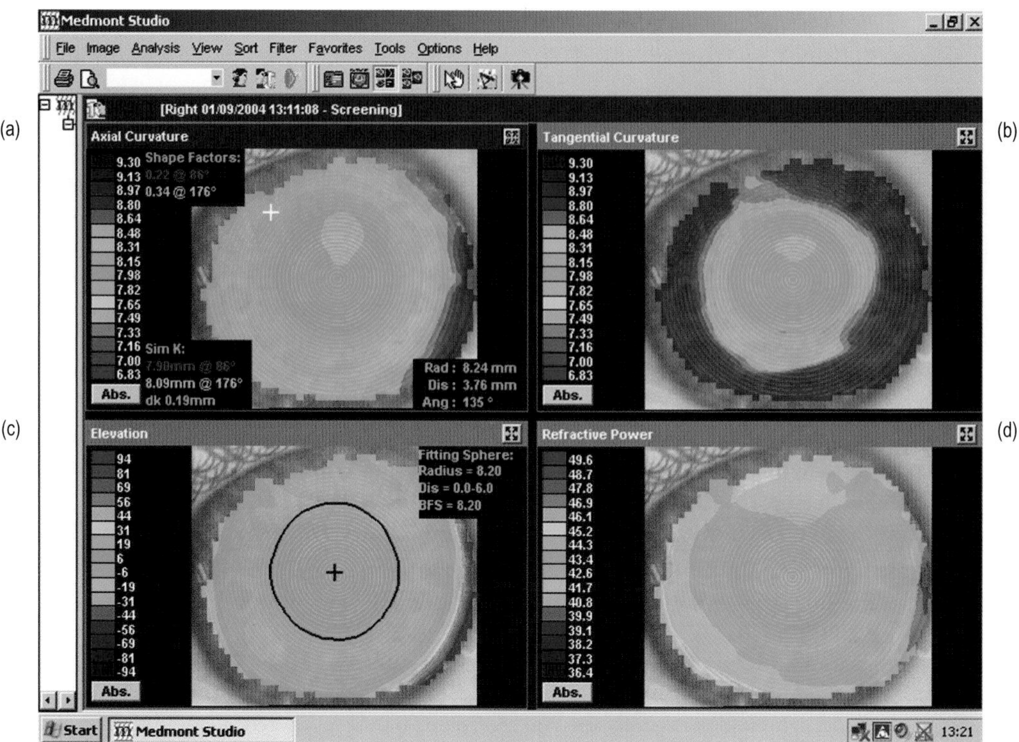

- a poor tear film.
- inaccurate instrument focusing.
- corneal disease or epithelial disorders.

- The number of points detected on each ring is usually the same, resulting in less sampling per unit area in the periphery than in the centre.
- Narrower, more closely spaced rings allow greater sampling but they are more difficult to detect in distorted corneas.
- Peripheral rings in bowl-based topographers are often limited by shadows from anatomical features such as nose or eyelashes. Cone-shape topographers avoid this problem, allowing larger areas of the cornea to be analysed (this is more relevant in orthokeratology). Orientation of the patient's head to the opposite side from the eye being measured assists in minimizing shadows in bowl topographers and allows cone-shaped topographers to be positioned sufficiently close to the eye.
- Ocular accommodation and vergence can also affect accuracy.
- The two principal meridia of a toric cornea are not imaged in the same plane.
- Alignment errors, often due to a patient's high prescription and/or poor visual acuity, can cause inaccuracy, although the magnitude may be limited if the working distance is sufficiently long (Nieves & Applegate 1992).
- More consistent and significant errors occur because the image is centred on the visual axis, which may not coincide with the geometric axis of the cornea. This results in nasal displacement of the mire image and measurement error, which affects nasal readings more than temporal ones, inducing errors in calculating the peripheral curvature of aspheric surfaces (McCarey et al. 1992).

Videotopography contour plots are particularly useful:

- In assessing irregular corneas, e.g. trauma and displaced apices.
- In advanced lens fitting such as orthokeratology (see Chapter 19).
- In keratoconus (see Chapter 20).
- Following postrefractive surgery (see Chapter 23).

Accuracy does reduce, however, with the irregularity of the cornea and varies between models (Dave et al. 1998, Hilmantel et al. 1999, McMahon et al. 2001, Cairns et al. 2002, Cho et al. 2002).

Most instruments have software to simulate the expected fluorescein patterns of specific lenses (either custom-made by the manufacturer or the practitioner's own design), allowing improved empirical fitting accuracy (Fig. 7.7) (see also Chapter 9).

An alternative approach of producing contour mapping of the cornea is by scanning a series of slit sections of the cornea (de Cunha & Woodward 1993) as in the Orbscan II (Bausch & Lomb, Rochester, USA). The Pentacam (Oculus, Giessen, Germany) uses a rotating Scheimplug camera. The Orbscan and the Pentacam are able to give corneal curvature data for the anterior and posterior cornea and are able to provide other anterior segment data such as anterior chamber angle, anterior chamber depth, anterior chamber volume and corneal pachymetry (Fig. 7.8).

SLIT-LAMP BIOMICROSCOPY

Careful observation of the eye and monitoring of ocular response to contact lens wear are prerequisites to successful contact lens fitting. The slit-lamp biomicroscope is the main tool used in this process, providing a magnified, illumination-controlled, binocular view of the ocular structures.

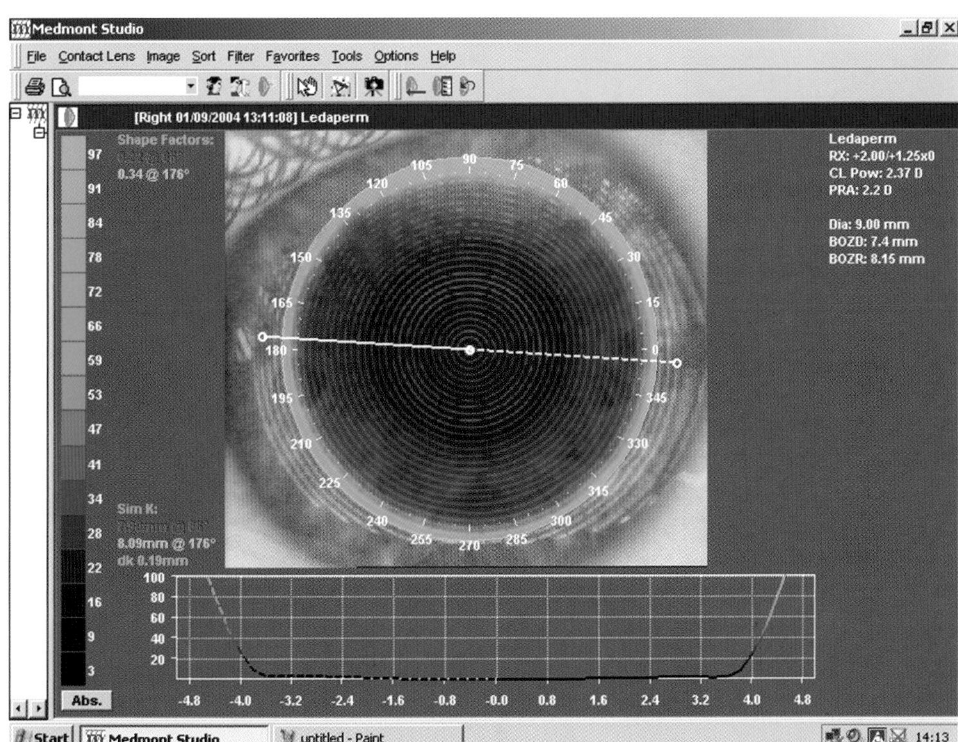

Figure 7.7 Simulated fluorescein pattern produced by the contact lens-fitting program of the Medmont Corneal topographer. (Reproduced with permission from Medmont International)

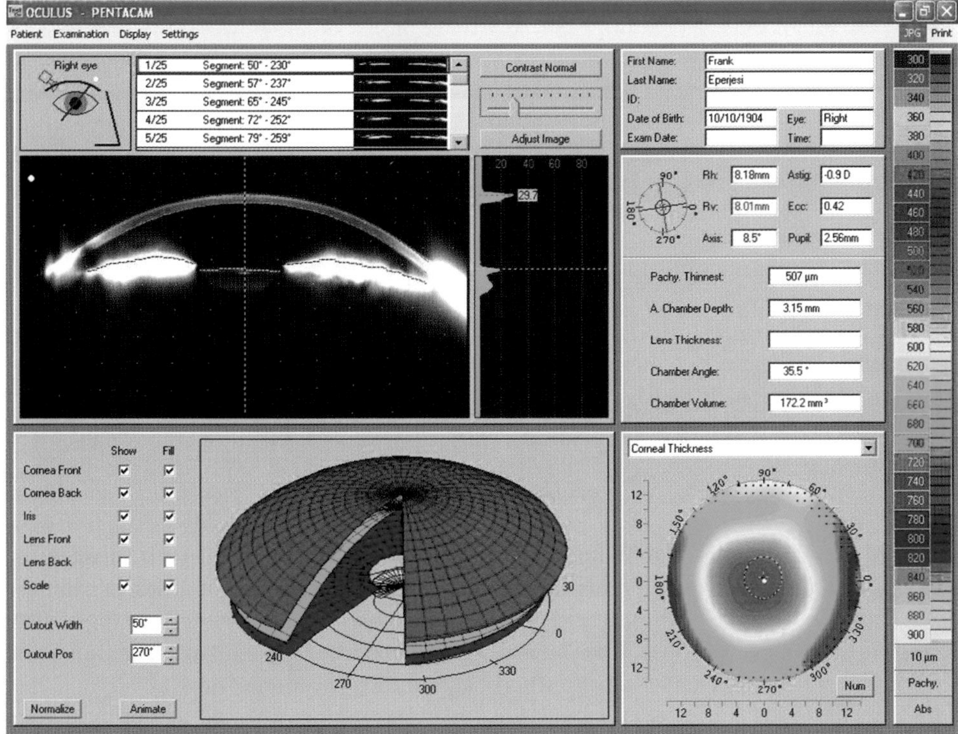

Figure 7.8 The Pentacam provides an array of useful anterior segment information

The principal components of the slit-lamp are an illumination system that provides a focused slit image of light, and a microscope with high resolution providing magnification typically between 7 and 40 times. Both systems can be moved around a common centre of rotation so that there is a common point of focus, which is constant as the system is moved over the curved surfaces of the eye. This can be uncoupled in order to employ special methods of illumination (see Fig. 7.12b).

Illumination system

To assess changes in the optically transparent media, a light source with clearly defined edges is needed. This ensures that

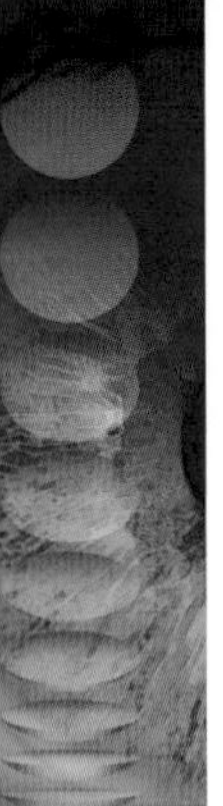

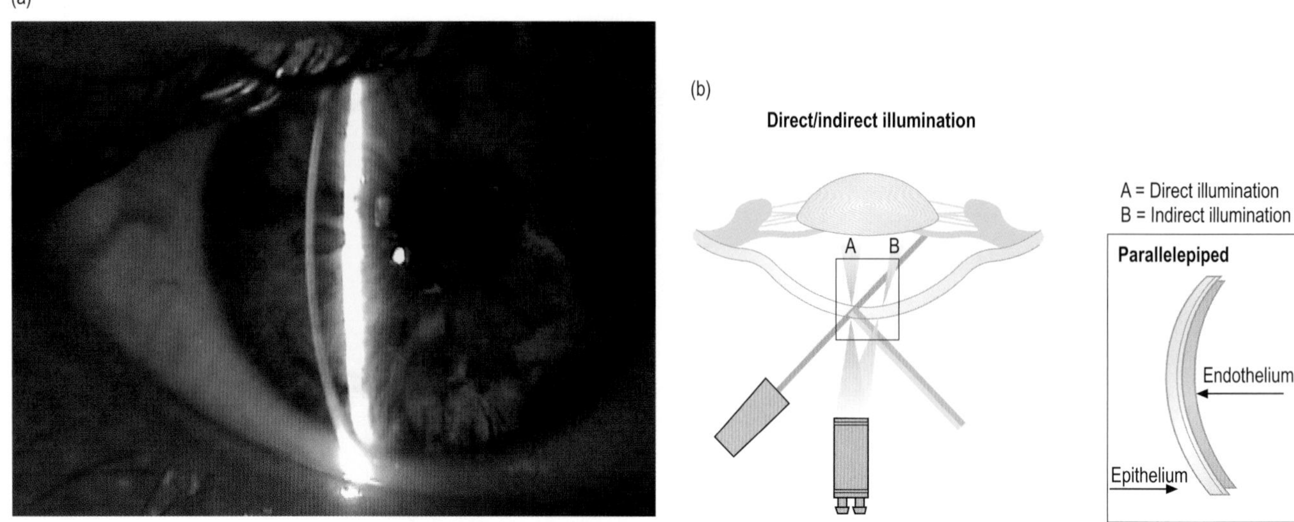

Figure 7.9 Illumination: (a) the beam on the left is direct illumination, the darker area to the right of the direct beam is indirect illumination, while the light coming back from the iris will retroilluminate the cornea. (b) Diagram showing illumination system on the left and microscope in the centre, with a cross-section of the cornea shown in the inset (Reproduced with permission from Vistakon, Synoptik and Tom Løfstrøm, Denmark)

light is not diffused away from the point of focus unless there is irregularity in the media. An optical system projects an image of a mechanical slit aperture, which can be varied in height and width, onto the surface being examined.

The slit illumination can be augmented by the use of filters, such as:

- Diffusing.
- Heat reducing (dichroic filters).
- Neutral density – less light so more comfortable for the patient.
- Red-free – enhances contrast between blood vessels and the cornea or sclera to render vascularization and hyperaemia more visible.
- Blue – used in conjunction with fluorescein to assess corneal damage or the fitting of rigid lenses. The exciter filter will cause fluorescein dye to fluoresce and the addition of a yellow barrier filter (e.g. Wratten 12) in the observation system will enhance the contrast and maximize the visibility of the fluorescence (Pearson 1984, 1986).

Observation system

This comprises a microscope with converging or parallel eyepieces. A turret of objectives allowing a greater range of magnification can be connected to the latter, without the need to change eyepieces. Eyepiece reticules can be used for measuring purposes although calibration is necessary for each magnification used.

Slit-lamp techniques

To ensure the slit image is produced in the same plane as the focus of the microscope, each eyepiece must be focused individually.

'Uncoupling' the illumination system from the observation system is necessary for certain types of viewing such as sclerotic scatter. This is achieved by physical rotation of the illumination system about a horizontal or a vertical plane.

There are a number of different methods of illumination, which can be isolated and described individually (Stockwell & Stone 1988, Morris & Stone 1992). However, in routine slit-lamp examination, the field-of-view of the observation system is always larger than the area illuminated by the slit, such that several types of illumination are evident at any one time. Scanning of the structures by moving both the illumination and the observation system across the surfaces under examination will allow objects of interest to pass from one method of illumination to another. It is the change in appearance of the objects as they are illuminated in different ways that makes them readily visible.

The conventional examination technique is to scan the whole cornea in three sweeps with the illumination system moved laterally so that it is always on the same side of the mid-line as the part of the cornea under examination (Stockwell & Stone 1988). Figure 7.9 highlights the different types of illumination that can be seen within the field-of-view.

- *A diffuser* is used when a focused slit in not needed for general examination of the external eye and adnexa and the assessment of a contact lens fit under white light (Fig. 7.10). This is more comfortable for the patient and does not flood the eye with light, resulting in reflex tearing.
- *Direct illumination* involves focusing and observing the slit of light directly on a structure. The slit is narrowed to produce an optic section and passed perpendicularly through the cornea (Fig. 7.9). A parallelepiped is a wider optic section that can be reduced in height to form a conical beam which is shone through the pupil at various angles to the visual axis; this is carried out in a dark room.
- *Indirect illumination* is observation to the side of a direct beam to highlight features otherwise obscured by direct bright light (Fig. 7.9). To focus accurately on the area under

(a)

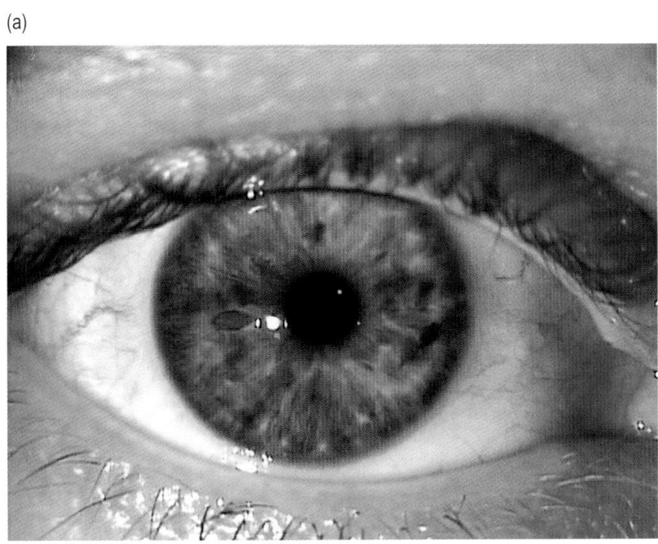

(b)

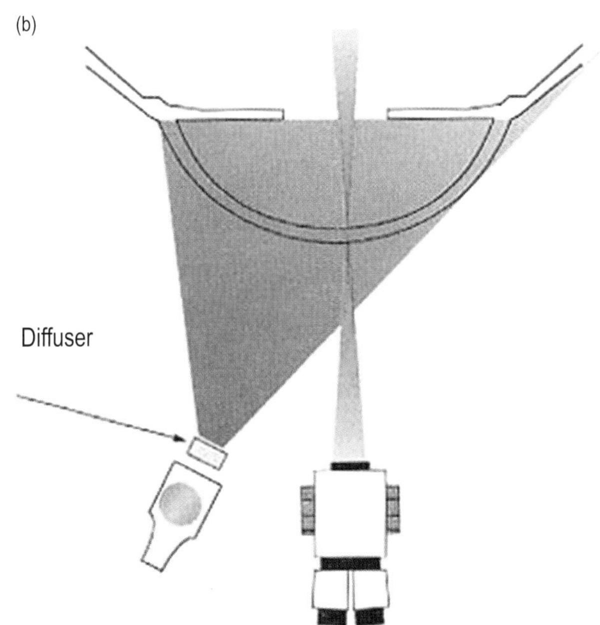

Figure 7.10 Diffuse illumination can be used to obtain a general overview of the adnexa and anterior structures of the eye: (a) image; (b) diagram (Reproduced with permission from Vistakon, Synoptik and Tom Løfstrøm, Denmark)

observation, the observation and illumination systems need to be uncoupled.

- *In retro-illumination* the illumination is reflected off (usually) the iris in order to view the cornea (Fig. 7.9). Again, the illumination needs to be uncoupled from the observation system for accurate focusing.
- *Specular reflection* occurs when the angles of illumination and observation are equal and opposite about the normal to the surface. This creates a Purkinje image wherever there is a change in refractive index:
  - Purkinje I is from the front surface of the tear film and, following a blink, the tears can be seen moving just to the side of the bright reflection.
  - Purkinje II is from the endothelium aqueous interface and the endothelial mosaic of hexagonal cells can be seen under high (~40×) magnification in the dimmer reflection.
  - Purkinje III is from the front surface of the lens and the dimpled appearance can be seen with quite a narrow angle between the observation and illumination systems (Fig. 7.11).
- *Sclerotic scatter* requires the light to be displaced to the limbus while the cornea is viewed. The magnification system can be ignored and the result viewed with the naked eye, but to view the central cornea with magnification requires uncoupling of the illumination and observation systems. Light incident on the limbus travels through the cornea by total internal reflection and will only be visible within the cornea if there is an irregularity or opacity that causes light to scatter outwards, such as rigid lens-induced oedema (Fig. 7.12).
- *Tangential illumination* can be used to inspect the iris for raised naevi. The illumination system is set parallel to the iris and the iris observed perpendicular to the visual axis.

Applications

Table 7.1 indicates some typical conditions and the preferred methods of illumination to render them most visible.

For measurements such as blood vessel encroachment, contact lens movement and opacity dimensions, the slit width or length scale on the slit-lamp can be used (although it is important to check this is calibrated). The slit can be turned through up to 180° in order to take measurements at the appropriate angle. Alternatively, a reticule can be incorporated into one of the eyepieces.

Grading

In order to make decisions based on slit-lamp microscope findings over a period of time or between clinicians, it is important to be able to make valid comparisons. Grading scales require a given ocular feature to be gauged relative to predetermined images chosen to represent different degrees of the condition of interest on an ordinal scale. Such scales vary in the number of images and condition of interest, but are usually descriptive, artistically rendered, photographic, or computer generated. Typically, the absence of a sign is given a grade zero on a five-point scale, such as the IER grading scale (see Appendix B) or the Efron scale. Expansion of the grading scale beyond five levels (such as by grading to 1/10th of a unit) increases discrimination.

Even using a pictorial grading scale as reference, there are wide discrepancies between the grade allocated to a particular image by different clinicians. Interobserver variability would appear to improve with practice. A number of computer-assisted objective grading techniques have been described to quantify retinal vasculature. Edge detection and colour extraction techniques have been shown to be the most stable to

(a)

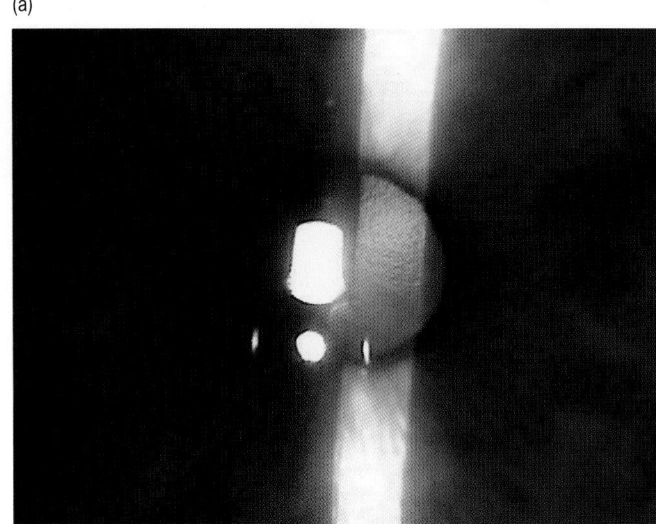

(b)

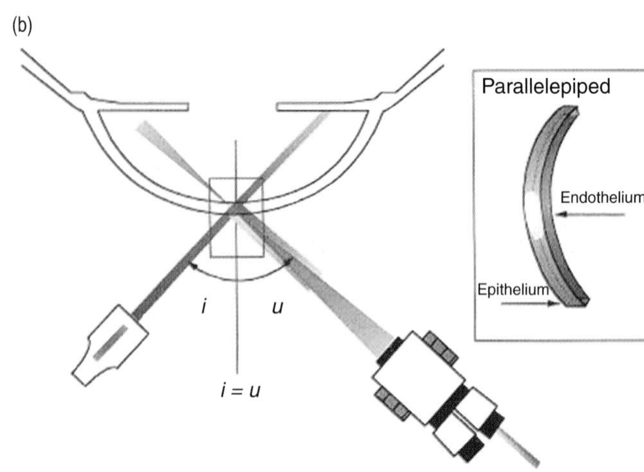

Figure 7.11 Specular reflection of the anterior surface of the crystalline lens: (a) image; (b) diagram, where *i* is the angle of incidence and *u* is the angle of reflection (Reproduced with permission from Vistakon, Synoptik and Tom Løfstrøm, Denmark)

(a)

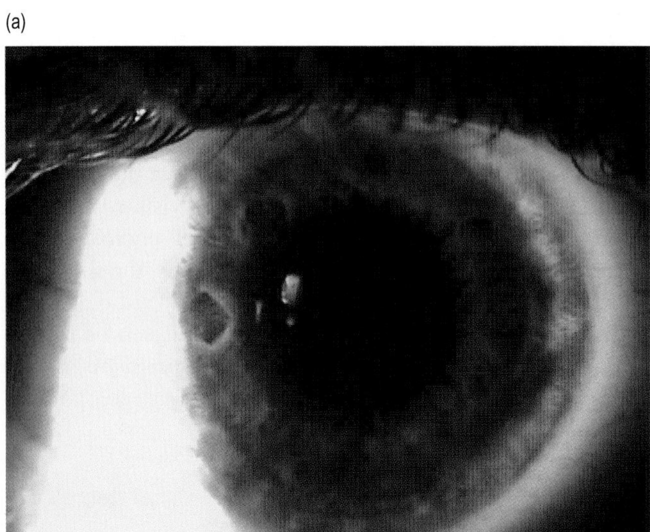

(b)

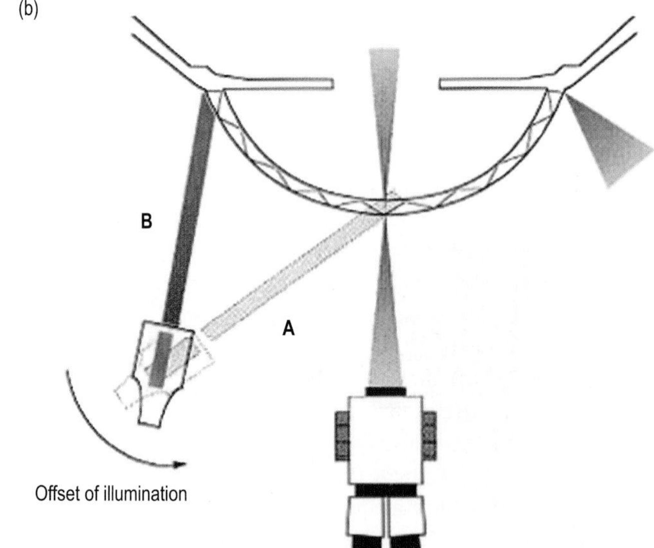

Figure 7.12 Sclerotic scatter using total internal reflection of the cornea: (a) image; (b) diagram; A = coupled; B = uncoupled (Reproduced with permission from Vistakon, Synoptik and Tom Løfstrøm, Denmark)

changes in image luminance and to correlate well to traditional grading scale images (Wolffsohn and Purslow, 2003).

PACHOMETRY (PACHYMETRY)

In response to physiological compromise, the normal hydration of the cornea can be upset, resulting in swelling (see Chapter 2), while in conditions such as keratoconus, there is progressive thinning of the central cornea. Pachometry provides a method by which corneal thickness can be measured.

In its simplest form, this can be achieved by directing a narrow slit-lamp beam normally at the corneal surface to provide a thin section of the central cornea. A variable prism introduced into half the field will permit the displacement of one half of the corneal image with respect to the other. This is viewed through a doubling system in the eyepiece. If the image of the cornea is displaced so that the endothelium of one image aligns with the epithelium of the second, the apparent thickness is equal to the amount of displacement (Figs 7.13, 7.14). Apparent thickness can be converted to real thickness by using a nominal refractive index for the corneal tissue.

This method of optical pachometry has limitations due to the need for accurate alignment of the slit-lamp beam both horizontally and vertically on the cornea and the need for the beam to be imaged normally to the corneal surface. Failure to obtain accurate alignment will lead to errors and poor precision of measurement.

Ultrasonic pachometry (Fig. 7.15) is more commonly used nowadays because of its simplicity of use. It offers an alternative approach without the need for a slit-lamp. At each major corneal interface, an echo will be evident on an ultrasound trace. Once calibrated, the distance between the epithelial and endothelial echoes will provide a measure of corneal thickness,

Table 7.1: Application of slit-lamp techniques to ocular examination

Area/abnormality to be observed	Magnification	Illumination method	Slit width	Filter accessory
Lids and general view of external eye	Low–medium	Diffuse	Wide	Diffuser
Lashes	Medium	Direct focal	Medium to wide	None
Localized oedema	Low	Sclerotic scatter	Medium	Uncoupled system
Corneal opacities/defects	Medium–high	Direct focal Indirect focal	Medium to narrow	None
Depth of opacity/defect within cornea	Medium–high	Direct focal	Narrow	None. Wide separation between illuminating and observation system
Microcysts	High	Indirect	Narrow	None
Striae	High	Indirect	Medium to narrow	None
Neovascular changes/ghost vessels	Medium–high	Indirect retro	Medium to narrow	None. Green filter may help if there is blood flow
Endothelium	High	Specular reflection	Medium	None
Dystrophies	Low Medium	Direct retro Direct focal	Wide Medium	Neutral density? None
Fluorescein staining	Low–medium	Direct focal or diffuse	Wide	Blue filter in illumination system; yellow filter in observation system

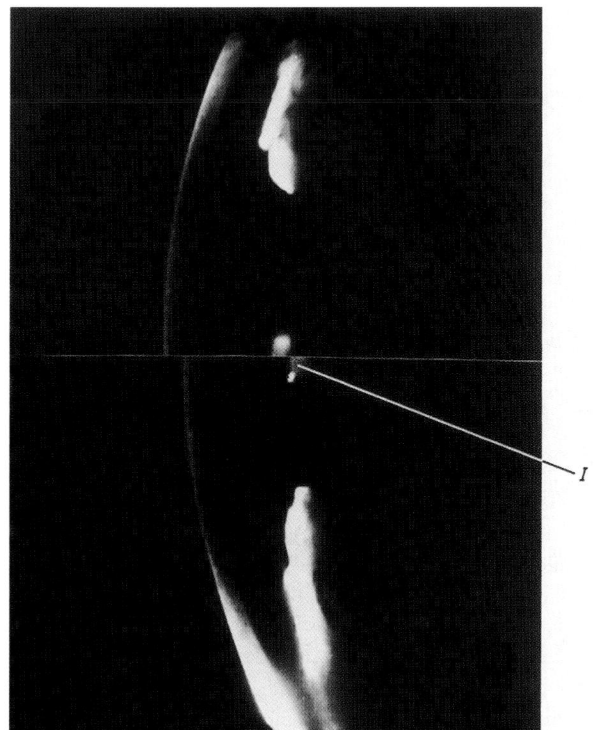

Figure 7.13 Appearance of slit section. *I* indicates Purkinje III which is also doubled: this aids centration of the slit section

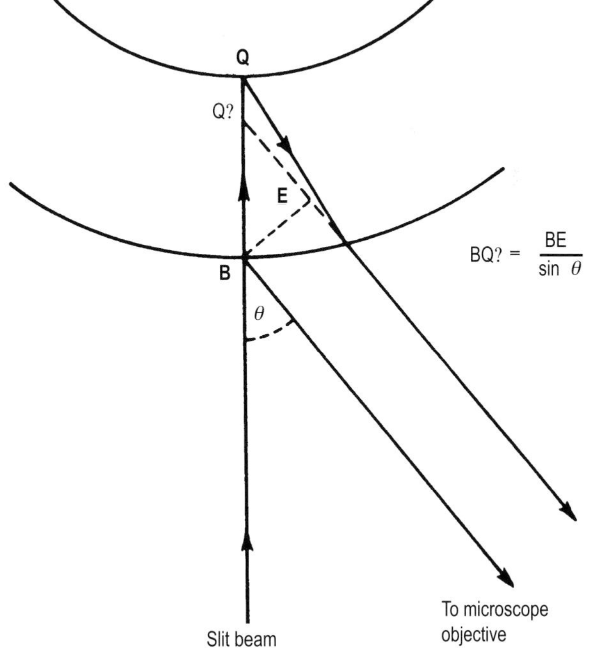

Figure 7.14 Optical principle of pachometry

and modern instruments give a digital read-out. (For a review of the use of ultrasound in optometry, see Storey 1988.) There are potential errors in this method due to the need to:

- Use appropriate ultrasound velocity for the tissue being measured.
- Hold the probe perpendicular to the cornea.

However, results from the ultrasonic pachometer provide good reproducibility (Miglior et al. 2004) and results comparing ultrasonic and optical pachometry show good correlation (Ling et al. 1986).

Pachometry is useful both as a clinical and a research tool, and is used particularly to assess corneal thickness prior to refractive surgery. It is also used to monitor keratoconus and, increasingly, as a correction factor in the calculation of intraocular pressure.

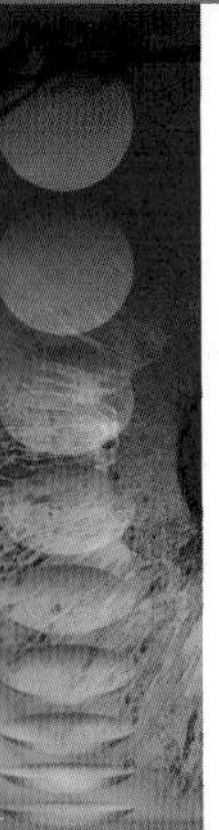

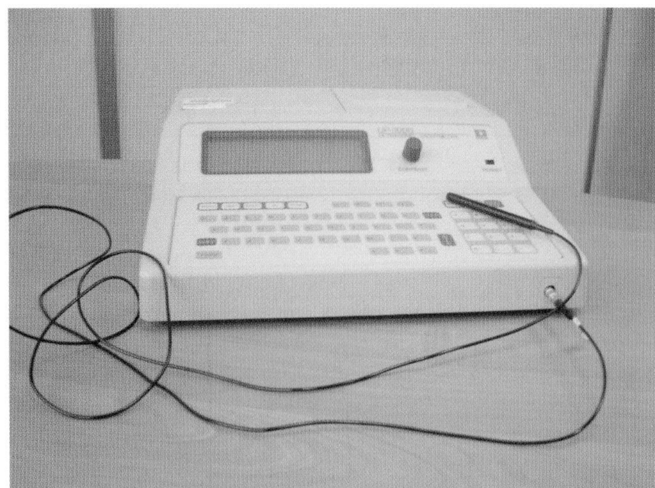

Figure 7.15 An ultrasonic pachometer (pachymeter)

Corneal sensitivity

Aesthesiometers have been used to assess corneal sensitivity and its variation with contact lens wear (Millodot 1976, 1978), and are comprised of nylon filaments which can be brought into contact with the cornea with a known force. Some slit-lamps facilitate attachments of this type. Touch thresholds can be established by using the microscope to assess when contact with the cornea is made, and the threshold level recorded when the subject indicates awareness of contact as the filament length is varied. Shorter filament lengths will apply greater force at contact (see also Chapter 2).

Pneumatic aesthesiometers are more commonly used nowadays, for example the Belmonte carbon dioxide aesthesiometer (Belmonte et al. 1999).

This technique is not a common clinical tool in general practice.

SLIT-LAMP PHOTOGRAPHY

There are two main options for anterior segment imaging with a slit-lamp biomicroscope. A camera system can be attached to the existing eyepieces of the slit-lamp (typically a C-mount screw fitting). The main advantage is the relatively low cost, although a computer image database storage program and image board are still required. The slit-lamp eyepieces have optics designed for the 60 D cornea/lens assembly which have to be adapted using the camera's optics to allow in-focus imaging by a camera. Therefore, the optical path is different from that of a purpose-dedicated photographic slit-lamp. Light loss occurs at the eyepiece lens assembly, but an internal beam splitter is unnecessary. The field of view of the image is also generally reduced and the camera obscures at least one eyepiece, so the advantages of a binocular system are lost in aligning and focusing an object of interest.

The more common format of photo-slit-lamp involves a beam splitter being inserted into the optical path of the slit-lamp when photography is required, but removed for general eye examination to maximize the image light intensity available. The use of a beam splitter still allows binocular viewing through the eyepieces and hence the camera only receives about 50% of the available light (depending on the reflectance of the beam splitter) (Fig. 7.16).

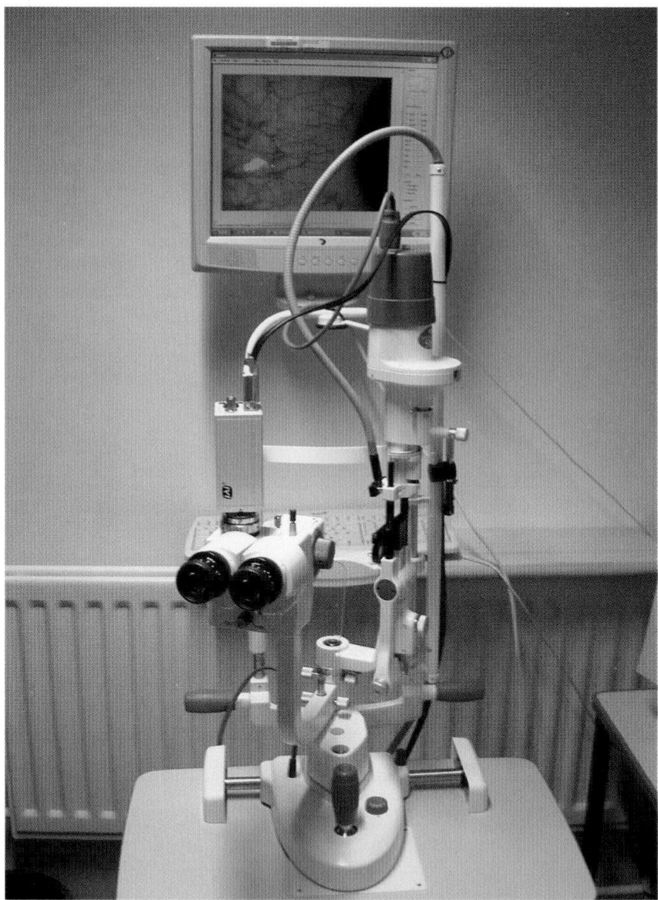

Figure 7.16 A video-based camera incorporating a beam splitter

A traditional analogue camera is a basic device, exposing a piece of film through a lens and shutter. The complexity is in the design of the film and the processing stage. In comparison, digital cameras (Fig. 7.17) are more complex, with the image processing undertaken internally by the camera's electronics. 'Digital' photo-sensors are smaller than the equivalent area of 35 mm film, so camera lenses have to be longer (typically 1.4–1.6×). Film cameras are becoming less common due to the delay in processing the film.

Digital cameras typically have one of two types of light-detection chip. The charged couple device (CCD) consists of an etched pixelated metal oxide semiconductor made from silicone, sensitive in the visible and near infrared spectrum. Light is converted into electrons, which sense the level of light rather than colour. Only the photon-to-electron conversion is conducted on the pixel, allowing the maximum amount of space to remain within each pixel for capturing light information. They have, therefore, a low signal-to-noise ratio. The electron-to-voltage conversion is done on the light detection chip, leaving the

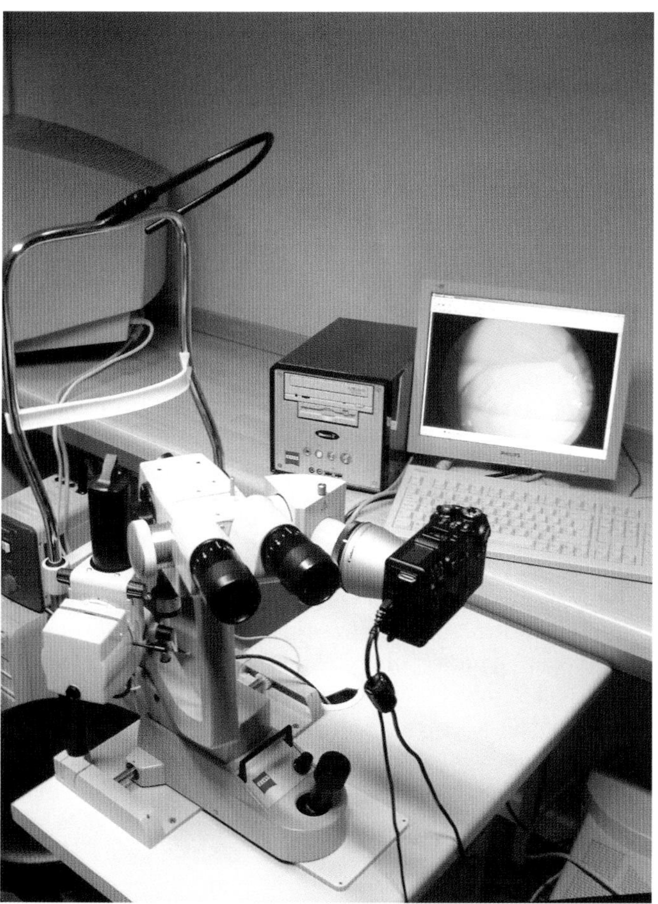

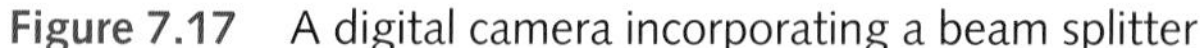

Figure 7.17 A digital camera incorporating a beam splitter

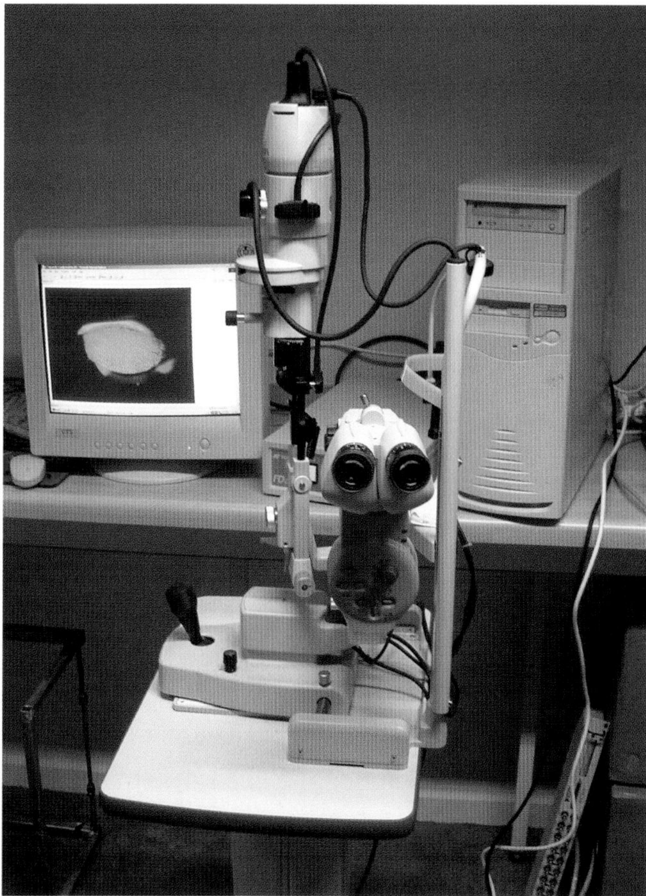

Figure 7.18 The Topcon DC-1 slit-lamp and integral camera

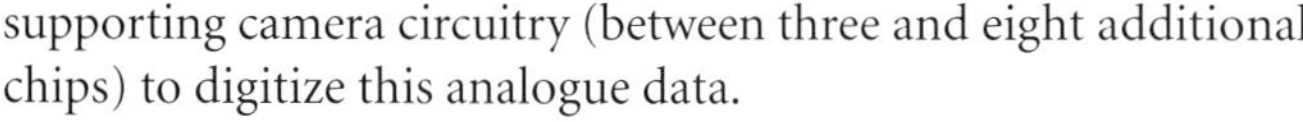

supporting camera circuitry (between three and eight additional chips) to digitize this analogue data.

Complementary metal-oxide semi-conductor (CMOS) chips are similar to CCDs but both photon-to-electron and electron-to-voltage conversions are conducted within the pixel, together with digitization of the signal, leaving less room for the light-sensitive part of the sensor. Normally a microlens is used to capture more light within the pixel area and bend it towards the light-sensitive part (the fill factor) of the pixel. CMOS chips have the advantage of being cheaper and less power hungry than CCDs, due to having fewer components, making them more reliable.

The capture technology is usually based on a single chip with each pixel coated in a different colour, spatially arranged in a mosaic pattern (providing twice as many green as red or blue pixels). The image is then processed (interpolation of colour data from the surrounding pixels) to an image with the full resolution of the chip, with 100% spatial, but only 90–95% spectral, efficiency (fidelity). This can result in colour fringing around sharp edges, although more modern interpolation algorithms have reduced this effect. Interpolation requires a significant amount of processing, which takes both time and power to accomplish. The alternative is the three-chip camera, with each chip capturing an image of the scene at its full resolution, but through a different filter (red, green or blue). Prisms behind the lens aperture allow green-filtered light to pass undiverted to their chip, whereas red and blue light is diverted to their respective chips on either side of the 'green' chip. The processing converts the image to resolution of one chip (not the resolution of one chip times three as is sometimes suggested), with absolute data for red, green and blue light allowing 100% spatial and spectral efficiency. These cameras are more expensive, delicate, heavier and bulkier than single-chip cameras and, due to the light loss from the two beam splitters, require a higher light output from the slit-lamp for equivalent performance.

Digital cameras are generally more expensive than analogue cameras and require complex, expensive, image capture cards. Although commercially available digital cameras often have a small built-in real-time monitor, this is inadequate to allow non-eye-piece focusing of the image. However, an analogue output is usually available and can be fed into a larger monitor to allow subjective manipulation of the slit-lamp to produce the optimum captured image. Features such as autofocusing must be disabled from commercial cameras, usually by selecting infinity ('mountain') viewing. More recent slit-lamp image capture systems, such as the Topcon DC-1, have incorporated the camera in the body of the slit-lamp system itself (Fig. 7.18). This creates a neater imaging solution, but restricts the owner to the manufacturer's own camera products.

There are a number of interfaces that are currently used to connect digital cameras or memory card readers direct to a computer:

- *Small computer system interface* (SCSI) – used more often with high-end scanners than digital cameras, offers reasonable transfer speed (Ultra 2 SCSI 40 MBps), but limited to a short cable length and difficult to set up. It must be turned on before the host computer and each device requires a unique number.
- *Firewire* – a high-speed transfer system that provides autoconfiguration and plug-and-play technology. It is robust and easy to use, allowing transfer speeds of ≥50 MBps.
- *Universal serial bus* (USB) – allows autoconfiguration and plug-and-play technology and also providing a small external power source (500 mA). The slow transfer speed of USB1 (1.5 MBps) has been improved with USB2 (up to 60 MBps).

The speed of transfer will affect the ability to display and the temporal resolution of a real-time image display.

File formats

Each bit of information can contain a 0 or 1, so 8-bit colour can code 2^8 = 256 colours (usually greyscales) for each pixel (1 byte). High colour (12-bit) can code 65,536 colours and true colour (24-bit) 16,777,216 colour shades (3 bytes per pixel). An uncompressed 800 × 600 pixel 24-bit, image takes up 1.44 Mb of storage space. Most imaging systems offer a selection of different file formats with which to save images and movies.

There are two types of graphic files: vectors and bitmaps. Vector files (Window Meta Files [*.wmf]) and Pict format (Macintosh computers) store images as a series of descriptions of simple shapes, such as lines and rectangles. They split the image into these shapes, describe the position and colour within the image, and reconstruct the image from these details when the file is opened. The image size can therefore be changed without any effect on image quality, but these files are not really suited to complex images such as real images of the eye.

The whole image of a bitmap file is divided into tiny squares (pixels) and the colour of each pixel recorded. The result is a relatively large file size and an image that cannot be enlarged without loss of resolution. Formats include:

- *TIF* (tagged information file) – a lossless format, storing all the data from the camera once its internal processing (such as colour interpolation) has taken place. It uses algorithms to make the file size smaller for storage, but all the compression is reversed on opening. However, the stored images are still relatively large, even larger than the RAW format (see below). For example, a 1600 × 1200 pixel image in 24-bit colour (3 bytes per pixel) would result in an ~5.8 Mb TIF.
- *RAW* – a newer option allowing the captured data to be stored in its raw form, before any processing has taken place. This results in a smaller image file than the TIF format and the archived data are always available for reprocessing. However, each camera captures its data in a different way, so there is no standardization of format, and proprietary software is needed to convert the image to a general readable format.
- *JPEG* (Joint Photographic Experts Group) – a compressed format, resulting in the loss of some image integrity. Non-lossy compression aims to reduce the storage space taken up by a file without losing any information. Although this works well when the number of colours is limited, it is generally ineffective with continuous tone pictures of high colour depth (such as photographs). JPEG compression attempts to eliminate redundant or unnecessary information (lossy compression). Red, green, blue (RGB) files are converted into luminance and chrominance components, merging pixels and utilizing compression algorithms to remove frequencies not utilized by the human eye, followed by rounding to integer values. Different compression levels can usually be selected. Using the example above, depending on content, a low-compression JPEG would be ~0.3 Mb. Some systems offer a modified JPEG file type known as an exchangeable image file (EXIF) which stores 'tags' onto the header of the image file containing technical data such as time, exposure settings and camera make. This feature allows documented proof of when an image was captured, should it be needed for litigation protection.
- *BMP* – Microsoft Windows native bitmap format. Although it supports run-length encoding it is most commonly used as an uncompressed format so file sizes can be large.

Image capture

The physical action necessary to capture an image differs between systems, with more advanced systems overriding the software or camera control in favour of a foot-pedal or joystick button.

Optical considerations

The optics of a slit-lamp is critical to good imaging, and features such as the type of zoom (continuous or fixed level) should also be considered. The quality of any camera image can only be as good as the lens system, which captures the light and focuses it on the light receptor. This is even more critical with a light receptor chip camera due to the smaller capture area compared to 35 mm film.

As well as stating the type of light receptor chip used (e.g. CCD or CMOS), the size of chip should also be recorded (normally 1/4 to 3/4 inch). Each pixel receptor will be larger on a larger chip of the same resolution as a smaller chip. The bigger the pixel receptor target, the more chance the photon has of hitting it. The latest digital cameras boasting resolutions of around 6 million pixels on a 1/2 inch chip have pixel receptors of <1 micron in diameter and therefore are limited by the size of a photon. The image looks good and takes up plenty of disk space, but, when zooming, appears blurred.

Illumination

Analogue cameras use mechanical shutters that physically expose the film to light for a predetermined period of time. Digital cameras have the advantage of being able to 'turn-on'

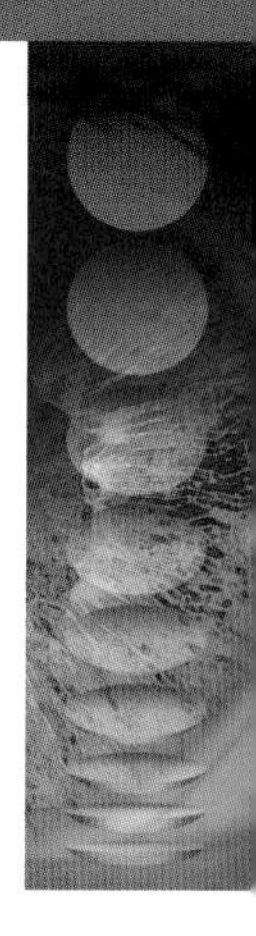

the light receptor for a set period of time (electronic shutter), which involves no moving parts. Additional lighting is essential for optometric imaging due to the loss of light from intervening beam splitters and lenses, incomplete fill factor of the sensor pixels and a reduced light sensitivity compared to the human eye. This is particularly the case for blue/ultraviolet illumination. CCD and CMOS photoreceptors are more responsive to the red end of the spectrum. Therefore they often have an infrared filter and compensate for the low blue sensitivity by amplifying blue signals within the image processing. Therefore, the blue channel is likely to exhibit more noise than the red or green channels and can be a good way to examine the quality of a digital camera (TASI 2003). External eye illuminators, not governed by the normal illumination controls, are particularly useful for slit-lamp imaging as they provide a brighter, diffuse light source to overcome the light lost by additional imaging components. Commercial lamps attached to flexible arms can provide cheaper alternatives.

Software

Purpose-designed systems usually allow not only the image to be captured, but also the image to be enhanced and annotated. Most allow connection to an anterior eye image capture device as well as a fundus camera and a patient management system. Further developments in this area could allow a less paper-based practice, with a fully integrated patient management, record keeping (including all instrumentation) and accountancy package. The compatibility of the software with existing database systems and its ability to connect to a network are important considerations.

References

Belmonte, C., Acosta, M., Schmeltz, M. and Gallar, J. (1999) Measurement of corneal sensitivity to mechanical and chemical stimulation with a CO_2 esthesiometer. Invest. Ophthalmol. Vis. Sci., 40(2), 513–519

Cairns, G., McGhee, C. N. J., Collins, M. J., Owens, H. and Gamble, G. D. (2002) Accuracy of Orbscan II slit-scanning elevation topography. J. Cataract Refractive Surg., 28(12), 2181–2187

Cho, P., Lam, A. K. C., Mountford, J. and Ng, L. (2002) The performance of four different corneal topographers on normal human corneas and its impact on orthokeratology lens fitting. Optom. Vis. Sci., 79(3), 175–183

Dave, T., Ruston, D. and Fowler, C. (1998) Evaluation of the EyeSys model II computerized videokeratoscope. Part I: Clinical assessment. Optom. Vis. Sci., 75(9), 647–655

de Cunha, D. A. and Woodward, E. G. (1993) Measurement of corneal topography in keratoconus. Ophthalmic Physiol. Opt., 13, 377–382

Guillon, M., Lydon, D. P. M. and Wilson, C. (1986) Corneal topography: a clinical model. Ophthalmic Physiol. Opt., 6, 47–56

Hilmantel, G., Blunt, R. J., Garrett, B. P., Howland, H. C. and Applegate, R. A. (1999) Accuracy of the Tomey Topographic Modeling System in measuring surface elevations of asymmetric objects. Optom. Vis. Sci., 76(2), 108–114

Hirji, N. K., Patel, S. and Callender, M. (1989) Human tear film pre-rupture phase time (TP-RPT). A non-invasive technique for evaluating the pre-corneal tear film using a novel keratometer mire. Ophthalmic Physiol. Opt., 9, 139–142

Ling, T., Ho, A. and Holden, B. A. (1986) Method of evaluating ultrasonic pachometers. Am. J. Optom. Physiol. Opt., 63, 462–466

McCarey, B. E., Zurawski, C. A. and O'Shea, D. S. (1992) Practical aspects of a corneal topography system. CLAO J., 18, 248–254

McMahon, T. T., Anderson, R. J., Joslin, C. E. and Rosas, G. A. (2001) Precision of three topography instruments in keratoconus subjects. Optom. Vis. Sci., 78(8), 599–604

Miglior, S., Albe, E., Guareschi, M., Mandelli, G., Gomarasca, S. and Orzalesi, N. (2004) Intraobserver and interobserver reproducibility in the evaluation of ultrasonic pachymetry measurements of central corneal thickness. Br. J. Ophthalmol., 88(2), 174–177

Millodot, M. (1976) Effect of the length of wear of contact lenses on corneal sensitivity. Acta Ophthalmol., 54, 721–730

Millodot, M. (1978) Effect of long term wear of hard contact lenses on corneal sensitivity. Acta Ophthalmol., 96, 1225–1227

Morris, J. and Stone, J. (1992) The slit-lamp biomicroscope in optometric practice. Optom. Today, 7 September, 26–28; 5 October, 16–19; 2 November, 28–30

Nieves, J. E. and Applegate, R. A. (1992) Alignment errors and working distance directly influence the accuracy of corneal topography measurements. Invest. Ophthalmol. Vis. Sci., ARVO supplement

Pearson, R. M. (1984) The mystery of the missing fluorescein. J. Br. Contact Lens Assoc., 7, 122–125

Pearson, R. M. (1986) The mystery of the missing fluorescein – a postscript. J. Br. Contact Lens Assoc., 9, 36–37

Stockwell, H. and Stone, J. (1988) Anterior eye examination. In Optometry, ed. K. H. Edwards. Oxford: Butterworth-Heinemann

Storey, J. (1988) Ultrasonography of the eye. In Optometry, pp. 342–352, eds. K. Edwards and L. Llewellyn. London: Butterworths

Technical Advisory Service for Images (TASI) (2003) Advice paper on digital cameras. Online. Available: www.tasi.ac.uk

Wolffsohn, J. S. and Purslow, C. (2003) Clinical monitoring of ocular physiology using digital image analysis. Cont. Lens Anterior Eye, 26, 27–35

Chapter 8

Assessment of patient suitability for contact lenses

Janet Stone and Robert Terry

CHAPTER CONTENTS

Since the early editions of this book were published, contact lenses have become a popular form of visual correction and their fitting has become largely soft lens orientated. However, there has been a renewal of interest in corneal lens fitting with the advent of more rigid gas-permeable (RGP) materials with increasing oxygen permeability and better wetting characteristics.

Scleral lens fitting is time consuming and costly, and is now rarely considered as a practical option outside hospital departments or specialist contact lens practices. There, scleral lenses are used for eyes with pathological or abnormal conditions unsuited to soft or corneal lenses (see Chapters 15, 20 and 26).

The advent of disposable and frequent-replacement soft lenses of various water contents and tints, including toric lenses and bifocals, has also extended the scope of contact lenses to cater for different patient requirements. Daily disposables have extended the options yet further as has the development of silicone hydrogel lenses, which now cater for both daily and extended-wear modalities.

Contact lenses are frequently the main form of optical correction although they are often requested for specific limited use and need to be interchangeable with spectacles. The contact lens practitioner not only has to assess patient suitability for contact lenses in general, but also the best form of lens and material to satisfy these more sophisticated requirements. There are therefore more factors to consider when assessing patients for contact lens fitting. Limitations still exist in the types of lens available as well as in the suitability of the prospective wearers. Careful selection benefits both patient and practitioner by avoiding time wasted attempting to fit unsuitable patients or in fitting patients with unsuitable lenses.

It is now possible to fit any ocular contour with a contact lens as long as the patient is motivated and there are no contraindications.

Certain pathological and abnormal conditions of the eye and adnexa are a definite indication for contact lenses (e.g. keratoconus).

INDICATIONS AND CONTRAINDICATIONS FOR CONTACT LENS WEARING

These may be considered broadly under three headings:

- Psychological influences.
- Pathological, anatomical and physiological factors.
- Personal and external factors.

Some overlap between the three is inevitable.

It is useful to consider these factors during after-care of contact lens wearers (see Chapter 17), and patients should not necessarily be rejected if they fail in one particular area.

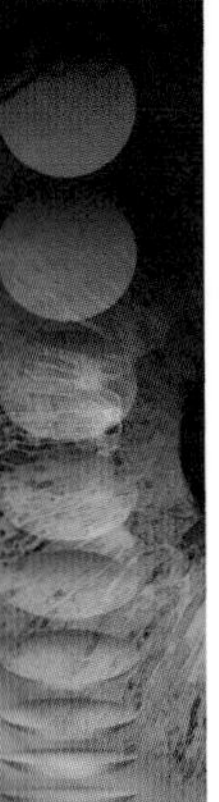

PSYCHOLOGICAL INFLUENCES

Seltzer (1988) suggested that factors such as motivation, coping abilities, willingness to set realistic goals and the degree of tolerance to pain and frustration should be considered as indicators of potential success with contact lens wear.

A small study by Nelson and West (1987) indicated that extroverted, well-adjusted, stable people were more likely to successfully adapt to contact lenses than anxious, introverted people. Practitioners need to keep this in mind and make their patients aware of the differences between the fitting and wearing of spectacles and contact lenses to avoid subsequent disillusionment.

From the legal standpoint, patients should be issued with a printed booklet containing general facts about contact lenses. This also helps patients who are not fully attentive at the initial interview and forget what they have been told (see also Chapter 32).

In the United Kingdom the College of Optometrists advises members that: 'Appropriate elements of the instructions are given in writing to comply with the Medical Devices Directive.' They also state that: 'Since the amount and complexity of information provided to patients at the time of contact lens dispensing is significant, it is appropriate for as much of this information as possible to be provided additionally in written form and advice about required changes in the type of lens, lens wearing pattern or recommended hygiene regimen should also be given in writing.'

So that the patient has the opportunity to reject lenses before being placed under any obligation, their attention should be drawn to the following.

Time taken for fitting

This varies and can depend on the skill of the practitioner and the type of lens to be fitted. It is up to each practitioner to say how long the entire fitting is likely to take. Including tuition of lens handling, some 2–3 hours may be needed with the practitioner and/or optometric assistant. Numerous visits to the practitioner may be necessary and, if the fitting proves complicated, a longer time may be involved.

Tolerance trials can add to the time spent by both patient and practitioner. The desirable minimum for a tolerance trial is about 4 hours but some may need to be as long as 2 weeks. Extended- or continuous-wear lenses should have a 24-hour tolerance trial, commencing early in the day, where possible, and seeing the patient again at the end of the day, and the following morning after the lenses have been worn all night. This may add another hour of 'chair' time to the fitting, and if more than one tolerance trial is necessary, the time spent with the patient during fitting may be extended.

When fitting silicone hydrogel lenses for extended or continuous wear it is advisable to start with a daily wear schedule for 2–3 weeks to determine suitability prior to converting to overnight wear. This may be considered as a tolerance test for extended wear and also enables the essential practice of inserting and removing lenses (see also Chapters 10, 11 and 13). A further examination is essential on the first morning following overnight wear.

Fitting children with contact lenses can be time consuming and parents should be advised of this (see Chapter 24). It is especially important that children are dealt with in an unhurried but reassuringly firm fashion. If less than 16 years, ideally the child should be fitted in the presence of one of the parents, both to give the child reassurance and to demonstrate lens handling to the parent who may be required to carry this out.

At the first visit, besides the preliminary examination and measurements, it may be enough to insert one lens and leave proper fitting for a further visit. A child may require a lot of time to perfect insertion and removal techniques, a few short visits being better than one long one, although children who are well motivated or whose parents wear contact lenses may learn quickly, often managing better than adults.

Time is also needed for continuing clinical care at regular after-care check-ups.

Initial discomfort – physical and visual

Patients may be totally unprepared for the initial difficulties with contact lenses and should be warned about corneal and lid sensation, photophobia, flare and after-wear blur with spectacles (more noticeable with rigid lenses than with soft); however, these aspects should not be overly stressed or the patient may be too nervous to continue!

Gradual wearing procedure

Wearing time, particularly with rigid lenses, should be built up gradually. Extended or continuous wear lenses do not usually require a build-up time but, as mentioned above, a period of daily lens wear is advisable prior to commencing a new patient with overnight contact lens use.

Special storage

Contact lenses must be handled and stored carefully and hygienically. Because of their wetting and hydration properties and the danger of transferring harmful organisms on to the eye, specific solutions are used during handling and storage. Patients must be warned of the risks and advised which solutions are suitable for their lenses and which may come into contact with the eye.

Only daily disposable lenses do not require cleaning and soaking solutions, although even with these lenses, sterile saline and/or rewetting drops may be necessary.

Extra hygiene

Patients often fail to maintain good hygiene regimes, and older lenses with poor surfaces are more likely to become soiled. Lenses should be checked daily to avoid wearing damaged lenses. Rigorous care is important throughout the lens life: by contrast, spectacle wearers spend very little time cleaning their spectacles.

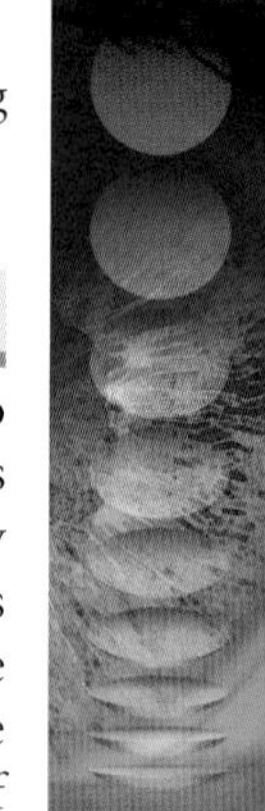

When handling contact lenses, hands should be washed to remove traces of grease and nicotine. Contamination of the lenses with make-up must be avoided and special types of make-up may be necessary. Eye make-up is known to be a source of potentially serious infection (Bruch 1973, Wilson et al. 1973), and cases of conjunctival-embedded pigment from mascara and eye-liner have been reported, both of which cause long-term discomfort and excessive lacrimation (Stewart 1973, Davis et al. 1992, Pesudovs & Phillips 1992). It is helpful to issue patients with a leaflet explaining the safest methods of using eye and other make-up with contact lenses (see also Chapters 5 and 11).

Cleaning and disinfection unfortunately add to the time and cost of lens maintenance and for patients who are unwilling or unable to look after their contact lenses properly, either daily disposable lenses should be considered or the patient should continue with spectacles.

Stringent after-care at regular intervals

Contact lenses can cause corneal abrasion from:

- Foreign bodies beneath them.
- Adherent deposits.
- Trauma from the edge of a rigid lens during insertion or removal.
- Finger nails.

Usually the ensuing discomfort is minimal, but patients have been known to reject lens wear as a result.

Patients must understand the need for after-care and the possibility of minor emergencies. Examination of the eyes and lenses at intervals of no greater than 1 year is advisable, so that the practitioner may detect any changes and advise accordingly. Some patients require more frequent after-care checks because of recurrent symptoms or pathology, or type of lens.

The after-care check is, of necessity, longer and more detailed than that given to a normal spectacle wearer.

Lack of protection from foreign bodies

Spectacle wearers who transfer to contact lenses miss the protection afforded by their spectacles initially and should be warned of possible difficulties in windy or dusty atmospheres.

Soft and scleral lenses provide more protection from foreign bodies than corneal lenses, the degree of protection being related to the size of the lens, its edge clearance, and the close fit of soft lenses. Sunglasses can provide some protection from foreign bodies, and increase the comfort for someone adapting to contact lens wear for the first time.

Cost of lenses, examination fees and accessories

Practitioners should include up to 1 year of after-care in the initial fitting fee, which should be adequate to cover the time likely to be spent with the average patient during that time. Patients should be advised of other costs that they are likely to incur, such as solutions, accessories and even travelling expenses.

Need for and cost of insurance

All contact lenses can be lost or damaged. This is most likely to occur during the initial wearing period before the patient is fully adapted and before handling has been completely mastered. Patients should be advised, therefore, to insure lenses for their replacement value plus the estimated cost of the practitioner's fee at the time of replacement. The insurance premium may be up to 20% of the original fee plus the cost of the lenses. Disposable lenses do not need insurance. Some lens manufacturers run insurance or replacement schemes of their own, which can be helpful to both patient and practitioner, but practitioners should be aware of the legal implications of being involved in these schemes.

Fear of lenses

Another barrier to be overcome is the fear of having anything put in the eye. A practitioner who inspires confidence is usually able to help a patient overcome this quickly (see also Chapter 11).

Apart from these possible 'psychological' disadvantages, there are many definite indications for contact lenses which have a psychological background, as will be seen from the following.

SAFETY

Fear of injury from spectacles during sport is removed. Contact lenses can afford protection from a blow that might have resulted in both external and internal ocular damage. However, special safety spectacles or goggles for sports use provide better protection and should be worn over contact lenses.

SECURITY AND CLARITY OF VISION

A feeling of safety is engendered by contact lenses instead of spectacles for certain sports such as horse riding, cycling (especially in the rain) and sailing. Spectacles may steam up or become coated with spray and contact lenses provide a distinct advantage. Again, safety spectacles or goggles designed to avoid these problems are a viable alternative or addition to contact lenses.

Cosmetic reasons

Intense dislike of spectacles, especially with thick lenses, can result in a marked cosmetic improvement when contact lenses are fitted. This can lead to a beneficial personality change from introvert to extrovert. To some patients, spectacles are an advertisement of a personal disability, which is relieved by wearing contact lenses.

Restoration of normal appearance

Similar psychological benefits occur when a disfigured eye is fitted with a prosthetic lens to give a normal appearance (see Chapters 24 and 25).

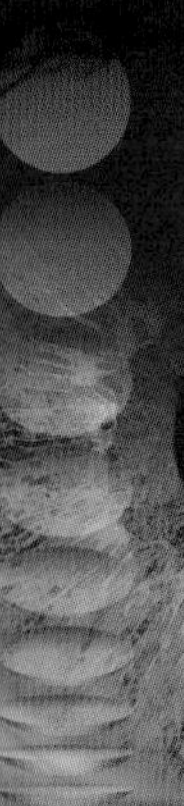

Children

Children who wear spectacles occasionally suffer taunts from their classmates. If children are keen to wear contact lenses, they usually adapt readily and thereby avoid such problems. However, it is not desirable to force children to wear contact lenses because the parents are keen. Fitting lenses can be traumatic if it is carried out against the will of the child and can lead to upset and possible long-lasting psychological disturbance.

PATHOLOGICAL, ANATOMICAL AND PHYSIOLOGICAL FACTORS

Some patients are fitted with lenses because no other form of correction is as good or even suitable. Others may be rejected due to the presence of an abnormal anatomical feature or because of the existence of a pathological condition.

Contact lenses for pathological reasons

Patients with certain pathological conditions may be referred by a medical practitioner to a contact lens practitioner. If this is not the case, a medical opinion may be necessary before fitting lenses in certain situations (see Chapters 11 and 26). A few points are considered here.

NON-TOLERANCE OF SPECTACLES

Spectacles may not be tolerated due to:

- Trauma.
- Skin disease.
- Allergies.
- Nervous troubles.
- Absence of one or both external ears.

Contact lenses may then be suitable, but some skin diseases may be made worse by their wear.

Epidermolysis bullosa (see p. 178), a rare inherited skin disease in which blisters appear at sites of mechanical trauma, makes both spectacle and contact lens wear hazardous. Rubinstein (1984) reported success using high water content (extended wear) soft lenses on a daily wear basis.

People who 'cannot bear' spectacles may not tolerate the difficulties of contact lenses and should not be advised to wear them when a lighter-weight non-allergic spectacle frame may be all that is required. However, because soft lenses are usually easy to adapt to, they may be of benefit in such cases if the patient is otherwise suitable.

PARTIAL SIGHT

Visually impaired patients may benefit from wearing a telescopic aid to provide magnification. A contact lens can form the eyepiece of such a system, with a spectacle lens as the objective (see Chapter 29). Generally, soft lenses perform better than corneal lenses, as they are more stable as an 'eyepiece'. While, in theory, such systems can be used to assist any person with low visual acuity, in practice the system only works in rare instances. Elderly people usually find it extremely difficult to use.

Pathological defects found during examination

If any previously unsuspected pathological condition is found during the preliminary examination, or if the history reveals the existence of pathology, contact lenses should not be fitted until medical advice has been sought. Both general and ocular conditions requiring referral are considered below.

GENERAL CONDITIONS

General debility

Tolerance of contact lenses is likely to be poor unless the general health is good.

Diabetes

O'Donnell and Efron (1998) described some of the potential difficulties in fitting diabetics. These include:

- Blepharitis.
- Dry eye.
- Epithelial fragility and reduced rate of healing.
- Keratitis.
- Unstable refraction.

Where the diabetes is poorly controlled there are also other risks (Rubinstein 1987), including:

- Lowered corneal sensitivity.
- Higher risk of bacterial and fungal infections.

Soft lenses can be fitted but all types of extended-wear lens should be avoided. RGP corneal lenses are more commonly fitted due to the lower risk of infection, but care should be taken to prevent '3 and 9 o'clock' corneal desiccation with its attendant risks. Reduced wearing schedules should be considered.

Skaff et al. (1995) showed that thick soft lenses appeared to cause less swelling of the corneas of insulin-dependent diabetics than normal healthy controls. However, the corneas of the diabetic subjects were thicker (and therefore probably oedematous) to start with.

O'Donnell et al. (2001) found that the clinical response of the diabetic eye to contact lens wear does not differ appreciably from that of the non-diabetic eye. This suggests that the current generation of soft contact lens materials offers a viable mode of vision correction for diabetics.

Hyperthyroidism

The disturbed metabolism, which results in exophthalmos and lack of blinking, can make contact lens wear difficult as there is likely to be insufficient tear flow.

Chronic catarrh and sinusitis

Patients with these conditions are at greater risk of ocular infection if corneal abrasions occur. The associated mucus in the tears also causes visual problems and deposits on the lens surfaces. In scleral lens wearers, strings of mucus may collect

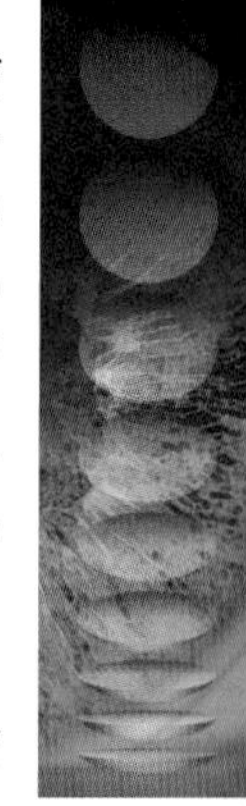

behind the lens. If the nasolacrimal drainage channels become blocked, epiphora can result, which is exacerbated by contact lens wear.

Herpes simplex of the mouth

There is a danger of corneal infection from 'cold sores' when contact lenses are worn. Cold sores on the mouth may be transferred to the eye, either from licking the lenses or by hand. The resultant corneal dendritic ulcers frequently recur and contact lens wear must be discontinued. Once the virus becomes quiescent, it may be possible to refit RGP lenses, which can improve visual acuity but this should only be resumed on medical advice.

Skin conditions and allergic reactions (see also Chapter 18)

Ocular allergies can involve:

- Cornea.
- Conjunctiva (both bulbar and palpebral).
- Limbus.
- Eyelids (skin and margins).

Jennings (1990) produced an excellent summary of the mechanisms involved, their diagnosis and management. Some patients may be hypersensitive to certain plastics (or the residual monomer therein) used in contact lens materials. However, there is a greater risk of hypersensitivity or delayed hypersensitivity to the preservatives in some contact lens solutions and to deposits which form on the lens surface during wear.

Careful questioning about allergies is advisable before fitting (Larke 1985) and the upper tarsal conjunctiva should be examined for any signs of papillary conjunctivitis likely to be of allergic origin.

Atopic individuals are said to be five times more likely to be contact lens intolerant than non-atopic wearers, and should reduce contact lens wearing time during periods of seasonal allergy (Kari & Haahtela 1993).

Hingorani (1999) suggested that patients with seasonal or perennial allergic conjunctivitis may experience more problems with contact lens wear but can obtain satisfactory wearing time with appropriate management.

During lens wear, patients with atopic eye disease may benefit from:

- More rigorous lens hygiene.
- Materials with less tendency to deposition.
- Frequent replacement of lenses.
- Unpreserved artificial tears and lens solutions.

Backman and Bolte (1974) showed that desensitization treatment for chronic allergic conjunctivitis, although lengthy, was successful in most cases and useful for contact lens patients. However, the Committee on Safety of Medicines in the UK (1986) reported a disturbing number of deaths from anaphylaxis during such treatment and it is therefore now undertaken much less frequently.

If there is serious concern that a patient may react to a contact lens material or a solution preservative whose use cannot be avoided, then the patient should be referred for a patch test to be carried out. Wilson (as reported by Rengstorff 1986) stated that patch testing is positive where a hypersensitivity reaction (a gradual build-up of signs and symptoms which is slow to resolve) is likely or has previously occurred. Conversely, patch testing is negative if there has been a toxic reaction where the onset and resolution of signs and symptoms are both rapid.

To minimize allergy/hypersensitivity problems for lenses other than daily disposables (see also Chapter 4), the following are necessary:

- Strict hygiene, to avoid deposit formation.
- Soft lens disinfection systems that avoid the use of preservatives.
- Rinse off cleaning solutions containing preservatives using sterile non-preserved saline.
- Select rigid lens soaking and wetting solutions containing minimum preservatives.
- Rinse off storage solutions prior to lens insertion.
- Clean with non-ionic surfactants to reduce the risk of preservatives binding to the lens surfaces.
- Initiate regular use of protein-removing systems from the outset and ensure that the protein remover is itself thoroughly cleaned and rinsed off, as patients sometimes react to the enzymes used.

SKIN CONDITIONS

Where there are infections of the eye or its adnexa, soft lenses should not be fitted except under medical supervision because of the likelihood of material contamination and the risk of extending the infection.

Instillation of one drop of 1% Rose Bengal shows up desquamated conjunctival and corneal epithelium and mucus, indicative of active or subclinical conditions, which may be irritated by contact lenses (see Chapter 5).

Typical of such conditions are the following, and extra care and prolonged tolerance trials should be undertaken during fitting. If the skin condition worsens or the eye becomes involved during fitting, contact lenses may have to be abandoned.

Acne vulgaris

- Occurs around the age of puberty.
- Not markedly aggravated by contact lens wear.
- Greasing and frothing of the tears may prevent satisfactory wear of any type of lens.
- Prolonged tolerance trials are useful.
- Wetting and soaking solutions containing polyvinyl alcohol minimize greasing of rigid lenses.
- Fit corneal lenses within the palpebral aperture to reduce the massaging effect on the lids, which increases the output of sebum.
- Soft lenses may be satisfactory but lens surfaces rapidly deteriorate due to contamination by sebum from the eyelids (see 'Lid hygiene', Chapter 17).

Acne rosacea

- This is accentuated as the foreign body reaction to contact lenses increases the blood vessel dilatation of the skin of the face and conjunctiva.

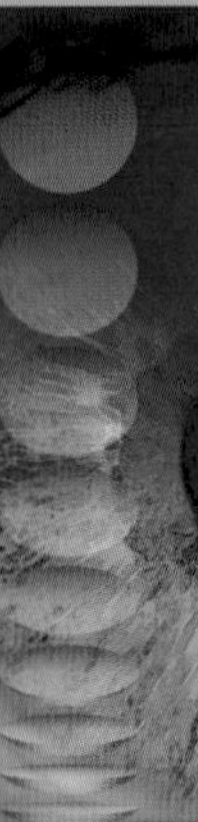

- Punctate keratitis associated with the condition may be exacerbated by contact lens wear.
- In the absence of keratitis, daily wear silicone hydrogel, high water content soft or RGP corneal lenses may be tolerated.
- Alternatively, if contact lenses are essential, scleral lenses, fitted to avoid any corneal touch, may succeed.

Atopic eczema – associated with asthma and hay fever

- Contact lenses may cause an urticarial reaction, less so with soft lenses but the lens surfaces may degrade rapidly due to excessive protein deposits.
- A low wetting angle is more important than oxygen permeability in RGP lens materials. Fluoropolymers (see Chapters 3 and 9) having a high Dk value and also wetting well can be recommended for such patients, although careful temperature-controlled manufacture is necessary to ensure good surfaces. Excess polishing creates a high temperature and can reduce the surface wetting properties. Polymethylmethacrylate (PMMA) and moulded cellulose acetate butyrate (CAB) lenses, although rarely fitted now, have good wetting properties and some PMMA materials were developed to enhance the surface wetting characteristics. These may still be the best materials for some patients, provided that a suitable fit is selected to ensure adequate oxygen supply to the cornea via the retrolens tears.
- Lid irritation from rigid lens edges should be avoided by fitting with minimum peripheral clearance and as large a lens as is practicable, with thin (0.12 mm radial edge thickness) and well-rounded edges (see Chapter 9).

Epidermolysis bullosa (EB)

As already mentioned, EB may necessitate the correction of any refractive error with high water content soft or daily wear silicone hydrogel lenses. Other types of lens are likely to exacerbate the effects of the condition on the eye (Rubinstein 1984). These depend on severity and range from mild blepharitis and conjunctivitis to pronounced vesicle formation over the anterior eye.

Keratoconjunctivitis sicca (Sjögren's syndrome) – associated with rheumatoid arthritis

- There is a lack of tear secretion and filamentary keratitis is common (see Fig. 26.7).
- The lens of choice is a high Dk rigid corneal lens used with artificial tear supplements, and, if necessary, occlusion of the puncta with plugs (O'Callaghan & Phillips 1994).
- Soft lenses are not recommended but silicone hydrogels may prove successful, together with regular instillation of saline solution or artificial tear drops. If lenses dehydrate, they will become unwearable.
- Sealed RGP scleral lenses used with a suitable artificial tear solution (see Chapter 15) also prove satisfactory and assist in protecting the cornea.
- Silicone rubber lenses can be used but are only available currently in aphakic prescriptions.

Psoriasis

Although not directly aggravated by contact lenses, psoriasis may be associated with a nervous disposition, which may lead to a worsening of symptoms during contact lens adaptation. For this reason soft lenses are likely to perform best.

Seborrhoeic eczema

- Manifests as dandruff, blepharitis (see Fig. 18.11) and otitis externa.
- Contact lens wear may exacerbate the problem.
- Contact lenses are contraindicated in the presence of blepharitis (see Chapters 17 and 18).
- If blepharitis can be resolved, soft or silicone hydrogel lenses cause less irritation than rigid lenses.
- Patients should be advised to discontinue lens wear during attacks because of the risk of associated staphylococcal keratoconjunctivitis (Catania 1987).

Xerophthalmia (vitamin A deficiency), congenital ichthyosis (dry skin) and sarcoidosis

The approach to these conditions is similar to that of keratoconjunctivitis sicca. Success is possible with all options but more likely with high Dk RGP corneal lenses or silicone hydrogel lenses.

Voke (1986) reported a case of keratomalacia – the corneal manifestation of xerophthalmia – in a vegan (an extreme vegetarian) whose diet lacked vitamin A and carotenoids. It would therefore seem wise to question all dry-eyed patients about possible dietary causes of their symptoms (see 'Diet', p. 186). Artificial tear drops containing vitamin A may be beneficial.

OCULAR EXAMINATION

A number of different examination techniques must be employed prior to contact lens fitting to assess the suitability of the eyes to lens wear. Some of these techniques are now discussed.

SLIT-LAMP EXAMINATION (see also Chapter 7)

The anterior segment of the eye and adnexa should be examined. Magnification of ×20 is recommended for routine use, with ×40 for examination of detail.

NORMAL SIGNS, USING BROAD OR DIFFUSE ILLUMINATION

Using broad or diffuse illumination with white, red-free and blue light after fluorescein instillation (see below) check the following.

Cornea and limbus

- Dust or eye make-up particles in the tear film which move with blinking. The amount of debris in the tear film is an indicator of the amount of deposit formation likely to occur on contact lenses, and the patient can be forewarned.
- Cell bodies making up the granular structure of the cornea.
- Several very fine nerve fibres. The radial arrangement of myelinated nerve fibres around the limbus usually ceases

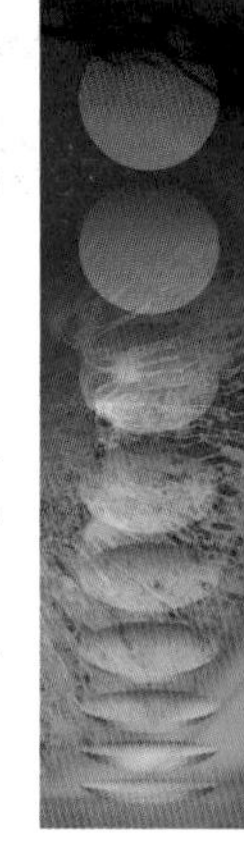

about 1 mm in from the limbus but may extend to the centre of the cornea.

- Limbal blood vessel loops normally encroach into the cornea about 0.25 mm, and a little more than this at the upper limbus.
- Aqueous veins (usually in the horizontal meridian).
- A ring or crescent of more opaque corneal tissue separated from the limbus by a narrow, transparent band more pronounced at the upper limbus. This is normally associated with advancing age (arcus senilis) and consists of cholesterol deposits. If seen at a younger age (less than 50 years), particularly if xanthelasma is also present, it may be indicative of familial hypercholesterolaemia (FHC) associated with heart disease (Winder 1981, Cantle 1988). All such patients should be referred for measurement of blood cholesterol levels and medical advice.
- A fairly common finding is posterior embryotoxon – a narrow, semi-opaque, linear structure situated at the posterior corneal surface about 2 mm from the limbus and running parallel to it, mainly in the horizontal meridian.
- The termination of the endothelium at the anterior chamber angle (Schwalbe's line) is not usually visible except by gonioscopy. However, if tags of endothelium extend into the anterior chamber, or the endothelium is raised at that point, it becomes visible by normal direct illumination with the slit-lamp. When visible like this, the anterior chamber angle is likely to become blocked more easily. Care should be exercised when fitting soft or scleral lenses to avoid corneal oedema near the limbus and the intraocular pressure (IOP) should be regularly checked and compared with pre-fitting values.
- The endothelium should have a uniform hexagonal pattern but pigment cells or fine striate lines may be evident. These might later, subsequent to soft lens wear, be attributed to corneal oedema (see Fig. 13.13).

Bulbar conjunctiva and sclera

- Conjunctival blood vessels appear to move with respect to deeper scleral vessels during blinking and eye movements. Most conjunctival blood vessels are normally almost empty and the conjunctiva is transparent (see Appendix B for reference scale of conjunctival hyperaemia; after McMonnies & Chapman-Davies 1987).
- Pigment, mainly near the limbus, is normal in dark-skinned races but not in those with fair skin.
- The irregularity of the conjunctiva and its looseness at the limbus increase with age.

While these findings are normal, irregularities of the conjunctiva such as those described may encourage xerosis of the conjunctiva and contribute to limbal desiccation of the corneal epithelium at the 3 and 9 o'clock positions during corneal lens wear (see Fig. 17.29).

Plica semilunaris and caruncle

- Fine hairs are normally visible on the caruncle.
- The blood vessels should not appear unduly engorged.
- Both tissues should appear smooth and not granular.

Iris

This should exhibit a fine meshwork of fibres, often with areas of pigment within the fibres.

Pupil

- Small pigment deposits of normal chromatophores and xanthophores are frequently visible on the anterior lens surface.
- Pupillary remnants may be present, arising from the region of the collarette.
- The pupil should be round and reactions normal.

Anterior lens surface

- Epicapsular pigment stars, often associated with pupillary remnants, may be seen.
- 'Orange peel' effect of the anterior capsular epithelium should be visible.

Lid margins

By slightly everting the lids, their margins may be seen under magnification. Any abnormalities, such as blocking of the orifices of the meibomian glands, can be detected. Small marginal cysts, which disappear after a few days, are often visible. They give rise to discomfort when corneal lenses are worn. Slight pressure just above or below the lid margins should result in a clear fluid being expressed.

Lashes

These should be clean and regular.

NORMAL SIGNS, USING A CORNEAL SECTION OR PARALLELIPIPED

The microscope should be centred and the illumination arm eyepieces moved to one side.

Cornea

- Slightly granular in cross-section, with a brighter reflex from both the front surface (lacrimal layer and epithelium) and back surface (endothelium).
- With age, a few iris pigment cells are deposited on the endothelium.
- Corneal guttatae (or Hassall–Henle endothelial warts) appear in old age. Large numbers of guttatae can be an early sign of corneal decompensation, or Fuchs' dystrophy. High Dk lens materials should be used.

Anterior chamber

- Optically empty except for normal pupillary remnants and, with age, a few pigment granules.
- Its depth can be assessed and the chamber angle estimated (van Herick et al. 1969). It is important to rule out patients with shallow anterior chamber angles if highly minus soft lenses, which may cause corneal oedema, are to be fitted, because in soft lens wear the cornea is thought to swell backwards slightly, into the anterior chamber. In such cases,

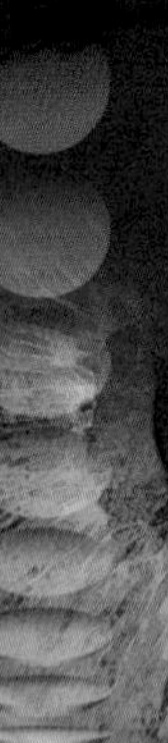

carry out gonioscopy or refer for medical advice before fitting, as there is a small risk of angle closure.

STAINING (see also Chapter 5)

Diagnostic stains may be employed to detect abnormality.

Fluorescein

Cornea

- A drop of 1 or 2% sterile sodium fluorescein solution should be instilled into the conjunctival sac or applied from an impregnated paper strip moistened with sterile saline solution. The excess may be rinsed out with sterile physiological saline solution if necessary.
- Examine the cornea using a suitable blue filter or long-wavelength ultraviolet light (short-wavelength ultraviolet rays are dangerous). Magnification of ×20 will show any staining of the cornea (e.g. see Fig. 17.35).
- Staining is abnormal unless caused by a foreign body (the presence of which may usually be elucidated by questioning the patient), although a few punctate dots of stain, increasing in number with age, are normal in about 20% of the population (Norn 1970).
- Staining of the inferior cornea may indicate poor lid closure during blink or sleep. This is not necessarily a contraindication to contact lens wear but care must be taken.
- More extensive staining indicates the probable need for referral. However, following an illness or head cold, more punctate epitheliopathy may be evident and the cornea absorbs some fluorescein as permeability is increased. This gives only a slight green haze, unlike the bright green stain of an abraded area. When the corneal permeability is grossly increased, some fluorescein may enter the anterior chamber.

Lacrimal drainage

- The patency of the puncta and lacrimal drainage channels may be demonstrated by asking the patient to blow their nose on to a paper tissue, which should stain green and fluoresce from the sodium fluorescein. Each side should be checked separately.
- It is unwise to proceed with fitting if the nasolacrimal passages are blocked, as the conjunctival sac may not be sterile. In addition, the excess tear production caused by some contact lenses may lead to epiphora in such a case.
- Decongestant eye and/or nasal drops should be used or, if necessary, the nasolacrimal passages should be irrigated.
- Epithelial debris, blocking the nasolacrimal passages, is common in catarrh and hay fever sufferers, and in those with dry eyes. This may help dry-eyed patients, permitting the available tears to be retained on the eye.
- Where contact lens fitting is essential, but the nasolacrimal drainage channels remain blocked, fitting should proceed with extra care and the patient advised about risks of eye infection.

Rose Bengal

- Not commonly used in routine practice (see Chapters 5 and 17).
- A drop of 1% solution or impregnated paper strips should not reveal any marked corneal or conjunctival staining.
- Where such staining is apparent, it is best observed using red-free illumination and low magnification with the slit-lamp microscope. As this indicates that tear output may be reduced or an abnormal skin condition may exist, contact lens fitting should be undertaken with caution.
- The mucus strip along the lid margins normally stains red. If mucus detaches from the lid margin during contact lens wear and adheres to the lens or floats in the precorneal film it may interfere with vision.
- Heavy staining of the lid margin may indicate a posterior blepharitis.
- Rose Bengal stings, particularly in dry eyes, and should be instilled after fluorescein, otherwise it may cause the appearance of punctate staining with fluorescein. Well-moistened impregnated strips sting significantly less.

SENSITIVITY

- An anaesthetic cornea is abnormal and contact lenses should only be fitted under medical supervision (for fitting anaesthetic corneas, see Chapter 26).
- People with insensitive corneas readily accept contact lenses, as abrasions caused by poorly fitting lenses do not cause discomfort, so extra care is needed and the patient must be warned of the risks.
- Sensitivity may be quickly checked by gently holding the lids apart and, avoiding the lashes, touch a wisp of sterile cotton wool on to the cornea from one side, so that its approach is not seen by the patient. A normal blink reflex response should result from both apical and limbal touch. More refined measurements of sensitivity are useful if there is any doubt (see Chapter 7).
- Reduced sensitivity follows corneal grafting as well as interstitial keratitis or past ulceration of the cornea.
- Refractive surgery techniques such as photo-refractive keratectomy (PRK) and laser-assisted in situ keratomileusis (LASIK) can cause a reduction in corneal sensitivity.
- Following low Dk rigid and soft contact lens wear, sensitivity is reduced but recovery rapid (Millodot 1976).

PACHOMETRY (PACHYMETRY) (see Chapter 7)

- An optical pachometer (pachymeter) used in conjunction with the slit-lamp measures corneal thickness. Nowadays ultrasound pachometers are generally used.
- Corneal thinning or irregularity as in keratoconus should, if marked, be noted prior to fitting.
- Corneal thickening indicates oedema, so baseline measurements can be useful as a reference for future measurements.
- The majority of normal corneas lie between 0.50 and 0.60 mm.

CLASSIC KERATOMETRY (see Chapter 7)

Keratometry measures:

- Curvature of the anterior surface of the central cornea – normal corneas measure within the range 7.2–8.6 mm. Radii

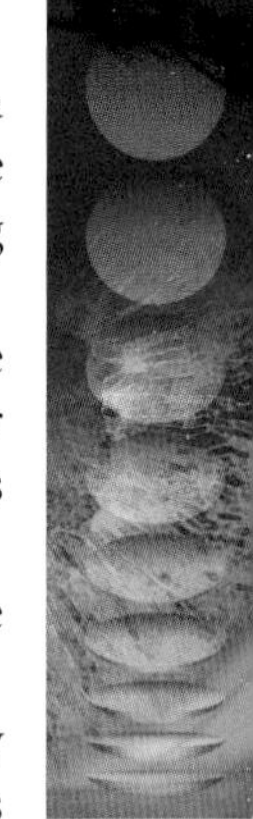

outside this range may indicate abnormalities. Steep radii may indicate keratoconus and flat radii possibly megalocornea (large cornea), Marfan's syndrome or cornea plana (flat radii).
- Corneal astigmatism. A toric cornea may prove difficult to fit and require extra fitting time. A difference between ocular and corneal astigmatism indicates uncorrected astigmatism with a rigid spherical lens, possibly requiring a bi-toric design (see Chapters 6, 9 and 12). Where rigid lenses are unsuitable, toric soft lenses may be better.

Any surface irregularities seen with the keratometer should be investigated prior to fitting.

CORNEAL ANALYSIS OR TOPOGRAPHY (see also Chapters 7, 9 and 19)

Computerized corneal topography analyses almost the entire front surface of the cornea. This is useful:

- When fitting contact lenses to normal corneas to assess the amount of peripheral corneal flattening in order to estimate eccentricity.
- Where the peripheral topography is irregular.

Refractive surgical techniques such as radial keratotomy and laser keratectomy (see Chapter 23) result in the peripheral cornea becoming steeper than the central cornea (oblate shape). Contact lenses may be required afterwards to eliminate residual refractive errors. Oblate corneas are also created by orthokeratology (see Chapter 19). It is important, therefore, to be able to map the entire corneal contour (Sanders & Koch 1992).

Instruments for corneal analysis (video-keratoscopes) (Mandell 1992) such as the Medmont Topographer, the EyeSys Corneal Topography system and the TMS (Topographic Modelling System) have evolved from the Placido disc, a flat disc composed of alternate black and white concentric rings with a central viewing lens. This enables the radii of curvature of the peripheral cornea and the rate of flattening from apex to periphery to be determined and is still occasionally used. Any distortion of shape or continuity in the appearance of the rings reflected from the cornea indicates a surface defect; for example the rings appear oval by reflection from a highly astigmatic cornea and the central rings may appear crowded and displaced when reflected from a keratoconic cornea.

TEAR OUTPUT (see Chapter 5)

A normal tear output and precorneal film are essential for comfortable, trouble-free contact lens wear. When the tear output or constituents are abnormal, problems such as greasing and deposit formation on the lenses occur. Dry eyes or lenses may lead to desiccation and infection.

The presence of foam in the tear film at the outer canthus is fairly normal (Norn 1963), but foam along the lower lid margin may be associated with instability of the tear film due to reduced meibomian secretion (Larke 1985). Blinking and the presence of foreign bodies such as contact lenses increase its production. The production of excessive mucus during a tolerance trial is a contraindication to fitting, as is excessive meibomian activity, which may give rise to subsequent greasing problems.

Both insufficient and excessive tear output can indicate some abnormality of the lacrimal or conjunctival glands or their nerve supply, and diseases causing discomfort give rise to excess tears (Phelps-Brown 1987).

Tear output is also affected by diet and by certain drugs (see below).

To fit lenses to a dry cornea can be harmful: soft lenses may alter curvature considerably on dry eyes and all types of lens may only be fitted if saline solution or artificial tears are repeatedly instilled.

Excessive tears will increase lens movement and affect centration. If the tear excess is due to disease, any type of contact lens is contraindicated without medical investigation. Fitting a larger total diameter RGP or soft lens may help.

TEAR MEASUREMENT

In 1961, Schirmer and Mellor described a now commonly used test for the measurement of aqueous volume. Another simple test is the phenol-red thread (PRT) test developed by Hamano et al. (1983) whereby a phenol-impregnated cotton thread is used in place of a Schirmer test paper (see Chapter 5).

The break-up time (BUT test) of the precorneal film should also be carried out (see 'Precorneal film', below).

Normal and abnormal signs – effect on lens fitting

SCLERA AND BULBAR CONJUNCTIVA (see above)

Pingueculae (see Fig. 17.29) – fat deposited with age in the conjunctiva within the region of the palpebral aperture – appears as thickened yellow irregularities. These are also associated with exposure to hot, dry atmospheres and UV radiation, and are found in many people who lead an outdoor life, particularly in hot, dry countries when the pingueculae may progress to become pterygia. Pingueculae are apt to be irritated by any sort of contact lens and patients should be warned of potential conjunctival hyperaemia, which may detract from their cosmetic appearance. With corneal lenses, 3 and 9 o'clock drying of the cornea may result (see Chapters 9 and 17). Care should be taken when fitting any contact lens to an eye having a limbal nodule, elevation or pre-existing pannus.

Pterygia (see Fig. 17.30) or old operation scars may make contact lenses difficult to fit and may be irritated by the presence of the lens. When large corneal lenses are worn, which knock the limbus, any loose conjunctival tissue becomes easily injected, inviting new blood vessel growth.

LIDS

The upper palpebral conjunctiva comes into contact with almost the entire front surface of a contact lens during blinking and lid closure, while the lower lid barely covers the lower part of a lens. The following must be considered:

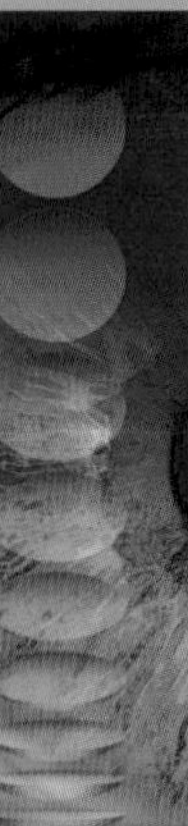

- Abnormal or excessive concretions or other elevations of the upper palpebral conjunctiva. The patient should be referred for treatment before fitting, although contact lenses may make the eye more comfortable in the presence of multiple concretions by protecting the cornea.
- Mild follicles and papillae (when blood vessels are present in the raised area) are normal nasally and temporally and along the sulcus but the area overlying the tarsal plate should be smooth (Larke 1985). If evident in this area, they are suggestive of allergy such as vernal conjunctivitis, and contact lens fitting should proceed with caution. Thin soft lenses are not advisable as the roughness of the lids may result in excessive movement.
- Check the depth of the fornices before fitting as past injury or surgery may restrict the limits of the conjunctival sac, making soft and scleral lenses either unsuitable or difficult to fit (see Chapters 15 and 26).

Due attention should be paid to hygiene and minimizing any possible irritants, such as surface deposits or poorly formed lens edges, or the preservatives of solutions, etc.

Ptosis

Special scleral lenses can be fitted where there is ptosis of the upper lid. The right and left eyelids should be compared and any slight tendency to ptosis noted in order to differentiate it later from possible contact-lens-induced ptosis. Levy and Stamper (1992) and Vanden Bosch and Lemij (1992) described ptosis following rigid lens wear, some in one eye only (see Chapter 9). This can also occur with soft lenses, when one eyelid swells and droops in association with contact-lens-induced papillary conjunctivitis.

Blepharospasm

If persistent, this can be a nuisance to corneal lens wearers as considerable discomfort ensues. In such cases scleral lenses may help. Soft lenses may be satisfactory but the excessive lid pressure may distort or move the lens.

The cause of the blepharospasm should be investigated before fitting, although people who are apprehensive about wearing lenses may exhibit excessive blepharospasm, due to nervousness, which subsequently disappears.

Blepharitis (see also Chapter 18 and Seborrhoeic eczema, p. 178)

Patients should not be fitted with lenses as there is a risk of corneal infection. Corneal lenses can give rise to discomfort and lid soreness if lid margins are sensitive.

Other lid conditions

- *Recurrent styes* or lid margin growths are a contraindication.
- *Absence of lashes* – a sign of eczema and/or alopecia – fitting should proceed with care: the patient (and practitioner) may have difficulty in gripping the lids during insertion and removal of lenses.
- *Parasites* may be encountered among the eyelashes and must be cleared before contact lenses are fitted:
  - *Demodex folliculorum* (Coston 1967), which breeds in the eyelash follicles, can be removed using a cotton bud soaked in alcohol carefully applied to the lashes.
  - Londer (1987) reported finding canine lice, which were cleared with liquid paraffin (Lacri-Lube) ointment. Parasite infestation gives the appearance of blepharitis.

Palpebral aperture size and lid tightness

These affect the size of any corneal lens fitted:

- Small palpebral apertures and tight lids need small lenses.
- Large palpebral apertures and loose lids need larger lenses.

Physiologically, small lid apertures have a greater temperature increase behind the contact lens (Hill & Leighton 1965) and a reduction in the tear pump efficiency, i.e. the amount of oxygen supplied to the cornea via the tears (Fink et al. 1990). Temperature increase raises metabolic rate, which, if not met by sufficient oxygen, leads to corneal oedema. Thus, for less oxygen-permeable materials, a smaller area of eye should be covered.

An excessive temperature rise leads to evaporation of tears and the formation of salt deposits at the canthi. This may be due to the foreign body sensation of an RGP lens leading to partial eyelid closure. Small, mid to high water content soft or silicone hydrogel lenses may be preferable as they are least likely to upset corneal metabolism.

Lacrimal gland

This should be checked for normal size, position and colour. If it is large and prominent and scleral lenses are to be fitted, the temporal portion of the lens must be made sufficiently thin to slide under the gland without bumping it.

Precorneal film (see Chapter 5)

A number of qualitative tests may be used to assess the normality of the precorneal film prior to fitting contact lenses. This area is covered in Chapter 5 but some aspects are discussed briefly here.

Even if one tear assessment test shows poor results, patients should not necessarily be rejected from lens wear as a different type of lens or modality of wear may be successful.

The wettability of the tear layer is a function of the mucoid layer, and its efficiency may be judged by observing through the biomicroscope the reflection of an ordinary movable lamp in the lacrimal fluid or tear prism at the lower lid margin (see Fig. 5.5). This prism has three zones:

- Upper convex zone against the lower cornea.
- Middle concave zone at the centre of the rivus.
- Lower convex zone at the limit of the tear layer on the rear of the lower lid.

As the lamp is slowly moved up and down, three bright reflections should be seen in the prism – the upper and lower zones giving a 'with' movement and the centre zone an 'against' movement. It may be necessary to ask the patient to look downwards to see all three, but if all or parts of these reflections are missing, the wettability of the tears is abnormal.

The quality of the surface lipid (oily) layer, which controls the rate of evaporation of the tears, can be judged by looking at

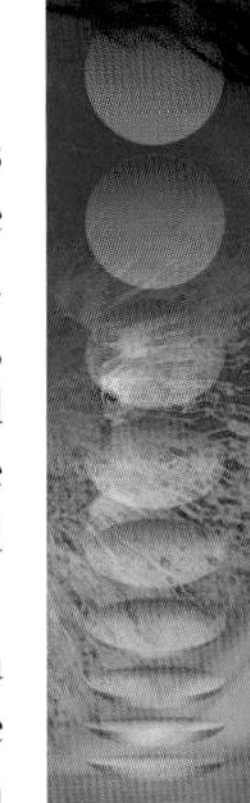

the corneal surface reflection of the lamp. The patient should blink normally about once every 4 seconds, and the reflection of the lamp should remain bright. If streaks of interference colours appear, the tear layer is too thin (or there is too great an evaporation rate). If the reflection is irregular and pocked, the surface is very dry.

The interference patterns and viscosity assessment indicate the quantity and quality of the tear film which in turn affects the fit and comfort of lenses, and what cleaning solutions are best for the particular patient.

A rolled oily deposit may be left on the lower third of the cornea after each blink, visible with a wide slit beam. Lowther et al. (1970) and Young and Hill (1973) found this was more noticeable after a high cholesterol intake and suggested that tear chemistry may be related to diet.

Polse (1975) suggested that a deficiency of mucus production results in corneal dry spots which show up when the tear film is seen to break up into droplets. The test is known as the BUT (break-up-time) test. It is seen most easily by applying fluorescein below the cornea and observing with the slit-lamp, using blue light and the largest possible circular aperture to illuminate the entire cornea. The patient is instructed to make one complete blink and then hold the eyes wide open. In Caucasians, dry spots, which show up as black areas within the fluorescein-covered corneal surface (see Fig. 5.3), usually only appear if the lids are held apart for 20 seconds or more after a complete blink, whereas they appear within 10 seconds after a complete blink in certain pathological and dry-eye conditions and if there is a mucus deficiency (Lemp et al. 1970, 1971, Koetting 1976). Cho and Brown (1993) showed that Hong Kong Chinese have an acceptably shorter non-invasive break-up time (NIBUT) (mean 7.6 seconds) than Hong Kong Caucasians (mean 10.8 seconds).

Guillon (1986) stated that instillation of fluorescein upsets stability of the tear film and that it is preferable to observe the lipid layer using the Tearscope (see Chapter 5).

Other non-invasive tests include the tear thinning time (TTT) when, following a few blinks, the time taken for the keratometer mire images to become distorted or out-of-focus in any way while the eye remains open, is recorded (Patel et al. 1988, Patel & Farrell 1989), and similar tests for NIBUT using grid patterns reflected in the tear film such as the Mengher grid (Mengher et al. 1985) and the Loveridge grid – a modified Klein keratoscope (Loveridge 1993).

Puncta

The puncta should be examined and their apposition to the globe checked. Abnormalities which result in poor tear drainage contraindicate contact lens wear.

Punctum plugs can be used for dry-eyed patients to prevent existing tears from draining. Dissolvable collagen plugs can be used to determine whether more permanent silicon plugs are likely to be successful. Tomlinson and Giesbrecht (1993) suggested that reduced tear production with age is at least partially offset by a reduced drainage facility, probably caused by some obstruction, as they found no change in evaporation rate of the tear film with age.

Pupil size and reactions

Reactions should be normal. The maximum pupil size is measured in ultraviolet illumination in a dark room when the fluorescence of the crystalline lens shows up the pupil size. Large pupils create difficulties for some corneal lens wearers, particularly motorists who drive at night, when flare around headlights may be annoying if the optic zone is smaller than the pupil size. Wearers of bifocal contact lenses may suffer flare and monocular diplopia if pupils are large.

Deeper anterior chambers require larger optic zones for a given pupil diameter (Stone 1959). Modern RGP lenses are fitted with large back optic zones and total diameters, and with minimum peripheral corneal clearance, all of which help to reduce flare (see Chapter 9).

Soft lenses should give rise to fewer problems of flare, although the problem may still occur with bifocals and lenses with poor surfaces.

Iris

Normality should be established. Special lenses may be fitted if the iris is wholly or partially absent, to occlude the unwanted iris apertures. This can result in a considerable improvement in vision. Soft, corneal or scleral lenses may be used depending on the severity of the condition (see Chapter 25).

Exophthalmos or enophthalmos

After any pathology has been medically reviewed, lenses can be fitted. Corneal lenses may have to be fitted slightly steep in order to be retained on the cornea in exophthalmos and there is a risk of reduced tear flow behind the lens.

Scleral lenses may improve the cosmesis in enophthalmos, but it is rare that they would be fitted for this reason alone and would need to be made small to facilitate insertion and removal.

OPHTHALMOSCOPY

This is carried out to check the media and fundi to establish absence of abnormalities. Any persistent disturbance of the normal red fundus reflex should be noted in case it is later mistaken for the after-effects of contact lens wear.

VISUAL FIELDS

These should be checked if there are any doubts about their normality. In general, contact lenses improve the visual field compared to spectacles (see Chapter 6), especially in higher prescriptions.

TONOMETRY

This is usually carried out if raised IOP is suspected, and routinely in the over-40 age group.

There is a possible risk that some soft lenses might increase IOP by pressing on the anterior ciliary veins (see above). Tonometry should therefore be checked both before and after fitting whenever there is any concern.

VISUAL ACUITY AND REFRACTION

In theory, contact lenses should give better visual acuity than spectacles as there are no oblique aberrations or distortion with contact lenses. However, this is not always the case:

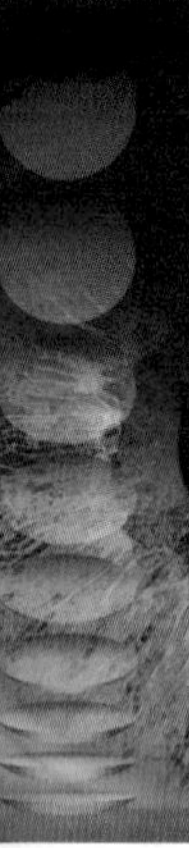

- Contact lenses frequently suffer from surface contamination, which leads to reduced visual acuity and veiling glare.
- Soft lenses may alter power while on the eye, and rigid lenses may flex (see Chapter 9).
- High-power lenses have steeply curved front surfaces and the slightest movement of the lens on the eye may effect a power change due to spherical aberration, affecting the acuity.
- The back vertex distance of the spectacle lens from the eye increases the retinal image size, which improves acuity in hypermetropes. Unfortunately, the better spectacle acuity may not be compatible with good binocular vision, and the weight of the spectacle lenses and reduced field may be unacceptable.

Myopes (see also Chapter 21)

Effects are all proportional to the power of the lenses.

- Contact lenses produce a bigger retinal image than spectacles, which can lead to initial disorientation with contact lenses but should give better visual acuity.
- More accommodation and convergence are required than with spectacles (see Chapter 6) so myopes tend to experience near-vision difficulties not encountered with spectacles, although the accommodation–convergence relationship remains the same (Stone 1967).
- In contact lenses, myopes must move their eyes more as objects appear further from the central point of fixation.
- Myopes' eyes look bigger in contact lenses as the reduced magnification of spectacles has been removed.

Hypermetropes

In hypermetropia, the effects of contact lenses are the opposite of those for myopes. Smaller retinal images are obtained than with spectacles, and the eyes look smaller than in spectacles. Less accommodation and convergence are required and the eyes have to move less than with spectacles.

Astigmats

Spectacle wearers learn to compensate for the distortion of the retinal image afforded by an astigmatic spectacle correction. This compensation by the brain is continued when contact lenses are first worn, and gives rise to a feeling of distortion which usually soon disappears.

Residual astigmatism in rigid lenses can be predicted by comparing ocular (spectacle) astigmatism with corneal (keratometry) astigmatism and a suitable lens construction chosen (see Chapters 6 and 12).

Ocular astigmatism greater than 1 D indicates that a toric lens may be necessary. Where corneal astigmatism neutralizes crystalline lens astigmatism, soft lenses are optically ideal, provided the corneal astigmatism is not so great as to affect the fit.

Anisometropes (see also Chapters 6, 21 and 24)

Most congenital anisometropia is axial (Sorsby et al. 1962) so, theoretically, retinal image sizes are more likely to be similar with a spectacle correction rather than contact lenses but in practice this is not the case. Contact lenses often give rise to better binocular vision than spectacles (Winn et al. 1986).

Crystalline lens changes, which cause a myopic shift (nuclear sclerosis) may be greater in one eye, leading to refractive anisometropia: contact lenses are then ideal – especially disposable or frequent replacement lenses – as they give better binocular vision and can be altered as the nuclear sclerosis worsens.

Contact lenses are likely to be optically satisfactory for young anisometropes and refractive anisometropes, but where a spectacle correction affords good binocular vision in high anisometropia and has done so for many years, contact lenses may cause aniseikonia and a tolerance trial should be carried out.

BINOCULAR VISION

It may be found that non-comitant heterophorias are noticed when contact lenses are first fitted, as the brain continues to compensate for the ocular movements made with the anisometropic spectacle correction.

Unilateral aphakia is an example in which a contact lens correction may give binocular vision where spectacles will not. However, a contact lens is worn some distance in front of the nodal point of the eye and residual aniseikonia may preclude binocular vision. The patient may then prefer monocular vision to the asthenopic symptoms of disturbed binocularity.

Heterotropias

Contact lenses perform as well as spectacles in the treatment and correction of squints.

- A full prescription will correct a fully accommodative squint in the same way as spectacles and the cosmetic advantage of contact lenses may encourage their wear.
- Disposable lenses permit variations in negative additions for exotropes to be made.
- Where bifocals would be prescribed, contact lenses can be worn for general purposes with additional spectacles for close work.
- Difficulties arise where there is a vertical element or a residual high heterophoria requiring prismatic correction (see below).
- Most patients requiring refractive corrections for heterotropias are children. Soft lenses are quicker to adapt to and cause less discomfort and, if used in combination with spectacles, the latter can provide any necessary cylindrical or prism correction.

High heterophorias

- Only about 4 prism dioptres (Δ) can be satisfactorily incorporated into a contact lens.
- With soft and corneal lenses, the base always rotates downwards, which limits any prismatic correction to 4 Δ base-down.
- In practice, 2 Δ is a more reasonable figure because, with too much prism, the lower edge is thick, leading to discomfort.
- The prism base usually takes up a slightly nasal position due to lid action.

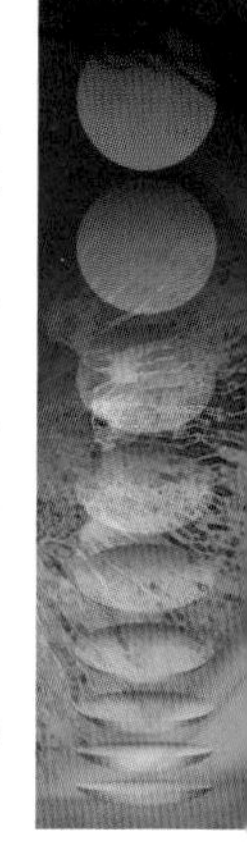

- Only with scleral lenses can the prism base be put in any direction, as long as the scleral zone is a good fit and the lens does not rotate.
- Myopes often require less prism in contact lenses than in spectacles, presumably because the bigger retinal image size with contact lenses affords a better binocular lock.
- The minimum prism to eliminate any fixation disparity and/or symptoms should be prescribed.

Amblyopia

Care is needed to ensure that any improved visual acuity given by contact lenses does not give rise to insuperable diplopia. As visual acuity improves, orthoptic exercises may help consolidate any potential binocular vision.

Eye movements

Pareses of extraocular muscles give rise to diplopia with contact lenses as with spectacles. As already mentioned, contact lenses can affect the amount of eye movement required because they remove the prismatic effects of spectacle lenses, so that both version and vergence movements may be affected.

Aniseikonia

A combination of spectacles and contact lenses can be used to create size differences to relieve symptoms due to aniseikonia. The principles are those of a Galilean telescope system, similar to the type used as an aid to the partially sighted (see Chapter 29 and p. 176).

Uniocularity

Contact lenses are a hazard – even if a very slight one – and it may be in the best interest of a uniocular patient, or one with intractable amblyopia in one eye, not to fit contact lenses for purely cosmetic reasons. If patients are to be fitted, they should be warned of the risk. Spectacles should have toughened lenses.

PERSONAL AND EXTERNAL FACTORS

Age and gender

Incentive, enthusiasm and handling ability are generally better in younger people, although there are exceptions. Presbyopic patients need bifocal lenses or monovision (although these have certain limitations – see Chapter 14) or to wear reading spectacles over their single vision lenses.

Andres et al. (1987) found the tear film BUT insignificantly greater (i.e. better) in men than in women, but they did find a significant reduction in BUT with age.

Corneal sensitivity reduces with age (Millodot 1977). In women, it is affected by the menstrual cycle, reducing considerably during the premenstruum and menstruation (Millodot & Lamont 1974, Guttridge 1994), although the beneficial effect on contact lens wear from the slight loss of sensitivity may be offset by other changes (see below).

The eyelid tissue slackens with age providing less support to a corneal lens. Other changes associated with ageing lead to less-efficient tear drainage from the conjunctival sac, which in some people is beneficial (see 'Puncta', above). Each case must be assessed individually.

Women undergoing the menopause may experience difficulties with their lenses as xerosis sometimes occurs.

Occasionally hormonal changes during pregnancy or menopause can lead to psychological disturbances and consequent loss of motivation to wear lenses. Pregnancy can also disturb contact lens wear, presumably due to metabolic changes in the cornea (Imafidon et al. 1993).

The change in hormone balance alters the water content of all tissues, including the cornea and lids, which may result in a corneal thickness or curvature change and a consequent alteration in lens fit. Lenses can become dramatically tighter, with little peripheral clearance where plenty existed before. Although modifications or refitting can be carried out, it should be borne in mind that, at the end of the pregnancy, the cornea will return to its original state and the new fitting will become loose and uncomfortable.

Soft lenses cause different problems from rigid lenses. Tear output is often reduced during periods of water retention and this, coupled with corneal curvature and thickness changes, can make soft lens wear difficult. Similar effects were recorded in women taking oral contraceptives (Koetting 1966), although with modern drugs, the effects are minimal. Tomlinson et al. (2001) found no effect on tear physiology for serum hormone changes induced by oral contraceptives or in normal cyclic variations in healthy young females.

Guttridge (1994) discussed the ocular changes associated with the menstrual cycle, most of which may affect contact lens wear to a greater or lesser extent as all the ocular tissues and adnexa may be involved.

Skin, hair and eye colouring

Millodot (1975) showed that, in general, corneal sensitivity was greater in people with blue eyes and fair skin, although Henderson et al. (2005) refuted this and Simpson et al. (2003) found no association between eye colour and corneal sensitivity to either mechanical or chemical stimuli.

The authors find that auburn-haired patients with fair freckled skin may be sensitive to rigid lenses and, if appropriate, soft lenses may be preferable.

Ability to handle lenses

Contact lenses should not be supplied unless the patient can handle them properly. A light (neutral) handling tint may help. In cases such as aphakia, a spectacle frame can be supplied, glazed to a suitable prescription on one side only, the other being left empty and the lower rim removed. The first contact lens is then inserted through the empty 'eye' of the frame, which enables the patient to see it with the other eye. The frame is then removed, as the patient is able to see the second lens with the first in place.

Patients with clumsy or shaky hands may be better with extended wear lenses, provided they are otherwise suitable. Someone close to the patient should, if possible, be taught

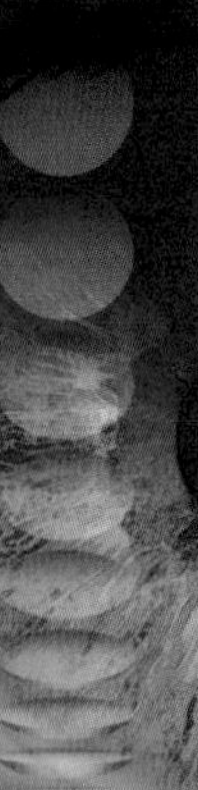

insertion and removal and be given all the necessary information, so that the lenses may be removed and cleaned periodically (see Chapter 11).

Some soft lenses are easier to handle than others, thin and ultrathin being most difficult.

Working and living conditions

Certain conditions make lens wear difficult:

- Dusty and smoky atmospheres.
- Hot or cold temperatures.
- Windy weather.
- Dry or humid atmospheres.

Some examples of difficult conditions include the following:

- Aircraft cabins have low humidity, leading to lens dehydration and discomfort. By contrast, hot, humid conditions do not seem to affect soft lenses (Fatt & Rocher 1994).
- People working in rarefied atmospheres or at high altitudes may suffer corneal oedema due to lack of oxygen.
- Soft lenses are contraindicated for people coming into contact with noxious fumes such as workers in the chemical industry.

Lighting

- In poor light, the pupil dilates and flare may result (see 'Pupil size and reactions', p. 183).
- In bright light, a tint may be helpful although tinted spectacles worn over the contact lenses may be more practical.
- The tint depends on the absorption required and the colour rendering, as the wavelength of some monochromatic illumination may not be transmitted by the tinted contact lens, which is dangerous. A neutral density tint is therefore preferable (Fletcher & Nisted 1963).
- Tints affect dark adaptation.
- Some countries have a legal limit on the maximum light absorption permissible for night driving.

UV-inhibiting lenses

The types of UV radiation are:

- UV-A – 315–400 nm.
- UV-B – 280–315 nm.
- UV-C – 100–280 nm.

with some overlap of wavelength between them.

According to Pitts (reported by Kerr 1987), those particularly at risk include:

- Aphakics and pseudophakics.
- Cataract patients suffering glare due to lenticular scatter.
- Those taking photosensitizing drugs such as sulphonamides, tetracyclines and oral contraceptives.
- People who spend hours in bright sunlight (e.g. when sunbathing, skiing or mountaineering).
- Those suffering from pingueculae, pterygia and macular degeneration.
- Workers in vocations which expose them to large amounts of UV-B, such as welders, electronics workers and graphic artists.

Contact lenses are readily available in soft and rigid materials, and manufacturers can supply details of the transmission curves of materials which absorb ultraviolet radiations below about 400 nm (see also Chapters 9 and 29).

Some RGP lenses develop surface cracking (see Fig. 9.25) and fracture spontaneously. Silk (1987, 1988) attributed this to the build-up of static on the lenses, which may affect the polarity of the material and its surfaces. Some people are more static sensitive than others, and many artificial fibres encourage the build-up of static charges. In extreme cases, this may cause epithelial damage. The effects are worse in cold, dry conditions than wet or humid ones. Thus people wearing synthetic clothing or walking on synthetic carpets, or even playing football on synthetic pitches, may experience more problems with their RGP lenses than at other times.

Drugs

Drugs can influence metabolism, which in turn may influence contact lens wear, and extended tolerance trials may be advisable before prescribing. Examples include:

- Women on hormone treatment and people on steroids, both of which can affect tear output and result in corneal oedema (see 'Age and gender', above).
- Thyroxine treatment has been reported to cause intolerance to contact lenses (Marsh 1975).
- Tear output may be reduced and lysozyme concentration altered with:
  - beta-blockers (Mackie et al. 1977).
  - diuretics (Bergman et al. 1985).
- Antihistamines and tricyclic antidepressants have also been found to cause dry eyes.

Check on the side-effects of any regular medication taken by a patient. Those reported to cause a dry mouth are also likely to cause dry eyes. Reference to the Data Sheet Compendium produced annually by the Association of the British Pharmaceutical Industry (ABPI), or similar publication, is recommended.

Diet

As already indicated (see 'Xerophthalmia', p. 178 and 'Precorneal film', p. 182), diet can affect the state of the eye and in particular the quality of the tears and their output (see Chapter 5).

- A high-cholesterol diet, as well as obesity, can increase cholesterol levels in the tears (Terry & Hill 1975, Hill & Terry 1976).
- A deficiency in potassium and sodium was found in patients with coated lenses (Lane 1985). Increasing folic acid, ascorbic acid, vitamin B6 and potassium, and decreasing sugar intake (which reduces potassium in the body) succeeded, within 1 month, in treating those with coated lenses, and many of the dry-eyed patients improved after several months.

Habits

Hygiene is essential when handling contact lenses. Eye rubbing should be discouraged, and preferably both active and passive smoking avoided as soft lenses may become discoloured, and nicotine on the fingers can cause eye irritation if transferred via contact lenses.

Hobbies

Although most RGP corneal lenses can be fitted to give minimum peripheral clearance, making them relatively difficult to dislodge, they are still less stable than soft or scleral lenses. Soft lenses are the lens of choice for virtually all sports including high-altitude mountaineering. However, in order to avoid such infection as acanthamoeba, patients should be advised, where possible, to swim without lenses or to use swimming goggles.

Neither the Sports Council in the United Kingdom nor the Sports Vision Association issues specific advice about contact lens wear. The regulating authority of each particular sport must be consulted regarding permission to wear contact lenses for professional sports.

When wearing contact lenses on stage, arc lights can produce photophobia. Various tints are available, as are lenses having artificial iris patterns (see Chapters 25 and 29).

Some rigid lens wearers, before they are fully adapted, find certain head postures and eye movements cause discomfort; for example looking up when playing snooker or making rapid lateral eye movements when copy typing.

Looking down continuously (e.g. doing embroidery) reduces the palpebral aperture size. This may lead to corneal oedema (see 'Palpebral aperture size and lid tightness', above).

Special occupations

Restrictions regarding the wearing of contact lenses may apply while driving, piloting an aircraft and serving in the armed forces or emergency services as well as in certain other occupations. Such restrictions may vary from country to country and regulations regarding the use of contact lenses should be requested from the appropriate vehicle or driver/pilot licensing authority in that country or from the prospective employer.

SUMMARY

Sufficient has now been said about indications, contraindications and selection of patients and contact lenses, as well as the factors to be considered in the choice of the best type of lens to fit. The reader must realize that both frustration and satisfaction are to be the lot of the contact lens practitioner at different times and with different patients.

References

Andres, S., Henriquez, A., Garcia, M. L., Valero, J. and Valls, O. (1987) Factors of the precorneal tear film break-up time (BUT) and tolerance of contact lenses. Int. Contact Lens Clin., 14, 103–107

Backman, H. and Bolte, C. (1974) Chronic allergic conjunctivitis and its effect on contact lenses. Optom. Wkly, 65(31), 26–30

Bergmann, M. T., Newman, B. L. and Johnson, N. C. (1985) The effect of a diuretic (hydrochlorothiazide) on tear production in humans. Am. J. Ophthalmol., 99, 473–475

Bruch, C. W. (1973) Eye products: handle with care. Optician, 166(4297), 22, 27

Cantle, S. (1988) Cholesterol and the eye. Optician, 195(5141), 29

Catania, L. J. (1987) Contact lenses, staphylococcus, and 'Crocodile OD'. Int. Contact Lens Clin., 14, 113–115

Cho, P. and Brown, B. (1993) Review of the tear break-up time and a closer look at the tear break-up time of Hong Kong Chinese. Optom. Vis. Sci., 70, 30–38

Committee on Safety of Medicines (1986) Desensitising vaccines. BMJ, 293, 948

Coston, T. O (1967) Demodex folliculorum blepharitis. Trans. Am. Ophthalmol. Soc., 65, 361–392

Davis, L. J., Paragina, S. and Kincaid, M. C. (1992) Mascara pigmentation of the bulbar conjunctiva associated with rigid gas permeable lens wear. Optom. Vis. Sci., 69, 66–71

Fatt, I. and Rocher, P. (1994) Contact lens performance in different climates. Optom. Today, 34(2), 26–31

Fink, B. A., Carney, L. G. and Hill, R. M. (1990) Influence of palpebral aperture height on tear pump efficiency. Optom. Vis. Sci., 67, 287–290

Fletcher, R. J. and Nisted, M. (1963) A study of coloured contact lenses and their performance. Ophthalmol. Opt., 3, 1151–1154, 1161–1163, 1203–1206, 1212–1213

Guillon, J-P. (1986) Observing and photographing the pre-corneal and pre-lens tear film. Contax, November, 15–22

Guttridge, N. M. (1994) Changes in ocular and visual variables during the menstrual cycle. Ophthalmic Physiol. Opt., 14, 38–48

Hamano, H., Hori, M., Hamano, T. et al. (1983) A new method for measuring tears. CLAO J., 9, 281–289

Henderson, L., Bond, D. and Simpson, T. (2005) The association between eye color and corneal sensitivity measured using a Belmonte esthesiometer. Optom. Vis. Sci., 82(7), 629–632

Hill, R. M. and Leighton, A. J. (1965) Temperature changes of human cornea and tears under a contact lens. Part II: Effects of intermediate lid apertures and gaze. Am. J. Optom., 42, 71–77

Hill, R. M. and Terry, J. E. (1976) Human tear cholesterol levels. Arch. Ophthalmol., 36, 155–160

Hingorani, M. (1999) The compromised eye: tear film abnormalities and atopic disease. Optom. Today, 39(19), 28–34

Imafidon, C., Akingbade, A., Imafidon, J. and Onwudiegwu, U. (1993) Anterior segment adaptations in gestation. Optom. Today, 33(7), 25–29

Jennings, B. (1990) Mechanisms, diagnosis and management of common ocular allergies. J. Am. Optom. Assoc., 61(Suppl), S32–S41

Kari, O. and Haahtela, T. (1993) Is atopy a risk factor for the use of contact lenses? Allergy, 47, 295–298

Kerr, C. (1987) The UV debate: symposium report. Optician, 193(5087), 14–18

Koetting, R. A. (1966) The influence of oral contraceptives on contact lens wear. Am. J. Optom., 43, 268–274

Koetting, R. A. (1976) Tear film break-up time as a factor in hydrogel lens coating – a preliminary study. Contacto, 20(3), 20–23

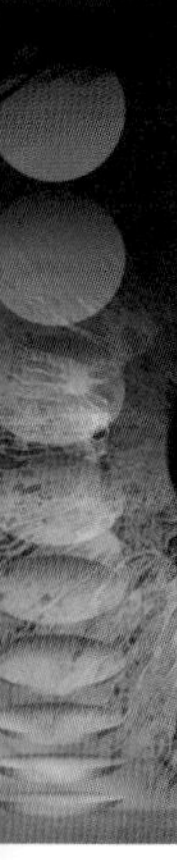

Lane, B. C. (1985) Newsbriefs: Hair it is. Int. Contact Lens Clin., 12(2), 72

Larke, J. (1985) The Eye in Contact Lens Wear. London: Butterworths

Lemp, M. A., Dohlman, C. H. and Holly, F. J. (1970) Corneal desiccation despite normal tear volume. Ann. Ophthalmol., 2, 258–261, 284

Lemp, M. A., Dohlman, C. H., Kuwabara, T., Holly, F. J. and Carroll, J. M. (1971) Dry eye secondary to mucus deficiency. Trans. Am. Acad. Ophthalmol. Otolaryngol., 75, 1223–1227

Levy, B. and Stamper, R. L. (1992) Acute ptosis secondary to contact lens wear. Optom. Vis. Sci., 69, 565–566

Londer, C. (1987) Canine lice in the lashes. Optician, 193(5094), 26

Loveridge, R. (1993) Breaking up is hard to do? J. Br. Contact Lens Assoc., 16(2), 51–55

Lowther, G. E., Miller, R. B. and Hill, R. M. (1970) Tear concentrations of sodium and potassium during adaptation to contact lenses. 1. Sodium observations. Am. J. Optom., 47, 266–275

Mackie, I. A., Seal, D. V. and Pescod, J. M. (1977) Beta-adrenergic receptor blocking drugs: tear lysozyme and immunological screening for adverse reaction. Br. J. Ophthalmol., 61, 354–359

Mandell, R. B. (1992) The enigma of the corneal contour. CLAO J., 18, 267–273

Marsh, R. (1975) Thyroxine and contact lenses. In 'Points from Letters'. BMJ, 2, 689

McMonnies, C. W. and Chapman-Davies, A. (1987) Assessment of conjunctival hyperaemia in contact lens wearers. Parts I and II. Am. J. Optom. Physiol. Opt., 64, 246–255

Mengher, L. S., Bron, A. J., Tonge, S. R. and Gilbert, D. J. (1985) Effect of fluorescein instillation on the pre-corneal tear film stability. Curr. Eye Res., 4, 9–12

Millodot, M. (1975) Do blue-eyed people have more sensitive corneas than brown-eyed people? Nature, 255(5504), 151–152

Millodot, M. (1976) Effect of the length of wear of contact lenses on corneal sensitivity. Acta Ophthalmol., 54, 721–730

Millodot, M. (1977) Influence of age on the sensitivity of the cornea. Invest. Ophthalmol., 16, 240–243

Millodot, M. and Lamont, A. (1974) Influence of menstruation on corneal sensitivity. Br. J. Ophthalmol., 58, 752–756

Nelson, D. M. and West, L. (1987) Adapting to lenses: the personality of success and failure. J. Br. Contact Lens Assoc., 10, 36–37

Norn, M. S. (1963) Foam at outer palpebral canthus. Acta Ophthalmol., 41, 531–537

Norn, M. S. (1970) Micropunctate fluorescein vital staining of the cornea. Acta Ophthalmol., 48, 108–118

O'Donnell, C. and Efron, N. (1998) Contact lens wear and diabetes mellitus. Cont. Lens Anterior Eye, 21, 19–26

O'Donnell, C., Efron, N. and Boulton, J. M. (2001) A prospective study of contact lens wear in diabetes mellitus. Ophthalmic Physiol. Opt., 21, 127–138

O'Callaghan, G. J. and Phillips, A. J. (1994) Rheumatoid arthritis and the contact lens wearer. Clin. Exp. Optom., 77, 137–143

Patel, S., Bevan, R. and Farrell, J. C. (1988) Diurnal variation in pre-corneal tear film stability. Am. J. Optom. Physiol. Opt., 65, 151–154

Patel, S. and Farrell, J. C. (1989) Age-related changes in pre-corneal tear film stability. Optom. Vis. Sci., 66, 175–178

Pesudovs, K. and Phillips, A. J. (1992) Mascara pigmentation of the palpebral conjunctiva in rigid contact lens wear. Clin. Exp. Optom., 75, 153–155

Phelps-Brown, N. (1987) The watering eye. Optician, 193(5095), 47–49

Polse, K. A. (1975) Observation of corneal dry spots. Optom. Wkly., 66(18), 20–21

Rengstorff, R. H. (1986) University of Maryland 2nd annual contact lens symposium, solutions cited as causing complications. Contact Lens Forum, 11(5), 50–51

Rubinstein, M. P. (1984) Epidermolysis bullosa – report of a case with contact lens implications. J. Br. Contact Lens Assoc., 7, 218–221

Rubinstein, M. P. (1987) Diabetes, the anterior segment and contact lens wear. Contact Lens J., 15, 4–11

Sanders, D. R. and Koch, D. D. (1992) An Atlas of Corneal Topography. New Jersey: Slack

Schirmer, K. E. and Mellor, L. D. (1961) Corneal sensitivity after cataract extraction. Am. Med. Assoc. Arch. Ophthalmol., 65, 433–436

Seltzer, R. L. (1988) Spotting probable contact lens failures. Contact Lens Forum, 3, 40–45

Silk, A. A. (1987) Puzzle of the polymers. Trans. BCLA Conference 1987, pp. 57–61

Silk, A. A. (1988) Nissel Memorial Lecture. J. Br. Contact Lens Assoc. (Scientific Meetings), 18–22

Simpson, T., Henderson, L. and Bond, D. (2003) The association between eye colour and corneal sensitivity. J. Am. Acad. Optom., 80(12), 256

Skaff, A., Cullen, A. P., Doughty, M. J. and Fonn, D. (1995) Corneal swelling and recovery following wear of thick hydrogel contact lenses in insulin-dependent diabetics. Ophthalmic Physiol. Opt., 15(4), 287–297

Sorsby, A., Leary, G. and Richards, M. J. (1962) The optical components in anisometropia. Vision Res., 2, 43–51

Stewart, C. R. (1973) Conjunctival absorption of pigment from eye make-up. Am. J. Optom., 50, 571–574

Stone, J. (1959) Factors governing the back central optic diameter of a micro-lens. Optician, 138, 20–22

Stone, J. (1967) Near vision difficulties in non-presbyopic corneal lens wearers. Contact Lens, 1(2), 14–16, 24–25

Terry, J. E. and Hill, R. M. (1975) Cholesterol: blood and tears. J. Am. Optom. Assoc., 46, 1171–1174

Tomlinson, A. and Giesbrecht, C. (1993) The ageing tear film. J. Br. Contact Lens Assoc., 16(2), 67–69

Tomlinson, A., Pearce, E. I., Simmons, P. A. and Blades, K. (2001) Effect of oral contraceptives on tear physiology. Ophthalmic Physiol. Opt., 21, 9–16

Vanden Bosch, W. A. and Lemij, H. G. (1992) Blepharoptosis induced by prolonged hard contact lens wear. Ophthalmology, 99, 1759–1765

van Herick, W., Shaffer, R. N. and Schwartz, A. (1969) Estimation of width of angle of anterior chamber. Am. J. Ophthalmol., 68, 626–629

Voke, J. (1986) A case of keratomalacia on a healthy diet (Research review). Optician, 192(5075), 41

Wilson, L. A., Kuehne, J. W., Hall, S. W. and Ahearn, D. G. (1973) Microbial contamination in ocular cosmetics. Optician, 166(4298), 4, 6, 12

Winder, A. F. (1981) Relationship between corneal arcus and hyperlipidaemia is clarified by studies in familial hypercholesterolaemia. Br. J. Ophthalmol., 67, 789–794

Winn, B., Ackerley, R. G., Brown, C. A. et al. (1986) The superiority of contact lenses in the correction of all anisometropia. Trans. BCLA Conference 1986, pp. 95–100

Young, W. and Hill, R. M. (1973) Cholesterol levels of human tears: case reports. J. Am. Optom. Assoc., 45, 424–428

Chapter 9

Rigid gas-permeable corneal lens fitting

Anthony J. Phillips

CHAPTER CONTENTS

INTRODUCTION

With the advent of inexpensive, easy-to-fit hydrophilic lenses, some practitioners have abandoned or see little need to learn the art of rigid gas-permeable (RGP) fitting. There are, in fact, many reasons why practitioners attempting to do contact lens practice with any degree of seriousness should have a detailed knowledge of RGP lens fitting:

- Some patients will get better visual acuity with RGPs
  - astigmats
    a. irregular astigmats.
    b. low levels of astigmatism left uncorrected in hydrophilic lenses but are corrected by the tear lens with an RGP fit.
  - build-up of deposits or surface dryness on soft lenses leading to poor acuity.
- Some conditions can *only* be fitted with RGPs
  - keratoconus.
  - traumatized corneas.
  - post-grafts.
- RGP lenses may be easier to handle
  - narrow interpalpebral apertures.
  - enophthalmics.
- RGP lenses perform better physiologically and there are fewer adverse corneal reactions because there is:
  - less corneal coverage.
  - greater oxygen permeability.
  - better retro-lens tear flow.

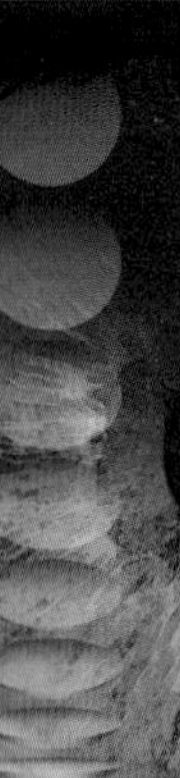

- For the above reasons, since silicone hydrogel soft lenses are not available in higher prescriptions at the time of writing, patients with higher prescriptions or borderline acceptable physiology (e.g. traumatized corneas) are more safely fitted with RGP lenses.
- Former polymethylmethacrylate (PMMA) and RGP wearers usually need refitting at some stage.
- RGP lenses may provide a better, and sometimes the only alternative to hydrophilic lenses in some clinical situations; for example, giant (GPC) or contact-lens-induced papillary conjunctivitis (CLPC), superior epithelial arcuate lesions (SEALS) (see Chapter 17) or in certain other cases such as marginal dry eyes.
- As well as affecting the acuity, the better deposit resistance makes RGP lenses easier to maintain and last longer.
- Lenses are more economic for the patient because of
  - greater deposit resistance.
  - greater resistance to breakage.
- RGP lenses can be modified
  - power – up to ±0.75 D.
  - peripheral curves – flattened to increase the edge lift.
  - total diameter (TD) – reduced.
  - edges – reshaped or repolished.
  - front surface – repolished if moderately abraded.

  The inability to modify hydrophilic lenses makes them unsuitable for patients whose prescriptions are changing and who are not in the parameter or affordable range of disposable lenses, e.g. young myopes.
- Compliance is easier and quicker, and RGP lenses carry significantly reduced contamination risk and should be considered for the following patients:
  - generally non-compliant with lens maintenance.
  - out of the range of daily disposable lenses.
  - lifestyle such that they are unlikely to devote sufficient time to lens maintenance.
- Because patients appreciate the higher level of skill involved in fitting RGP lenses, they are often more loyal to their practitioner and refer more new patients.
- The inherent ability of hydrophilic lenses to absorb and concentrate substances into the lens matrix means that they may be unsuitable for some patients using long-term topical preserved medication such as steroids or glaucoma drugs. Although this has not been found to be a problem in the large majority of cases, if drug absorption is suspected the patient should be refitted with RGP lenses.
- The above point may also apply to patients working in environments where gaseous or suspended droplets or aerosols may be absorbed into the lenses; for example, hairdressers, industrial chemists, etc.
- Although controversial, there is some evidence at least to indicate that the wearing of RGP lenses may retard the progression of myopia (see Chapter 30).
- In certain specialized areas, such as orthokeratology, a high degree of knowledge and experience with RGP lens fitting is an absolute prerequisite.

BASIC REQUIREMENTS

The student new to contact lens practice is often confused by the multitude of different lens materials and fitting techniques, each claiming its own special advantages. The basic requirements of a well-fitting contact lens are often forgotten and should be stressed from the outset. These are simply:

- Maintenance of corneal integrity (including integrity of the related ocular and extraocular tissues).
- Maintenance of normal tear flow behind and over the lens.
- Adequate vision.
- Patient comfort.
- Invisibility.

It follows, therefore, that the best fitting technique or lens construction to use in any one particular instance is the one which most readily satisfies these criteria. For many patients, several different techniques may all perform adequately; in others, the use of a specific technique may give improved results.

The ideal corneal lens material should have a high degree of the following properties:

- Oxygen permeability.
- Surface wettability.
- Low surface reactivity.
- Dimensional stability.
- Flexure resistance and recovery.
- Surface hardness.
- Machine and polishing capability.
- Fracture resistance.
- Material and quality control, i.e. different batches of the material should have the same chemical and physical characteristics and should behave in an identical manner during the lens fabrication process.
- A range of tints and depths of tints.

With the exception of oxygen permeability, the original hard lens material, PMMA, satisfied all these requirements to a good or acceptable degree. Indeed, the first few RGP materials were forced to sacrifice several material considerations in order to gain oxygen permeability. Fortunately, over the last few years, materials have developed that now satisfy almost all the above desiderata including excellent oxygen permeability.

RGP LENS MATERIALS (see also Chapter 3)

Early materials to replace the non-oxygen-permeable PMMA, such as cellulose acetate butyrate (CAB), are no longer in use, generally being replaced with materials of greater stability and oxygen permeability. Although new materials and material improvements are constantly appearing, the majority of modern lenses are made of silicone-acrylate or fluorosilicone-acrylate. These are discussed in brief as follows.

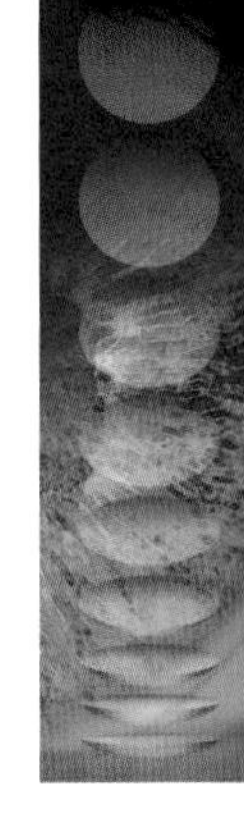

Silicone-acrylate (or siloxanyl-acrylate)

Although highly permeable to oxygen, pure silicone polymers are soft and hydrophobic. They are therefore combined with PMMA to enhance the hardness and stability of the material. To ensure adequate wettability, hydrophilic monomers (e.g. methacrylic acid) are also incorporated into the polymer so that surface treatment or special solutions are required to maintain adequate wettability. This allows subsequent laboratory and practitioner modification or repolishing of the lens. Different additives such as dimethacrylate may be used to enhance tensile strength and resistance to deformation.

The ratio of PMMA to silicone is generally 65% PMMA to 35% silicone. The greater the proportion of silicone, the higher the oxygen permeability, but the poorer the wettability, stability and strength. Similarly, the greater the proportion of wetting agent, the greater the surface wettability, but the poorer the dimensional stability and the greater the affinity for surface deposition due to increased surface reactivity.

The range of Dk values of the materials commonly available is limited (generally 9–30 units*), although some laboratories have achieved higher values by the incorporation of proprietary compounds without sacrificing other desirable properties.

As with all RGP materials, care is needed during manufacture although there is less susceptibility to distortion than with earlier materials such as CAB. Warpage often indicates excessive overheating during the button blocking or lathing procedures (see Chapter 27). Ammoniated polishes are best avoided and alcohols, esters, ketones and aromatic hydrocarbons will damage the material.

ADVANTAGES

- PMMA acts as a thermal insulator. Not only does the lack of oxygen create corneal hypoxia but, by insulating the cornea, it raises the basal metabolic rate and increases the oxygen demand of the corneal epithelium. However, silicones, either in the pure form or polymerized with PMMA, are thermal conductors which remove the heat of metabolism away from the corneal surface, thereby decreasing oxygen requirements. Silicone-acrylates are approximately twice as good thermal conductors as PMMA and CAB which is useful for patients living or working in hot environments.
- The oxygen permeability of the silicone-acrylate group ranges from 50% to several hundred per cent greater than CAB.
- The material is less susceptible to warpage and hydration–dehydration changes than CAB.

DISADVANTAGES

- The silicone-acrylate group of materials are softer and more flexible than PMMA and thus scratch more easily and flex on astigmatic corneas (see below). Most RGP materials break more easily than PMMA.
- The hydrophobic nature of silicone and the relatively high surface charge provide a propensity to attract protein deposits and to bind these tenaciously.
- As a rough guide, there is a manufacturing trade-off with increasing oxygen permeability. Thus, increased permeability is often traded for poor optical quality, poor wettability, etc. Most manufacturers now incorporate proprietary ingredients to counteract these problems. Certain of the original high Dk value silicone-acrylate materials were also prone to surface cracking (see p. 213).

Fluorosilicone-acrylate (fluoropolymers)

As stated earlier, attempts to increase the oxygen permeability of silicone-acrylate polymers, particularly for extended wear, resulted in compromises in dimensional stability, flexure resistance and/or surface interaction with tear components.

Fluorocarbon gases have been widely used since the early 1900s as a form of refrigerant (e.g. Freon) and gaseous propellant for aerosol sprays. Fluoroplastics include high-temperature cable insulation, heat-resistant plastics for piping and gaskets, low-friction and anti-stick applications for non-lubricated bearings and coating of cooking utensils (e.g. Teflon). In more recent years, elaborate uses of fluorine-based compounds have been investigated. Researchers have discovered that liquid fluorochemicals are highly efficient carriers of oxygen and carbon dioxide. These properties have led to the use of fluorochemicals in physiological salt solution as a form of artificial blood. The newly created 'blood' supplies oxygen to the body tissues while carrying away waste products such as carbon dioxide.

Early reference to fluoroplastics for contact lenses appeared in patents by the Dupont Corporation in 1970 and Gaylord in 1974. These early contact lens materials never reached the commercial stage of development, partly due to the poor wetting characteristics, softness, high specific gravity (1.60) and low index of refraction (1.388) (Caroline & Ellis 1986).

Polymer Technology were the first to attempt to avoid these problems in the 'Boston Equalens' by using a polymer incorporating a fluorinated monomer and combining it with a silicone-acrylate moiety. The fluorinated component enhances the material's capability of resisting mucus adhesion and deposit formation while promoting its affinity for tear mucin and soluble proteins for superior wettability in vivo.

Many materials now incorporate an ultraviolet absorber within the polymer matrix in response to the growing concern over the potential cataractogenic and retinal toxic effects of ultraviolet light.

Fluorosilicone-acrylates (and a small number of silicone-acrylates) now make up the majority of RGP lenses currently being fitted.

ADVANTAGES

- High oxygen permeability.
- Resistance to mucus and deposit formation.
- Dimensional stability equal to silicone-acrylate materials and significantly better than CAB.
- Effective ultraviolet light filtration when required.
- Suitability for daily, flexi- or extended wear.

---

* Oxygen permeability units or Dk units are expressed as units of 10^{-11}(cm ml O_2)/(cm^2s mmHg). See also Chapters 3 and 31.

DISADVANTAGES

Compared to silicone-acrylate lenses

- Breakage – many materials are less resistant.
- Flexure – materials may be more vulnerable and slower to recover.
- Hardness – may be worse so lenses scratch more easily.
- Modifications – the response of the material is quicker and should therefore be carried out by skilled technicians. Polishing compounds containing ammonia, alcohol or organic solvents should not be used.
- The lenses are generally more prone to lipoidal deposits.

The incorporation of an ultraviolet absorber in some materials means that conventional hand ultraviolet lamps cannot be used for assessing fluorescein patterns. A white light with blue filter or the blue light of a slit-lamp must be used (see Fluorescein patterns, p. 196).

Siloxanylstyrene-fluoromethacrylate

This material represents a further modification to the fluorosilicone-acrylates. Currently only available as the Menicon Z lens, this polymer is composed of siloxanylstyrene, fluoromethacrylate and benzotriazol UV absorber. The surface is modified to improve wettability (see below). The result is a material with good structural integrity and hyper-oxygen transmissibility.

Modified surface materials

Some lenses have their surfaces modified in order to optimize the surface wettability. These lenses claim to have the physical characteristics (durability, flexure resistance and oxygen transmissibility) of RGP lenses but the wettability and easier adaptability of hydrophilic lenses. This is achieved either by surface treatment or incorporation of hydrophilic monomers into the lens material.

The Novalens (Ocutec Ltd) is composed of rosilfocon A, a hydrophilic stryl-silicone material. The lens consists of a rigid core and a surface polymer that has hydrophilic properties. Aquasil (Aquaperm) is a silicone-acrylate copolymer, which, immersed in a weak acidic solution, produces a thin layer of pHEMA on the surface 15–20 µm thick. The hydroxyl groups of pHEMA that are permanently bonded to the polymer are claimed to be non-reactive. Solution uptake is less than 2%, making solution sensitivity unlikely, provided that the correct cleaning regime is used. The hydrophilized surface can be re-treated if worn off or removed by repolishing or modification.

A different technique is used in the Menicon's Super-EX which is a surface-modified fluorosilicone acrylate material. In this case the very high Dk value has been gained at the expense of surface wettability, hence the surface treatment. Lens modifications are not possible with this design and the lens is contraindicated for patients with a dry-eye problem. The lens is mainly indicated for those patients with a high physiological demand or for extended wear.

The SEED S-1 (Seed Co., Japan) uses polyethylene glycol, a hydrophilic monomer, grafted onto the surface of a fluorosilicone-acrylate RGP material by plasma treatment and polymerization. Improved hydrophilicity and the ability to resist contamination and spoiling are claimed.

The Hybrid FS Plus (Contamac), Innovations 50 (ACL Ltd), Tyro-97 (Lagado Corporation) and Harmony 56 and 98 (Gelflex Labs) incorporate small amounts of hydrophilic monomer into a fluorosilicone-acrylate RGP material during the polymerization process. Surface treatment is therefore unnecessary and the material can be machined, processed and modified as with any other RGP material. Water uptake is less than 0.85% in the Hybrid FS Plus so that the material displays great stability. Conventional RGP solutions can be used.

The Comfort O_2 lens (David Thomas, UK) is a rigid silicone–hydrogel polymer claimed to hydrate on the surface like a soft silicone–hydrogel while remaining rigid in the lens interior. It has a Dk of 56 and can be made to any prescription.

Opinions vary as to the value of these modified materials. Hatfield et al. (1993) found no difference in initial comfort or wettability between the Novalens and two other RGP materials. Of 20 patients fitted by the author with an Aquasil material lens in one eye and a conventional FSA material in the other, only one could detect any improvement in comfort or wettability. On the other hand, Watt (1993) reported improvements using the Aquasil material in patients over 35 years of age, in patients showing GPC, dry-eye and PMMA refit cases. Osterland (1992) reported similar good results using the Novalens, and Brown (1991), using Aquasil.

ADVANTAGES

- Possible improved surface wettability and initial comfort.
- Possible deposit resistance.
- Good oxygen permeability and extremely high permeability in the case of the Menicon Super-EX and Z materials.

DISADVANTAGES

- Many of the advantages claimed for improved surface wettability (in the appropriate materials) are disputed.
- The advantages may only apply to certain wearers.
- Specific cleaners or disinfecting regimens may be necessary.
- Abrasive cleaners should not be used for surface-treated materials.
- In some types (e.g. Menicon's Super EX), reapplication of the hydrophilic coating is not possible should this either wear off or be removed by modification or repolishing.
- Practitioners other than the prescribing practitioner may not appreciate that a surface-modified material has been used and may inadvertently repolish the lens.
- Some lenses may be vulnerable to parameter changes.
- The lenses are often more expensive than conventional RGP lenses.

Material and design classification

The International Organization for Standardization (ISO) has produced a new method of classification of both soft and rigid

Table 9.1: Classification of RGP materials by group code

Group code	Dk units	Examples
1	1–15	Boston ES/IV
2	16–30	B & L Quantum 1
3	31–60	Boston EO/7, Equalens
4	61–100	Boston XO, Quantum 2, Paragon HDS100
5	101–150	Europerm 120, CIBA Aquila
6	151–200	FluoroPerm 151
7	200+ (in 50s)	Menicon Z

Table 9.2: Differentiation of RGP materials by chemistry

Group suffix	Content	Examples
I	No silicone or fluorine	Persecon E (CAB)
II	Silicone but no fluorine	Boston IV
III	Silicone and fluorine	Lamda Europerm
IV	Fluorine but no silicone	

CAB, cellulose acetate butyrate.

lenses which differs from the US Food and Drug Administration (FDA) 'Approved Names' system (USAN). The objective is to identify each material more accurately (Table 9.1).

Material names, therefore, indicate the polymer (whether it is a first or subsequent development of that polymer), the constituents and the Dk. Nowadays, nearly all new materials will be Group III lenses (Table 9.2).

For example: Paragon HDS is called Paflufocon B III 3:

- *Paflu* – name of polymer mix.
- *focon* – rigid lens material.
- *B* – second generation of this polymer.
- *III* – fluorosilicone-acrylate.
- *3* – ISO Dk is between 31 and 60 units.

CORNEAL SHAPE

The use of modern computerized videotopography has led to an understanding of corneal shape and its variations. Figure 9.1 shows the variations of the conicoids in Cartesian coordinates.

Almost all corneas show as a flattening or prolate ellipse. The degree of flattening, or asphericity, may be expressed in several ways: *e*, *p*, *Q* value, or 'shape factor' (SF). The relationship between the various terms is as follows:

$$p = 1 - e^2$$
$$\text{SF} = 1 - p = e^2$$
$$e = \sqrt{1 - p} = \sqrt{\text{SF}}$$
$$Q = -e^2$$

Table 9.3 gives a summary of the mean asphericity data for the anterior surface of the cornea.

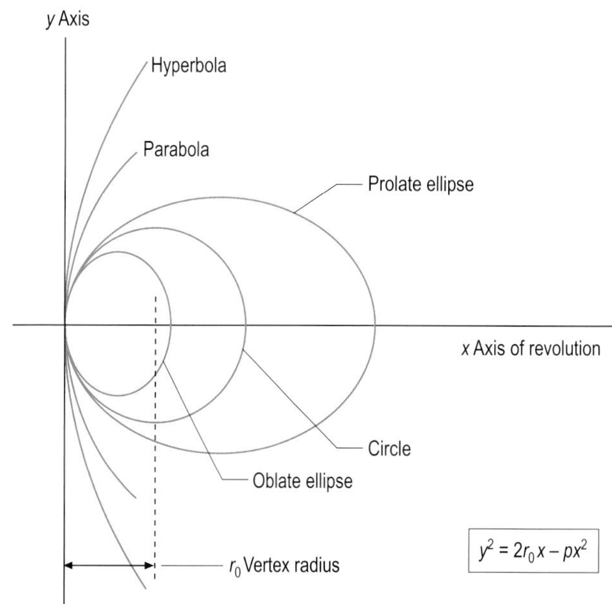

Figure 9.1 The conicoids in Cartesian coordinates with a circle shown as reference. The cornea and most aspheric lens designs are prolate ellipses

Table 9.3: Summary of the mean asphericity data for the anterior surface of the cornea

	e	*p*	*Q*	SF
Townsley (1967)	0.54	0.70	–0.30	0.30
Mandel & St Helen (1971)	0.48	0.77	–0.23	0.23
Kiely et al. (1982)	0.51	0.74	–0.26	0.26
Guillon et al. (1986)	0.42	0.82	–0.18	0.18
Patel et al. (1993)	0.17	0.97	–0.03	0.03
Eghbali et al. (1995)	0.42	0.42	–0.18	0.18
Carney et al. (1997)	0.57	0.67	–0.33	0.33
Douthwaite et al. (1999)	0.49	0.76	–0.24	0.24
Chui (2004)	0.66	0.56	–0.44	0.44

SF, shape factor.

The most commonly used term in corneal topography is the eccentricity or '*e*' value. The *e* value of a sphere is zero and, as the rate of corneal flattening increases away from a true sphere, its *e* value will increase. An extreme example of this would be in keratoconus.

If we ignore the results from Patel et al. (1993) in Table 9.3 (since they vary considerably from those found by all other workers), we find an average *e* value of 0.51. Douthwaite et al. (1999) gave a range of *e* values from 0.14 ($p = 1.02$) to 0.75 ($p = 0.50$) in the near horizontal meridian but found no difference in asphericity between steep and flat corneas in the normal range. Chui (2004) also found no difference in *e* values between steep and flat corneas.

Both Douthwaite et al. (1999) in Caucasian subjects and Chui (2004) in Chinese subjects, found no significant difference in *e* values with either gender or age. Chui did note, however, that the average *e* value taken across a 7.20 mm chord (0.59 ± 0.10 mm) was less than across a 9.80 mm chord (0.66 ± 0.10 mm). Douthwaite et al. (1999) noted that the *e* value varied between the horizontal meridian (0.49) and the vertical (0.42), i.e. the near-horizontal cornea is more aspheric than the near-vertical cornea.

When examining *e* values (or any other measurement of corneal shape), the figure derived will depend upon:

- The instrument used.
- How many readings are taken (i.e. the repeatability of the instrument and whether the result given is from a single measurement or an average of several measurements).
- The algorithm used to calculate the eccentricity.
- Whether the calculated *e* value is from along a single meridian or if it is a global measurement, i.e. the average of the eccentricities from all meridians.
- From Douthwaite's results, the direction of any astigmatism and its effect on any measurement given.
- The chord width being measured. Unfortunately most topographers do not use chord widths of greatest value for RGP fitting or do not allow practitioner choice of the chord width.

Thus, while current topography methods have given us a significantly better understanding of the corneal shape, they do have certain limitations which will have an effect on the calculation of lens design and subsequent fitting (see below).

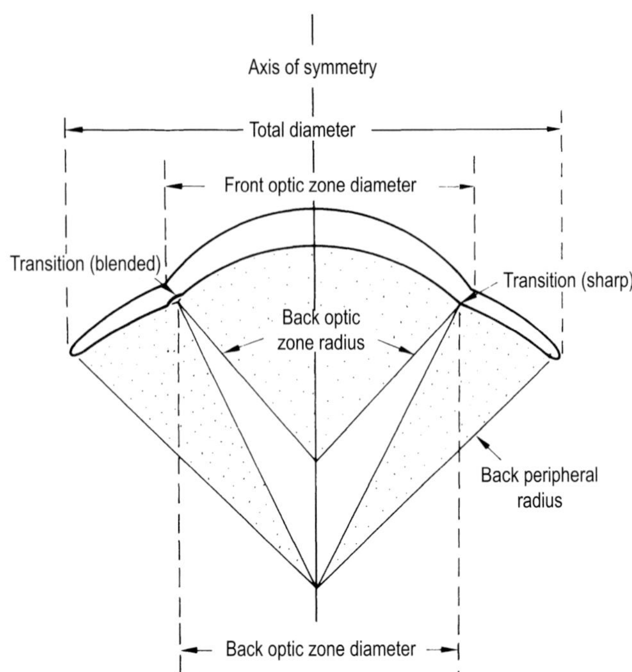

Figure 9.2 Corneal lens dimensions as recommended by the International Organization for Standardization

TERMS RELATING TO CORNEAL LENSES

Detailed terminology relating to corneal lenses is summarized in the Glossary of terms at the beginning of the book. For ease of reference the major terms are summarized in Figure 9.2 (see also Chapter 31).

FORCES AFFECTING THE LENS ON THE EYE

For a lens to fit correctly, a balance is needed between the forces acting to hold the lens against the cornea and those acting to move the lens or eject it from the eye.

Capillary attraction/post-lens tear layer forces

The force of attraction between the lens and the cornea varies inversely with the distance between the two surfaces (Wray 1963), i.e. the more closely a lens surface matches the corneal contour, the greater the force of attraction. Because the cornea is not spherical, the posterior lens surface is made either of multiple flattening curves or aspherical curves. In practice, however, while it is desirable to achieve a reasonable area of corneal 'alignment' to aid capillary attraction and prevent corneal insult, a lens that conformed exactly to the corneal contour over the whole of its surface would not be comfortably tolerated. The capillary attraction would be so great that there would be minimal lens movement or tear circulation beneath the lens.

Tear fluid squeeze pressure (TFSP)

Since the lens does not exactly match the shape of the eye, capillary attraction is not a major force holding the lens in place – it is the tear fluid squeeze pressure (TFSP). This is the pressure that develops behind the optic zone in the post-lens tear film. It centres the lens by opposing the gravity force (see below) that acts to decentre the lens inferiorly and the eyelid force that acts to decentre the lens superiorly at equilibrium. During blinking, the TFSP is the main recentration force as its dynamic action creates a symmetrical force on the contact lens (Guillon & Sammons 1994).

This force is proportional to the irregularity of the post-lens tear layer in that region and directly proportional to the tear layer thickness (TLT): the greater the TLT, the greater the TFSP. Manipulation of the fitting affects the TLT in conventional RGP fitting (see below) and this pressure is utilized in orthokeratology (see Chapter 18).

Hayashi (1977) showed that if a lens with zero apical tear thickness is placed on the cornea, the lack of TFSP allows the lid to manipulate the lens position until a tear layer develops. This occurs as the lens decentres, usually superiorly, and continues until the surface tension forces around the lens edge balance the squeeze force so that a quasistatic state re-emerges.

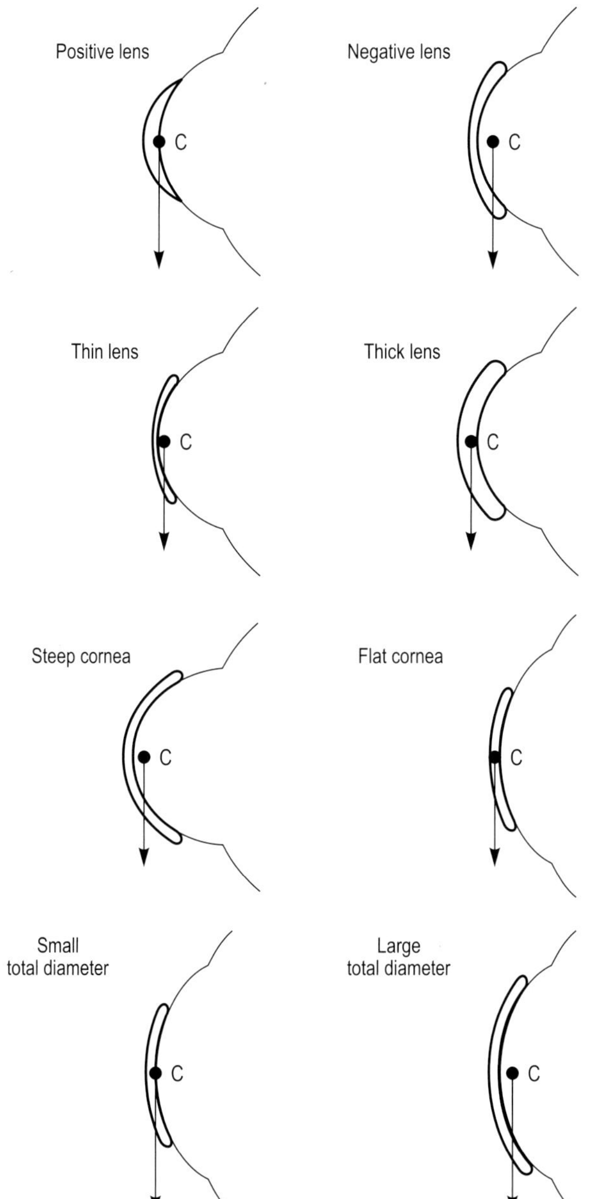

Figure 9.3 Centre of gravity (C) with lenses of differing power, thickness, BOZR and TD

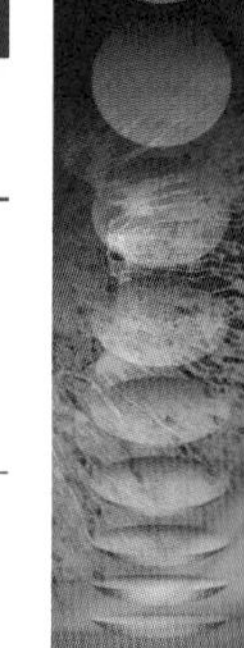

Gravity

The effects of gravity on the lens are best envisaged using the concept of the centre of gravity. This has the property that the object acts as though all of its weight were concentrated at that one point. For a corneal lens, the position of the centre of gravity is near the back surface or actually behind the lens. The further the centre of gravity moves behind the lens the greater the area of support above it. As the centre of gravity moves towards the front surface of the lens, there is less support for the lens and it tends to drop or 'lag' more readily under the effect of gravity.

The position of the centre of gravity is affected by the lens total diameter, back vertex power, thickness and back optic zone radius (BOZR) (Fig. 9.3). Thus the effects of gravity are lessened for lenses with negative powers, minimal centre thickness, steep corneal curvature and larger total diameters (TD).

Carney and Hill (1987) summarized the relative effects of various changes in lens parameters and the effect that these have on the movement of the lens centre of gravity. These are shown in Table 9.4. This shows the markedly superior effect achieved by increasing the total diameter in comparison to other design changes.

Table 9.4: The effect of lens parameter changes in shifting the centre of gravity to enhance lens stability*

	Centre of gravity change/parameter change	Relative effect
Negative lenses		
Total diameter	0.018 mm/0.1 mm	× 4.5
Back central radius	0.004 mm/0.05 mm	× 1
Centre thickness	0.006 mm/0.01 mm	× 1.5
Positive lenses		
Total diameter	0.014 mm/0.1 mm	× 7
Back central radius	0.004 mm/0.05 mm	× 2
Centre thickness	0.002 mm/0.01 mm	× 1

* Derived from the altered centre of gravity resulting from the smallest parameter change of clinical relevance. The change in centre of gravity is based on the total parameter ranges encompassed in the figures; the exact values will vary slightly depending on position within those ranges.
After Carney and Hill (1987).

For example, if a practitioner wishes to stabilize a –3.00 D lens of 9.00 mm TD, 7.40 mm back optic zone diameter (BOZD) and 7.80 mm BOZR, the following options are realistically available:

- Increase diameter by 0.10 mm steps to shift the centre of gravity back by 0.018 mm.
- Steepen the BOZR by 0.05 mm steps to shift the centre of gravity back by 0.004 mm.
- Reduce the centre thickness by 0.01 mm steps to shift the centre of gravity back by 0.006 mm.

In conclusion, it is therefore apparent that changes in lens thickness, total diameter and power are those parameter changes most likely to affect lens position on the eye.

Specific gravity

The specific gravity of a material affects the lens mass. Table 3.1 shows the range of specific gravities in some current RGP materials. In a study on a small group of wearers exhibiting poor lens centration, Quinn and Carney (1992) found no major effect by changing to materials of differing specific gravity but made the following recommendations:

- If a patient consistently exhibits a high-riding lens, material changes to manipulate specific gravity will probably not significantly improve centration. However, refabricating a lens in a thinner design may provide some benefit.
- If a patient consistently exhibits a low-riding lens, selection of a low specific gravity material and/or thinning the lens should prove beneficial.

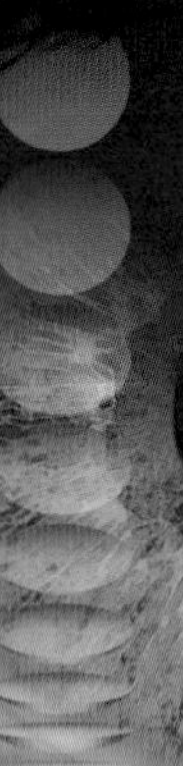

Tear meniscus/edge tension force

The existence of a tear meniscus under the edge of a corneal lens, producing an edge tension force (ETF), is essential for lens centration (Kikkawa 1970, Mackie et al. 1970, Mackie 1973). This force acts to hold the lens against the cornea whenever the lids do not cover the edge.

For any given lens, the greater the circumference of the meniscus, the better the lens centration. If the peripheral curve of the lens is too close to the cornea, the tear meniscus will be ineffective in holding the lens on the eye and will reduce tear interchange. If the clearance is too great, the meniscus will be inverted and will reduce the adhesion causing possible 3 and 9 o'clock staining (see p. 211) or bubbles under the edge.

The ETF depends on the radius of the tear meniscus: the smaller the radius the stronger the force (Hayashi 1977, Hayashi & Fatt 1980). Altering the edge clearance and edge thickness can vary this (see p. 210).

The ETF has a secondary effect on mechanical performance but plays a key role in maintaining a continuous tear film at the edge of the lens (Guillon 1994). Here again, the shorter the radius, the more likely the tear film is to remain contiguous.

Eyelid force (ELF) and position

The eyelids exert the principal role in RGP lens mechanical performance.

- During blinking, the lens may displace 2–3 mm.
- The lens may be supported by the lower lid.
- Between blinks the eyelid force affects extrapalpebral fitting lenses by acting normally to the contact lens to hold it against the cornea. This results in negative pressure which keeps the lens centred or riding high, counteracting gravity which is forcing the lens to ride low.
- Where TFSP and ETF are inadequate, gravity forces excessive or the lens edge too thick, the lids may push the lens down on the cornea where it may 'bind'.

To increase ELF (for low-riding lenses)

- Increase the TD of the lens, thereby increasing the area of contact between lens and eyelid and reducing the effect of gravity (see p. 194).
- Reshape the lens front edge into a negative carrier (see The edge shape, p. 220).

To reduce ELF (for high-riding lenses)

- Decrease the TD (and therefore eyelid contact).
- Reshape the lens front edge to produce a positive carrier.

FLUORESCEIN PATTERNS

Fluorescein patterns (see Figs 9.7–9.11) are used to estimate lens fit and are produced when a small drop of 2% sodium fluorescein is instilled in the lower fornix or onto the bulbar conjunctiva in order to colour the tears. The lens fit is then viewed under ultraviolet light, which renders the tears fluorescent. A different pattern is obtained as the lens moves following each blink and as the fluorescein drains from behind the lens. It is thus a dynamic picture and not easily represented pictorially.

The fluorescein picture depends on several factors (see below), especially tear flow and lens fit. A few moments should be allowed for excess fluorescein to drain from the front surface in order to see the retro-lens picture. However, excess tearing may rapidly wash all fluorescein from behind the lens, leaving the 'black' appearance of an aligning zone or lens. Conversely, lack of blinking or tearing may leave fluorescein on the lens front surface, thereby mimicking fluorescein trapped under the back optic zone (BOZ) of a steep-fitting lens. If the fluorescein is not allowed to dilute enough, it will not fluoresce and the fit of the lens cannot be assessed.

With a tight-fitting lens where the BOZ transition or lens edge indent the cornea, preventing retro-lens tear flow, fluorescein cannot enter behind the lens. Tight-fitting lenses do not usually move on normal blinking but digital manipulation of the lens using the lid margin will allow lens movement and an influx of fluorescein underneath. This might also indicate a very dry eye (see also Lens adhesion phenomenon, p. 211). A lens that is too flat may move excessively and cause lens edge irritation, resulting in excess tearing and loss of fluorescein from under the lens.

The experienced practitioner can quickly judge corneal 'alignment' (where the appearance is almost black), small degrees of corneal clearance (where fluorescence pools) or poor edge clearance. On astigmatic corneas (see Fig. 9.19) the difference in the degree of fluorescence between the two meridians can be seen.

Figure 9.4 (and other figures in this chapter and on the disk accompanying this book) shows the layer of tears trapped between the lens back surface and the eye. The corneal surface is shown as a straight line along the X axis and the tear layer thickness (TLT) is in microns along the Y axis.

For simplicity, the whole tear layer is shown in green. In reality the degree of fluorescence becomes increasingly less visible below around 20 microns. This is shown diagrammatically in Figure 9.5a (a modified Fig. 9.4) with the 'real life' picture shown in Figure 9.5b for comparison.

Carney (1972) showed that, between 10 and 40 microns, the degree of fluorescence was related linearly to the TLT between lens and eye. At the typical fluorescein tear concentration of 0.025%, there is maximum saturation at around 60 microns so that TLTs above this thickness cannot be judged by appearance alone (Young 1988). Hence, the experienced practitioner can judge the degree of fluorescence of TLT between 15 and 60 microns but lenses which are centrally slightly flat, or show edge clearances above 60 microns, cannot be judged on fluorescein appearance alone.

Some RGP materials contain UV absorbers for ocular protection. These are particularly useful for

- Aphakes who have lost their UV-absorbing crystalline lens.
- Children whose crystalline lenses have little natural UV-absorbing properties.
- Those working outdoors much of the time.

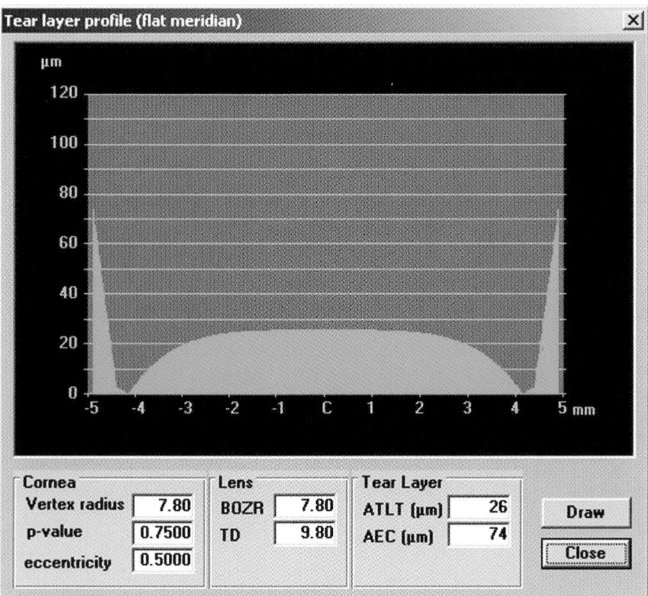

Figure 9.4 Tear layer thickness (TLT) with the corneal back surface represented by the straight line of the *x* axis and the tear layer thickness shown in microns on the *y* axis

However, the fluorescein pattern of these lenses cannot be viewed with a normal hand UV (Burton) lamp, and the cobalt blue filter of a slit-lamp, set at low magnification, or a white hand lamp with a Wratten No. 47 filter over the light emitter and a Wratten No. 12 filter over the viewing aperture, should be used instead. The No. 12 filter can also be used over the viewing microscope end of a slit-lamp to enhance the fluorescence. These filters may be available from lens material manufacturers or their suppliers.

Photochromatic RGP material is also available; for example, Eclipse (ACL Ltd), Varichrome Plus (Gelflex), etc. The main difficulty with these materials is that the thinness of the lenses precludes a significant photochromatic effect. Nevertheless, they have found value in certain cases such as rod monochromats and some albinoids and aniridics. Lens fitting assessment may again be difficult with hand UV lamps.

In summary, the degree of fluorescence of the tear layer between the lens and the cornea is a useful guide to the fit but has certain limitations that need to be understood. The degree of fluorescence will depend upon:

- Concentration of fluorescein.
- Tear flow.
- Wavelength of emitter light.
- Presence of appropriate filters in the viewing system.
- Fluorescein on the lens front surface (which may obscure the fluorescence of the tear layer behind the lens).
- Any UV absorber in the lens material.
- pH of the saline used (fluorescence is more effective in an alkaline pH).
- Tear layer thickness.
- Possibly the brand of fluorescein used.

THE GENERAL PRINCIPLES OF RIGID LENS FITTING

In the simplest form these may be listed as follows:

- As large an area of corneal alignment as possible in order to spread the weight of the lens and pressure of the eyelids against the lens and also to minimize lens-induced trauma

(a)

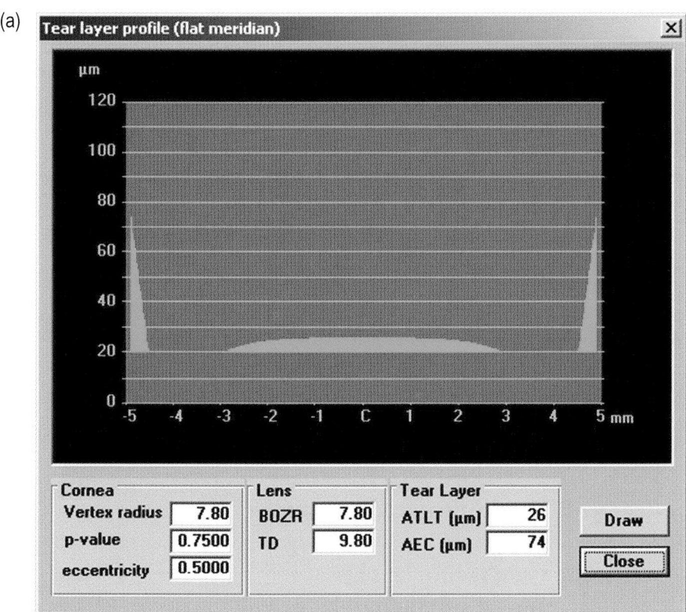

(b)

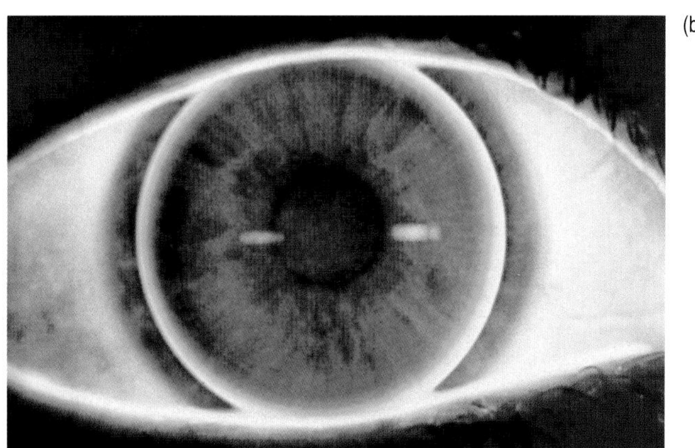

Figure 9.5 (a) Figure 9.4 modified to remove the 'invisible' part of the TLT, i.e. to show the visible part of the fluorescein pattern as seen under UV light (b)

through localized pressure (e.g. from a sharp transition or too steep a BOZR).

- Back surface peripheral curve(s) flat enough to prevent lens indentation on movement to the flatter corneal periphery, but not such excess edge clearance as to cause lid margin or perilimbal irritation. Also, the peripheral back surface configuration should encourage good retro-lens tear flow and allow easy lens removal.
- BOZD large enough to prevent flare from the peripheral curves when the pupil is dilated at night but not so large as to prevent adequate alignment of the aspheric corneal shape.
- Lens material
  - adequate Dk to allow normal corneal physiological function for each eye and wearing time required.
  - lens thickness to optimize transmissibility but not so thin that the lens warps, distorts or is easily fractured.
- Back surface design to encourage good retro-lens tear flow and no pressure points on the cornea.
- Lens edge should be thin enough and correctly shaped for comfort, but not so thin that it effectively becomes sharp or may chip.
- TD large enough to
  - encompass the chosen BOZD.
  - allow adequate width for the peripheral curve configuration.
  - provide minimal lid irritation.
  - assist good centration.
- TD too large may
  - reduce retro-lens tear flow.
  - increase the lens mass.
  - possibly allow limbal 'bumping' on lateral eye movements.

It is now pertinent to enlarge on these points individually once a picture of the overall lens fitting has been understood.

Selection of BOZR and BOZD in spherical or near-spherical corneas

Because the cornea is aspherical in shape, as stated earlier, a small amount of tear liquid must exist between the cornea and spherical back optic zone of the lens. This volume will tend to increase when the lens is decentred and thereby tend to recentre the lens after lens movement by the negative pressure thus induced. In the case of an aspheric back surface lens, negative pressure can only be induced if the lens fit creates a positive tear layer between the lens centre and the point of contact with the cornea.

Thus, although practitioners commonly refer to 'lens alignment' of the cornea, in reality there will always be a very thin layer of tears between the lens and cornea as discussed earlier. This is shown diagrammatically in Figure 9.6.

TLT = sag of BOZR – sag of cornea at BOZD

Sag of the contact lens $= r - \sqrt{r^2 - y^2}$ (r = BOZR and y = BOZD/2) and the sag (x) of the cornea (assumed elliptical) can be determined from

$y^2 = 2r_0x - px^2$ (see Fig. 9.1)

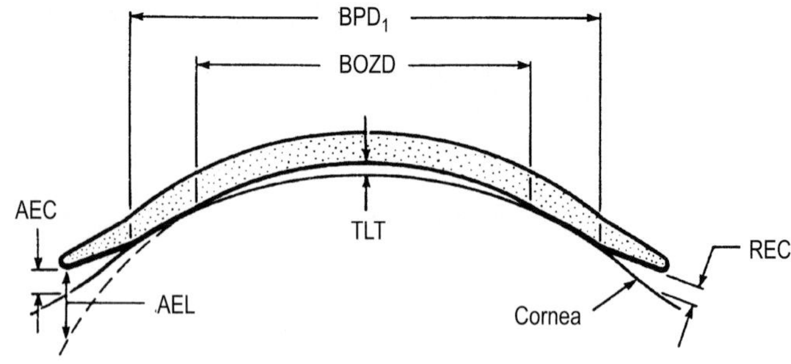

Figure 9.6 Tear layer trapped between the back optic zone of the lens and cornea. The central clearance between lens and cornea is known as the tear layer thickness. Also shown is the axial and radial edge clearance from the cornea and axial edge lift between the lens edge and extended BOZR (dotted). AEC, axial edge clearance; BOZD, back optic zone diameter; BPD_1, first back peripheral curve diameter; REC, radial edge clearance; TLT, tear layer thickness

where y = BOZD/2, r_0 = apical corneal radius and p = asphericity. Also, $r_0 = b^2/a$ and $p = b^2/a^2$ where a and b are the semi-major and semi-minor axes of the corneal ellipse (Baker 1943, Bennett 1988).

Fortunately, these calculations can be done easily using suitable lens design programs such as the one on the CD-ROM accompanying this book. The examples listed below can thus be reproduced and neophyte practitioners are urged to do this.

Clinical experience has shown that the ideal central TLT to give apparent alignment is between 10 and 25 microns with a typical value of around 20 microns (Atkinson 1985). Increasing the TLT beyond this will show increasing lens clearance (Fig. 9.7).

As the BOZD increases, the BOZR should be flattened on the normal prolate cornea. Thus the choice of BOZR will depend not only on the apical radius and the degree of flattening (e or p value), but also on the BOZD selected, which, in turn, will depend upon the lens TD. The practitioner must look not at one parameter in isolation but at the overall lens design and fitting philosophy. However, it is logical to examine the selection of BOZR first and how typical changes in corneal and lens parameters will affect this.

Keratometry typically measures the corneal curvature approximately 1.50–1.75 mm from the corneal apex, i.e. a diameter of around 3.0–3.5 mm across. Fortuitously this gives an approximate average mid value curvature for the 7.00 mm BOZD which historically was a common value in early fitting set lenses. In order to create a TLT of 15–20 microns, practitioners then simply fitted lenses 0.05 mm steeper than the flattest K reading. This is shown in Figure 9.8 for a typical cornea with K readings of 7.80 mm at 180° and 7.60 mm at 90°, an e value of 0.5 and BOZR of 7.75 mm.

With the advent of gas-permeable materials, practitioners have mostly moved to larger TDs, which allow:

- Larger BOZDs for reduced flare and better vision.
- Greater capillary attraction and edge tension force to improve centration and reduce lens loss.
- Greater comfort by commonly tucking the upper lens edge under the upper lid so that there is reduced lens edge sensation.

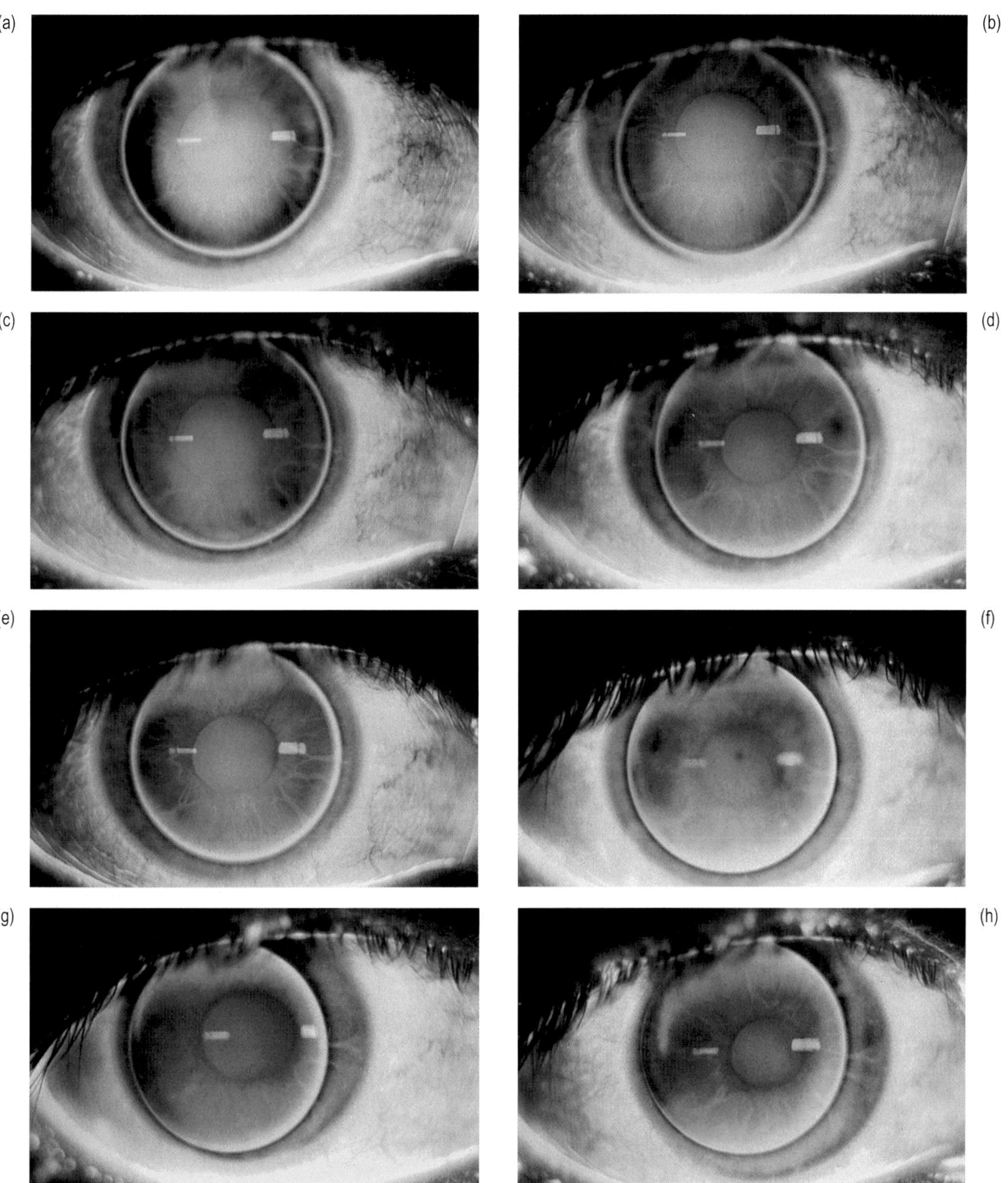

Figure 9.7 This series of pictures shows lenses of various BOZR on the same eye, *K* readings 7.90 at 180°, 7.70 at 90°. The lens TD is 9.60 mm and BOZD 7.50 mm. The horizontal visible iris diameter is 11.50 mm. (Courtesy of The Institute for Eye Research, Sydney). (a) BOZR 7.65 mm: the central fit is grossly steep with accumulation of fluorescein under the whole back optic zone. (b, c) BOZR 7.70 and 7.75 mm, respectively: the steep central fit is still obvious, with the depth and intensity of fluorescence reducing as the fitting approaches central alignment. (d) BOZR 7.80 mm: the BOZR is still slightly steeper than the flattest horizontal corneal meridian and the slight fluorescence centrally can just be seen. There is more peripheral clearance in the vertical meridian. (e) BOZR 7.85 mm: the BOZR is now in good compromise alignment over most of its area. The lack of fluorescence from the tear film over the back optic zone is apparent. (f) BOZR 7.90 mm: by assessment of the fluorescein pattern the lens still appears in good alignment with the cornea. A BOZR of 7.85 and 7.90 mm may indeed give a good fit but it is extremely difficult to judge the very slightly flat fit that could possibly result from the 7.90 mm BOZR, although the peripheral clearance is now greater. (g) BOZR 8.00 mm: a slightly flat fitting lens is now apparent. The lens cannot balance on the corneal apex and so tilts to (in this instance) the temporal cornea so that central and temporal contact becomes apparent. (h) BOZR 8.05 mm: a definite flat-fitting lens can now be seen rocking from the apex to the temporal corneal zone

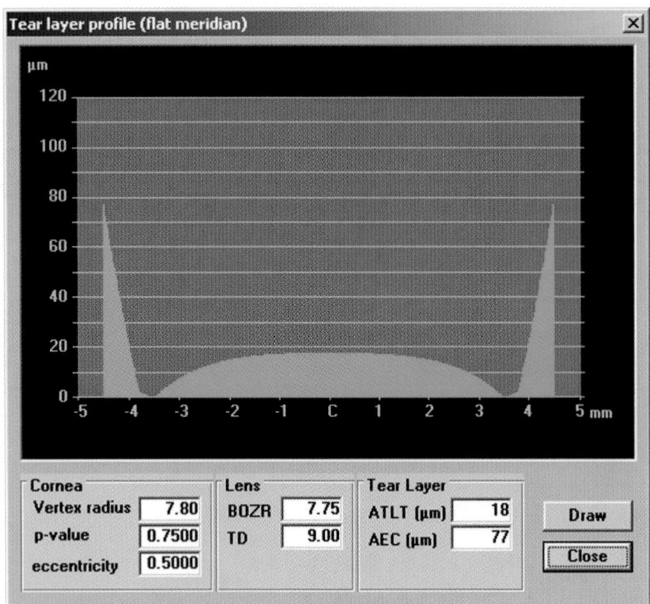

Figure 9.8 The TLT of a lens C3/7.75:7.00/8.10:7.60/9.40:9.00 on a cornea of *K* reading 7.80 at 180°, 7.60 at 90° and *e* value 0.50, i.e. the BOZR (7.75 mm) is 0.05 mm steeper than the flattest *K* and gives a TLT of 18 microns. If a BOZR of 7.80 mm had been chosen, the TLT would have been only 12 microns, i.e. imperceptibly 'flat'

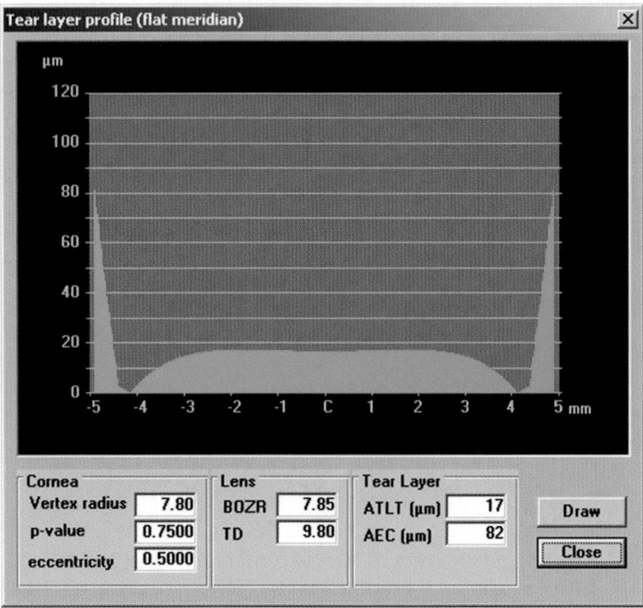

Figure 9.9 The TLT for the same cornea as shown in Figure 9.8 but with the BOZD increased to 8.30 mm and the TD increased to 9.80 mm. To give a similar TLT, the BOZR must now be flattened to 7.85 mm and the full lens prescription is C3/7.85:8.30/8.20:8.80/9.80:9.80

Figure 9.9 shows the change in parameters necessary to produce a similar central TLT to that in Figure 9.8 with the BOZD now increased to 8.30 mm (and the TD increased to 9.80 mm).

So far we have seen the effect of changing the BOZD and how this alters the BOZR for an equivalent fit. A rough rule of thumb is:

- *increasing (or decreasing) the BOZD by 0.5 mm requires an increase (or decrease) of the BOZR by 0.05 mm.*

However, using the CD-ROM computer program allows a much more accurate approach, for example when a suitable diameter trial lens is not available for a specific patient (see also Effects of variations in the BOZD, p. 217).

Next we need to examine the effect of varying corneal eccentricities and how these affect the choice of BOZR.

In the example given above in Figure 9.9 we have assumed an average *e* value of 0.5. Let us now examine the typical extreme values of 0.3 and 0.7. Figures 9.10 and 9.11 give the TLTs of the lenses necessary to produce a theoretical 'ideal' fit for these values.

We can therefore see that for this typical cornea of 7.80 mm and this particular BOZD, the ideal BOZR can vary from 7.75 to 7.95 mm. Table 9.5 shows how the theoretical BOZR varies according to the flattest *K* reading (K_F) and *e* value.

Although a corneal topographic device is extremely helpful in selecting this 'ideal' BOZR, an experienced clinician can estimate the fluorescein pattern and judge an acceptable fit. However, neophyte practitioners should determine the first BOZR to show mild central fluorescence and then fit 0.05 mm flatter since a borderline flat fit can be difficult to determine. Even topographical devices have limitations (see Chapter 7), and two BOZR may both produce central TLTs that are within the acceptable range.

In conclusion, the initial BOZR for a nearly spherical cornea is chosen as the flattest *K* reading but it may need to be modified depending on:

- The BOZD chosen (which in turn may be governed by the TD selected).
- The patient's corneal eccentricity. The higher the *e* value, the flatter the compromise spherical BOZR should be.

Thus, the final BOZR selected will typically vary by 0.10 mm steeper than the flattest *K* reading to 0.20 mm flatter, and possibly 0.25 mm flatter for patients at the steep end of corneal curvature and with high *e* values.

Selection of the BOZR in astigmatic corneas

The majority of contact lens patients will show some degree of corneal astigmatism. If this is under 1.00 D, most can be fitted with a spherical BOZR. As the astigmatism increases, a steeper (0.05 mm) BOZR may centre better. If a topographical device is available, corneas showing central astigmatism only (as opposed to a limbus-to-limbus astigmatic pattern) are more likely to be able to be fitted with a spherical BOZR. As the corneal astigmatism approaches 1.50 D an astigmatic BOZR becomes more essential for a good fit.

A spherical lens can be adequately fitted to 'with-the-rule' corneal astigmatism of values greater than 'against-the-rule'. This is because a lens on a with-the-rule cornea often decentres upwards where it is comfortable, whereas a lens on an against-the-rule cornea displaces sideways where it is less comfortable.

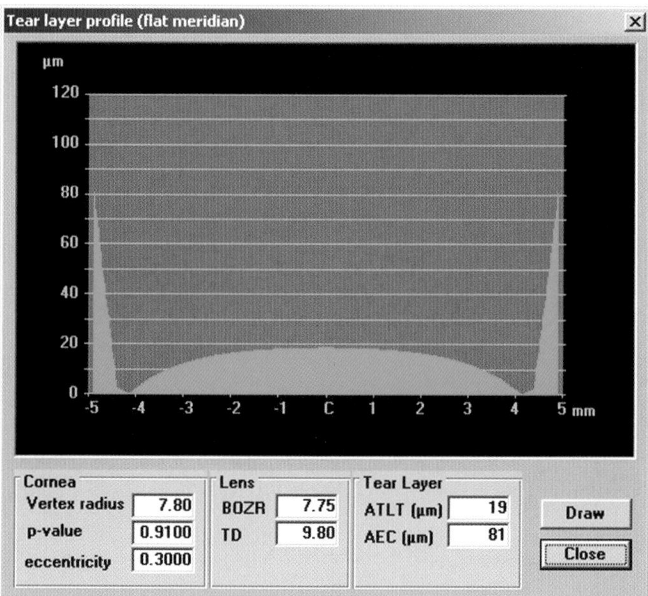

Figure 9.10 For the same patient as used in Figures 9.8 and 9.9 and the lens prescription as used in Figure 9.9, an *e* value of 0.3 would give a central TLT of just 10 microns. It is therefore necessary to *steepen* the BOZR from 7.85 to 7.75 mm to now give a TLT of 19 microns

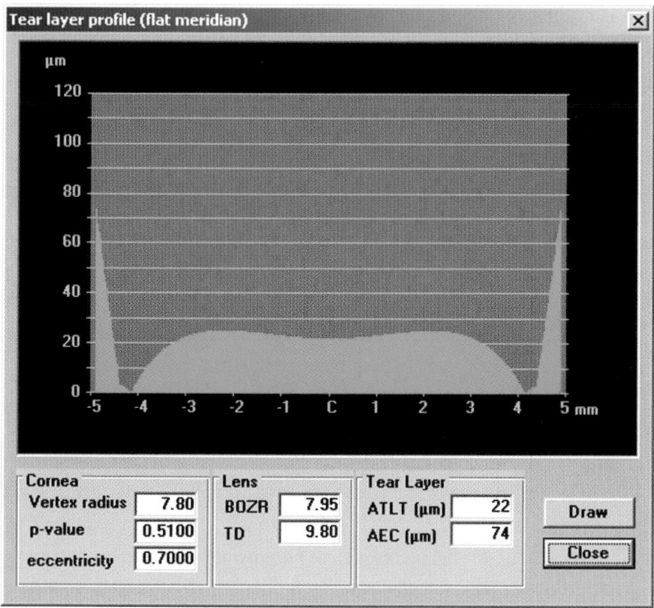

Figure 9.11 Following Figure 9.10, if the corneal *e* value is now increased to 0.7, the TLT for the same lens prescription as in Figure 9.9, the TLT would become too steep with a TLT of 29 microns and show slight central fluorescein pooling. In this instance the BOZR must be *flattened* to 7.95 mm to now give a central TLT of 22 microns

Because of the differences in sag between the two meridians, an astigmatic back surface will become necessary in larger TD lenses before the same level of astigmatism in a cornea requiring a smaller TD lens.

As Douthwaite et al. (1999) have shown that the steeper corneal meridian has a slightly lower *e* value than the flatter meridian, trial set fitting becomes essential in most cases. Fitting sets with meridional differences of 0.4–0.6 mm are extremely useful.

Table 9.5: The theoretical BOZR required for the normal extremes of K_F and *e* values

K_F (mm)		*e* =	0.3	0.5	0.7
7.20	BOZR (mm)	=	7.15	7.30	7.45
7.80			7.75	7.85	7.95
8.40			8.35	8.45	8.55

The decision to use an astigmatic lens will depend upon:

- Lens centration, i.e. stable vision.
- Patient comfort.
- Acceptable corneal and limbal physiology.

The optical implications of astigmatic lenses are discussed in Chapter 13 and under 'Assessment of fit', below.

Selection of the BOZD

This should be at least 1.50 mm larger than the pupil diameter in average room illumination, and larger still if the lenses are to be frequently used for such examples as night driving.

As already mentioned, if the BOZD is changed, a corresponding alteration to the BOZR should be made to maintain the same lens sag.

Selection of the edge curve (see also Tear meniscus, p. 196)

The purpose of the edge curve is to:

- Prevent lens edge indentation on lens movement.
- Assist in lens centration by providing a tear meniscus.
- Not be so excessive as to allow lens movement onto the perilimbal area.
- Not be so excessive as to cause edge awareness.
- Be adequate enough to encourage good retro-lens tear flow.
- Be adequate enough to allow easy lens removal.

The axial edge clearance (AEC) will be dictated by the radii and width of peripheral curve(s). There are a number of fitting philosophies regarding the optimal AEC which is generally agreed should range from 60 to 90 microns.

In patients with 3 and 9 o'clock staining, a small (40–60 microns) AEC may be preferred (Bennett 1985, Businger et al. 1989). In such cases, providing the lens remains mobile and does not bind to the cornea, by keeping the lens edge closer to the corneal surface there is better contact between the superior palpebral conjunctival surface and the cornea and limbal conjunctiva, reducing desiccation. A small AEC has also been suggested as a way of promoting greater lens comfort with RGP lenses as a lens edge that is close to the cornea causes less irritation of the upper lid margin during blinking.

However, where the AEC is too small, the periphery may cause discomfort when it moves to a flatter part of the cornea,

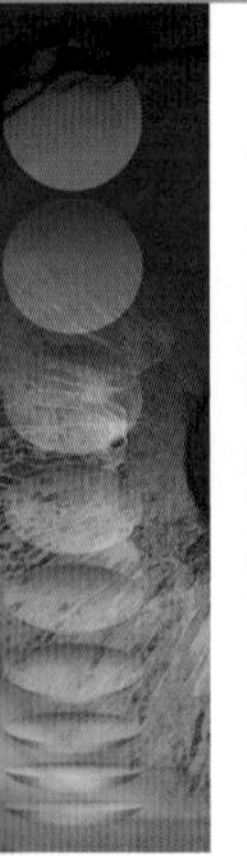

Figure 9.12 The fluorescein edge pattern of an RGP lens with axial edge clearance of 80 microns

as the lens edge will exert greater pressure on the corneal surface. It will also be more difficult to remove. It is necessary, therefore, to weigh the advantages and disadvantages of fitting with reduced AEC for each patient.

Conversely, excessive AEC can result in a thinning of the corneal tear layer adjacent to the lens edge, resulting in punctuate staining. A large AEC will also destabilize the lens fitting, resulting in excessive movement. This is partly due to a reduction in the surface tension force caused by a change in the tear meniscus around the edge of the lens and partly to the effect of the lid action on blinking. Another consequence is formation of bubbles under or adjacent to the lens edge.

The ease and extent of lens movement is largely controlled by the peripheral zone width and the AEC. A small change in the width of the peripheral zone will generally not have as great an effect on the fitting characteristics as an increase or decrease in the AEC (by changing the peripheral curve radius). However, a narrow peripheral zone combined with an average AEC may cause a problem when the lens moves towards the flatter corneal periphery. In this situation the peripheral zone fluorescein pattern will quickly disappear (see Fig. 9.7b) resulting in the edge indenting the cornea and causing discomfort. Conversely, an excessively wide edge curve may move too far to the corneal periphery and may accumulate large amounts of debris in the tear reservoir which can be a source of foreign body irritation.

Bibby (1979) showed that the ideal width of the peripheral curve is approximately 0.50–0.60 mm. For smaller widths of peripheral curve, a large change in radius is necessary to change the AEC significantly but a small error in diameter during manufacture would change the edge clearance considerably. Similarly, at large peripheral curve widths, a small error in radius would be significant but a large error in diameter less significant. Examples of curve changes are given below and can be worked out from the accompanying CD-ROM.

It is necessary, therefore, when fitting a patient, to assess the performance of trial lenses with a known peripheral curve radius and width, and then to modify the design of the lens to ensure that the peripheral curve is neither inadequate nor excessive. A typical edge curve fluorescein pattern is shown in Figure 9.12.

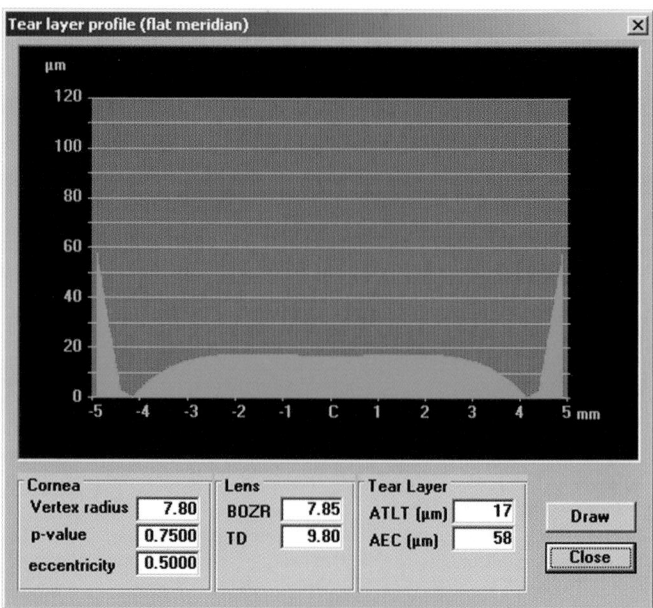

Figure 9.13 The TLT and fluorescein picture of a lens with the borderline adequate axial edge clearance of 66 microns

For typical back optic zone radii and diameters, a change of 0.05 mm in radius may produce a clinically significant change in AEC. For the flatter and narrower edge curves a much larger change in radius is necessary to produce a clinically significant change, as illustrated in the following example:

- A patient has a lens prescription of : C3/7.85:8.30/8.20:8.80/**9.20**:9.80
- Working from the CD-ROM, if the corneal *e* value is 0.50 (and K_F is 7.80 mm), the axial edge lift (AEL) is 58 microns, i.e. the edge may be considered borderline tight. This is shown in Figure 9.13.
- Changing the edge curve from 9.20 to 9.40 mm increases the AEL from 58 to only 66 microns, i.e. clinically insignificant.
- If the edge curve is now changed to 9.60 mm, the AEC increases to 74 microns (Fig. 9.14).
- Thus, in contrast to the relatively small change necessary to show a clinically significant change in BOZR (0.05–0.10 mm), *relatively large changes are commonly necessary to the (narrow) edge curve radius/ii (0.20–0.40 mm) to show clinical significance.*

Selection of the TD

Modern RGP materials have eliminated the need in most cases for the minimal corneal coverage necessary in older design PMMA or early low Dk materials. The use of larger TD lenses has allowed for the lens to be fitted in such a way that the superior lens edge is positioned under the upper lid. Such a fitting can provide better comfort for the patient as the interaction between the lens edge and the lid margin will be reduced. Nevertheless, each case should be judged on its own merits.

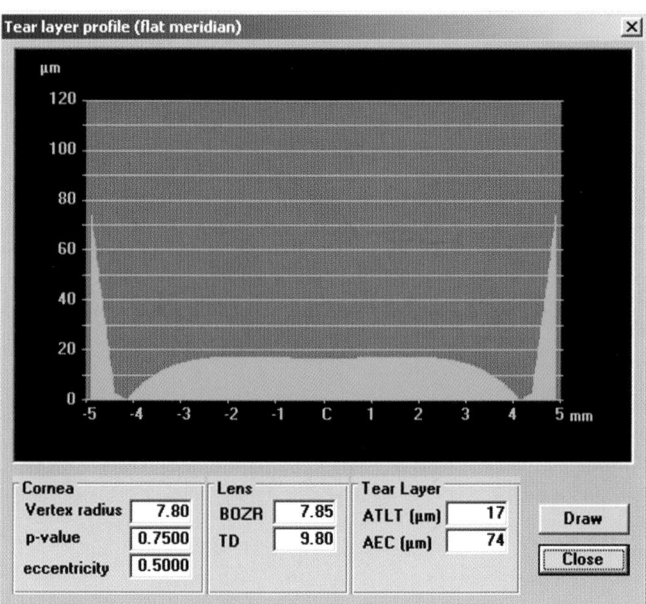

Figure 9.14 The TLT and fluorescein picture of the same lens shown in Figure 9.13 but with the edge curve now flattened to 9.60 mm to give an AEC of 74 μm

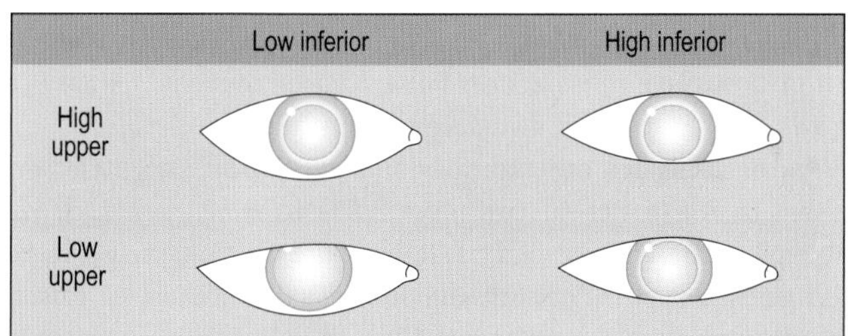

Figure 9.15 Suggested lens TD depending upon the relative position of the eyelids in relation to the cornea

Too large a TD may allow limbal bumping on ocular excursion and, in the case of moderately astigmatic corneas, may precipitate the need for an astigmatic fitting lens due to excess edge clearance along the steeper corneal meridian.

In cases where the upper lid margin lies above the lens, factors dictating comfort will be the design and shape of the edge of the lens. Lindsay and Bruce (personal communication, 2004) have devised a schema for the selection of the lens TD depending upon the relative position of the two eyelids. This is shown in Figure 9.15.

As most eyes show 'low' upper lids (i.e. covering the upper part of the cornea) and lower lids level with or slightly covering the lower limbal area, a relatively large TD is possible for the majority of patients. Thus, while TDs of 8.00–9.00 mm were historically the norm, most lenses now have TDs of 9.50–10.50 mm.

Selection of the intermediate curve(s)

These curve(s) merely serve to provide a transition between the BOZR and edge curves. A minimum width of 0.25 mm should be allowed for, with a radius that is between the BOZR and edge curve, and showing a small edge lift. Commonly only one intermediate curve is necessary but, if there is a relatively large distance between the edge of the BOZ and edge curve, more than one curve may be necessary to follow the corneal contour. Examples of intermediate curves have been given above in Figures 9.8–9.14.

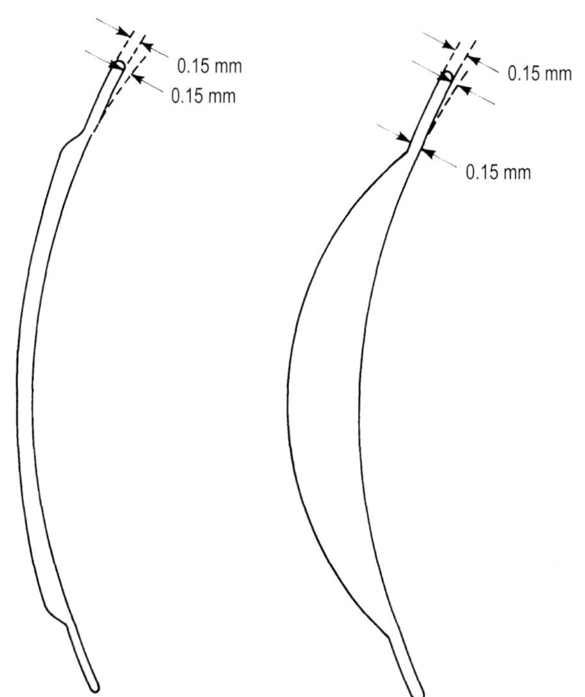

Figure 9.16 Cross-section of parallel-surfaced peripheral zone lenses: negative (left) and positive (right). The carrier zone is held by the upper lid

SPECIAL LENS DESIGNS

Lens-lid (parallel-surfaced or negative carrier peripheral zone attachment) lenses

Because almost all precorneal film movement is the result of upper lid action, and because the precorneal film may in effect be considered as attached to the upper lid, Korb and Korb (1974) argued that the ideal contact lens should be effectively 'attached' to the upper lid. This concept of lens performance, in which the lens remains immobile without upper lid action or eye version movements, but moves during blinking as if the lens were attached to the upper lid, facilitates the movement of tears during the acts of blinking and eye movement, and permits the successful training of blinking. The technique is particularly useful in patients with poor centring lenses, peripheral desiccation, or low lower lids.

The main technique of 'lid attachment' is achieved by arranging that 0.75–1.00 mm of the most peripheral portion of the lens has parallel front and back surfaces or is even slightly negative in cross-section (i.e. slightly thicker at the very edge) (Figs 9.16 and 9.28). This may be done by simply requesting from the laboratory, by tables (Korb & Korb 1974) or by using the CD-ROM supplied with this book.

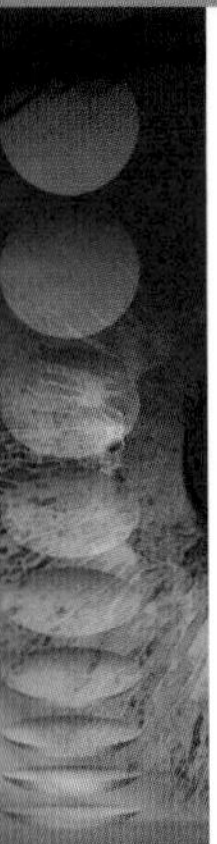

Unlike all other fitting techniques, Korb and Korb recommend that the lens is fitted flatter than the central cornea to give an approximate alignment fit when riding superiorly on the cornea and actually moving some 3 mm on to the inferior sclera during blinking. The lens edge is made more blunt and rounded than normal to increase the tear meniscus. This is acceptable because the upper lid does not have to pass over the lens edge. Lens mass is kept to an absolute minimum.

During primary gaze, upward gaze and between blinks, the upper edge of the lens should be retained under the upper lid. The bottom edge of the lens should be above the lower lid but below the inferior pupillary margin in order to prevent flare. During primary gaze, the lens should not intrude upon the temporal or nasal limbus. The lens should move with the upper lid during blinking. To achieve this, a lens BOZR approximately 0.1–0.3 mm flatter than the flatter *K* reading is usually necessary, together with a larger BOZD than used with more conventional designs. TDs vary between 10.30 and 11.00 mm, typically around 10.50 mm.

For *K* readings of 7.80 at 180°, and 7.60 at 90°, the back curves of such a lens might be: 8.00:8.20/9.60:9.50/11.00:10.50.

Aspheric design lenses

It has already been stated that the cornea is typically a prolate ellipse, i.e. it flattens away from the apex. It seems logical therefore to design lenses to match the true corneal shape for the following reasons:

- Better capillary attraction between lens and eye.
- Less flare as the BOZD should, in theory, be the whole lens back surface.
- No pressure from transition indentation.
- Reduced thickness and better vision with aspheric front surfaces.
- Easier to fit.
- Less spectacle blur/corneal moulding.
- The small edge clearance (20–60 microns) in some designs is helpful in decreasing lens edge sensation. Three and 9 o'clock staining may also be reduced for the same reason by allowing better lid contact with the cornea as long as lens movement is not compromised.

Aspheric surfaces can be defined by mathematical equations and describe a surface of revolution having continuously variable curvature from vertex to edge, these equations being used to derive the principal radii of curvature and AEL at any given point on the lens. Aspheric surfaces essentially consist of two 'families' of curves, the conicoids (see Fig. 9.1) and the polynomials (Fig. 9.17).

The x and y co-ordinates of conicoids are linked by the equation

$$y^2 = 2r_0x - px^2$$

where p is a number (termed the p value; see Corneal shape, p. 193) which describes each conic and its related conicoids, and r_0 is the central radius.

Polynomial theory is based on the formula

$$x = \mathrm{A}y^2 + \mathrm{B}y^4 + \mathrm{C}y^6 + \mathrm{D}y^8 + \mathrm{E}y^{10} \text{ etc.}$$

and from the Cartesian convention

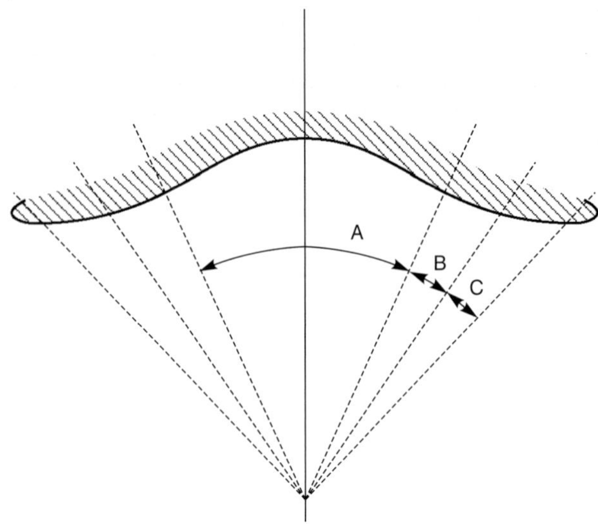

Figure 9.17 An example of a triple zone polynomial back surface lens shown diagrammatically. The asphericity changes across each of the three zones (A, B and C) according to the polynomial formula

$$x = y^2/r_0 + r_0 + py^2$$

In the first formula, y^3 and y^5 etc. are not used because these do not give positive numbers on both sides of the axis. Figure 9.17 shows a triple zone back surface polynomial lens design.

Aspheric lenses are typically made with an eccentricity (e value) in the order of 0.40 ($p = 0.84$) to 0.50 ($p = 0.75$). An aspheric lens which exactly followed the corneal shape to the lens periphery would both dig in on lens movement and be almost impossible to remove. For this reason a variety of modifications to a true asphere have been produced:

- Full aspheric back surfaces, e.g. Boston *Envision* (central ellipse and peripheral hyperbola joined tangentially) and No. 7 Laboratory's *Quasar*.
- Spherical BOZDs with an aspheric periphery, e.g. Bausch & Lomb's *Quantum*, Cooper's *Reflex 60*, and CIBA's *Astrocon*.
- Aspherical BOZDs with narrow spherical peripheral curves, e.g. CIBA's *Aspothericon*.
- Bi-aspherics where both back and front surface are aspheric.

Generally speaking, the conicoid aspherics will give inadequate edge clearance without the addition of narrow spherical peripheral curves to give an edge clearance of 60–80 microns. In some lenses, a bi-elliptical design – which has a periphery with a differing e number from the central area – is used to generate a greater flattening in the periphery. Bausch & Lomb's Quantum is of polynomial design but only after a 3.5–4.0 mm central spherical optical zone.

The fitting of aspheric lenses is described below.

DISADVANTAGES OF ASPHERIC DESIGNS

- Without a computerized topographical device, corneal asphericity is not easily measured nor considered totally accurate. Arbitrary values have therefore to be chosen and fitting done by the use of trial lenses and observation.

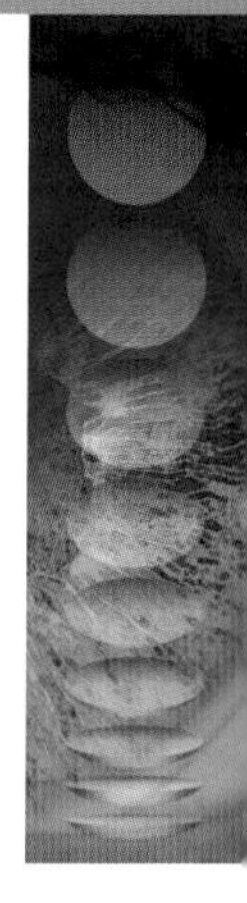

- Spherical lenses rely on the negative pressure of the tear layer trapped between the lens and the cornea to centre the lens. This facility is absent in aspheric designs unless fitted slightly steep centrally. The advantage of matching the corneal shape is therefore partly lost and the back surface design compromised.
- For the above reason, lenses may need to be fitted larger than normal or by lid attachment to assist centration. The variation in corneal shape over the normal population has been referred to earlier.
- Optical properties can be a problem in designs with aspheric central zones where lenses show poor centration. Lens profiles tend to flatten quite quickly away from the lens apex. This peripheral flattening creates an increase in plus power in both the sagittal and tangential meridians at each elliptical point from the apex onwards. In general, the radius change in the tangential meridian is about three times the corresponding change in the sagittal meridian and therefore the mean extra positive power change is accompanied by an astigmatic power of approximately the same magnitude. In practical terms this causes extra negative and/or unexplained residual astigmatism during over-refraction with lenses of this design that show poor centration (Meyler & Ruston 1994). Some manufacturers produce lenses of front surface asphere design to compensate for the induced astigmatism resulting from the rear surface when the lens decentres.
- There is no freedom of manoeuvre in fitting. Practitioners must use the eccentricity value(s) chosen by the laboratory.
- Aspheric lenses cannot be modified other than by adding spherical peripheral curves to loosen the fit.
- Lenses are difficult to check. A radiuscope can be used to check the back central optic radius (BCOR), sometimes referred to as the posterior apical radius (PAR), but the degree of flattening is almost impossible to measure in general practice. A keratometer cannot be used.
- Most aspheric designs are not available in astigmatic form.
- The practitioner is forced to use the laboratory that produced the fitting set.
- Aspheric lenses are not easily identified by other practitioners seeing the patient.
- Aspheric lenses may be more difficult to manufacture. For example, overpolishing will change the degree of asphericity.

Front surface aspheric lenses have been used to reduce the lens thickness, especially in aphakic designs, to provide presbyopic corrections (see Chapter 14), to reduce spherical aberration (Kerns 1984, Oxenberg & Carney 1989) and to improve acuity with residual astigmatism (Evans & Morrison 1984).

Selection of the first aspheric trial lens

Because the aspheric surface flattens away from the lens apex, the sagittal depth of an aspheric lens is considerably less than a spherical lens with the same central radius. An aspheric lens must therefore be fitted steeper than a spherical lens to obtain the same corneal clearance. However, the degree of steepening will depend upon the design of the trial lens in use and also its *e* value. For example, a lens with a spherical BOZR and an elliptical periphery may be treated much the same way as any other spherical lens. Conversely, a full aspheric lens with a high *e* value of, say, 0.6, will require a nominal BCOR possibly 0.2–0.3 mm steeper than *K*.

Depending upon the specific design selected, there are only two parameters that the practitioner can vary to modify the central fit, lens positioning and edge clearance. These are the BCOR (or PAR) and TD. Thus if a lens shows excess AEC the practitioner should steepen the BCOR or reduce the TD; or choose a lens design with a lower *e* value. In the event of too little AEC, the practitioner must:

- Flatten the BCOR.
- Increase the TD.
- If necessary, add a small spherical edge curve.
- Choose a lens with a higher *e* value.

In lens designs with spherical back optic zones, the same allowances as for normal spherical designs should be made to the BOZR if the BOZD is changed. However, this is commonly not allowable as the lens parameters are fixed. For example, in an aspheric central design the flattening of the BCOR with increases in TD is built into the asphericity itself and should not therefore be amended.

In conclusion practitioners must:

- Understand the design and eccentricity of the trial lens in use.
- Be guided by the manufacturer's literature in the choice of the first lens.
- Understand how to modify the particular design in use to manipulate the lens fitting.
- Be prepared to use a different aspheric design or a multicurve, if the particular one in use does not give an acceptable fit.

Front optic zone diameter

Reducing the front optic zone is an effective strategy in reducing the centre thickness in positive-powered lenses and the edge thickness in negative-powered lenses. For example, if a lens of TD 9.80 mm and BVP +7.00 D does not have a reduced front optic zone diameter (FOZD), the lens centre thickness would be around 0.41 mm. With a FOZD of 7.00 mm, the centre thickness would be around 0.26 mm, i.e. nearly 60% thinner and the oxygen transmission would improve by a similar amount. Nowadays, computer-generated lathes reduce the FOZD in all powers.

Where computer-generated lathes are not used, all lenses above −5.00 D or +4.00 D should be lenticulated. The practitioner can request a different FOZD from standard and this is determined by the pupil size in dull illumination, the size of the BOZD and the lens TD. For small lenses, the FOZD should be around 0.2 mm larger than the BOZD to allow for junction blending; for example, if the BOZD is 7.00 mm, the FOZD should be specified as 7.20 mm. In larger lenses, the diameter of the FOZD is judged by the size of the pupil; for example, a BOZD of 8.30 mm may have a FOZD of 7.40 mm in a patient with a pupil diameter of 5.00 mm in low-level illumination. In this case a FOZD of 8.50 mm would produce a negligible lenticulation and a thick lens would still result.

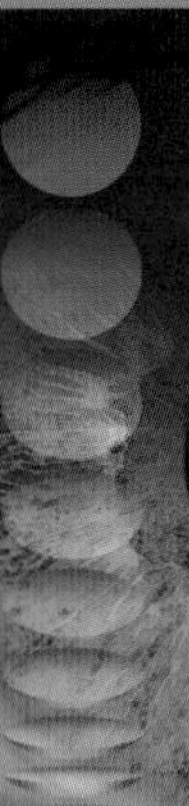

In conclusion:

- BOZD and FOZD must cover the cornea consistently throughout lens movements associated with blinking.
- Inadequate optic zones will cause flare, especially when the pupil is dilated.
- Non-lenticulated higher-powered lenses will be thick, uncomfortable and tend to lag or sit low or high.
- Oxygen permeability will be reduced.
- The most common cause of flare is poor centration, which may be related to other fitting factors.

Lens material

A general discussion of lens materials has already been given earlier in this chapter and in more detail in Chapter 3. In summary, when selecting a lens material, practitioners must ensure that the material selected:

- Satisfies the oxygen demand of that particular patient.
- Remains biocompatible with the eye.
- Is durable on the eye, maintaining a stable shape to correct vision.

The important material properties include permeability to oxygen, wettability, hardness and modulus of elasticity.

OXYGEN PERMEABILITY

The Cooperative Research Centre for Eye Research and Technology in their CD (see note at the end of this chapter) make the following general recommendations:

Not suitable for extended wear (EW) or prolonged day wear (DW) (Dk <20)	Boston II, SGP 1, Paraperm O_2, Optacryl 60
Suitable for DW but not EW (Dk 20–50)	Boston ES, Boston IV, Boston RXD, FluoroPerm 30, FluoroPerm 60, Paragon HDS, Boston EO, Boston 7, Boston Equalens I, Quantum 1, SGP III, Menicon EX, Paraperm EW
Suitable for DW (high Rx) and occasionally overnight (Dk 50–100)	Boston Equalens II, FluoroPerm 92, FluoroPerm 151
Suitable for DW and overnight (Dk >100)	Boston XO, Quantum II, Menicon SFP, Menicon Z

This list is by no means exhaustive and new materials constantly appear. Practitioners should update themselves by reading current literature and talking to the companies involved.

WETTABILITY

Wettability is defined as the ability of a fluid to spread and remain over the surface. The tear film on a contact lens must be smooth and stable between blinks for good vision, comfort and lubrication of the ocular surface.

Typical methods for measuring wettability are the sessile drop, the captive bubble and Wilhelmy plate methods. Practitioners should check the method of testing used by the laboratory and the relative results using the same method by competitors. However, the laboratory-determined wetting angle does not necessarily predict the wettability performance of the final lens on the eye. The effect of polishing (and especially overpolishing) during manufacture, lens surface deposition (biofilm) and contamination of the surface by hydrophobic substances such as oils and moisturizers from make-up will all affect the in vivo lens wettability. Tear film coverage is best evaluated with a slit-lamp using relatively dim, diffuse illumination with moderate magnification.

HARDNESS

This is defined as the ability of the surface of the material to resist compression or penetration.

The Roswell hardness test uses a round head probe to exert pressure on an RGP button to determine the amount of compression it will withstand. The Shore D Test determines the resistance of a lens surface to penetration by a sharp probe.

Hardness has implications for lens manufacture and clinical performance.

- A softer lens surface
  - is more difficult to manufacture.
  - can lead to problems with wettability and subsequent deposition problems from surface damage during manufacture.
- A harder material is
  - easier to manufacture.
  - more brittle.
  - less resilient to breakage.

MODULUS OF ELASTICITY

The modulus of elasticity is a stiffness constant reflecting the ability of a material to resist deformation in tension.

The higher the modulus of elasticity of a material, the more rigid or less flexible will be the lens made from that material. Conversely, the lower the modulus of elasticity, the more flexible the lens, especially with thinner lenses and, following a blink, there is more chance of a lens distorting on the eye, producing variable vision.

- Softer lens materials are more likely to
  - scratch.
  - conform to an astigmatic cornea producing residual astigmatism.
- Harder or more rigid materials are more likely to crack or break.

Hardness and rigidity may therefore be a determinant as to the minimum thickness of a lens but should not be the major factors in choosing a lens material.

EASE OF MANUFACTURE

For ease of manufacture, a lens material should be homogeneous and have consistent mechanical properties so it is:

- Stress free.
- Durable.

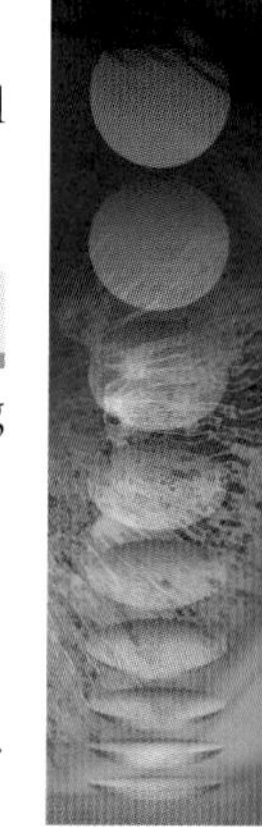

- Resistant to local heating.
- Easy to polish.
- Has predictable hydration characteristics.

When choosing a lens material it is often helpful to talk to the laboratory making the lens. They will not only have all the technical information available but will also be aware of any manufacturing difficulties that may influence the clinical decision.

In summary, the ideal RGP material will supply adequate oxygen for the wearer's needs, be readily wettable on the eye, have a high modulus of elasticity to resist flexure, have resilience to compression for durability and ease of manufacture, and not be susceptible to breakage.

COMPUTERIZED LENS DESIGN AND FITTING

A lens design CD-ROM is supplied with this book. Many topographical devices also include an RGP design program.

ADVANTAGES

- The ability to customize lens designs, particularly for unusually shaped corneas, and assess the fitting without taking up prolonged chair time. The simulated fluorescein pattern can also be inspected if this facility is available.
- Where legislation may prevent the reuse of trial lenses, the first lens can be ordered from the laboratory with reasonable confidence. By using laboratories that allow 'warranty exchanges' the ideal fitting can then be ordered by observation of this first, calculated, diagnostic lens.
- Less patient discomfort is involved as fewer trial lenses are necessary.
- Where lenses of a differing TD are needed (e.g. to match a lost lens) and where the practitioner does not have a trial lens of the required diameter, the correct fitting can be calculated from the nearest correct trial lens.
- As modifications are made to the fit (e.g. changing a BOZD), alterations in the lens parameters can be assessed in order to examine the effect on the overall fit.
- Post-fitting analysis of the effect of a patient's contact lens can be accomplished from videokeratographs taken pre-fitting and compared to subsequent videokeratographs taken at follow-up visits.
- As an aid to teaching; for example, to demonstrate the effect of various parameter changes.

DISADVANTAGES

- Lid tension, lid position and tear dynamics are not taken into account.
- Lens mass and centre of gravity cannot be assessed.
- Subtle aspects of post-lens fluorescein cannot always be detected on the VDU screen.
- Change in fit on lens decentration is difficult to assess.
- Accuracy of lens design and fluorescein patterns cannot be greater than the accuracy with which the original topographical plot has been made.
- For all the above reasons, a trial lens fitting is still essential wherever possible.

Advanced RGP fitting program

The *advanced fitting module* on the CD-ROM accompanying this book allows more experienced practitioners to feed in the:

- Desired TLT.
- BOZD and TD.
- *e* or *p* value over the BOZD.*
- Peripheral curve widths and the desired *e* or *p* value over each diameter.*
- AEC required at each curve diameter.

Ideally, a topographical device such as the Medmont E300 is desirable in order to measure the *e* or *p* values over the different diameters. In countries where concern over Creutzfeldt–Jakob disease precludes or makes difficult the reuse of trial lenses, this program allows practitioners the facility to order the first lens with a high likelihood of success.

A more mathematical approach to lens design is given in Chapter 6 and in more detail on the accompanying CD-ROM.

FITTING ROUTINE FOR RGP LENSES

Most RGP fitting is still carried out in the conventional manner without the aid of topographical devices. Even where such equipment is available, the following are required before fitting commences:

- General discussion with the patient on advantages and disadvantages of contact lenses, patient suitability, motivation etc., as discussed in Chapter 8.
- Corneal, lid and limbal integrity using a slit-lamp (see Chapters 7 and 8).
- Tear film assessment (see Chapter 5).
- Measurements to decide initial trial lens parameters
  - accurate keratometer reading and/or corneal topography – BOZR (see Chapter 7).
  - horizontal and vertical visible iris diameters (which approximately equal the corneal diameters) – total diameter (TD).
  - interpalpebral aperture size and lid positions – TD.
  - pupil size in average and low illuminations – BOZD.
- Accurate spectacle refraction and calculation of ocular refraction, so a subsequent check on the liquid lens power can be made. This is approximately zero in a true alignment fit.
- Decision of lens type to be used (e.g. multicurve, aspheric, toric, bifocal).

Assessment of the fit

At least 5 minutes should be allowed after insertion of the first lens for lacrimation to subside. This may be reduced if a local anaesthetic is used. Subsequent lenses settle more quickly whether an anaesthetic is used or not. Patients usually comment

* If not known, assume an average *e* value of 0.5.

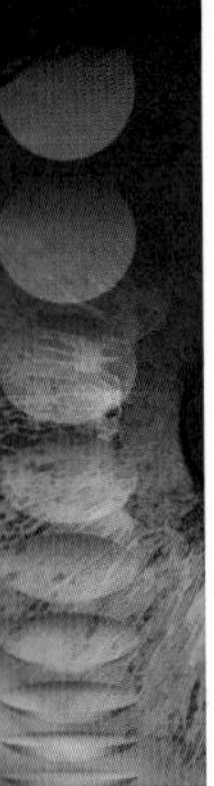

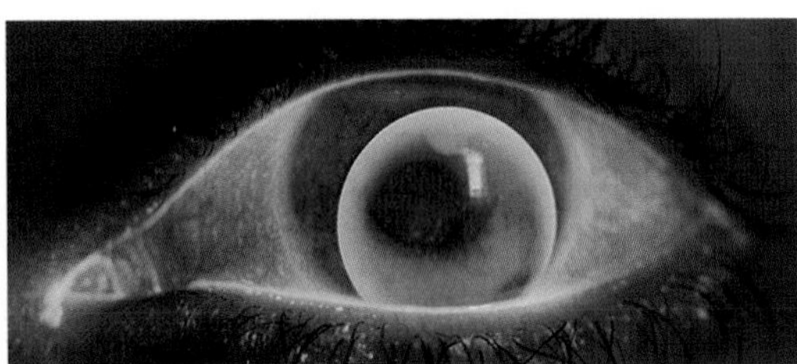

Figure 9.18 The pentacurve lens C5/8.10:7.00/8.60:7.60/9.60:8.20/10.80:8.80/12.25:9.20 on a cornea with *K* readings 7.91 at 180° and 7.81 at 90°. The fluorescein pattern shows a central flat fit with bearing on the apex of the cornea and a slight epithelial abrasion as a result. The lens is riding lower-temporally. The lens periphery appears to have excessive clearance, partially due to the central flat fit. (Courtesy of M. Wilson)

that the lens is more comfortable than expected and the practitioner should maintain conversation to reassure them and take their mind off any irritation produced by the lens. While adapting to the lens it is often helpful to instruct the patient to look downwards (where the lids are at their most relaxed) and to blink normally.

WHITE LIGHT ASSESSMENT (Table 9.6)

- *Lids in the normal position*: as the lids move, the lens should remain within the limbal area and the superior lens edge ideally positioned under the upper lid.
- *Lids separated*: the lens should drop slowly when pushed to the top of the cornea. A flat-fitting lens falls more quickly and often drops in a curved path as it pivots around the apex of the cornea (Fig. 9.18). A steep-fitting lens falls more slowly and often remains at the corneal apex.
- The lens should promptly return to the same position after each blink. Post-blink movement should be 1.5–2.0 mm, smooth, medium to fast and vertical.

ULTRAVIOLET LIGHT ASSESSMENT (Table 9.7)

One drop of 2% fluorescein is applied from a wetted impregnated strip or unit dose container on to the superior conjunctiva with the patient looking down and the lids retracted (see Fig. 9.7).

- *Lens centred*: Table 9.7 supplements the fluorescein patterns in Figure 9.7 and elsewhere in this chapter. The fluorescein picture of aspheric lenses is generally the same but without any obvious transitions.
- *Lens displaced upwards*: fluorescein will disappear from under the upper periphery of the lens, except at the extreme edge, and will collect under the lower periphery and lower part of the back optic zone – this can be mistaken for a steep lens. Care should be taken to ensure that the extreme edge of the lens does not indent the peripheral cornea.
- *Movement*: with fluorescein present, the movement of the lens is observed with the lids in the normal position, during blinking and normal eye rotations. The BOZD, or the TD in the case of aspheric lenses, is checked relative to the pupil size as the lens moves. The lens should centre itself after each blink and eye movement. Whenever a lens consistently takes up an incorrect position, the transitions or edges may bear on the cornea: these should be blended.

Table 9.6: White light assessment of lens fit

Lens position	Possible cause
Continually high, not dropping after blinks	Flat peripheral zone; too large a lens; too wide a peripheral zone; lens too thin; thick edges; lens slightly steep occasionally; lens too light in weight due to small TD, or too thin, or both; negative lens
Continually low, with rapid dropping after blinks	Too small a lens; too thick a lens; lens fit slightly flat; (prism) ballasted lens; too heavy a lens due to large TD or thickness, or both; positive lens
Continually to one side	Apex of cornea displaced; lens too small or too flat; spherical lens on an 'against-the-rule' cornea
Hardly any movement from the centre	Lens too steep; inadequate edge clearance
Lens moving about too much and beyond limbus	Profuse lacrimation due to foreign body or poor lens edge; lens too flat, allowing excess movement; lens too flat or too steep causing irritation and lacrimation; spherical lens on toroidal cornea

TD, total diameter.

Table 9.7: Fluorescein assessment of lens fit

Fit		
Central	Peripheral	Fluorescein picture
Ideal alignment	–	Even dark blue of BOZD with a 0.5–1.0 mm wide green band at edge of lens. A central trace of fluorescein is acceptable
–	Flat	Bright green under the entire peripheral zone, possibly with bubbles at or under the edge
Flat	–	Dark blue centrally with green encroaching under periphery of back optic zone
–	Steep	Narrow blue touch band at extreme edge, green within this. Possible blue transition touch with wide peripheral curves
Steep	–	Blue transition with green under back optic zone and bubble if very steep

ASTIGMATIC CORNEAS (see also Chapter 12)

When fitting a spherical lens to an astigmatic cornea, a compromise is needed (see p. 200). If a with-the-rule cornea (i.e. flatter meridian horizontal) is fitted with a lens showing

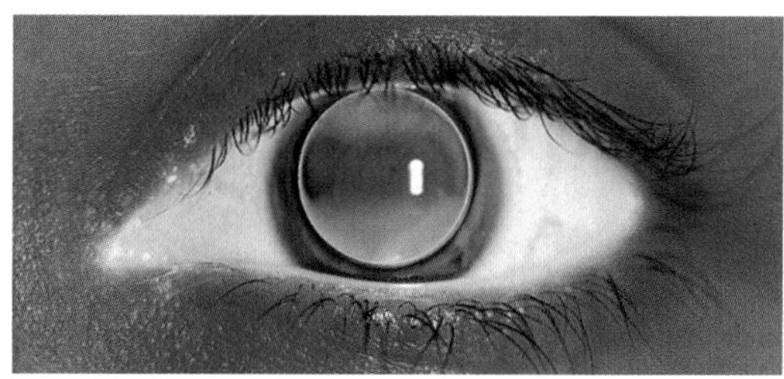

Figure 9.19 An interpalpebral spherical corneal lens with the back optic zone in alignment with the horizontal meridian of a toroidal cornea having 'with-the-rule' astigmatism. (Courtesy of M. Wilson)

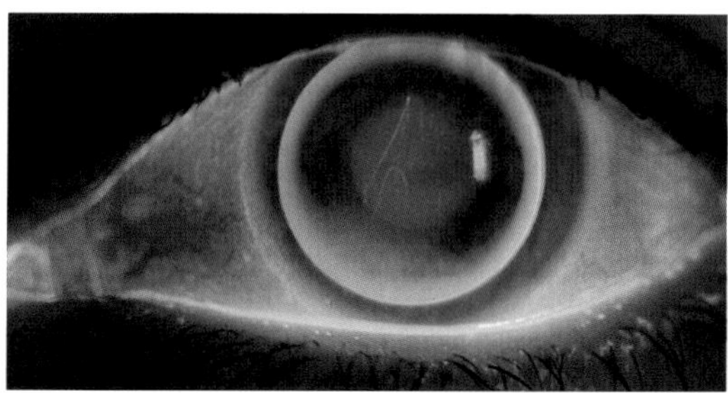

Figure 9.20 A spherical lens fitted with slight apical clearance to a 'with-the-rule' toroidal cornea, the steeper meridian being along 70°. The peripheral zone has been fitted slightly steep to prevent too much edge clearance at the top and bottom in order to minimize discomfort when blinking. There are two crescentic bands of corneal touch on either side of the 160° meridian and fluorescein shows on the front surface of the top of the lens. Slight central clearance can just be seen along the 70° meridian. (Courtesy of M. Wilson)

central alignment of the flattest meridian and a peripheral zone also showing near alignment in this meridian, then the fluorescein picture should show:

- *Centrally*: an elongated 'H' or dumb-bell-shaped blue touch area as wide as the BOZD (Figs 9.19, 9.20).
- *Peripherally*: blue touch in the horizontal meridian and green stand-off in the vertical. The peripheral alignment should not occupy more than one-third of the lens circumference. Vertical stand-off is liable to cause discomfort when blinking. This can be minimized by making the lens as small as possible and the peripheral zone narrow (Fig. 9.19).

A fully aligning astigmatic lens will show the same fluorescein pattern as a spherical lens on a spherical cornea.

Due to the reduced sagittal depth of aspheric lenses, higher degrees of astigmatism can be fitted with these lenses but back toric lens fittings may still be necessary for corneas showing more than 1.50 D astigmatism in order to maintain good lens centration and comfort.

REFRACTION

This should be performed with the patient wearing the lens whose BOZR is the nearest to the correct fitting. The contact lens over-refraction is a means of checking the fit because with exact alignment the liquid lens power would be zero and the over-refraction (plus any power of the trial contact lens) equal to the ocular refraction after allowing for the back vertex distance. In reality, the lens BOZR is often slightly different from the flattest *K* reading and the allowance for this is discussed later. However, if the over-refraction shows less negative or more positive power than the calculated ocular refraction, then a flat fitting should be suspected. A steep fitting (positive liquid lens) gives a more negative or less positive contact lens refraction.

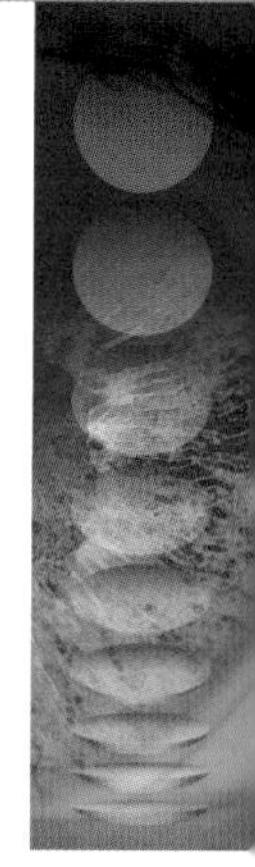

FITTING SETS

Most laboratories produce their own fitting sets. Where these are used, the following pertain:

- What lens design is used – for example, 'constant axial lift' or 'constant axial edge clearance' design? The latter is preferable as relating to a more 'real world' situation.
- Is every lens marked with its BOZR to prevent lens mix-up?
- What *e* value has been assumed in the lens design? It should be around 0.45–0.50.
- Are the transitions lightly, moderately or heavily blended? A moderately blended lens will be more like the finished lens but will still allow easy differentiation of the curves when assessing the lens fit or when checking the lens.
- What material has been used? PMMA may retain its parameters longer than an RGP trial set but the lens material will affect its possible flexure on the eye as discussed below.
- What manufacturing tolerance has been accepted? This should be better than normal standards as small errors can affect the final lens ordered. Ideally, practitioners should regularly re-measure all trial lens parameters.
- Are the *full* lens parameters supplied with the set? *No* fitting set should be accepted without complete details of every curve, diameter, etc., being available.

The CD-ROM supplied with this book now allows practitioners to design their own fitting sets. It is useful to have sets with at least three TDs (e.g. 9.0, 9.50 and 10.00 mm). Ideally, each set should be duplicated in differing *e* values (e.g. 0.3, 0.5 and 0.7), although this may be impractical and unnecessary as, with experience, eccentricity differences can be estimated by visual observation. The following may give a useful guide.

As shown earlier, the average *e* value tends to remain around the same whether the cornea is steep or flat. However, steeper corneas usually have a smaller visible iris diameter. Practitioners doing little RGP work may therefore select a single fitting set with a smaller TD up to, say, 7.60 mm BOZR and a larger TD above this. As can be seen from Tables 9.8 and 9.9, this also enables the initial BOZR to approximate the flattest *K* reading for the initial lens selection. Practitioners doing greater volumes of RGP work will require several different sets. Many of these may be eclectic, accumulated from unsuitable lenses collected over the years.

Lens–cornea relationship and lens flexibility

The following factors should be taken into account.

- When the eyelid moves over the cornea during blinking it presses the eye back about 1.25 mm (Holden 1984). Clearly

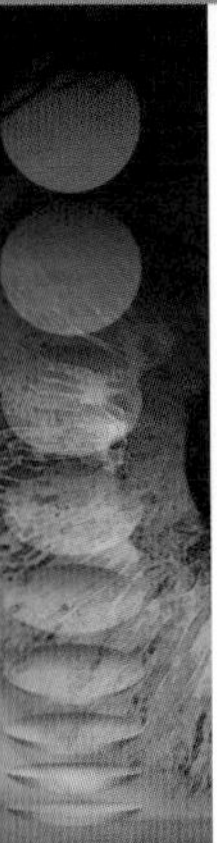

Table 9.8: A partially illustrated three-curve fitting set showing the nominal flattest keratometer reading (K_F), the tear layer thickness (TLT) and axial edge clearance (AEC) for a 9.80 mm TD lens fitting set and for corneas with nominal *e* values of 0.5

K_F (mm)	Lens prescription	TLT (μm)	AEC (μm)
7.15	7.20:8.30/7.55:8.80/8.60:9.80	24	75
7.25	7.30:8.30/7.65:8.80/8.75:9.80	23	75
7.35	7.40:8.30/7.75:8.80/8.90:9.80	16	82
7.55	7.60:8.30/7.95:8.80/9.10:9.80	14	76
7.80	7.80:8.30/8.20:8.80/9.50:9.80	21	76
8.00	8.00:8.30/8.40:8.80/9.90:9.80	19	78
8.20	8.20:8.30/8.60:8.80/10.20:9.80	18	77
8.40	8.40:8.30/8.80:8.80/10.60:9.80	16	78

Table 9.9: A partially illustrated three curve fitting set in 0.20 mm steps showing the nominal flattest keratometer reading (K_F), the tear layer thickness (TLT) and axial edge clearance (AEC) for a 9.30 mm TD lens fitting set and for corneas with a nominal *e* value of 0.5

K_F (mm)	Lens prescription	TLT (μm)	AEC (μm)
7.15	7.20:7.80/7.50:8.30/8.80:9.30	17	77
7.40	7.40:7.80/7.70:8.30/9.20:9.30	23	77
7.60	7.60:7.80/7.95:8.30/9.50:9.30	21	76
7.80	7.80:7.80/9.90:8.30/9.90:9.30	19	77
8.00	8.00:7.80/8.35:8.30/10.20:9.30	18	76
8.20	8.20:7.80/8.60:8.30/10.70:9.30	23	77
8.40	8.40:7.80/8.80:8.30.11.00:9.30	21	76

the front surface of the contact lens is subjected to considerable force. With PMMA lenses this resulted in distortion of the shape of the cornea over years of wear producing considerable blur when spectacles were subsequently worn. In the case of the more flexible RGP materials, the eyelid may succeed in distorting the shape of the lens itself. The lens does not then return to its original shape but stays flexed because the surface tension in the tear meniscus around the contact lens edge is sufficient to hold it in place. For PMMA, the critical centre thickness at which flexure on the eye could be observed was about 0.12 mm. For many RGP lenses, flexure is still obvious at 0.15 mm (greater for CAB materials).

- One would expect to find that, if an RGP lens is placed on a with-the-rule astigmatic cornea, then with-the-rule flexure of the lens on the eye would occur. In practice, not only will the degree of flexure depend upon the rigidity and thickness of the lens being used, but it will also depend upon the lens–cornea relationship. Stone and Collins (1984), Herman (1984) and others showed that, in the case of with-the-rule astigmatic corneas, as the lens BOZR becomes flatter than the flattest keratometer reading (K_F), the lens flexes in an against-the-rule fashion. Conversely, as the lens BOZR becomes steeper than K_F, the lens flexes in a with-the-rule direction.
- Herman (1984) explained that, as the lens is fitted flatter, corneal adhesion is minimized, whereas the influence of the upper lid is maximized. The pressure exerted by the upper lid is then largely against the flat front periphery of the horizontal meridian of the lens (since the lens will have rocked to align the upper half of the corneal vertical meridian). This causes the horizontal meridian of the lens to steepen, accompanied by a corresponding flattening of the vertical meridian, i.e. the lens will flex against-the-rule. Correspondingly, as a lens is fitted steeper, corneal adhesion is maximized and the influence of the upper lid minimized. Tear film adhesion then causes the lens to flex in the same direction as the corneal toricity, i.e. with-the-rule on a with-the-rule cornea. Herman found mathematically that at approximately 0.14 mm flatter than *K*, zero flexure (±0.25 D) was observed, i.e. lid compression and tear film adhesion cancel out or negate each other, allowing lens rigidity to dominate. Thus, if a lens is actually required to flex with-the-rule (and sometimes this may be desirable to neutralize internal ocular astigmatism), it might be preferable to fit the lens slightly steep. This should allow the lens to centre so that it is not totally affected by the upper lid and is therefore allowed to flex somewhat with-the-rule. If, after the relationship of the *K* reading and refractive spectacle correction has been examined, it seems more desirable to minimize or create an against-the-rule effect, then the lens should be fitted flatter, allowing it to ride high, behind the upper lid, maximizing lid compression to minimize with-the-rule flexure.
- The numerical BOZR/*K* reading relationship should only be used as a guideline. Fluorescein patterns should be observed for individual cases. Such factors as peripheral corneal flattening and corneal diameter can make a significant difference. The fluorescein pattern should be coordinated with the measured flexure (by keratometry over the lens) and over-refraction to produce both an optimal fit and visual result. It should be emphasized that, although the lens BOZR may be nominally flatter than *K*, large BOZDs are now commonly used and the fluorescein picture may still be that of corneal alignment.
- The foregoing explanation applies only to with-the-rule corneas. In the case of against-the-rule corneas, both the tear film adhesion factor and the upper lid forces are additive. Both act in an against-the-rule direction, causing significant flexure in the against-the-rule direction of almost any BOZR placed on the eye. In such cases, toric fitting lenses are preferable. The only possible exception is the higher values of hyperopic astigmatism where lens thickness may prevent flexure on the eye with the thicker/more rigid material.
- The increased flexibility of some RGP lenses reduces their capability of resisting the compression forces created during reflex blinking. If the lens is fitted even slightly on the steep

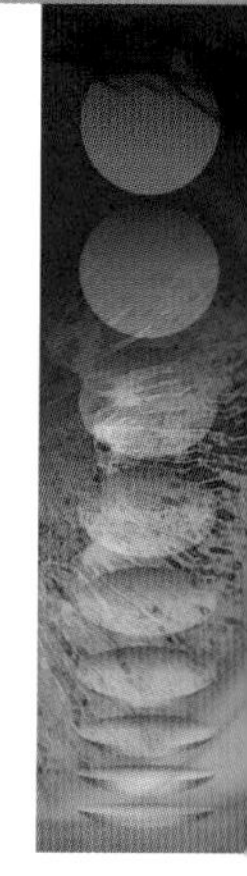

side of alignment, blink-induced compression may create a temporary seal between the periphery of the lens and the underlying cornea. As the lens decompresses during the opening phase of each blink cycle, the resulting hydrodynamic forces can create a transient negative pressure at the corneal surface that will cause increasing lens awareness as well as unstable vision. The final fitting of lenses should therefore err slightly on the flatter side of alignment (see also 'Lens adhesion phenomenon', below).

- The amount of lens flexure may be influenced not only by peripheral corneal flattening, lid pressure and capillary attraction of the tears, but also by the back surface geometry of the lens and its cross-sectional thickness distribution which influence lid pressure and tear meniscus. For example, an elliptical lens may flex slightly differently from a multicurve lens and a lenticular construction may differ from a non-lenticular construction.
- With early RGP materials, flexure was found to be greater as the material Dk increased. More modern materials are now largely independent of their Dk value with regard to their tendency to flexure (Blehl et al. 1991, Cornish et al. 1991, Sorbara et al. 1992).
- Astigmatism: It can now be appreciated that a different approach to dealing with astigmatism is needed with RGP lenses than the typically used PMMA trial lenses. Ideally, a short tolerance trial should be carried out with lenses of the same material, thickness and diameter as the final lens, and practitioners are well advised to stockpile old or non-prescribed lenses for this purpose. As the centre thickness decreases, the fitting of the BOZR should approach the flatter K reading to slightly flatter than K_F in cases of with-the-rule astigmatism. In the case of against-the-rule astigmatism, the practitioner will fairly quickly require a toroidal back surface lens.
- Sevigny and Bennett (1984) advised increasing the centre thickness by 0.02 mm/D of corneal astigmatism or decreasing the BOZD by 0.2–0.4 mm to minimize flexure in cases of with-the-rule astigmatism. However, increasing lens centre thickness will reduce oxygen transmissibility.

Lens adhesion phenomenon

The intermittent adhesion of high Dk lenses to the cornea during sleep is a phenomenon mainly associated with overnight wear, although it can occur with daily wear. Such lenses are found fixed to the cornea, partially overlapping the limbus and with the patient usually asymptomatic. In most instances the lens adhesion disappears spontaneously shortly after awakening, leaving a compression ring that resolves after a few hours. This ring is identified by the instillation of fluorescein, which collects in the circular groove (Fig. 9.21). Too steep a fit or poor blending of the peripheral curves should be suspected if the base of the compression groove stains with fluorescein and causes discomfort. Some patients are more susceptible to this phenomenon than others (Swarbrick & Holden 1989) and should be advised to check that the lenses move freely on waking. Patients experiencing occasional adhesion should be instructed to free the lens by compressing the lid margin just above or below the lens to release the suction. Additionally, the centre thickness of the lens may be increased by at least 0.03 mm to reduce lens flexure, or the edge clearance increased slightly if the problem persists (Kenyon et al. 1989). Logically it might be expected that the lens BOZR should be flattened to prevent binding and this may be correct in lenses fitted borderline tight. However, Swarbrick and Holden (1996) demonstrated that *steepening* the lens will often reduce binding. This is because a slightly flat-fitting lens tends to decentre to the corneal periphery where movement is restricted and lens binding more likely. Nevertheless, some patients seem prone to lens binding and overnight wear should be discouraged if this problem resists all corrective measures (see Chapters 14 and 17).

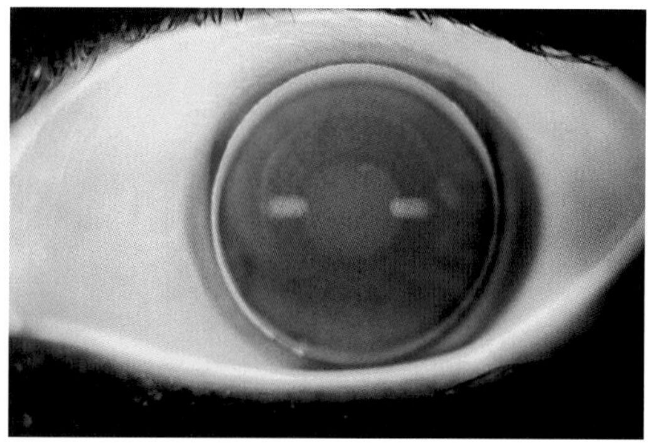

Figure 9.21 Lens binding can occur with extended wear RGP lenses after overnight wear. The lens fails to move with normal blinking for 1–5 hours in 10–50% of wearers. On lens removal the epithelium typically displays some central punctuate staining and often a prominent indentation or compression ring corresponding to the lens edge as shown above. The compression ring may itself stain with fluorescein although more typically there is pooling rather than true staining. (From Swarbrick and Holden (1987), *Am. J. Optom. Physiol. Opt.*, 64, 815, with kind permission. © The American Academy of Optometry, 1987)

Swarbrick (1988) showed that fenestrating RGP lenses has little effect on lens binding, indicating that lens flexure or tight fitting is not necessarily the causative factor. Sodium fluorescein also penetrates only very slowly under a bound lens, spreading in a fern-like pattern. From these observations Swarbrick postulated that the lens preferentially expresses the aqueous layer of the tear film overnight, leaving the mucus layer to act as an adhesive between lens and cornea.

Three and 9 o'clock staining

Although 3 and 9 o'clock staining of the exposed peripheral cornea was often seen in PMMA lens wearers (see Chapter 17 and Fig. 17.43), it is more commonly observed in RGP wearers for the following reasons:

- The reduced edge clearance techniques used to reduce lid awareness and lens movement.
- The larger TDs generally used increase edge thickness for negative-powered lenses.

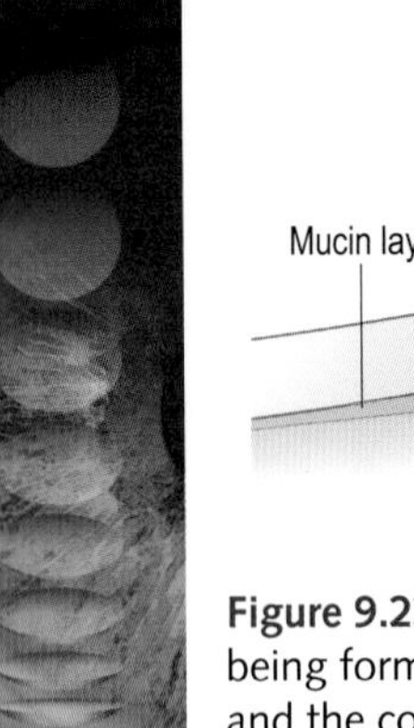

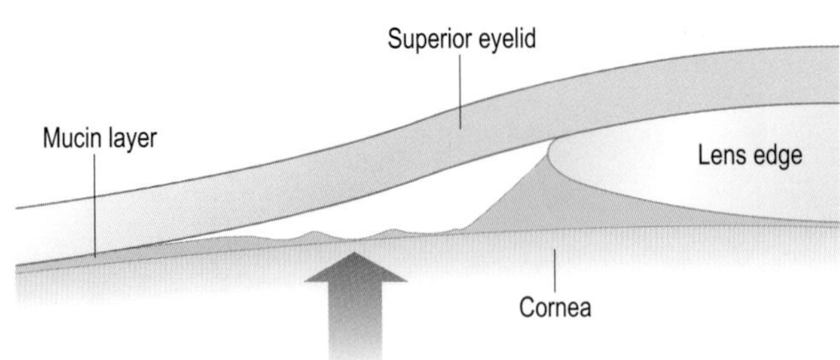

Figure 9.22 Bridge effect or lid gap theory. Due to a bridge being formed by the upper eyelid between the edge of the lens and the cornea during blinking, a gap is created under the eyelid, and mucin coverage (arrow) of the area under the 'bridge' may be inadequate. (After van der Worp et al. 2003)

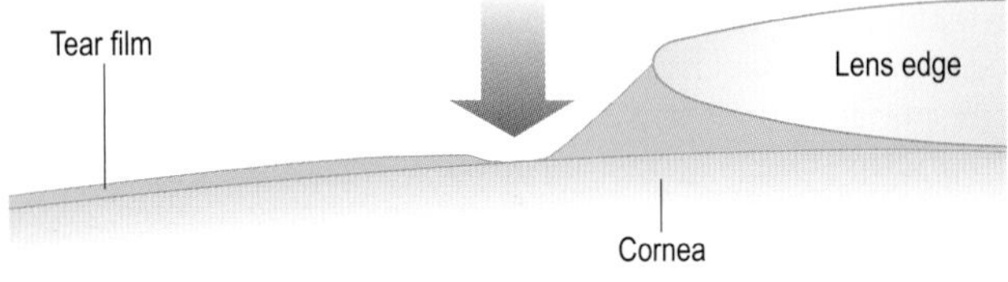

Figure 9.23 Tear meniscus theory. Localized thinning (arrow) of the tear film in the area immediately adjacent to the tear meniscus at the lens edge. (After van der Worp et al. 2003)

- Many gas-permeable materials, because of their tendency to attract deposits, cause reduced surface wettability and hence tear film disruption.

The effect of these creates an inadequate tear film in the exposed 3 and 9 o'clock areas which leads to corneal desiccation. The two common theories for 3 and 9 o'clock staining are therefore the 'bridge effect' (or 'lid gap') theory (Fig. 9.22) and the 'tear meniscus' theory (Fig. 9.23).

While minor 3 and 9 o'clock staining may be acceptable, a persistent or marked condition may lead to dellen (thinning of the epithelium), erosions and eventually local neovascularization or ulceration. The lateral conjunctiva adjacent to the 3 and 9 o'clock staining may also become hyperaemic. Where necessary, the following action should be taken:

- Thin the edges if considered thick.
- Check the lens has not been fitted too steeply.
- Give blink exercises and lateral eye movement exercises. Decreased blinking due to the discomfort associated with interaction of the lens edge and the upper eyelid in the early adaptive phase of lens wear is thought to result in increased tear evaporation. Blink exercises should hopefully restore a normal pattern (see Blink efficiency, Chapter 17).
- Flatten the peripheral curves to create more lens movement.
- Increase the lens TD if considered too small or decrease the TD if considered too large.
- Steepen the peripheral curves if considered excessively flat, i.e. reduce the AEC. Holden et al. (1987) demonstrated that, as the AEC was gradually increased from 100 to 120 μm (and beyond), all subjects showed increased 3 and 9 o'clock staining. The AEC should therefore be kept to around 70–80 μm as recommended earlier, and possibly less.
- Flatten the fitting to utilize the lid attachment technique, i.e. create more lens movement.
- Try a better wetting material.
- Use in-eye lubricant drops.
- Consider a trial of temporary, collagen, punctal occlusion in recalcitrant cases.
- Refit with a soft lens.

Algorithms for the treatment of recalcitrant 3 and 9 o'clock staining cases have been produced by Businger et al. (1989) and Jones et al. (1989).

Changes in BOZR

Lenses made from PMMA absorb 1–2% by weight of water and as they hydrate or dehydrate, undergo cyclic changes in BOZR depending upon their centre thickness and BVP (Gordon 1965, Phillips 1969). The classic work of Gordon is shown in Figure 9.24. All PMMA lenses flatten with hydration.

CAB materials are known to be at least as, if not more, sensitive to hydration–dehydration changes as PMMA, with the degree of flattening increasing as the lens centre decreases and high minus lenses being very unstable.

The incorporation of wetting agents, such as methacrylic acid, into silicone-acrylate polymer can be responsible for the BOZR flattening observed when this group of lens materials is hydrated. Kerr and Dilly (1988) reported increased flattening of –10.00 D lenses made from this material from 0.08 mm after 24 hours to 0.11 mm after 3 months. For –15.00 D lenses, the flattening increased from 0.09 mm after 24 hours to 0.15 mm after 3 months. With fluoropolymers the flattening effect was greater, a –10.00 D lens typically flattening 0.08 mm after 24 hours to 0.19 mm after 3 months, and a –15.00 D lens flattening by 0.12 mm after 24 hours to 0.34 mm after 3 months.

If these changes are modest, consistent and limited to the higher minus powers, they may be acceptable. Because of the lower water uptake than either PMMA or CAB, the silicone-acrylate and fluorosilicone groups generally undergo smaller hydration changes than these other two groups of materials. Significant and unpredictable fluctuation in BOZR measurements that occur after hydration are undesirable and may reflect a weakness in the design or polymerization of the material. Because of its potential to alter the anticipated fit and visual correction of the lens, the dimensional stability of all new products should ideally be evaluated by measuring the BOZR of a series of negative-powered lenses before and after 24 hours of hydration.

Occasionally, flattening of a lens BOZR will be observed that cannot be explained by normal hydration changes (e.g. 0.05–0.20 mm flattening on low-powered lenses). The common cause would appear to be stress put on the lens during the lathe-cutting process in the form of heat transfer (Schwartz 1986). If the laboratory technician runs the cutting lathe too fast, makes the cuts too fast or too deep, polishes the lens too long or does not use enough coolant, then stress is induced into the lens which will cause subsequent lens flattening. This stress may be cumulative and is also more likely if the practitioner orders a

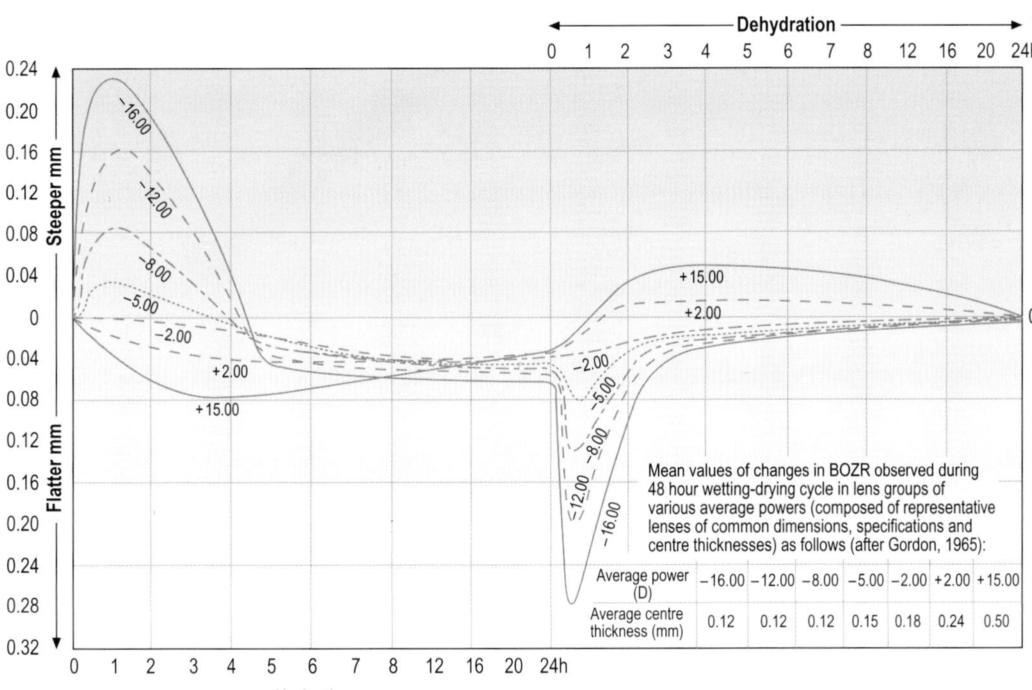

Figure 9.24 The wetting–drying cycle of polymethylmethacrylate corneal lenses

lens too thin for a particular material. Finally, stress-induced flattening is more likely in larger-diameter and higher minus-powered lenses due to the difference in thickness between lens edge and centre. To minimize this effect, front surface lenticulation may be ordered from BVPs of –3.00 D and +1.00 D upwards if necessary as opposed to the ±5.00 D upwards of PMMA lenses.

Walker (1988) reported BOZR flattening with hydration of the order of 0.10 mm for –7.50 D and 0.25 mm for –15.00 D lenses made from Paraperm EW, and 0.17 mm for –15.00 D lenses made from Boston IV and Equalens. Unlike PMMA, high positive-powered lenses (+15.00 D) were steepened by 0.05 mm for Paraperm EW and Equalens and 0.03 mm for Boston IV materials. By using photokeratograms, Walker showed that these curvature changes were largely restricted to the central 3–4 mm so that the effect on fitting (but not vision) may not be as great as expected. Nevertheless, as the lens centre flattens, the mid-periphery will steepen, producing an unexpected fluorescein pattern. This may also be a factor in lens binding (see above) with higher-powered negative lenses.

Changes with hydration cannot be assumed to happen: some materials may show no clinically significant changes with hydration. Pearson (1989) found BOZR changes of less than 0.05 mm over 6 weeks with a range of BVPs up to –14.00 D using Quantum material. Ideally, all RGP materials should be hydrated before being dispensed and the BOZR periodically monitored.

Surface crazing and cracking phenomenon

Over a period of time, many patients show deposit build-up on the lens surface. This appears as plaques or areas of deposit or as surface lines or patterns. In this situation of surface crazing, better cleaning or extra or more frequent use of proteolytic enzymes is necessary. Surface crazing is also amenable to repolishing by the laboratory.

The more serious appearance of surface cracking is seen rarely nowadays (Fig. 9.25). These are deep fissures within the lens surface appearing largely in certain early higher Dk silicone-acrylate materials.

Research by the author did not appear to show causative factors such as either ultraviolet or preservative exposure. It may have originated from either surface stress introduced during lens manufacture, which ultimately showed cracking from repeated flexure during blinking, or from constant hydration–dehydration changes or poor polymer material design. Seidner (1987) postulated the cause to be the incorporation of too high a percentage of methacrylic acid in the material formulation.

Surface cracking is often not visible to the patient, who may present with symptoms of slight loss of comfort and visual deterioration, especially if the cracking is central. Only rarely was it reported on the lens back surface (Grohe et al. 1987). Cracking is visible to the practitioner either by slit-lamp examination or hand-held magnifier and cannot be removed by repolishing: lens replacement is the only answer.

McLauglin et al. (1988) and Moody et al. (1989) reported pseudomonal and staphylococcal infections, respectively associated with the wearing of surface-cracked RGP lenses.

While surface cracking has not been reported in more recent materials it is occasionally seen in older 'emergency' or spare lenses. It is nevertheless an example of potential problems that practitioners should always be aware of with any new lens material.

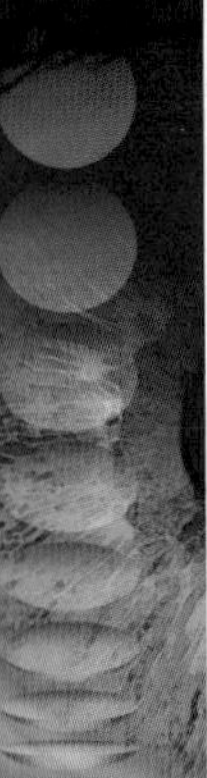

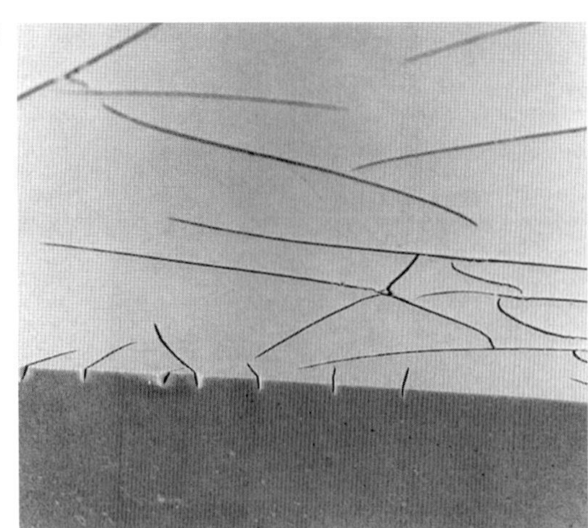

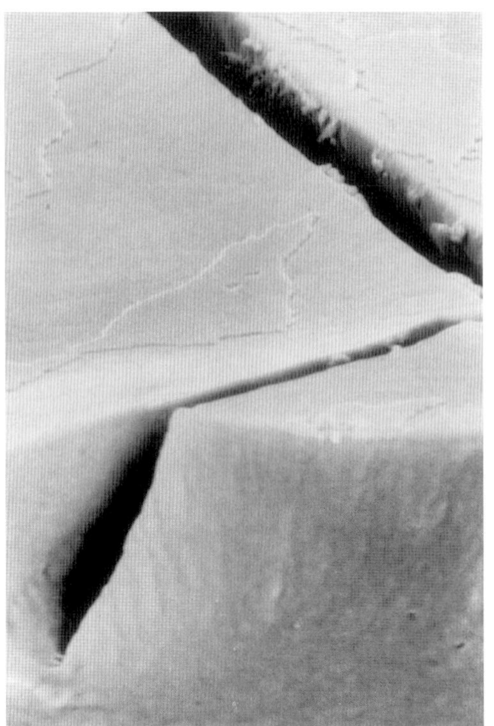

Figure 9.25 Surface cracking of an RGP lens. (a) Low magnification in cross-section showing both the surface pattern and depth of crack. (b) High magnification showing debris accumulating in the crack. Surface protein deposits are also visible. (c) Slit-lamp appearance of surface cracking on the eye

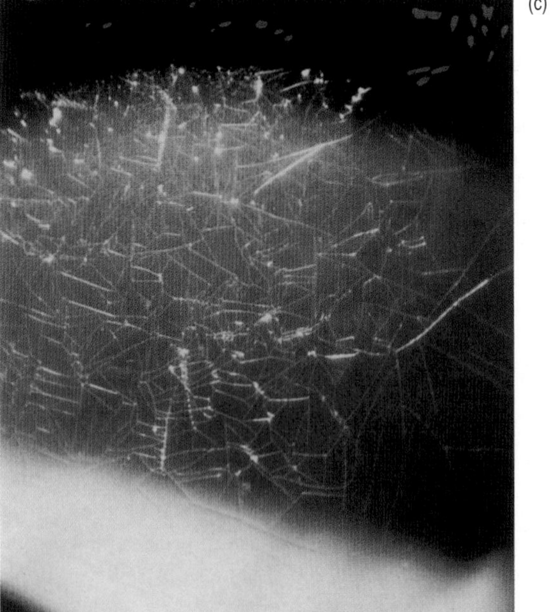

LENS CARE AND MAINTENANCE

The solutions used with RGP lenses are discussed in Chapter 4. Patients who have been previous PMMA wearers must be warned of the greater fragility of RGP materials, their greater vulnerability to scratching and distortion, and the greater emphasis necessary on cleaning. Specifically these patients should be advised to:

- Exercise care when retrieving lenses from the storage case, especially if the lens has been inadvertently placed in its compartment convex side up.
- Minimize lens compression during cleaning and handling.
- Clean lenses in the palm of the hand as with a soft lens rather than between the thumb and fingers.
- Avoid handling lenses by opposing edges.
- Avoid dropping lenses onto hard surfaces and exercise care when retrieving a dropped lens.
- Be sure that the lens is centred in the storage compartment before closing to avoid edge breakage.
- Use only solutions advised by the practitioner as being suitable for the lens material prescribed.
- Regularly check the lens for deposit build-up after drying and observing against a good light. Most patients will benefit from the use (typically monthly) of an enzymatic or periodic cleaner (e.g. Menicon's 'Progent').

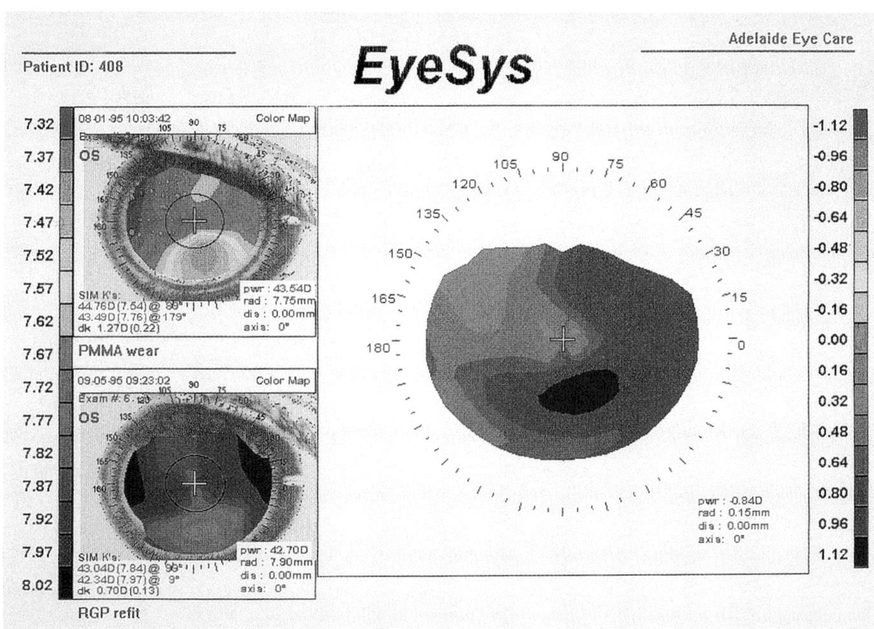

Figure 9.26 The corneal topographical plot (top left) was taken immediately after removal of a PMMA lens. The PMMA lens had been worn for approximately 15 years. The steepness of the corneal apex can be seen in the top left-hand plot giving a picture of apparently keratoconus. Sixteen weeks after wearing fluorosilicone-acrylate RGP lenses, the cornea (bottom left) resembles a now near-normal shape and the *K* readings have flattened by 0.15 mm. The right-hand 'difference map' shows a change in apical power of over 1.00 D. Lens refitting was necessary at the new corneal shape

- Not be over-zealous with the use of abrasive ('friction enhanced') cleaners. Boltz (1989), Bennett and Henry (1990) and Carrell et al. (1992) found that the over-zealous use of these cleaners can lead to an increase in lens thinning, lens warpage and the addition of minus power.
- These same cleaners should not be used with surface-treated materials (see above).

Piccolo et al. (1990) found no significant change in RGP parameters of both silicone-acrylate and fluorosilicone-acrylate lenses stored in 3% hydrogen peroxide although a small amount of warpage was found in some cases (mean 0.04 mm). This is important as hydrogen peroxide is recommended as disinfecting lenses against the HIV virus (see Chapter 4).

REFITTING THE FORMER PMMA WEARER

Although RGP lenses have become the material of first choice for all patients requiring a rigid lens, small numbers of former PMMA wearers still require refitting with RGP lenses. The change of material is advisable for patients with marked spectacle blur, persistent corneal staining, decreased wearing time (the so-called 'corneal exhaustion syndrome') or endothelial changes. Methods of refitting long-term PMMA wearers include reduced wearing time, or immediate refitting. The advantages of immediate refitting with RGP lenses are that patients are not inconvenienced because they can continue full-time lens wear and, in most cases, experience no significant drop in visual acuity or inhibition of corneal recovery with the new lenses. However, the decision as to the optimum method of refitting depends upon the state of the patient's corneas.

To make an adequate assessment of corneal physiology (staining, oedema, etc.) and post-wear spectacle refraction and acuity, a preliminary evaluation of the patient's eyes should be scheduled after a minimum of 4 hours of their PMMA wear. If the induced changes are minimal, the patient can be refitted at that time. If excessive corneal staining, oedema, significant spectacle refractive or acuity changes, or keratometric mire distortion is present, a more feasible option would be to gradually decrease the patient's lens wear, possibly one eye at a time if that is helpful, to the minimum number of hours possible or refit one eye at a time. Spectacles, if available, usually fail to provide adequate visual acuity so that decreasing lens wear to 8–12 hours is the minimum most patients will accept.

The patient should then maintain a limited wearing schedule until the dispensing visit of the refitted RGP lenses. Although the patient's progress should be closely monitored, immediate full-day wear or rapid readaptation can be instructed. Spectacles can also be prescribed once the patient's refraction has stabilized, although this may be several weeks after dispensing the RGP lenses, depending on the severity of the corneal changes. With greatly distorted corneas, patients should be warned that further refitting may be necessary as corneal regularity and curvature stabilize following the first refitting (Fig. 9.26). A return to the original pre-PMMA-fitting keratometer readings often indicates when stability has been reached. If these are not available, a request to the patient's original practitioner may provide the necessary information.

Patients refitted with RGP lenses may initially complain of lens awareness even though the fit is excellent and corneal physiology improved. This occurs because corneal sensation improves when gas-permeable lenses are worn. Thus a PMMA lens-wearing patient who tolerates corneal oedema, erosions or epithelial infiltrates because of corneal hypoaesthesia, may be quite irritated by new RGP lenses even though the corneal state is much improved. Symptoms of increased sensation last about 3 weeks and the patient *must* be warned in advance to accept this.

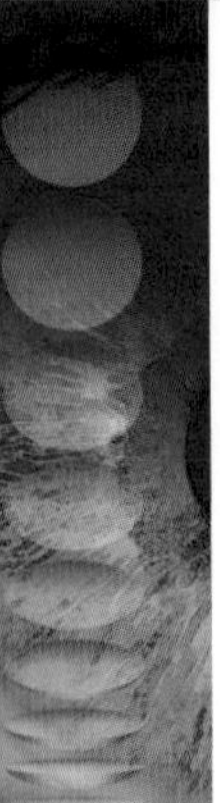

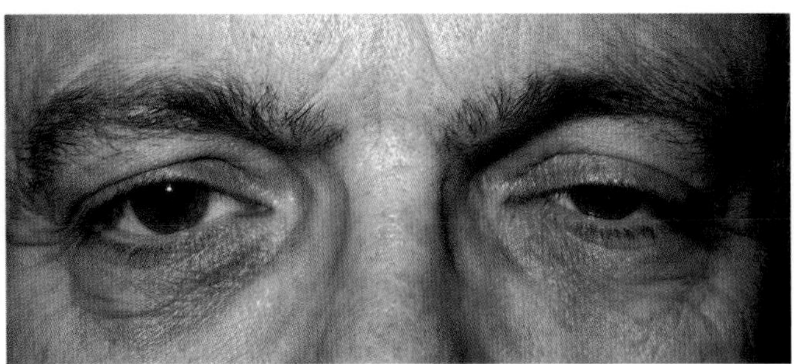

Figure 9.27 A long-term monocular RGP wearer showing slight ptosis of the left lens-wearing eye after some 20 years of wear

Finally, due to the softer and more flexible nature of RGP materials, former PMMA wearers are more likely to break or distort their new lenses. Apart from the appropriate warnings, practitioners should use stronger, mid-Dk materials, such as Boston ES, to minimize problems.

BLEPHAROPTOSIS IN CORNEAL LENS WEARERS

A small percentage of long-term corneal lens wearers will show mild to moderate ptosis of the eyelids (Fig. 9.27). Good levator function is maintained and an elevated lid crease typically present. The problem may take many years to develop.

Vanden Bosch and Lemij (1992) postulated the following mechanisms as causation:

- Simultaneous, antagonistic action of the orbicularis and levator muscles while squeezing the eyelids to remove the lens.
- Forceful rubbing of the lens and subsequent stretching of the upper eyelid structures during failed attempts at lens removal.
- Repeated and similar although less forceful rubbing of the lens during blinking.
- Irritation, leading to oedema.
- Irritation, leading to blepharospasm.

Ptosis is sometimes seen during the early adaptive phase of corneal lens wear and is presumably due to lid oedema resulting from the mechanical effects of the lid edge. This usually disappears on further adaptation (or cessation of lens wear). However, in long-term wearers the condition is often persistent, even upon cessation of wear. Kersten et al. (1995) and Thean and McNab (2004) have confirmed from surgical results that in many cases the problem is due to thinning and disinsertion of the levator aponeurosis from chronic manipulation of the upper lid during lens removal.

In the latter case, cessation of lens wear does not, of course, help. Ptosis-repair surgery is necessary only if cosmetically unacceptable or if vision is affected. Changing to a soft lens is the next best clinical step where feasible, as Fonn et al. (1996) have demonstrated that some cases do recover upon cessation of RGP wear. Alternatively, as soon as any early sign of ptosis is noticed, the patient should be instructed to change their removal technique; for example, from the 'stare-blink' method to the 'lid-squeeze' or suction holder methods (see Chapter 11).

IDENTIFICATION OF RGP MATERIALS

Occasionally, patients present with complications, wearing corneal lenses of unknown material. If the lenses were fitted elsewhere, the practitioner must first establish what the material is, so that correct management can be facilitated. This may constitute refitting with a more oxygen permeable material.

There are several ways of identifying the material (see also Chapter 16):

- *Ask the patient*: they may know whether the lenses are PMMA or RGP if not the specific material
  - specific solutions or cleaning techniques may give clues.
  - the patient may have a copy of their lens prescription. In some countries the issuing of a contact lens prescription, including lens material, is now mandatory.
  - the former practitioner should be able to supply relevant information.
- *Check the lens*: some practitioners engrave a code to identify the lens material.
- *Spectroscopy*: in theory, lens materials may be identified by spectroscopy, principally in the infrared region (Pearson 1986). While materials may be identified in terms of their general groups (e.g. silicone-acrylate), batch variations of materials and even variation along rods of materials, make specific identification difficult. Dain and Pye (1993) showed that combined ultraviolet and visible transmission curves can also be used to identify RGP materials.
- *Specific gravity*: Refojo and Leong (1984) used a series of 21 solutions of calcium chloride with concentrations ranging from 18 to 38%. Specific gravity was established by noting the solution in which the lens neither floated nor sank upon immersion. Materials of higher oxygen permeability were associated with lower values of specific gravity (see Table 3.1 for values).
- *Densitometry*: Arce et al. (1999) utilized a similar method to the specific gravity technique above but with a saturated salt solution and hydrometer to measure density.
- *Refractometry*: Hodur et al. (1992) suggested the use of the Atago N3000 refractometer (see Fig. 16.15) to identify RGP material refractive index. This instrument is normally used to measure the water content of hydrogel lenses (see Chapter 16) but since the refractive index of RGP materials is commonly available, the instrument can be used for identification of the RGP material or its grouping. The method is as follows.

  Place a clean dry PMMA trial lens, convex side down, on the refractometer and a drop of saline on the concave side of the lens to neutralize the air space between lens and prism cover. Taking care not to crack the contact lens by closing the prism cover too firmly, hold the cover plate firmly enough to produce full optical contact and alignment of the lens with the prism. Hold up to a suitable light or pale-coloured wall to view the boundary line denoting the refractive index. The reading of the refractive index is taken from the internal scale and calibrated to 1.49 (for PMMA) using the screw ring. The unknown lens can now be measured in the same manner.

Typical refractive indices for some commonly used materials are shown in Table 3.1.

ORDERING

During the fitting routine a single lens may not be available which is correct in all its specifications. It may be necessary to combine specifications from more than one lens or to extrapolate a dimension from the nearest trial lens. Often these can be checked by using the CD-ROM supplied with this book and other information such as corneal eccentricity if available. The following provides notes and 'rules of thumb' which may be helpful.

BOZR

EFFECT OF VARIATIONS IN THE BOZD

As mentioned earlier, since the cornea flattens towards its periphery as the BOZD is increased, the BOZR must be flattened to maintain the nearest to an alignment fit. The opposite applies on reducing the BOZD. It has been found from clinical experience that:

- *for every 0.50 mm increase in BOZD the BOZR must be flattened by approximately 0.05 mm, and vice versa.*

Atkinson (1990) pointed out that, in terms of tear layer optics, a 0.7 mm increase in the BOZD for a 0.05 mm flattening of the radius, and vice versa, is technically more correct and leaves the central tear layer thickness the same in most average cases.

EFFECT OF HYDRATION

RGP lenses generally appear to flatten less with hydration than PMMA lenses. Nevertheless, higher-powered negative lenses are still sometimes vulnerable to this effect. Practitioners may prefer to order lenses a few hundredths of a millimetre steeper initially to allow for this (depending upon the lens thickness and BVP) but detailed information on the specific material being ordered should be sought from the manufacturer or current literature. Lenses should be rechecked after hydration prior to being issued to the patient and at periodic intervals thereafter. At after-care examinations any apparent indication that negative lenses, which were previously of the correct power, are now too strong would suggest that the BOZR has flattened.

Back peripheral radius (BPR)

The same allowances apply as for the BOZR, both for alterations in the total diameter and hydration flattening (usually taken to the nearest 0.05 mm owing to the difficulty of accurately manufacturing and checking peripheral curves).

BOZD and TD

See BOZR and BPR.

BVP

COMPARISON OF SPECTACLE AND CONTACT LENS CORRECTION

The initial spectacle refraction is best written in negative cylindrical form because the tear lens acts as a negative cylinder in a lens aligning the flattest corneal meridian and corrects most of the corneal astigmatism (see Chapter 6). Thus the power of these two negative cylinders can be compared and, where spectacle astigmatism approximates to keratometer astigmatism, it should be corrected by the tear lens so the cylinder in the spectacle correction may be ignored. The spherical component of the spectacle refraction referred to the corneal plane should then equal the liquid lens power along the flattest corneal meridian plus the BVP of the trial contact lens. If there is more than 0.50–0.75 D difference between spectacle and keratometer astigmatism, depending on the visual acuity and visual tolerance of each patient, it may be necessary to incorporate a front surface cylindrical correction. Because of possible lens flexure, residual astigmatism should be checked more than once before proceeding to incorporate a front surface cylinder or supplying any form of toric lens. To maintain lens orientation in these cases, a prism-ballasted lens or double truncation may be used where the cornea is close to spherical, or preferably a toroidal back surface lens should be fitted where the cornea is toroidal (see Chapter 12).

VERTEX DISTANCE

A refraction is carried out over the trial contact lens and provided adequate visual acuity is achieved, the 'best sphere' power is used.

The BVP of the trial contact lens is then added to the power of the spectacle spherical power, having allowed for vertex distance, to give the BVP of the lens to be ordered.

A table of vertex distance allowances is given in Appendix A and on the CD-ROM or may be determined by calculation. It can be seen that for spectacle corrections of less than 4.00 D the effects of vertex distance may be ignored provided that the latter lies within normal limits.

EFFECTS OF VARIATIONS IN THE BOZR

It may be necessary to carry out the refraction with a contact lens whose BOZR differs from that ordered on the final lens. Altering the BOZR affects the power of the tear liquid lens, so the power of the final lens must be adjusted accordingly. It can be calculated that, for small amounts and for corneas of average curvature:

- *an alteration of 0.05 mm in the BOZR requires an alteration in BVP of 0.25 D.*

Thus, if the BOZR is 8.00 mm and the BVP –3.00 D, ordering a BOZR of 8.05 mm produces a more negative liquid lens. The BVP of the final lens must therefore be ordered as –2.75 D to compensate.

No alteration to the BVP should be made where the BOZR is altered to compensate for flattening with hydration. This allowance normally disappears when the lens becomes fully hydrated.

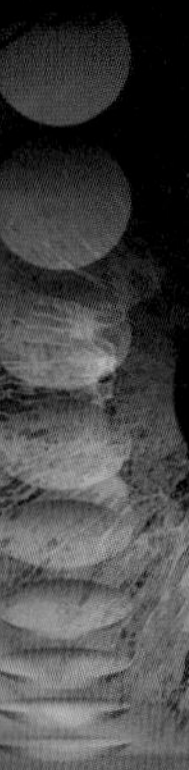

Table 9.10: Corneal lens thickness chart

Negative-powered lenses BVP (D)	Total diameter (mm) 8.50 to 8.80	8.90 to 9.20	9.30 to 9.60	9.70 to 10.00	10.10 to 10.30	10.40 and over
Afocal to −0.50	0.215	0.210	0.210	0.210	0.200	0.180
−0.75 to −1.00	0.215	0.210	0.200	0.190	0.190	0.170
−1.25 to −1.50	0.210	0.200	0.190	0.190	0.175	0.160
−1.75 to −2.00	0.200	0.200	0.190	0.180	0.165	0.155
−2.25 to −2.75	0.190	0.190	0.175	0.170	0.155	0.150
−3.00 to −3.25	0.180	0.180	0.160	0.155	0.150	0.145
−3.50 to −4.25	0.170	0.160	0.150	0.145	0.140	0.130
−4.50 to −5.00	0.160	0.155	0.140	0.135	0.125	0.115
−5.25 to −5.50	0.150	0.145	0.130	0.120	0.110	0.105
−5.75 to −6.00	0.140	0.135	0.120	0.105	0.100	0.100
−6.25 to −7.00	0.130	0.120	0.110	0.105	0.100	0.100
−7.00 and over	0.100	0.100		Make in lenticular form		
Positive-powered lenses BVP (D)	**Total diameter (mm) 8.40 to 8.70**	**8.80 to 9.20**	**9.30 to 9.70**	**9.80 to 10.00**	**10.50 (approx.)**	**11.00 (approx.)**
Afocal to +1.00	0.210	0.220	0.230	0.235	0.240	0.245
+1.25 to +2.00	0.230	0.240	0.250	0.255	0.265	0.270
+2.25 to +3.00	0.260	0.270	0.280	0.290	0.310	0.330
+3.25 to +4.00	0.280	0.295	0.310	0.325	0.350	0.370
+4.25 to +5.00	0.305	0.315	0.330	0.360	0.395	0.450
+5.25 to +6.00	0.330	0.345	0.365	0.385	0.420	0.470
+6.25 to +7.00	0.350	0.370	0.395	0.440	0.470	0.520
+7.00 and over			Make in lenticular form			

The figures given above for centre thickness (mm) are the average for the power and total diameter groups and generally give an edge thickness of about 0.14–0.18 mm for an average tri-curve lens (P. Bryant, 1975, personal communication). Lens thicknesses should be ordered to two decimal places only.

Note: Lenses with a BVP of about ±5.00 D should be made in lenticular form (see also p. 205). In general, centre thicknesses of greater than 0.40 mm should be avoided where possible by the use of lenticulation. Some practitioners advocate lenticular construction for all positive lenses to minimize centre thickness but give adequate edge thickness and similarly for very low minus lenses, down to −2.00 D.

Centre and edge thickness

Although the centre thickness of a lens should normally be specified, the edge thickness is just as important clinically. An edge which is either too thick or too thin may give rise to lid irritation. An edge thickness of around 0.16–0.18 mm appears to be the ideal.

A lens which is too thin centrally flattens excessively with hydration and may become distorted or damaged if handled incorrectly. Cornish and Sulaiman (1996) demonstrated that, surprisingly, a very thin lens (less than 0.08 mm centre thickness) was less comfortable than a lens of centre thickness 0.12 mm (but comfort decreased again as the thickness increased further), presumably due to lens flexure on the eye. Conversely, a lens which is too thick is relatively heavy and constantly positions low on the cornea. A list of suggested centre thicknesses for variations in BVP and TD is given in Table 9.10.

Higher powers should be made in lenticular form to reduce the lens weight. This aids lens centration, gives easier control of edge thickness and reduces the effects of hydration. When a lens is ordered in lenticular form, the FOZD and desired final edge thickness should be specified. The FOZD is generally around 0.20 mm larger than the BOZD or 2.0 mm larger than the pupil in average illumination, whichever is the smaller. Junction thickness may also be specified.

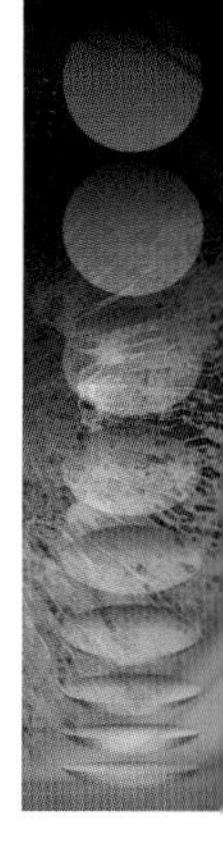

Transitions

These may be left sharp or blended lightly, moderately or heavily. Although a heavily blended transition lessens any risk of corneal abrasion caused by this area, there are two possible disadvantages. First, it is difficult to check if the BOZD has been made correctly; if incorrect, it effectively alters the fit of the back optic zone. Second, the transition, if polished well into the BOZD, reduces its effective diameter, often causing flare under conditions of low illumination. Ideally, the transition should be ordered lightly blended and the blending increased later by the practitioner as necessary.

If blending is carried out, a tool should be chosen whose radius lies one-third to mid-way between the BPR and BOZR so that most of the lens substance is removed from the peripheral curve (see Chapter 20).

Lens engraving and distinguishing marks for right and left lenses

Right and left lenses should be distinguished by the letters R and L or by small dots – one for the right lens and two for the left (British Standard, BS 5562:1989). If dots are used for identification marks, often only the right lens is so marked because the drilling of two small marks in the lens surface may weaken the lens. A hole filled with black pigment shows less against a dark iris background. A small painted dot on the lens front surface is also possible and does not involve drilling into the lens surface. A dot is more easily visible to hyperopes and presbyopes without their correction. All marks should be positioned near the lens edge so that there is no risk of visual interference and, ideally, both lenses should be engraved. Lens engraving marks may be inadvertently removed when power alterations are carried out and, like scratches, they may encourage deposits. For some patients, the simple expedient of using two different handling tints is a simple way of determining left and right lenses, as long as the same or similar material is available for both eyes.

With the plethora of materials currently available, it is strongly recommended that all RGP lenses are engraved with a simple code to identify the material prescribed. Thus Boston XO may be engraved 'BXO' or even 'XO'. This is useful, not only when patients are seen elsewhere but also in the identification of old lenses, confirming that lenses are suitable for extended wear etc. It may help in more difficult cases to number lenses consecutively as the fitting is refined, to ensure that the correct lens is being worn for after-care visits; for example, the third right lens in an ongoing fitting procedure may be engraved 'R3'.

Toroidal lenses should have a dot or line marked at each end of the flattest meridian. This not only identifies the lens as toroidal but also allows the practitioner to check if the lens has orientated correctly or rotated.

Material selection

The choice of lens material has been dealt with above. PMMA is now considered the material of last choice, used only for:

- Trial lenses.
- Recalcitrant GPC sufferers where a high surface polish, good deposit resistance and thin edges are necessary.
- Some 3 and 9 o'clock sufferers where a small lens with a thin edge is the only design that helps.
- Patients who are allergic to all RGP materials.

Lens tint

Tinted lenses can be prescribed:

- For photophobia.
- To alter or enhance iris colour within limits.
- As a handling tint which aids location of a clear lens on the sclera or in a bowl of water.

If the contact lens wearer is more light sensitive than when wearing spectacles, there are three possible reasons (Phillips 1968):

1. Increased light transmission of the contact lens since there is only one air–lens surface, which causes the greatest light loss by reflection. However, the wearing of plano spectacle lenses over the contact lenses does not relieve this photophobia (Bergevin & Millodot 1967).
2. The small amount of corneal oedema sometimes present in new wearers while adapting to their lenses, which causes increased scattering of light.
3. The foreign body sensation of the lens edge, again present in new wearers, which probably causes reflex iris blood vessel dilatation, iris congestion and pain on sphincter constriction.

Because both (2) and (3) are normally temporary in nature, the temptation to prescribe a deeper tint should be avoided. However, in the case of a badly fitting lens, the photophobia may be excessive and prolonged. The lens design or construction then needs improving, not a deeper tint.

Many modern materials are, unfortunately, made in only one tint (or no tint!). Others are available in several colours. Only a very few are available in the deeper tints necessary to help the severe photophobic or to significantly change the iris appearance. In these cases a second, duplicate clear or lightly tinted pair should be prescribed for night-time use.

Fenestration

With the excellent gas transmissibility of modern RGP materials, fenestrating lenses is rarely necessary. Fenestrations are now only used either to rescue a slightly tight-fitting lens (e.g. in a teenager whose cornea has flattened rapidly) or in irregular corneas (e.g. trauma, keratoconus, etc.) where fenestrations may be used to prevent tear stagnation.

Fenestrations should only be used in those areas which are definitely clear of the cornea, otherwise an additional tear meniscus is formed between lens and cornea which tends to reduce lens movement. In addition, there is a greater risk of epithelial trauma from the edge of the fenestration.

Central fenestrations are typically 0.10 mm in diameter but it is more usual to position a 0.25 mm fenestration near the edge of the back optic zone. Occasionally a 0.50 mm diameter fenestration is used.

Atkinson and Phillips (1971) listed the proposed advantages of fenestrations in PMMA lenses. Hill and Uniacke (1968)

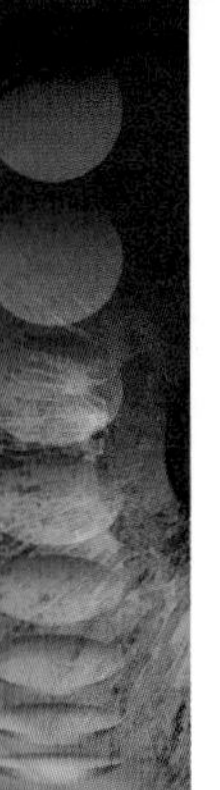

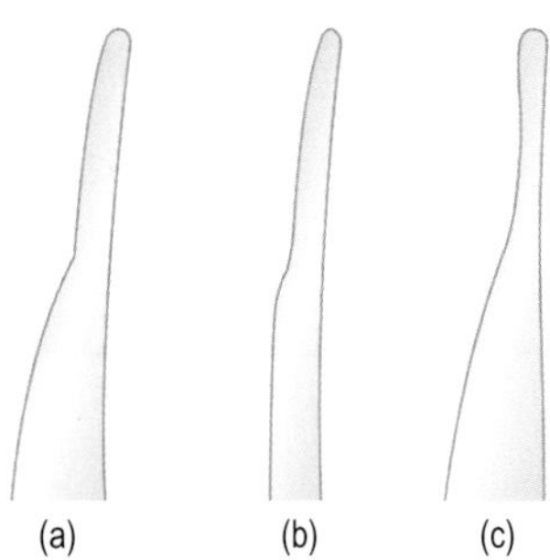

Figure 9.28 Three typical carrier portion shapes: (a) parallel or plano; (b) positive; (c) negative

showed that there is little oxygen movement (via the tears) through the fenestration itself but that any physiological improvement is more likely to be due to the prevention of negative pressure under the lens.

Methods of lens fenestration by the practitioner are described in Chapter 20. Lenses fenestrated by a laser beam permit multiple well-finished holes of 0.10 mm diameter.

The edge shape

The lens edge shape is important for both patient comfort and, to a lesser extent, in lens movement and centration. La Hood (1988) showed that a well-rounded edge, particularly on the front surface, is essential for comfort. Too thick or square an edge may be uncomfortable whereas too thin an edge may be sharp or chip easily. Lens edge shapes may be checked as explained in Chapter 16 or modified as in Chapter 28.

An ideal edge thickness has been found clinically to be around 0.16–0.18 mm although this may depend upon the lens BVP. Lens edges thinner than 0.14 mm are vulnerable to lens flexure, particularly on astigmatic corneas with tight lids.

The carrier portion of the lens edge was discussed earlier (see Front optic zone diameter, p. 205). This band should not be less than 0.5 mm wide and its shape can influence the lens position (Fig. 9.28).

Because of their shape, low-powered negative lenses are gripped by the upper lid and usually centre well. A negative carrier lens therefore helps give lid attachment with low-riding or positive-powered lenses. Conversely, a positive carrier helps reduce a high-riding tendency. Because negative carrier lenses require a minimum junction thickness at the inner edge of the carrier, these lenses can sometimes be thicker than normal and have relatively thick edges. Great skill is therefore necessary on the part of the laboratory in fabricating these designs.

THE WRITTEN PRESCRIPTION

The most useful form of the written prescription is that recommended by the International Organization for Standardization in ISO 8320:1986.

The radius of each zone is given in turn from the centre outwards, immediately followed by its external diameter. Dimensions are invariably to be given in the following order:

(i) The letter C followed by the figure 1 for a single back curve, 2 for a double curve, 3 for a triple curve, etc. This is optional but avoids confusion.
(ii) Radius of the back optic zone surface followed by its diameter or the total diameter, whichever applies.
(iii) Radius of each surrounding back surface followed by external diameter or the total diameter, whichever applies.
(iv) Displacement of the optic zone (if applicable).

EXAMPLES

(1) Please supply one corneal lens
R C3/7.70:8.00/8.30:8.50/9.50:9.50/D1
(i) (ii) (iii) (iii) (iv)
BVP –6.00 D
Material RXD
T_c 0.12 mm, T_e 0.16–0.18 mm
Transitions left sharp
Mark one dot (black) and RXD
Light blue tint

(2) Please supply one pair corneal lenses
R C3/7.80:8.30/8.40:8.80/9.70:9.80
BVP –6.25 D
T_c 0.11 mm
FOZD 7.40 mm
L C3/7.95:8.30/8.55:8.80/10.00:9.80
BVP –1.00 D
T_c 0.19 mm, T_e 0.16 ±0.02 mm
Material: FluoroPerm 90
Transitions lightly blended
Engrave R & L and F90
Light blue tint

THE FINAL LENS

Whatever the lens material, the final lens should be fully hydrated and then checked (and preferably rechecked) as described in Chapter 16. The lens fit is then assessed. A gradual transition across the lens from touch to clearance is ideal for most fitting philosophies. If any hard blue arcuate-bearing areas (possibly indicative of a relatively sharp transition or too steep a peripheral curve) are apparent, either with the lens centred or as it moves on the cornea, the lens transitions or peripheral curves should be modified.

The patient is instructed in lens wear and handling as described in Chapter 11, and the period of after-care then begins.

SUMMARY

Although RGP lenses suffer from certain disadvantages, such as foreign bodies under the lens, 3 and 9 o'clock staining, greater initial sensation than soft lenses, etc., many of the disadvantages of early RGP materials have been solved and their usage in contact lens practice remains essential.

Finally, in understanding the work of this chapter, it is worth quoting the conclusion of van der Worp et al. (2002) who compared RGP lenses ordered empirically based on traditional fitting rules versus lenses modified to obtain the best possible fit from all available data. They concluded that:

> *Even small improvements in RGP fits influenced comfort of wear significantly. It should also be noted that this could potentially lead to drop out among patients with acceptable but not optimal fits.*

FURTHER INFORMATION

Readers are urged to obtain and view the CD entitled 'Fitting RGP Lenses – An Interactive Educational Program' developed by the Cooperative Research Centre for Eye Research and Technology of the University of New South Wales, Australia, and available through local agents of the Polymer Technology Corporation Inc.

A useful website can also be found at www.rgpli.org, an RGP lens institute based in the USA.

Acknowledgements

The author wishes to acknowledge the help and constructive comments made in the preparation of the original chapter by Janet Stone and in this updated chapter by Lynne Speedwell and John Mountford. Also to my two colleagues, René Malingré and Dipika Mistry for their critical comments on the manuscript. Angela Chappell is thanked for her invaluable help with many of the illustrations.

References

Arce, C. G., Schuman, P. D. and Schuman, W. P. (1999) Qualitative identification of rigid gas permeable contact lens materials by densitometry. CLAO J., 24(4), 204–208

Atkinson, T. C. O. (1985) A computer assisted and clinical assessment of current trends in gas permeable design. Optician, 189(4976), 16–22

Atkinson, T. C. O. (1990) The 'ideal' RGP back surface design for daily wear. Optician, March, 34–36

Atkinson, K. W. and Phillips, A. J. (1971) Fenestrations in corneal lenses. Br. J. Physiol. Opt., 26, 1–14

Baker, T. Y. (1943) Ray tracing through non-spherical surfaces. Proc. Phys. Soc., 55, 361–364

Bennett, E. S. (1985) Silicone acrylate lens design. Int. Contact Lens Clin., 12, 45–52

Bennett, A. G. (1988) Aspherical and continuous curve contact lenses. Optom. Today, 28, 11–14, 140–142, 238–242, 433–444

Bennett, E. S. and Henry, V. A. (1990) RGP lens power change with abrasive cleaner use. Int. Contact Lens Clin., 17(3), 152–153

Bergevin, J. and Millodot, M. (1967) Glare with ophthalmic and corneal lenses. Am J. Optom., 44, 213–221

Bibby, M. M. (1979) Factors affecting peripheral curve design. Part II. Am. J. Optom., 56, 618–627

Blehl, E., Lowther, G. E. and Benjamin, W. J. (1991) Flexural characteristics of Softperm, Boston IV, and RXD contact lenses on toric corneas. Int. Contact Lens Clin., 18(2), 59–62

Boltz, K. D. (1989) The overzealous contact lens cleaner. Contact Lens Spectrum, December, 53–54

Brown, J. (1991) A year with Aquasil. Contact Lens J., 20(4), 20–21

Businger, U., Treiber, A. and Flury, C. (1989) The etiology and management of 3 and 9 o'clock staining. Int. Contact Lens Clin., 16(5), 136–139

Carney, L. G. (1972) Luminance of fluorescence solution. Am. J. Optom. Arch. Am. Acad. Optom., 59, 200–204

Carney, L. G. and Hill, R. M. (1987) Center of gravity of rigid lenses: some design considerations. Int. Contact Lens Clin., 14(11), 431–435

Carney, L. G., Mainstone, J. C. and Henderson, B. A. (1997) Corneal topography and myopia. A cross-sectional study. Invest. Ophthalmol. Vis. Sci., 38, 311–320

Caroline, P. J. and Ellis, E. J. (1986) Review of the mechanisms of oxygen transport through rigid gas permeable lenses. Int. Eyecare, 2(4), 210–213

Carrell, B. A., Bennett, E. S., Henry, V. A. and Grohe, R. M. (1992) The effect of rigid gas permeable lens cleaners on lens parameter stability. J. Am. Optom. Assoc., 63(3), 193–198

Chui, V. (2004) Corneal topography in Chinese eyes. Paper read at the 1st Asian Cornea and Contact Lens Conference, Hong Kong

Cornish, R. and Sulaiman, S. (1996) Do thinner rigid gas permeable contact lenses provide superior initial comfort? Optom. Vis. Sci., 73, 139–143

Cornish, R., Sulaiman, S., Shiobara, M. et al. (1991) Relationship between material Dk, flexibility and correction of astigmatism. Optom. Vis. Sci., 68(Suppl), 145

Dain, S. J. and Pye, D. C. (1993) Identification of rigid gas permeable contact lens materials by means of ultraviolet-visible spectrophotometry. Optom. Vis. Sci., 70(6), 517–521

Douthwaite, W. A., Hough, T., Edwards, K. and Nolay, H. (1999) The EyeSys videokeratoscopic assessment of apical radius and p-value in the normal human cornea. Ophthalmic Physiol. Opt., 19(6), 467–474

Eghbali, F., Yeung, K. K. and Maloney, R. K. (1995) Topographic determination of corneal asphericity and its lack of effect on the refractive outcome of radial keratotomy. Am. J. Ophthalmol. 199, 233–236

Evans, T. C. and Morrison, I. (1984) Sensitivity to retinal defocus with aspheric soft lenses – predictions and clinical validation. Am. J. Optom. Physiol. Opt., 61, 729–736

Fonn, D., Pritchard, N., Garnett, B. and Davids, L. (1996) Palpebral aperture sizes of rigid and soft contact lens wearers compared to nonwearers. Optom. Vis. Sci., 73, 211–214

Gordon, S. (1965) Contact lens hydration: a study of the wetting–drying cycle. Optom. Wkly, 56, 55–62

Grohe, R. M., Caroline, P. J. and Norman, C. (1987) Rigid gas permeable surface cracking. Contact Lens Spectrum, May, 37–45

Guillon, M. and Sammons, W. A. (1994) Contact lens design. In Contact Lens Practice, pp. 87–103, eds. M. Ruben and M. Guillon. London: Chapman and Hall Medical

Guillon, M., Lydon, D. P. M. and Wilson, M. (1986) Corneal topography: a clinical model. Ophthalmic Physiol. Opt., 6, 47–56

Hatfield, R. O., Jordan, D. R., Bennett, E. S. et al. (1993) Initial comfort and surface wettability: a comparison between different contact lens materials. J. Am. Optom. Assoc., 64(4), 271–273

Hayashi, T. (1977) Mechanics of Contact Lens Motion. PhD Thesis. School of Optometry, U.C. Berkeley

Hyashi, T. and Fatt, I. (1980) Forces retaining a contact lens on the eye. Am. J. Optom. Physiol. Opt., 57(8), 485–507

Herman, J. P. (1984) Lens flexure: clinical rules. J. Am. Optom. Assoc., 55, 169–171

Hill, R. M. and Uniacke, N. P. (1968) Lacrimal fluid and lens design. Contacto, 12, 59–61

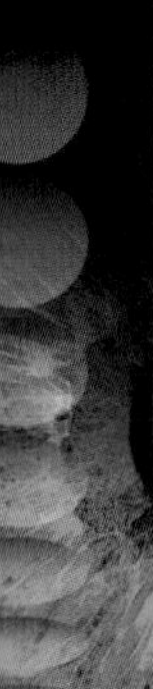

Hodur, N. R., Jurkus, J. and Gunderson, G. (1992) Rigid gas permeable lens identification using refractometry. Int. Contact Lens Clin., 19(2), 71–74

Holden, B. A. (1984) Predicting contact lens flexure from in-vitro tests. J. Am. Optom. Assoc., 55, 171

Holden, T., Oxnard, C. A., Bahr, K. et al. (1987) The effect of secondary curve liftoff on peripheral corneal desiccation. Am. J. Physiol. Optom., 64, 108P

Jones, D. H., Bennett, E. S. and Davis, L. J. (1989) How to manage peripheral corneal desiccation. Contact Lens Spectrum, May, 63–66

Kenyon, E., Mandell, R. B. and Polse, K. A. (1989) Lens design effects on rigid lens adherence. J. Br. Contact Lens Assoc., 12(2), 32–36

Kerns, R. L. (1984) Clinical evaluation of the merits of an aspheric front surface contact lens for patients manifesting residual astigmatism. Am. J. Optom. Physiol. Opt., 51, 750–757

Kerr, C. and Dilly, P. N. (1988) Problems of dimensional stability in RGPs. Optician, February, 21–23

Kersten, R. C., deConciliis, C. and Kulwin, D. R (1995) Acquired ptosis in the young and middle-aged adult population. Ophthalmology, 102, 924–928

Kiely, P. M., Smith, G. and Carney, L. G. (1982) The mean shape of the human cornea. Optica Acta, 29, 1027–1040

Kikkawa, Y. (1970) The mechanism of contact lens adherence and centralization. Am. J. Optom Arch. Am. Acad. Optom., 47(4), 275–281

Korb, D. R. and Korb, J. E. (1974) Fitting to achieve a normal blinking and lid action. Int. Contact Lens Clin., 1(3), 57–70

La Hood, D. (1988) Edge shape and comfort of rigid lenses. Am. J. Optom. Physiol. Opt., 65(8), 613–618

Mackie, I. A. (1973) Design compensation in corneal lens fitting. In Symposium on Contact Lenses: Transactions of the New Orleans Academy of Ophthalmology. St Louis: Mosby

Mackie, I. A., Mason, D. and Perry, B. J. (1970) Factors influencing corneal contact lens centration. Br. J. Physiol. Opt., 25, 87–103

Mandell, R. B. and Helen, St R. (1971) Mathematical model of the corneal contour. Br. J. Physiol. Opt., 26, 183–197

McLaughlin, R., Kelly, C. G. and Karns, L. J. (1988) Pseudomonas ulcer observed with surface crazed RGP. Contact Lens Spectrum, August, 58–60

Meyler, J. and Ruston, D. (1994) Rigid gas permeable aspheric back surface contact lenses – a review. Optician, 5467(208), 22–30

Moody, K., Mannarino, A., Tanner, J. and Hannash, S. (1989) Staphylococcal ulceration with RGP contact lens wear. Contact Lens Spectrum, March, 61–64

Osterland, G. (1992) Novalens: a 160-patient one-year retrospective study. Contact Lens Spectrum, September, 26–28

Oxenberg, L. D. and Carney, L. G. (1989) Visual performance with aspheric rigid contact lenses. Optom. Vis. Sci., 66, 818–821

Patel, S., Marshall, J. and Fitzke, F. W. (1993) Shape and radius of the posterior corneal surface. Refract. Corneal Surg., 9, 173–181

Pearson, R. M. (1986) The clinical performance of hard gas-permeable lenses. Clin. Exp. Optom., 69, 98–102

Pearson, R. M. (1989) Stability of hydrated curvature of Quantum lenses. Int. Contact Lens Clin., 16, 178–182

Phillips, A. J. (1968) Filters used by drivers at night. Ophthal. Opt., 8, 707–713, 756–763

Phillips, A. J. (1969) Alterations in curvature of the finished corneal lens. Ophthal. Opt., 9, 980–986, 1043–1054, 1100–1110

Piccolo, M. G., Leach, N. E. and Boltz, R. (1990) Rigid lens base curve stability upon hydrogen peroxide disinfection. Optom. Vis. Sci., 67, 19–21

Quinn, T. G. and Carney, L. G. (1992) Controlling rigid lens centration through specific gravity. Int. Contact Lens Clin., 19(2), 84–88

Refojo, M. F. and Leong, F. L. (1984) Identification of hard contact lenses by their specific gravity. Int. Contact Lens Clin., 11, 79–82

Schwartz, C. A. (1986) Radical flattening and RGP lenses. Contact Lens Forum, 11(8), 49–53

Seidner, L. (1987) Balance: the key to RGP. Contact Lens Spectrum, October, 32–34

Sevigny, J. and Bennett, E. (1984) Trouble shooting with silicone acrylate lenses. Rev. Optom., 122(12), 24–30

Sorbara, L., Fonn, D. and MacNeill, K. (1992) Effect of rigid gas permeable lens flexure on vision. Optom. Vis. Sci., 69(12), 953–958

Stone, J. and Collins, C. (1984) Flexure of gas-permeable lenses on toroidal corneas. Optician, 188(4951), 8–10

Swarbrick, H. A. (1988) A possible etiology for REP lens binding (adherence). Int. Contact Lens Clin., 15, 13–19

Swarbrick, H. A. and Holden, B. A. (1989) Rigid gas permeable lens adherence: a patient dependent phenomenon. Optom. Vis. Sci., 66(5), 269–275

Swarbrick, H. A. and Holden B. A. (1987) Rigid gas permeable lens binding: significance and contributing factors. Am. J. Optom. Physiol. Opt., 64(11), 815–823

Swarbrick, H. A. and Holden, B. A. (1996) Effects of lens parameter variation on rigid gas-permeable lens adherence. Optom. Vis. Sci., 73(3), 144–155

Thean, J. H. J. and McNab, A. A. (2004) Blepharoptosis in RGP and PMMA hard contact lens wearers. Clin. Exp. Optom., 87(1), 11–14

Townsley, M. (1967) New equipment and method for determining the contour of the human cornea. Contacto, 11(4), 72–81

Vanden Bosch, W. A. and Lemji, H. G. (1992) Blepharoptosis induced by prolonged contact lens wear. Ophthalmology, 99, 1757–1765

Walker, J. (1988) Radical flattening – a laboratory enigma. Optician, April, 21–23

Watt, T. J. (1993) Improved wettability and deposit resistance from surface treated gas permeable materials – fact or fiction? Contact Lens J., 20(8), 6–9

Worp, van der E., Brabander, de J., Lubberman, B., Marin, G. and Hendrikse, F. (2002) Optimising RGP lens fitting in normal eyes using 3D topographic data. Cont. Lens Anterior Eye, 25, 95–99

Worp, van der E., Brabander, de J., Swarbrick, H., Nuijts, R. and Hendrikse, F. (2003) Corneal desiccation in rigid contact lens wear: 3- and 9-o'clock staining. Optom. Vis. Sci., 80, 280–290

Wray, L. (1963) An elementary analysis of the forces retaining a corneal contact lens on the eye. Optician, 146, 239–241, 373–376

Young, G. (1988) Fluorescein in rigid lens fit evaluation. Int. Contact Lens Clin., 15, 95–100

Chapter 10

Soft contact lens fitting

Lyndon W. Jones and Kathy Dumbleton

CHAPTER CONTENTS

INTRODUCTION

Soft lenses were initially introduced in the early 1970s and are now the most prescribed lens type worldwide (Morgan et al. 2004), used by over 80% of contact lens patients. Over the past 30 years there have been numerous improvements in materials and manufacturing techniques. Hydrogel lenses can now be worn successfully on both a daily and overnight basis and replaced frequently at intervals ranging from 1 day to 1 month. The last 6 years have seen the most significant change in soft lens materials with the introduction of silicone hydrogel lenses.

Over the years a number of names or descriptions have been used for soft lenses, including hydrophilic, hydrogel, gel, flexible and pliable. The term 'soft' has become the most acceptable and widely used term.

Soft lenses, when hydrated, can be readily folded and manipulated without damage and drape across the cornea, resting on the conjunctiva. The term 'hydrogel' signifies a polymer that absorbs and binds water into its molecular structure and describes contact lenses that have a certain percentage water content.

Prior to hydration these hydrogels are referred to as 'xerogels', a state that is rigid in nature. When manufactured by a lathe-cutting procedure, lenses are lathed in the xerogel state and then placed in saline to hydrate and become soft and flexible (Davies 1992). If they dehydrate, they become rigid and inflexible.

This chapter will review the development and properties of soft contact lens materials, their classification, indications and contraindications for fitting, and the fitting process required to ensure that such lenses perform in an optimal fashion.

HISTORICAL OVERVIEW

For a review of the development of soft lenses, readers are referred to Chapter 1 and to more expansive reviews (Efron & Pearson 1988, Pearson & Efron 1989, Mertz 1997, Jones 2002).

In the early 1950s, Professor Otto Wichterle and Dr Drahoslav Lim, two polymer chemists based at the Prague Institute of Macromolecular Chemistry of the Czechoslovak Academy of Science (CSAS), were attempting to develop a

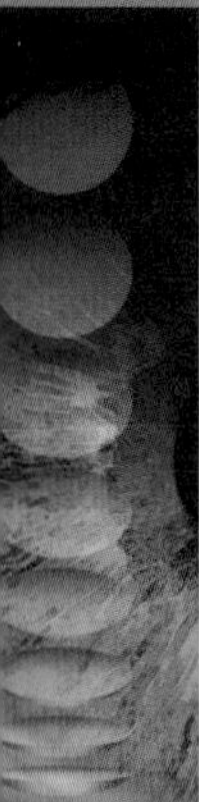

synthetic biomaterial for a variety of implant purposes and developed a water-absorbing polymer that absorbed 38% of its weight of water, which they termed poly-2-hydroxyethyl methacrylate (polyHEMA) (Wichterle & Lim 1960). They almost immediately began to conceive of its applicability to produce a thin, transparent membrane to correct myopia and produced the first hydrogel contact lenses in December 1961 using a simplistic spin casting process developed from a child's construction set.

Limited numbers of lenses were distributed in Europe in the early 1960s under the name 'Spofalens' and received US patents in 1962 and 1965 (Mertz 1997). Unfortunately, the CSAS inexplicably (and without Wichterle's knowledge) sold the patent rights to the United States National Patent Development Corporation in 1965 and later even consented to the cancellation of the licence agreements.

In 1966 a sublicensing agreement was reached with Bausch & Lomb (B&L), who significantly improved the manufacturing technology. B&L gained approval from the US Food and Drug Administration (FDA) in March 1971 for spun-cast lenses ('Soflens'), and thus began the huge proliferation of new materials and lenses. Soon after this, production of lenses was started in various other countries by the more usual method of lathing or 'lathe-cutting' buttons of polymer cut from solid rods (Davies 1992).

After extended wear was introduced in the 1970s, reports of hypoxic and inflammatory complications, and severe corneal ulceration with significant vision loss began appearing (Zantos & Holden 1978, Binder 1979, Larke & Hirji 1979, Lebow & Plishka 1980, Hassman & Sugar 1983, Weissman et al. 1984) and the safety of overnight wear was questioned (Smith & MacRae 1989). In Europe, awareness of these complications resulted in soft lenses being prescribed primarily for daily wear only.

By the mid 1980s, high water content materials had been developed and their use for daily wear grew (Jones 1988, 1990a–c). Rapid lens spoilage resulted in companies looking at the development of materials that could be replaced on a regular basis (Lowther 1984, Schwartz 1986, Jones 1994) and, as lathing was expensive, new manufacturing methods were required.

The first truly frequent replacement or 'disposable lens' was introduced in Denmark in the early 1980s (Vangsted et al. 1986, Mertz 1997) but poor reproducibility limited their commercial success. The technology, however, was purchased by Johnson and Johnson in 1984 and, after considerable refinement, resulted in the launch of the first true disposable lenses in June 1988 (Acuvue, Vistakon) (Mertz 1997).

This was such a success (Donshik et al. 1988, Grant & Holden 1988, Ivins 1988, Kaye et al. 1988, Gruber 1989, Krasnow 1989, Bergenske 1990, Lane 1990) that other manufacturers quickly released disposable lenses (e.g. B&L 'SeeQuence' and CIBA Vision 'NewVues') and the concept of frequently replacing lenses became entrenched in clinical practice.

In August 1994, the first daily disposable lenses became available (Kame et al. 1994, Nason et al. 1994, Mertz 1997), revolutionizing the way that clinicians manage patients (Hamano et al. 1994, Solomon et al. 1996). In some countries daily disposable lenses now account for almost 40% of new soft lens fits (Morgan et al. 2004).

The launch of a new family of hydrogel materials based on silicone technology in 1999 represented one of the most exciting developments for soft contact lenses since their initial introduction 30 years previously (Alvord et al. 1998, Grobe et al. 1999, Kunzler 1999, Nicolson & Vogt 2001, Jones 2002, Lopez-Alemany et al. 2002, Tighe 2004).

TERMINOLOGY

The terminology used to describe the wearing schedule or replacement period of soft lenses can be confusing (Doughman & Massare 1996, Mertz 1997). The following sections aim to clarify this.

Soft contact lens wearing modality

Soft contact lenses can be worn according to a number of different wearing modalities.

DAILY WEAR

Lenses worn on a daily wear basis are worn during waking hours, usually for periods of 8–16 hours. On removal they are either cleaned and disinfected in preparation for the next wearing period, or, in the case of single-use daily disposable lenses, discarded.

FLEXIBLE WEAR

Lenses worn on a flexible wear basis are typically worn on a daily wear basis, with occasional, infrequent overnight use. When removed, they should either be cleaned and disinfected or discarded.

EXTENDED WEAR

Extended wear lenses are worn constantly for up to 7 consecutive days and nights. When removed, they should either be cleaned and disinfected (reusable extended wear) or discarded (disposable extended wear).

Historically, reusable extended wear lenses were used in therapeutic applications or for patients who used their lenses for aphakia or other abnormally high refractive errors, with cosmetic lens wearers using their lenses on a disposable extended-wear basis. However, modern silicone hydrogel lenses are worn for four consecutive 1-week periods of extended wear and then discarded, making them reusable extended-wear lenses.

CONTINUOUS WEAR

In the late 1970s, high water content lenses such as Permalens (CooperVision) were frequently used for periods of up to 3 months, coining the phrase 'continuous wear'. The realization in the late 1980s that extended wear was responsible for an increased number of cases of microbial keratitis led to the Contact Lens Institute in the US sponsoring studies to investigate the relative risk and incidence of infectious keratitis.

The results were published in 1989 (Poggio et al. 1989, Schein et al. 1989) and clearly demonstrated that overnight wear carried a significantly increased risk of corneal infection, and that the risk increased with the number of consecutive nights of wear. The FDA immediately reduced the approved length of time for overnight wear without removal from 30 to 7 days, eliminating continuous wear as a concept.

Since the introduction of silicone hydrogel materials, however, continuous wear is once again becoming popular. In this modality, lenses are worn on a 24-hour basis for periods of up to 30 consecutive days and nights. Lenses may be removed before this time, but must be cleaned and disinfected before reinsertion. After 1 month of wear, with or without removal, the lenses are discarded.

Soft contact lens replacement schedule

When soft lenses were initially introduced in the 1970s, replacement was only felt to be necessary when the lenses were either permanently deposited or damaged. Frequently replacing lenses diminishes lens spoilage and complications and is considered to offer greater safety for contact lens wear on both a daily and overnight basis (Tripathi et al. 1980, Donshik et al. 1988, Grant & Holden 1988, Marshall et al. 1992, Gellatly 1993, Nason et al. 1993, Poggio et al. 1993, Hamano et al. 1994, Jones 1994, Nason et al. 1994, Nilsson & Montan 1994, Jones et al. 1996, Solomon et al. 1996, Jones et al. 2000, Keith et al. 2003). Lenses are now frequently classified according to their replacement schedule (Doughman & Massare 1996, Mertz 1997).

CONVENTIONAL REPLACEMENT

With a conventional replacement schedule, lenses are typically replaced every 6–18 months. Some patients wear their soft lenses for significantly longer periods, but this practice is not recommended.

PLANNED REPLACEMENT

The term 'planned replacement' describes lenses that are changed at intervals ranging from 2 weeks to 6 months.

DISPOSABLE LENSES

The term 'disposable' should be reserved for lenses which are discarded and replaced after a single wearing period, with no cleaning and disinfecting ever taking place (Doughman & Massare 1996). For daily disposable lenses this is a 1-day wearing period and for lenses worn on an extended- or continuous-wear regimen, timeframes range from 7 to 30 days (Mertz 1997). The term is, however, frequently synonymous with lenses which are removed for regular cleaning and disinfection and replaced after a period of 1–4 weeks (Mertz 1997).

SOFT CONTACT LENS PROPERTIES AND MATERIALS (see also Chapter 3)

OXYGEN PERMEABILITY AND TRANSMISSIBILITY

Oxygen permeability is an inherent property of a material and is independent of thickness. It is expressed as the 'Dk' value, where D represents the diffusion coefficient and k the solubility of oxygen (Peterson & Fatt 1973, Fatt 1979, 1986, Brennan et al. 1987). From a clinical perspective, oxygen transport to the cornea depends upon both the Dk of the material and the lens thickness (t), with thinner lenses allowing more oxygen to reach the cornea.

Table 10.1: 'Typical' examples of Dk/t for conventional lens materials

Hydrogels	Dk/t	RGPs	Dk/t
Low water content (38%)	15	Silicone-acrylates	27
Mid water content (55%)	27	Fluorosilicone acrylates	60
High water content (70%)	35	Fluoropolymers	130

The term Dk/t describes the 'oxygen transmissibility' of a lens and gives a quantitative indication of the amount of oxygen that a lens-wearing eye will receive through the lens. It is more clinically useful than Dk, which gives no indication of the effect of lens thickness or design.

Ideally, hydrogel lenses would have both a high Dk, as the oxygen is transported in the water, and a thin centre thickness. Such lenses are, however, impractical because they rapidly dehydrate, resulting in corneal staining (Holden et al. 1986, Orsborn & Zantos 1988). Thin high water content lenses are also difficult to manufacture, so, in practice, lens thickness is greater, which limits the Dk/t clinically obtainable.

Table 10.1 details typical Dk/t values available for conventional hydrogel materials and commonly encountered rigid gas permeable (RGP) materials, at centre thicknesses normally found for –3.00 D lenses. It is clear that conventional hydrogel materials have relatively low Dk/t compared with RGP materials.

Materials

All contact lens materials are polymers made up of repeating chains of monomers arranged in patterns with cross-linking between the polymer chains. These afford strength and further govern the characteristics of the materials. The lens materials have water contents ranging from 24 to 85% (Tighe 2002). The monomer most commonly employed in conventional contact lenses is poly-2-hydroxyethyl methacrylate (polyHEMA).

PolyHEMA is:

- Easily fabricated into contact lenses.
- Relatively cheap.
- Highly flexible.
- Dimensionally stable to changes in pH and temperature.
- Very successful as a contact lens material.

The principal disadvantage of polyHEMA is that it relies on water to transport oxygen across the material. Water has a limited ability to dissolve and transport oxygen, having an approximate oxygen permeability of around 80 Dk units (Fatt 1986).

In order to increase the Dk of a conventional hydrogel material beyond that of polyHEMA, it is necessary to

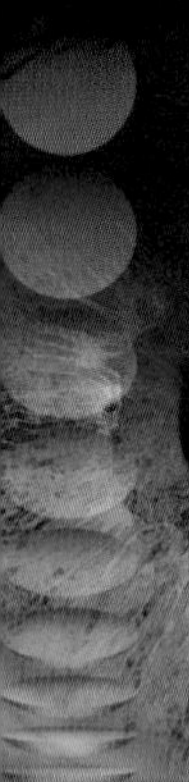

Table 10.2: Silicone hydrogel lens materials

Proprietary name	Focus Night & Day	AIR OPTIX	PureVision	Acuvue OASYS	Acuvue Advance
United States Adopted Name	lotrafilcon A	lotrafilcon B	balafilcon A	senofilcon A	galyfilcon A
Manufacturer	CIBA Vision	CIBA Vision	Bausch & Lomb	Vistakon	Vistakon
Centre thickness (@ –3.00 D) (mm)	0.08	0.08	0.09	0.07	0.07
Water content	24%	33%	36%	38%	47%
Total diameter (mm)	13.8	14.2	14.0	14.0	14.0
Back optic zone radius (mm)	8.4; 8.6	8.6	8.6	8.4	8.3; 8.7
Prescription range (D)	+6.00 to –10.00	+6.00 to –10.00	+6.00 to –12.00	–0.50 to –6.00	+ 8.00 to –12.00
Recommended replacement schedule	4 weeks	2 weeks	4 weeks	1–2 weeks	2 weeks
Oxygen permeability ($\times 10^{-11}$) (Dk)	140	110	91	103	60
Oxygen transmissibility ($\times 10^{-9}$) (Dk/t)	175	138	101	147	86
Modulus (psi)*	238	Unpublished	148	Unpublished	65
Surface treatment	25 nm plasma coating with high refractive index	25 nm plasma coating with high refractive index	Plasma oxidation process	No surface treatment. Internal wetting agent (PVP) throughout the matrix that also coats the surface	No surface treatment. Internal wetting agent (PVP) throughout the matrix that also coats the surface
FDA group	I	I	III	I	I
Principal monomers	DMA + TRIS + siloxane macromer	DMA + TRIS + siloxane macromer	NVP + TPVC + NCVE + PBVC	mPDMS + DMA + HEMA + siloxane macromer + TEGDMA + PVP	mPDMS + DMA + EGDMA + HEMA + siloxane macromer + PVP

* Modulus data taken from Steffen & McCabe (2004).
DMA (*N,N*-dimethylacrylamide); EGDMA (ethyleneglycol dimethacrylate); HEMA (poly-2-hydroxyethyl methacrylate); mPDMS (monofunctional polydimethylsiloxane); NVP (*N*-vinyl pyrrolidone); TEGDMA (tetraethyleneglycol dimethacrylate); TPVC (tris-(trimethylsiloxysilyl) propylvinyl carbamate); NCVE (*N*-carboxyvinyl ester); PBVC (poly[dimethysiloxy] di [silylbutanol] bis[vinyl carbamate]); PVP (polyvinyl pyrrolidone).

incorporate monomers that will bind more water into the polymer (Jones 2002, Tighe 2002). These higher water content materials typically use polyHEMA or methyl methacrylate (MMA), in conjunction with more hydrophilic monomers such as *N*-vinyl pyrrolidone (NVP) or methacrylic acid (MA) (Tighe 2002). The constituent monomers determine the various physical and chemical properties of the material, with MA-containing materials having a significant degree of negative surface charge.

Another method of increasing Dk is to incorporate silicone into the polymer (Morrison & Edelhauser 1972, Refojo 1979). Silicone-rubber-based flexible contact lenses have been used for therapeutic and paediatric applications for many years (Gurland 1979, Rogers 1980, Martin et al. 1983, Cutler et al. 1985). Although the lenses offer exceptional oxygen transmission and durability, they do have limitations for clinical use:

- Fluid is unable to flow through these materials, leading to possible lens binding to the ocular surface (Rae & Huff 1991).
- Lens surfaces are hydrophobic, resulting in marked lipid and mucous deposition (Dahl & Brocks 1978, Huth & Wagner 1981).

Silicone hydrogel materials combine silicone rubber with conventional hydrogel monomers (Tighe 2004). The silicone component provides high oxygen permeability, while the hydrogel facilitates flexibility, wettability and fluid transport, which aids lens movement.

Combining conventional hydrogel monomers with silicone proved to be an enormous challenge, being likened to combining oil with water, while maintaining optical clarity (Tighe 2004).

An additional problem with silicone-based materials is their decreased wettability, increased lipid interaction and accentuated lens binding. To overcome this, a variety of methodologies are used to enhance the wettability of the surfaces (Grobe 1999, Nicolson & Vogt 2001, Nicolson 2003, Jones & Dumbleton 2004, Steffen & Schnider 2004, Tighe 2004). Five silicone hydrogel lens materials currently available are compared in Table 10.2 (see also Table 3.3).

The differences between silicone hydrogel lens materials and conventional hydrogels are considerable and may be attributed to both their bulk and their surface properties (Jones & Dumbleton 2004, Tighe 2004).

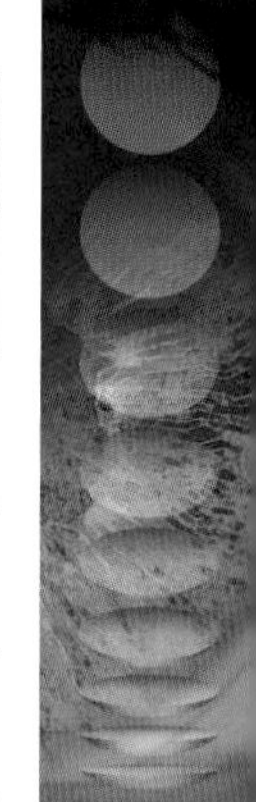

Water content and thickness

Soft lenses are frequently categorized according to their water content:

- 20–44% – 'low' water content
- 45–59% – 'mid' water content
- Greater than 60% – 'high' water content.

PolyHEMA has a water content of 38% and is obtainable in varying thicknesses; thinner lenses having increased transmissibility (Dk/t) and improved corneal physiology. Hypoxic complications with low water content lenses resulted in increasing numbers of mid and high water content lenses being fitted, since increasing the water content is a more efficient means of improving corneal oxygenation than reducing lens thickness (Brennan & Efron 1987, Efron & Brennan 1987, Fatt 1995).

In silicone hydrogel materials, the oxygen is mainly transmitted through the silicone component of the lens material, resulting in a dramatic increase in oxygen permeability with very low water content materials (Tighe 2004). These lenses have an inverse relationship between water content and Dk, with the highest Dk values corresponding with the lowest water contents (Tighe 2004).

Manufacturing methods (see also Chapter 19)

Soft lenses may be manufactured using several different techniques, including lathing, spin-casting, dry-moulding or the newer techniques of wet or 'stabilized soft' moulding (Davies 1992, Mertz 1997). Certain lenses, such as the Bausch & Lomb Optima lens, are hybrid in character, being lathe-cut on the back surface after initially spin-casting the front surface (Mertz 1997).

Moulding and spin-casting are ideal for mass production of lenses and a number of manufacturers have streamlined their moulding technologies to reduce production costs and allow more frequent replacement of lenses (Mertz 1997). Lathing is better suited to the production of individual lenses and specialized designs but, with modern automatic lathes, it is increasingly successful in mass production.

SOFT CONTACT LENS CLASSIFICATION

With such a wide variety of soft contact lens materials available, some form of classification system is needed. To complicate matters, four systems currently exist to subdivide and classify hydrogel materials (Jones 2002).

Commercial name

This is the name given to the lens by the manufacturer and is the brand name by which they are known, for example Acuvue and Focus Night & Day.

United States Adopted Name (USAN)

This is the unique name for a material consisting of a certain fixed monomer composition (e.g. etafilcon or tetrafilcon).

Table 10.3: FDA classification of hydrogel contact lens materials

		Water content (%)	Methacrylic acid (% m/m)
Group I	Low water content, non-ionic	<50	<0.2
Group II	High water content, non-ionic	>50	<0.2
Group III	Low water content, ionic	<50	>0.2
Group IV	High water content, ionic	>50	>0.2

Polymacon is a generic term for polyHEMA and several commercial names are given to lenses with the same USAN – for example Acuvue, 1-Day Acuvue, Acuvue Bifocal and Surevue, all of which are etafilcon-based lenses. Some historic anomalies to this system do exist, with the same USAN being assigned to materials of differing water content. Examples include bufilcon and phemfilcon (Tighe 2002).

FDA categorization

The United States Food and Drug Administration uses a simple subdivision of lens materials based upon water content and ionic charge. Materials with water contents greater than 50% are classified as 'high water content', and those with greater than 0.2% ionic material (invariably methacrylic acid) are termed 'ionic' (Table 10.3). This classification is useful to describe the way in which materials interact with both lens solutions and the tear film. Low water content non-ionic lenses (Group I) are generally the most stable and least affected by the tear film and environment. High water content lenses (Group IV) are the most reactive and readily deposit with positively charged proteins such as lysozyme. Groups II and III lenses fall between these two extremes of behaviour and performance. Silicone hydrogel lenses have been classified into FDA Groups I and III, although the properties of these materials are not suitably described within the current classification system. A fifth group may be required to adequately describe hydrogel lenses that incorporate silicone.

ISO classification

This system is outlined in International Standards EN ISO 11539:1999. Rigid lens materials are given a suffix of 'focon' and hydrogels a suffix of 'filcon', followed by a series of letters and a group suffix (Table 10.4).

INDICATIONS FOR SOFT CONTACT LENSES (see also Chapter 8)

The major indications for, and advantages of, soft contact lenses relate to their inherent flexibility and deformability. Below is an overview of the principal indications for soft lenses.

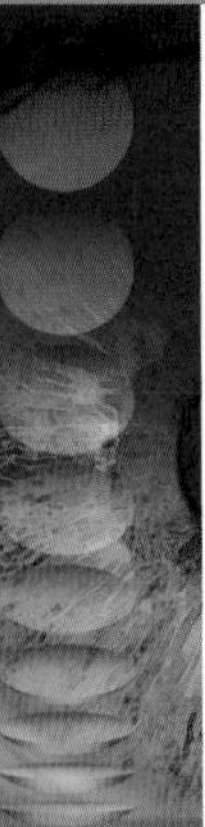

Table 10.4: ISO classification of lens materials

Group suffix	Rigid lenses – focon	Soft lenses – filcon
I	Does not contain silicone or fluorine	<50% water content, non-ionic
II	Contains silicone but not fluorine	≥50% water content, non-ionic
III	Contains both silicone and fluorine	<50% water content, ionic
IV	Contains fluorine but not silicone	≥50% water content, ionic

Examples include Filcon 1a (polyHEMA) and Focon 1a (polymethyl methacrylate) (Kerr & Meyler 2001).

Comfort

Low tensile modulus and a high degree of elasticity, together with a total diameter (TD) extending beyond the limbus, result in good initial comfort and little lid sensation compared with rigid lenses. This makes them ideal for patients with sensitive eyes and those who have previously failed with rigid lenses due to discomfort. The photophobia and lacrimation often encountered when adapting to rigid lenses is generally absent with hydrogels.

Rapid adaptation

The comfort of soft lenses makes these the lens of choice in cases where slow adaptation with rigid lenses is difficult due to constraints of work or study. While abnormal head posture and unnatural facial expressions may be seen with rigid lens wearers in the early stages of adaptation, soft lens wearers generally look quite natural from the beginning.

Occasional wear

Many patients only require social or part-time wear (e.g. sports once or twice a week). The ease of adaptation to soft lenses makes alternating between spectacles and contact lenses straightforward.

Low refractive errors

Patients with less than 1.00 D of ametropia are often poorly motivated to wear lenses and the comfort of soft lenses is preferable to the adaptation required for rigid lenses.

Uniocular wear

Patients who only require a lens in one eye for unilateral ametropia frequently find it easier to adapt to a soft lens than a rigid one. This does not apply to unilateral lens wear for ocular pathology such as injury or keratoconus, where optimum visual acuity would require that the eye be fitted with a rigid lens.

Sports

The excellent stability and initial comfort of soft lenses has made them the lens of first choice for many sporting activities, particularly contact sports. Well-fitting soft lenses are not easily ejected from the eye by rubbing or lid tension and are not normally dislodged onto the sclera.

Occupational

The size of a soft lens and the way in which it conforms to the shape of the eye means that there are few problems with dust and foreign bodies. For patients who work in windy or dusty atmospheres, soft lenses are generally the lens of choice.

Flare with rigid lenses

Patients with large pupils who wear rigid lenses may suffer from 'flare' in reduced illumination. The large diameter and reduced movement of soft lenses usually eliminates this.

Persistent '3 and 9' staining

Patients with poor quality or quantity of tears, low/high-riding lenses, incomplete blinking, wide palpebral apertures or high negative prescriptions may be predisposed to '3 and 9 o'clock' staining with RGP lenses (see Chapter 9). If all attempts to optimize the rigid lens fit and blinking have proved unsuccessful, then a soft lens may resolve the problem.

Paediatric wear (see Chapter 24)

The comfort associated with soft lenses makes them ideal for paediatric use in cases of, for example, aphakia or anisometropia.

Therapeutic wear (see Chapter 26)

Soft lenses are used as bandage lenses in many pathological cases in order to relieve pain, promote stable epithelialization, maintain epithelial hydration and provide mechanical protection. Soft lenses are also occasionally used as drug delivery systems.

Cosmetic lenses (see Chapter 25)

Tinted lenses are generally soft lenses, whether for prosthetic purposes in cases of scarred or unsightly corneas, or to cosmetically enhance or change eye colour.

CONTRAINDICATIONS FOR SOFT CONTACT LENSES

Despite their many advantages, soft lens wear is associated with a number of disadvantages. The use of frequent replacement and disposable lenses has overcome many of these but potential drawbacks should be carefully evaluated for each patient.

Variable vision

Visual acuity can vary with soft lenses as a result of blinking and changes in the tear film. Changes in the environment may affect the level of hydration, resulting in fluctuating vision. Unacceptable vision with low levels of corneal astigmatism may also indicate that the patient would be better fitted with spherical rigid lenses, which would neutralize the corneal astigmatism and may result in a better quality of vision.

Breakage and tearing

Soft lenses can suffer from tearing, breakage and edge nicks. Patients who repeatedly damage lenses should be fitted with lenses which are disposed of frequently.

Deposition

Soft lenses deteriorate with age. Their surfaces may become deposited with substances from the tear film, including protein, mucin, calcium and lipids. Deposited lenses eventually become uncomfortable, their fitting characteristics may change, and visual acuity may be reduced, particularly at low contrast levels (Gellatly et al. 1988). Frequent replacement of soft lenses has dramatically reduced this problem.

Lens care

With the exception of daily disposable and single-use continuous-wear lenses, soft lenses must be cleaned and disinfected after wearing to avoid the risk of contamination by microorganisms. Although this process has been simplified with the introduction of new care regimes (see Chapter 4), it is still seen to be expensive and time consuming by patients, and there are frequently problems with non-compliance.

Inability to modify soft lenses

It is not feasible to modify either the power or the fitting parameters of soft lenses. If the patient's refractive error should alter, it is necessary to supply a new lens. This is less of an issue with frequent-replacement lenses than with custom-designed conventional lenses.

Verification difficulties (see Chapter 16)

Soft lenses cannot be verified as readily as rigid lenses. In many cases it is difficult to confirm the back vertex power and other lens parameters. When soft lenses are verified, a number of factors including temperature and storage solution must be taken into account.

Chemical contamination

It is possible for soft lenses to absorb chemicals into their naturally porous structure – for example, if worn in a polluted environment or while swimming in chlorinated water. Chemicals may be retained and become a future source of ocular irritation. Eye drops not specifically formulated for use while wearing soft lenses should be avoided. Even those formulated for use with contact lenses need careful observation to ensure that there is no allergic or hypersensitivity reaction to the preservatives used in the product.

Patients on long-term topical agents such as glaucoma and steroid medications should be advised to instil their drops, where possible, before inserting and after removing their lenses, and to use frequent-replacement lenses.

BASELINE OCULAR ASSESSMENTS AND MEASUREMENTS

A number of measurements and baseline data are required before a suitable lens type and form can be chosen.

Ocular integrity

A thorough slit-lamp assessment should be carried out. Factors affecting lens choice include examination of the eyelids (including lid eversion), lashes and margins, integrity of the limbal region, and a detailed examination of the conjunctiva and cornea (see Chapters 7 and 8).

Corneal diameter

This may be estimated by measuring the horizontal visible iris diameter (HVID) with either a pupillary distance (PD) rule or a slit-lamp reticule. The true corneal diameter is approximately 1.25 mm larger than the HVID (Martin & Holden 1982). Soft lenses are generally chosen with a diameter 1.5–2.5 mm larger than the measured HVID. There is no set rule on this parameter, the judgement being based on clinical experience, individual preferences and available diameters. Although corneal diameter varies widely, disposable soft lenses are typically only available within a limited total diameter (TD) range, usually 13.8–14.5 mm.

Corneal curvature

Keratometry measurements of central corneal curvature have traditionally been used to predict the optimum soft contact lens back optic zone radius (BOZR) or base curve, particularly of thicker hydrogel lenses. More recently, other parameters such as corneal diameter, asphericity and sagittal height have been shown to be more useful when predicting the fit of modern, thinner lens designs, with corneal asphericity and sagittal height being the most important (Garner 1982, Young 1992b).

Corneal topography

Corneal topography is usually unnecessary to optimize the fit of soft lenses as the centration and movement is little influenced by corneal contour, except in cases of very steep central curvature, where lenses may have a tendency to decentre (Bruce 1994).

Refractive error

Two basic assumptions can be made when assessing the potential success of astigmatic patients being fitted with spherical soft lenses.

- Total ocular astigmatism = corneal astigmatism + lenticular and/or retinal astigmatism.

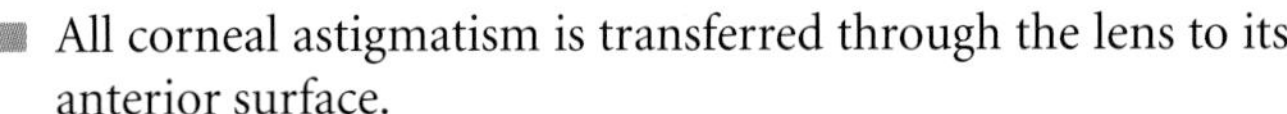

- All corneal astigmatism is transferred through the lens to its anterior surface.

Patients may therefore be divided into the following four groups at their initial examination by reference to their refractive error and keratometry (K) readings:

- Spherical cornea with spherical refraction, e.g.
  Rx: –3.00 DS
  K: 7.85 mm along 180° (43.00 D)
  7.85 mm along 90° (43.00 D)
  This is the ideal optical situation for contact lens fitting. Vision should be equally good with either rigid or soft lenses.
- Spherical cornea with astigmatic refraction, e.g.
  Rx: –2.00/–1.75 × 90
  K: 7.85 mm along 180° (43.00 D)
  7.90 mm along 90° (42.75 D)
  The astigmatism is almost entirely lenticular, so that the visual result is the same with either a rigid or a soft lens. In both cases, a front surface toric lens is required to correct the 1.50 D of residual astigmatism. However, due to orientation difficulties with an RGP lens, a toric soft lens is more practical in this case.
- Astigmatic cornea with astigmatic refraction, e.g.
  Rx: –2.00/–1.75 × 180
  K: 7.80 mm along 180° (43.25 D)
  7.50 mm along 90° (45.00 D)
  All of the astigmatism is corneal, so that a spherical RGP lens, or a toric soft lens, should be fitted.
- Astigmatic cornea with spherical refraction, e.g.
  Rx: –3.00 DS
  K: 7.80 mm along 180° (43.25 D)
  7.50 mm along 90° (45.00 D)
  In this last example, there is 1.75 D of with-the-rule corneal astigmatism together with an equivalent degree of against-the-rule lenticular astigmatism, resulting in a spherical refraction. A spherical rigid lens form would leave a residual cylinder of –1.75 D × 90. A soft lens, because it transfers all the corneal astigmatism through to its front surface without optically neutralizing it, is the lens of choice.

INSERTION AND REMOVAL TECHNIQUES FOR THE PRACTITIONER

Lens insertion and removal (see Chapter 11)

For patients who have not worn soft lenses previously, the practitioner should insert and remove the initial trial lenses. The majority of disposable lenses are now packaged in blister packs and removal of lenses from the packaging is relatively straightforward.

A number of manufacturers have incorporated inversion marks on their lenses as an aid to lens handling (Fig. 10.1). If these are not available, balance the lens on the index finger and examine the profile and check the orientation.

- A lens correctly orientated will have the appearance of a 'bowl' (Fig. 10.2); if pinched gently, the edges turn inwards.

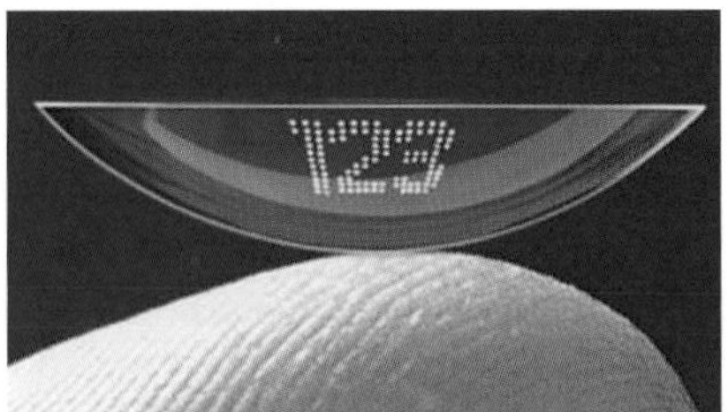

Figure 10.1 Example of an inversion marker on a soft lens (Acuvue)

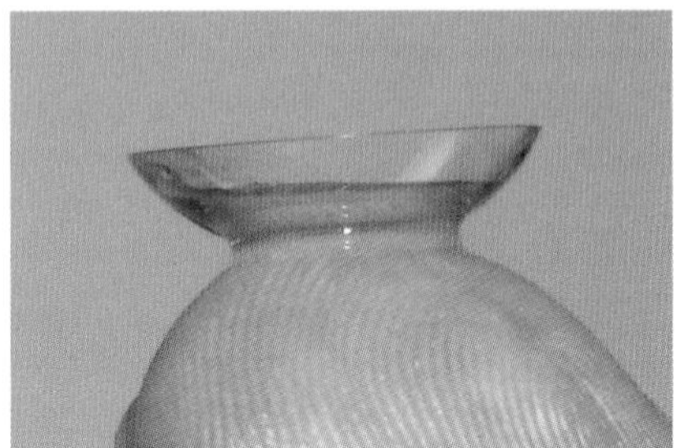

Figure 10.2 Correct orientation of a soft lens for insertion, demonstrating a 'bowl'-type appearance

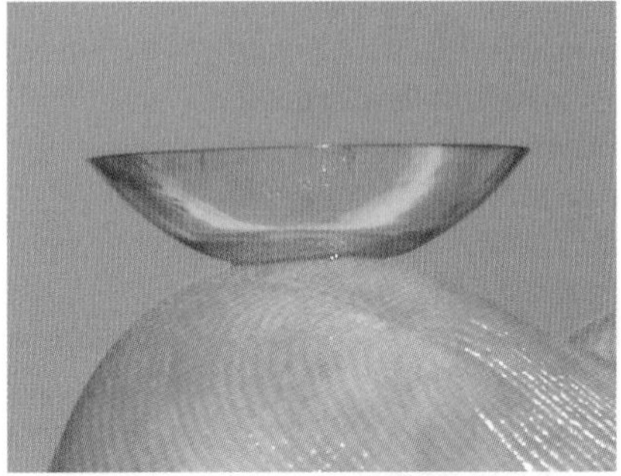

Figure 10.3 Incorrect orientation of a soft lens for insertion, demonstrating a 'dish'-type appearance

- An inverted lens will turn outwards slightly, resembling a 'dish' (Fig. 10.3); if pinched gently, the edges will turn out towards the fingers.

The lens can be inserted directly onto the cornea but it is usually easier to insert it onto the sclera (Fig. 10.4).

To remove the lens secure the eyelids and direct the patient to look nasally. Slide the lens onto the temporal sclera (Fig. 10.5) and gently pinch the lens with the thumb and index finger, breaking the capillary action and removing it from the eye (Fig. 10.6).

FITTING PROCEDURES

Suboptimal fitting lenses can compromise ocular integrity and result in higher levels of conjunctival and corneal staining and ocular hyperaemia (Young & Coleman 2001). Trial fitting should be undertaken before the commencement of wear so that alternatives can be found should problems occur.

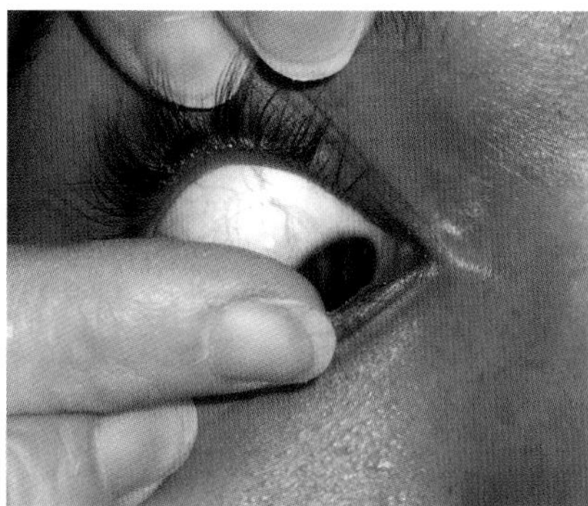

Figure 10.4 Suggested technique for soft lens placement on insertion

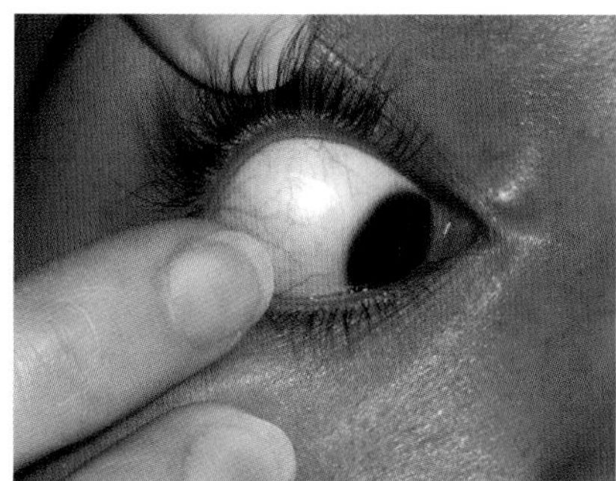

Figure 10.5 Sliding soft lens onto the inferior temporal sclera for lens removal

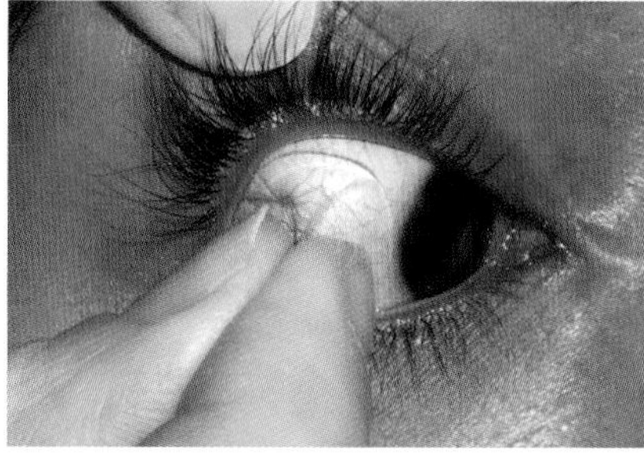

Figure 10.6 Soft lens removal from the sclera by 'pinching' the lens from the eye

Initial comfort during trial fitting influences the patient's perception of contact lenses (Efron et al. 1986, McMonnies 1997) and affects their ultimate success. Therefore, increasing the probability of achieving an optimal lens fit with the first trial lens can benefit both patient and practitioner. Over the last decade hydrogel trial lens fitting has become simplified, with many soft lenses now only available in one or two BOZRs.

Silicone hydrogel lens fitting may be more exacting since the increased 'stiffness' of these materials does not allow the lenses to drape over the cornea, as is often the case with traditional, thin soft lenses (Tighe 2004). Non-optimal fitting may result in reduced comfort and a variety of clinical complications (Dumbleton et al. 2002, Dumbleton 2003, Sweeney et al. 2004).

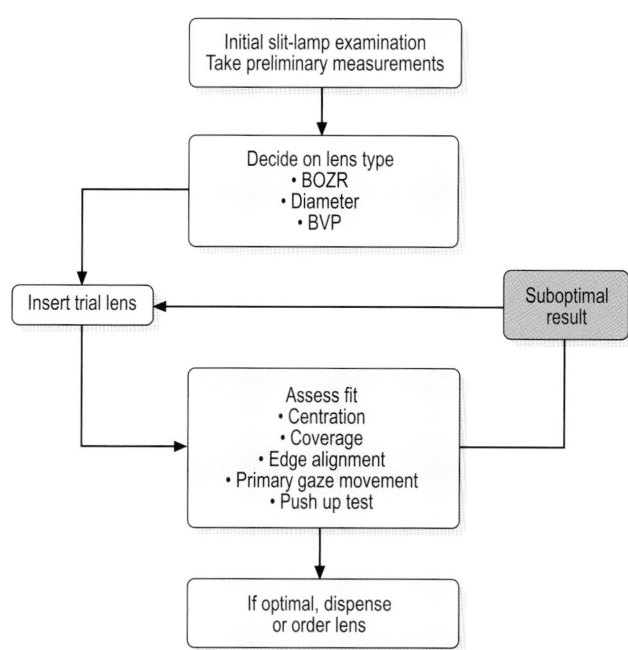

Figure 10.7 Steps taken in soft lens fitting

Initial trial lens selection (Fig. 10.7)

Since the introduction of frequent replacement and disposable lenses, the primary factor for choosing the initial trial lens generally relates to the available parameters in the required lens type. 'Good' soft contact lens fitting involves finding a well-fitting lens in the most appropriate material with optimal wearing regimen, and then reviewing the options of diameter and BOZR in that material. Most lens types are only available in one diameter and limited base curves, making lens fitting relatively easy.

Lenses across a wide range of BOZR can show similar amounts of movement, while those with similar BOZR but different designs can show markedly different fitting characteristics (Martin et al. 1989, Young 1992b,c, 1997, Young et al. 1993). This is because the key biometric factor controlling soft lens movement and fit is not central keratometry readings, which is often the factor used to select the BOZR of the lens, but the sagittal height of the eye (Young 1992a–c, 1998). Variations in corneal shape factor and diameter have a much greater influence on ocular sagittal height than variations in central corneal curvature (Young 1992b).

Once the appropriate material has been chosen, diagnostic lenses of the desired BOZR, diameter and prescription are inserted. After a suitable period to allow the lenses to settle, the overall fit is assessed.

In most cases practitioners will then dispense the lenses from a stock inventory. Occasionally, the optimal lens parameters need to be ordered from the information gathered at this fitting examination.

If trial soft lenses are not dispensed to the patient they should be discarded and not disinfected and reused for another patient. This is particularly important given the concerns relating

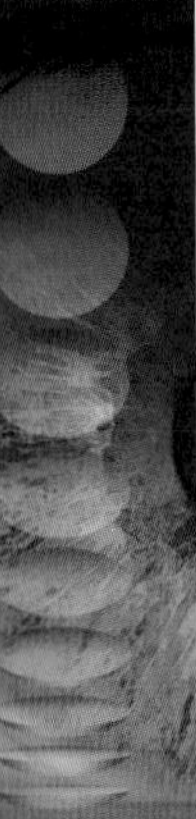

to transmission of a number of diseases including the prion diseases or transmissible spongiform encephalopathies (TSEs).

Back vertex power (BVP)

Back vertex powers of soft lenses can range from approximately +35.00 to −35.00 D. Many disposable lenses are available in a limited power range, typically +6.00 to −10.00 D, and very high ametropes often need custom-made soft lenses.

The BVP of the contact lens should closely approximate the patient's spectacle prescription, corrected for vertex distance. In cases of astigmatism, the equivalent sphere is usually chosen. It is recommended that for astigmatism of 0.75 D or more a toric lens design is considered (see Chapter 12), although some patients with astigmatism of up to 1.00 D may do well with a spherical lens design.

Back optic zone radius (BOZR)

The BOZR of soft lenses can be custom-made from approximately 7.00 to 9.50 mm but is generally available in a limited range from 8.3 to 9.2 mm.

When more than one BOZR is available for a given lens type, manufacturers will provide a fitting guide to indicate which BOZR to try first. These fitting guides usually make recommendations based on central keratometry readings, which, as explained previously, is not appropriate for most soft lens fitting, and variations in fit are frequently unrelated to large variations in BOZR (Lowther & Tomlinson 1981, Young 1992b, Young et al. 1993). Despite this, central keratometry readings remain the primary method used to choose the BOZR, if more than one BOZR is available.

For most conventional polyHEMA-based materials, a suitable BOZR will be 0.7–1.0 mm flatter than the flattest keratometry reading. However, a more appropriate choice for most patients would be to insert the lens with the middle base curve (if three options are available) or the flatter base curve (if two are available) and assess the fit of that lens, choosing to fit flatter or steeper based upon the fit of the first lens.

For silicone hydrogel lenses this theory does not hold true as their increased rigidity means that typically a lens with a steeper base curve will provide a more comfortable fit, with fewer mechanical complications (Dumbleton et al. 2002, Dumbleton 2003, Sweeney et al. 2004). In the case of silicone hydrogel lenses it is suggested that the initial BOZR should be the steepest available, with a flatter lens chosen if that lens appears to show insufficient movement.

Total diameter (TD)

The lens diameter must allow full corneal coverage in all directions of gaze. Soft lens TDs generally range from 13.8 to 14.5 mm, although larger and smaller diameters are available.

Choosing a trial lens based upon diameter may not be very valuable, since most lenses are temperature sensitive and become slightly smaller on the eye. Differences in materials and water content therefore restrict comparison between labelled lens diameters. In most cases the lens diameter is chosen according to availability of the diameter for the lens material and frequency of replacement required.

Thickness (centre and edge)

Central thickness (*ct*) for negatively powered soft lenses ranges from 0.035 to 0.15 mm and may be more than 0.35 mm for positively powered lenses.

High water content lenses are thicker than low water content lenses due to problems of dehydration and associated corneal staining that occur when high water content lenses are made too thin (Holden et al. 1986, Orsborn & Zantos 1988).

Spherical soft lenses are divided according to centre thickness:

- <0.06 mm are termed 'ultra-thin'.
- 0.06– 0.10 mm are termed 'thin'.
- >0.10–0.15 mm are termed 'standard'.

Lens thickness has implications for ocular physiology, with thick lenses transmitting less oxygen than thin lenses of identical water content (see Oxygen permeability and transmissibility, p. 225). While *ct* can influence lens fit, edge thickness appears to have relatively little impact on lens movement or comfort (Young et al. 1993, Young 1996) except for very high minus prescriptions.

Lens rigidity

This describes the 'stiffness' of lens materials as it relates to the modulus of elasticity of the material. Silicone hydrogel materials are considerably stiffer than conventional soft materials which can affect their fitting characteristics and ability to drape over the cornea (see Table 10.2) (Dumbleton et al. 2002).

Tint

Many soft lenses incorporate a handling tint, which can be helpful for lens location in the contact lens case. Cosmetic or colour-enhancing tints may appeal to some patients and, where a radical change in iris colour is required, opaque tints are used (see Chapter 25).

CHARACTERISTICS OF A WELL-FITTING LENS

The major objectives for any successful soft lens fit should be to provide:

- Good, stable vision (ideally comparable with spectacle acuity).
- Sufficient movement to allow 'flushing' of any debris from under the lens.
- Constant corneal coverage in all directions of gaze.
- No impingement of the limbal vasculature.
- Adequate comfort to allow a wearing time consistent (where possible) with the patient's requirements.

The measurements and observations of lens fit described below should not be considered in isolation. The characteristics of

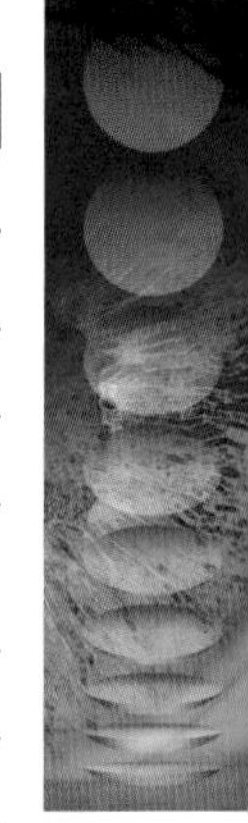

Table 10.5: Fitting characteristics of soft contact lenses

Characteristic	Optimal fit	Steep fit	Flat fit
Comfort	Good	Good initially	Poor
Vision	Good	Variable; may improve on blinking	Variable; often worse after a blink
Centration	Good	Often good	Poor
Corneal coverage	Complete in all directions of gaze	Often good	Poor, particularly on peripheral gaze
Edge alignment	Good	Conjunctival indentation	Edge stand-off or 'fluting'
Movement on blinking	0.25–0.50 mm	<0.2 mm	>0.8 mm
Movement on upgaze	<1.0 mm	<0.3 mm	>1.5 mm
Push up test	Easily moved; good recentration	Difficult to move; slow recentration	Easily moved; poor recentration
Retinoscopy reflex	Clear before and after blinking	Poor quality and distorted; marginally better after blinking	Variable; may be better just before blinking
Keratometer mires	Sharp before and after blinking	Poor quality and distorted; marginally better after blinking	Variable; may be better just before blinking

optimal, tight and loose lens fits are summarized in Table 10.5. A well-fitting lens should be associated with minimal physiological response over both the short and long term.

ASSESSMENT OF LENS FIT

After lens insertion, check the fit immediately. If the lenses are only slightly loose and fully cover the cornea, then allow them to settle for about 20–30 minutes. Lenses tighten and shrink following insertion, particularly during the first 5 minutes, showing approximately 20% reduction in lens movement (Martin & Holden 1983, Golding et al. 1995), which reaches equilibrium about 20 minutes after insertion (Brennan et al. 1992, Golding et al. 1995).

The reason for this reduction in lens movement remains under debate. Historically, it was assumed to be due to steepening of the lens, either from on-eye dehydration (Janoff 1982) or osmotically driven loss of water from the lens into the tears (Lovsund et al. 1980, Diefenbach et al. 1988).

Golding et al. (1995) questioned these theories and there is increasing evidence that, as the lens settles on the eye, the tear film between the cornea and the lens is gradually 'squeezed out' by blinking, resulting in thinning of the tear film, reduced lubrication and a subsequent reduction in lens movement (Bruce & Brennan 1988, 1992, Little & Bruce 1994a,b, Golding et al. 1995).

Judging the overall lens fit involves evaluating both static and dynamic criteria (Young 1998).

Centration and corneal coverage

Lens centration and corneal coverage are assessed using a slit-lamp biomicroscope employing diffuse illumination and low magnification. For record-keeping purposes:

- Centration can be measured using a slit-lamp graticule within the eyepiece or a slit of known width or length.
- Centration is recorded as half the difference between the distance of the lens edge from the limbal position in both the 180° and 90° meridians (Young et al. 1993).
- Plus values are assigned for nasal and superior decentration and minus values for temporal and inferior decentration.

Soft lenses should be centred on the cornea with an overlap of 1–2 mm in all meridians in primary gaze, and decentre only minimally on peripheral gaze (Fig. 10.8). Small amounts of decentration in the primary position are acceptable and most soft lenses show a small amount of inferior temporal decentration (Young et al. 1993).

If there is any corneal exposure on blinking or eye excursions, or if the lenses centre poorly, they should be replaced with lenses of a larger diameter or steeper BOZR. However, a lens that is very large may be difficult to insert and prove to be uncomfortable.

Lens movement

Adequate movement is required to remove trapped debris from underneath the lens in order to prevent inflammatory and infective complications (Mertz & Holden 1981, Zantos 1984, Cheng et al. 1999). It also provides freshly oxygenated tears to the cornea, assisting with corneal oxygenation.

With soft lenses, the movement is less than that seen with rigid lenses, resulting in only 1–2% of the tears under the lens being exchanged with each blink, while rigid lenses exchange some ten times this value (Polse 1979, 1981, Wagner et al. 1980, Veys & Davies 1995). Thus, increased oxygenation to the cornea via a tear pumping mechanism is negligible with soft lenses, but can be a significant factor with rigid lenses (Fink et al. 1990a,b, 1991).

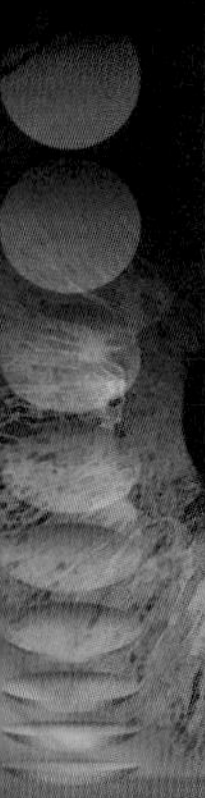

Figure 10.8 Lens centration for 'steep', 'optimal' and 'loose' lens fits

Gaze position	Tight fit	Optimal fit	Loose fit
Primary gaze			
Superior gaze			
Lateral gaze			

Direct focal illumination with a wide illuminating beam (0.5–2.0 mm) is used to assess lens movement in primary and superior gaze, and a graticule or vertical slit of known length is used to measure it.

With the eye in primary gaze, the patient should blink and the lens movement measured from a chosen reference point on the inferior conjunctiva. Movement in superior gaze is measured in a similar manner, with the patient looking up approximately 30° and then blinking. If the lower lid covers the inferior edge of the lens in primary gaze, a position slightly nasally or temporally may be used.

With earlier generations of soft lenses, 1.0 mm of movement on blink was advised (Kame 1979, Lowther 1982). With modern lenses the ideal movement in primary gaze should be 0.25–0.50 mm although it is easy to overestimate lens movement when looking with a slit-lamp (Martin et al. 1989, Young et al. 1993, Little & Bruce 1994b, Veys & Davies 1995, Le et al. 1996, Maldonado-Codina & Efron 2004). This is demonstrated in Figure 10.9, which shows an eye with a 1 mm and a 0.3 mm bar superimposed on the lens. If a lens with a TD of 14.00 mm were to truly move 1 mm on a 12.0 mm cornea, then the edge of the lens would cross the limbus with each blink (Young 1992c).

Lens movement with silicone hydrogels is greater than with conventional thin soft lenses, averaging 0.3–0.6 mm in the primary and superior gaze positions due to the increased modulus or stiffness of the materials (Tighe 2004).

Lenses worn overnight move little on eye opening, possibly due to transient hypotonicity of the tears creating an osmotic gradient that temporarily adheres the lens to the cornea (Begley et al. 1993). Hydrogel lenses worn overnight were fitted loose in an attempt to improve tear flushing and minimize lens binding on eye opening. However, if silicone hydrogel lenses are fitted flat, they may cause reduced comfort and clinical complications such as localized papillary conjunctivitis, superior epithelial arcuate lesions (SEALs) and corneal erosions (Dumbleton et al. 2001, Dumbleton 2003, Sweeney et al. 2004). Better clinical success may be obtained with silicone hydrogel lenses with BOZR slightly steeper than those fitted with hydrogel lenses (Dumbleton et al. 2002).

Back vertex power and back surface design also play a role in lens movement, although water content appears not to affect lens movement (Brennan et al. 1994). Plus lenses move more than minus lenses (Cedarstaff et al. 1983, Young et al. 1993), and back surface design can be manipulated to enhance lens movement (Young et al. 1993).

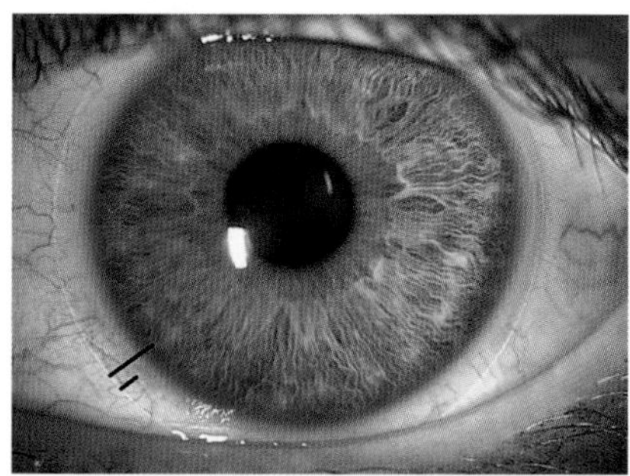

Figure 10.9 A well-centred lens with good corneal coverage. The two superimposed bars are of 1 mm and 0.3 mm in length. Optimal movement for soft lenses is 0.25–0.60 mm dependent on lens type. Movement in excess of this would result in exposure of the limbus on blinking

Tightness

The tightness of lenses is assessed with a push up test (Young 1992c, Young et al. 1993). The lens is gently dislodged upwards by digital manipulation of the lower lid against the lower edge of the lens and then released (Fig. 10.10). This assessment, which has been shown to be the most accurate single test of lens fit (Young 1992a, 1996), will determine both tight and loose fits, and is recommended for use in all soft lens fitting assessments.

When measuring both resistance to decentration and the recentration movement:

- 0% represents the lens being held by lid tension only (very loose) which drops rapidly on release.
- 100% represents a lens which is almost impossible to dislodge (very tight) and does not recentre.
- 50% is optimal although 40–60% is acceptable.

To loosen a tight lens, flatten the BOZR or reduce the TD; to tighten a loose lens, steepen the BOZR or increase the TD.

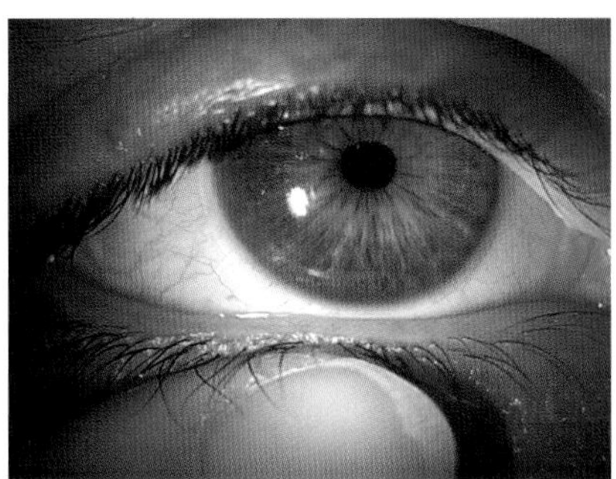

Figure 10.10 The 'push up' technique used to assess soft lens tightness

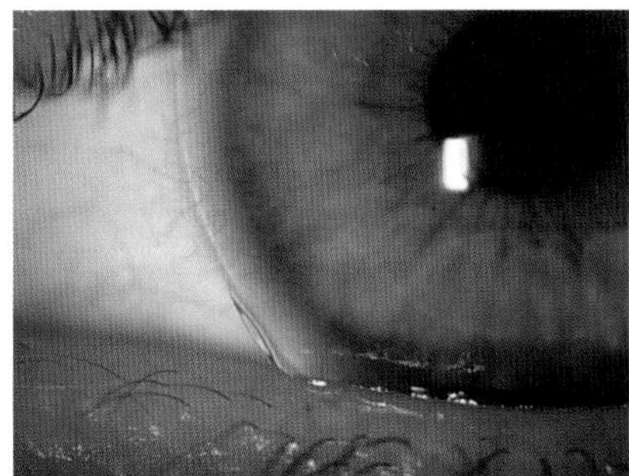

Figure 10.11 Edge fluting seen in a loose-fitting silicone hydrogel contact lens

Lens alignment

Direct focal illumination with a wide illuminating beam (0.5–2.0 mm) can be used to assess alignment of the lens in the peripheral cornea. A well-fitting lens should not produce any conjunctival indentation, crimping of conjunctival blood vessels or edge stand-off. The stiffer silicone hydrogel lenses require more critical lens-to-cornea alignment for comfortable fitting (Tighe 2004).

Buckling or 'fluting' of the lens edge due to excessive edge lift (Fig. 10.11) is observed more often with silicone hydrogel lenses than conventional soft lenses (Dumbleton et al. 2002, Sweeney et al. 2004). This may occur constantly or intermittently and is best detected by observing the lens edge moving over the temporal limbal area near the lower lid. It usually causes a foreign-body-like discomfort to the patient and, in extreme cases, the lens will ride onto the lower lid margin causing a varying degree of discomfort. Unfortunately, fluting does not reduce with time and an alternative base curve or design must be fitted (Dumbleton et al. 2002).

Bubbles under a soft lens:

- In the optic zone, indicate a steep central fit requiring a flatter BOZR.
- In the peripheral region, indicate poor alignment requiring a tighter lens.

Bubbles appearing under the periphery of stiffer silicone hydrogel lenses may be transient and should not be considered problematic (Fig. 10.12).

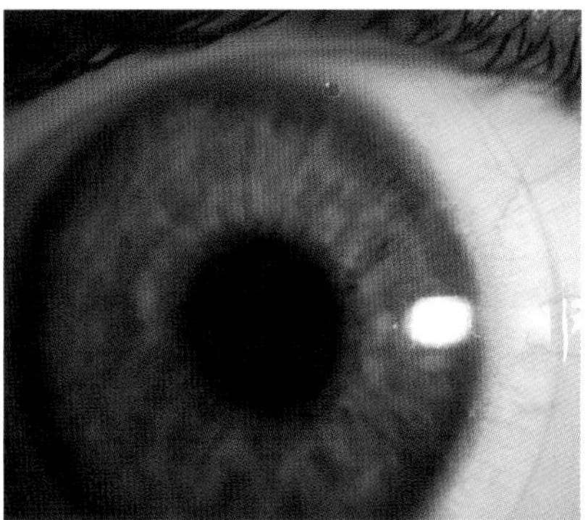

Figure 10.12 Transient appearance of a bubble under a silicone hydrogel contact lens

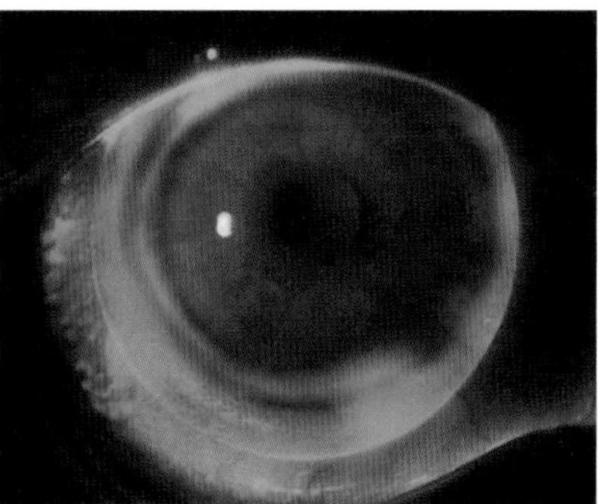

Figure 10.13 Assessment of a loose-fitting silicone hydrogel lens using high-molecular-weight fluorescein (Fluorexon)

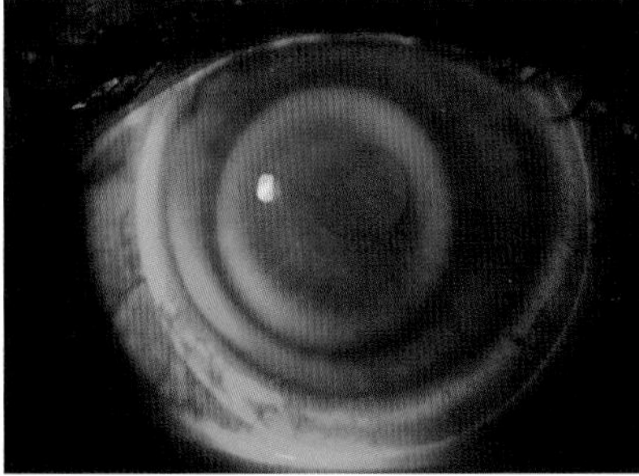

Figure 10.14 Assessment of silicone hydrogel lens fit using high-molecular-weight fluorescein (Fluorexon) with an inverted lens

The use of fluorescein in assessing lens fit

High-molecular-weight fluorescein dye (e.g. Fluorexon; see Chapter 5) may be used to assess the static and dynamic lens-fitting characteristics of soft lenses (Figs 10.13, 10.14) (Dumbleton et al. 2002). A cobalt blue excitation filter and yellow enhancement filter, placed in the illumination and observation systems, respectively, will improve the contrast. For optimal visibility, the dye should be instilled on the back surface of the contact lens before insertion. Minimal dosage is important because the dye can irritate, resulting in excessive tearing which alters the fit of the lens. Conventional fluorescein should be avoided as it will discolour the lens.

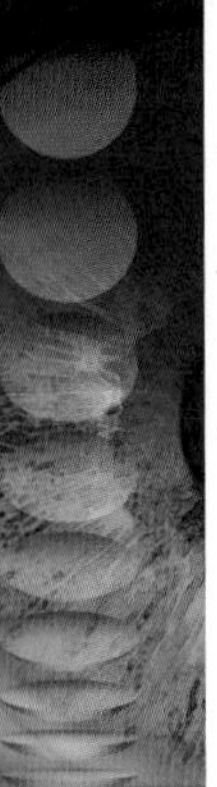

Table 10.6: Remedies to optimize fit of soft contact lenses

	Variation from 'optimal' requirement	Possible cause	Remedy
Comfort	Continual discomfort	Foreign body (FB) Thick lens	Remove lens, clean and reinsert Refit with thinner lens
	Discomfort on blinking	Loose lens Edge standoff	Refit with tighter lens Change design Refit with steeper base curve Refit into lens with lower modulus
Vision	Blurred vision	Incorrect power Uncorrected astigmatism	Over-refract and adjust BVP Refit with toric lens
	Variable vision after blinking	Loose lens	Tighten lens
	Variable vision before blinking	Steep lens	Flatten BOZR
	Variable over-refraction	Loose lens	Tighten lens
Centration	Greater than 2 mm overlap at limbus	Lens too large	Refit with smaller diameter
	Corneal exposure	Lens too small Lens too flat	Refit with larger diameter Refit with steeper BOZR
Edge alignment	Edge stand-off or 'fluting'	Modulus too high Lens too flat	Refit with lens with lower modulus Refit with steeper BOZR
	Conjunctival indentation	Lens too tight	Refit with looser lens
Movement on blinking	<0.25 mm	Lens too tight	Refit with looser lens
	>0.50 mm	Lens too loose Excessive lacrimation	Refit with tighter lens Check for FB or split in lens
Push up test	Resistance to movement	Tight lens	Refit with looser lens
	Excessive movement/erratic recovery	Lens too loose Excessive lacrimation	Refit with tighter lens Check for FB or split in lens

Adapted from Veys & Davies (1995).

Vision

- Visual acuity is measured using Snellen or LogMAR charts.
- Assessment is generally made using high-contrast charts only, but low-contrast measurements may be valuable.
- A binocularly balanced best sphere and spherocylindrical over-refraction should be performed, and the vision should be clear and stable.
- The combination of trial lens power and the best sphere over-refraction should be very close to the predicted final lens power.
- Patients may notice initial differences in their peripheral vision and in image size.
- Poorly fitting lenses can result in reduced visual acuity and fluctuations in vision.
- A retinoscopic reflex or mire appearance from keratometry performed over the lens surface can be helpful in evaluating visual problems relating to lens fit (see Table 10.5).

Comfort

Patients may notice mild discomfort initially on lens insertion due to differences between the pH of the packaging solution and their tears. Once settled, lenses should be comfortable with blinking and eye movement. If not, the lenses should be slid onto the sclera and then recentred. If still uncomfortable, remove the lens and examine for small nicks or tears, debris beneath the lens or whether the lens has been inserted inside out. Thicker toric lenses may take longer to become comfortable.

Final lens design

If the diagnostic lenses do not fit well, the lens fit can be altered by varying a number of parameters (Table 10.6). Different designs of lens should be tried until an optimal fit is obtained, then the final lens can be ordered or, more commonly, dispensed to the patient from the practitioner's stock lenses.

WEARING SCHEDULE AND ADAPTATION

Patients should be given clear instructions, both verbally and in writing, regarding their contact lens wear and care. Patient management and instruction are described in detail in Chapter 11; however, the most important points are summarized here.

Adaptation

Historically, patients were advised to build up their wearing time gradually from an initial period of 4 hours to the full wearing time over a 1- to 2-week period. With new lens materials and designs, this is considered unnecessary and many patients are advised to commence wear of up to 8–10 hours immediately, as long as the lenses feel comfortable. A follow-up examination is recommended before the wearing time is increased further, particularly if the lenses are to be worn on an extended- or continuous-wear basis (see Chapter 14).

Lens care and handling

Patients must be able to demonstrate effective handling techniques before they are allowed to leave the premises wearing soft contact lenses. The importance of cleaning lenses daily (with the exception of daily disposables) and the distinction between cleaning and disinfection must be explained. Recommended replacement frequency and importance of regular case replacement should be stressed.

Expectations

Comfort and vision with soft lenses should remain good throughout the wearing time until replacement is recommended.

Information and advice given to patients should include:

- Contacting the practitioner if they experience any unusual ocular redness, discomfort or visual disturbance.
- Appropriate cleaning and disinfection regime, together with instructions for use.
- Avoiding environments containing fumes, chemicals or sprays.
- Taking care with creams applied to the hands and face.
- Not using topical ocular treatments without first discussing these with the practitioner.
- If they are wearing disposable lenses, how often to insert a new pair of lenses and how many pairs they will receive at one time.
- The date of their first after-care appointment (see also Chapter 17) when they should:
  - bring both their lens case and spectacles with them.
  - arrive having worn the lenses for as long as possible on that particular day.

ABERRATION-CONTROLLED LENSES

Aberration of the eye acts to introduce additional blur into both in-focus and out-of-focus images (see Chapter 6). It is commonly expressed in terms of the wavefront aberration. If there are aberrations in the system, the image rays fail to intersect at a single image point and similarly the wavefronts, which are perpendicular to the rays, are not spherical.

The perfect optical system would have rays radiating from an object point and then converging at the image point. Standard contact lens designs focus on the correction of sphero-cylindrical errors but these corrections are accompanied by a significant increase in higher-order optical aberrations, such as coma and spherical aberration.

Higher-order aberrations of the eye are not constant and vary with factors such as increasing age. The manipulation of these aberrations is now the goal of some new aspheric designs called aberration-controlled lenses. These are targeted especially at either correcting low degrees of astigmatism or in the design of multifocal lenses but they may also prove useful in correcting failed refractive surgery patients.

Positive lenses exhibit positive longitudinal spherical aberration while negative lenses exhibit negative longitudinal spherical aberration. When considering straightforward aberration-blocking contact lenses (as they are often called), it is important to remember that a standard rigid lens may cancel the eye aberration and an aberration-controlled lens may actually *enhance* the difference (Douthwaite 2006). It is therefore vital to understand the underlying optics in order to use the manipulation of aberrations appropriately. This is done with aspheric multifocal rigid and soft lenses.

In the astigmat, correcting the spherical aberration in the lens/eye system has been shown to produce a better visual performance due to the reduction in size of the total blur circle even though the eye remains astigmatic (Charman & Chateau 2003). The visual performance will depend on the optical characteristics of a particular lens design interacting with the aberrations of the particular eye. Consequently, variations in ocular aberrations between individuals will mean that certain aberration-controlled designs will work for some patients and not for others.

Many companies now produce aberration-controlled lenses in both soft and rigid materials. Examples of soft lenses include Bausch & Lomb's PureVision and Ciba Vision's Night & Day.

Acknowledgements

The authors would like to acknowledge Andrew Gasson and Martin Lloyd, who wrote the chapter on soft lens fitting in the fourth edition of *Contact Lenses*, some of the text of which has been used in this chapter.

References

Alvord, L., Court, J., Davis, T. et al. (1998) Oxygen permeability of a new type of high Dk soft contact lens material. Optom. Vis. Sci., 75(1), 30–36

Begley, C., Metzger-Romatz, M., Simmons, D. and Lecher, C. (1993) The movement of soft contact lenses following eye closure. Optom. Vis. Sci., 70(12s), 123

Bergenske, P. (1990) The winning combination: disposable lenses for daily wear. Contact Lens Spectrum, 5(6), 72–74

Binder, P. S. (1979) Complications associated with extended wear of soft contact lenses. Ophthalmology, 86(6), 1093–1101

Brennan, N. and Efron, N. (1987) Strategies for increasing the oxygen performance of hydrogel contact lenses. Contax, July, 12–18

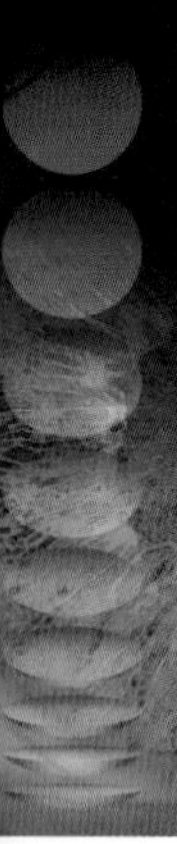

Brennan, N. A., Efron, N., Holden, B.A. et al. (1987) A review of the theoretical concepts, measurement systems and application of contact lens oxygen permeability. Ophthalmic Physiol. Opt., 7(4), 485–490

Brennan, N., McCraw, K., Young, L. et al. (1992) Soft lens movement. Optom. Vis. Sci., 69(12s), 24–25

Brennan, N. A., Lindsay, R. G., McCraw, K. et al. (1994) Soft lens movement: temporal characteristics. Optom. Vis. Sci., 71(6), 359–363

Bruce, A. (1994) Influence of corneal topography on centration and movement of low water content soft contact lenses. Int. Contact Lens Clin., 21(3/4), 45–49

Bruce, A. and Brennan, N. (1988) Clinical observations of the post-lens tear film during the first hour of hydrogel lens wear. Int. Contact Lens Clin., 15(10), 304–310

Bruce, A. and Brennan, N. (1992) Hydrogel lens binding and the post-lens tear film. Clin. Eye Vis. Care, 4(3), 111–116

Cedarstaff, T. H., Tomlinson, A. and Bibby, M. (1983) Validation of a model describing soft lens movement as a function of lens specification. Am. J. Optom. Physiol. Opt., 60(4), 292–296

Charman, W. N. and Chateau, N. (2003) The prospects for super-acuity: limits to visual performance after correction of monochromatic ocular aberration. Ophthalmic Physiol. Opt., 23(6), 479–493

Cheng, K. H., Leung, S. L., Hoekman, H. W. et al. (1999) Incidence of contact-lens-associated microbial keratitis and its related morbidity. Lancet, 354(9174), 181–185

Cutler, S. I., Nelson, L. B., Calhoun, J. H. et al. (1985) Extended wear contact lenses in pediatric aphakia. J. Pediatr. Ophthalmol. Strabismus, 22(3), 86–91

Dahl, A. A. and Brocks, E. R. (1978) The use of continuous-wear silicone contact lenses in the optical correction of aphakia. Am. J. Ophthalmol., 85(4), 454–461

Davies, I. (1992) The manufacture of soft contact lenses. Contact Lens J., 20(2), 16–21

Diefenbach, C. B., Soni, P. S., Gillespie, B. J. et al. (1988) Extended wear contact lens movement under swimming pool conditions. Am. J. Optom. Physiol. Opt., 65(9), 710–716

Donshik, P., Weinstock, F. J., Wechsler, S. et al. (1988) Disposable hydrogel contact lenses for extended wear. CLAO J., 14(4), 191–194

Doughman, D. J. and Massare, J. S. (1996) Defining contact lens terminology. CLAO J., 22(4), 228–229

Douthwaite, W. A. (2006) Contact Lens Optics and Lens Design (3rd edn). Oxford: Butterworth-Heinemann, Elsevier

Dumbleton, K. (2003) Noninflammatory silicone hydrogel contact lens complications. Eye Contact Lens, 29(1 Suppl), S186–189, discussion S90–91, S92–94

Dumbleton, K., Chalmers, R., Bayer, S., Fonn, D. and McNally, J. (2001) Lens base curve and subjective comfort with silicone hydrogel continuous wear lenses. Optom. Vis. Sci., 78(12s), 227

Dumbleton, K. A., Chalmers, R. L., McNally, J. et al. (2002) Effect of lens base curve on subjective comfort and assessment of fit with silicone hydrogel continuous wear contact lenses. Optom. Vis. Sci., 79(10), 633–637

Efron, N. and Brennan, N. (1987) How much oxygen? In search of the critical oxygen requirement of the cornea. Contax, July, 5–18

Efron, N. and Pearson, R. M. (1988) Centenary celebration of Fick's Eine Contactbrille. Arch. Ophthalmol., 106(10), 1370–1377

Efron, N., Brennan, N. A., Currie, J. M. et al. (1986) Determinants of the initial comfort of hydrogel contact lenses. Am. J. Optom. Physiol. Opt., 63(10), 819–823

Fatt, I. (1979) The definition of thickness for a lens. Am. J. Optom. Physiol. Opt., 56(5), 324–337

Fatt, I. (1986) Now do we need 'effective permeability'? Contax, July, 6–23

Fatt, I. (1995) Oxygen transmission. In Contact Lenses – The CLAO Guide to Basic Science and Clinical Practice, pp. 113–183, ed. P. Kastl. Dubuque, Iowa: Kendall/Hunt Publishing

Fink, B. A., Carney, L. G., Hill, R.M. et al. (1990a) Influence of palpebral aperture height on tear pump efficiency. Optom. Vis. Sci., 67(4), 287–290

Fink, B. A., Hill, R. M., Carney, L. G. et al. (1990b) Influence of rigid contact lens overall and optic zone diameters on tear pump efficiency. Optom. Vis. Sci., 67(8), 641–644

Fink, B., Carney, L., Hill, R. M. et al. (1991) Rigid lens tear pump efficiency: effects of overall diameter/base curve combinations. Optom. Vis. Sci., 68(4), 309–313

Garner, L. F. (1982) Sagittal height of the anterior eye and contact lens fitting. Am. J. Optom. Physiol. Opt., 59(4), 301–305

Gellatly, K. W. (1993) Disposable contact lenses: a clinical performance review. Can. J. Optom., 55(3), 166–172

Gellatly, K. W., Brennan, N. A., Efron, N. (1988) Visual decrement with deposit accumulation of HEMA contact lenses. Am. J. Optom. Physiol. Opt., 65(12), 937–941

Golding, T. R., Harris, M. G., Smith, R. C. et al. (1995) Soft lens movement: effects of humidity and hypertonic saline on lens settling. Acta Ophthalmol. Scand., 73(2), 139–144

Grant, T. and Holden, B. (1988) The clinical performance of disposable (58%) extended wear lenses. Trans BCLA Conference, 63–64

Grobe, G. L. 3rd. (1999) Surface engineering aspects of silicone-hydrogel lenses. Contact Lens Spectrum, 14(8 Suppl), 14–17

Grobe, G., Kunzler, J., Seelye, D. et al. (1999) Silicone hydrogels for contact lens applications. Polymeric Materials Science and Engineering, 80, 108–109

Gruber, E. (1989) The best reasons to include disposable contact lenses in your practice. Spectrum, 4(12), 31–36

Gurland, J. E. (1979) Use of silicone lenses in infants and children. Ophthalmology, 86(9), 1599–1604

Hamano, H., Watanabe, K., Hamano, T. et al. (1994) A study of the complications induced by conventional and disposable contact lenses. CLAO J., 20(2), 103–108

Hassman, G. and Sugar, J. (1983) Pseudomonas corneal ulcer with extended-wear soft contact lenses for myopia. Arch. Ophthalmol., 101, 1549–1550

Holden, B., Sweeney, D. and Seger, R. G. (1986) Epithelial erosions caused by thin high water content lenses. Clin. Exp. Optom., 69(3), 103–107

Huth, S. and Wagner, H. (1981) Identification and removal of deposits on polydimethylsiloxane silicone elastomer lenses. Int. Contact Lens Clin., 8(7/8), 19–26

Ivins, P. (1988) Early impressions of a disposable system. Optician, 195(5147), 27–35

Janoff, L. E. (1982) The consequence of temperature change on hydrophilic lens base curve in gels of varying water content. Int. Contact Lens Clin., 9(10), 228–232

Jones, L. (1988) The use of high water content lenses on a daily wear basis. J. Br. Contact Lens Assoc., Scientific Meetings, 26–31

Jones, L. (1990a) Daily wear high water content lenses. Optician, 199(5235), 17–23

Jones, L. (1990b) Daily wear high water content lenses (part 2). Optician, 199(5240), 15–23

Jones, L. (1990c) Daily wear high water content lenses (part 3). Optician, 199(5245), 31–39

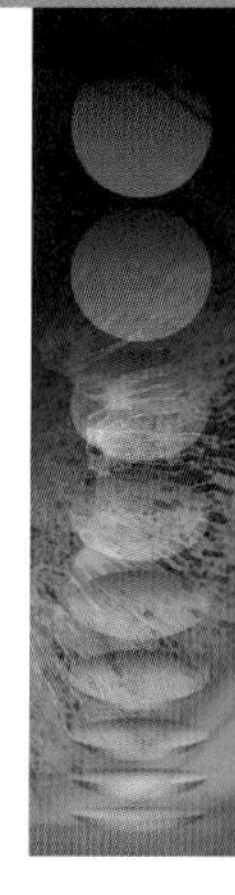

Jones, L. (1994) Disposable contact lenses: a review. J. Br. Contact Lens Assoc., 17(2), 43–49

Jones, L. (2002) Modern contact lens materials: a clinical performance update. Contact Lens Spectrum, 17(9), 24–35

Jones, L. and Dumbleton, K. (2004) Silicone hydrogels: will they displace conventional lenses? Optom. Today, Aug 20, 34–41

Jones, L., Franklin, V., Evans, K. et al. (1996) Spoilation and clinical performance of monthly vs three monthly group II disposable contact lenses. Optom. Vis. Sci., 73(1), 16–21

Jones, L., Mann, A., Evans, K. et al. (2000) An in vivo comparison of the kinetics of protein and lipid deposition on group II and group IV frequent-replacement contact lenses. Optom. Vis. Sci., 77(10), 503–510

Kame, R. (1979) Basic considerations in fitting hydrogel lenses. J. Am. Optom. Assoc., 50(3), 295–298

Kame, R., Farkas, B., Meltor, J. W. et al. (1994) Are your patients ready for daily disposables? Contact Lens Spectrum, 9(9), 26–31

Kaye, D., Hayashi, M., Schenkei, J. B. et al. (1988) A disposable contact lens program: a preliminary report. CLAO J., 14(1), 33–37

Keith, D. J., Christensen, M. T., Barry, J. R. et al. (2003) Determination of the lysozyme deposit curve in soft contact lenses. Eye Contact Lens, 29(2), 79–82

Kerr, C. and Meyler, J. (2001) The ISO system of contact lens materials classification. In The ACLM Contact Lens Year Book, pp. 7–8, eds. C. Kerr and J. Meyler. ACLM. Online. Available: www.aclm.org.uk/practitioner/ybol/index.php

Krasnow, D. (1989) Problem solving with the Acuvue disposable contact lens. CL Forum, 8, 41–44

Kunzler, J. (1999) Silicone-based hydrogels for contact lens applications. Contact Lens Spectrum, 14(8 Suppl), 9–11

Lane, I. (1990) Disposables increase patient compliance and referrals. Contact Lens Forum, 15(12), 32–36

Larke, J. and Hirji, N. (1979) Some clinically observed phenomena in extended contact lens wear. Br. J. Ophthalmol., 63, 475–477

Le, A., Liem, S., Su, J. L. et al. (1996) Fitting characteristics of 1-day and 14-day Acuvue disposable contact lenses. Optom. Vis. Sci., 73(12), 750–753

Lebow, K. and Plishka, K. (1980) Ocular changes associated with extended wear contact lenses. Int. Contact Lens Clin., 7, 49–55

Little, S. and Bruce, A. S. (1994a) Postlens tear film morphology, lens movement and symptoms in hydrogel lens wearers. Ophthalmic Physiol. Opt., 14(1), 65–69

Little, S. A. and Bruce, A. S. (1994b) Hydrogel (Acuvue) lens movement is influenced by the postlens tear film. Optom. Vis. Sci., 71(6), 364–370

Lopez-Alemany, A., Compan, V. and Refojo, M. F. (2002) Porous structure of Purevision versus Focus Night & Day and conventional hydrogel contact lenses. J. Biomed. Mater. Res. (Appl. Biomat.), 63, 319–325

Lovsund, P., Nilsson, S. E. and Oberg, P. A. (1980) The use of contact lenses in wet or damp environments. Acta Ophthalmol. (Copenh.), 58(5), 794–804

Lowther, G. (1982) In Contact Lenses: Procedures and Techniques, p. 148, London: Butterworths

Lowther, G. (1984) Truly disposable contact lenses: how close are we? Int. Contact Lens Clin., 11, 584

Lowther, G. E. and Tomlinson, A. (1981) Critical base curve and diameter interval in the fitting of spherical soft contact lenses. Am. J. Optom. Physiol. Opt., 58(5), 355–360

Maldonado-Codina, C. and Efron, N. (2004) Impact of manufacturing technology and material composition on the clinical performance of hydrogel lenses. Optom. Vis. Sci., 81(6), 442–454

Marshall, E., Begley, C. and Nguyen, C. (1992) Frequency of complications among wearers of disposable and conventional soft contact lenses. Int. Contact Lens Clin., 19(3/4), 55–59

Martin, D. K. and Holden, B. A. (1982) A new method for measuring the diameter of the in vivo human cornea. Am. J. Optom. Physiol. Opt., 59(5), 436–441

Martin, D. and Holden, B. (1983) Variations in tear fluid osmolality, chord diameter and movement during wear of high water content hydrogel contact lenses. Int. Contact Lens Clin., 10(6), 332–341

Martin, N. F., Kracher, G. P., Stark, W. J. and Maumenee, A. E. (1983) Extended-wear soft contact lenses for aphakic correction. Arch. Ophthalmol., 101(1), 39–41

Martin, D. K., Boulos, J., Gan, J. et al. (1989) A unifying parameter to describe the clinical mechanics of hydrogel contact lenses. Optom. Vis. Sci., 66(2), 87–91

McMonnies, C. (1997) The critical initial comfort of soft contact lenses. Clin. Exp. Optom., 80(2), 53–58

Mertz, G. (1997) Development of contact lenses. In Corneal Physiology and Disposable Contact Lenses, pp. 65–99, ed. H. Hamano. Edinburgh: Butterworth-Heinemann

Mertz, G. and Holden, B. (1981) Clinical implications of extended wear research. Can. J. Optom., 43(4), 203–205

Morgan, P., Efron, N., Woods, C. A. et al. (2004) International contact lens prescribing in 2003. Contact Lens Spectrum, 19(1), 34–37

Morrison, D. R. and Edelhauser, H. F. (1972) Permeability of hydrophilic contact lenses. Invest. Ophthalmol., 11(1), 58–63

Nason, R. J., Vogel, H., Tarbel, B. J. et al. (1993) A clinical evaluation of frequent replacement contact lenses on patients currently wearing premium reusable daily wear soft contact lenses. J. Am. Optom. Assoc., 64(3), 188–195

Nason, R. J., Boshnick, E. L., Cannon, W. M. et al. (1994) Multisite comparison of contact lens modalities. Daily disposable wear vs. conventional daily wear in successful contact lens wearers. J. Am. Optom. Assoc., 65(11), 774–780

Nicolson, P. C. (2003) Continuous wear contact lens surface chemistry and wearability. Eye Contact Lens, 29(1 Suppl), S30–32, discussion S57–59, S192–194

Nilsson, S. E. and Montan, P. G. (1994) The annualized incidence of contact lens induced keratitis in Sweden and its relation to lens type and wear schedule: results of a 3-month prospective study. CLAO J., 20(4), 225–230

Nicolson, P. C. and Vogt, J. (2001) Soft contact lens polymers: an evolution. Biomaterials, 22(24), 3273–3283

Orsborn, G. N. and Zantos, S. G. (1988) Corneal desiccation staining with thin high water content contact lenses. CLAO J., 14(2), 81–85

Pearson, R. M. and Efron, N. (1989) Hundredth anniversary of August Muller's inaugural dissertation on contact lenses. Surv. Ophthalmol., 34(2), 133–141

Peterson, J. F. and Fatt, I. (1973) Oxygen flow through a soft contact lens on a living eye. Am. J. Optom. Arch. Am. Acad. Optom., 50(2), 91–93

Poggio, E. C. and Abelson, M. (1993) Complications and symptoms in disposable extended wear lenses compared with conventional soft daily wear and soft extended wear lenses. CLAO J., 19(1), 31–39

Poggio, E. C., Glynn, R. J., Schein, O. D. et al. (1989) The incidence of ulcerative keratitis among users of daily-wear and extended-wear soft contact lenses. N. Engl. J. Med., 321(12), 779–783

Polse, K. A. (1979) Tear flow under hydrogel contact lenses. Invest. Ophthalmol. Vis. Sci., 18(4), 409–413

Polse, K. A. (1981) Factors controlling oxygen tension under a hydrogel contact lens. J. Am. Optom. Assoc., 52(3), 203–208

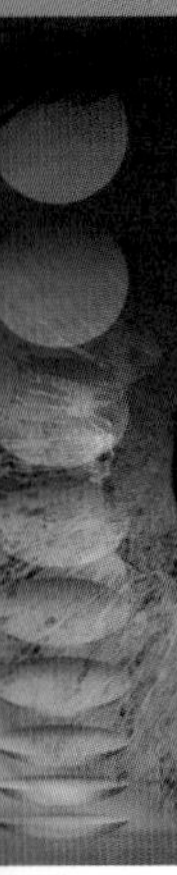

Rae, S. and Huff, J. (1991) Studies on initiation of silicone elastomer lens adhesion in vitro: binding before the indentation ring. CLAO J., 17(3), 181–186

Refojo, M. F. (1979) Mechanism of gas transport through contact lenses. J. Am. Optom. Assoc., 50(3), 285–287

Rogers, G. L. (1980) Extended wear silicone contact lenses in children with cataracts. Ophthalmology, 87(9), 867–870

Schein, O. D., Glynn, R. J., Poggio, E. C. et al. (1989) The relative risk of ulcerative keratitis among users of daily-wear and extended-wear soft contact lenses. A case-control study. Microbial Keratitis Study Group. N. Engl. J. Med., 321(12), 773–778

Schwartz, C. (1986) Contact lens update 1986. Contact Lens Forum, 11(1), 23

Smith, R. E. and MacRae, S. M. (1989) Contact lenses – convenience and complications. N. Engl. J. Med., 321(12), 824–826

Schein, O. D., Glynn, R. J., Poggio, E. C. et al. (1989) The relative risk of ulcerative keratitis among users of daily-wear and extended-wear soft contact lenses. A case-control study. Microbial Keratitis Study Group. N. Engl. J. Med., 321(12), 773–778

Steffen, R. and McCabe, K. (2004) Finding the comfort zone. Contact Lens Spectrum, 13(3), Suppl 1–4

Steffen, R. and Schnider, C. (2004) A next generation silicone hydrogel lens for daily wear. Part 1: Material properties. Optician, 227(5954), 23–25

Sweeney, D., du Toit, R., Keay, L. et al. (2004) Clinical performance of silicone hydrogel lenses. In Silicone Hydrogels: Continuous Wear Contact Lenses, pp. 164–216, ed. D. Sweeney. Edinburgh: Butterworth-Heinemann

Tighe, B. (2002) Soft lens materials. In Contact Lens Practice, pp. 71–84, ed. N. Efron. Edinburgh: Butterworth-Heinemann

Tighe, B. (2004) Silicone hydrogels: Structure, properties and behaviour. In Silicone Hydrogels: Continuous Wear Contact Lenses, pp. 1–27, ed. D. Sweeney. Edinburgh: Butterworth-Heinemann

Tripathi, R. C., Tripathi, B. J., and Ruben, M. (1980) The pathology of soft contact lens spoilage. Ophthalmology, 87(5), 365–380

Vangsted, P., Brincker, P., Prause, J. U. et al. (1986) Short term clinical trial of Danalens, a new disposable contact lens. Contactologia, 8(3), 129–132

Veys, J. and Davies, I. (1995) Soft contact lens fitting. Optician, 209(5504), 20–27

Wagner, L., Polse, K. and Mandell, R. (1980) Tear pumping and edema with soft contact lenses. Invest. Ophthalmol. Vis. Sci., 19(11), 1397–1400

Weissman, B. A., Mondino, B. J., Pettit, T. H. et al. (1984) Corneal ulcers associated with extended-wear soft contact lenses. Am. J. Ophthalmol., 97(4), 476–481

Wichterle, O. and Lim, D. (1960) Hydrophilic gels for biological use. Nature, 185, 117–118

Young, G. (1992a) How to fit soft contact lenses. J. Br. Contact Lens Assoc., 15(4), 179–180

Young, G. (1992b) Ocular sagittal height and soft contact lens fit. J. Br. Contact Lens Assoc., 15(1), 45–49

Young, G. (1992c) Soft lens fitting reassessed. Spectrum, 7(12), 56–61

Young, G. (1996) Evaluation of soft contact lens fitting characteristics. Optom. Vis. Sci., 73(4), 247–254

Young, G. (1997) Common contact lens misconceptions. Optician, 213(5587), 20–24

Young, G. (1998) Advanced soft CL fitting. Optician, 215(5654), 18–23

Young, G. and Coleman, S. (2001) Poorly fitting soft lenses affect ocular integrity. CLAO J., 27(2), 68–74

Young, G., Holden, B. and Cooke, G. (1993) Influence of soft contact lens design on clinical performance. Optom. Vis. Sci., 70(5), 394–403

Zantos, S. (1984) Ocular complications – corneal infiltrates, debris, and microcysts. J. Am. Optom. Assoc., 55(3), 196–198

Zantos, S. and Holden, B. (1978) Ocular changes associated with continuous wear of contact lenses. Aust. J. Optom., 61, 418–426

Chapter 11

Patient management

Kerry W. Atkinson

CHAPTER CONTENTS

INTRODUCTION

Patient management is a process of careful investigation before a patient starts to wear contact lenses. It is a means of informing, examining and selecting potential wearers, and anticipating or looking for possible causes that may prevent or modify successful contact lens wear. Patient management is also a procedure by which patients are re-examined at intervals and their wearing problems anticipated or dealt with. This includes a routine for regular after-care, dealing with emergencies and treating problems successfully.

Patient management is all the processes by which a non-contact lens wearer is changed into a successful lens wearer. It is necessary to:

- Establish patient suitability for wearing contact lenses.
- Record a set of baseline appearances of the anterior eye.
- Have a systematic approach to screening potential contact lens wearers to minimize unforeseen problems. Look for areas of potential difficulty and anticipate these with warnings to the patient of possible limitations of contact lens performance, or use special lenses or special techniques to overcome them.
- Establish a system of training, instruction and information for the future contact lens wearer.
- Have a system for dealing with potential, real or future emergencies and be able to diminish the risk by having systems in place to minimize adverse effects should an emergency occur.

Thorough examination and careful and comprehensive recording are absolute prerequisites.

Although contact lens wear is common (McMahon & Zadnik 2000), it is necessary to provide a background of accurate information to a prospective wearer in order to correct any misconceptions (Liesegang 2002, Holden et al. 2003).

Discussion should start with a consideration of what the patient wants from the lenses. There are also a series of 'frequently asked questions' that need answers.

Frequently asked questions

- Do they hurt?
- Is it difficult for me to put the lenses in?
- How long does it take to get used to them?
- Can I sleep in them?
- Will they fall out?
- Can I wear them in the shower, or in the rain?

- Can I swim in them?
- How much will they cost?
- Will they change the colour of my eye?

Comfort

SOFT LENSES

Once the lenses are on the eye there is little sensation from them. However, having the first lens put onto the eye by the practitioner can be stressful and may be uncomfortable. Getting a lens onto the eye reasonably quickly and holding the top lid up until it is correctly in place will make the first insertion as comfortable as possible.

RIGID LENSES

Rigid lenses hold their shape. Their total diameter is usually less than the corneal diameter, making them more liable to be dislodged and produce more sensation. Initial sensation can be reduced by directing the patient to look down to relax the top lid.

Corneal anaesthetics may help with initial lens insertion (Bennett et al. 1998a,b), especially with sensitive patients such as children or those with keratoconus, and can make assessment of lens fit easier. Corneal anaesthetics make the corneal epithelium more fragile and more likely to take up fluorescein. Assessment of the rigid lens fit may then be more difficult, and compromised corneal epithelium is more susceptible to infection.

The time taken to adapt to the lenses depends on:

- Lens material.
- Patient confidence.
- Practitioner confidence and experience.

Wearing schedules

Soft lens wearers should restrict their wearing time on the first day to about 8 hours and, after that, wear the lenses for as long as they are comfortable. Rigid lens wearers need more time: with a well-fitting lens they can start at 4–6 hours and add 2–3 hours daily. Slower adaptation may be needed for compromised corneas but if too extended may diminish the patient's confidence or motivation.

Retention

Soft lenses are flexible and larger than the cornea so they mould to the shape of the eye and stay on the eye for most activities. In body contact sports, rigid lenses can occasionally dislodge, although with soft lenses, fingers or other parts of an opponent can move a lens off-centre or wipe it from the eye. Fortunately, lens loss is fairly infrequent for the large majority of activities.

Sleeping in lenses

Sleeping in conventional hydrogel lenses is not recommended as the lenses may feel dry and uncomfortable on waking. During sleep the tear constituents are altered (Stapleton et al. 1998) and less watery tears are produced. Wearers may have to wait up to half an hour after waking before the lenses are mobile enough to be removed comfortably.

The risk of infection is significant when low water content lenses are regularly worn during sleep. Silicone hydrogel materials are much safer to sleep in although some people experience drying and need to instil lubricating eye-drops upon waking, especially during the early stages of lens wear (Sweeney et al. 2002). Rigid lenses may be less comfortable to sleep in and may also need lubricating.

Swimming

Swimming in clean seawater does not present a greater risk of lenses being lost or moving off-centre. However, it has been shown to increase the risk of infection with silicone hydrogel lenses (Willcox & Holden 2001), so it is safer to wear swimming goggles.

Swimming in pools, fresh water or in spa pools is not advisable as there is a small but real risk of *Acanthamoeba* keratitis (see Chapter 18). In addition, the hypotonic solution makes lenses fit more loosely and the risk of loss is increased. Swimming pool disinfectants are retained in soft lens material and can have toxic effects.

PRELIMINARY DIAGNOSTIC TESTING

Tests carried out prior to lens insertion can make a significant difference to their potential success. The following may all have an effect on successful contact lens wear:

- Degree of ametropia.
- Uncorrected astigmatism.
- Binocular vision.
- Existing pathology.
- Risks of unsafe patients.

Choice of lenses

Contact lenses are available to correct most degrees of ametropia. The choice of lens material and design depends upon the patient's:

- Motivating factor (e.g. cosmesis or sport).
- Prescription.
- Tear flow and quality.

Disposable soft contact lenses are the lens of choice in most soft contact fittings (Ehlers et al. 2003) because they:

- Provide better patient comfort, safety, and long-term eye health compared to conventional soft lenses (Dumbleton et al. 2001).
- Produce less giant papillary conjunctivitis (GPC), limbal blood-vessel extensions, chronic red eyes and minor infections.
- Are usually comfortable at first insertion and the patient is soon unaware of having a lens in the eye.

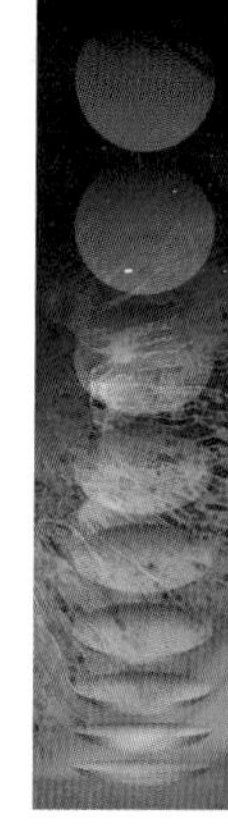

- Can be used for occasional wear or part-time wear if the lenses are uncomfortable towards the end of the day.
- Can be replaced quickly and easily if one is lost or damaged or if the vision alters.

There are relatively few patients for whom non-stock lenses are necessary – for example, those with high degrees of astigmatism or very high powers.

Rigid lenses are usually made to order, although some stock rigid lenses are available. They have many advantages (McMahon 2003), especially for fitting irregular corneas (Szczotka & Lindsay 2003). Rigid lenses can be used to alter the shape of the cornea, as in orthokeratology, but may also induce spectacle blur if they are poorly fitted. Those wearers who wish to have refractive surgery will need to be without lenses for at least 3 months prior to surgery or until they have attained a stable refraction. High-Dk soft lenses can be worn during that period.

ASTIGMATISM

Moderate astigmatism can be corrected using stock soft toric lenses but larger amounts may require custom-made toric lenses (either soft or rigid – see Chapter 12). Irregular astigmatism may indicate keratoconus, which will require a more careful fitting (see Chapter 20).

Where corneal and spectacle astigmatism differ, the practitioner must assess whether a compensated rigid toric lens or a non-stock toric soft lens would provide a better correction. Some patients (e.g. those with keratoconus) may need an astigmatic spectacle overcorrection if the astigmatism is not fully corrected by the contact lens.

BINOCULAR VISION

It is difficult to successfully incorporate horizontal prismatic correction into most contact lenses but small amounts of vertical prism can be corrected.

EXISTING PATHOLOGIES

The eyes should be examined carefully prior to lens fitting to check for pre-existing pathology (see Chapter 8). Where possible the condition should be treated before embarking on lens wear (see below).

DRY EYES (see also Chapters 5 and 18)

- Tear insufficiency is the most common problem of lens wearers and the most common reason for discontinuing lens wear.
- Causes include poor lid mechanics, insufficient tear volume and infrequent blinking.
- Careful consideration of these factors is vital (Foulks 2003, Glasson et al. 2003).
- Consider using:
  - a dry eye questionnaire (Nichols et al. 2002).
  - tear supplements.

CHRONIC LID PATHOLOGY (see also Chapters 8, 17 and 18)

- Most cases of blepharitis are recurring and, when active, increase the risk of corneal infection.
- Signs of blepharitis include red lid margins and flaky skin (see Fig. 18.10). The tear prism on the lower lid will have a scalloped or irregular appearance (Lemp 2003, McCulley & Shine 2003).

Treatment includes:

- Hot compresses and attention to lid margin hygiene.
- Baby shampoo or specially made solutions such as Lid Care (CIBA) or Supranettes (Alcon).

ALLERGIES AND PAPILLARY CONJUNCTIVITIS (see also Chapter 18)

Triggers for ocular allergies may be pollens or plant material, household dust or dust mites, animal fur or dander (particularly cats and horses) and some dietary allergies, which may sensitize people generally. Sufferers often have some idea what causes their allergies, but may need to be made aware of the linkage between their eye problems and their general allergies. Systemic antihistamines are not normally successful in treating ocular allergies.

- Eye allergies reduce the comfort of contact lenses as normal tear function is altered and ocular tissues swollen.
- During the active period (e.g. hay fever season), reduce or cease lens wear.
- Rigorous hygiene is essential.
- Daily disposable lenses can help.
- Mast cell stabilizers may be necessary.
- Steroid eye drops if severe.

LID EVERSION

The upper lid is more difficult to evert than the lower lid. Pull the lashes down and away from the eye while at the same time pushing behind the upper tarsal plate with a finger or cotton bud.

UNSAFE OR NON-COMPLIANT PATIENTS

Unsafe patients need to be identified as early as possible. Non-compliant patients place at risk their own eye health and also the reputation of the contact lens practitioner. Unsafe patients are those who will not listen to or follow instructions, and are not compliant with lens care. Wearers of coloured lenses, whose motivation is only to change their appearance and not to correct their vision, as a group are less likely to be compliant. Swapping lenses with others, and not discarding lenses as instructed, increase the likelihood of eye problems.

Unfortunately, many non-compliant patients are not detected until they have been wearing contact lenses for some time. A robust system of instruction and information may protect a contact lens practitioner from legal difficulties, but it may become necessary to refuse to supply more lenses to these patients.

PRELIMINARY EXAMINATION

The preliminary examination is the time to:

- Establish baseline appearances to provide a standard against which to measure subsequent changes.

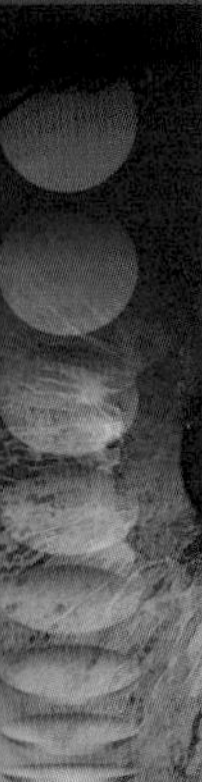

- Decide which lenses and lens materials will be most suitable for the patient and the most appropriate wearing schedule.
- Talk about the limitations of contact lenses (see also Chapter 32).
  Lens considerations could include:

- Rigid or soft lenses.
- The need for toric lenses.
- Ionic or non-ionic material.
- High or low water content material.
- The ease of handling, i.e. lens insertion and removal.
- The cost and availability of optimum lenses.
- Special types of lens.
- Extended wear versus daily wear.
- Special lens designs – for example, those appropriate for Asian eyes (Chui et al. 2000, Hamano et al. 2002).
- Replacement schemes.

Grading scales

Using grading scales and having the experience to define values in a consistent fashion is important. There are several grading scales available, the best known of which are those from the IER (see Appendix B and the CD-ROM accompanying this book) or the Efron grading scale (Efron 1998). Because these grading scales supply a consistent reference image (Efron et al. 2003a,b), they are better than word descriptions. Digital photography can also be used to grade, but its use is not widespread at present.

SLIT-LAMP EXAMINATION

A thorough examination of the cornea, anterior eye and lids is vital to the preliminary examination (see Chapter 8).

The following appearances should be viewed, graded and/or measured:

- Limbal redness.
- Epithelium.
- Endothelium.
- Tear prism height.
- Precorneal tear film.
- Lid margins, lashes and meibomian glands.
- Upper lid eversion for examination of the palpebral conjunctiva (see above). The ease or difficulty of lid eversion is often a useful clue about patient sensitivity and level of relaxation, and how simple or difficult lens insertion is likely to be.
- Tear break-up times.
- Iris, anterior angle and crystalline lens.
- Examine a corneal section from the side to assess regularity of corneal curvature.
- Keratometry.
- Corneal topography.
- Pupil diameter in bright and dim light.

The health of the posterior segment of the eye should always be assessed before any lenses are fitted.

SELECTING THE FIRST LENS

The first lens should:

- Be straightforward to insert.
- Settle quickly once it is on the eye.
- Be comfortable to wear.
- Give a reasonable standard of vision.

Use the spectacle refraction to arrive at an estimated power, allowing for back vertex distance. A useful rule of thumb is to ignore cylinders of less than 0.75 D unless acuity is affected.

As far as possible, trial lenses should be disposable lenses, used once and thrown away or directly dispensed to the patient. Any trial lenses that are not disposable should be cleaned carefully and disinfected in hydrogen peroxide. Rigid lenses should be cleaned with an appropriate solution, disinfected with 2% sodium hypochlorite solution for 1 hour, rinsed in normal saline and stored dry. As trial lenses have the potential to carry viruses or prions, reusing them may be risky (www.college-optometrists.org, Feys 2004).

A well-equipped practice should have a variety of spherical soft and silicone hydrogel lenses, toric soft lenses with variable cylinder powers and axes, and rigid lenses of different designs and total diameters. It is also useful to have some bifocal contact lenses and reverse geometry rigid lenses so that an appropriate first lens can be selected most times.

Inserting the first lens

The need for care with hygiene when using contact lenses should be discussed with the patient and demonstrated.

- Wash your hands before touching a person's eye or eyelids (Ly et al. 1997).
- Remove the lens from the package and rinse with appropriate solutions where necessary. Blister-packed lenses do not need rinsing.
- Place the lens on the index finger of the hand used to insert the lens. Where possible, insert the right lens from the right hand while approaching on the patient's right side and vice versa for the left lens. This is more comfortable for the patient.
- Check the lens is not inside out (see Figs 10.1, 10.2 and 10.3). This is a good time to demonstrate to the patient the lens flexibility.
- The lens should be slightly wet and the fingers dry to aid insertion.
- Ask the patient to look up and pull the lower lid down with the middle finger of the hand holding the lens.
- With the patient looking slightly down and nasally, pull up the upper eyelid close to the margin using the middle or index finger of the other hand. If patients are apprehensive and find looking down too difficult, they can be directed to keep looking up or nasally once the eyelids have been secured.
- Place the lens on the superior or temporal sclera (see Fig. 10.4). The lens will usually centre itself but, if necessary, use the eyelids to gently push the lens onto the cornea.

- Hold the lids until the lens centres and then gently release them otherwise the lens may fall out again.
- Once the lens is in the eye, allow it to settle for a moment before checking for bubbles or comfort.
- If the comfort and vision are satisfactory (e.g. 6/9 or 6/6), then leave any final adjustments until the next visit.
- Allow the lenses up to half an hour to settle (depending on the manufacturer's recommendations).
- Carry out an over-refraction.

Be reasonably firm inserting the first lenses in order to reduce the discomfort of waiting. Some patients find it difficult for someone else to put a lens in; teaching them to insert the lens themselves may be less stressful.

For lens removal, see 'Insertion and removal', below and Addendum 1.

DISPENSING CONTACT LENSES

Lenses can be dispensed at the initial appointment but the practitioner may prefer to leave the lenses to settle for longer and to teach care and handling at a collection appointment.

Dispensing is the time when the practitioner hands over responsibility for the contact lenses to the patient who must learn to wear the lenses successfully and safely. Instruction must be given about how the patient should wear and care for the lenses discussed (Claydon et al. 1997). One way to do this is to talk through the contact lens wearer's day.

The practitioner inserts the lenses and checks their appearance and fitting. The patient removes the lenses, reinserts them and leaves the practice, wearing the lenses or, alternatively, removes them again, cleans them and places them in the storage case.

Insertion and removal

This is done in a similar fashion by either the patient or the practitioner.

Common causes of failure are not having the lids wide enough or not placing the lens on centre. Self-insertion may initially be best done in front of a mirror. This helps to keep fixation central. Myopes may be better to watch their finger approaching the eye.

For full instructions on lens insertion and removal, see Addendum 1.

SUCTION HOLDERS

The use of suction holders to remove rigid contact lenses is controversial, but is worth considering where difficulty is encountered with other methods. For those wearing semi-scleral rigid lenses, using a suction holder may be the only method of removing them. The risk with suction holders is of applying it directly to the corneal surface, where it may not be removed easily without damaging the epithelium.

The lens should always be centred before removal is started and after any unsuccessful attempt (normally by checking for clarity of vision). The suction holder should be cleaned with contact lens storage solution every time it is used, then air-dried and stored in an appropriate container.

Care by the practitioner

Practitioner care should be demonstrated to encourage good care by the patient. The following points are important:

- Wash hands before handling lenses, examining eyes or demonstrating insertion and removal.
- Use current solutions and recap bottles after each use.
- Use the same solutions that the patient will be given and use them appropriately, as suggested by the manufacturer.
- Take time to emphasize the importance of the cleaning process.
- Cleaning must be carried out on lens removal and every time the lenses are worn.

Care of lens case

- Once the lenses are inserted, the case should be rinsed with saline, shaken dry then left open to dry while the lenses are being worn.
- Disinfect weekly using boiling water (if suitable) or by scrubbing with soap and saline rinse or using a contact lens solution.
- Replace the case on a regular basis (maximum 3 months).

Patient lens handling

Most people are apprehensive about lens insertion and removal.

- They need to be encouraged to relax.
- Lens handling must be reasonably comfortable if it is to be successful.
- Check that the patient's fingernails are short and clean. Short nails make handling easier and are less likely to scratch the eye or damage the lens.
- Asking the patient to wash their hands before they start to handle the lenses should reinforce the need for care with hygiene.

Full instructions for lens insertion and handling are given in Addendum 1 at the end of this chapter.

Take-home messages

Either written material or an instructional video or CD should be provided to remind patients of what they have been told. This material should cover insertion and removal, cleaning and storage of the lenses, and likely problems.

CLEANING AND STORING CONTACT LENSES

The system will vary depending on the solution used (see also Addendum 1).

The choice of care regimen depends on:

- The type of lens being used, i.e. rigid or soft.
- The material prescribed – for example, a hydrogen peroxide system may be indicated for a high water conventional hydrogel.
- The wearing modality – for example, an enzymatic cleaner may not be considered necessary for a monthly disposable soft lens.
- Any previous problems with particular products.
- Cost and availability.
- Patient compliance – some patients are unlikely to follow a three-step system.

End of initial appointment

An appointment should be made for the next visit. A new wearer often needs reassurance and encouragement while at the same time ensuring that the instructions are being followed correctly.

When the novice contact lens wearer leaves your practice, they should have with them:

- Their lenses.
- Instructions on lens handling and care.
- A solution starter kit to clean and store the lenses.
- In appropriate cases (e.g. with extended-wear silicone hydrogel lenses or monovision lenses), the patient should have their part of the informed consent form to take away.
- A practitioner contact phone number in case of emergency or if they need extra information.
- A follow-up appointment.

Appropriate fees should be paid at this stage.

AFTER-CARE (see also Chapter 17)

The after-care appointment is the time to note and deal with contact lens-related conditions and complications. It is the time to check compliance with instructions for safe contact lens wear – for example, daily wearing times, the proper use of solutions and care systems, and the timely discarding and replacement of lenses.

Timing of after-care appointments is important. The following intervals are only a guide and will vary depending on the type of lenses fitted and whether the patient is having problems.

- 2 weeks after dispensing.
- 2–3 months later.
- Annually thereafter.
- More frequently in the case of difficult fittings or if there are complications.

Extended-wear patients need careful monitoring and should be seen:

- After 24 hours' continuous wear.
- 1 week later.
- 3 weeks later.

Where patients fail to attend their after-care appointments, they should be threatened with no further lens supply, although this is not always effective as most lenses can now be bought over the internet. Reminders should be sent and follow-up telephone calls if appointments are missed. From a legal point of view it is essential that all this is noted on the patient's record (see also Chapter 32).

Patients must be given strict instructions to remove the lenses at any sign of a problem and to seek help immediately.

The after-care appointment

Look, listen and record the patient's comments carefully.

Likely problems could be any of the following:

- Loss of confidence
  - handling difficulties.
  - cannot see well.
  - lenses are uncomfortable.
- Poor comfort or discomfort
  - lens damage.
  - lenses in wrong eyes.
  - using the lenses or solutions incorrectly.
  - lens over-wear response or sleeping in lenses.
  - accidental contamination or using an inappropriate solution.
- Poor vision/unclear vision or less clear than glasses
  - lenses in wrong eyes.
  - wearing two right or two left lenses.
  - refraction is different.
  - uncorrected astigmatism.
  - an incorrect lens has been supplied.

A thorough examination using the slit-lamp and careful inspection for minute signs should provide the necessary information to solve problems and to reassure the practitioner that the patient is safe to continue.

The first after-care appointment is also a good time to check the visual clarity of lenses and to modify as necessary.

REFRACTION THROUGH CONTACT LENSES

- Spectacle refraction and contact lens refraction are not always the same.
- Always refract through the contact lenses.
- Carry out binocular refraction to relax accommodation and reduce errors (e.g. the Humphriss technique).
- Prescribe a toric lens, if necessary. If already wearing a toric lens, check the cylinder axis both by observation of any markings and by over-refraction (see Chapter 12 and also the CD-ROM).

POOR-QUALITY TEARS

- A soft lens tends to dehydrate on the eye (Thai et al. 2002).
- The lens may decentre.
- The lens surface may become coated or spoiled, thereby affecting comfort and vision.
- Refit RGP lenses with a better wetting material.
- Refit soft lenses with a different material – lower water content, silicone hydrogel or one with 'bound' water. Consider refitting with an RGP lens.

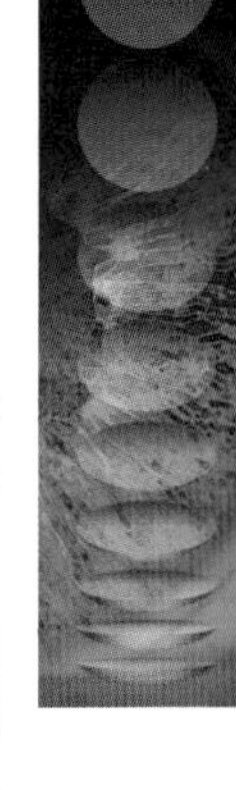

Annual after-care

There are two parts to the annual after-care:

- The contact lens assessment.
- A routine eye examination.

CONTACT LENS ASSESSMENT

Ask about any symptoms. Check the wearing time(s) and replacement schedule (if relevant).

Ask direct questions about the patient's care and compliance. Emphasize:

- Care.
- Compliance.
- Safety.

Reinforce these aspects and the proper use of the lenses and associated care systems (Ky et al. 1998). Simpler care systems should enhance compliance by making it easier to be compliant (Levey & Cohen 1996, Rakow 2003); however, those who are careless will modify their systems and become less safe. Direct questions will make them think about the difference between their actual use and the correct way of doing things. The risk of infection for contact lens wearers is ongoing (Willcox & Holden 2001, Giese & Weissman 2002, Driebe 2003).

Care systems compliance

Questions on the use of care systems should reiterate:

- The need for hand-washing every time before the lenses or eyes are touched.
- Cleaning the lenses every time they are worn and before they are put away in the storage case.
- Changing the storage solution daily.
- Cleaning the case weekly and replacing it every 1–3 months.
- Capping the solution bottles after use.
- Avoidance of tap water in the care regime.

Contact lens use compliance

- How many hours are the lenses worn each day/week?
- How often are the disposable lenses changed? Remind them of the correct interval – daily, weekly, etc.
- How many nights a week do they sleep in the lenses? (This is a leading question designed to pick up those who sleep in lenses that are not of the appropriate material for overnight wear.)
- Do they have an up-to-date pair of spectacles?
- Remind them of the need for continuing regular check-ups.

Contact lens routine

Problems may be encountered at any stage during the assessment (see 'Emergency after-care' below). Most of the visual checks are carried out with the contact lenses in situ (see 'Routine eye examination' below) and it is important to test the vision binocularly as well as monocularly. Once the visual acuity has been fully checked, the lenses are assessed using a Burton/UV lamp and a slit-lamp for:

- Fit – centration, coverage, movement.
- Condition.
- Tear film over lenses.

The lenses are then removed and the eyes examined.

ROUTINE EYE EXAMINATION

A complete eye examination should be carried out. Be aware that the contact lens patient may need referral to an ophthalmologist for treatment of a condition unrelated to their contact lenses.

Emergency after-care (see also Chapter 17)

Such issues are often complicated and test the practitioner's problem-solving ability. They can vary from minor problems with comfort and red eyes to major eye infection and consequent visual loss. The following could be areas of difficulty.

POOR COMFORT

- Old lenses.
- Lenses coated with tear proteins.
- Use of incorrect solutions.
- Not using the care system competently.
- Lens damage.
- Poor handling skills.
- Lens surface changes.
- Overwear response or overnight wear of low Dk lenses.
- GPC or CLARE (see Chapter 17).
- Infection.
- Other eye problems (e.g. closed angle glaucoma).

POOR VISION

- Sight has changed.
- Needs an astigmatic correction.
- Patient becoming presbyopic and requiring an appropriate correction.
- Lenses coated with tear protein.
- GPC leading to excess mucus.
- Other eye problems (e.g. retinal detachment).

RED EYES (see also Chapters 17 and 18)

Of most concern are those who present with red eyes. Is it an infection and, if so, what is the cause?

Possible causes could be:

- Infectious.
- Allergic.
- Toxic or chemical.
- Mechanical.

INFECTIONS

Infections of the eye, allergies, blepharitis and toxic reactions are dealt with in Chapters 8, 17 and 18.

Contact lens wear should always be halted until the eye is healed. Lenses and cases should not be discarded as they may be sent for culture to help diagnose the infection. Once the eyes have returned to normal, new lenses, case and/or solutions should be substituted.

CRISIS MANAGEMENT

Managing crises or risk management is best done with forethought. The following should be considered:

- Accurate note taking and records are essential for both patient and practitioner protection.
- Careful preparation, selection and instruction of patients.
- Verbal and written information sheets (see below).
- Keeping up to date with current trends – continuing education is vital.
- Protocols or routines should be available for all procedures.
- Staff should be trained to recognize emergencies, make appropriate appointments and give advice where they are competent.

If a crisis occurs, the practitioner needs to be able to:

- Diagnose the condition causing the emergency.
- Plan the appropriate treatment.
- Supervise a treatment plan to a successful conclusion.

Information

Written or electronic material should be available to give to contact lens wearers to reinforce the verbal information they have been given. These should:

- Answer questions that may arise.
- Help to solve problems occurring during adaptation or subsequent lens wear.
- Provide consistency of information.

Topics could include the following:

- Information for new contact lens wearers.
- Insertion and removal techniques.
- Cleaning and care regimes.
- Adaptation schedules.
- Lens replacement schedules.
- Normal symptoms.
- What to do in an emergency.

Informed consent

There are a number of occasions when informed consent forms should be used. These relate to special lenses, which may have some risks to the wearer if they are not used properly. The following are examples of such lenses:

- Extended wear.
- Orthokeratology.
- Bifocal or monovision.
- Keratoconus, post-graft or post-LASIK lenses.

Well-designed informed consent material will include a form giving:

- Background information on the lenses used.
- A list of possible risks and how they are being minimized.
- A statement of the responsibilities of the practitioner.

Patients will be less upset when they have problems if they have been warned in advance, and informed patients are generally more compliant. The form will demonstrate practitioner commitment to caring for their patients.

Some patient instruction material is available from contact lens or care system manufacturers. Two samples are included: one for new soft lens wearers with a modification for RGP wearers (Addendum 1) and the other an informed consent form for silicone hydrogel wear and which can be modified for extended wear of high-Dk RGP materials (Addendum 2).

Acknowledgements

I wish to acknowledge the contribution of Margaret Tibbles, University of Auckland, for help with references, and Fiona Cottam and Alinga and Russell Wackrow for help with photography.

References

Bennett, E. S., Smythe, J., Henry, V. A. et al. (1998a) Effect of topical anesthetic use on initial patient satisfaction and overall success with rigid gas permeable contact lenses. Optom. Vis. Sci., 75(11), 800–805

Bennett, E. S., Stulc, S., Bassi, C. J. et al. (1998b) Effect of patient personality profile and verbal presentation on successful rigid contact lens adaptation, satisfaction and compliance. Optom. Vis. Sci., 75(7), 500–505

Chui, W. S., Cho, P. and Brown, B. (2000) Soft contact lens wear in Hong Kong-Chinese: predicting success. Ophthalmol. Physiol. Opt., 20(6), 480–486

Claydon, B. E., Efron, N. and Woods C. (1997) A prospective study of the effect of education on non-compliant behaviour in contact lens wear. Ophthalmol. Physiol. Opt., 17(2), 137–146

Driebe, W. T. Jr. (2003) Present status of contact lens-induced corneal infections. Ophthalmol. Clin. North Am., 16(3), 485–494, viii

Dumbleton, K. A., Chalmers, R. L., Richter, D. B. and Fonn D. (2001) Vascular response to extended wear of hydrogel lenses with high and low oxygen permeability. Optom. Vis. Sci., 78(3), 147–151

Efron, N. (1998) Grading scales for contact lens complications. Ophthalmol. Physiol. Opt., 18(2), 182–186

Efron, N., Morgan, P. B., Farmer, C., Furuborg, J., Struk, R. and Carney L. G. (2003a) Experience and training as determinants of grading reliability when assessing the severity of contact lens complications. Ophthalmol. Physiol. Opt., 23(2), 119–124

Efron, N., Morgan, P. B. and Jagpal, R. (2003b) The combined influence of knowledge, training and experience when grading contact lens complications. Ophthalmol. Physiol. Opt., 23(1), 79–85

Ehlers, W. H., Donshik, P. C. and Suchecki, J. K. (2003) Disposable and frequent replacement contact lenses [review]. Ophthalmol. Clin. North Am., 16(3), 341–352

Feys, J. (2004) [Rules and regulations concerning contact lens-related infection] [review]. J. Fr. Opthalmol., 27(4), 420–423

Foulks, G. N. (2003) What is dry eye and what does it mean to the contact lens wearer? Eye Contact Lens: Sci. Clin. Pract., 9(1 Suppl), S96–100; discussion S115–118, S192–194

Giese, M. J. and Weissman, B. A. (2002) Contact lens associated corneal infections. Where do we go from here? [review]. Clin. Exp. Optom., 85(3), 141–148

Glasson, M. J., Stapleton, F., Keay, L., Sweeney, D. and Willcox, M. D. (2003) Differences in clinical parameters and tear film of tolerant and intolerant contact lens wearers. Invest. Ophthalmol. Vis. Sci., 44(12), 5116–5124

Hamano, H., Jacob, J. T., Senft, C. J. et al. (2002) Differences in contact lens-induced responses in the corneas of Asian and non-Asian subjects. CLAO J., 28(2), 101–104

Holden, B. A., Sweeney, D. F., Sankaridurg, P. R., Carnt, N., Edwards, K., Stretton, S. and Stapleton, F. (2003) Microbial keratitis and vision loss with contact lenses [review]. Eye Contact Lens: Sci. Clin. Pract., 29(1 Suppl), S131–134; discussion S143–144, S192–194

Ky, W., Scherick, K. and Stenson, S. (1998) Clinical survey of lens care in contact lens patients [see comment in: CLAO J., 24(4):194]. CLAO J., 24(4):216–219

Lemp, M. A. (2003) Contact lenses and associated anterior segment disorders: dry eye, blepharitis, and allergy [review]. Ophthalmol. Clin. North Am., 16(3), 463–469

Levey, S. B. and Cohen, E. J. (1996) Methods of disinfecting contact lenses to avoid corneal disorders [review]. Surv. Ophthalmol., 41(3), 245–251

Liesegang, T. J. (2002) Physiologic changes of the cornea with contact lens wear [review]. CLAO J., 28(1), 12–27

Ly, V. T., Simmons, P. A., Edrington, T. B., Wechsler, S. and De Land, P. N. (1997) Efficacy of hand washing procedures on bacterial contamination of hydrogel contact lenses. Optom. Vis. Sci., 74(5), 288–292

McCulley, J. P. and Shine, W. E. (2003) Eyelid disorders: the meibomian gland, blepharitis, and contact lenses [review]. Eye Contact Lens: Sci. Clin. Pract., 29(1 Suppl), S93–95; discussion S115–118, S192–194

McMahon, T. T. (2003) The case for rigid lenses [review]. Eye Contact Lens: Sci. Clin. Pract., 29(1 Suppl), S119–121; discussion S143–144, S192–194

McMahon, T. T. and Zadnik, K. (2000) Twenty-five years of contact lenses: the impact on the cornea and ophthalmic practice. Cornea, 19(5), 730–740

Nichols, J. J., Mitchell, G. L., Nichols, K. K., Chalmers, R. and Begley C. (2002) The performance of the contact lens dry eye questionnaire as a screening survey for contact lens-related dry eye. Cornea, 21(5), 469–475

Rakow, P. L. (2003) Current contact lens care systems [review]. Ophthalmol. Clin. North Am., 16(3), 415–432

Stapleton, F., Willcox, M. D., Morris, C. A. and Sweeney, D. F. (1998) Tear changes in contact lens wearers following overnight eye closure. Curr. Eye Res., 17(2), 183–188

Sweeney, D. F., Keay, L., Carnt, N. and Holden, B. A. (2002) Practitioner guidelines for continuous wear with high Dk silicone hydrogel contact lenses. Clin. Exp. Optom., 85(3), 161–167

Szczotka, L. B. and Lindsay, R. G. (2003) Contact lens fitting following corneal graft surgery [review]. Clin. Exp. Optom., 86(4), 244–249

Thai, L. C., Tomlinson, A. and Ridder, W. H. (2002) Contact lens drying and visual performance: the vision cycle with contact lenses. Optom. Vis. Sci., 79(6), 381–388

Willcox, M. D. and Holden, B. A. (2001) Contact lens related corneal infections [review]. Biosci. Rep., 21(4), 445–461

ADDENDUM 1

Instructions for soft contact lens wearers

BEFORE STARTING

- Always wash your hands before handling the lenses.
- Get into the habit of working with one lens at a time, so that they are not mixed up.
- Is it the right way out? To make sure, sit the lens on your finger and view from the side (Fig. 11.1). If the edge tends to go outwards, the lens is inside out.
- A drop of multipurpose solution can be placed on the lens before starting as this may aid easier insertion.

INSERTION

- With the lens on the index finger, use the middle finger(s) of the other hand to pull up the upper lid.
- Use the other hand to pull down the lower lid.
- Place the lens centrally on the eye (Fig. 11.2).
- Look down to position the lens properly. Remove the index finger and gently let go of the eyelid.

IF THE LENS IS UNCOMFORTABLE

- Look in the mirror and gently place a finger on the edge of the lens.
- Slowly slide the lens away from your nose while looking in the opposite direction (Fig. 11.3).
- Slide the lens right off, onto the white part of the eye and then back on.
- If it is still uncomfortable, remove the lens, clean it and start again. If discomfort persists, remove the lens and consult your eye-care practitioner.

LENS REMOVAL

- Look up, and pull down the lower lid with your middle finger. Hold the top lid up with the other hand.
- Slide the lens onto the white of the eye below the cornea.

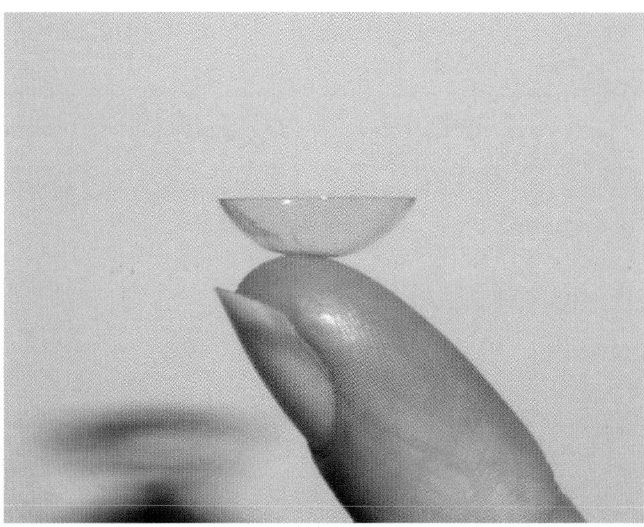

Figure 11.1 Checking a soft lens profile for the correct way out

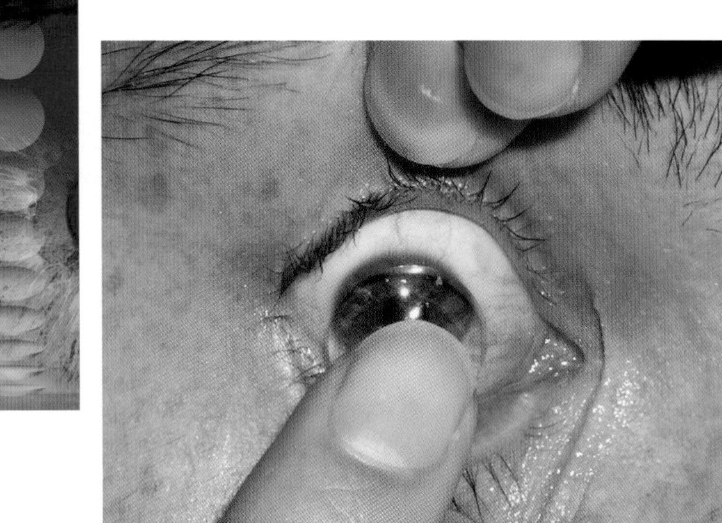

Figure 11.2 Soft lens insertion. Note how both lids are held apart

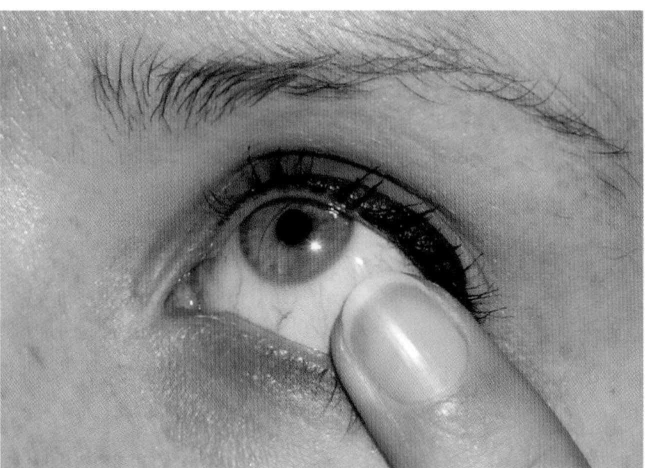

Figure 11.3 Sliding a soft lens off-centre to release a foreign body

- Pinch the lens lightly between the thumb and index finger. Lift it gently off the eye (Fig. 11.4). With practice the lens can be slid onto the lower sclera and gently pinched out without the need to hold the upper lid (Fig. 11.5).
- Alternatively, use the ends of the fingers to pull the lids wide apart vertically. Then push the lid edges firmly together to scoop the lens out (Fig. 11.6).
- Clean the lens according to your care system and put it away before you remove and clean the other lens.

Caring for your lenses

CLEANING

- After removing the right lens from your eye, place it in the palm of the hand.
- Add three drops of multipurpose solution (or soft lens cleaner).
- Supporting the lens on your index finger, rub the lens gently for about 10 seconds.

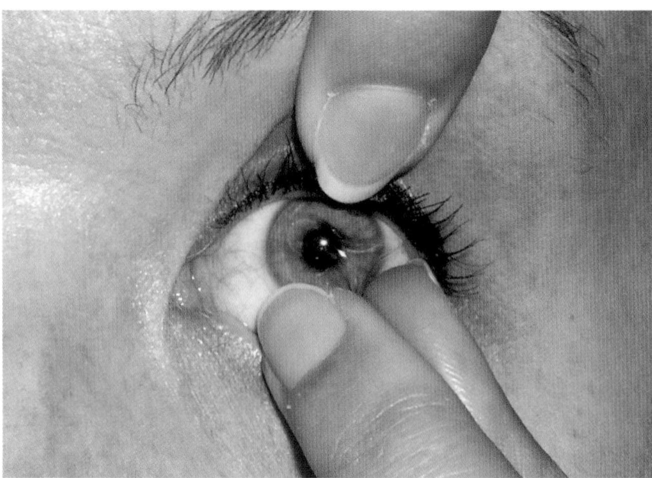

Figure 11.4 Gently folding and pinching a soft lens to remove it

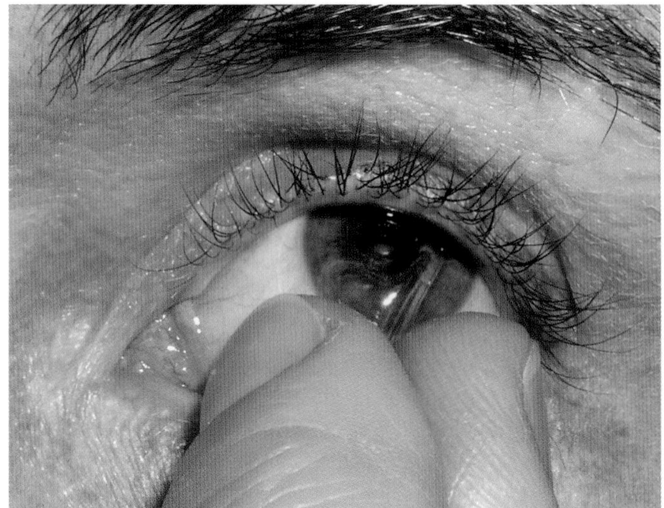

Figure 11.5 Soft lens removal without holding the upper lid

- Turn the lens over and clean the other side.
- Rinse both sides of the lens in the palm of your hand with a steady stream of multipurpose solution.
- If you prefer to not rub your lens to clean, it must be rinsed in a steady stream of solution for at least 10 seconds.
- Fill each lens well two-thirds full with multipurpose solution and place in the correct lens well. Twist the cap on until finger tight.
- Repeat these steps with the left lens, and leave to soak for at least 4 hours.

REMEMBER! – CLEAN – RINSE – DISINFECT

Special hints and warnings

LISTEN TO YOUR PRACTITIONER

- Dispose of the lenses every month or as advised.
- Be sure to use the lens products recommended to you by your practitioner. Follow the instructions carefully.
- Do not substitute products without checking.
- Make sure you keep your after-care appointments. These are essential to ensure long-term safety of your eyes.

(a)

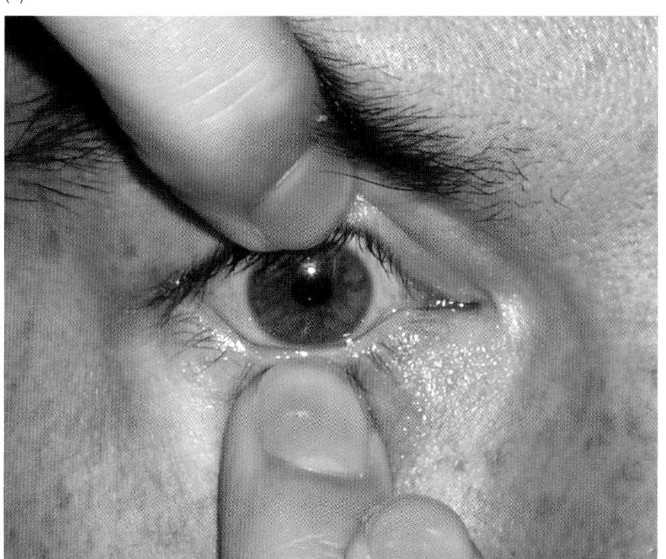

(b)

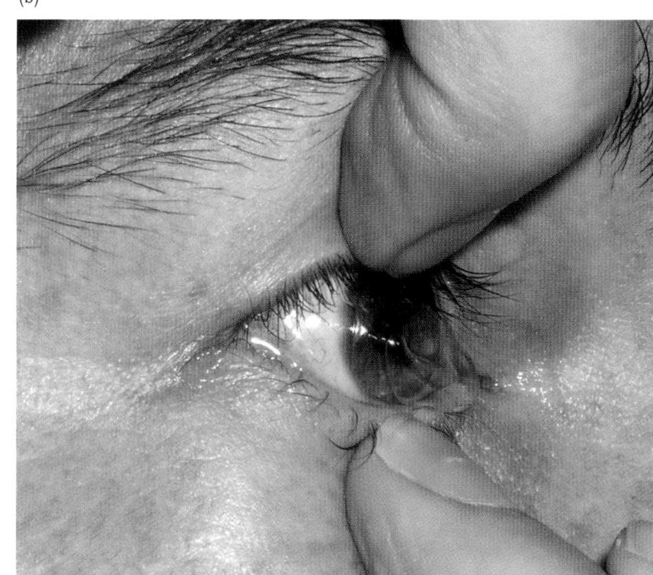

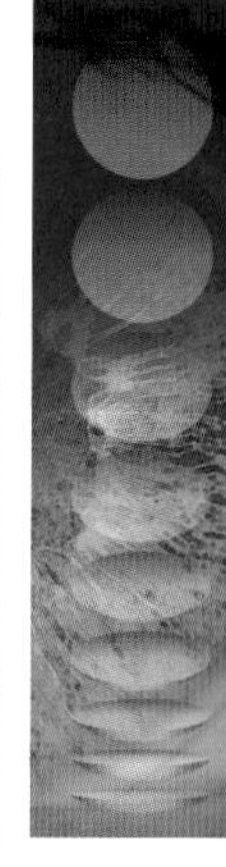

Figure 11.6 (a) Scissor removal of a soft lens showing the lid positions; (b) showing the lids scooping the lens out

DRY EYES

Your soft contact lenses may dry out slightly in dry, air-conditioned buildings or when you blink less often (e.g. when using a computer).

- Soft lens rewetting agents can be used to help rewet the lenses and relieve discomfort.
- If you find yourself using a lubricant frequently, contact your eye-care practitioner for advice.

CASE CARE

The lens case also needs regular cleaning. After a while the bacteria in cases can produce a biofilm (bacterial 'slime'). Biofilm can allow bacteria to survive your cleaning routine, increasing the risk of eye infections.

To reduce any risk:

- Rinse the used solution from the case daily using fresh multi-purpose solution, shake it to dry and leave with the caps off while wearing the lenses.
- Digitally (or with a soft, clean toothbrush) clean your case weekly with multipurpose solution. Let the case dry in air.
- Alternatively, pour boiling water over the open case once a week. Check first that the case material is suitable for this.
- Replace your lens case every 1–3 months.

COSMETICS

- Always insert lenses before applying make-up or using a moisturizer. Use a water-resistant mascara to reduce flaking and smudging. Waterproof mascara is oil-based and may cause eye irritation.
- Never use saliva to thin a cosmetic product or to rewet a lens – this could lead to serious eye infection.
- Close your eyes when using aerosols, and leave the room as soon as you have finished spraying.

SORENESS AND IRRITATION

- If you experience any redness, itchiness, soreness, blurred vision or excessive tearing that persists while wearing the lenses, remove them and consult your eye-care practitioner.
- Keep the lenses wet at all times. When not worn, store in the carrying case.
- Replace lenses as advised. Old lenses can be uncomfortable to wear and may reduce the amount of oxygen getting to the eye.
- Unless stated on the bottle, eye medication or eye drops should not be used while wearing your lenses. Wait at least 15 minutes after using the drops before putting the lenses on your eyes.

EMERGENCIES

In case of any emergency, our phone numbers are:

Office numbers: ....
Other contact numbers: ....

If we are unobtainable, you should report to the Accident or Emergency Department of your local hospital.

Instructions for rigid contact lens wearers

Instructions for RGP patients are similar to those for soft lenses. RGP lens insertion is shown in Figure 11.7. The main difference is the method of lens removal as follows.

LENS REMOVAL

Use the stare–pull–blink method to remove the lens:

- Open the eye widely so the lids are further apart than the lens, pull the lids tightly in the direction of the top of the ear, and then blink strongly (Fig. 11.8).
- The released lens can be caught in the other hand, or removed from the lids or face.

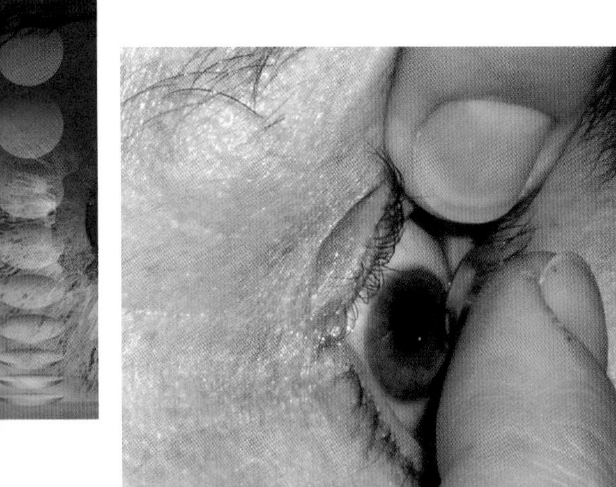
Figure 11.7 Inserting a rigid lens

- If the lens goes off-centre it should be massaged around the eye and the bottom eyelid used to push the lens back on centre and removed from there (Fig. 11.9).

A suction holder is an alternative for removing a lens (either centred or off-centre):

- Clean and moisten the suction holder as for the lens itself.
- Always check that your vision is clear before attempting lens removal, i.e. that the lens is in place.
- Press gently against the lens centre and remove (Fig. 11.10).
- If this does not work then either:

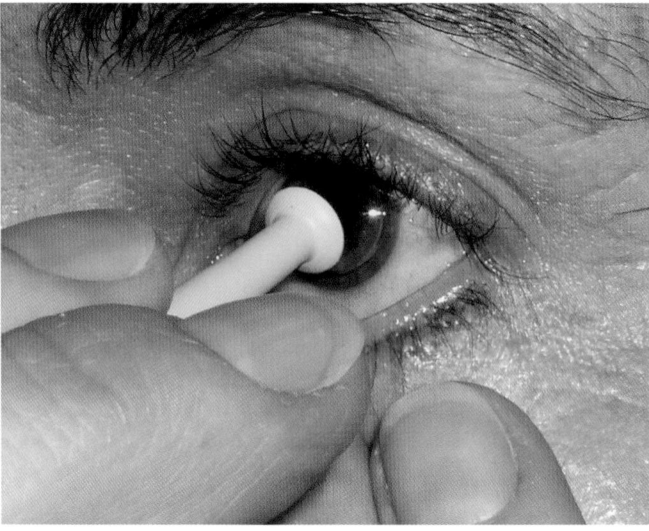
Figure 11.10 Removing a rigid lens with a suction holder

  - the lens has come out or been displaced (Fig. 11.11).
  - the suction holder is slightly tilted, i.e. it is at an angle to the lens surface.

Additional instructions for extended or continuous wear

Wearers of these lens types should, in addition to the above, be warned of:

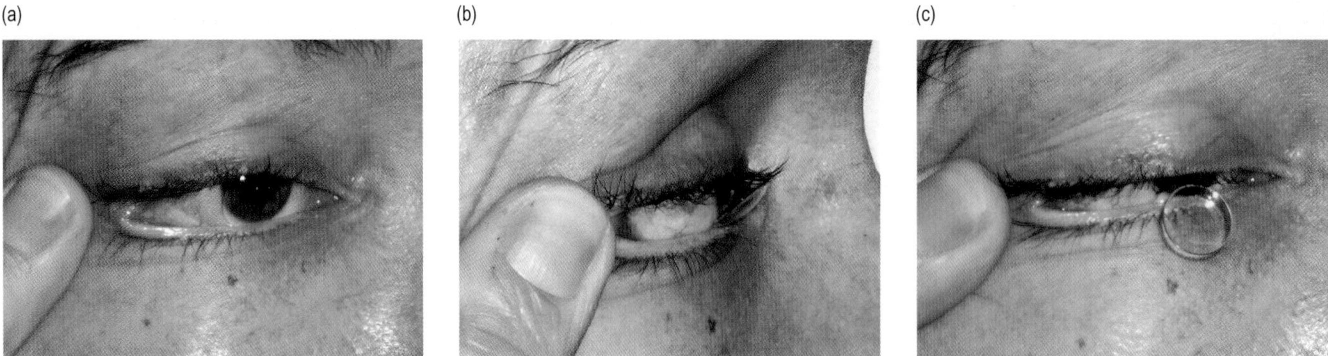

Figure 11.8 (a) Removal of a rigid lens; (b) just coming off the eye; (c) tumbling onto the face

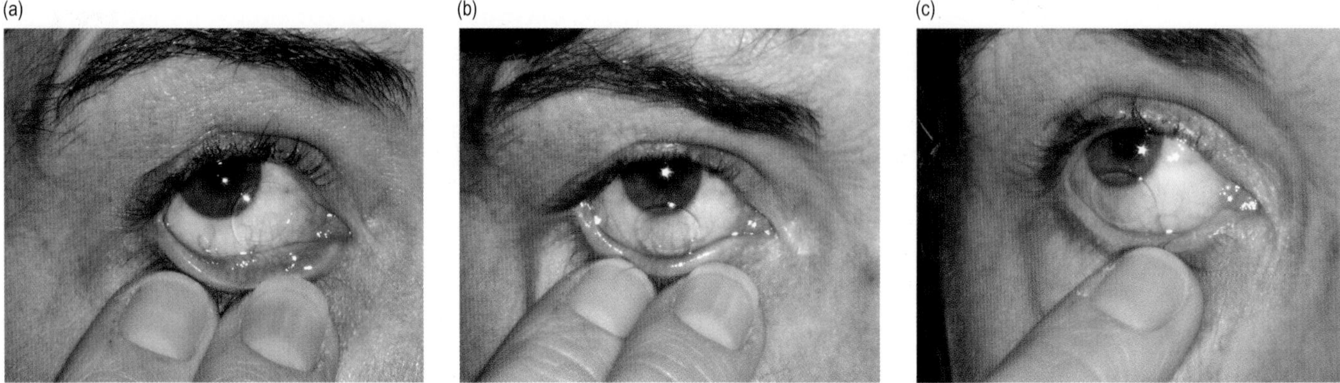

Figure 11.9 Moving the lens in the eye using the lower lid (a); recentring a rigid lens using (b) two fingers and (c) one finger

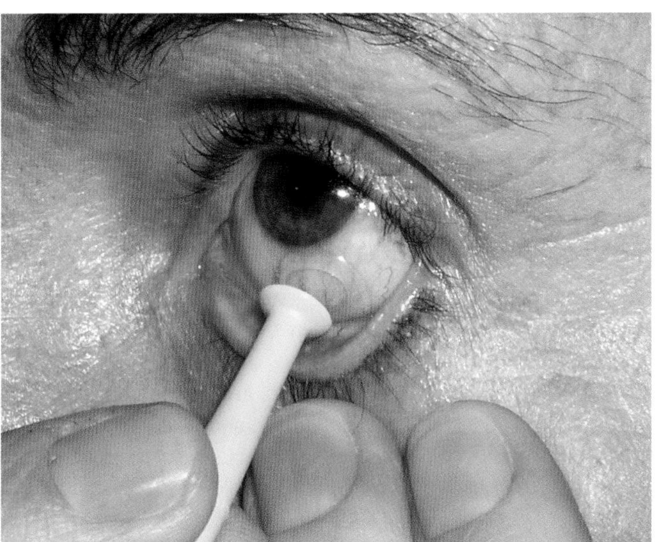

Figure 11.11 Removing an off-centre rigid lens with a suction holder

- The need for additional after-care visits.
- To cease lens wear if there is any sign of redness, foggy vision, discomfort or discharge from the eye.
- The need to report for immediate care if any of the former persists for more than an hour or two.
- The initial possible need for ocular lubricant drops before sleep and on waking.
- The need to drop back to daily wear if they are less than 100% physically well.
- In the case of RGP extended wear, to ensure that the lenses move on or shortly after waking.

ADDENDUM 2

Informed consent for extended wear of silicone hydrogel lenses

Silicone hydrogel is a relatively new contact lens material which has taken many years of research and several hundred million dollars to develop. It transmits several hundred per cent more oxygen through to the cornea than conventional soft lenses. The US Food and Drug Administration (FDA) has approved these materials as being safe to wear 24 hours a day over a 30-day period.

The new material still has some water in it but not as much as the older hydrogel materials. It does not dry as much, for example, in aircraft or on waking after sleeping.

Previous materials did not always allow sufficient oxygen through to maintain the eye in a completely normal state for those who slept in their lenses regularly. This resulted in an increased risk of eye infection of 20 in 10,000 people wearing them overnight compared with 4 in 10,000 wearing them only while awake. Silicone hydrogels have been used worldwide for several years now, and the risk factor for infection has been found to be very low and only slightly more than that for daily wear hydrogel lenses. Nevertheless, it is vital to maintain normal hygiene, to report back for after-care visits as advised, and to cease lens wear and seek help if there are any abnormal signs.

There are alternative forms of treatment to consider. These are refractive surgery, daily wear conventional hydrogel materials and orthokeratology. Refractive surgery is the process whereby the shape of the front of the eye is changed surgically, but this is not a reversible process. Refractive surgery is expensive, there is a risk of permanent eyesight loss, and a number of people suffer from regression where their sight goes back towards the original refraction. Daily wear, conventional hydrogel materials are safe but lenses need to be taken in and out every day which may be inconvenient. Orthokeratology is the reshaping of the eye's surface using rigid gas-permeable lenses worn overnight. This gives clear vision during the day without any form of correction but does not work for everyone and generally only for lower focusing errors.

ADVERSE EFFECTS

There are some possible risks from wearing contact lenses overnight:

- Irritation or discomfort.
- Dry eyes.
- An allergic eye response.
- Reduced comfort or tolerance, or inability to wear overnight.
- Chances of abrasions or changes to the cornea (the front of the eye).
- Infection, which, if severe, could lead to permanent loss of vision.

Most adverse effects are rare and can be minimized or avoided by following your practitioner's instructions carefully.

RISK FACTORS

Some people are more at risk of having problems or an eye infection. These include:

- Smokers.
- People who swim without goggles.
- Those with persistent dry eyes or chronic lid or eye infections, or blepharitis.
- Young men.
- People with poor personal hygiene.

THE CONTACT LENS WEARER/PATIENT AGREES TO

- Check/look at their eyes daily.
- Remove lenses if the eyes are red or persistently uncomfortable.
- Seek help within 24 hours if problems persist.
- Discard the lenses every calendar month.
- Have checkups when advised to do so.

THE OPTOMETRIST/CONTACT LENS PRACTITIONER AGREES TO PROVIDE

- Appointments as necessary to supervise safe wearing of the lenses.
- Checks and care in an emergency and speedy referral to medical care where necessary.

- Continuing care and supervision of overnight wear.
- A system of continuous care so that in their absence from work there will be someone else available to provide care or advice.

RED EYES

Redness is a sign of inflammation, which is potentially serious. It can also be due to irritation, dry eyes, and dirty or old lenses.

Every day, look at your eyes in the mirror, cover one eye and then the other, and ask yourself:

- Do my eyes look good?
- Do my eyes feel good?
- Do I see well?

WHAT TO DO IF PROBLEMS ARISE

- If your vision is blurred, try rewetting the lenses. If that does not help, remove them, clean them and put them back in.
- Use wetting/comfort drops if your eyes are uncomfortable or a bit red.
- If your eyes stay red, take the lenses out, clean them and leave them out overnight before wearing them again.
- If your eyes remain red and sore for more than 12 hours, stop wearing the lenses and contact us straight away.
- *Normal rules for hygiene apply even if the lenses are worn overnight.*
- Hand-washing and reasonable personal hygiene will reduce the risk of problems with your lenses.
- *If you are unwell*, the risk of getting an eye infection is increased
  - only wear the lenses while you are awake.
  - if you are ill enough to go to bed, leave your lenses out.

If you do have problems do not hesitate to contact us and come and see us. We have short times available every day for urgent appointments.

A list of contact phone numbers is given below. If no-one is available, attend the Accident or Emergency Department of the nearest hospital if you suspect an infection or damage to the eye(s).

Office numbers: ....
Other contact numbers: ....

Disclaimer: It should be stressed that advice given in this Addendum is of a general nature only and may vary from country to country. Practitioners should always seek advice from their own professional body.

Chapter 12

Toric contact lens fitting

Richard G. Lindsay

CHAPTER CONTENTS

Fitting rigid toric lenses

INDICATIONS FOR THE USE OF RIGID TORIC LENSES

Rigid toric lenses are indicated in preference to rigid spherical lenses under the following circumstances:

- To improve vision in cases where a lens employing spherical front and back optic zone radii is unable to provide adequate refractive correction.
- To improve the physical fit where a lens with a spherical back optic zone radius (BOZR) and spherical back peripheral zone radii fails to provide an adequate physical fit.

These two situations are not always distinct and a toric lens may be used for both physical and optical reasons. For example, when fitting an eye with both a high degree of residual astigmatism and a large amount of corneal toricity, a toric lens is required optically, to correct the residual astigmatism, and physically, to optimize the lens fit (Lindsay 1996).

FORMS OF TORIC LENS

Toric corneal lenses, most commonly with a toroidal back optic zone and peripheral zone, are generally used to obtain a good physical fit on a cornea that is too toroidal to allow a good fit with a completely spherical lens. There are several varieties of these lenses:

- Toroidal back surface lenses can be produced with a spherical front optic surface.
- A toroidal back surface with a toroidal front surface. These lenses therefore have a bitoric construction.
- If the principal meridians are not parallel, the lens is of oblique bitoric construction.
- A spherical back optic zone and a toroidal peripheral zone are used in an attempt to improve the physical fit of a lens on an astigmatic cornea, while avoiding the optical complications inherent in the use of lenses with toroidal back optic zones (this form of lens can also be produced with a toroidal front surface).

- Occasionally, a lens is produced with a toroidal back optic zone and a spherical peripheral zone, with the intention of improving the circulation of tears beneath the lens. However, this can cause the lens to become less stable to resisting rotation. One limitation on the spherical peripheral radii is that they have to be greater than or equal to the flatter radius for the preceding toroidal curve (this form of lens can be made with or without a toroidal front surface).
- A spherical back optic zone and spherical peripheral zone combined with a toroidal front optic surface. This type of lens is required where there is significant residual (non-corneal) astigmatism but minimal corneal astigmatism. The residual astigmatism needs to be corrected with a toroidal front surface and a spherical back optic zone due to the negligible corneal astigmatism. Some form of orientation mechanism will, of course, be required such as prism ballast or truncation (see later).

CRITERIA FOR USE OF RIGID TORIC LENSES

Corneal lenses with both spherical BOZR and peripheral radii are often used successfully on corneas with medium to high degrees of astigmatism. It is important, therefore, to decide what degree of corneal astigmatism should indicate the use of toroidal back optic zones. In general, these should only be used when a lens with a spherical BOZR cannot be made to fit successfully. It is rare to find that toroidal back optic zones are necessary, unless the corneal astigmatism exceeds 2.0–2.50 D (i.e. the difference in the corneal radii, as measured with a keratometer, exceeds approximately 0.4–0.5 mm).

In cases of uncertainty (e.g. where the corneal astigmatism is between 1.50 and 2.50 D), a toroidal back optic zone would be used in preference to a spherical back surface curve when:

- A spherical lens exhibits poor centration or excessive movement.
- Excessive lens flexure is noted with a spherical lens.
- Fluorescein patterns with a spherical lens reveal excessive bearing along the flatter corneal meridian, regardless of what BOZR is fitted.
- Significant 3 and 9 o'clock staining occurs with a spherical lens.
- There is marked corneal distortion and spectacle blur upon removal of the spherical lens from the eye. This occurs as a result of poor alignment between the spherical lens and the toric cornea, with the spherical lens subsequently having a moulding effect on the toric cornea.
- There is significant residual astigmatism. In this case, a spherical back surface may provide an adequate fit but a toric back surface will stabilize the lens, prevent rotation, and allow correction of the residual astigmatism.

A great deal depends on factors other than corneal astigmatism (e.g. lid positions and tension). For an eye with high with-the-rule corneal astigmatism and a low, loose lower lid, a toroidal back optic zone may be needed to obtain a good physical fit and centration. A similar eye with a firm, high lower lid may well be successful with a spherical lens.

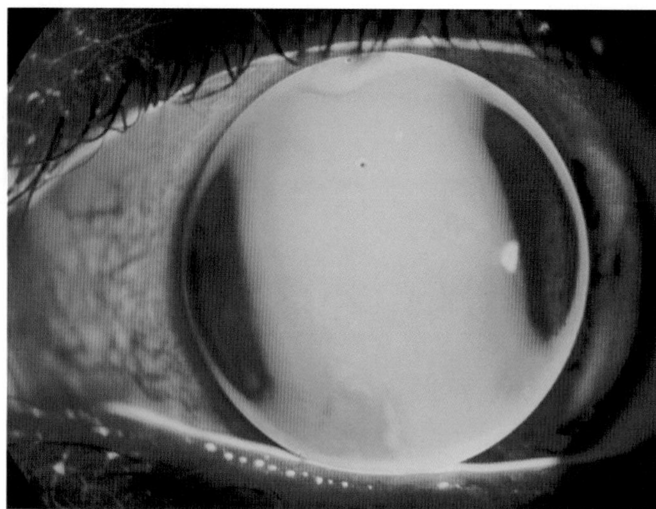

Figure 12.1 Left eye with high corneal astigmatism. Keratometer reading 8.14 mm along 11, 7.12 mm along 101. Fitting with spherical (7.50 mm) BOZR reveals harsh bearing along the horizontal (flatter) meridian and poor centration

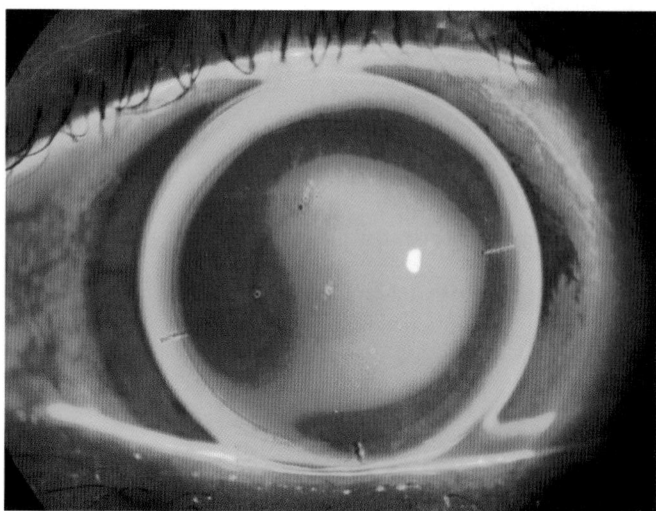

Figure 12.2 Same left eye as in Figure 12.1 wearing a rigid lens using a toroidal back optic zone of BOZR 8.10 × 7.20 mm. Although too steep, the lens now shows a more spherical fit

The majority of cases of corneal astigmatism are found with the steeper corneal curve in the vertical meridian (with-the-rule). If an attempt is made to fit such an eye with a spherical BOZR, the lens may exhibit heavy bearing along the flatter (horizontal) meridian of the cornea and poor centration (Fig. 12.1), causing physical discomfort and/or poor vision.

If the same eye is fitted using a lens with toroidal back optic and peripheral curves, then the physical fit and centration are usually much improved (Fig. 12.2).

The presence of against-the-rule corneal astigmatism (steeper axis horizontal) usually necessitates fitting a toroidal back optic zone earlier than would be required with an equivalent amount of with-the-rule corneal astigmatism because rigid spherical lenses tend to decentre laterally with moderate amounts of against-the-rule astigmatism (1.50–2.00 D).

DESIGN CONSIDERATIONS

Toroidal back optic zone lenses should be fitted on or near alignment. The fluorescein pattern will be similar to that seen with a well-fitted spherical lens on a spherical cornea.

A toric lens aligning too closely to the cornea can lead to poor tear interchange. Consequently, it is advisable to use a toroidal back optic zone with the steeper radius fitted slightly flatter (longer radius) than the corresponding corneal radius so as to assist the interchange of tears. The flatter radius will generally be fitted 'on K' or else a little steeper than its corresponding corneal radius.

Example 1

Keratometry reading: 7.90 mm (42.72 D) along 180
7.35 mm (45.91 D) along 90

Prescribed lens: C3 Toric/$\frac{7.85}{7.40}$:7.50/$\frac{8.45}{8.00}$:8.50/$\frac{9.25}{8.80}$:9.50

Many practitioners use spherical trial lenses when fitting rigid toric lenses. However, even a limited set of diagnostic fitting lenses with both toroidal back optic and peripheral curves can be extremely valuable. A suggestion for a minimum set is one covering the range 7.50 × 7.00 mm to 8.50 × 8.00 mm BOZR in 0.1 mm increments in both meridians.

The BOZR should be chosen with at least 0.3 mm (1.50 D) meridional difference in radii. Otherwise, the toroidal BOZR may not position properly on the toroidal cornea, leading to lens rotation and possible visual disturbance. (Note that BOZR indicates back optic zone radius for a spherical surface and back optic zone radii for a toroidal surface.)

Each meridian is considered separately and the peripheral fittings in the two principal meridians are selected to provide the same difference between back optic and peripheral radii most commonly used by the practitioner in fitting spherical corneas. The peripheral curves usually have the same degree of toricity as the BOZR.

- For example, if the back peripheral radius (BPR) is 0.9 mm flatter than the BOZR for a spherical lens, then for a lens with toroidal BOZR of 7.90/7.40, the BPR ordered would be 8.80/8.30.

For lenses with a spherical back optic zone and a toroidal peripheral zone, the width of the peripheral curve should be as large as possible to increase the likelihood of alignment with the toric cornea. The meridional difference in the peripheral curves should be at least 0.6 mm to help minimize lens rotation (Ruston 1999). These lenses have a small total diameter (TD) to minimize meridional sag differences and are fitted steeper centrally than the flatter corneal meridian to achieve a compromise fit.

Example 2

Keratometry reading: 7.90 mm (42.72 D) along 180
7.30 mm (46.23 D) along 90

BOZR chosen: 7.70 mm
BOZD chosen: 6.50 mm
TD chosen: 9.50 mm

Prescribed lens: C4/7.70:6.50/$\frac{8.50}{7.90}$:7.50/$\frac{9.20}{8.60}$:8.50/$\frac{10.00}{9.40}$:9.50

While this type of lens can be useful where a fully spherical lens fits poorly, the toroidal peripheral zones are, at best, a compromise. They usually rotate more than lenses with all toroidal back surfaces and the steeper peripheral radii occasionally end up in close proximity to the flatter corneal meridian, causing problems.

It is possible to see if the lens is rotating by observing the peripheral fluorescein fit. It may be helpful to have the flatter or steeper peripheral meridian marked with two dots, one at each edge of the lens. Two dots are more useful than one for this purpose.

Lenses with spherical back optic zones and toroidal peripheral zones can also be used in keratoconic eyes to enhance lens centration and eradicate inferior lens stand-off, and will often stabilize reasonably well as the BPR_1 is the main bearing surface (see Chapter 20).

OPTICAL CONSIDERATIONS (see Chapter 6)

The complexity of calculations to determine the necessary radii and power of toric lenses is often exaggerated. However, the fundamentals of the optics of contact lenses must be understood in order to appreciate some of the complications (Douthwaite 1995).

CORNEAL ASTIGMATISM AND THE EFFECT OF THE TEAR LENS

Front surface corneal astigmatism is only partly neutralized by the back surface astigmatism of the resultant tear lens when a rigid lens with spherical back surface is placed on the eye. The refractive index (RI) of tears is 1.336, while that of the cornea is 1.376. The amount neutralized is thus 336/376, almost 90%. It is assumed that the back surface of the cornea neutralizes the remaining 10% of its front surface astigmatism and the RI of calibration of most keratometers (1.3375) is chosen to take this effect into account. This gives the user a guide to the total refractive effect of the cornea. Hence, keratometers measure front surface corneal radii but give *total* corneal power on the assumption that the back surface has –10% of the power of the front surface.

The RI of 1.3375 is very close to that of the tears (1.336). Thus, the corneal astigmatism measured with the keratometer should be completely corrected by the tear lens between the cornea and contact lens, provided the back of the contact lens is spherical.

REFRACTION WITH TOROIDAL BACK OPTIC ZONES

Calculating the back vertex powers (BVPs) for a rigid lens with toroidal back optic zone is more complex than determining the BVP for a spherical lens, yet the two processes involve the same basic principles. For spherical lenses:

- Contact lens power in air plus tear lens power in air should add up to ocular refraction.

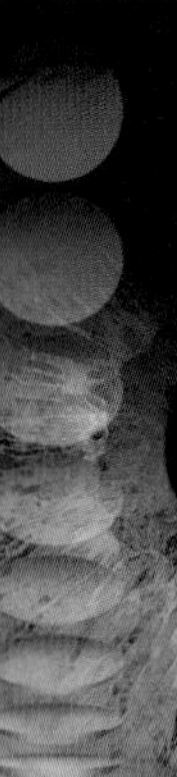

- With toric lenses, the same rule applies, but here the two separate meridians must be considered.

Example 3: Calculating the BVP for a rigid lens with a toroidal back optic zone

Spectacle refraction (vertex distance ignored): +2.50/–3.00 × 180.
(*Note*: the effect of the vertex distance must be taken into account if this distance is great or if the refractive power in either meridian exceeds 4.00 D.)

Keratometry reading: 8.04 mm (42.00 D) along 180
7.50 mm (45.00 D) along 90

A rigid spherical trial lens with BOZR 7.95 mm and BVP +1.00 D is placed on the cornea. Refraction with this lens in situ gives +1.00 DS (no residual astigmatism) and 6/6 acuity. (*Note*: the over-refraction is best performed over a spherical trial lens aligned along the flattest meridian of the cornea and only *one* over-refraction is required to calculate both BVPs.)

Based on the keratometry readings, BOZR of 8.00 and 7.55 mm are chosen to fit the horizontal and vertical meridians, respectively. The BVP of the contact lens (BVP_{CL}) is determined as with a rigid spherical lens, except that two meridians need to be considered instead of one.

$$BVP_{CL} = BVP_{trial} + OR$$

where BVP_{trial} = back vertex power of the trial lens along each meridian and OR = over-refraction.

For a spherical lens, if the BOZR of the trial lens is different from the BOZR to be ordered, the change in resultant tear lens power must then be considered.

Based on a tear lens refractive index of 1.336, this change in tear lens power is given by the formula:

$$\left(\frac{336}{BOZR_{final}} - \frac{336}{BOZR_{trial}}\right)$$

where $BOZR_{final}$ is the back optic zone radius of the lens to be ordered and $BOZR_{trial}$ is the back optic zone radius of the trial lens. Thus:

- For every 0.05 mm that the BOZR is flattened, approximately –0.25 D must be added to the BVP of the contact lens.
- Likewise, for every 0.05 mm that the BOZR is steepened, approximately +0.25 D must be added to the BVP of the contact lens.

This approximation only holds for relatively small differences in BOZR and, if in doubt, it is safer to use the above formula.

The back vertex power that needs to be ordered (BVP_{CL}) when calculated in full is then:

$$BVP_{CL} = BVP_{trial} + OR - \left(\frac{336}{BOZR_{final}} - \frac{336}{BOZR_{trial}}\right)$$

There will also be a change to the trial lens BOZR in at least one meridian. In this example, the back optic zone radii to be ordered are both different from the trial lens BOZR and so it will be necessary to allow for the change in tear lens power in both meridians.

$$\text{Along 180: } BVP_{CL} = +1.00 + 1.00 - \left(\frac{336}{8.00} - \frac{336}{7.95}\right) = +2.25\text{ D}$$

$$\text{Along 90: } BVP_{CL} = +1.00 + 1.00 - \left(\frac{336}{7.55} - \frac{336}{7.95}\right) = -0.25\text{ D}$$

(When calculating BVP, values are rounded off to the nearest 0.25 D.)

The final prescription (Rx) of lens is therefore:

BOZR 8.00 mm along 180: +2.25 D
BOZR 7.55 mm along 90: –0.25 D

Alternatively, the BVPs of the contact lens can be calculated empirically, firstly by using the required BOZR and the keratometry reading of the patient to calculate the tear lens power (BVP_{tears}) and then using the formula:

$$BVP_{CL} = \text{ocular refraction} - BVP_{tears}$$

to calculate the back vertex powers along both meridians.

The power of the tear lens is obtained from the following formula:

$$BVP_{tears} = \left(\frac{336}{BOZR} - \frac{336}{K}\right)$$

where K is the corneal front surface radius of curvature (in millimetres) along that respective meridian.

Once again, it can be approximated (for very small differences) that there is 0.25 D of tear lens power for every 0.05 mm difference between the BOZR and the corneal front surface radius of curvature.

$$\text{Along 180: } BVP_{tears} = \left(\frac{336}{8.00} - \frac{336}{8.04}\right) \sim +0.25\text{ D}$$

$$BVP_{CL} = +2.50 - 0.25 = +2.25\text{ D}$$

$$\text{Along 90: } BVP_{tears} = \left(\frac{336}{7.55} - \frac{336}{7.50}\right) \sim -0.25\text{ D}$$

$$BVP_{CL} = -0.50 - (-0.25) = -0.25\text{ D}$$

While the empirical method is probably simpler, more accurate results are obtained when the BVP is calculated from a refraction over a trial lens.

RESIDUAL ASTIGMATISM

Residual astigmatism is frequently confused with induced astigmatism or corneal astigmatism. Residual astigmatism has been variously defined (Goldberg 1964), including the simplistic definition which states that residual astigmatism is the component of the spectacle (ocular) astigmatism which is not due to the cornea.

In the context of rigid lens fitting:

Definition: Residual astigmatism is the astigmatic component of a lens required to correct fully an eye wearing a spherical powered rigid contact lens with a spherical BOZR.

Example 4: Calculating the BVP for a rigid lens with a toroidal back optic zone when there is residual astigmatism present

Spectacle refraction (vertex distance ignored): +2.50/–2.00 × 180

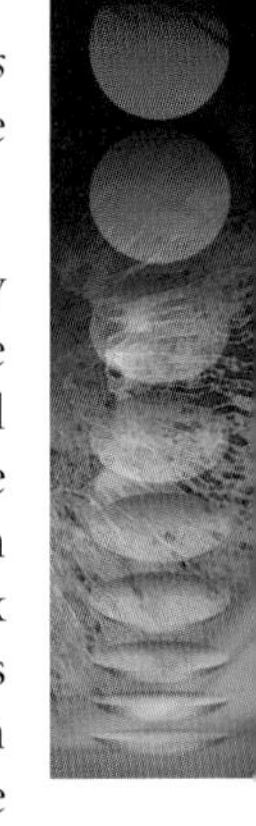

Keratometry reading: 8.04 mm (42.00 D) along 180
7.50 mm (45.00 D) along 90

A rigid spherical trial lens with BOZR 7.95 mm and BVP +1.00 D is placed on the cornea. Refraction with this lens in situ gives +2.00/–1.00 × 90 and 6/6 acuity.

Based on the keratometry readings, BOZR of 8.00 and 7.55 mm are chosen to fit the horizontal and vertical meridians, respectively.

In this case, the residual astigmatism is equal to –1.00 DC × 90. If the patient is to be given the best possible vision, it is necessary to incorporate the correction for this residual cylinder into the BVP to be ordered.

The method for determining the BVPs is the same as used in the previous example:

$$\text{Along 180: } BVP_{CL} = +1.00 + \mathbf{1.00} - \left(\frac{336}{8.00} - \frac{336}{7.95}\right) = +2.25\text{ D}$$

$$\text{Along 90: } BVP_{CL} = +1.00 + \mathbf{2.00} - \left(\frac{336}{7.55} - \frac{336}{7.95}\right) = +0.75\text{ D}$$

(*Note*: the values for the over-refraction are in bold to emphasize the fact that there is residual astigmatism present in this case.)

Final Rx of the lens:

BOZR 8.00 mm along 180: +2.25 D
BOZR 7.55 mm along 90: +0.75 D

In Examples 3 and 4, the powers specified are the BVPs of the toric lens in the appropriate meridians. These are the powers read by the laboratory when checking the lens on a focimeter (vertometer).

It is useful, in considering bitoric lenses, to draw a representation of meridional powers to avoid confusing axes and meridians (Fig. 12.3).

The incorporation of the correction for residual astigmatism into the toric lens prescription is not difficult.

- If residual astigmatism, in negative cylinder form, has its axis *parallel* to the negative cylinder axis in the spectacle prescription, then the *spectacle astigmatism is greater than corneal astigmatism* by an amount equal to the residual astigmatism.
- Alternatively, if residual astigmatism, in negative cylinder form, has its axis *perpendicular* to the negative cylinder axis in the spectacle prescription, then the *corneal astigmatism is greater than spectacle astigmatism* by an amount equal to the residual astigmatism.

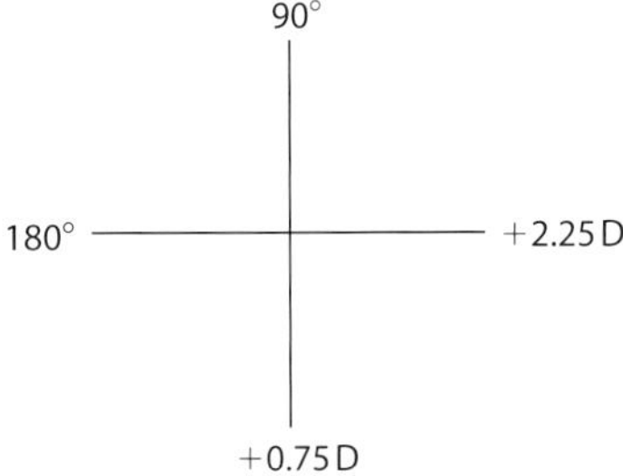

Figure 12.3 Meridional powers required in Example 4. This shows the powers and directions as they will be measured by the contact lens laboratory

The axis of the residual astigmatism may not correspond exactly with one of the principal corneal meridians. If the difference between the axes of the spectacle refraction and the principal meridians of the cornea is less than 20°, one can assume that the axes of the spectacle refraction over the lens *do* correspond with the principal meridians of corneal curvature and complex oblique cylinder calculations are obviated. The resulting error is usually not significant (Lindsay 1996). If the difference between the axes is more than 20°, an oblique bitoric lens (where the principal meridians of the toroidal front and back surfaces are not parallel) will be required.

The information provided so far on refraction with toroidal back optic zones is sufficient to be able to calculate the BVPs of rigid toric lenses, yet no mention has been made of terms such as 'induced astigmatism' and 'bitoric lenses'. These elements are important but power calculations for rigid toric lenses can be carried out without them and are relatively straightforward. Factors such as induced astigmatism arise from the specified back optic zone radii and calculated BVPs, such that they are incidental to the determination of the toric lens prescription.

INDUCED ASTIGMATISM

Definition: Induced astigmatism is the astigmatic effect created in the contact lens/tear lens system by the toroidal back optic zone bounding two surfaces of different RI, namely the lens and the tears.

Example 5

Consider the lens designed in Example 3.

Back surface toric curves of 8.00 and 7.55 mm, and n = 1.47. The surface powers of these curves in air are –58.75 and –62.25, giving a back surface cylinder of –3.50 DC × 180.

On the eye, where the back surface is against tears (n = 1.336), the powers of the back surface interface are –16.75 and –17.75, respectively and the back surface cylinder in tear fluid is –1.00 DC × 180. This 1.00 D back surface cylinder ('induced astigmatism') must be compensated by generating a +1.00 DC × 180 on the front surface (Sarver et al. 1985).

The front surface cylinder correction for the induced astigmatism is automatically incorporated into the lens prescription when the practitioner calculates the BVPs for the rigid toric lens. Once again, consider the lens designed in Example 3, where BOZR = 8.00/7.55 mm and n = 1.47, ct = 0.25 mm, BVP is +2.25 and –0.25 as calculated. The front surface powers (calculated using thick lens formulae) would be +60.37/+61.35, respectively. Specification of the appropriate BOZR and BVP therefore results in the front surface incorporating the required compensating cylinder of +1.00 DC × 180.

Consequently, once the practitioner has calculated the required BVP, it is *not* necessary to perform the additional calculations to determine what cylinder is needed on the front

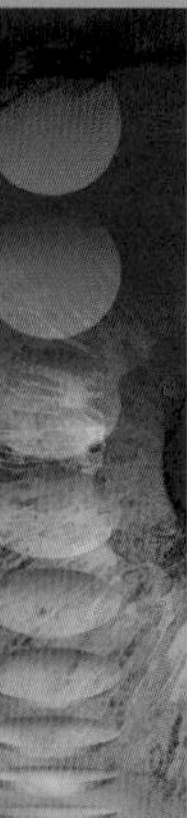

surface of the lens to correct for the induced astigmatism. This arises from the specified BOZR and calculated BVPs. In other words, the ascertained toric lens prescription determines the degree of induced astigmatism, not the other way around. This important point is demonstrated in Example 6.

Example 6

Spectacle refraction (vertex distance ignored):	+3.00/–6.00 × 180
Keratometry reading:	8.00 mm (42.19 D) along 180 7.00 mm (48.21 D) along 90

A rigid spherical trial lens with BOZR 8.00 mm and BVP +1.00 D is placed on the cornea. Refraction with this lens in situ gives +2.00 DS (no residual astigmatism) and 6/6 acuity.

Based on the keratometry readings, BOZR of 8.00 and 7.00 mm are chosen to fit the horizontal and vertical meridians, respectively.

$$\text{Along 180: } BVP_{CL} = +1.00 + 2.00 + \left(\frac{336}{8.00} - \frac{336}{8.00}\right) = +3.00\text{ D}$$

$$\text{Along 90: } BVP_{CL} = +1.00 + 2.00 + \left(\frac{336}{8.00} - \frac{336}{7.00}\right) = -3.00\text{ D}$$

Specification of these BVPs (+3.00 D and –3.00 D) along with the respective BOZR (8.00 mm and 7.00 mm) will *automatically* bring about the incorporation of the front surface cylinder to correct for the induced astigmatism. This can be demonstrated by calculating the resultant front surface powers based on the BVPs and BOZR to be ordered.

Assume the refractive index for the rigid lens material is 1.47 and the lens centre thickness is 0.30 mm:

Along 180: Back surface power of the contact lens

$$= \frac{1000(1 - 1.47)}{8.00} = -58.75\text{ D}$$

BVP = +3.00 D

Using thick lens formula for the front surface power (see Chapter 6), F_1:

$$F_1 = \frac{F_{v'} - F_2}{1 + (F_{v'} - F_2)\frac{t}{n}}$$

Front surface power of the contact lens = +60.98 D

Along 90: Back surface power of the contact lens

$$= \frac{1000(1 - 1.47)}{7.00} = -67.14\text{ D}$$

BVP = –3.00 D

Again, using thick lens formula:

Front surface power of the contact lens = +63.31

Hence, the total power of the front surface is +60.98 DS with +2.33 DC × 180. This front surface cylinder represents the correction for the induced astigmatism.

The correction for the induced astigmatism is always a plus cylinder with the *same axis as the flatter principal meridian of the cornea* (in other words, the same axis as the corneal cylinder). The magnitude of the induced astigmatism is directly proportional to the degree of contact lens toricity and the refractive index of the lens material.

A quick way to calculate the induced astigmatism is to use the appropriate radii as they change from the rigid lens to tears. That is:

$$\text{Power of the RGP lens/tear boundary} = \frac{1000(1.336 - 1.47)}{r} = \frac{-134}{r}$$

where r = radius (in millimetres) and assuming n = 1.47 for the rigid lens material.

By subtracting this value for one principal meridian from the other, the value for the induced astigmatism may be obtained directly. For rigid lens materials with a different refractive index, –134/r no longer applies; for example, a refractive index of 1.45 would yield a figure of 114/r for determining the surface power at the lens/tear boundary.

SPHERICAL POWER EQUIVALENT OR COMPENSATED BITORIC LENSES

These are lenses which, like spherical lenses, do not correct for any residual astigmatism (Sarver 1963). They are bitoric because the front surface contains a cylinder solely for the correction of the induced astigmatism. The lens designed in Example 3 would be classed as a compensated bitoric lens.

> *Definition: A compensated bitoric is a lens designed to correct all of the refractive cylinder created due to the corneal toricity* (Lowther 1990).

If the corneal toricity is equal to the spectacle astigmatism, when a compensated bitoric is placed on the cornea the cylinder will be fully corrected. It can rotate on the eye without visual disturbance because the effect of the rotation is counteracted by an equal change in the cylinder power of the tear lens.

Regarding the front surface cylinder, the correction for induced astigmatism is only necessary because the toroidal back optic zone creates the induced astigmatism along its principal meridians. Consequently, it does not matter if the lens does rotate as it carries its correction for induced astigmatism with it when it moves away from its intended position.

CYLINDRICAL POWER EQUIVALENT TORIC LENSES

All other types of rigid toric lens come under this classification, and the unifying feature of these lenses is that they incorporate a correction for residual astigmatism. This category can be further subdivided as follows.

Alignment bitoric lenses

These are also known as 'parallel bitoric' lenses. Both the front and back surfaces are toroidal. The front surface incorporates correction for residual astigmatism as well as for the induced astigmatism. In addition, the axes of the spectacle refraction over the lens correspond with the principal meridians of corneal curvature, so the correction for the residual astigmatism will be along one of the principal meridians of the lens (hence the name 'alignment bitoric'). As such, the use of the term alignment bitoric here should not be confused with alignment in regard to lens fitting. The lens in Example 4 is an alignment bitoric lens.

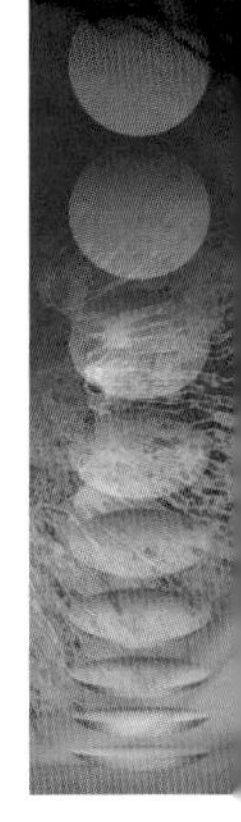

Back surface toric lenses

These have a toroidal back surface but a spherical front surface. The design principle is similar to that for alignment bitoric lenses. As with alignment bitoric lenses, the front surface incorporates correction for residual astigmatism as well as for the induced astigmatism and the axes of the spectacle refraction over the lens correspond with the principal meridians of corneal curvature, so the correction for the residual astigmatism is along one of the principal meridians of the lens.

In the case of a back surface toric lens, however, the correction for the residual astigmatism is equal and opposite to the correction for the induced astigmatism. Hence the two required cylindrical corrections cancel each other out, meaning that the front surface can be left spherical.

Very occasionally, a case of induced and residual astigmatism cancelling out one another is encountered in practice, as in the following example.

Example 7

Spectacle refraction (vertex distance ignored):	+3.00/–4.00 × 180
Keratometry reading:	8.04 mm (42.00 D) along 180
	7.50 mm (45.00 D) along 90

A rigid spherical trial lens with BOZR 7.95 mm and BVP +1.00 D is placed on the cornea. Refraction with this lens in situ gives +1.50/–1.00 × 180 and 6/6 acuity. Hence there is residual astigmatism present of –1.00 DC × 180.

Based on the keratometry readings, BOZR of 8.00 and 7.55 mm are chosen to fit the horizontal and vertical meridians, respectively.

The induced astigmatism can be determined using the method described previously of calculating the change in power of the RGP lens/tear boundary. By subtracting the values found of –134/r for one principal meridian from the other (assuming a lens refractive index of 1.47), the value for the induced astigmatism is obtained.

$$\text{Induced astigmatism} = \frac{-134}{8.00} - \frac{-134}{7.55} = +1.00\text{ D}$$

The induced astigmatism, expressed in negative cylinder form, will always have the same axis as the corneal astigmatism. Hence, the induced back surface cylinder here is –1.00 DC × 180.

The correction for the residual astigmatism is –1.00 DC × 180, so the residual astigmatism and the induced astigmatism should cancel each other out. This can be confirmed by calculation of the BVPs and the front and back surface powers of the lens (assuming a lens centre thickness of 0.25 mm):

$$\text{Along 180: } BVP_{CL} = +1.00 + 1.50 + \left(\frac{336}{7.95} - \frac{336}{8.00}\right) = +2.75\text{ D}$$

$$\text{Back surface power of the contact lens} = \frac{1000(1-1.47)}{+8.00}$$

$$= -58.75\text{ D}$$

Front surface power of the contact lens = +60.86 D

$$\text{Along 90: } BVP_{CL} = +1.00 + 0.50 + \left(\frac{336}{7.95} - \frac{336}{7.55}\right) = -0.75\text{ D}$$

Back surface power of the contact lens

$$= \frac{1000(1-1.47)}{+7.55} = -62.25\text{ D}$$

Front surface power of the contact lens = +60.86

The front surface is spherical (same power along both principal meridians) so the residual and induced astigmatism have indeed cancelled each other out. (When calculating surface powers, for clinical purposes a difference in power of ≤0.12 D between the principal meridians constitutes a spherical surface.)

Many practitioners believe that most rigid toric lenses can be made to correct residual and induced astigmatism utilizing a back surface toric design only and yet the preceding discussion clearly demonstrates the absurdity of this position. A back surface toric design is only possible if the correction for the residual astigmatism is *equal* and *opposite* to the correction for the induced astigmatism. A back surface toric design is therefore only worth considering if the patient's ocular astigmatism is greater than the corneal astigmatism (Meyler & Ruston 1995). The residual astigmatism must also then be of a magnitude whereby it will be neutralized by the resultant induced astigmatism. The likelihood of both of these requirements being met is low, so only in a small percentage of cases will a back surface toric design alone be appropriate. Indeed, in most cases the induced astigmatism usually exaggerates the effect of the residual astigmatism.

Front surface toric lenses

Residual astigmatism frequently needs to be corrected where a spherical back optic zone fits well. Such a lens requires a toroidal front surface but must avoid lens rotation, otherwise visual disturbance will result. When the corneal astigmatism is less than 2.00 D, a toric back surface will not always prevent lens rotation and so another form of lens stabilization is required, such as prism ballast or truncation.

Prism ballast is the most commonly used method of lens stabilization and can be used in combination with a toroidal back surface where the corneal astigmatism is not enough (<2.00 D) to maintain the proper position of a bitoric lens but is large enough (>1.00 D) to cause a front toric lens to become unstable (Gonce & Kastl 1994):

- Prescribe the lens in the normal manner with the addition of between 1 and 3 Δ.
- Record the location as 270 or 280 to ensure accuracy rather than 'down along 90' or 'down along 100'.

Truncations can also be added if prism ballasting is insufficient to stabilize the lens.

- Prescribe the lens in the usual way with the addition of the front surface cylinder at the correct angle relative to the estimated or observed position of the lens base.
- Observe the relationship of the lower lid to the edge of the lens.
- Cut the truncation to align with the lower lid (Fig. 12.4).

Prism ballasting can result in lenses sitting inferiorly, causing symptoms of discomfort and flare. Truncations can also be uncomfortable and are not always successful in preventing lens rotation. Consequently, a soft toric lens is generally preferred (see below) when fitting patients who have significant residual astigmatism but negligible corneal astigmatism.

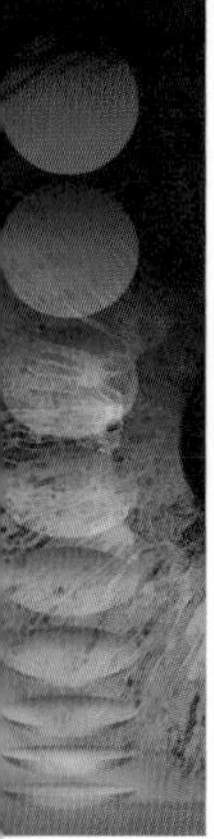

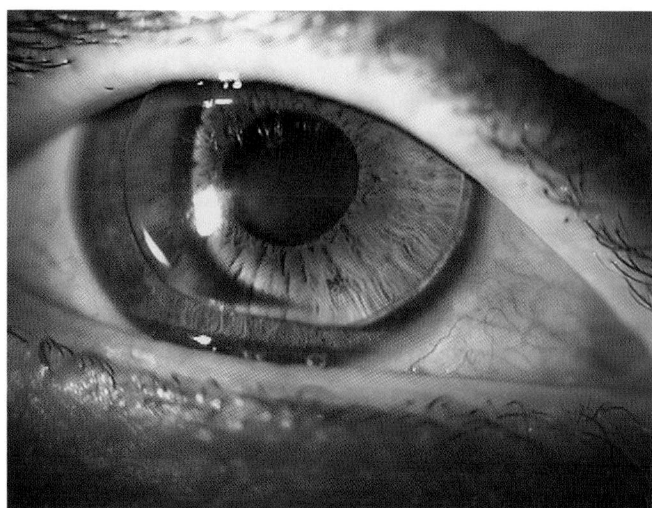

Figure 12.4 A prism-ballasted rigid toric lens with single truncation

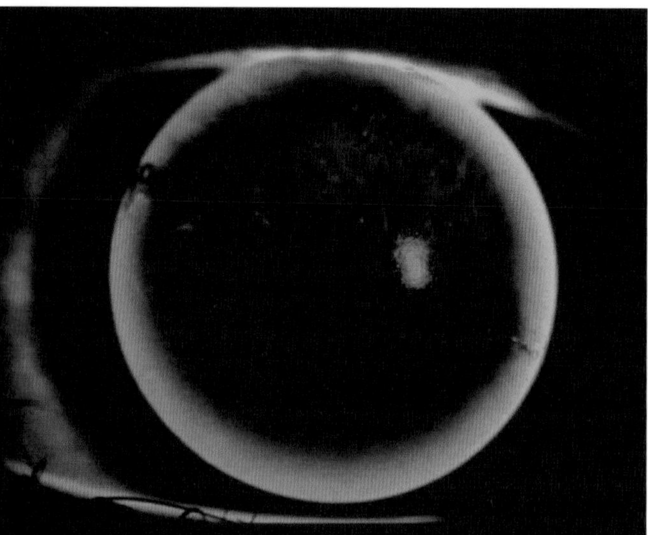

Figure 12.5 A right lens with a toroidal back optic zone fitted in alignment. Keratometer reading 8.13 mm along 160, 7.62 mm along 70. Lens BOZR 8.10 × 7.70 mm. The 8.10 meridian is marked with grease pencil and can be seen aligning well with the 160 meridian. There is no significant rotation, thus permitting accurate correction of residual astigmatism, as well as induced astigmatism, with a front surface cylinder

Oblique bitoric lenses

As with alignment bitorics, these have both a toroidal front and back surface. With oblique bitoric lenses, however, the principal meridians of the toroidal back and front surfaces are not parallel, due to a difference between the axes of the spectacle refraction and the principal meridians of corneal curvature. The specification and manufacture of these lenses is difficult. One solution is to use a fitting set of lenses, all of which have a toroidal back optic zone and a spherical front surface. Refraction is performed over the appropriate trial lens and the oblique cylinder obtained is incorporated onto the front surface of the lens. These lenses are rarely prescribed.

Effect of lens rotation

With all cylindrical power equivalent bitoric lenses, some visual disturbance will occur with rotation as the lenses incorporate a correction for residual astigmatism. The axis of correction for the residual astigmatism remains fixed in relation to the eye.

Because of the limitation on rotation, when there is a small amount of residual astigmatism, it is not worthwhile incorporating its correction. If the residual astigmatism is clinically significant, it should be incorporated into the lens, but lens rotation must be kept to a minimum (Figs 12.5, 12.6).

With lenses incorporating a toroidal back surface, rotation is generally not a problem due to the stabilizing effect of the toric back surface on the toric cornea (provided there is sufficient corneal toricity).

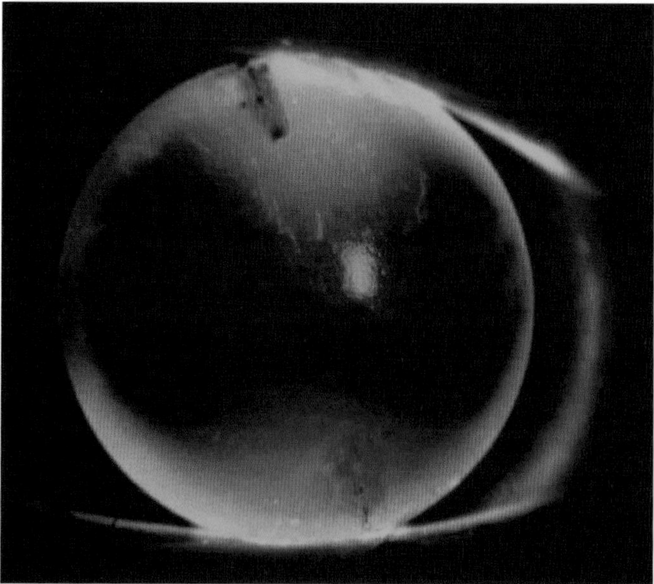

Figure 12.6 Same right eye as in Figure 12.5. Lens BOZR 8.05 × 7.75 mm with 8.05 meridian marked with grease pencil. This should be located along the 160 meridian, but, as shown, this lens rotates badly, thus permitting only the accurate correction of induced astigmatism with a front surface cylinder

Fitting soft toric lenses

For many years it was held that prospective contact lens wearers with clinically significant astigmatism could not be fitted successfully with soft lenses. However, current soft toric lens technology allows the majority of these patients to now be corrected.

INDICATIONS FOR THE USE OF SOFT TORIC LENSES

Soft toric lenses (in preference to soft spherical lenses) can correct both corneal and non-corneal astigmatism. Soft lenses do not mask corneal astigmatism but rather conform to the shape of the cornea. Consequently, the cylinder must be incorporated into the BVP of the lens.

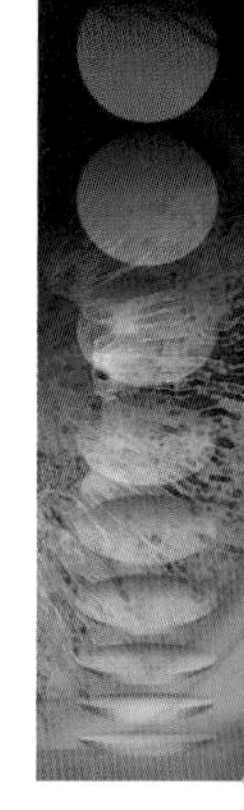

Numerous manufacturers have claimed that their spherical soft lenses were able to correct, satisfactorily, astigmatism of between 1 and 2 D: rarely is this achieved. Bernstein et al. (1991) showed that there was no statistically significant masking of corneal cylinder even with standard thickness soft spherical lenses. Indeed, the most likely residual astigmatism found while wearing a soft spherical contact lens is the ocular astigmatism determined from an accurate subjective spectacle refraction.

CRITERIA FOR USE OF SOFT TORIC LENSES

Practitioners should avoid using criteria such as 'all patients with cylinders greater than a certain amount should be fitted with soft toric lenses'. Instead, each patient should be assessed individually, taking into account the following:

- *Degree of astigmatism*: There is no simple answer as to how much astigmatism should be left uncorrected. As a generalization, 1.00 D or more of astigmatism should be corrected, although there will be significant variability between patients. Holden (1975), in discussing the criteria for the prescribing of toric lenses, showed that 45% of the population required a cylindrical correction of up to 0.75 D and 25% of the population required a correction of 1.00 D or more.
- *Cylinder axis*: An uncorrected cylinder with an oblique axis will cause greater degradation of visual image compared with an equivalent amount of uncorrected with-the-rule or against-the-rule astigmatism (Lindsay 1998).
- *Ocular dominance*: Uncorrected astigmatism is more likely to be accepted by the patient if it is in the non-dominant eye. Patients may tolerate an uncorrected cylinder of up to 2.00 D in their non-dominant eye, while at the same time requiring that a cylinder as small as 0.50 D be corrected in their dominant eye. Where a patient has unequal visual acuities, higher degrees of uncorrected astigmatism will usually be tolerated in the eye with the poorer acuity.
- *Viability of other alternatives*: Are soft toric lenses the best option or would the patient be better off with spectacles or rigid lenses? A patient with high degrees (>5.00 D) of both corneal and spectacle astigmatism would most likely achieve better acuities with a rigid toric lens.
- *Assessment of the patient's visual needs*: Usually the less critical the visual task, the greater the amount of astigmatism that can be left uncorrected (and vice versa). For example, a musician may require that a cylinder as small as 0.50 D be corrected to enable music to be read, while a person with no critical visual requirements may be happy with a cylinder as high as 2.00 D left uncorrected, as long as the spherical component of their refractive error is corrected.

DESIGN OF SOFT TORIC LENSES

Satisfactory visual performance depends on two key design components: surface optics and lens stabilization.

SURFACE OPTICS

A soft toric lens will always be bitoric in lens form on the eye due to the wrapping of the front and back surfaces onto the cornea.

There are two principal categories of surface optics:

- Toroidal back surface with a spherical front surface.
- Spherical back surface with a toroidal front surface.

The optical considerations for soft toric lenses are different from those encountered when using rigid lenses. A soft toric lens tends to wrap onto the cornea such that there is a negligible tear lens between the back surface of the lens and the front surface of the cornea. Consequently, the optical principles of rigid toric lenses do not apply. There are no tear lens calculations to perform and, as discussed above, the ocular astigmatism will be corrected by incorporation of a cylinder into the BVP of the lens.

The choice of design (i.e. toric back surface versus toric front surface) is generally based more on considerations relating to manufacture, lens stability and physiological performance. Currently, the majority of soft toric lenses prescribed globally are of a planned replacement form and virtually all of these lenses are mass produced by a process of cast moulding. All other soft toric lenses are custom made for the patient by a process of either crimping or generating, the latter being a specific form of lathe-cutting devoted to the production of toric surfaces. As a general rule, generated toric lenses will be thinner and show better reproducibility than those made from crimping techniques.

STABILIZATION TECHNIQUES

All forms of soft toric lens need to be stabilized to minimize rotation, so that the toric optics of the lens can be maintained in the desired orientation to correct the ocular astigmatism. The orientation must be predictable and consistent, otherwise suboptimal vision will result.

Toroidal back surface

Some practitioners and laboratories believe that a soft toric lens with a toric back surface will generally locate better than a front surface toric lens, because it is believed that the back toric surface is more likely to align, or 'lock on', to the matching toroidal corneal surface. However, experience has shown that a toroidal back surface alone is insufficient to achieve lens stabilization.

Prism ballast

Prism ballast has long been used as a technique for stabilizing toric lenses but it does have certain disadvantages when applied to soft lens designs.

- The additional thickness of a prism can be a problem in that it reduces oxygen transmissibility in the thick prism zone.
- The prismatic area can cause discomfort in patients with sensitive lids.
- These lenses often sit low on the eye.
- If a prism is prescribed monocularly it may cause unwanted vertical prismatic effects. This can be overcome by prescribing a similar prism for the other eye, although this can prove difficult if the other eye requires a spherical lens or is

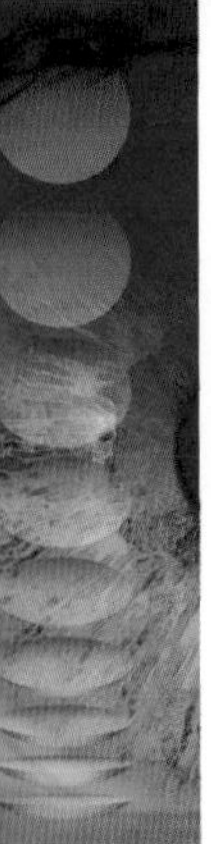

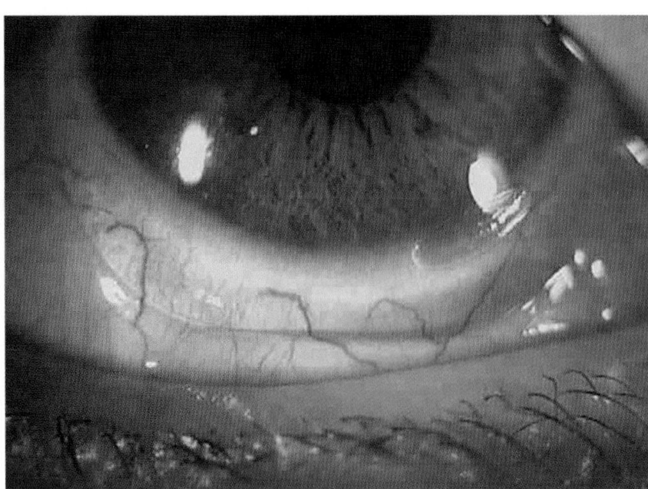

Figure 12.7 A prism-ballasted soft toric lens with a single (inferior) truncation. The truncation has been cut at the angle of the middle third of the lower lid, but in this photograph the patient had to look up in order to bring the truncation near the lower lid. The lid margin may thus only have a limited effect on the truncation. Note the prominent bubble under the lens near the truncation – a common problem with these lenses

emmetropic. Fortunately, prism ballast does not often give rise to binocular problems (Gasson 1977).

The thicker edge in the region of the prism base can be thinned during the manufacturing stage to form a 'comfort' chamfer (Edwards 1999), although this will slightly negate the intended thickness differential along the vertical axis of the lens. The problem here is finding an acceptable compromise between comfort and lens stability.

The underlying principle of prism ballast is to balance the forces acting on the lens in order to stabilize it. Originally it was thought that the major locating force was provided by displacing the centre of gravity away from the geometric centre of the lens – this was subsequently shown not to be the case (Hanks 1983).

Peri-ballast

With this method, the lens is manufactured with a minus carrier, with the carrier being thicker inferiorly. Therefore, the prismatic thickness profile changes are confined to the lens edge only, i.e. outside the optic zone. This design is fabricated simply by removing the high minus lenticular carrier from the superior portion of the lens, leaving a prism ballast effect inferiorly.

Truncation

Truncation is reasonably successful in stabilizing lenses with thick edges, especially when combined with prism ballast (Fig. 12.7).

Either a single or a double truncation can be used (Strachan 1975). With the former, the truncation can be anywhere between 0.5 and 1.5 mm and is usually inferior so that the lower lid acts as a stabilizing force.

Truncation does have disadvantages:

- The truncated edge can make the lens uncomfortable to wear.
- The measurement of the lid angle can be difficult and imprecise.
- Quite often the truncation does not work, with the lid angle appearing to have no effect on the positioning or location of the lens.
- Lens instability can occur with oblique cylinders (see below) because of their uneven construction.

For these reasons, soft toric lens truncation is rarely used nowadays.

Dynamic stabilization

Dynamic stabilization was initially developed by Fanti (1975) and is currently the most commonly used method of stabilization for soft toric lenses. The lens is orientated by pressure primarily from the upper lid, but also from the lower lid. Hanks (1983) used the analogy of the 'watermelon seed' to illustrate how dynamic stabilization works. Simply put, pressure applied to the thin end of a watermelon seed by the fingers (i.e. the pressure exerted on the thin zone of a lens between the upper lid and globe) causes the watermelon seed to move away from the fingers (i.e. causes the lens to orientate away from the squeezing force of the eyelid and globe). Hanks (1983) therefore demonstrated that the effect of the thickness profile interaction with the upper lid is the dominant stabilizing component and that gravity has little effect.

With dynamic stabilization, the contact lens toricity is confined to the central portion of the lens. The superior and inferior 'dynamic stabilization' zones of the lens incorporate a thickness differential and the action of the lids on these superior and inferior lens chamfers stabilizes the lens (Fig. 12.8). Many such designs – referred to as 'double slab-off', 'thin-zone' or 'reverse prism' – are manufactured throughout the world.

Dynamic stabilization avoids the complications of truncation and prism ballast. Oxygen transmissibility is not reduced as additional thickness is minimal. The excessive thickness of prism ballast lenses can be avoided and, by producing toroidal back surfaces, the average lens thickness is only slightly greater than that of equivalent spherical designs.

The main disadvantage of the dynamic stabilization design is that the thickness differential at the edge of the lens is dependent on the spherical power of the lens. Lower-powered lenses have a reduced thickness differential and, therefore, a design incorporating prism ballast is often more effective in stabilizing a soft toric lens with a low spherical power component (Snyder 1998).

The orientation in which such a lens is inserted into the eye is generally not important since the lid action during blinking will quickly stabilize the lens to the correct orientation. With some designs, the upper half of the lens is larger and thinner than the lower half to utilize the greater blink action of the upper eyelid. With these designs it is more important that the lens is inserted the correct way up. To facilitate this – and to assist the practitioner in determining the degree of in-eye lens rotation – such lenses will generally have some form of marking at the 6 or 12 o'clock position.

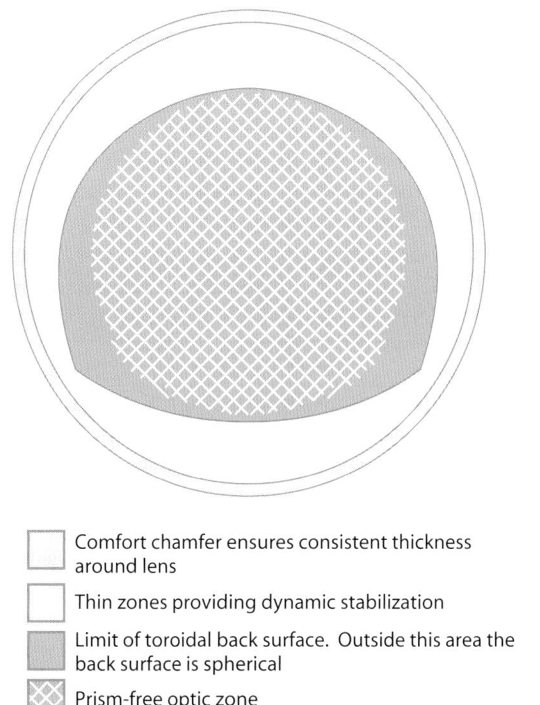

Figure 12.8 Soft toric lens showing the design features that help to minimize lens rotation. Note the prism-free optic zone in the toroidal region of the lens

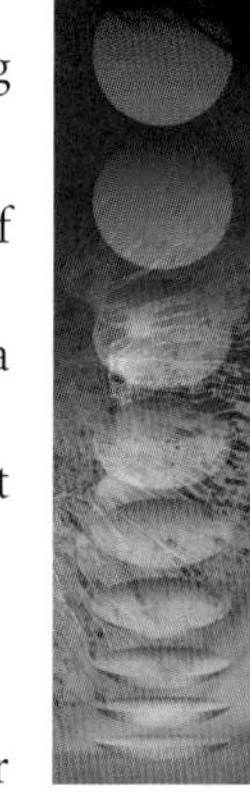

PRINCIPLES OF CORRECTION

It is clear that to produce a stable ocular correction for the astigmatic eye, the lens must:

- Align closely over the central cornea in front of the pupil.
- Provide the correct power while in situ.
- Stabilize effectively to prevent the rotation of the meridional powers away from their intended orientation.

FITTING

The fitting principles for soft toric lenses are similar to those for all soft spherical lenses (see Chapter 10). A well-fitting lens is comfortable in all directions of gaze, gives complete corneal coverage and centres well. On blinking there should be approximately 0.25–0.5 mm of vertical movement when the eye is in the primary position. On upwards gaze or lateral movements of the eye, the lens should lag by no more than 0.5 mm.

The TD of the lens influences both lens centration and lens stability. Generally, when specifying the lens diameter, the practitioner should err on the large side, as a larger diameter means that more area is available for the stabilization zones to take effect in the periphery of the lens.

Current soft toric lens designs will not stabilize on the eye if they are fitted tight, as the locating forces designed to stabilize orientation are ineffective (Holden 1976). Consequently, a steeply fitting lens may actually decrease stability and lead to limbal indentation and fluctuating vision, the latter being caused by the soft lens vaulting the corneal apex.

- A well-fitting lens will be stable and quickly return to axis if mislocated.
- A tight-fitting lens will show stable lens orientation but a slow return to axis if mislocated.
- A loose-fitting lens will demonstrate unstable and inconsistent lens orientation (Hanks & Weisbarth 1983).

BACK VERTEX POWER DETERMINATION

The determination of BVP for a soft toric lens is much easier than that for a rigid toric lens. Due to the absence of a tear lens, the BVP should be similar to the spectacle refraction (or ocular refraction if the vertex distance effect is significant). This is determined either empirically by using the patient's spectacle refraction or by carrying out a spherocylindrical over-refraction (SCO) over either a spherical or a toric trial lens.

Use of a spherical trial lens is preferable, as an SCO with a toric trial lens may require complex calculations involving oblique cylinders in order to determine the required lens power. When using a spherical trial lens, the resultant toric lens power is simply calculated by adding the SCO to the BVP of the trial lens. With both methods, some arbitrary allowance for lens rotation may have to be incorporated into the final lens prescription.

EFFECT OF LENS ROTATION

A considerable degree of cylindrical error can be induced when a soft toric contact lens does not stabilize satisfactorily and rotates away from the intended orientation (Lindsay et al. 1997); this phenomenon is demonstrated in Table 12.1.

For example, if the contact lens incorporates a cylindrical correction of –2.00 DC × 180, a mislocation of the axis by 10° results in a spherocylindrical error of +0.35/–0.69 × 40.

A useful rule-of-thumb here is that:

A lens made to specification but mislocating on the eye will produce an over-refraction with a spherical equivalent equal to zero.

Where the sphere or cylinder power is also incorrect, the spherical equivalent of the over-refraction will not equal zero (Long 1991).

PREDICTING LENS ROTATION

Hanks and Weisbarth (1983) showed that soft toric lenses tend to rotate nasally by approximately 5–10°, where nasal rotation is designated as rotation of the inferior aspect of the lens towards the nose. However, there is significant variability in the actual amount and direction of lens rotation. This is due to the following.

Lid anatomy

Lid tension (tightness), position, angle and symmetry can all affect the location and stability of a toric lens on the eye. For example, tight lids are more likely to affect lens movement and location than loose lids.

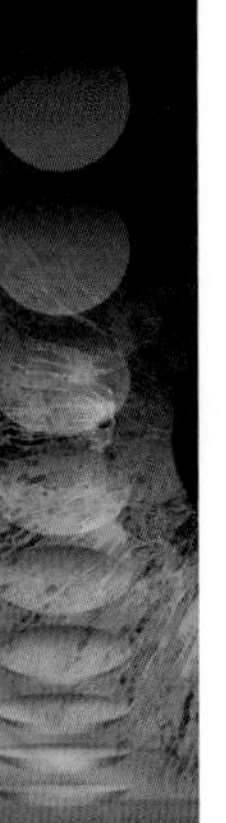

Table 12.1: Residual refractive error induced by mislocation of toric lenses of various cylindrical powers

Example

- Ocular refraction (required refractive correction) is: plano/−1.00 × 180
- A lens is placed on the eye of back vertex power: plano/−1.00 × 180
- An over-refraction yields a residual error of: +0.34/−0.68 × 35
- From the table, a mislocation is indicated of: −20°
- The lens back vertex power in situ is therefore: plano/−1.00 × 160

Mislocation (−)	−1.00 cylinder	−2.00 cylinder	−3.00 cylinder
5°	0.09/−0.17 × 42.5	0.17/−0.35 × 42.5	0.26/−0.52 × 42.5
10°	0.17/−0.35 × 40.0	0.35/−0.69 × 40.0	0.52/−1.04 × 40.0
15°	0.26/−0.52 × 37.5	0.52/−1.04 × 37.5	0.78/−1.55 × 37.5
20°	0.34/−0.68 × 35.0	0.68/−1.37 × 35.0	1.03/−2.05 × 35.0
25°	0.42/−0.85 × 32.5	0.85/−1.69 × 32.5	1.27/−2.54 × 32.5
30°	0.50/−1.00 × 30.0	1.00/−2.00 × 30.0	1.50/−3.00 × 30.0
35°	0.57/−1.15 × 27.5	1.15/−2.29 × 27.5	1.72/−3.44 × 27.5
40°	0.64/−1.29 × 25.0	1.29/−2.57 × 25.0	1.93/−3.86 × 25.0
45°	0.71/−1.41 × 22.5	1.41/−2.83 × 22.5	2.12/−4.24 × 22.5
50°	0.77/−1.53 × 20.0	1.53/−3.06 × 20.0	2.30/−4.60 × 20.0
55°	0.82/−1.64 × 17.5	1.64/−3.28 × 17.5	2.46/−4.91 × 17.5
60°	0.87/−1.73 × 15.0	1.73/−3.46 × 15.0	2.60/−5.20 × 15.0
65°	0.91/−1.81 × 12.5	1.81/−3.63 × 12.5	2.72/−5.44 × 12.5
70°	0.94/−1.88 × 10.0	1.88/−3.76 × 10.0	2.82/−5.64 × 10.0
75°	0.97/−1.93 × 7.5	1.93/−3.86 × 7.5	2.90/−5.80 × 7.5
80°	0.98/−1.97 × 5.0	1.97/−3.94 × 5.0	2.95/−5.91 × 5.0
85°	1.00/−1.99 × 2.5	1.99/−3.98 × 2.5	2.99/−5.98 × 2.5
90°	1.00/−2.00 × 0.0	2.00/−4.00 × 0.0	3.00/−6.00 × 0.0

Adapted from Bruce (2002).

Lens–eye relationship

The type of fit (steep, alignment or flat) has a significant bearing on lens position. As mentioned above, a tight lens will not be influenced by the locating forces designed to stabilize lens orientation (Holden 1976).

Lens thickness profile

It has been noted previously that with dynamic stabilization the thickness profile interaction with the upper lid is the dominant stabilizing force. While most soft toric lenses manufactured today have the contact lens toricity confined to the central portion of the lens, a thickness differential due to the astigmatic correction can still have a significant effect on lens location.

The lens thickness profile is determined by the power of the lens – in particular, the axis and magnitude of the astigmatic correction. For soft toric lenses incorporating dynamic stabilization, Gundel (1989) showed that rotational influence is greatest for lenses with cylinders at oblique axes (either between 30 and 60 or 120 and 150), followed by lenses incorporating correction for with-the-rule astigmatism (between 150 and 30), and is least for lenses with against-the-rule axes (between 60 and 120).

Gundel (1989) postulated that the principal factor affecting lens rotation is the initial point of contact between the upper lid and the thicker meridian of the lens. For toric lenses with oblique axes, the implication is that there will be notable rotational effects as contact from the upper lid will always affect one edge of the thicker meridian before the other. As the upper lid comes down, it will force the lens down at this first point of contact, causing it to rotate in a certain direction (Fig. 12.9).

A mislocating effect also occurs with lenses correcting for with-the-rule astigmatism as the lid contraction angle will usually be at a slight angle to the thickest axis of the lens (Holden 1975). For toric lenses incorporating a correction for against-the-rule astigmatism, upper lid contact with the thicker (horizontal) meridian will be fairly symmetrical and so the rotational effect is minimal.

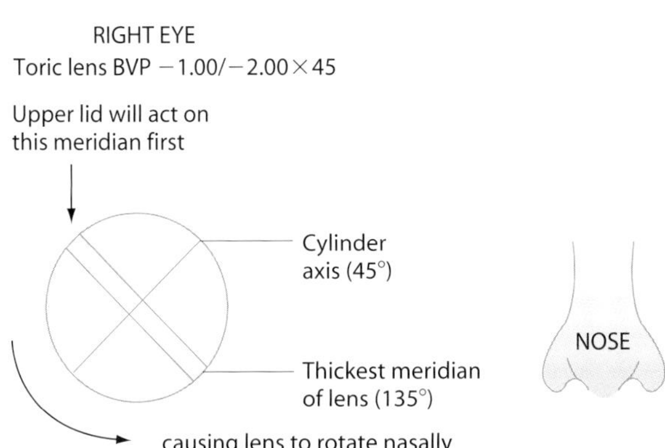

Figure 12.9 The effect of lid action on lens rotation for a soft toric lens with the prescription −1.00/−2.00 × 45 being worn in the right eye. As the upper lid comes down, it will first act on the lens (and the 135° meridian) at around the 10 o'clock position on the cornea. The downward motion on the lens at this point will cause it to rotate nasally

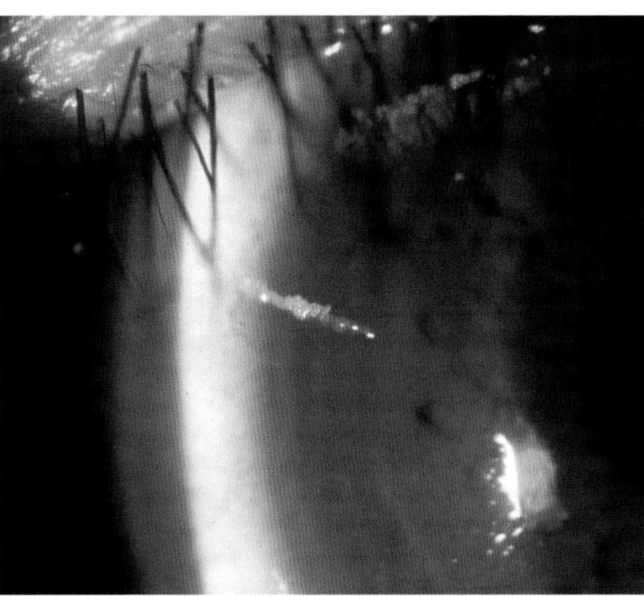

Figure 12.10 Scribe line on a soft toric lens. This lens has two scribe lines as markers with the reference points at the 3 and 9 o'clock locations (only the 9 o'clock mark is visible here). Debris has accumulated in the scribe line – a common site for deposit formation

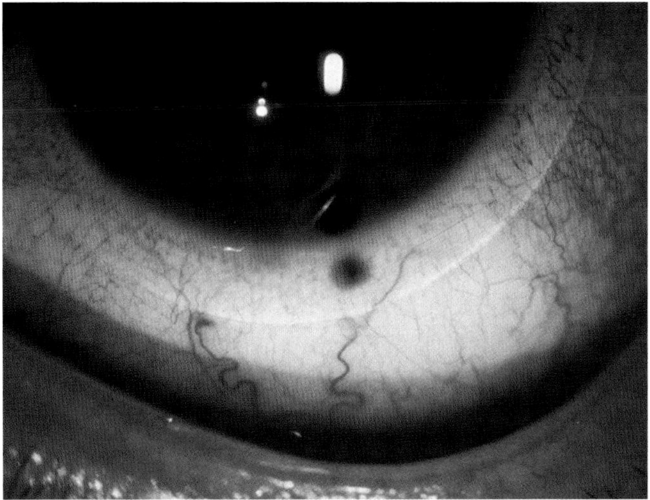

Figure 12.11 Soft toric lens with ink dots – one above the other – as markers for the 6 o'clock reference point. The upper ink dot is only just visible against the dark iris. Two dots are used to help with lens identification; the lens in the other (R) eye has just one ink dot. This lens is exhibiting about 10° temporal rotation

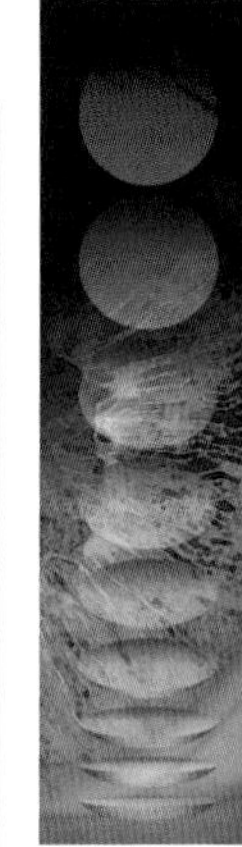

ALLOWING FOR LENS ROTATION

If the soft toric lens being ordered is expected to rotate on the eye, an allowance must be made for this rotation, otherwise the cylinder axis of the lens in situ will not coincide with the axis of the cylinder in the patient's ocular correction. When allowing for nasal rotation in the right eye, the amount of rotation should be subtracted from the required cylinder axis and vice versa for the left eye. When allowing for temporal rotation in the right eye, the amount of rotation should be added to the required cylinder axis and vice versa for the left eye.

Hence:

- If left eye and nasal rotation – add.
- If left eye and temporal rotation – subtract.
- If right eye and nasal rotation – subtract.
- If right eye and temporal rotation – add.

The acronym 'LARS' (left add, right subtract) – relating to nasal rotation of the inferior aspect of the lens – can be quite useful.

Many practitioners work on the principle that clockwise rotation necessitates adding the allowance for rotation to the required cylinder axis and counter-clockwise rotation requires subtracting the allowance for rotation to determine the final cylinder axis.

Hence:

- If clockwise rotation – add.
- If counter-clockwise rotation – subtract.

If, at the dispensing or after-care visit, the lens rotation is not as expected (but the lens location is stable), simply reorder the lens with the revised allowance for lens rotation. Rotational stability is generally more important than the degree of rotation. Lenses which give suboptimal, but stable acuity are more likely to be acceptable than lenses that give moments of clear vision followed by moments of poor vision as the lens rotates.

MEASUREMENT OF LENS ROTATION

Most soft toric lenses have markings at specific reference points so the degree of rotation can be assessed on the eye. The markings may be in the form of laser trace, scribe lines (Fig. 12.10), engraved dots or ink dots (Fig. 12.11). These markings are a point of reference by which the rotation of the lens can be assessed and do not represent the cylinder axis. They may either be at the 6 o'clock position of the lens or in the horizontal lens meridian at the 3 and 9 o'clock positions, the latter being

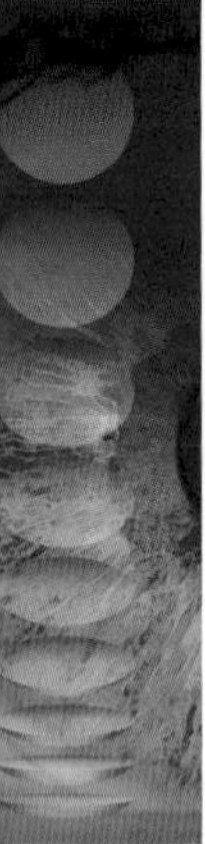

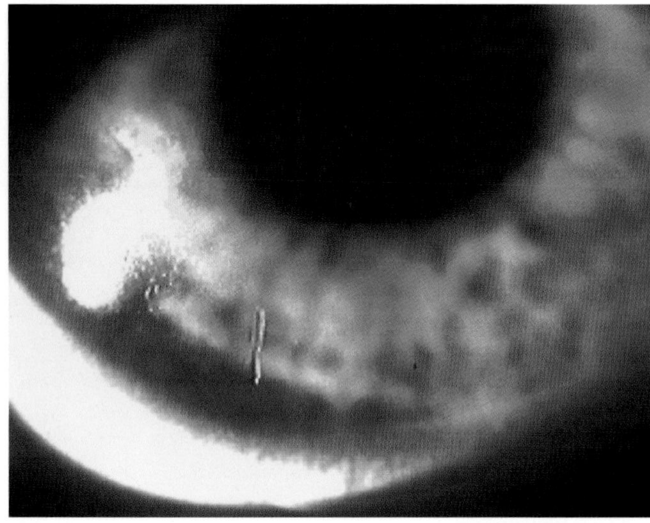

Figure 12.12 Misleading lens rotation resulting from a decentred contact lens

preferable as the markings can be observed without having to retract the lower eyelid (which would interfere with the dynamic stabilizing forces). In addition, having two widely spaced markings about 14 mm apart makes it easier to quantify the angle of rotation. When the markings on the lens are at the 6 o'clock position, they often comprise three lines, each separated by the same known angle, thus also facilitating the degree of lens rotation. Generally, lenses with markings at the 6 o'clock position are those with asymmetrical dynamic stabilization where it is important for the larger, thinner peripheral zone to be orientated superiorly for optimal lid interaction.

The angular position of the marker on the lens is significant and not the position of the marker on the cornea. Figure 12.12 shows a soft toric lens on a left eye with the marker indicating that the lens is rotating nasally by about 20° (given that the reference point for the marker is the 6 o'clock position). However, a closer look at the marker reveals that it is vertically orientated, the expected orientation if the lens was not rotating. In this case, the apparent nasal rotation is due to a nasal decentration of the contact lens.

Estimation is straightforward and is a reasonable technique for assessing the degree of lens rotation, made simpler if the practitioner remembers that there is 30° between each hour on a clock face. Clinical experience has shown that this is a satisfactory method of assessing lens rotation, with errors more likely to occur when evaluating higher amounts of lens rotation (Snyder & Daum 1989).

DETERMINING LENS MISALIGNMENT

The usual method of determining lens misalignment is to estimate the degree of lens rotation by observing the location of the lens on the eye. This value is compared with the expected lens rotation incorporated into the BVP of the contact lens. The difference between the actual and expected values represents the degree of lens misalignment.

A spherocylindrical over-refraction can also be used to determine the degree of lens misalignment. The lens misalignment is deduced by calculating the effective back vertex power of the lens on the eye ($BVP_{in\ situ}$). This, in turn, is done by subtracting the SCO obtained over the mislocating soft toric lens from the ocular refraction (Oc Rx) of the patient (Lindsay et al. 1997).

i.e. $BVP_{in\ situ} = Oc\ Rx - SCO$

Calculating the $BVP_{in\ situ}$ will require the resolving of obliquely crossed cylinders and this is best done by matrix optics (Long 1976, Keating 1980) using the following method:

1. Express both the spherocylindrical ocular refraction and the spherocylindrical over-refraction in dioptric power matrix form (F), whereby:

$$F = \begin{matrix} S + C\sin^2\theta & -C\sin\theta\cos\theta \\ -C\sin\theta\cos\theta & S + C\cos^2\theta \end{matrix}$$

where S is the sphere power, C is the cylinder power and θ is the axis (in radians) of the cylinder.

2. Subtract the dioptric power matrix for the over-refraction from the dioptric power matrix for the ocular refraction, to obtain the dioptric power matrix, F_r, for the $BVP_{in\ situ}$.

$$F_r = \begin{matrix} S_r + C_r\sin^2\theta_r & -C_r\sin\theta_r\cos\theta_r \\ -C_r\sin\theta_r\cos\theta_r & S_r + C_r\cos^2\theta_r \end{matrix}$$

3. Convert the matrix form of the $BVP_{in\ situ}$ back to spherocylindrical notation using the following formulae:

If the lens power matrix is $\begin{matrix} a_{11} & a_{12} \\ a_{21} & a_{22} \end{matrix}$

trace (t) = $a_{11} + a_{22}$ and determinant (d) = $(a_{11}a_{22}) - (a_{12}a_{21})$

To convert the matrix form of the $BVP_{in\ situ}$ back to spherocylindrical notation, S_r, C_r and θ_r (the sphere power, cylinder power and cylinder axis, respectively, of the $BVP_{in\ situ}$) can be determined as follows:

$$S_r = \frac{(t - C_r)}{2}$$

$$\theta_r = \text{atan}\,\frac{(S_r - a_{11})}{a_{12}} \times \frac{180}{\pi} \quad \text{(where } \theta_r \text{ is in degrees)}$$

$$C_r = -\sqrt{t^2 - 4d}$$

(The minus sign prior to the radical symbol simply means that the final solution will be in minus cylinder form.)

These formulae can easily be incorporated into a spreadsheet (Fig. 12.13) which can then be quickly utilized in clinical practice. Alternatively, the CD-ROM supplied with this book allows simple calculation of mislocation measurement.

Once the $BVP_{in\ situ}$ has been determined, any degree of lens misalignment can then be identified along with any errors in the power of the manufactured lens by comparing the $BVP_{in\ situ}$ with the BVP specified for the contact lens.

Example 8: Consider a soft toric lens being fitted to the left eye of a patient

- The ocular refraction of the patient is –3.00/–2.00 × 10.
- The specified BVP of the contact lens is –3.00/–2.00 × 20, so this prescription incorporates an allowance for 10° nasal rotation.

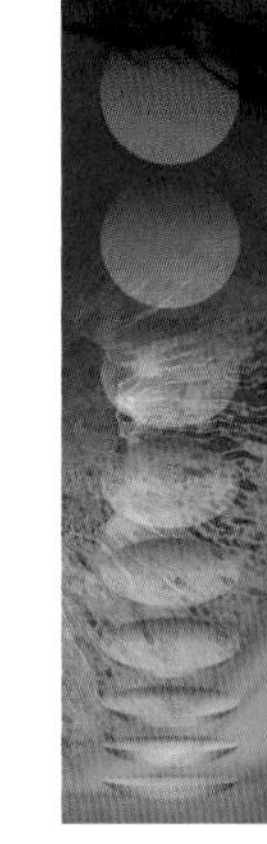

	A	B	C	D	E
1		SPHERE	CYLINDER	AXIS	
2					
3	Oc Rx	−3	−2	10	=D3/57.2958
4	MATRIX	=B3+C3*(SIN(E3)^2)	=−C3*SIN(E3)*COS(E3)		
5		=−C3*SIN(E3)*COS(E3)	=B3+C3*(COS(E3)^2)		
6	OR	0.5	−1	47.5	=D6/57.2958
7	MATRIX	=B6+C6*(SIN(E6)^2)	=−C6*SIN(E6)*COS(E6)		
8		=−C6*SIN(E6)*COS(E6)	=B6+C6*(COS(E6)^2)		
9	SUM	=B4-B7	=C4-C7		
10		=B5-B8	=C5-C8		
11	TRACE	=B9+C10			
12	DET	=(B9*C10)−(B10*C9)			
13	BVPin situ	=(B11-C13)/2	=−SQRT((B11^2)−4*B12)	=IF(57.2958*ATAN((B13-B9)/C9)>0, 57.2958*ATAN((B13-B9)/C9), 180+57.2958*ATAN((B13-B9)/C9))	
14					

Figure 12.13 Spreadsheet for determining soft toric lens misalignment

- A SCO with this lens yields +0.50/–1.00 × 47.5.
- Solving for $BVP_{in\ situ}$ (using matrix optics) gives –3.00/–2.00 × 175.

Although the specified cylinder axis was 20°, the effective cylinder axis on the eye is 175°. Therefore the lens is exhibiting 25° nasal rotation on the eye (instead of the expected 10° nasal rotation).

To allow for this 25° nasal rotation, the contact lens would now have to be reordered with a cylinder axis of 35° to achieve the target cylinder axis on the eye of 10°.

If visual acuity is not improved by the SCO, the cause of the suboptimal acuity may be a poorly fitting lens, a lens of poor quality (possibly due to significant deposition on the lens surface) or some form of ocular pathology (Myers et al. 1990).

PLANNED REPLACEMENT OF SOFT TORIC LENSES (see also Chapter 10)

Virtually all disposable soft toric lenses are produced as a stock range of lenses encompassing a certain number of cylindrical powers (e.g. –0.75 D, –1.25 D and –1.75 D), a set choice of spherical powers (e.g. from +6.00 to –9.00) and cylinder axes in 5 or 10° steps – usually the latter – most often ranging from zero to 180°. The choice of BOZR and TD for these lenses is also limited.

With the ongoing expansion of the types and parameters of disposable lenses, the need for prescribing custom-made soft toric lenses on a non-replacement basis is diminishing (Efron 2002). However, as there will always be patients requiring cylindrical corrections that are not covered by these ranges, it is essential to have access to a custom laboratory which can produce lenses to any required parameter.

It is possible for practitioners to hold a selection of disposable soft toric lenses in their own inventory. This allows for a more accurate assessment of the effects of lens rotation, by using a lens of almost the correct power and axis on the eye while carrying out a tolerance trial (see Chapter 11).

LIMITATIONS OF SOFT TORIC LENSES

There will be a certain number of cases encountered in practice where soft toric lenses are either less likely to be successful or do not represent the best option for the prospective contact lens patient.

LOW SPHERICAL COMPONENTS

Patients who are fitted with soft toric lenses with a low spherical component (e.g. +0.25/–2.50 × 180) are often critical of any axis misalignment because the astigmatism is the most significant component of their refractive error. As discussed above, prism ballast lenses may prove more stable for these prescriptions. In addition, with some of the older soft toric lens designs, the thickness differentials (to aid lens location) that can usually be achieved are reduced with small spherical components (Hanks & Weisbarth 1983).

LARGE CYLINDRICAL COMPONENTS

Lens rotation also becomes more significant as the degree of cylinder is increased. For example, a patient with a toric lens incorporating a 1.25 D cylinder may be able to tolerate a 5° rotation from the expected lens location, whereas someone with a 3.50 D cylinder will notice a significant drop in vision for the same degree of rotation off axis.

OBLIQUE CYLINDERS

As previously discussed (Holden 1975, Gundel 1989), soft toric lenses incorporating oblique cylinders (e.g. –2.00/–2.00 × 45) may show poorer stability due to complex lid–lens interactions.

IRREGULAR ASTIGMATISM

No form of soft toric lens is able to correct irregular astigmatism. Patients with astigmatic errors of this nature are usually corrected with some form of rigid contact lens.

PHYSIOLOGICAL CONSIDERATIONS

Improvements in design have led to an overall decrease in the thickness of most soft toric lenses and a reduction in the number of physiological problems encountered during lens wear. However, these lenses are still significantly thicker than spherical soft lenses because of the addition of cylinder and the creation of thickness differentials throughout the toric lens form. Oxygen transmissibility is reduced and mechanical irritation increased from the thicker regions of the lens, and may lead to the following:

- Corneal oedema – especially in patients with hyperopic astigmatism.
- Corneal neovascularization (Fig. 12.14) – usually inferior and superior and more likely in myopic patients.
- Superior limbic keratoconjunctivitis – especially with large lenses.
- Conjunctival indentation – especially with tight-fitting lenses.

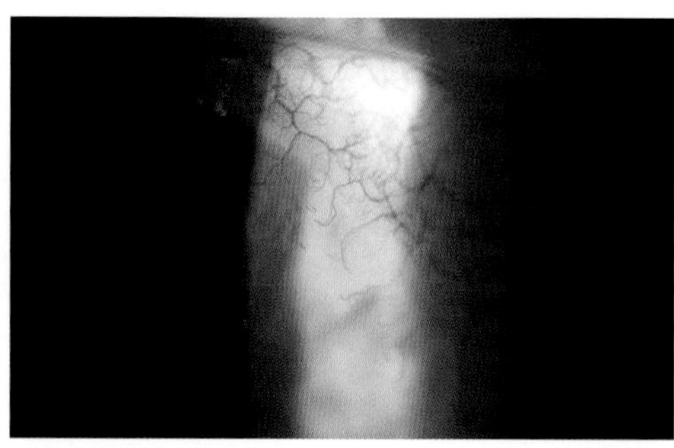

Figure 12.14 Marked superior corneal vascularization caused by wear of a low (38%) water content soft toric contact lens

If corneal hypoxia is suspected, the material of the lens should, if possible, be changed to silicone hydrogel or a material with a higher water content.

SUMMARY

With the wide range of toric RGP, soft and disposable lenses available, almost all cases of astigmatism can now be corrected. Although greater care and time are necessary, the end result of a happy patient with good acuity more than justifies the additional effort required.

References

Bernstein, P. R., Gundel, R. E. and Rosen, J. S. (1991) Masking corneal toricity with hydrogels: does it work? Int. Contact Lens Clin., 18, 67–70

Bruce, A. (2002) Soft toric lens misalignment demonstrator. In Contact Lens Practice, Appendix I, p. 483, ed. N. Efron. Oxford: Butterworth-Heinemann

Douthwaite, W. A. (1995) Contact Lens Optics and Lens Design. London: Butterworth-Heinemann

Edwards, K. (1999) Problem-solving with toric soft contact lenses. Optician, 217(5695), 18–19, 22, 24–25, 27

Efron, N. A. (2002) Unplanned lens replacement. In Contact Lens Practice, Chapter 19, ed. N. Efron. Oxford: Butterworth-Heinemann

Fanti, P. (1975) The fitting of a soft toroidal contact lens. Optician, 169(4376), 8–9, 13, 15–16

Gasson, A. P. (1977) Back surface toric soft lenses. Optician, 174(4491), 6–7, 9, 11

Goldberg, J. B. (1964) The correction of residual astigmatism with corneal contact lenses. Br. J. Physiol. Opt., 21, 169–174

Gonce, M. A. and Kastl, P. R. (1994) Bitoric rigid contact lens with prism fitting in rare cases of moderate corneal and residual astigmatism. Contact Lens Assoc. Ophthalmol. J., 20, 176–178

Gundel, R. E. (1989) Effect of cylinder axis on rotation for a double thin zone design toric hydrogel. Int. Contact Lens Clin., 16, 141–145

Hanks, A. J. (1983) The watermelon seed principle. Contact Lens Forum, 9, 31–35

Hanks, A. J. and Weisbarth, R. E. (1983) Troubleshooting soft toric contact lenses. Int. Contact Lens Clin., 10, 305–317

Holden, B. A. (1975) The principles and practice of correcting astigmatism with soft contact lenses. Aust. J. Optom., 58, 279–299

Holden, B. A. (1976) Correcting astigmatism with toric soft lenses – an overview. Int. Contact Lens Clin., 3, 59–61

Keating, M. P. (1980) An easier method to obtain the sphere, cylinder, and axis from an off-axis dioptric power matrix. Am. J. Optom. Physiol. Opt., 57, 734–737

Lindsay, R. G. (1996) Toric rigid gas-permeable contact lenses: indications, fitting principles and prescription calculations. Pract. Optom., 7, 218–224

Lindsay, R. G. (1998) Toric soft contact lens fitting. Optician, 216(5671), 18–20, 22, 24

Lindsay, R. G., Bruce, A. S., Brennan, N. A. and Pianta, M. J. (1997) Determining axis misalignment and power errors of toric soft lenses. Int. Contact Lens Clin., 24, 101–107

Long, W. F. (1976) A matrix formalism for decentration problems. Am. J. Optom. Physiol. Opt., 53, 27–33

Long, W. F. (1991) Lens power matrices and the sum of equivalent spheres. Optom. Vis. Sci., 68, 821–822

Lowther, G. E. (1990) Toric RGPs: should they be used more often? Int. Contact Lens Clin., 17, 260–261

Meyler, J. and Ruston, D. (1995) Toric RGP contact lenses made easy. Optician, 209(5504), 30–35

Myers, R. I., Jones, D. H. and Meinell, P. (1990) Using over-refraction for problem solving in soft toric fitting. Int. Contact Lens Clin., 17, 232–234

Ruston, D. (1999) The challenge of fitting astigmatic eyes: rigid gas-permeable toric lenses. Cont. Lens Anterior Eye (Suppl), 22, S2–S13

Sarver, M. D. (1963) A toric base corneal contact lens with spherical power effect. J. Am. Optom. Assoc., 34, 1136–1137

Sarver, M. D., Kame, R. T. and Williams, C. E. (1985) A bitoric gas permeable hard contact lens with spherical power effect. J. Am. Optom. Assoc., 56, 184–189

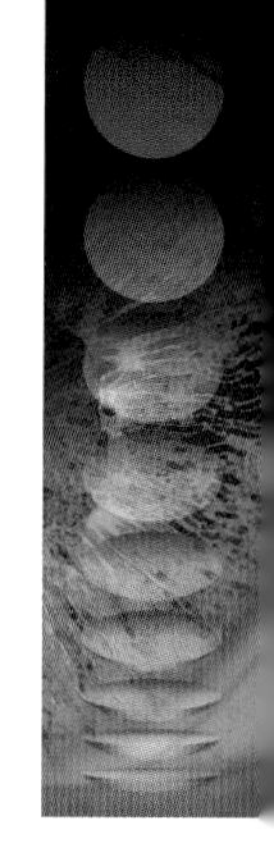

Snyder, C. (1998) Overcoming toric soft lens challenges. Contact Lens Spectrum (Suppl), 2–4

Snyder, C. and Daum, K. D. (1989) Rotational position of toric soft contact lenses on the eye – clinical judgements. Int. Contact Lens Clin., 16, 146–151

Strachan, J. P. F. (1975) Correction of astigmatism with hydrophilic lenses. Optician, 170(4402), 8–11

Chapter 13

Extended- and continuous-wear lenses

Deborah F. Sweeney, Serina Stretton, Desmond Fonn, Helen A. Swarbrick and Brien A. Holden

CHAPTER CONTENTS

INTRODUCTION

Lenses for extended wear (up to 1 week) and continuous wear (up to 1 month) have always held considerable attraction for contact lens wearers because of the possibility of normal vision without glasses. However, as well as being convenient, they must be safe, effective and extremely comfortable.

New-generation contact lenses made from silicone hydrogel and rigid gas-permeable (RGP) materials of high oxygen permeability (Dk) have reawakened the concepts of extended and continuous wear because they have sufficient oxygen transmissibility (Dk/t) to meet the oxygen requirements of the closed eye and eliminate the hypoxic effects traditionally associated with extended wear.

At the end of 2004, it was estimated that there were close to two million silicone hydrogel lens wearers. Silicone hydrogels provide comparable levels of comfort to hydrogels but their oxygen transmissibilities are making them the lens of choice for all wear modalities: daily wear, flexi-wear, extended wear and continuous wear.

THE OCULAR ENVIRONMENT

Oxygen needs and supply

When the eye is open, oxygen is supplied to the cornea directly from the atmosphere (Smelser & Ozanics 1952, Hill & Fatt 1964a). At sea level, the concentration of oxygen in the atmosphere is approximately 21%, corresponding to a partial pressure (PO_2) of 155 mmHg (21 kPa*). When the eye is closed, oxygen is provided to the cornea almost exclusively from the capillary plexus of the palpebral conjunctiva, but at much reduced levels (PO_2 = 60 mmHg or 8 kPa) (Efron & Carney 1979, Holden & Sweeney 1985).

An adequate supply of oxygen is essential to maintain normal epithelial aerobic metabolism. When the level of oxygen at the anterior corneal surface is reduced, the rate of aerobic metabolism in the epithelium decreases, and consequently the rate of anaerobic metabolic activity increases. One major metabolic waste product of anaerobic glycolysis is lactate, which is usually oxidized in the presence of oxygen. Under hypoxic conditions, lactate remains unoxidized and accumulates in the epithelium and stroma as it gradually moves towards the aqueous where it is eliminated from the tissue. According to Klyce (1981), the increased concentration of lactate in corneal tissue during hypoxia osmotically induces an influx of fluid into the stroma, leading to corneal swelling or oedema.

Polse and Mandell (1970) originally found that an atmospheric level of only 1.5–2.5% oxygen (11–19 mmHg or 1.5–2.5 kPa) was required to avoid corneal oedema. This was later increased to 3.5–5.5% oxygen (Mandell & Farrell 1980)

* kPa = kiloPascals, where 1 Pascal = 10 millibars

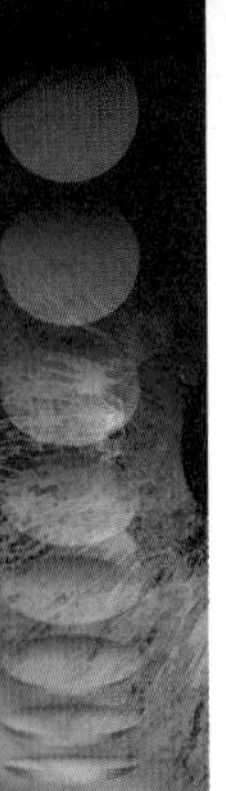

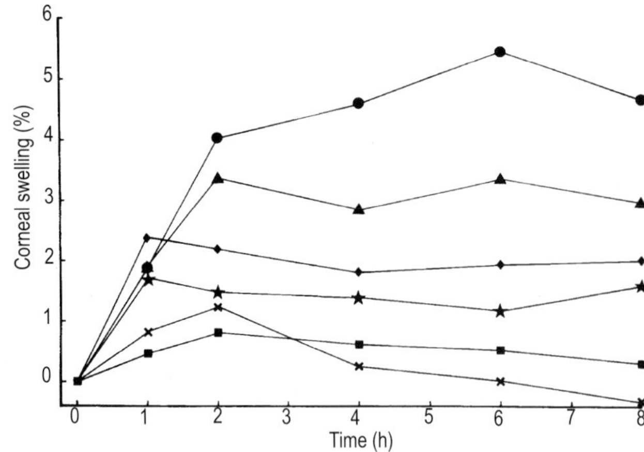

Figure 13.1 To determine the minimum oxygen requirements of the cornea to avoid oedema, average corneal swelling was measured for a range of precorneal oxygen concentrations. Gas-goggles were used to expose the cornea to gases of various oxygen tensions over an 8-hour period. Eight human subjects were used. On average, a precorneal oxygen concentration of 10.1% was required to avoid corneal oedema in this group of subjects. (×) 21.4% O_2; (■) 10.1% O_2; (★) 7.5% O_2; (◆) 4.9% O_2; (▲) 2.5% O_2; (●) 1.0% O_2. (From Holden et al. 1984, with permission)

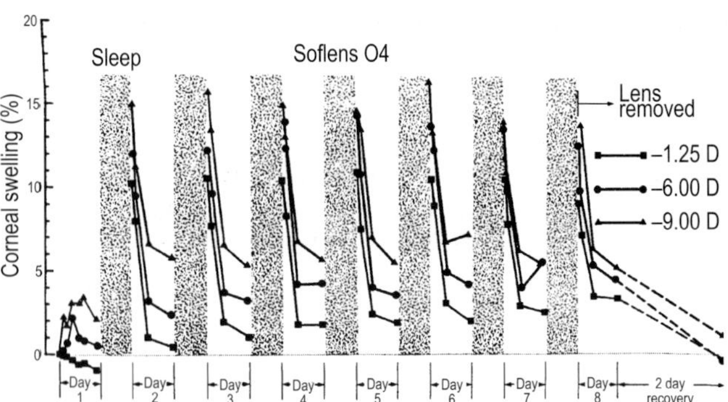

Figure 13.2 The typical 'oedema cycle' associated with hydrogel extended wear is shown in this graph of average corneal swelling versus time for ten unadapted subjects wearing Bausch & Lomb Soflens O4 series contact lenses continuously for a period of 1 week. All subjects wore −1.25 D lenses on one eye, half wore −6.00 D lenses and half wore −9.00 D lenses on the other eye. (■) −1.25 D; (●) −6.00 D; (▲) −9.00 D. (From Holden et al. 1983, with permission)

but we now know that even higher levels are necessary with considerable individual variations.

Using eight subjects, Holden et al. (1984) found that at least 10% oxygen must be available to the cornea to prevent oedema (Fig. 13.1) and that the level of oxygen required can range from 7.5 to 21%. Parallel work by Mizutani et al. (1983) found the figure to be approximately 15% oxygen. These results are supported by other laboratory studies. Hamano et al. (1983) found that the rate of epithelial mitosis was reduced, and lactate began to accumulate in the aqueous if less than 13% oxygen was supplied to the anterior corneal surface; Millodot and O'Leary (1980) reported that corneal sensitivity is decreased when the eyelids are closed and oxygen availability falls to 8% oxygen, and Williams (1986) reported that an endothelial bleb response is generally induced if oxygen levels fall below 15%. In addition, equivalent oxygen percentage (EOP), which is an indirect measure of the amount of oxygen behind a contact lens, has been used to estimate the amount of oxygen required during lens wear (Hill & Fat, 1964b; Hill 1965). EOP is obtained by sliding a lens off the eye and immediately measuring the oxygen uptake rate. This rate is then compared to calibration curves of corneal swelling to gases of known oxygen concentration.

Contact lenses impede the passage of oxygen to the anterior corneal surface. This causes problems during overnight sleep when less oxygen is available. Oxygen reaches the cornea by circulation of oxygen-rich tears behind the lens, mediated by a lid-activated tear pump, or by diffusion of oxygen through the lens material. The tear pump is active only when the eye is open and possibly during rapid eye movement (REM) sleep, although this is unlikely to supplement oxygen availability to any significant extent (Benjamin & Rasmussen 1985).

Both soft and RGP materials provide oxygen to the cornea during closed-eye wear by diffusion through the lens material, and lenses of comparable Dk/t will induce similar levels of overnight oedema. However, the lid-activated tear pump mechanism is considerably more efficient with RGP lenses than with soft lenses. An estimated 10–20% tear exchange occurs under an RGP lens with each blink (Cuklanz & Hill 1969, Fatt & Hill 1970) whereas Polse (1979) estimated a tear exchange per blink of only 1% under soft lenses. When the eye is opened after overnight wear, oxygen is provided to the anterior cornea more efficiently with RGP corneal lenses than soft, facilitating rapid corneal recovery from overnight hypoxic stress. Andrasko (1986) and Holden et al. (1988) demonstrated that the cornea de-swells more rapidly as a result and that this is also partly due to the smaller size of RGP lenses.

The cornea can eliminate approximately 8% corneal oedema during the day following overnight wear of hydrogel lenses (Holden et al. 1983). Extended-wear soft lenses, which cause more than 8% overnight oedema, will induce residual low-level daytime oedema leading to an 'oedema cycle' of high overnight swelling, followed by partial recovery (Fig. 13.2).

The amount of oedema eliminated by the cornea following overnight wear with RGP lenses is uncertain and depends on the relative efficiency of the tear pump. This in turn is a function of lens fit and blink frequency (Fatt 1969, Fink et al. 1990). Holden et al. (1988) suggested that approximately 10% oedema is eliminated because of the supplementation of corneal oxygenation by the tear pump. However, RGP lenses can also lead to an oedema cycle similar to that of extended-wear soft lenses.

Oxygen transmissibility

Fatt and co-workers (Fatt & Bieber 1968, Fatt & St Helen 1971, Fatt & Wiessman 1992) devised a model for oxygen distribution across the cornea based on Fick's law of diffusion. This model took into account the Dk (oxygen permeability) of a lens material, thickness of the lens (t) and rates of oxygen consumption for each layer of the cornea, and led the way for the use of Dk/t as a simple benchtop measurement for comparing the performance between hydrogel and silicone elastomer lenses. The Holden and Mertz (1984) criteria followed, which outlined ideal levels of Dk/t (oxygen transmissibility) required to prevent lens-induced oedema during daily and extended wear.

The Holden–Mertz criteria for overnight wear (87.3×10^{-9} (cm ml O_2)(s ml mmHg)$^{-1}$) and daily wear (24.1×10^{-9} (cm ml O_2)(s ml mmHg)$^{-1}$) were based on published nominal Dk values for hydrogel lenses and on 4% swelling immediately after sleep in non-lens wearers (Mertz 1980). The criterion for extended wear was later recalculated to be even higher after La Hood et al. (1988) revised the level of overnight swelling after sleep to 3.2% using a greater number of subjects than originally used by Mertz (Holden, personal communication). This was supported by Harvitt and Bonanno (1999) in their mathematical model of oxygen diffusion across the cornea and also by the Papas (1998) model of the impact of peripheral lens Dk/t on limbal hyperaemia, which estimated that the level of peripheral Dk/t required to prevent limbal hyperaemia is 125×10^{-9} (cm ml O_2)(s ml mmHg)$^{-1}$.

Although Dk/t enables practitioners to compare the transfer of oxygen across contact lenses, it does not provide a measure of the amount of oxygen that enters the cornea over time (corneal oxygen flux) and gives no indication of corneal metabolic activity during lens wear (oxygen consumption). Most importantly for practitioners, although the relationship between Dk/t and the corneal response to oxygen supply is linear for hydrogel lenses, it does not remain so for hyperoxygen-transmissible lenses such as silicone hydrogels, so that an increase in Dk/t does not mean an equivalent increase in oxygen supply (Fatt 1996). Some researchers therefore suggest that the flux of oxygen through a contact lens may be a better index for comparison of the physiological performance of highly oxygen-transmissible contact lenses (Brennan 2001).

Irrespective of which method is used to calculate oxygen needs or what levels are calculated, there will always be a demand for hyperoxygen-transmissible lenses because it is impossible to predict the oxygen requirements of individual patients before lens wear commences, and because some patients such as astigmats and high ametropes require thicker than average lenses.

Elimination of waste products

As well as impeding the supply of oxygen to the anterior corneal surface, contact lenses may also provide a barrier to the elimination of waste products from the anterior cornea, in particular carbon dioxide and cellular debris.

CARBON DIOXIDE

Because the permeability of hydrogel materials to carbon dioxide is approximately 20 times that of oxygen (Fatt et al. 1969, Ang & Efron 1989), it was thought that they did not restrict carbon dioxide efflux from the cornea. However, Holden et al. (1987a) demonstrated that even thin (0.035 mm) hydrogel lenses provide a significant barrier to carbon dioxide efflux. Hence, during extended lens wear, the cornea may experience chronically raised levels of carbon dioxide, or hypercapnia, with little opportunity for recovery to normal open-eye levels.

Increased carbon dioxide concentration is likely to lead to an increase in the concentration of carbonic acid in the tissue and associated stromal acidosis. Such an effect has been demonstrated during eye closure and contact lens wear (Bonanno & Polse 1987a–c) and may be responsible for the endothelial bleb response (Holden et al. 1985a).

CELLULAR DEBRIS

The corneal epithelium continually replenishes its cells by mitosis. Epithelial stem cells located in the basal layer of the epithelium, in the limbal zone, move towards the corneal surface where they exfoliate and are washed away in the tears. Most cells proliferate at the corneal periphery adjacent to the limbus (Kruse 1994, Zieske 1994, Ren et al. 1999a, Ladage et al. 2001a,b) while exfoliation occurs mostly at the centre of the cornea (Yamamoto et al. 2002) and is driven by apoptosis (Ren & Wilson 1996, Estil et al. 2000). This centripetal movement of epithelial cells is still being explored (see Chapter 2).

Cellular debris and exfoliated cells are readily flushed out from behind an RGP lens but are more likely to become trapped behind a soft lens because of the larger diameter and lower rate of tear exchange. Accumulation of host cell enzymes and other products released during breakdown of this cellular material have the potential to provoke a toxic reaction from the epithelium. This mechanism has been implicated in contact lens-associated acute red eye (CLARE) which is observed immediately after a prolonged period of eye closure in some extended wearers of soft contact lenses (Zantos & Holden 1978, Sweeney et al. 2003). RGP extended-wear lenses have less potential to provoke such a response because debris is more rapidly removed after eye opening due to the greater tear exchange. However, RGP lenses may occasionally provoke a CLARE reaction if the lens remains bound to the cornea after the eye is opened (Schnider et al. 1988) (see Chapters 9 and 17).

Environmental changes under the closed lid

OVERNIGHT CORNEAL OEDEMA (NO LENS)

After 8 hours of overnight eye closure without contact lenses, the cornea swells by 3–4% corneal oedema (Mandell & Fatt 1965, Mertz 1980, La Hood et al. 1988, Fonn et al 1999). It is reasonable to assume that hypoxia contributes to this swelling as the level of oxygen provided by the capillary plexus of the palpebral conjunctiva (8%) is lower than the average level of atmospheric oxygen (10%) required to avoid swelling (Holden et al. 1984).

Holden et al. (1984) found that a gas mixture containing 7.5% oxygen (the approximate level of oxygen available during eye closure) induced an average of approximately 2% corneal oedema over 8 hours of exposure to the gas. This suggests that other factors, such as changes in temperature, tear pH and tonicity under the closed lid, may also contribute to overnight corneal swelling.

TEMPERATURE

The temperature of the anterior corneal surface of the open eye is approximately 34.5°C (Fatt & Chaston 1980, Martin & Fatt 1986). When the eye is closed, the cornea is exposed to the

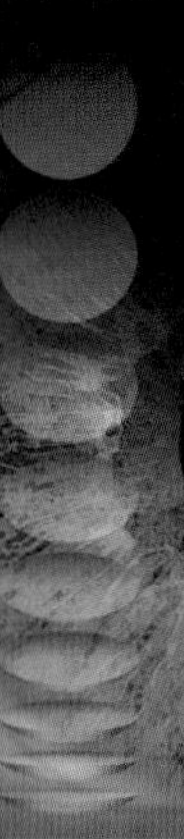

palpebral conjunctiva, which is 36.2°C (Holden & Sweeney 1985). This increases the temperature of the corneal surface by approximately 2°C (Fatt & Chaston 1980, Martin & Fatt 1986), influencing the rate of epithelial metabolism (Freeman & Fatt 1973) and increasing epithelial oxygen consumption. Temperature may thereby contribute to overnight corneal swelling accompanying both sleep and overnight lens wear.

TEAR pH

Tear pH usually exhibits a pattern of diurnal variation about a mean of 7.45 ± 0.16 in the open eye, with a general increase in alkalinity during the day (Carney & Hill 1976). When the eye is closed, there is an acid shift in tear pH to approximately 7.25, with recovery to average open-eye levels within 3–4 hours.

Tear pH may also be low in neophyte contact lens wearers (Hamano 1978), although attempts to determine long-term changes in tear pH with contact lens wear have been less conclusive. It is probable that reductions in tear pH with eye closure and contact lens wear are due in part to the restriction of carbon dioxide efflux from the cornea, and reflect parallel changes in stromal pH under these conditions (Bonanno & Polse 1987b,c).

Changes in ambient pH can alter the ion transport properties of the epithelium (Fischer et al. 1978), affecting corneal hydration. Thus the normal acid shift in tear pH during eye closure, possibly compounded by reduced pH accompanying contact lens wear, could contribute to the overnight swelling of the cornea. Carney and Efron (1980) suggested, however, that an acidic environment might decrease corneal oxygen consumption. Furthermore, a number of authors (Carney 1974, Holden et al. 1985a, Sweeney 1991) have reported that exposure of the cornea to gas mixtures containing oxygen and carbon dioxide, which would be expected to lower tear film and corneal pH, does not induce corneal oedema.

TEAR OSMOLARITY

Terry and Hill (1978) found a shift in tear tonicity from 0.97 ± 0.02% NaCl in the open eye to 0.89 ± 0.01% NaCl following 6–8 hours of sleep. This may be explained by reduced tear evaporation during eye closure. Recovery in corneal thickness from induced oedema at 100% humidity is significantly impeded compared to a normal (60% humidity) environment (O'Neal & Polse 1985), apparently confirming the role of tear evaporation in the control of normal corneal thickness as suggested by Mishima and Maurice (1961).

Rigid lens wear can induce a hypotonic shift in tear tonicity, particularly due to reflex tearing during adaptation (Harris & Mandell 1969). In comparison, soft lenses induce only small, transient changes in tear osmolarity (Martin & Holden 1983), probably due to better comfort. A decrease in the tonicity of the tears may osmotically increase corneal thickness and may contribute to the overall closed-eye swelling response.

Sweeney (1991) examined the separate effects of hypoxia, temperature, osmolality, humidity and carbon dioxide on corneal oedema and demonstrated that hypoxia during eye closure accounts for approximately half of the normal overnight oedema. Changes in temperature, osmolality and humidity approximating those found during overnight eye closure induced low and similar levels of oedema, accounting for the remaining normal overnight oedema. Increases in ambient carbon dioxide partial pressure, which would be expected to influence tear and stromal pH, did not induce corneal swelling.

SOFT CONTACT LENSES

Historical review of extended and continuous wear

Hydrogel lenses became available commercially in 1971, just over a decade after the first report of the development of a hydrophilic material suitable for contact lens applications (Wichterle & Lim 1960). Although initially used for daily wear, it soon became apparent that hydrogel lenses could be worn as bandage lenses 24 hours a day in the treatment of ocular diseases such as bullous keratopathy, recurrent corneal erosions, corneal ulcers and perforation, and dry eye syndromes (Gasset & Kaufman 1970, Dohlman et al. 1973, Ruben 1976).

At about the same time, John de Carle pioneered development of high water content hydrogel lenses for continuous wear (de Carle 1972). In spite of reported complications (Hodd 1975, Cooper & Constable 1977, Ruben 1977, Zantos & Holden 1978, Zantos 1981), cosmetic extended wear of hydrogel lenses gained FDA approval in 1981, and, by 1985, approximately 4 million people in the US were wearing extended-wear lenses.

Warnings of severe corneal complications went largely unheeded until Barry Weissman raised the issue in 1983. Subsequent clinical and media reports of corneal infections and litigation led to a re-evaluation of the safety of extended wear and a down-turn in pressure for this modality.

The concept of regular lens replacement was pioneered by Klas Nilsson (1983) and Ake Gustafsson, leading to increased success and low complication rates (Holden et al. 1985b, Nilsson & Persson 1986, Kotow et al. 1987a,b, Ames & Cameron 1989). Replacement every 1–2 weeks soon followed and, in 1989, the FDA issued a recommendation that extended wear should be for a maximum of six nights.

Even this modality led to reports of serious infections (e.g. Dunn et al. 1989, Ficker et al. 1990), as did improper care of disposable lenses during daily wear (Efron et al. 1991). A 1989 survey of disposable-lens wearers found that only 54% always replaced their lenses according to their prescribed schedule, while 22% usually wore the lenses longer than recommended (Anon 1989).

Extended-wear lenses must transmit considerably more oxygen than daily wear lenses in order to minimize disruption to corneal physiology during eye closure. This led to the formulation of a wide range of high water content and very thin low water content hydrogel lenses aimed at optimizing Dk/t. However, with hydrogels, the maximum Dk/t was insufficient to overcome the long-term hypoxic consequences of overnight wear.

Interest in continuous wear has increased dramatically since the launch of high Dk silicone hydrogel lenses in the late 1990s.

The first of these lenses were approved for 30 nights of continuous wear in Australia and Europe in 1999 and in the United States in 2001. High Dk silicone hydrogel lenses have the Dk/t to overcome the subtle long-term effects traditionally associated with extended wear of low Dk hydrogel lenses, and are rapidly becoming the lens of choice for all wear modalities. In 2003, silicone hydrogels accounted for over 90% of extended-wear fits, including continuous wear, in Australia, Norway and the United Kingdom, and over 50% in Canada, Singapore and the United States (Morgan et al. 2004).

The principal advantage of continuous wear over daily wear is convenience. Lenses do not have to be inserted and removed each day and patients see well immediately on awakening and there is no daily maintenance. This is beneficial to wearers who have difficulty handling lenses, particularly the elderly and children. After 12 months of continuous wear with silicone hydrogel lenses, subjects at the Cornea and Contact Lens Research Unit (CCLRU) – now the Institute for Eye Research (IER) – overwhelmingly nominated convenience as the major reason for their satisfaction with this wear modality (Skotnitsky et al. 1999).

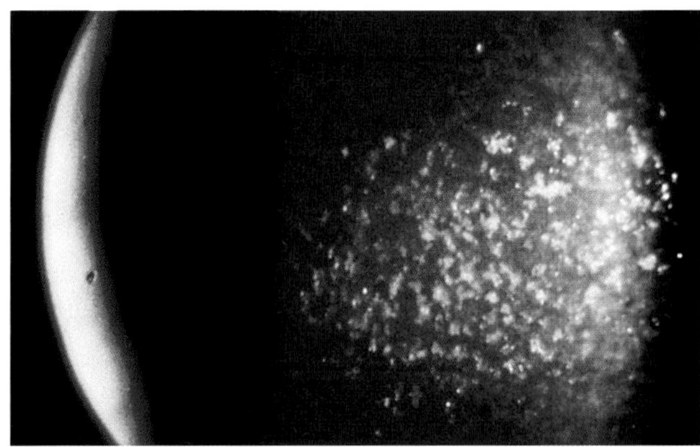

Figure 13.3 Epithelial erosions may occur when soft lenses dehydrate on the eye, such as this case of multiple confluent erosions following short-term wear of a very thin high water content hydrogel lens. It is postulated that small areas of dehydrated epithelial tissue become attached to the lens and are torn away when the lens is removed. Erosions may also occur when mild degrees of punctate stain remain untreated for long periods or when debris builds up under a lens or adheres to its back surface. (From Holden et al. 1986a, with permission)

Advantages and disadvantages

While Dk/t is of major importance, lens material and design is important in maintaining corneal health and improving wearer acceptance. In particular:

- Clearing of debris from behind the lens.
- Minimizing deposit formation.
- Providing tear-carried metabolites essential for the maintenance of epithelial growth and repair.
- Minimizing complications from mechanical interaction between lenses and ocular surfaces.

CONVENTIONAL HYDROGEL LENSES

The major parameters that determine the characteristics of hydrogel materials are:

- Water content.
- Ionicity.

The main component of hydrogels is poly 2-hydroxyethyl methacrylate (HEMA), with other monomers being added to improve wettability and oxygen transport. The Dk of hydrogel lenses is dependent on the water content because the hydrophilic monomers incorporated into the material attract and bind water into the polymer. Oxygen dissolved in the water is transported through the lens to the cornea; therefore, the higher the water content, the higher the level of oxygen transport.

Early research on extended wear focused on maximizing Dk/t by combining highly oxygen-permeable lens materials with a range of lens thicknesses. Relatively thick (0.12 mm centre thickness) high water content lenses retained their shape and were easier to handle but were associated with lens contamination and deposits, leading to ocular irritation and poor visual acuity.

Relatively thin (0.035 mm centre thickness) low water content lenses reduced problems with deposit accumulation and were more durable, but were difficult to handle and more vulnerable to tearing. In addition, the tendency of these lenses to 'drape' the cornea resulted in less lens movement compared to thicker, high water content lenses.

Thin, high water content lenses were investigated because, in theory, high water content (70–75%) combined with reduced centre thickness (0.03–0.08 mm) would enhance Dk/t but, as well as being fragile and difficult to handle, they potentially induced epithelial erosions (Fig. 13.3) due to on-eye dehydration which causes epithelial desiccation (Holden et al. 1986a, Orsborn & Zantos 1988).

The maximum Dk that can be achieved with a hydrogel lens material is limited by the Dk of water, which is 80 barrers. This means that even if a 100% water content lens were possible, this lens could never satisfy the Holden–Mertz criterion for extended wear. Current hydrogel lenses for extended wear are made from medium water content materials (45–60%) with moderate centre thickness in the range 0.05–0.12 mm. The oxygen permeabilities of these lens materials range from 20 to 40 barrers, and on average the lenses induce between 10 and 14% overnight corneal swelling (La Hood et al. 1988, Grant 1991). They result in long-term hypoxia with:

- Epithelial microcysts.
- Reduced epithelial adhesion.
- Endothelial polymegethism.

(Donshik et al. 1988, Grant & Holden 1988, and others).

SILICONE ELASTOMER LENSES (see also Chapter 3)

Silicone-based lenses have been available since the 1970s, but a number of unique and frustrating drawbacks have limited these

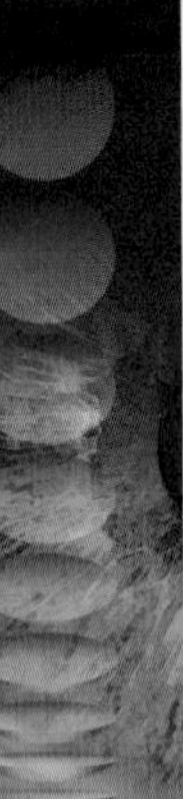

lenses to paediatric and therapeutic applications. Silicone elastomer lenses became available for aphakic and cosmetic extended wear in Japan and Europe in the mid-1970s but only gained FDA approval in the USA for paediatric and aphakic use (see also Chapter 24).

Compared to hydrogel lenses, silicone elastomer lenses are more durable and easier to handle, and are made from more highly oxygen-permeable materials. The high level of oxygen provided to the eye during overnight wear induces significantly less overnight oedema than actually occurs during sleep without lenses (Sweeney & Holden 1987) and endothelial polymegethism does not increase during extended wear (Schoessler et al. 1984). Silicone elastomer lenses are also able to promote wound healing (Sweeney et al. 1987).

Unfortunately, silicone elastomers have several disadvantages:

- Problems with manufacturing cause poor edge shape and fitting difficulties.
- The lenses are prone to accumulate excessive levels of lipid deposits.
- Unless fitted flat, lenses tend to adhere to the cornea, causing infections and inflammation.
- Lens manufacturing difficulties and poor wettability can cause discomfort.

(Ruben & Guillon 1979, Fanti 1980, Fanti & Holly 1980, Josephson & Caffery 1980, Blackhurst 1985, Mannarino et al. 1985, Nelson et al. 1985).

SILICONE HYDROGEL LENSES

Silicone hydrogel lenses incorporate the high Dk of silicone with the benefits of hydrogel materials. The main difference is that, unlike hydrogels, Dk is not dependent on water content but on the level of silicone incorporated into the material. Several silicone hydrogel lenses are currently approved for six or 30 nights' continuous wear and more are expected.

High Dk/t silicone hydrogel lenses allow sufficient oxygen to the anterior corneal surface to maintain normal epithelial functioning when worn on a continuous-wear basis (Covey et al. 2001, Brennan et al. 2002, Stern et al. 2004). Long-term pre-market clinical trials indicate that 90% of subjects can wear their lenses for 21 to 30 consecutive nights (n = 815) with a high level of satisfaction, comfort and good vision (Sweeney et al. 2002b, Stern et al. 2004). Their use has expanded to therapeutic applications (Ambroziak et al. 2004, Szaflik et al. 2004) and made piggyback contact lens systems a viable correction system for highly ametropic and keratoconic RGP lens wearers (O'Donnell & Maldonado-Codina 2004).

The differences observed between non-lens-wearing eyes and those with continuous-wear high-Dk silicone hydrogel lenses are not associated with hypoxia but are mechanical in nature (Covey et al. 2001). Comfort with silicone hydrogel lenses is comparable to that with other disposable lenses (Brennan et al. 2002, Fonn & Dumbleton 2003, Aakre et al. 2004, Stern et al. 2004); comfort is lowest on waking and improves during the day.

Adverse responses do occur with silicone hydrogel lenses:

- The level of corneal inflammatory events is similar to the levels seen with hydrogels (Nilsson 2001, Brennan et al. 2002, Sweeney et al. 2002a).
- Microbial keratitis has not been eliminated (Morgan et al. 2005a, Schein et al. 2006).
- Contact lens papillary conjunctivitis (CLPC) remains a significant cause of discontinuation from lens wear (Stern et al. 2004).

Impact of soft contact lens wear on the cornea

The chronic changes that have been observed in all layers of the cornea during long-term extended wear with hydrogel lenses signal potentially detrimental effects to corneal structure and function. Holden et al. (1985b) examined the corneas of 27 subjects from Göteborg, Sweden, who had been wearing a hydrogel lens in one eye (because of amblyopia or anisometropia) on an extended-wear basis for an average of 5 years. Compared to the non-lens-wearing fellow eye, the lens-wearing eye showed:

- Significant reductions in epithelial thickness and oxygen uptake rate.
- More epithelial microcysts.
- Stromal thinning.
- Increased endothelial polymegethism (variation in endothelial cell area).

No interocular differences in endothelial cell density were found.

In order to investigate the recovery from these corneal changes, subjects were asked to discontinue lens wear for 1 month. During this time epithelial thickness and oxygen uptake rate returned to levels found in non-lens-wearing eyes and the number of epithelial microcysts eventually decreased in number. This recovery of normal epithelial function (Fig. 13.4) is thought to reflect a resurgence in epithelial metabolic activity, which was depressed by chronic lens-induced hypoxia. The stromal and endothelial changes, however, were more long lasting; continued follow-up of several of the study subjects over 6 months without lens wear showed little recovery in stromal thickness or endothelial cell regularity (Holden et al. 1985c).

The clinical significance of these subtle alterations in corneal structure and function is yet to be clarified. Most studies examining long-term performance of contact lenses present average responses, not the range of individual responses. It is possible that some lens wearers show greater susceptibility to corneal stress and have increased risk of lens-induced complications. This is highlighted by the subset of wearers who develop high levels of oedema after overnight wear even with high-Dk silicone hydrogels (Comstock et al. 1999, Mueller et al. 2001).

Another complication associated with long-term wear of low-Dk contact lenses is 'corneal exhaustion' (see Chapters 9 and 17), first described by Sweeney (1992) in long-term polymethylmethacrylate (PMMA) and low-Dk hydrogel lens

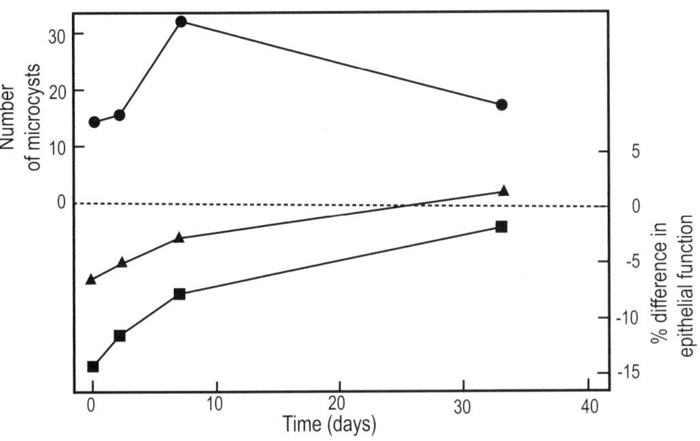

Figure 13.4 Long-term hydrogel extended wear causes significant changes in corneal physiology. This graph, taken from a study of unilateral hydrogel extended lens wearers, traces the recovery of epithelial oxygen uptake rate (■), epithelial thickness (▲) and epithelial microcysts (●) after cessation of long-term extended wear of high water content hydrogel contact lenses. Data on day 0 were obtained within 2 hours of lens removal. The dotted line represents the control (non-lens-wearing) eye data. (From Holden et al. 1985b, with permission)

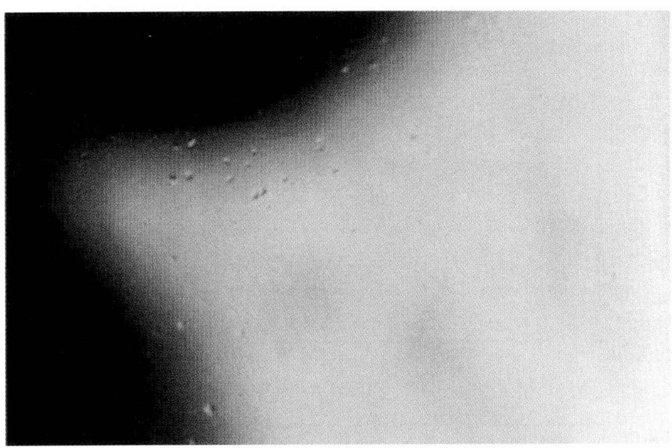

Figure 13.5 Epithelial microcysts are small inclusions displaying reversed illumination, i.e. the distribution of light within the inclusion (darker on the left side) is opposite to that of the background (darker on the right side). Microcysts are seen best by indirect illumination at the highest magnification possible. (From Swarbrick & Holden 1993, with permission)

wearers. Sweeney hypothesized that after many years of chronic hypoxic stress the endothelium was functionally compromised and unable to adjust to the sudden increase in oxygen. This phenomenon seems to occur more often in lens wearers with higher than average requirements for oxygen and in those such as moderate to severe hypermetropes who effectively have lenses of lower Dk/t.

Hypoxia impairs wounds healing (Mauger & Hill 1992); therefore lens-induced hypoxia may predispose the cornea to a greater rate of infection and inflammation. Several authors have found a relationship between the Dk/t of contact lenses and adherence of bacteria to epithelial cells (Imayasu et al. 1994, Cavanagh et al. 2002, 2003, Ladage et al. 2003a).

Hypoxia also causes:

- Reduced epithelial cell turnover (Lemp & Gold 1986, Ladage et al. 2003a).
- Reduced corneal sensitivity (Millodot 1974).
- Increased fragility (O'Leary & Millodot 1981).
- Reduced epithelial adhesion to basement membrane (Madigan et al. 1987).

EPITHELIUM

In general, contact lens wear significantly slows epithelial cell turnover (see above) by suppressing epithelial cell proliferation (Ladage et al. 2003c) and migration (Ladage et al. 2003b), and by decreasing the rate of exfoliation (O'Leary et al. 1998, Ren et al. 1999b, Ladage et al. 2001a). These effects are dependent in part on lens Dk/t and by the mechanical interaction of a lens with the ocular surface.

Epithelial surface cells taken from high-Dk silicone hydrogel lens wearers after 3 months of continuous wear are indistinguishable in size, morphology or viability from cells taken from non-lens wearers, whereas those taken from wearers of hydrogels are significantly bigger (Stapleton et al. 2001). Using confocal microscopy, Jalbert (2004) found that the regularity of the basal epithelium was similar between those who wore silicone hydrogels and non-lens wearers, but was less regular in wearers of hydrogels. Epithelial changes from low-Dk lenses indicate potential impairment of normal corneal homeostasis, which may contribute to the greater rate of epithelial thinning observed with extended wear of hydrogels compared to silicone hydrogels (Holden et al. 1985b, Cavanagh et al. 2002, Ren et al. 2002, Pérez et al. 2003).

EPITHELIAL MICROCYSTS

Epithelial microcysts are common in hydrogel lens wearers. They are best detected with the slit-lamp using high magnification and marginal retro-illumination (see Chapter 7) (Zantos & Holden 1978, Zantos 1983, Holden & Sweeney 1991). They appear as tiny translucent irregular dots, approximately 10–50 μm in diameter (Fig. 13.5), and are usually distributed in an annulus in the corneal mid-periphery. Because they display reversed illumination, it is thought that microcysts comprise pockets of disorganized cellular material (Bergmanson 1987) or dead (apoptotic) cells (Tripathi & Bron 1972, Madigan 1989). Microcysts are thought to form in the deeper layers of the epithelium and move gradually towards the epithelial surface in response to changes in metabolic activity.

The level of microcysts that develop during contact lens wear is a reliable index of chronic hypoxic stress and gives an indication of the degree of compromise to epithelial metabolism (Holden et al. 1987b, Holden & Sweeney 1991). Fewer than ten microcysts are observed in non-lens wearers and daily lens wearers and indicates lens wear that is free from hypoxia (Holden et al. 1987b, Terry et al. 1993, Hickson & Papas 1997) whereas more than 50 microcysts or marked epithelial disruption is a sign of severe chronic hypoxic stress (Zantos 1983).

Typically, microcysts develop within 3 months of commencing extended wear with hydrogels, and their numbers

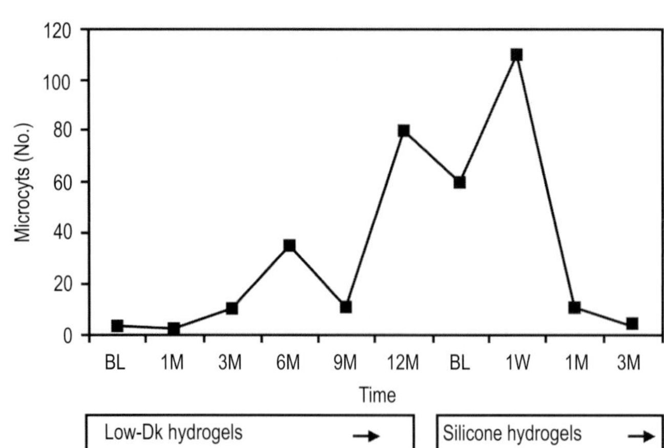

Figure 13.6 Rebound effect in the microcyst response observed when a patient is refitted with silicone hydrogel lenses after 12 months of extended wear with low-Dk conventional hydrogels. (From Sweeney et al. 2004, with permission of Butterworth-Heinemann)

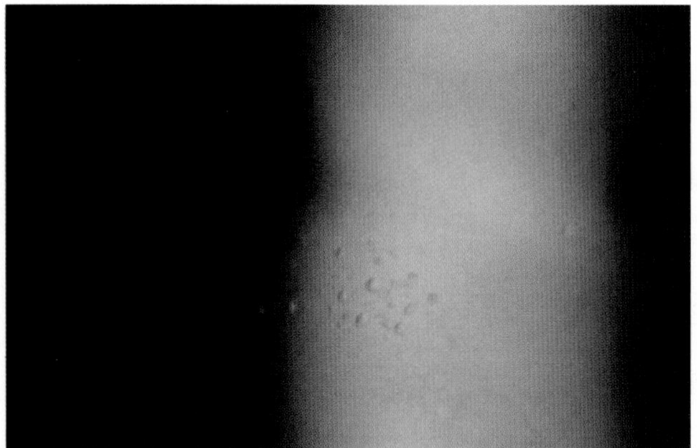

Figure 13.7 Epithelial vacuoles can be distinguished from microcysts by their more rounded shape, and their unreversed illumination, i.e. the light distribution within is the same as the background, which suggests that they represent fluid-filled inclusions. (From Terry et al. 1993, with permission of Lippincott Williams & Wilkins)

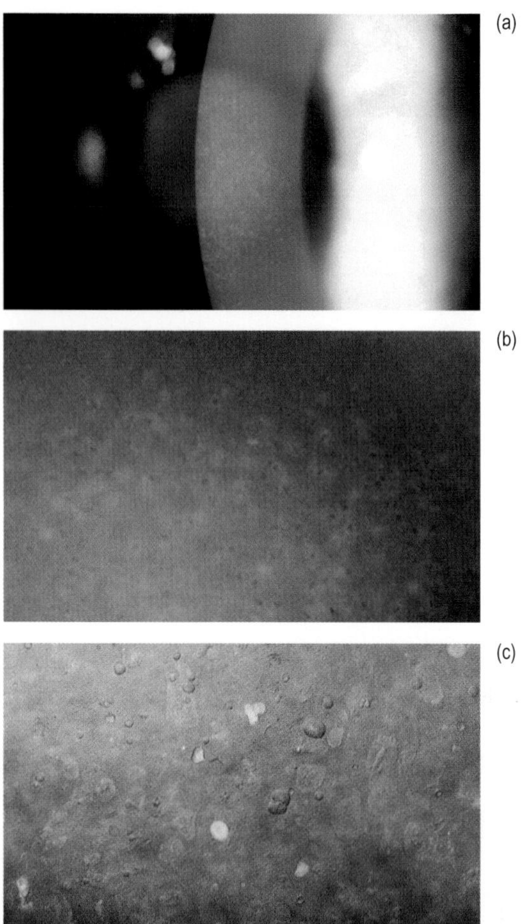

Figure 13.8 In acute localized epithelial oedema, fluid collects in intracellular spaces throughout the epithelial layer. These 'cysts' move rapidly towards the surface where they rupture. (a) The general appearance of this response, sometimes called microcystic oedema, can be similar to superficial punctate keratitis. However, at high magnification (b) the small ruptured and non-ruptured 'cysts' can be clearly seen. (c) Empty (clear) and filled 'cysts' can be seen by using an endothelial camera but focusing at the level of the epithelium. (Courtesy of A. J. Phillips)

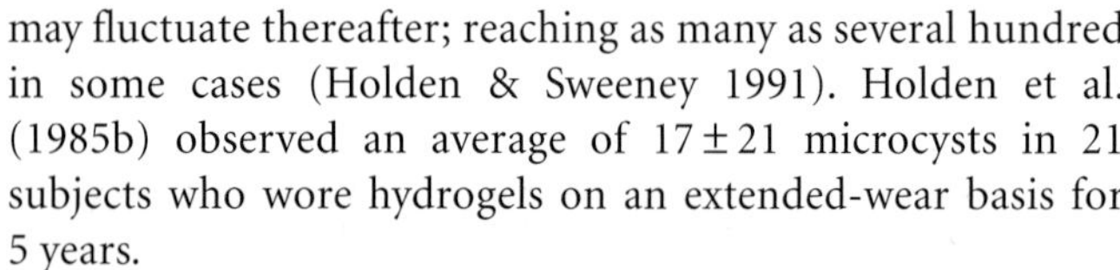

may fluctuate thereafter; reaching as many as several hundred in some cases (Holden & Sweeney 1991). Holden et al. (1985b) observed an average of 17 ± 21 microcysts in 21 subjects who wore hydrogels on an extended-wear basis for 5 years.

If normal levels of oxygen are supplied to the cornea by removing lenses, or by refitting with high-Dk silicone hydrogel lenses, the number of microcysts *increases* within a week and gradually subsides over 1–3 months to non-lens wear levels (Fig. 13.6) (Holden et al. 1985b, Keay et al. 2000). This transitory increase in number, known as the rebound effect, is accompanied by a recovery in epithelial thickness and oxygen uptake rates (see Fig. 13.4) and therefore is an indication that normal metabolic activity has been restored to the epithelium (Holden et al. 1985b). It does not necessitate removal of silicone hydrogel lenses.

Microcysts should not be confused with epithelial vacuoles which are fluid-filled vesicles that also occur during soft contact lens wear (Zantos 1983). Although similar in size, vacuoles can be distinguished from microcysts by their more rounded shape and unreversed illumination (Fig. 13.7). Although the aetiology of vacuoles is unclear, they occur more frequently during extended-wear compared to daily wear, and are noted less frequently with high-Dk silicone hydrogel lenses. Management of vacuoles parallels that for microcysts, with temporary discontinuation of lens wear a recommended strategy if the epithelial barrier is compromised.

Acute epithelial oedema, or microcystic oedema (Fig. 13.8), should also be distinguished from the more chronic microcystic

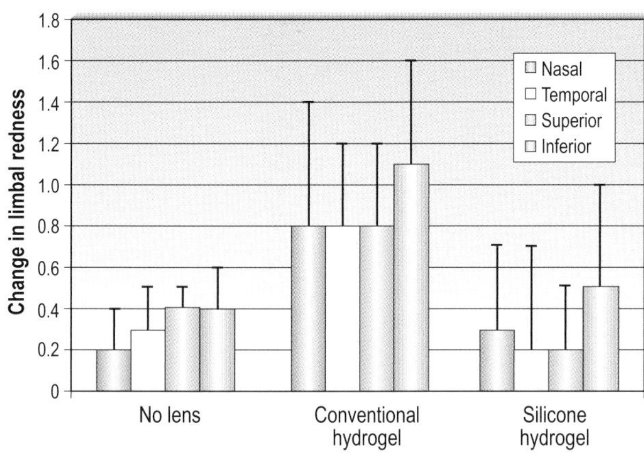

Figure 13.9 Change in limbal redness from baseline after 16 hours. The change in limbal redness was measured using CCLRU decimalized grading scales where 0.0 = absent, 1.0 = very slight, 2.0 = slight, 3.0 = moderate and 4.0 = severe

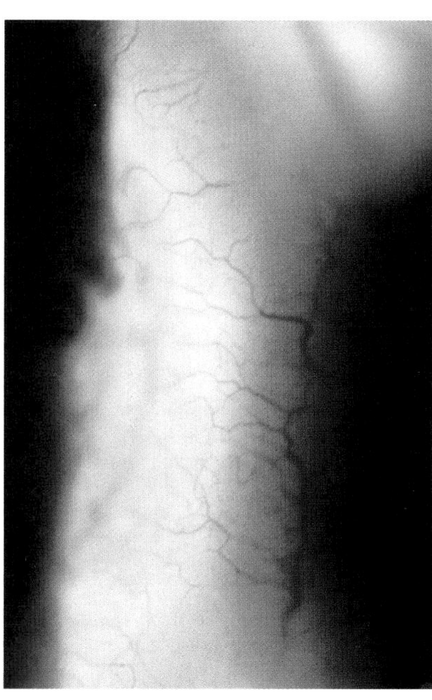

Figure 13.10 Increased limbal vessel proliferation and hyperaemia in association with extended hydrogel lens wear and certain other conditions. (Courtesy of C. McMonnies)

response. It is characterized by more than 200 clear cysts surrounded by epithelial haze and occurs in response to a toxic stimulus, usually within 12 hours of exposure. It resolves rapidly once the stimulus is removed.

LIMBAL HYPERAEMIA

Increased limbal hyperaemia is a common finding with both short-term and extended wear of hydrogel lenses (Holden et al. 1986b) but it does not occur in most high-Dk silicone hydrogel wear (Papas et al. 1997, Brennan et al. 2002, Fonn et al. 2002). Studies by Covey et al. (2001) and Dumbleton et al. (2001) established that the level of redness induced by silicone hydrogels is comparable to no lens wear.

The work of Papas (Papas et al. 1997, Papas 1998, 2003) established that the level of limbal hyperaemia induced by soft lenses correlated with the Dk/t, with the strongest effect in the periphery, and that reduced oxygen concentration at the ocular surface in non-lens wearers induces more blood flow in limbal vessels (Fig. 13.9). Epithelial stem cells rely on the limbal blood vessels to provide nutrients, immunoglobulins and systemic defence components (Zieske 1994). Inflammation at the limbus is therefore a potential cause of damage to the renewal process of the corneal epithelium.

Chronic increased limbal vessel injection and proliferation has the potential to progress to corneal neovascularization (Cogan 1948, Collin 1973) because of the active vascular plexus immediately adjacent to the corneal tissue. Long-term wearers of hydrogel lenses have significantly more limbal vessel penetration compared to non-lens wearers (Holden et al. 1986b) or wearers of high-Dk silicone hydrogels (Holden et al. 1986b, Dumbleton et al. 2001).

Limbal vessels may be distinguished from corneal vessels by locating the translucent limbal transition zone (Fig. 13.10) using marginal retro-illumination with the slit-lamp (McMonnies et al. 1982). Vessels that extend beyond this zone, particularly if unlooped, threaten tissue integrity. Switching from hydrogel to high-Dk silicone hydrogel causes established vessels to empty (Sweeney et al. 2004) (Fig. 13.11); however, these ghost vessels rarely regress and may refill rapidly if low-Dk lens wear resumes (McMonnies 1983).

A variety of predisposing or triggering mechanisms have been proposed for corneal neovascularization, including:

- Peripheral corneal oedema, which reduces stromal tissue compactness at the limbus (Cogan 1949).
- Hypoxia (Knighton et al. 1983).
- By-products of altered corneal metabolism under hypoxic conditions, such as lactate (Imre 1972).
- Vasostimulatory factors released by damaged epithelial cells (Eliason 1978).
- Inflammatory cells (Fromer & Klintworth 1976, Sholley et al. 1978).
- Locally released vasoproliferative factors associated with inflammation (Klintworth & Burger 1983), such as plasminogen activator (Berman et al. 1982, van Setten et al. 1990).

Stroma

STROMAL SWELLING (see also Chapter 17)

Contact lens-induced corneal oedema has been suggested as an aetiological factor in corneal neovascularization (Cogan 1949), limbal injection (Tomlinson & Haas 1980) and changes in corneal curvature (Mandell 1975). In addition, chronic hypoxia, of which stromal oedema is an important index, can have a significant effect on corneal structure and function in the long term (Holden et al. 1985b).

Stromal oedema induced by soft contact lenses is evenly distributed across most of the cornea, although there is

(a)

(b)

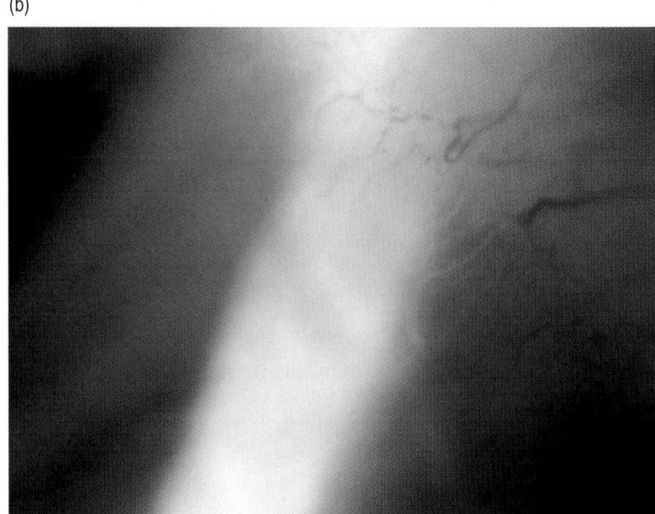

Figure 13.11 Limbal vascularization in a patient after 15 years of low-Dk conventional lens wear (a). After 6 months of silicone hydrogel lens wear a significant reduction in filling of the limbal vessels was observed (b). (From Sweeney et al. 2004, with permission of Butterworth-Heinemann)

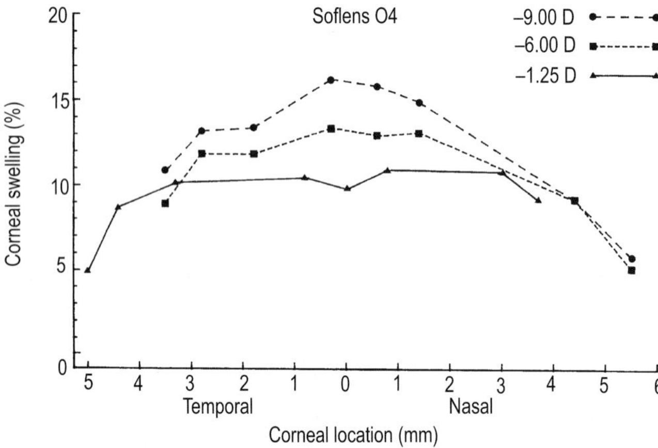

Figure 13.12 Topographical distribution of hydrogel lens-induced corneal oedema of average overnight corneal swelling versus horizontal corneal location. Ten unadapted subjects wore Bausch & Lomb Soflens O4 series contact lenses continuously for a period of 1 week. All subjects wore −1.25 D lenses on one eye; half wore −6.00 D lenses and half wore −9.00 D lenses on the other eye. Significantly less swelling occurred in the peripheral cornea compared to the centre. (●) −9.00 D; (■) −6.00 D; (▲) −1.25 D. (From Holden et al. 1985d, with permission of Blackwell Publishing)

significantly less swelling in the extreme periphery than in the centre (Bonanno & Polse 1985, Holden et al. 1985d) (Fig. 13.12). This is thought to reflect physical restraints at the limbal region.

As discussed previously, estimates for the amount of overnight swelling that occurs in the central cornea of non-lens wearers range from approximately 3 to 4% (Mertz 1980, Koers 1982, La Hood et al. 1988, Cox et al. 1991, Fonn et al. 1999). Extended wear with hydrogels leads to overnight corneal swelling of between 10 and 15% (Holden et al. 1983, La Hood et al. 1988, Fonn et al. 1999), whereas high-Dk silicone hydrogel lenses show no difference from levels in non-lens wearers. Fonn et al. (1999) observed that corneal swelling in lens-wearing eyes is associated with smaller but concomitant increases in swelling in fellow non-lens-wearing eyes. This sympathetic response was repeated by Guzey et al. (2002) in rabbits and also by Drubaix et al. (1997) who found concomitant changes in fellow control eyes after surgery or injury.

Although the absence of corneal swelling with high-Dk silicone hydrogel lenses indicates that hypoxia has been eliminated during overnight wear for most wearers, practitioners should be aware of the variation in oxygen consumption between individuals and the reduced Dk/t of higher-power lenses. Two studies of subjects wearing high-Dk silicone hydrogels demonstrated that although overnight oedema does not occur in most wearers, a small proportion can still experience swelling at levels similar to those seen with low-Dk hydrogels (Comstock et al. 1999, Mueller et al. 2001). In Comstock et al.'s (1999) examination of 30 subjects wearing balafilcon A lenses, 11% experienced overnight corneal swelling greater than 7.7%, the amount that the cornea can eliminate during the day (Holden et al. 1983).

The diffuse nature of lens-induced stromal oedema makes it difficult to visualize with the slit-lamp, as there is minimal light scatter in the stroma unless oedema is severe, and moderate levels are unlikely to give rise to significant symptoms. However, when the stroma swells more than 4–6%, fine striae appear at the posterior stroma and Descemet's membrane (Sarver 1971, Polse & Mandell 1976). These are usually vertical, but may be horizontal or oblique (Fig. 13.13). If stromal oedema is severe (>12–15%), dark lines resembling folds in Descemet's membrane may also be observed (Holden 1977) (Fig. 13.14). La Hood and Grant (1990) devised an easy method for estimating corneal oedema. In this system:

- One stria correlates with a mean of 5% stromal oedema.
- Five striae with 8% oedema.
- Ten striae with 11% oedema.
- One fold suggests 8% oedema.
- Five folds indicate 11% oedema.
- Ten folds indicate 14% oedema.

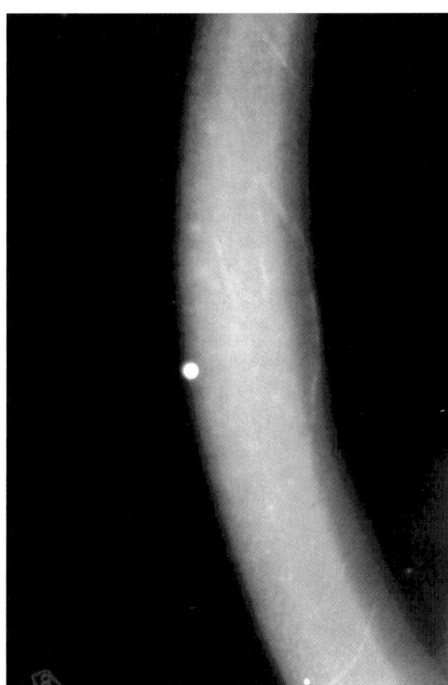

Figure 13.13 Striae begin to appear when approximately 5–6% corneal oedema occurs. They appear as fine, usually vertically oriented, greyish-white, wispy lines in the posterior stroma. They need to be differentiated from nerve fibres, the latter being more regular in appearance and with obvious bifurcations. Striae are thought to represent a refractile effect due to fluid separation of fine, vertically oriented collagen fibrils in the posterior stroma. (From Zantos & Holden 1978, with permission of Optometrists Association Australia)

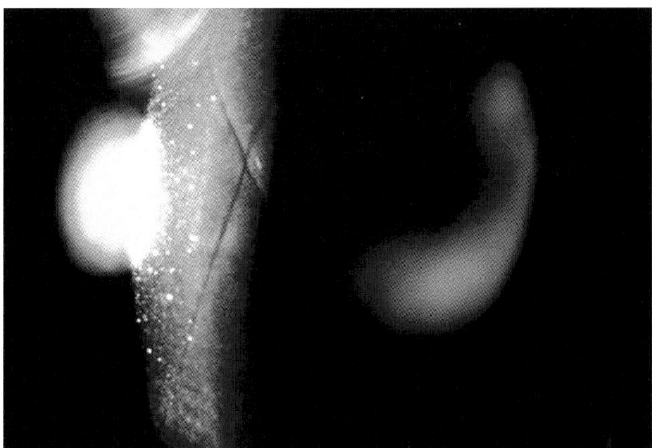

Figure 13.14 Stromal folds form in the posterior stroma and Descemet's membrane when corneal oedema reaches more than 10–12%. They are thought to represent a physical buckling of the posterior corneal layers, as in this case of a patient with 19.6% central corneal oedema induced by a tightly fitted soft lens. (From Zantos & Holden 1978, with permission of Optometrists Association Australia)

Striae and folds are uncommon with continuous wear of high-Dk silicone hydrogels and, if present, indicate a patient with higher than average oxygen demands.

STROMAL THINNING

There have been a series of conflicting reports of the effect of low-Dk lens wear on stromal thickness, showing either a small decrease in thickness (Fig. 13.15) or no apparent change (Holden et al. 1985b, Liu & Pflugfelder 2000, Patel et al. 2002). The differences found between these studies probably reflect the difficulties in isolating the direct effects of contact lens wear on stromal thickness from those caused by residual oedema and by the differences in methodology between the groups.

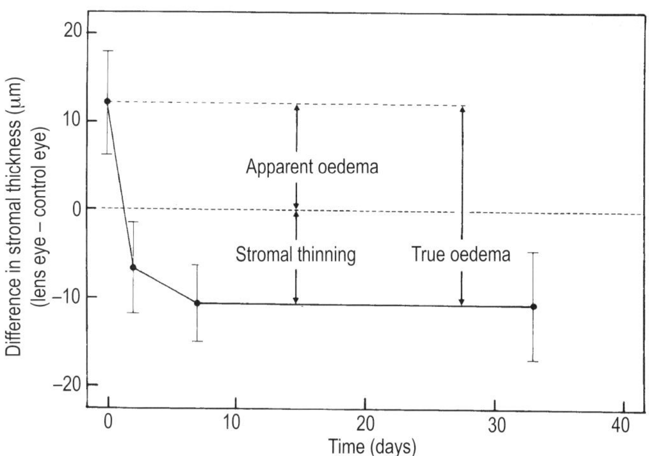

Figure 13.15 Stromal thinning is induced by long-term hydrogel lens wear, but may be masked immediately on lens removal by stromal oedema. This graph, taken from a study of unilateral hydrogel extended lens wearers, shows the change in stromal thickness of the lens-wearing eye relative to the control (non-lens-wearing) eye (top dotted line), after cessation of long-term extended wear of high-water-content hydrogel contact lenses. Data on day 0 were obtained immediately following lens removal. Error bars represent the standard error. The apparent oedema on lens removal, stromal thinning and true oedema are indicated. (Adapted from Holden et al. 1985b, with permission)

Keratocytes comprise up to 10% of the volume of the stroma and help maintain stromal structure. Lens-induced changes to the stroma may be caused by a loss of keratocytes. Although Jalbert and Stapleton (1999) and Efron et al. (2002) reported a reduction in keratocyte density with extended wear of soft lenses, Patel et al. (2002) found no differences in keratocyte density between long-term daily hydrogel wearers and non-lens wearers. Several mechanisms have been suggested to explain the loss of keratocytes, including hypoxia-mediated cell death and/or the pressure-induced effects of lens wear (Jalbert & Stapleton 1999, Kallinikos & Efron 2004, Jalbert et al. 2005).

REFRACTIVE ERROR

Increased myopia (myopic shift) with daily and extended hydrogel lens wear has been reported since the 1970s, in some cases with concurrent steepening of the curvature of the cornea (Grosvenor 1975, Hill 1975, Barnett & Rengstorff 1977, Miller et al. 1980, Binder 1983). High-Dk silicone hydrogels can result in 'hypermetropic shifts' soon after lens wear commences. Jalbert et al. (2004) found an average hyperopic shift (mean = 0.18 ± 0.33 D) with concurrent corneal flattening

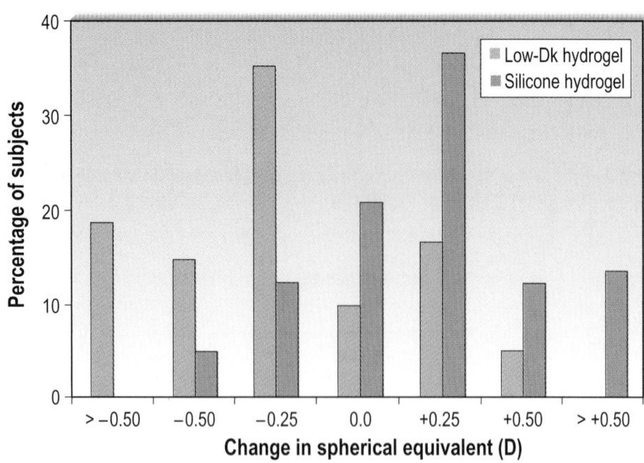

Figure 13.16 Frequency distribution of the progression in myopia after 6 months of extended wear with low-Dk conventional hydrogels or continuous wear with silicone hydrogels. (From Jalbert et al. 2004, with permission of Lippincott Williams & Wilkins)

(mean = −0.24 ± 0.20 D) after 6 months of extended wear. Approximately 26% of the 41 subjects had a hyperopic shift of 0.50 D or more whereas 5% of subjects had a myopic shift of −0.50 D or less (Fig. 13.16). Usually the change in refraction occurs within the first few months of commencing extended wear, and does not worsen afterwards (Dumbleton et al. 1999, Fonn et al. 2002, Jalbert et al. 2004).

Myopic shifts and associated changes in corneal curvature are hypothesized to result from hypoxia-driven corneal oedema leading to an increase in corneal thickness (Høvding 1983a,b, Dumbleton et al. 1999). However, there is little correlation between increases in corneal thickness induced by oedema and changes in shape of the anterior cornea (Carney 1975, Mandell 1975, Rom et al. 1995). Mathematical models indicate that corneal oedema mostly affects the posterior surface of the cornea and is only associated with very small shifts in myopia (Erickson et al. 1999).

Jalbert et al. (2004) propose that lens-induced hypoxia causes corneal steepening through different rates of thinning between the central cornea and the periphery, and that changes in refractive error and corneal flattening associated with high-Dk silicone hydrogel lenses, may be related to pressure-induced changes in corneal shape. They hypothesize that the central cornea is flattened by an orthokeratology-like effect of the silicone hydrogel materials. These effects would be more pronounced in prolate corneas and/or with the increased lens central thickness of high hyperopic corrections.

Practitioners should fully refract their patients before lenses are fitted and carry out corneal topography and central corneal thickness measurements where possible. These should be regularly reviewed during the first months of wear, especially in high hyperopes.

Endothelium

ENDOTHELIAL BLEBS

Endothelial blebs appear as small, dark, non-reflective areas scattered over the endothelial mosaic (Fig. 13.17) and can be easily distinguished from guttata which appear as 'holes' (Fig. 13.18). Blebs have been observed within minutes of inserting both low-Dk soft and RGP lenses (Zantos & Holden 1977a, Barr & Schoessler 1980, Kamiya 1980, Vannas et al. 1981, Schoessler et al. 1982, Inagaki et al. 2003) and also in eyes exposed to atmospheric anoxia (Holden & Zantos 1981) or carbon dioxide (Holden et al. 1985a) and occasionally in non-lens wearers after eye closure (Khodadoust & Hirst 1984, Inagaki et al. 2003). Hamano et al. (2002) found that Asian eyes are more susceptible to the formation of endothelial blebs with low-Dk lenses.

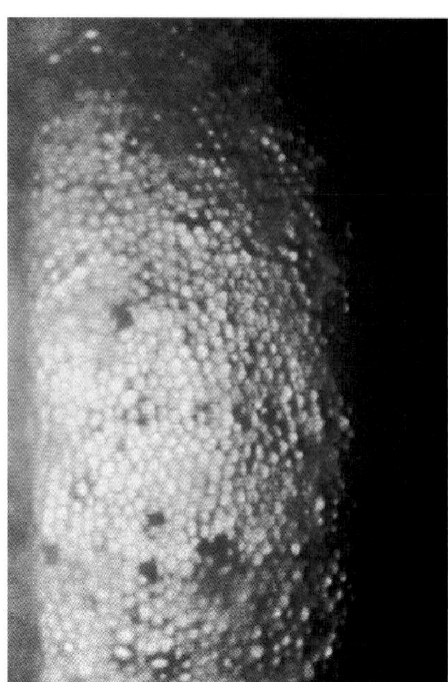

Figure 13.17 Endothelial blebs appear as black, non-reflecting areas of the endothelium, and are best observed using the highest slit-lamp magnification and looking to one side of the specularly reflected light source. (From Holden et al. 1985a, with permission)

Endothelial blebs increase in size and number immediately after exposure to a hypoxic stimulus, then disappear rapidly following removal. In non-lens-wearing eyes, endothelial blebs cover less than 2% of the endothelium after 20 minutes of eye closure and disappear within 15 minutes after eye opening (Inagaki et al. 2003). Bleb formation and disappearance is the same for high-Dk silicone hydrogel lenses and high-Dk RGP lenses of similar Dk (Inagaki et al. 2003). During extended wear with hydrogels, the bleb response occurs in a biphasic diurnal cycle; the number of blebs reduces after eye opening and increases in late afternoon and evening (Williams & Holden 1986).

Endothelial blebs have little clinical significance but are thought to indicate corneal stress from an acid shift under hypoxic conditions (Holden et al. 1985a). As intracorneal pH decreases, endothelial cells become oedematous, causing bulging of the posterior endothelial cell membrane.

ENDOTHELIAL POLYMEGETHISM

Endothelial polymegethism is a normal age-related process; in association with contact lens wear (Fig. 13.19), however, it is believed to be a permanent effect of chronic lens-induced

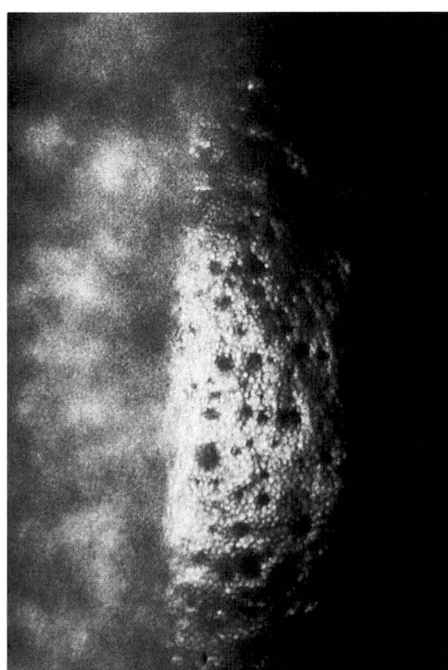

Figure 13.18 Endothelial guttata can be easily distinguished from blebs by their characteristic appearance which resembles 'holes' in the endothelial mosaic and by their persistence even without a contact lens on the eye. Guttata may occur as a congenital deformity, in certain dystrophic conditions, and associated with anterior segment inflammation

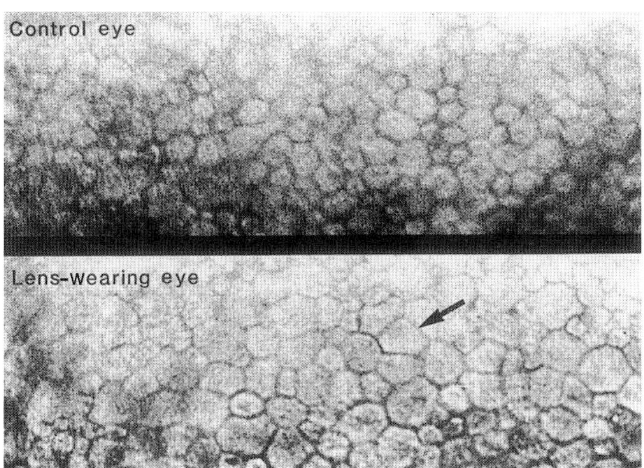

Figure 13.19 Endothelial photograph of the non-lens-wearing eye (top) and lens-wearing eye (bottom) of a patient who had worn a hydrogel lens on an extended-wear basis in one eye only for 79 months. A greater variation in endothelial cell size (polymegethism) is evident in the lens-wearing eye. Also evident in that eye are a number of rosette formations (arrow); these are thought to occur following injury of a single endothelial cell, whereby neighbouring cells radiate towards the centre of the damaged cell. (Adapted from Holden et al. 1985b, with permission)

hypoxia. First reported by Schoessler (1983), it has been observed with long-term daily and extended wear of hydrogel, RGP and PMMA lenses (Schoessler et al. 1982, Hirst et al. 1984, Stocker & Schoessler 1985, MacRae et al. 1986) but not in subjects wearing silicone elastomer (Schoessler et al. 1984) or high-Dk silicone hydrogel lenses (Covey et al. 2001).

Although Sibug et al. (1991) found this effect subsided in long-term wearers, 5 years after discontinuation from lens wear, other evidence indicates that it is irreversible (Holden et al. 1985c, MacRae et al. 1986, Yamauchi et al. 1989).

An association has been reported between significant increases in endothelial polymegethism and pleomorphism and a reduction in endothelial cell density in long-term lens wearers (MacRae et al. 1994, Lee et al. 2001) but it is not confirmed whether endothelial polymegethism and pleomorphism are precursors to the reduction in cell density. Rao et al. (1984) reported that lens wearers with high levels of preoperative endothelial polymegethism are significantly more likely to experience complications following intraocular surgery, suggesting that the changes compromise the functioning of the endothelium. However, Bates and Cheng (1988) failed to substantiate these findings.

Complications associated with soft lens extended wear

CORNEAL INFLAMMATION

Corneal infiltrative events are acute inflammatory responses in which inflammatory cells are released from the limbal vasculature and invade corneal tissue. Infiltrates are thought to comprise predominantly polymorphonuclear leucocytes, although macrophages and lymphocytes may also be present. The chemotactic stimulus to leucocyte invasion may be:

- Traumatic.
- Viral.
- Allergic.
- Toxic.
- Associated with:
  - solution preservatives.
  - poor lens fit or condition.
  - toxic environmental stimuli.
  - bacterial degradative products or toxins (e.g. in chronic blepharitis due to *Staphylococcus* spp.).

Asymptomatic infiltrative reactions also occur in the absence of a contact lens or other obvious stimuli. Up to 30% of the population is reported to exhibit asymptomatic infiltrates upon examination (Josephson & Caffery 1979, Sweeney et al. 1996, Hickson & Papas 1997), indicating that normal protective cellular processes exist in the absence of contact lens wear.

Tears in the closed eye are relatively stagnant, rich in secretory IgA (Sack et al. 1992), increased albumin, activated complement and plasminogen with recruitment of polymorphonuclear cells (Wilson et al. 1989, Sack et al. 1992, Vannas et al. 1992, Tan et al. 1993) and expression of a range of inflammatory mediators (Thakur & Willcox 1998, 2000). These changes are suggestive of a state of subclinical inflammation. The introduction of a contact lens and associated inflammatory stimuli can precipitate an acute inflammatory reaction.

Classification of infiltrative events associated with contact lens wear in the past has focused on whether an event is infectious or sterile (Catania 1987, Stein et al. 1988, Bates et al. 1989, Snyder 1995). Collating data from 10 years of clinical experience at the CCLRU, Sydney, Australia, and the LV Prasad

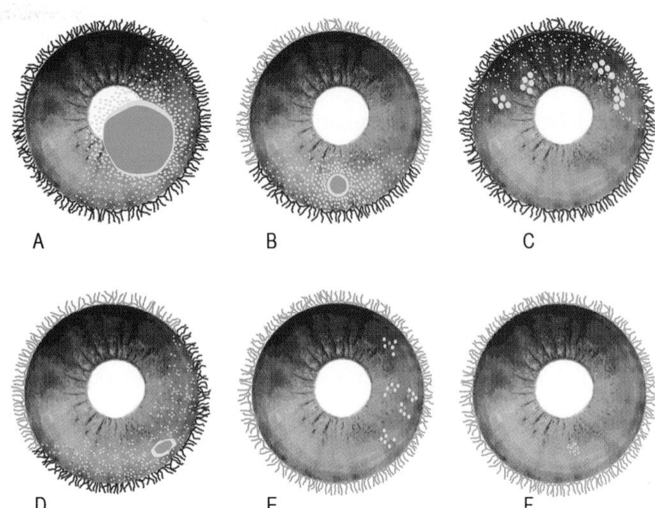

Figure 13.20 The six categories of infiltrative events seen with soft contact lens wear: (A) microbial keratitis, (B) contact lens-induced peripheral ulcer, (C) contact lens-induced acute red eye, (D) infiltrative keratitis, (E) asymptomatic infiltrative keratitis, (F) asymptomatic infiltration. Small yellow dots represent areas of diffuse infiltration, larger yellow dots represent focal infiltration, and green areas represent corneal staining. (From Sweeney et al. 2003, with permission of Lippincott Williams & Wilkins)

Eye Institute (LVPEI), Hyderabad, India, Sweeney et al. (2003) enabled a system to be devised whereby infiltrative events associated with soft contact lens wear can be categorized as serious, clinically significant and clinically insignificant. Microbial keratitis is the only serious event because of the potential for vision loss. Clinically significant events are symptomatic and include contact lens-induced peripheral ulcer (CLPU), CLARE and infiltrative keratitis; clinically insignificant events include asymptomatic infiltrative keratitis and asymptomatic infiltrates (Fig. 13.20).

With the exception of microbial keratitis, most corneal infiltrative events resolve soon after lenses are removed without the need for therapeutic treatment. However practitioners should always take a conservative approach to management and use appropriate therapy if uncertain. Patients should be monitored closely and can resume lens wear once the event has resolved, although some patients may be at greater risk of recurrence. Bates et al. (1989) found that sterile epithelial infiltrates are four times more likely to recur in contact lens-wearing patients compared to non-lens wearers. Sweeney et al. (2003) found recurrence rates of 12% for CLPU, 17% for CLARE and 13% for infiltrative keratitis in those who resumed extended wear.

The incidence of clinically significant corneal infiltrative events is similar with extended wear of both hydrogel and high-Dk silicone hydrogel lenses (Sankaridurg et al. 1999, Sweeney et al. 2002a) (Fig. 13.21), indicating that further lens improvements are still needed.

Pathogenic bacteria colonize soft lenses during extended wear (Sankaridurg et al. 2000). Gram-negative *Pseudomonas aeruginosa*, and the Gram-positive coagulase-negative *Staphylococcus aureus* and *Streptococcus pneumoniae* are the most common associated with microbial keratitis (Galentine et al. 1984, Schein et al. 1989). Less pathogenic strains of these

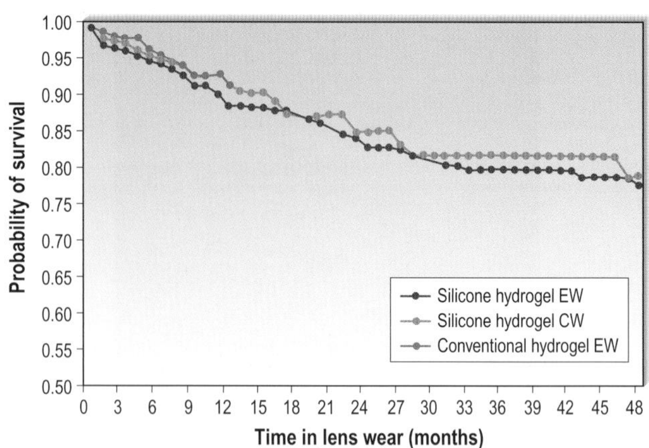

Figure 13.21 Probability of surviving contact lens wear without developing a corneal infiltrative event (CCLRU study data)

bacterial species are also isolated from patients with non-infectious inflammatory events (Cole et al. 1998, Cowell et al. 1998, Wu et al. 2000). Events of CLARE and infiltrative keratitis are most commonly associated with Gram-negative bacterial species, and Gram-positive bacteria are predominantly associated with CLPU (Table 13.1).

MICROBIAL KERATITIS (see Chapters 4, 17 and 18)

The spectrum of bacteria isolated from the known cases of microbial keratitis is the same with continuous wear of high-Dk silicone hydrogels and conventional hydrogels (Edwards et al. 2004). If microbial keratitis is suspected, contact lenses should be removed immediately and the patient treated or referred for treatment without delay. The contact lens, lens case and care solutions should not be discarded but sent for culture.

There is also a possibility that silicone hydrogel lens wearers are at increased risk of *Acanthamoeba* keratitis. In vitro analysis of the attachment of *Acanthamoeba* trophozoites (active and motile phase) to contact lenses indicates that the trophozoites attach in significantly greater numbers to silicone hydrogel lens materials (Beattie et al. 2003).

Epidemiological studies of microbial keratitis with soft lens extended wear show that the annual rates of infection with hydrogel and silicone hydrogel lenses are similar, ranging between 10 and 20 cases per 10,000 wearers (Poggio et al. 1989, Nilsson & Montan 1994, Cheng et al. 1999, Lam et al. 2002, Morgan et al. 2005a, Schein et al. 2005) and that the risk factors for infection remain essentially the same: overnight wear, male gender, smoking and lens care hygiene (Schein et al. 1989, Dart et al. 1991, Stapleton et al. 1993, Lam et al. 2002, Morgan et al. 2005b). Although not confirmed by epidemiological reports, microbial keratitis in silicone hydrogel lens wearers has also been associated with swimming without goggles prior to the event (Lim et al. 2004).

These data stress the importance of careful patient selection, rigorous instruction and continual education for all forms of extended lens wear as delay in removing lenses and in seeking treatment exacerbate the severity of infections (Cooper & Constable 1977, Salz & Slanger 1983, Lemp et al. 1984). Lenses must always be removed and the practitioner contacted

Table 13.1: Microorganisms associated with non-infectious symptomatic infiltrative events

Microbe	Event
Gram-negative bacteria	
Abiotrophia defectiva	Infiltrative keratitis
Acinetobacter spp.	CLARE, infiltrative keratitis
Aeromonas hydrophilia	CLARE
Alcaligenes xylosoxidans subsp. *denitrificans*	Infiltrative keratitis
Branhamella catarrhalis	Infiltrative keratitis
Enterobacter cloacae	Infiltrative keratitis
Escherichia coli	CLARE, infiltrative keratitis
Haemophilus influenzae	CLARE, infiltrative keratitis
Haemophilus parainfluenzae	CLARE, infiltrative keratitis
Klebsiella oxytoca	CLARE, infiltrative keratitis
Klebsiella pneumoniae	CLARE
Neisseria spp.	Infiltrative keratitis
Pseudomonas aeruginosa	CLARE, CLPU
Serratia liquefaciens	CLPU, infiltrative keratitis
Serratia marcescens	CLARE, infiltrative keratitis
Stenotrophomonas maltophilia	CLARE
Gram-positive bacteria	
Non-haemolytic *Streptococcus* spp.	Infiltrative keratitis
Staphylococcus aureus	CLPU, infiltrative keratitis
Streptococcus pneumoniae	CLARE, CLPU, infiltrative keratitis
Streptococcus viridans	CLARE, infiltrative keratitis
Fungi	
Yeast	Infiltrative keratitis
Mould	Infiltrative keratitis

CLARE, contact lens-induced acute red eye; CLPU, contact lens-induced peripheral ulcer.
Data from Holden et al. (1996); Sankaridurg et al. (1996); Sankaridurg et al. unpublished. Cultures returning normal microbiota (coagulase-negative staphylococci, *Propionibacterium* spp. and *Corynebacterium* spp.) are not included as these would have been cultured in the absence of an adverse event. (After Willcox et al. 2004, with permission of Butterworth-Heinemann)

immediately if any unusual redness, discomfort or blurred vision occurs, particularly in one eye only (see also Chapters 11 and 32).

Extended-wear lenses for therapeutic purposes carry an increased risk of corneal infection, due to the frequent presence of concomitant disease and epithelial compromise (Dohlman et al. 1973, Kent et al. 1990). Other factors that may increase the risk of corneal infection include:

- Concomitant immune disease (Chalupa et al. 1987).
- Lens wear in warm climates (Liesegang & Forster 1980, Sjöstrand et al. 1981).
- The initiation of inappropriate antibiotic (Galentine et al. 1984, Derick et al. 1989) or corticosteroid therapy (Eichebaum et al. 1982, Adams et al. 1983, Chalupa et al. 1987, Derick et al. 1989).

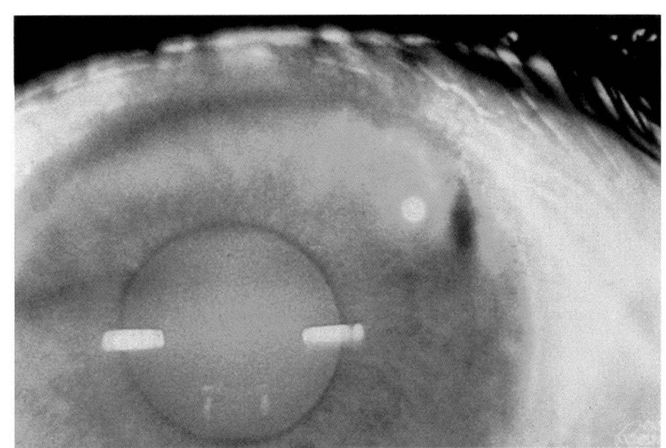

Figure 13.22 Contact lens-induced peripheral ulcer (From Swarbrick & Holden 1993, with permission)

- Diabetics have abnormal endothelial structure and function (Schulz et al. 1984, Weston et al. 1995, Roszkowska et al. 1999), increasing their risk of complications during extended wear (Eichebaum et al. 1982, Spoor et al. 1984). Practitioners should always exercise caution, therefore, when recommending lens wear to patients with diabetes.

CONTACT LENS-INDUCED PERIPHERAL ULCER (CLPU)

(see Chapter 18)

CLPU is associated mostly with extended wear of soft contact lenses (Long et al. 2000, Iruzubieta et al. 2001, Sweeney et al. 2003).

In its active stage, CLPU is characterized by limbal and bulbar redness with one, or very rarely two, small (<2 mm diameter), circular, well-circumscribed full-thickness epithelial lesions and occasionally multiple infiltrates (Sweeney et al. 2000). The lesions occur in the peripheral or mid-periphery of the cornea and are surrounded by diffuse infiltration (Fig. 13.22). Sometimes, CLPU is detected at routine after-care visits on the basis of residual scarring. This scarring is a small, white, circular anterior stromal opacity in the corneal periphery and appears as a 'bull's eye'.

When diagnosing CLPU, a conservative approach is needed. CLPU signs and symptoms are relatively benign compared to those observed with microbial keratitis, and they rapidly resolve after lenses are removed. CLPU lesions are always circular in shape, which is in contrast to microbial keratitis where lesions are usually irregular, larger (>1 mm) and may have smaller satellite lesions. The size of a lesion should not be used as a single differentiating feature as small infiltrates (<1 mm) may still be culture-positive (Stein et al. 1988). CCLRU and LVPEI have devised a probability index to guide practitioners in their diagnosis (Fig. 13.23). Central infiltrates and overlying epithelial loss or irregular, focal infiltrates with raised edges of satellite lesions should be treated as microbial keratitis until proven otherwise; all lesions should be closely monitored because of the potential for misdiagnosis.

CONTACT LENS-INDUCED ACUTE RED EYE (CLARE)

CLARE is an acute complication of extended wear of soft contact lenses that is alarming for both lens wearers and practitioners. Symptoms always manifest after overnight sleep and include conjunctival redness, tearing and ocular irritation or pain. About a third of patients are woken by severe pain (Sweeney et al. 2003).

Clinical signs include:

- Marked conjunctival and circumferential limbal hyperaemia.
- Multiple focal infiltrates with circumferential diffuse infiltration (Fig. 13.24).
- Epithelial staining not overlying the infiltrates, which often corresponds to the pattern of tear debris.
- A uveal response in severe cases with aqueous flare and keratic precipitates.
- Reduced vision if infiltration occurs in the central cornea.

Lens wearers should be advised to remove their lenses immediately and to consult their practitioner as soon as possible. Lens removal generally gives considerable relief from symptoms, although cold compresses may be helpful to relieve ocular discomfort. Patients should be seen as soon as possible in the morning, and again later in the day following the episode. Any sign of aqueous involvement requires prompt treatment.

The major discomfort of CLARE usually resolves within 3 days, although infiltrates may take up to 2 weeks (Sweeney et al. 2003) and complete resolution within 6 weeks. Once the cornea is clear, extended wear can recommence with a lens. If patients have repeat events they should be counselled on their risk of recurrences.

CLARE is considered to be:

- Associated with Gram-negative bacterial colonization of soft contact lenses especially *P. aeruginosa* (Baleriola-Lucas et al. 1991, Holden et al. 1996, Sankaridurg et al. 1996).

INFILTRATIVE KERATITIS (see also Chapters 17 and 18)

Infiltrative keratitis is a relatively mild inflammatory event in an otherwise quiet eye. Symptoms are not associated with sleep, rarely occur in the morning, and can include irritation and tearing. Events are usually associated with ocular redness and are characterized by dense diffuse corneal infiltration in the

(a)

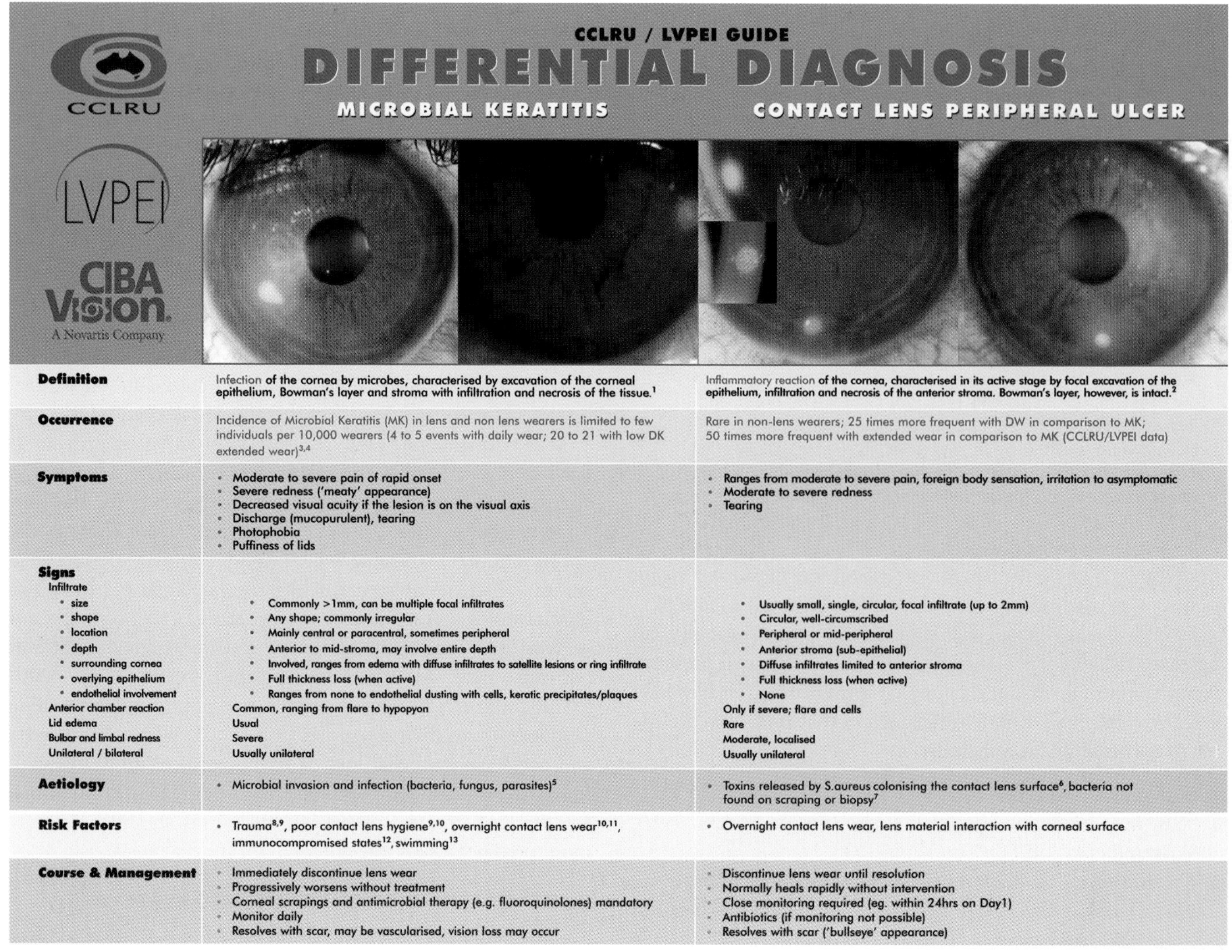

	MICROBIAL KERATITIS	CONTACT LENS PERIPHERAL ULCER
Definition	Infection of the cornea by microbes, characterised by excavation of the corneal epithelium, Bowman's layer and stroma with infiltration and necrosis of the tissue.[1]	Inflammatory reaction of the cornea, characterised in its active stage by focal excavation of the epithelium, infiltration and necrosis of the anterior stroma. Bowman's layer, however, is intact.[2]
Occurrence	Incidence of Microbial Keratitis (MK) in lens and non lens wearers is limited to few individuals per 10,000 wearers (4 to 5 events with daily wear; 20 to 21 with low DK extended wear)[3,4]	Rare in non-lens wearers; 25 times more frequent with DW in comparison to MK; 50 times more frequent with extended wear in comparison to MK (CCLRU/LVPEI data)
Symptoms	• Moderate to severe pain of rapid onset • Severe redness ('meaty' appearance) • Decreased visual acuity if the lesion is on the visual axis • Discharge (mucopurulent), tearing • Photophobia • Puffiness of lids	• Ranges from moderate to severe pain, foreign body sensation, irritation to asymptomatic • Moderate to severe redness • Tearing
Signs		
Infiltrate		
• size	• Commonly >1mm, can be multiple focal infiltrates	• Usually small, single, circular, focal infiltrate (up to 2mm)
• shape	• Any shape; commonly irregular	• Circular, well-circumscribed
• location	• Mainly central or paracentral, sometimes peripheral	• Peripheral or mid-peripheral
• depth	• Anterior to mid-stroma, may involve entire depth	• Anterior stroma (sub-epithelial)
• surrounding cornea	• Involved, ranges from edema with diffuse infiltrates to satellite lesions or ring infiltrate	• Diffuse infiltrates limited to anterior stroma
• overlying epithelium	• Full thickness loss (when active)	• Full thickness loss (when active)
• endothelial involvement	• Ranges from none to endothelial dusting with cells, keratic precipitates/plaques	• None
Anterior chamber reaction	Common, ranging from flare to hypopyon	Only if severe; flare and cells
Lid edema	Usual	Rare
Bulbar and limbal redness	Severe	Moderate, localised
Unilateral / bilateral	Usually unilateral	Usually unilateral
Aetiology	• Microbial invasion and infection (bacteria, fungus, parasites)[5]	• Toxins released by S.aureus colonising the contact lens surface[6], bacteria not found on scraping or biopsy[7]
Risk Factors	• Trauma[8,9], poor contact lens hygiene[9,10], overnight contact lens wear[10,11], immunocompromised states[12], swimming[13]	• Overnight contact lens wear, lens material interaction with corneal surface
Course & Management	• Immediately discontinue lens wear • Progressively worsens without treatment • Corneal scrapings and antimicrobial therapy (e.g. fluoroquinolones) mandatory • Monitor daily • Resolves with scar, may be vascularised, vision loss may occur	• Discontinue lens wear until resolution • Normally heals rapidly without intervention • Close monitoring required (eg. within 24hrs on Day1) • Antibiotics (if monitoring not possible) • Resolves with scar ('bullseye' appearance)

Figure 13.23 CCLRU/LVPEI guide to differential diagnosis of microbial keratitis from contact lens-induced peripheral ulcers

subepithelium in the corneal mid-periphery to periphery (Zantos & Holden 1977b, 1978, Josephson & Caffery 1979) (Fig. 13.25).

In mild cases, lenses should be removed until infiltrates resolve. More severe cases can occur and these should be treated as microbial keratitis until proven otherwise (see Chapter 18). Mild stromal infiltrates take approximately 2 weeks to resolve whereas more severe cases can take several months.

If the predisposing factor can be found, such as excessive lens deposition or solution preservatives, extended wear can be resumed with caution. In cases associated with chronic staphylococcal blepharitis, improved lid hygiene and treatment with antibiotics are recommended before resuming lens wear.

CONTACT LENS-INDUCED PAPILLARY CONJUNCTIVITIS (CLPC) (see Chapters 17 and 18 and Appendix B)

CLPC or giant papillary conjunctivitis (GPC) is characterized by pronounced papillary hypertrophy and hyperaemia of the upper tarsal conjunctiva (Fig. 13.26), with excess mucus discharge and ocular itching and discomfort.

CLPC is one of the most common reasons patients discontinue lens wear. The condition is precipitated by all lens modalities (Allansmith et al. 1978, Poggio & Abelson 1993, Nilsson 2001, and others), is more common with soft lenses than RGPs (Alemany & Redal 1991), and occurs more with extended wear than daily wear (Levy et al. 1997).

With soft lenses papillae occur either as small clusters localized to one area of the tarsal conjunctiva (local CLPC) or are randomly spread across the entire tarsus (general CLPC) (see Fig. 13.26). However, local CLPC is more commonly observed with silicone hydrogel lenses compared to conventional hydrogel lenses (Skotnitsky et al. 2000a,b, Sankaridurg et al. 2001b).

The aetiology of CLPC is not fully understood but is thought to involve delayed hypersensitivity (Allansmith et al. 1978) or IgE-mediated hypersensitivity (Donshik & Ballow 1983) predominantly to deposits on the lens surface rather than the lens material itself (Fowler et al. 1979) or from a mechanical

(b)

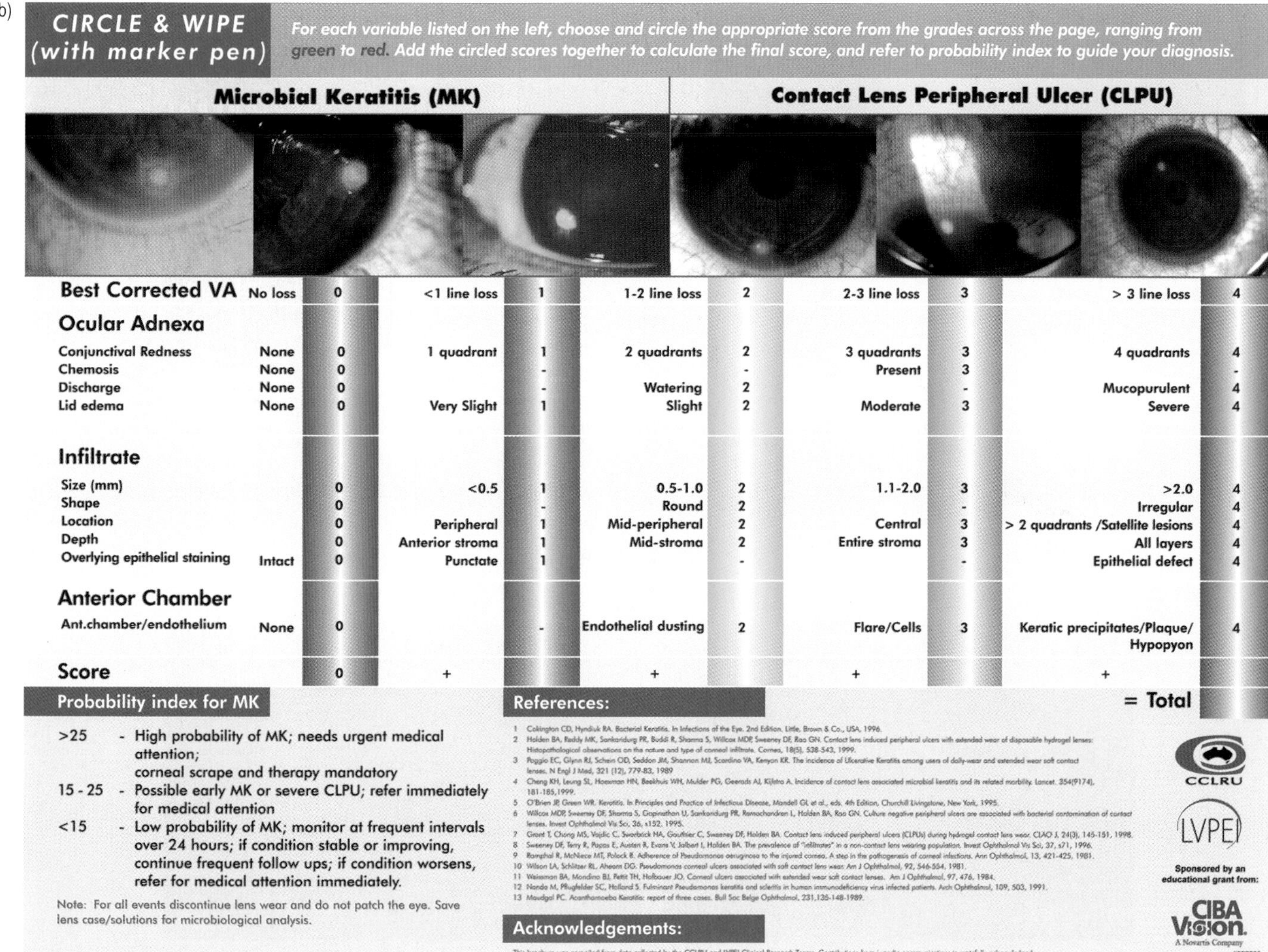

CIRCLE & WIPE (with marker pen)

For each variable listed on the left, choose and circle the appropriate score from the grades across the page, ranging from green to red. Add the circled scores together to calculate the final score, and refer to probability index to guide your diagnosis.

Microbial Keratitis (MK) | **Contact Lens Peripheral Ulcer (CLPU)**

Best Corrected VA	No loss	0	<1 line loss	1	1-2 line loss	2	2-3 line loss	3	> 3 line loss	4
Ocular Adnexa										
Conjunctival Redness	None	0	1 quadrant	1	2 quadrants	2	3 quadrants	3	4 quadrants	4
Chemosis	None	0		-		-	Present	3		-
Discharge	None	0		-	Watering	2		-	Mucopurulent	4
Lid edema	None	0	Very Slight	1	Slight	2	Moderate	3	Severe	4
Infiltrate										
Size (mm)		0	<0.5	1	0.5-1.0	2	1.1-2.0	3	>2.0	4
Shape		0		-	Round	2		-	Irregular	4
Location		0	Peripheral	1	Mid-peripheral	2	Central	3	> 2 quadrants /Satellite lesions	4
Depth		0	Anterior stroma	1	Mid-stroma	2	Entire stroma	3	All layers	4
Overlying epithelial staining	Intact	0	Punctate	1		-		-	Epithelial defect	4
Anterior Chamber										
Ant.chamber/endothelium	None	0		-	Endothelial dusting	2	Flare/Cells	3	Keratic precipitates/Plaque/ Hypopyon	4
Score		0	+		+		+		+	
									= Total	

Probability index for MK

>25 - High probability of MK; needs urgent medical attention; corneal scrape and therapy mandatory

15 - 25 - Possible early MK or severe CLPU; refer immediately for medical attention

<15 - Low probability of MK; monitor at frequent intervals over 24 hours; if condition stable or improving, continue frequent follow ups; if condition worsens, refer for medical attention immediately.

Note: For all events discontinue lens wear and do not patch the eye. Save lens case/solutions for microbiological analysis.

References:

1 Cokington CD, Hyndiuk RA. Bacterial Keratitis. In Infections of the Eye. 2nd Edition. Little, Brown & Co., USA, 1996.
2 Holden BA, Reddy MK, Sankaridurg PR, Buddi R, Sharma S, Willcox MDP, Sweeney DF, Rao GN. Contact lens induced peripheral ulcers with extended wear of disposable hydrogel lenses: Histopathological observations on the nature and type of corneal infiltrate. Cornea, 18(5), 538-543, 1999.
3 Poggio EC, Glynn RJ, Schein OD, Seddon JM, Shannon MJ, Scardino VA, Kenyon KR. The incidence of Ulcerative Keratitis among users of daily-wear and extended wear soft contact lenses. N Engl J Med, 321 (12), 779-83, 1989
4 Cheng KH, Leung SL, Hoekman HN, Beekhuis WH, Mulder PG, Geerards AJ, Kijlstra A. Incidence of contact lens associated microbial keratitis and its related morbility. Lancet. 354(9174), 181-185,1999.
5 O'Brien JP, Green WR. Keratitis. In Principles and Practice of Infectious Disease, Mandell GL et al., eds. 4th Edition, Churchill Livingstone, New York, 1995.
6 Willcox MDP, Sweeney DF, Sharma S, Gopinathan U, Sankaridurg PR, Ramachandran L, Holden BA, Rao GN. Culture negative peripheral ulcers are associated with bacterial contamination of contact lenses. Invest Ophthalmol Vis Sci, 36, s152, 1995.
7 Grant T, Chong MS, Vajdic C, Swarbrick HA, Gauthier C, Sweeney DF, Holden BA. Contact lens induced peripheral ulcers (CLPUs) during hydrogel contact lens wear. CLAO J, 24(3), 145-151, 1998.
8 Sweeney DF, Terry R, Papas E, Austen R, Evans V, Jalbert I, Holden BA. The prevalence of "infiltrates" in a non-contact lens wearing population. Invest Ophthalmol Vis Sci, 37, s71, 1996.
9 Ramphal R, McNiece MT, Polack R. Adherence of Pseudomonas aeruginosa to the injured cornea. A step in the pathogenesis of corneal infections. Ann Ophthalmol, 13, 421-425, 1981.
10 Wilson LA, Schlitzer RL, Ahearn DG. Pseudomonas corneal ulcers associated with soft contact lens wear. Am J Ophthalmol, 92, 546-554, 1981.
11 Weissman BA, Mondino BJ, Pettit TH, Hofbauer JO. Corneal ulcers associated with extended wear soft contact lenses. Am J Ophthalmol, 97, 476, 1984.
12 Nanda M, Pflugfelder SC, Holland S. Fulminant Pseudomonas keratitis and scleritis in human immunodeficiency virus infected patients. Arch Ophthalmol, 109, 503, 1991.
13 Maudgal PC. Acanthamoeba Keratitis: report of three cases. Bull Soc Belge Ophthalmol, 231,135-148-1989.

Acknowledgements:

This brochure was compiled from data collected by the CCLRU and LVPEI Clinical Research Teams. Contributions from i-media communications is gratefully acknowledged.

Figure 13.23 Cont'd

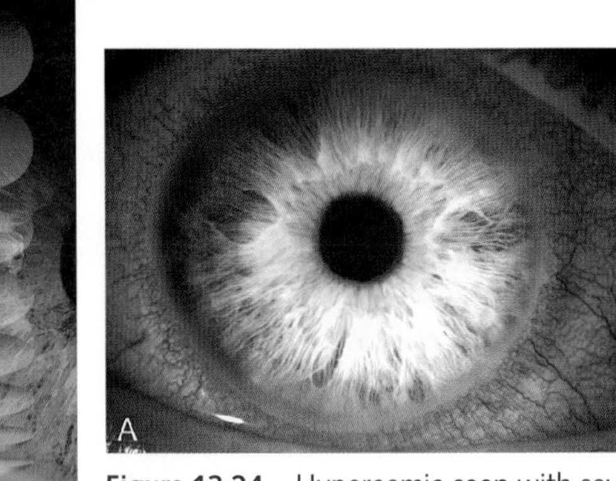

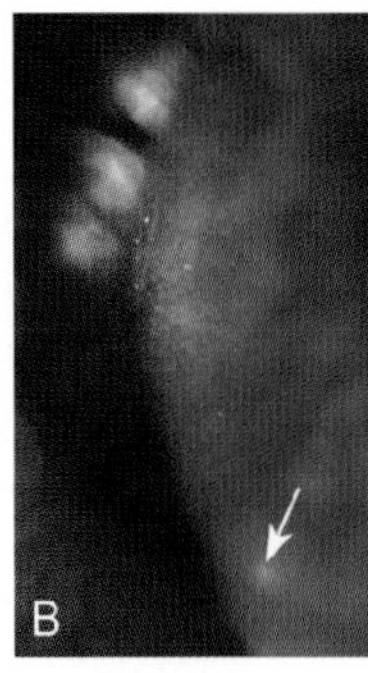

Figure 13.24 Hyperaemia seen with severe contact lens-induced red eye (A). An example of diffuse and focal infiltration is indicated by the arrow (B). (From Sweeney et al. 2003, with permission of Lippincott Williams & Wilkins)

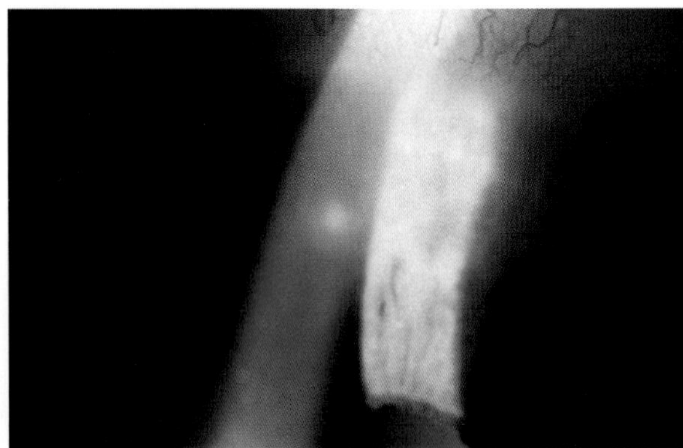

Figure 13.25 Stromal infiltrates appear as hazy, grey areas which may be focal, as shown here, or diffuse. (Courtesy of H. Rypdal)

component such as trauma (Reynolds 1978, Sankaridurg et al. 2001a, and others). The irritation of a lens or suture may allow access of the antigen to the mucous membrane, initiating a hypersensitivity reaction in susceptible individuals (Molinari 1983).

Once CLPC has resolved (for treatment strategies, see Chapters 17 and 18), patients can resume extended wear with a different lens material, but if there is a recurrent event the patient should be refitted with either a daily disposable or frequent replacement hydrogel lens, or an RGP lens.

SUPERIOR EPITHELIAL ARCUATE LESIONS (SEALS) (see Chapter 17)

Sometimes reported as epithelial splits (Malinovsky et al. 1989) or superior arcuate keratopathy (Young & Mirejovsky 1993), SEALs occur with all types of soft lenses (Holden et al. 2001). SEALs are whitish, arcuate-shaped lesions usually found between the 10 and 2 o'clock positions of the superior cornea with clear cornea between lesion and limbus in the area covered by the upper eyelid. Patients with continuous-wear silicone hydrogels can also develop SEALs in the paracentral region of the cornea (O'Hare et al. 2000) (Fig. 13.27). Most patients are asymptomatic or experience minor discomfort or foreign body sensation; lesions in the paracentral region are more likely to cause symptoms.

Risk factors include:

- Tight upper lids.
- Oriental race.
- Low-positioned upper lids.
- Steep corneas.
- Lens material and design characteristics (Kline & De Luca 1977, Josephson 1978a,b, Horowitz et al. 1985, Young & Mirejovsky 1993, and others).
- Poor tear film characteristics.
- Tighter-fitting lenses (O'Hare et al. 2002).

Most factors indicate a mechanical aetiology with inadequate lens flexure causing misalignment of the lens in the superior cornea where pressure from the lid forces the lens against the cornea (Young & Mirejovsky 1993). Localized pressure from the lens may thin the tear film in the superior region which would exacerbate the existing frictional forces. Silicone hydrogel lenses are made from slightly stiffer lens materials and when first introduced were associated with an increased risk of SEALs; however, the improved designs of current lenses have eliminated this risk.

SEALs resolve quickly once lenses are removed and require minimal intervention (Hine et al. 1987, Malinovsky et al. 1989, Gerry 1995, Sankaridurg et al. 1999). Patients can resume lens wear with a new lens once staining and infiltration have resolved but unless the type of lens is changed, there is a greater risk of a

(a)

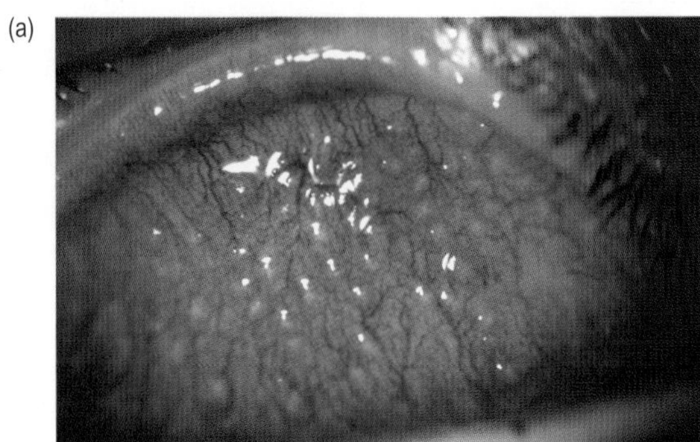

(b)

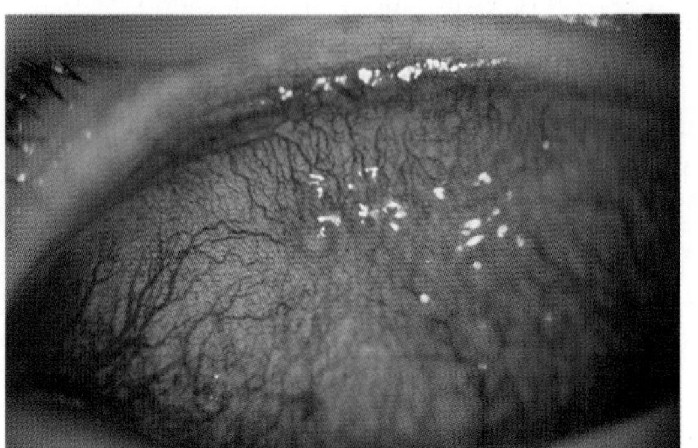

Figure 13.26 Contact lens-induced papillary conjunctivitis (CLPC). Papillae are scattered over the entire tarsus in general CLPC (a) or are localized to one or two zones in local CLPC (b)

(a)

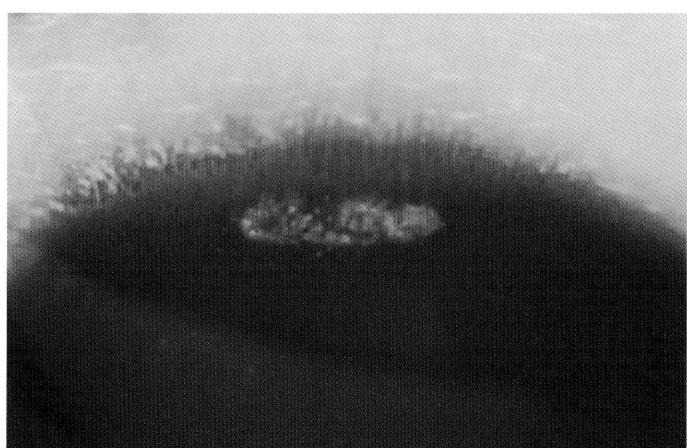

(b)

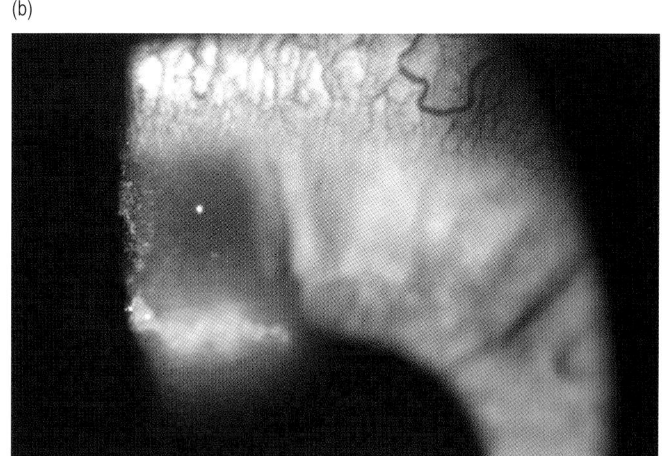

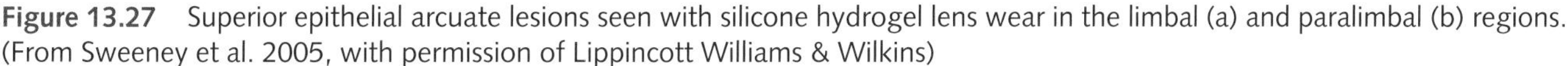

Figure 13.27 Superior epithelial arcuate lesions seen with silicone hydrogel lens wear in the limbal (a) and paralimbal (b) regions. (From Sweeney et al. 2005, with permission of Lippincott Williams & Wilkins)

recurrence (Hine et al. 1987, Malinovsky et al. 1989). Patients who experience more than two events may be predisposed to this condition and should be refitted with new silicone hydrogel, conventional hydrogel or RGP lenses.

Patient selection and lens fitting

PATIENT SELECTION (see Chapter 8)

Selection of suitable candidates for contact lens wear is critical for achieving success with any contact lens type or wear modality, including extended wear. It involves avoiding patients with potential for adverse events and discouraging those whose expectations are unrealistic for the product.

As discussed above, convenience is the primary reason for patients wanting extended wear. It offers advantages for all, in particular those with specific occupations, such as military personnel or those on call, and for certain leisure pursuits such as camping or ocean sailing where daily lens removal is awkward or inconvenient.

Overall, patients find hydrogels and silicone hydrogel lenses comfortable (Nilsson 2001, Brennan et al. 2002, Fonn & Dumbleton 2003). There are some indications for patients who experience symptoms of dryness and discomfort with hydrogels to be refitted with silicone hydrogel lenses (Brennan et al. 2002, du Toit et al. 2003, Aakre et al. 2004) and they may also be beneficial for patients who complain of dryness or who work in highly air-conditioned or dry environments.

Continuous wear with silicone hydrogel lenses is well tolerated by those who require contact lenses for therapeutic purposes, and also in piggyback systems where the combination of high-Dk/t with a soft lens material promotes corneal healing and the alleviation of ocular discomfort (see Chapter 26).

Contraindications for extended- or continuous-wear lenses include:

- Compromised immunity.
- Severe allergies.
- Patients on systemic medication such as steroids.
- Repeated episodes of mechanical or inflammatory events.
- Difficulties with daily wear.
- Inability to maintain an extended-wear schedule.

LENS FITTING

There are no major differences in the approach to fitting hydrogel lenses compared to silicone hydrogel lenses or any other soft lens type (see Chapter 10). The main aim is to optimize lens movement and centration, maximize tear exchange and avoid discomfort and lens awareness. Trial lens fitting should be carried out before extended or continuous wear commences and alternative products tried if difficulties or abnormalities are encountered. The lens should not fit tightly or tighten with wear, and should move across the cornea with ease when pushed up by the eyelid. Lenses should be slightly loose (45–50% tightness using the push-up test; Young et al. 1993) with 0.2–0.3 mm lens movement and good limbal coverage in all gaze positions.

The proportion of patients who can be successfully fitted with hydrogel and silicone hydrogel lenses is similar, but the reasons for failure are different. Unsuccessful lens fitting with conventional hydrogel lenses is primarily caused by insufficient limbal coverage and decentration, whereas lens fluting – an intermittent buckling at the lens edge (Fig. 13.28) – is the main cause of failure with silicone hydrogels (Sweeney et al. 2002b).

Patients who experience discomfort during the trial fit may not adapt to this discomfort over time, although fitting a steeper BOZR may solve the problem (Dumbleton et al. 2002). If this does not resolve lens fluting, an alternative lens type is necessary.

After-care and patient management

New lens wearers should be adapted to their lenses with a short period of daily wear (minimum of 1 week). If no problems are encountered they can proceed to extended wear over several nights using a new pair of lenses and, if successfully using

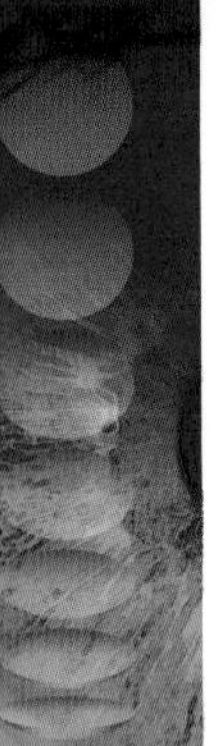

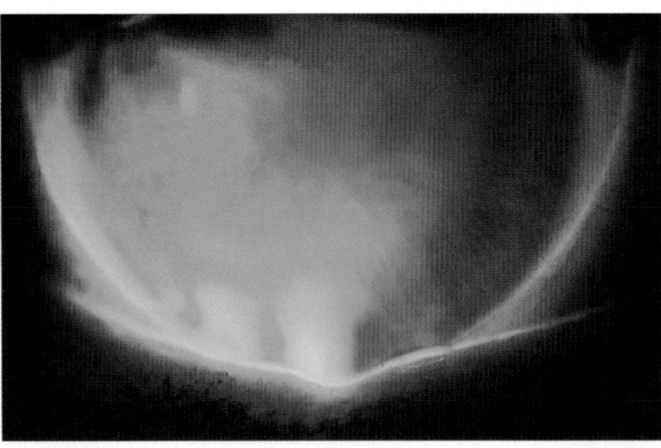

Figure 13.28 Lens fluting indicating an unsuccessful fit with a silicone hydrogel lens. Visualization is improved with fluorexon, a high-molecular-weight fluorescein. (From Sweeney et al. 2005, with permission of Lippincott Williams & Wilkins)

silicone hydrogels, move on to 30-night continuous wear once they have demonstrated success with extended wear. This allows the practitioner to assess a patient's suitability for lens wear and allows patients to become accustomed to lens insertion and removal as well as care and maintenance regimens.

Patients should be seen early in the morning following the first month, then every 3 to 6 months thereafter. Practitioners who are new to continuous wear may wish to see their patients more frequently in the initial stages of lens wear. Patients should be encouraged to bring their lens solutions and case to each after-care visit to discuss and reinforce lens-handling techniques, and care and maintenance procedures. Patients must be advised to consult their practitioner if problems arise between scheduled after-care visits and must have access to a practitioner 24 hours a day.

For details of after-care assessments, see Chapters 10 and 17. Table 13.2 outlines recommended guidelines for assessing successful wear of high-Dk silicone hydrogel lenses.

Table 13.2: Guidelines for successful continuous wear with high-Dk silicone hydrogels

Characteristic	Requirement
Wear time	Ability to wear lenses for ≥6 consecutive nights
Comfort	Grade 3 (comfortable) or better
Subjective vision rating	Grade 3 (good) or better
Visual acuity	Within one line of best spectacle acuity
Biomicroscopy	
Hypoxic effects	≤10 microcysts/vacuoles No striae 1 hour after wakening No endothelial folds
Vascularization	≤0.5 mm vessel penetration
Endothelial polymegethism	≤ one grade increase
Change in corneal curvature/refractive error	≤ ± 0.50 D flat *K* and/or ± 0.75 D steep *K* ≤ ± 0.50 D sphere and/or ± 0.75 D cylinder with spectacles
Corneal staining	Macropunctate staining (≤ Grade 2) Superficial epithelial involvement (≤ Grade 1) ≤1–15% surface involvement (Grade 1)
Lens adherence	No signs 1 hour after awakening
Eyelid changes	≤ one grade increase in papillae or redness of the superior palpebral conjunctiva
Bulbar redness	≤ one grade increase
Lens fit	
Tightness	45–50%
Movement	0.2–0.3 mm
Limbal coverage	Good in all gaze positions and no fluting
Lens deposition	≤ Grade 1
Wettability	Equivalent to hydrogel lenses

Grading scales refer to those outlined in CCLRU/IER Standards for Success of Daily and Extended Wear Contact Lenses (Terry et al. 1993). From Sweeney et al. (2002b), with permission of the Optometrists Association of Australia.

Lens care and maintenance

Although silicone hydrogel lenses can be worn for up to 30 nights without removal, patients should be encouraged to be flexible in their wearing schedule and remove lenses as often as necessary to reduce the potential risk of adverse events. Patients should be discouraged from wearing contact lenses:

- During upper respiratory tract infections.
- During hospitalization.
- While swimming (or to wear watertight swimming goggles).

If lenses are removed overnight or for long periods of time, they should be cleaned and disinfected before they are reinserted. Lenses can be disinfected with a peroxide system with a 4- to 6-hour soak before wear or thoroughly rubbed and rinsed with multipurpose solution followed by a 4- to 6-hour soak in fresh solution before wear. Lenses that are removed for brief periods should be rubbed and rinsed with sterile unit dose unpreserved saline before reinsertion.

Some silicone hydrogel wearers may develop unacceptable levels of corneal staining with their lens care solution. Little or no solution staining occurs with hydrogen peroxide-based or polyquaternium-1-based systems but different silicone hydrogel lenses vary in their interaction with polyaminopropyl biguanide (PHMB)-based multipurpose solutions. PHMB may not be the only factor contributing to this staining as the same silicone hydrogel can interact differently with PHMB multipurpose solutions made from different formulations (see Chapter 4).

Practitioners should ensure that all patients are confident with lens handling and care and maintenance regimens, and are prepared at any time should they need to remove their lenses. This includes keeping a pair of up-to-date spectacles and

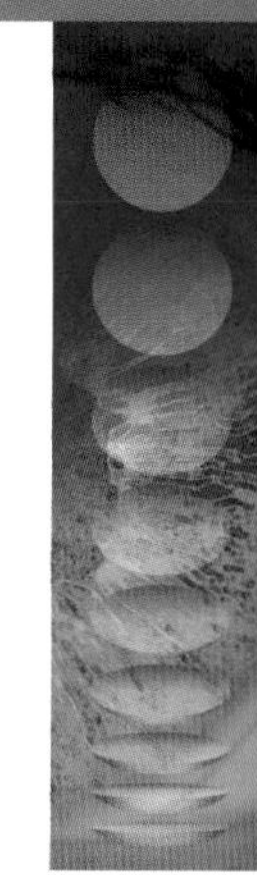

ensuring that solutions have not expired. Continuous-wear patients must understand that contact lens care solutions are still necessary.

Lens surface performance

The lens surface is assessed by examining a range of variables that contribute to the biocompatibility of contact lenses.

WETTABILITY (see Chapters 3, 5 and 17)

Wettability is a subjective measure of tear film quality during lens wear that takes into account the:

- Pattern in which tears break over a lens.
- Speed of tear break-up.
- Stability of the tear film.
- Appearance of the lipid layer.
- Non-invasive break-up time (NIBUT).

The CCLRU/IER scale for assessing wettability ranges from 0 to 5, where:

- 0 corresponds to a non-wettable surface.
- 1 is non-wetting patches immediately after blinking.
- 2 is the appearance equivalent to a HEMA surface.
- 3 is more wettable than HEMA.
- 4 is an appearance approaching that of a normal healthy cornea.
- 5 corresponds to the wettability of a normal healthy cornea.

Typically, a normal healthy cornea has a NIBUT of more than 30 seconds and a stable, even, lipid layer. The CCLRU/IER scale also uses the wettability of HEMA lenses as a benchmark midway in the scale. HEMA lenses usually have a NIBUT from 5 to 7 seconds (Guillon & Guillon 1993) and correspond to grade 2.0. The surface wettability of silicone hydrogel lenses during continuous wear remains relatively constant over time, irrespective of whether they are worn on a 6- or 30-night lens wear schedule, and is similar to the levels seen with extended wear of hydrogels (grade 2.0) (Stern et al. 2004).

Front and back surface deposit accumulation is low during extended wear of soft lenses for both 6- and 30-night wear (Stern et al. 2004). However, the deposits that do accumulate vary in the ratio of protein to lipid, with less protein but more lipid usually being found on silicone hydrogel lenses compared to conventional hydrogels (McKenney et al. 1998, Jones et al. 2003). Some soft contact lens wearers develop 'haze' and 'globular' lens deposits over several days, which can interfere with vision (Stern et al. 2004) (Fig. 13.29). These appear to be patient specific and are likely to be lipid (Tighe et al. 2000). Occasionally, these deposits will accumulate several hours after lenses are inserted. They can be removed easily by cleaning with a surfactant.

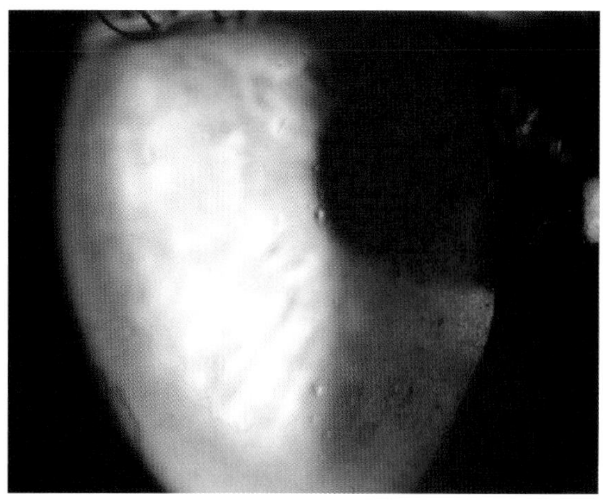

Figure 13.29 Haze and globule-type deposits seen during continuous wear with silicone hydrogel lenses. (From Sweeney et al. 2005, with permission of Lippincott Williams & Wilkins)

MUCIN BALLS

These precorneal deposits or lipid plugs are spherical structures that are found embedded in the epithelium during contact lens wear (Figs 13.30 and 17.27a,b) (see also Chapter 17). They are:

- Quite rigid and can indent both the overlying contact lens and the underlying epithelium into the anterior stroma (Jalbert et al. 2003).
- Predominantly composed of mucin (Millar et al. 2003).
- Typically translucent.
- Range in size from 10 to 50 μm in diameter (Tan et al. 2000).
- Usually evident in the superior quadrant of the cornea with both hydrogel and silicone hydrogel lenses (Dumbleton et al. 2000, Tan et al. 2003).
- Static when the lens moves.

Mucin balls can form within minutes of lens insertion and increase in size and number over time. Once lenses are removed, the mucin balls dislodge, leaving indentations in the corneal surface which resolve rapidly. However, practitioners should closely monitor patients with this condition to discount any potential negative effects on corneal integrity.

Mucin balls are different from corneal staining and other lens-related conditions such as corneal blotting, micro-deposits and dimple veiling. They can be differentiated from epithelial microcysts and vacuoles as they are generally larger and do not require marginal retro-illumination to be seen. The indentations left behind after they have dislodged usually disappear within a few blinks and show pooling of fluorescein dye although not frank staining.

Mucin balls develop at similar frequencies irrespective of the type of soft contact lens worn, but occur in higher numbers in wearers of silicone hydrogel lenses and those with steep corneas (Dumbleton et al. 2000, Tan et al. 2003). The suggested hypothesis for the aetiology of mucin balls is that they occur as the result of a collapse in ocular mucin which then coalesces into spherical structures as a contact lens moves over the surface of the epithelium (Millar et al. 2003).

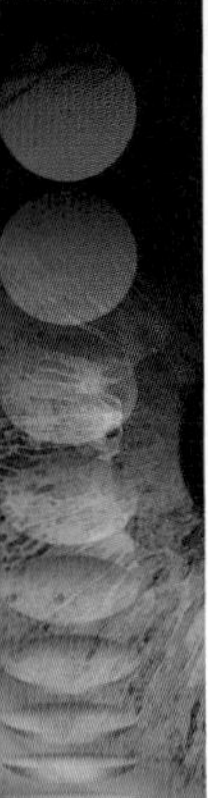

(a)

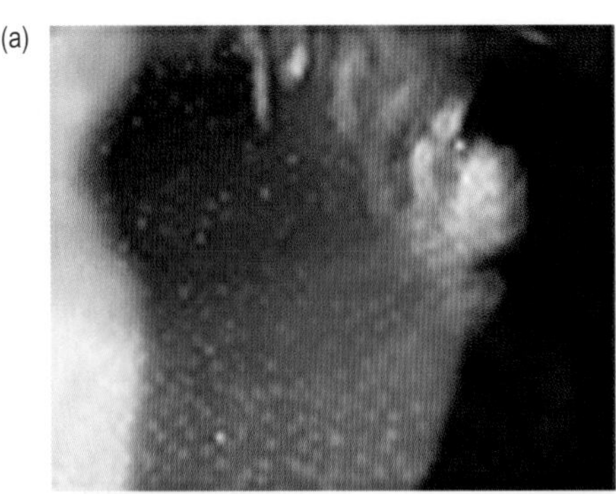

(b)

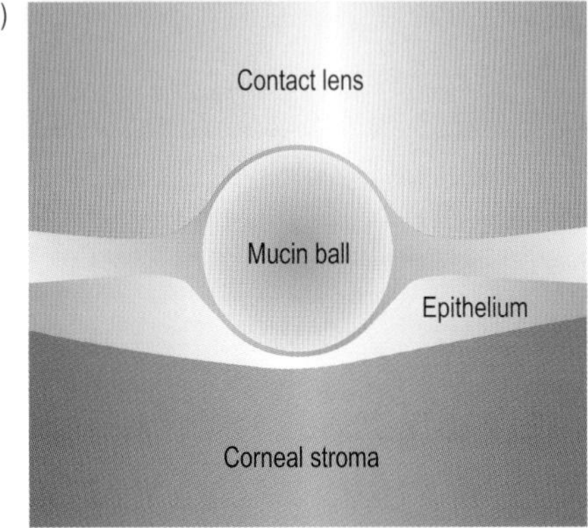

Figure 13.30 (a) High numbers of mucin balls in a silicone hydrogel lens wearer; (b) localization of mucin balls in the corneal epithelium

PATIENT ADVICE (see Chapters 11, 17 and 32)

The primary responsibility of the contact lens practitioner is to educate patients about the risks, benefits and realities of their chosen wear modality. Patients with extended- or continuous-wear lenses differ from those wearing daily wear lenses. Potential acute complications and long-term effects should be clearly explained. Patients at greater risk of adverse events should be advised accordingly. These patients include smokers and those who are non-compliant with lens care and wear schedules. Patients with a history of non-infectious corneal infiltration with contact lens wear should be advised of the risk of developing recurrent events (Bates et al. 1989, Sweeney et al. 1993, 2003).

Emphasis should be placed on the need for regular overnight lens removal and replacement, and meticulous lens hygiene and disinfection procedures. In addition, patients should be encouraged to instil sterile unpreserved saline drops on waking and before retiring to sleep. If there is any unusual redness, discomfort or blurred vision at any stage, lenses should be removed and the patient should consult their practitioner.

The preliminary discussion should be reinforced with a written summary detailing the patient's responsibilities and the risks involved, and these responsibilities should be reiterated at each after-care visit. Brennan and colleagues (2001, 2004) recommend a documentation kit comprising an information brochure, practitioner–patient agreement, instruction sheet, question and answer sheet, informed consent and documentation for what to do in an emergency as a useful way to outline what patients can expect form their lens wear (Fig. 13.31). This kit also serves to formalize the necessity for compliance, particularly with continuous wear (see also Chapter 32).

RIGID GAS-PERMEABLE LENSES

Historical review

Rigid gas-permeable (RGP) lenses have been available for daily wear since the mid-1970s but only received approval for extended wear by the US FDA in 1986. The lag in the development of RGP lenses for extended wear was caused in part by the popularity of soft contact lens extended wear and the lack of suitable lens materials.

Garcia (1976) was the first to report extended wear with RGP lenses for the correction of aphakia, but they were not used for cosmetic purposes until a few years later (Levy 1983). In 1984, Fonn (at the 8th European Research Symposium, Interlaken, Switzerland) reported comparative data from a small pilot study in which ten subjects were fitted for extended wear with a hydrogel lens in one eye and an RGP lens in the other. He found fewer acute adverse responses and less physiological effect in the RGP lens-wearing eyes, and these findings were confirmed in a follow-up study with a further 30 subjects (Fonn & Holden 1988).

The interest in RGP extended wear was spurred primarily by the potential of RGP lenses to transmit more oxygen to the cornea than was possible with hydrogel materials. The oxygen transmissibility of the earliest RGP lenses was equivalent to those provided by hydrogel extended-wear lenses and unsurprisingly induced similar levels of overnight corneal oedema (Sweeney & Holden 1983, Kenyon et al. 1985, Zantos & Zantos 1985). Developments in the field of polymer chemistry soon resulted in RGP lenses with higher Dk/t, which reduced the incidence of hypoxia-induced corneal changes relative to hydrogel lenses (Henry et al. 1987, Polse et al. 1988, Key & Mobley 1989, Levy 1991, Rivera & Polse 1991, Young & Port 1992) but these lenses did not meet the oxygen requirements of the cornea during overnight wear and were not approved for continuous wear.

The more recently developed fluorosilicone-acrylate materials incorporate fluorinated monomers within silicone acrylate materials. The addition of fluorine, an efficient oxygen-transmitting substance, reduces the need for silicone to attain high Dk and therefore, in addition to enhanced Dk, it enhances the wettability and resistance of a polymer to deposit accumulation. Other co-monomers are added to enhance strength and wettability, and the ratio of these co-monomers can be manipulated to alter the physical and physiological properties of the material (see Chapters 3 and 9).

The measured Dk of the most common fluorosilicone-acrylate RGP lenses ranges from 27 barrers (Boston ES) up to 99 barrers (FluoroPerm 151) (Benjamin & Cappelli 2002). Menicon Z is the only RGP lens to attain approval for 30-nights continuous wear by the US FDA. This lens is made from a styrene-based fluoromethacrylate material with a Dk of 175 barrers (Benjamin & Cappelli 2002).

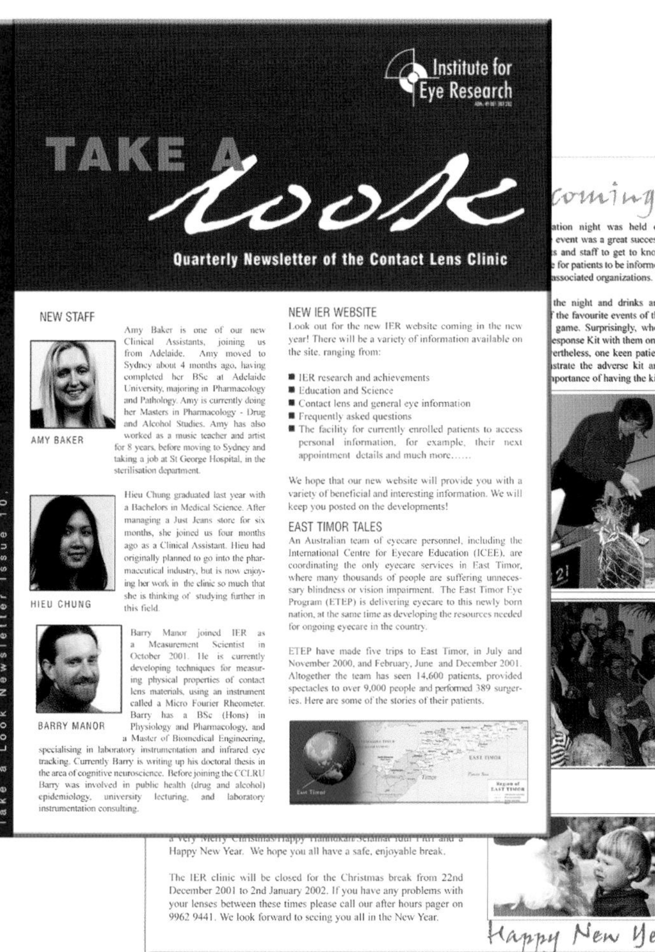

Institute for Eye Research

TAKE A look

Quarterly Newsletter of the Contact Lens Clinic

Take a Look Newsletter Issue 10.

NEW STAFF

AMY BAKER

Amy Baker is one of our new Clinical Assistants, joining us from Adelaide. Amy moved to Sydney about 4 months ago, having completed her BSc at Adelaide University, majoring in Pharmacology and Pathology. Amy is currently doing her Masters in Pharmacology - Drug and Alcohol Studies. Amy has also worked as a music teacher and artist for 8 years, before moving to Sydney and taking a job at St George Hospital, in the sterilisation department.

HIEU CHUNG

Hieu Chung graduated last year with a Bachelors in Medical Science. After managing a Just Jeans store for six months, she joined us four months ago as a Clinical Assistant. Hieu had originally planned to go into the pharmaceutical industry, but is now enjoying her work in the clinic so much that she is thinking of studying further in this field.

BARRY MANOR

Barry Manor joined IER as a Measurement Scientist in October 2001. He is currently developing techniques for measuring physical properties of contact lens materials, using an instrument called a Micro Fourier Rheometer. Barry has a BSc (Hons) in Physiology and Pharmacology, and a Master of Biomedical Engineering, specialising in laboratory instrumentation and infrared eye tracking. Currently Barry is writing up his doctoral thesis in the area of cognitive neuroscience. Before joining the CCLRU Barry was involved in public health (drug and alcohol) epidemiology, university lecturing, and laboratory instrumentation consulting.

NEW IER WEBSITE

Look out for the new IER website coming in the new year! There will be a variety of information available on the site, ranging from:

- IER research and achievements
- Education and Science
- Contact lens and general eye information
- Frequently asked questions
- The facility for currently enrolled patients to access personal information, for example, their next appointment details and much more……

We hope that our new website will provide you with a variety of beneficial and interesting information. We will keep you posted on the developments!

EAST TIMOR TALES

An Australian team of eyecare personnel, including the International Centre for Eyecare Education (ICEE), are coordinating the only eyecare services in East Timor, where many thousands of people are suffering unnecessary blindness or vision impairment. The East Timor Eye Program (ETEP) is delivering eyecare to this newly born nation, at the same time as developing the resources needed for ongoing eyecare in the country.

ETEP have made five trips to East Timor, in July and November 2000, and February, June and December 2001. Altogether the team has seen 14,600 patients, provided spectacles to over 9,000 people and performed 389 surgeries. Here are some of the stories of their patients.

…coming

…ation night was held on … event was a great success, …s and staff to get to know … for patients to be informed … associated organizations.

… the night and drinks and … the favourite events of the … game. Surprisingly, when … esponse Kit with them only … ertheless, one keen patient … strate the adverse kit and … portance of having the kits

… Happy New Year. We hope you all have a safe, enjoyable break.

The IER clinic will be closed for the Christmas break from 22nd December 2001 to 2nd January 2002. If you have any problems with your lenses between these times please call our after hours pager on 9962 9441. We look forward to seeing you all in the New Year.

Happy New Year

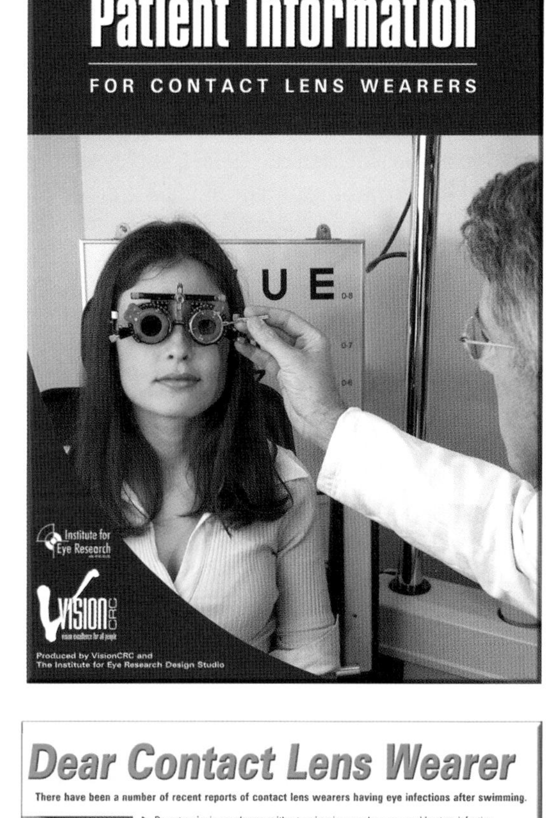

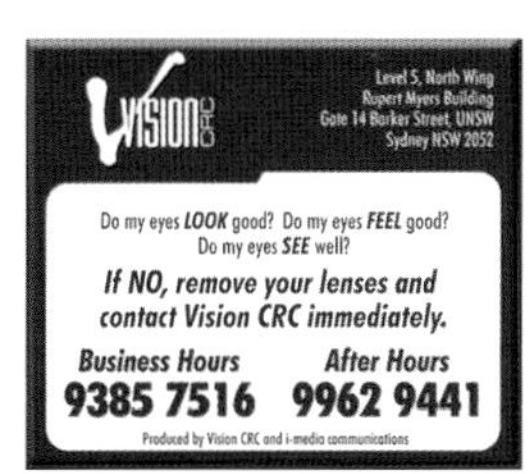

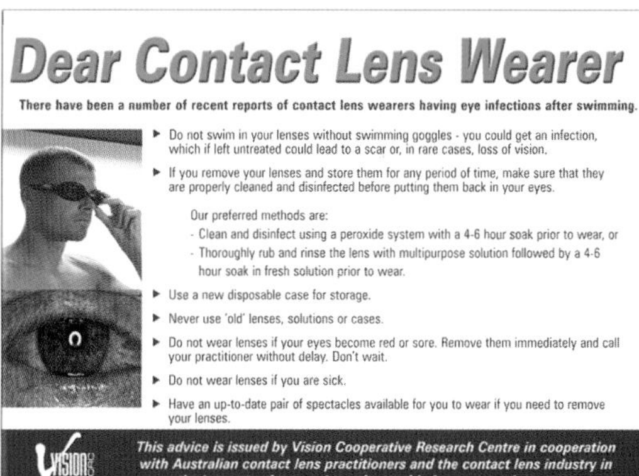

Dear Contact Lens Wearer

There have been a number of recent reports of contact lens wearers having eye infections after swimming.

- Do not swim in your lenses without swimming goggles - you could get an infection, which if left untreated could lead to a scar or, in rare cases, loss of vision.
- If you remove your lenses and store them for any period of time, make sure that they are properly cleaned and disinfected before putting them back in your eyes.

  Our preferred methods are:
  - Clean and disinfect using a peroxide system with a 4-6 hour soak prior to wear, or
  - Thoroughly rub and rinse the lens with multipurpose solution followed by a 4-6 hour soak in fresh solution prior to wear.
- Use a new disposable case for storage.
- Never use 'old' lenses, solutions or cases.
- Do not wear lenses if your eyes become red or sore. Remove them immediately and call your practitioner without delay. Don't wait.
- Do not wear lenses if you are sick.
- Have an up-to-date pair of spectacles available for you to wear if you need to remove your lenses.

This advice is issued by Vision Cooperative Research Centre in cooperation with Australian contact lens practitioners and the contact lens industry in the interests of promoting safe, trouble free contact lens wear.

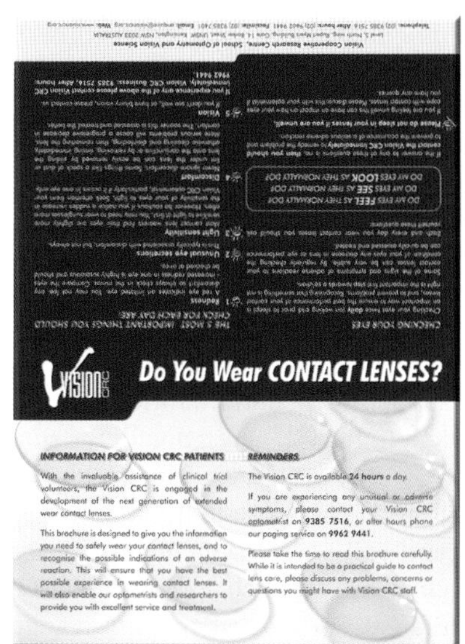

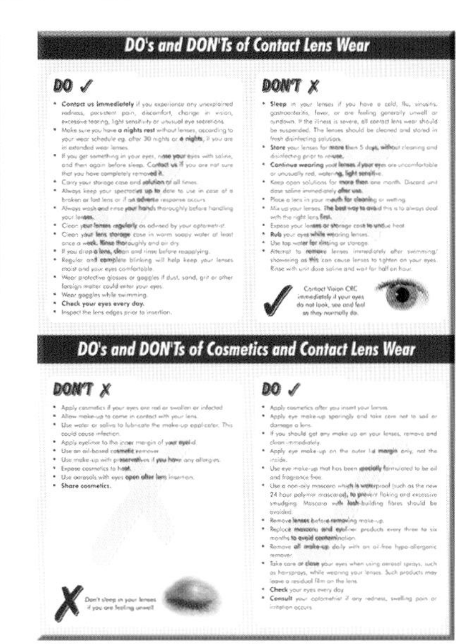

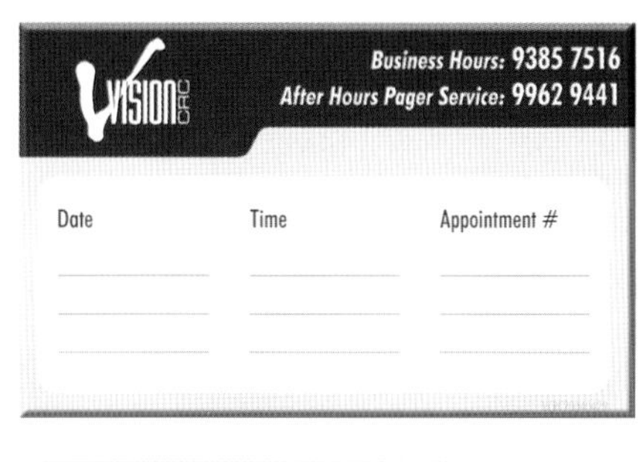

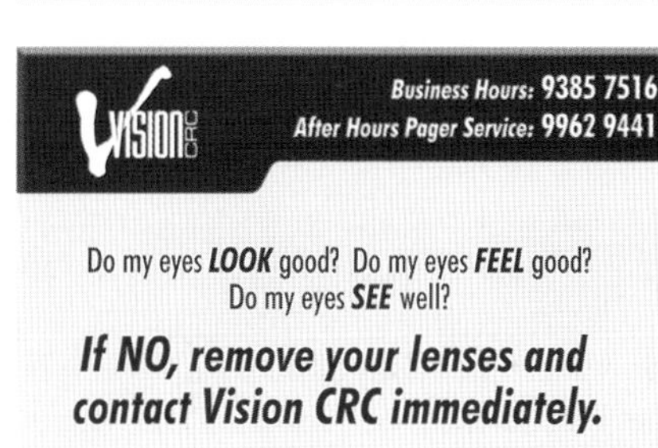

Figure 13.31 Patient education and support materials

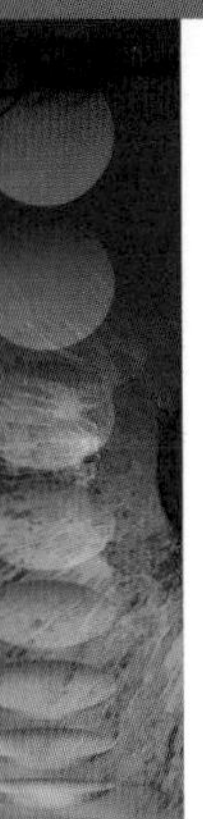

Advantages and disadvantages

The advantages of RGP lenses are the superior optics compared to soft contact lenses and the low rate of infection and inflammatory events during extended and continuous wear. However, despite these advantages, RGP lenses still only represent a small proportion of the contact lens market. Data from Morgan and colleagues' (2005c) survey of practitioner lens prescribing from 14 countries in 2004 indicate RGP lenses comprise only 11% of new contact lens fits and 15% of refits worldwide.

The Berkeley Contact Lens Extended Wear Study (Polse et al. 2001) compared clinical outcomes and success of RGP lenses in subjects wearing high- or low-Dk RGP lenses over 12 months. In this study, there were very few indicators of hypoxic stress in either group over the 12 months, and very few cases of corneal infiltrates or CLARE. The most common complications found in both groups were corneal staining, followed by redness and staining of the conjunctiva. More significantly, approximately 34% of subjects discontinued after the initial lens fitting and before the extended-wear phase because of discomfort.

Other studies comparing the performance of RGP lenses with hydrogels confirm these results. Compared with hydrogel extended wear, there appeared to be a much lower rate of serious complications such as CLARE and CLPC (Henry et al. 1987, Polse et al. 1987, Fonn & Holden 1988, Young & Port 1992), and the incidence of infection with RGP lenses is equivalent to or lower than with daily wear soft lenses (Poggio et al. 1989, Cheng et al. 1999, Lam et al. 2002). In most cases, corneal ulcers associated with RGP extended wear appear to be more benign than hydrogel-related infections, being typically peripheral in location and consequently less sight threatening.

There are a number of reasons for the lower incidence of acute complications:

- The efficient tear pump with rigid lenses, flushing tear debris and contaminants from behind the lens. This may explain the low rate of CLARE reactions, which are thought to be triggered in part by breakdown products of retained back surface debris.
- As RGP lenses attract less deposition and are more easily cleaned than hydrogel lenses, inflammatory reactions to lens deposits, such as CLPC, are minimized.
- Bacteria and other pathogens are also less likely to be retained on the lens surface. Ren et al. (2002) demonstrated that less *P. aeruginosa* binds to exfoliated corneal cells of subjects who have worn high-Dk RGP lenses on a continuous-wear schedule over 1 year than those wearing high- or low-Dk soft lenses on either extended- or continuous-wear schedules.

Because of their rigidity, RGP lenses have a number of other advantages over hydrogel lenses:

- Corneal astigmatism of up to 2.5 D can be corrected.
- The greater ease of cleaning and maintenance, combined with enhanced deposit resistance, provides better vision, comfort and convenience.
- They are more durable and stable.
- Lenses can be modified or polished.

RGP extended wear is not without its drawbacks, however. They can cause:

- Corneal distortion or moulding.
- Lens adherence or 'binding'.
- Corneal staining.
- Abrasions due to foreign bodies.

Gleason et al. (2003) compared the performance of continuous-wear Menicon Z lenses to a conventional hydrogel lens worn for extended wear and showed that the major adverse events to result in discontinuation over 1 year were foreign body abrasions in the RGP lens wear group, and infiltrative keratitis and bacterial conjunctivitis in the soft lens wear group. Three and 9 o'clock corneal staining occurred with a greater frequency in the RGP lens wearers (22.2%) compared to soft lens wearers (0.4%); lens adherence did not occur in any Menicon Z lens wearer.

Fonn and Holden (1986) and later Gauthier et al. (1992) and Fonn et al. (1996) reported the development of eyelid ptosis in association with RGP extended wear. It is thought that the ptosis is caused by lid oedema or inflammation due to chronic irritation of the eyelid by the lens edge (see also Chapter 9).

As previously discussed, initial lens discomfort and intolerance occurs in a substantial number of patients but once adaptation has been achieved, comfort is usually good, and, in some cases, superior to that with soft lenses (Fonn & Holden 1988). Morgan et al. (2003) compared the comfort response to RGP and silicone hydrogel lenses in groups of neophyte and experienced lens wearers. The level of comfort was similar between all experienced lens wearers and for the neophyte silicone hydrogel lens wearers from the beginning of the study. The discomfort experienced by neophyte subjects wearing RGP lenses steadily improved during the 1-week daily wear phase and increased to levels comparable with the other groups after 2 weeks of continuous wear. A rounded front edge is the most important factor in providing good subjective comfort (La Hood 1988) (see Chapters 9 and 17).

Acute complications of RGP extended wear

STROMAL OEDEMA

As with hydrogel extended wear, overnight wear of low- or moderate-Dk/t RGP lenses may give rise to significant levels of overnight corneal oedema. Because the oedema accompanying RGP lens wear is usually localized in the central 6 mm of the cornea (Fonn et al. 1984), it may be detected with the slit-lamp using sclerotic scatter (see Chapter 7). However, it resolves rapidly following eye opening due to circulation of oxygenated tears behind the lens and will not be evident on examination unless the patient is seen within 1 hour of eye opening. Striae or folds seen in the posterior stroma more than 2 hours following eye opening suggests clinically unacceptable levels of overnight corneal swelling.

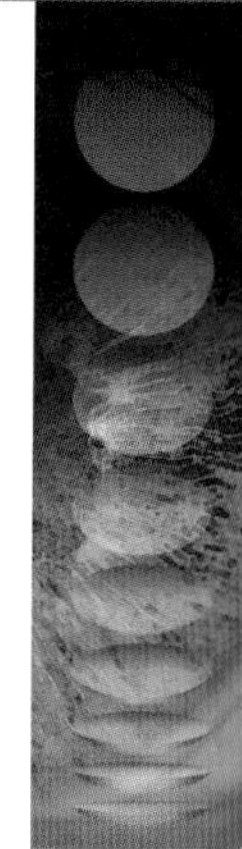

CORNEAL MOULDING AND DISTORTION

The greater rigidity of RGP lenses compared to hydrogel lenses may result in corneal distortion or moulding of corneal curvature after overnight wear. This is due to sustained pressure exerted by the eyelid on the lens and cornea and may be facilitated in a 'softened' or swollen cornea during closed-eye lens wear.

Corneal moulding appears to be towards a slight flattening of corneal curvature, especially in more astigmatic corneas but is reduced with higher-Dk/t materials. The steeper corneal meridian appears to be more affected, resulting in reduced corneal toricity (Benjamin & Simons 1984, Sigband & Bridgewater 1994, and others). Corneal moulding may be reduced with higher-Dk/t lenses (Polse et al. 1988). Slight corneal moulding does not appear to cause detectable structural changes in the cornea and, in general, corrected visual acuity is unaffected; however, long-term significance remains unclear.

Temporary localized corneal distortion and spectacle blur have been reported in association with lens adherence and other physiological disturbances such as corneal oedema, vacuoles and staining (Zabkiewicz et al. 1986, Young & Port 1992). Appropriate clinical management of the underlying condition is likely to eliminate this distortion.

LENS ADHERENCE

During sleep, rigid lenses can adhere tightly to the cornea (Zantos & Zantos 1985, Seger & Mutti 1986, Swarbrick & Holden 1987, and others). The lens is typically decentred, usually in the nasal position and often overlapping the limbus, and causes little discomfort or subjective symptoms (Swarbrick & Holden 1989). Spontaneous lens movement generally occurs within the first hour after eye opening due to increased tear secretion and lid action, although the lens may remain bound to the cornea for many hours (Swarbrick & Holden 1987). When lenses are removed, a complete or partial indentation or compression ring corresponding to the lens edge is usually observed (Fig. 13.32), and the epithelium may display some central punctate staining (Kenyon et al. 1988). The compression ring rarely stains with fluorescein; more typically fluorescein pools in the indented zone, or appears to thin in this area if the indentation is shallow. Lens adherence has been estimated to occur in approximately 50% of RGP extended wearers (Seger & Mutti 1986, Swarbrick & Holden 1987, and others), although higher incidence figures have been reported. Gleason et al. (2003) conducted a clinical trial of 317 Menicon Z wearers and found no instances of lens binding at any of six examinations up to 12 months of continuous wear.

Lens adherence causes several complications:

- Epithelial compression causes significant localized corneal distortion (Fig. 13.33), which may persist for some hours.
- Some patients bind lenses frequently (Swarbrick & Holden 1989), often in the same position (Swarbrick 1991), causing potential long-term compromise of the underlying epithelium and stroma, although the significance has yet to be determined.

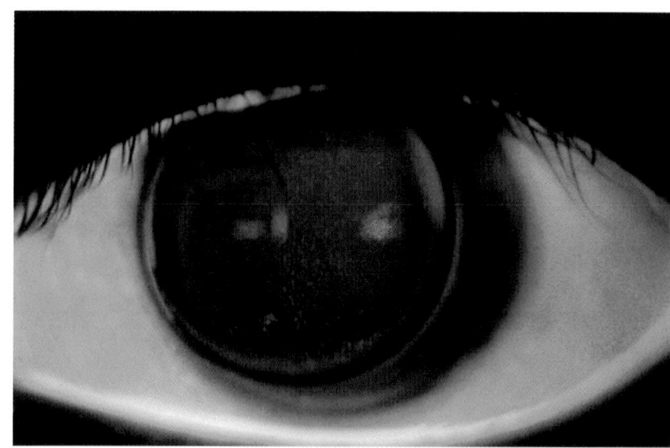

Figure 13.32 Lens adherence or binding occurs with extended-wear RGP lenses after overnight wear. (From Swarbrick 1988, with permission)

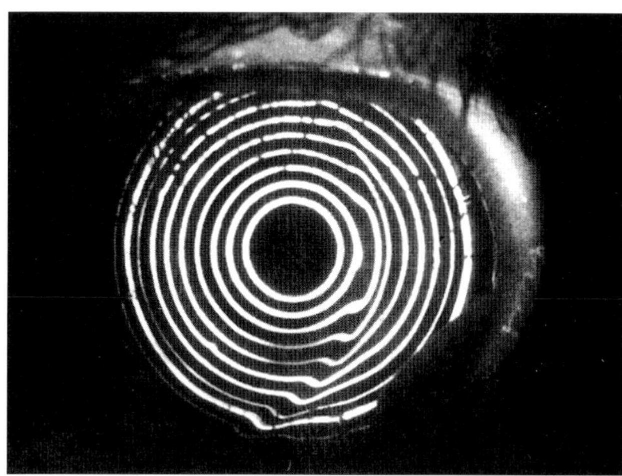

Figure 13.33 Photokeratoscopic image showing corneal distortion associated with a corneal indentation or compression ring induced by the edge of an adherent RGP lens. The photograph was taken immediately following lens removal. Recovery is usually complete within 8 hours. (From Swarbrick & Holden 1987, with permission)

- Exacerbation of peripheral 3 and 9 o'clock staining, which can show rapid progression to dellen formation and peripheral corneal ulceration (Levy 1985). This is only likely to occur if the lens is held in place for some time after eye opening (Swarbrick 1991). Swarbrick postulated that tear film disruption at the intersection of the limbus and the edge of the stationary lens is the major contributing factor.
- While the lens is adhered, tears cannot circulate behind it and corneal de-swelling may be impeded, although this may not cause significant problems with high-Dk/t lenses.
- Tear debris and mucus remain trapped behind the lens, typically collecting in a ring behind the mid-periphery of the lens (Fig. 13.34) (Zantos & Zantos 1985). This can provoke an acute inflammatory reaction and such a course of events has been noted in two RGP extended lens wearers

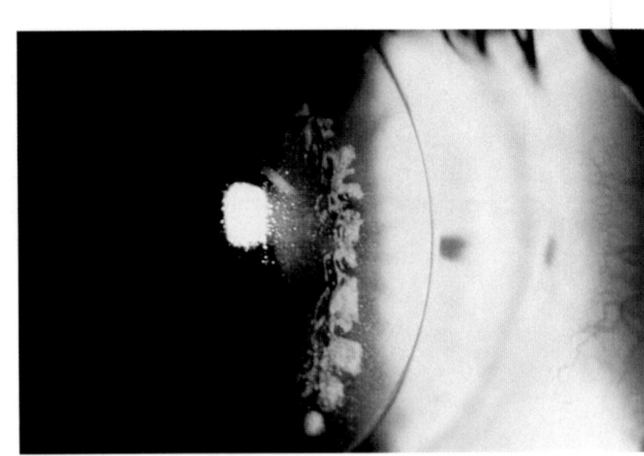

Figure 13.34 Tear debris and mucus remain trapped behind the lens, typically collecting in a ring behind the mid-periphery of an RGP lens, as shown here, and centrally under a soft lens. This trapped debris has the potential to provoke an acute inflammatory response, such as the CLARE reaction. (Courtesy of R. Terry)

participating in CCLRU/IER clinical studies (Schnider et al. 1988). Fortunately, however, this consequence appears to be rare.

In a retrospective study, Swarbrick and Holden (1987) found the factors likely to cause lens adherence were:

- Large diameter.
- Flat BOZR lenses with little edge lift.
- Lenses fitted on-K or slightly flatter than central K.
- Lenses which showed insufficient lens movement before eye closure.

Swarbrick and Holden (1996) also found that changing lens diameter and edge fitting did not influence the incidence of lens adherence. However, steeply fitted lenses bound with the same frequency as those fitted in alignment with the cornea, which negated Fatt's (1979) theory of a 'suction cup' effect of silicone elastomer lens adhesion. Further evidence against this theory is the high incidence of adherence of hydrogel lenses (which contain no silicone) immediately on eye opening after overnight lens wear (Kenyon et al. 1988, La Hood & Holden, personal communication). Lens fenestration, which would be expected to reduce any suction effect, appears to have little effect on lens adherence (Polse et al. 1987, Swarbrick 1988, Kenyon et al. 1989). (For a further explanation of this effect, see Fenestration, Chapter 9.)

Some patients have a markedly greater propensity to repeatedly bind lenses, suggesting that individual patient factors may influence this phenomenon (Swarbrick & Holden 1987, 1989, 1993). In particular, ocular rigidity may be a significant factor (Swarbrick 1991), although this was not predictive in identifying those prone to frequent adherence. Corneal flexure or moulding towards the back surface of the adhered lens during eye closure may contribute to the phenomenon.

Swarbrick (1988, 1991) proposed that lens adherence is precipitated by gradual expulsion of the aqueous phase of the tear layer from between the lens and cornea due to light, but prolonged pressure of the eyelid on the lens during eye closure. The resulting very thin, highly viscous layer of mucus-rich tears then acts as an adhesive between the lens and the cornea. When the eye opens, the force required to initiate lens movement may exceed that exerted by the eyelid on blinking, and the lens will remain adhered until the retained mucus layer is thickened and diluted by gradual penetration of aqueous tears behind the lens. Corneal moulding towards the back surface of the rigid lens during sleep may also play a role in thinning the tear film between the lens and cornea.

Examination of RGP extended-wear patients should take place early in the morning following overnight lens wear. Although an adhered lens will rarely be observed, as spontaneous lens movement after eye opening is generally rapid, the presence of a corneal indentation ring should be considered a positive diagnostic sign (Kenyon et al. 1988).

Various strategies can be tried to prevent lens binding but the problem can recur. These include:

- Avoiding flat-fitting lenses.
- Manipulating the edge design (Quin 1990).
- Increasing or decreasing optic zone diameter.
- Changing lens back surface design.
- Blending the peripheral curves.
- In-eye wetting drops (Bennett & Egan 1986, Henry et al. 1987).
- Increasing lens thickness to reduce lens flexure (Bennett & Egan 1986, Morgan & Bennett 1989), although this will reduce the Dk/t value of the lens (Polse et al. 1987) and appears to be relatively ineffective (Kenyon et al. 1989).
- Alerting the patient to the phenomenon so that lens movement can be initiated soon after eye opening, thereby avoiding complications, in particular progressive 3 and 9 o'clock staining. Irrigation with sterile saline solution and gentle lens manipulation with the lid margins may reduce the risk.
- Returning the persistent lens binder to a daily wearing schedule (see also Chapter 9).

CORNEAL STAINING

Persistent 3 and 9 o'clock staining (Fig. 13.35) has been discussed on page 297 and in Chapter 9. During extended wear, insufficient edge clearance may precipitate 3 and 9 o'clock staining due to reduced tear flow under the periphery of the lens or restricted lens movement (Andrasko 1990, Schnider et al. 1996). A compromise must be reached in lens edge design to avoid both excessive and insufficient edge clearance. Cornish et al. (1988) advocated an on-eye edge clearance of approximately 70–80 μm and edge width of approximately 0.4–0.5 mm for extended wear (Fig. 13.36).

Patients who are more prone to developing this type of staining tend to show:

- Higher levels of baseline conjunctival hyperaemia.
- More tear debris and lipid.
- Faster lens drying.
- Poor lens centration and movement (Schnider et al. 1996).

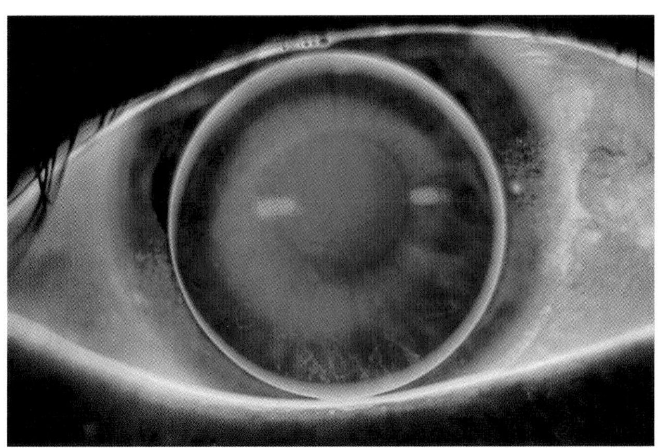

Figure 13.35 During extended wear, inadequate edge clearance and associated restricted lens movement may also induce 3 and 9 o'clock staining. (Courtesy of R. Terry)

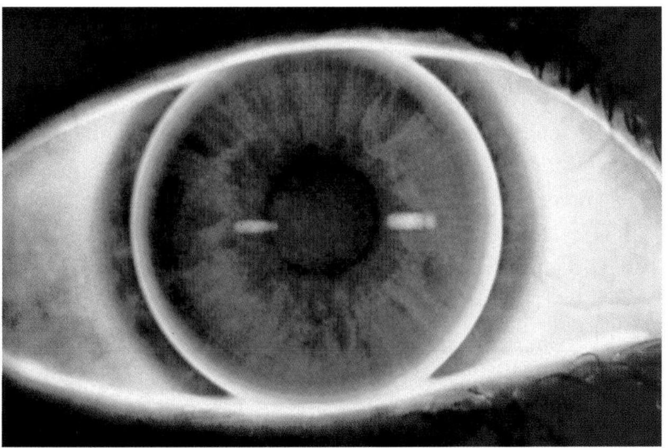

Figure 13.36 Fluorescein photograph of an acceptable RGP lens fitting for extended wear. Slight apical clearance is apparent, with light mid-peripheral bearing and a moderate edge width and clearance. (Courtesy of R. Terry)

Successful daily wear without the development of more than slight 3 and 9 o'clock staining should be a prerequisite for commencing RGP extended wear. Although mild 3 and 9 o'clock staining is not unusual during RGP extended wear, severe cases must be managed promptly by reducing wearing time until the staining resolves, and by altering the lens edge design to avoid peripheral desiccation. Avoiding persistent lens adherence following eye opening will also help to minimize 3 and 9 o'clock staining, as will altering lens design to maintain lens centration and adequate and sustained lens movement during open-eye lens wear (see also Chapters 9 and 17).

Another type of corneal staining, termed the Fischer–Schweitzer polygonal mosaic, is occasionally noted immediately upon lens removal following RGP extended lens wear (Benjamin & Simons 1984, Levy 1985, Zantos & Zantos 1985, Zabkiewicz et al. 1986). This phenomenon is not staining of the epithelium, but a polygonal meshwork of fluorescein pooling in the central or superior cornea. The aetiology of the phenomenon was described by Bron and Tripathi (1969), who considered that external pressure exerted on the cornea causes ridges to form in Bowman's layer as the cornea flattens. Following removal of the pressure, Bowman's layer regains its normal curvature, leaving grooves where epithelial cells have been compressed above the ridges during flattening. The corneal mosaic normally disappears within 10 minutes after lenses are removed. Although not of concern in itself, the appearance of this corneal mosaic pattern suggests that contact lenses may exert undue pressure on the cornea during wear, possibly indicating an excessively flat fit.

Corneal staining due to foreign bodies, lens mishandling or dislodgement, lens adherence or damaged lenses may also occur during RGP extended wear. In severe cases, it is wise to discontinue lens wear until the epithelial defect has resolved. Appropriate clinical management and patient education may reduce the incidence of these complications.

Long-term effects of RGP extended and continuous wear

The long-term corneal changes accompanying hydrogel extended wear are induced directly or indirectly by chronic hypoxic stress on the corneal tissue (Holden et al. 1985b). Therefore, similar changes might be anticipated with long-term extended wear of RGP contact lenses of comparable Dk/t. As RGP lenses of higher Dk/t become available, changes such as epithelial thinning and microcyst development, reduced epithelial oxygen uptake, stromal thinning and endothelial polymegethism should become less apparent.

Indeed, results from RGP extended-wear studies at the CCLRU/IER and elsewhere indicate that epithelial microcysts, which are invariably seen in hydrogel extended lens wear after 3 months, are infrequent with high-Dk/t RGP lenses (Terry et al. 1986, Holden et al. 1987b, and others). A number of investigators have also reported minimal induction of endothelial polymegethism with moderate- or high-Dk/t RGP lenses, although the periods of observation have generally been less than 12 months (Orsborn & Schoessler 1988, Polse et al. 1988, Rivera & Polse 1991). However, polymegethism accompanying hydrogel extended wear may be noted after as little as 2 weeks of lens wear (Holden et al. 1985c).

Long-term clinical studies of high-Dk RGP extended wear conducted at the CCLRU/IER (reported by Cornish et al. at the 7th International Contact Lens Congress in Queensland, Australia, 1990) provide some further information concerning the long-term viability and safety of this lens-wearing modality. A total of 135 patients were enrolled in these studies, and fitted with extended-wear lenses with oxygen transmissibilities greater than 50.3×10^{-9} units with overnight lens removal as desired by the patient. Lenses were to be cleaned as frequently as required, and there were no scheduled lens replacements. The cleaning regimen, which was tailored to each patient, included the use of an alcohol-based cleaner in cases of lipid deposition, and a textured cleaning pad for removing heavy deposition. An enzymatic cleaner was not used.

Lens-related discontinuations were highest in the first year, with 30% of patients leaving the study. By far the most frequent

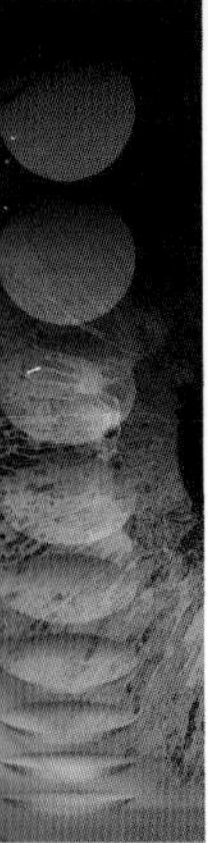

cause of discontinuation was discomfort (24%), and the majority of discontinuations for this reason (87%) occurred in the first month. In the first year, CLPC was confined to previous soft lens wearers with pre-existing upper lid changes. Discontinuations were less frequent in subsequent years. Notably, some patients developed CLPC associated with lens deposits in the third and fourth years of the study. However, after 3 years, 54% of patients entered in the study (excluding non-lens-related discontinuations) were still successfully wearing the lenses. Adverse responses during this period were rare. One patient developed idiopathic infiltrates, and another experienced an eruption of vacuoles; both successfully resumed extended wear after resolution. No CLARE reactions or corneal infections were recorded over the 3 years.

The development of CLPC during RGP extended wear was also reported by others including Zabkiewicz et al. (1986) and Douglas et al. (1988). The eyelid changes are different from those seen during hydrogel lens wear, being more localized in the central portion of the eyelid, and less marked than the typical hydrogel-induced CLPC in both extent and roughness.

Factors that may precipitate these eyelid changes include:

- Mechanical effect of the lens itself.
- Mechanical and/or antigenic effects of lens deposits.

Annual lens replacement and enzymatic cleaning may prove successful in the management of deposits, thus reducing the incidence of upper eyelid changes.

Clinical management

PATIENT SELECTION (see Chapter 8)

RGP lenses have been used successfully for both aphakic (Benjamin & Simons 1984, Garcia et al. 1990) and cosmetic extended wear (Levy 1985, Henry et al. 1987, and others). Kastl and Johnson (1989) reported success with this modality for patients with high astigmatism and keratoconus.

As with soft extended wear, the risk:benefit ratio for each patient should be considered carefully before proceeding. Thorough patient education and instruction are essential in order to emphasize the realities of extended wear, including the need for regular lens cleaning and maintenance, frequent overnight lens removal to rest the cornea, and prompt contact with the practitioner should unusual redness, discomfort or blurred vision occur.

More latitude is available for correcting corneal astigmatism with RGP lenses compared to soft lenses, although the centre thickness of the lenses may have to be increased to minimize on-eye flexure which may cause fluctuating vision on blinking (see Chapter 9). It must be remembered that increasing lens thickness will reduce the Dk/t of the lenses.

Contraindications for both soft and RGP extended wear are similar (see p. 291) and refitting unsuccessful soft lens wearers with RGP lenses is rarely a solution (Douglas et al. 1988, Schnider et al. 1988).

LENS FITTING

Techniques for fitting RGP lenses are discussed in Chapter 9, and therefore will not be considered in detail in this section. In general, RGP lens fitting for extended wear requires more care and expertise than soft lens fitting. Particular points of note are:

- For high-Dk materials, large-diameter lenses of 9.4–10.2 mm, with back optic zone diameters in the range 8.0–8.2 mm, can be used as less reliance needs to be placed on tear exchange for provision of oxygen to the anterior corneal surface.
- An alignment fit to minimize the bearing pressure on any particular corneal location, especially the mid-periphery, to encourage an even tear flow beneath the lens and minimize lens-induced corneal distortion. Multicurve back surface designs with well-blended transition zones, or aspheric lens designs, can be used.
- Flat-fitting lenses should be avoided.
- A tapered edge design incorporating two or three peripheral curves with an edge band approximately 0.4–0.5 mm wide and 70–80 μm deep (see above and Fig. 13.36). Excessive or insufficient edge lift may exacerbate 3 and 9 o'clock desiccation staining.
- Lens movement or lag following a blink should be smooth, without apical rotation or excessive lens–lid interaction, in the order of 0.75–1.50 mm in order to permit efficient flushing of debris and waste products from behind the lens.
- Good centration of the lens between blinks is also desirable; it may be necessary to steepen the BOZR slightly in some cases to achieve this.

Factors that need to be considered regarding lens material are Dk/t of the lens, lens wettability and deposit formation. Lens wettability and deposit formation appear to vary between patients, and should be evaluated carefully before a final decision on lens material is made. Lens centre thickness influences the physiological performance of the lens but a balance must be achieved between enhancing the Dk/t of the lens and minimizing on-eye flexure, particularly on astigmatic corneas. An increase in lens thickness of 0.02 mm for every dioptre of uncorrected corneal cylinder has been suggested as a rule of thumb (Bennett 1985) (see also Chapter 9).

PATIENT ADVICE AND MANAGEMENT

Patients should be advised to remove their lenses overnight at least once a week to rest the cornea, and encouraged to remove their lenses as often as they desire. Regular lens replacement is probably not as necessary as it is with soft lenses, because RGP lenses do not absorb contaminants or age as rapidly as soft lenses. Obviously, replacement of damaged, deposited or scratched lenses is essential to avoid corneal or lid trauma.

Patients must be able to handle their lenses competently before they are dispensed. Between 1 and 2 weeks of daily wear help to reinforce the patient's lens handling techniques and to ensure an optimal lens fit before extended or continuous wear begins. Problems with lens wettability and deposit formation may be identified during this period and changes in lens material or care and maintenance procedures can be made. Those patients prone to excessive peripheral desiccation staining can be identified and discouraged from progressing to extended or continuous wear, which will exacerbate this problem. Adaptation to RGP lenses is generally rapid, and full-time daily wear is often possible from the first day, although some discomfort or lens awareness is common during the first few days.

At the first review early in the morning following overnight wear, the practitioner should examine the cornea carefully for signs of residual corneal oedema (striae and folds) and lens adherence (compression ring). Follow-up visits after 3 days, 1 week, 2 weeks, 1, 2 and 3 months of extended or continuous wear are then advised; if no problems are apparent, 3-monthly after-care visits should follow.

Patient advice and management procedures are similar to those suggested for soft lens wearers. It is essential to emphasize that if unusual redness, discomfort or blurred vision develops, particularly in one eye only, the patient should remove their lenses and consult the practitioner immediately.

THE FUTURE FOR EXTENDED AND CONTINUOUS WEAR

Contact lenses with oxygen transmissibilities that far exceed the Holden–Mertz criterion for overnight wear are an important step forward in providing the majority of patients with the flexibility and convenience to wear their lenses for daily, extended or continuous wear with minimal long-term impact on corneal physiology. Despite these innovations, more highly oxygen-permeable lens materials may be required if contact lenses are to become available for complex prescriptions.

The new focus for continuous wear needs to be on improving comfort and biocompatibility, and on removing concern regarding infection and inflammation. A better understanding of the factors that influence comfort and the way in which contact lenses interact with ocular structures is instrumental in tackling biocompatibility. The quality of the tear film during lens wear is particularly important as it has the potential to impact on adverse reactions. Incorporation of novel antimicrobial compounds into lens surfaces or bulk materials will help reduce lens contamination and is likely to lower the risk of infection and inflammation.

References

Aakre, B. M., Ystenaes, A. E., Doughty, M. J. et al. (2004) A 6-month follow-up of successful refits from daily disposable soft contact lenses to continuous wear of high-Dk silicone-hydrogel lenses. Ophthal. Physiol. Opt., 24, 130–141

Adams, C. P. Jr, Cohen, E. J., Laibson, P. R. et al. (1983) Corneal ulcers in patients with cosmetic extended-wear contact lenses. Am. J. Ophthalmol., 96, 705–709

Alemany, A. L. and Redal, P. (1991) Giant papillary conjunctivitis in soft and rigid lens wear. Contactologica, 13, 14–17

Allansmith, M. R., Korb, D. R. and Greiner, J. V. (1978) Giant papillary conjunctivitis induced by hard or soft contact lens wear: quantitative histology. Ophthalmology, 85, 766–778

Ambroziak, A. M., Szaflik, J. P. and Szaflik, J. (2004) Therapeutic use of a silicone hydrogel contact lens in selected clinical cases. Eye Contact Lens, 30, 63–67

Ames, K. S. and Cameron, M. H. (1989) The efficacy of regular lens replacement in extended wear. Int. Contact Lens Clin., 16, 104–111

Andrasko, G. (1986) Corneal deswelling response to hard and hydrogel extended wear lenses. Invest. Ophthalmol. Vis. Sci., 27, 20–23

Andrasko, G. (1990) Peripheral corneal staining: edge lift and extended wear. Contact Lens Spectrum, 5, 33–35

Ang, J. H. B. and Efron, N. (1989) Carbon dioxide permeability of contact lens materials. Int. Contact Lens Clin., 16, 48–58

Anon. (1989) Disposable lens compliance monitored. Contact Lens Forum, 14, 15

Baleriola-Lucas, C., Grant, T., Newton-Howes, J. et al. (1991) Enumeration and identification of bacteria on hydrogel lenses from asymptomatic patients and those experiencing adverse responses with extended wear [ARVO Abstract]. Invest. Ophthalmol. Vis. Sci., 32, S739

Barnett, W. A. and Rengstorff, R. H. (1977) Adaptation to hydrogel contact lenses: variations in myopia and corneal curvature measurements. J. Am. Optom. Assoc., 48, 363–366

Barr, J. T. and Schoessler, J. P. (1980) Corneal endothelial response to rigid contact lenses. Am. J. Optom., 57, 267–274

Bates, A. K. and Cheng, H. (1988) Bullous keratopathy: a study of endothelial cell morphology in patients undergoing cataract surgery. Br. J. Ophthalmol., 72, 409–412

Bates, A. K., Morris, R. J., Stapleton, F. et al. (1989) 'Sterile' infiltrates in contact lens wearers. Eye, 3, 803–810

Beattie, T. K., Tomlinson, A., McFadyen, A. K. et al. (2003) Enhanced attachment of acanthamoeba to extended-wear silicone hydrogel contact lenses: a new risk factor for infection? Ophthalmology, 110, 765–771

Benjamin, W. J. and Cappelli, Q. A. (2002) Oxygen permeability (Dk) of thirty-seven rigid contact lens materials. Optom. Vis. Sci., 79, 103–111

Benjamin, W. J. and Simons, M. H. (1984) Extended wear of oxygen-permeable rigid lenses in aphakia. Int. Contact Lens Clin., 11, 547–560

Benjamin, W. J. and Rasmussen, M. A. (1985) The closed-lid tear pump: oxygenation? Int. Eyecare, 1, 251–256

Bennett, E. S. (1985) Silicone acrylate lens design. Int. Contact Lens Clin., 12, 45–53

Bennett, E. S. and Egan, D. J. (1986) Rigid gas-permeable lens problem solving. J. Am. Optom. Assoc., 57, 504–511

Bergmanson, J. P. G. (1987) Histopathological analysis of the corneal epithelium after contact lens wear. J. Am. Optom. Assoc., 58, 812–818

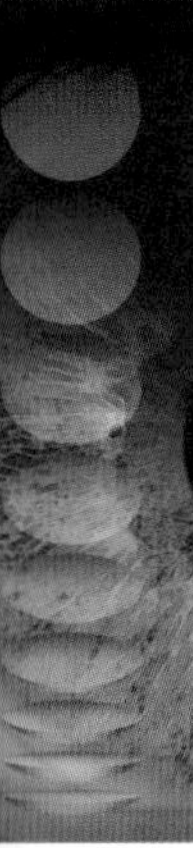

Berman, M., Winthrop, S., Ausprunk, D. et al. (1982) Plasminogen activator (urokinase) causes vascularisation of the cornea. Invest. Ophthalmol. Vis. Sci., 22, 191–199

Binder, P. S. (1983) Myopic extended wear with the Hydrocurve II soft contact lens. Ophthalmology, 90, 623–626

Blackhurst, R. T. (1985) Personal experience with hydrogel and silicone extended wear lenses. J. Contact Lens Assoc. Ophthalmol., 11, 136–137

Bonanno, J. A. and Polse, K. A. (1985) Central and peripheral corneal swelling accompanying soft lens extended wear. Am. J. Optom., 62, 74–81

Bonanno, J. A. and Polse, K. A. (1987a) Corneal acidosis during contact lens wear: effects of hypoxia and CO_2. Invest. Ophthalmol. Vis. Sci., 28, 1514–1520

Bonanno, J. A. and Polse, K. A. (1987b) Measurement of in vivo human corneal stromal pH: open and closed eye. Invest. Ophthalmol. Vis. Sci., 28, 522–530

Bonanno, J. A. and Polse, K. A. (1987c) Effect of rigid contact lens oxygen transmissibility on stromal pH in the living human eye. Ophthalmology, 94, 1305–1309

Brennan, N. A. (2001) A model of oxygen flux through contact lenses. Cornea, 20, 104–108

Brennan, N. A., Chantal Coles, M. L., Jaworski, A. et al. (2001) Proposed practice guidelines for continuous contact lens wear. Clin. Exp. Optom., 84, 71–77

Brennan, N. A., Chantal Coles, M. L., Comstock, T. L. et al. (2002) A 1-year prospective clinical trial of balafilcon A (PureVision) silicone-hydrogel contact lenses used on a 30-day continuous wear schedule. Ophthalmology, 109, 1172–1177

Brennan, N. A., Chantal Coles, M. L. and Dahl, A. K. (2004) Where do silicone hydrogels fit into everyday practice? In Silicone Hydrogels: Continuous-wear Contact Lenses, pp. 275–308, ed. D. F. Sweeney. Edinburgh: Butterworth-Heinemann

Bron, A. J. and Tripathi, R. C. (1969) Anterior corneal mosaic – further observations. Br. J. Ophthalmol., 53, 760–764

Carney, L. G. (1974) Studies on the basis of ocular changes during contact lens wear. PhD Thesis, University of Melbourne, Melbourne, Australia

Carney, L. G. (1975) Hydrophilic effects on central and peripheral corneal thickness and corneal topography. Am. J. Optom. Physiol. Opt., 52, 521–523

Carney, L. G. and Efron, N. (1980) [Environmental pH and corneal oxygen flux.] J. Fr. Ophthalmol., 3, 125–126

Carney, L. G. and Hill, R. (1976) Human tear pH. Arch. Ophthalmol., 94, 821–824

Catania, L. J. (1987) Sterile infiltrates vs. infectious infiltrates: worlds apart. Int. Contact Lens Clin., 14, 412–415

Cavanagh, H. D., Ladage, P. M., Li, S. L. et al. (2002) Effects of daily and overnight wear of a novel hyper-oxygen-transmissible soft contact lens on bacterial binding and corneal epithelium: a 13-month clinical trial. Ophthalmology, 109, 1957–1969

Cavanagh, H. D., Ladage, P. M., Yamamoto, K. et al. (2003) Effects of daily and overnight wear of hyper-oxygen transmissible rigid and silicone hydrogel lenses on bacterial binding to the corneal epithelium: 13 month clinical trials. Eye Contact Lens, 29, S14–S16

Chalupa, E., Swarbrick, H. A., Holden, B. A. et al. (1987) Severe corneal infections associated with contact lens wear. Ophthalmology, 94, 17–22

Cheng, K. H., Leung, S. L., Hoekman, H. W. et al. (1999) Incidence of contact-lens associated microbial keratitis and its related morbidity. Lancet, 354, 181–185

Cogan, D. G. (1948) Vascularisation of the cornea: its experimental induction by small lesions and a new theory of its pathogenesis. Trans. Am. Ophthalmol. Soc., 46, 457–471

Cogan, D. J. (1949) Vacularisation of the cornea. Arch. Ophthalmol., 41, 406–416

Cole, N., Willcox, M. D. P., Fleiszig, S. M. J. et al. (1998) Different strains of Pseudomonas aeruginosa isolated from ocular infections or inflammation display distinct corneal pathologies in an animal model. Curr. Eye Res., 17, 730–735

Collin, H. B. (1973) Limbal vascular response prior to corneal vascularisation. Exp. Eye Res., 16, 443–455

Comstock, T. L., Robboy, M. W., Cox, I. G. et al. (1999) Overnight clinical performance of a high Dk silicone soft contact hydrogel lens. Poster presented at the British Contact Lens Association Conference, Birmingham, May. Online. Available: www.siliconehydrogels.com

Cooper, R. L. and Constable, I. J. (1977) Infective keratitis in soft contact lens wearers. Br. J. Ophthalmol., 61, 250–254

Cornish, R., Holden, B. A., Terry, R. et al. (1988) Rigid gas permeable fitting philosophies for extended wear. Am. J. Optom., 65, 131P

Covey, M., Sweeney, D. F., Terry, R. L. et al. (2001) Hypoxic effects on the anterior eye of high Dk soft contact lens wearers are negligible. Optom. Vis. Sci., 78, 95–99

Cowell, B. A., Willcox, M. D. P., Hobden, J. A. et al. (1998) An ocular strain of Pseudomonas aeruginosa is inflammatory but not virulent in the scarified mouse model. Exp. Eye Res., 67, 347–356

Cox, I., Zantos, S. G. and Orsborn, G. N. (1991) The overnight corneal swelling response of non-wear, daily wear, and extended wear soft lens patients. Int. Contact Lens Clin., 17, 134–137

Cuklanz, H. D. and Hill, R. M. (1969) Oxygen requirements of corneal contact lens systems. Am. J. Optom., 46, 228–230

Dart, J. K. G., Stapleton, F. and Minassian, D. (1991) Contact lenses and other risk factors in microbial keratitis. Lancet, 338, 651–653

de Carle, J. (1972) Developing hydrophilic lenses for continuous wearing. Aust. J. Optom., 55, 343–346

Derick, R. J., Kelley, C. G. and Gersman, M. (1989) Contact lens related corneal ulcers at the Ohio State University Hospitals 1983–1987. Contact Lens Assoc. Ophthalmol. J., 15, 268–270

Dohlman, C. H., Buruchoff, S. A. and Mobilia, E. F. (1973) Complications in use of soft contact lenses in corneal disease. Arch. Ophthalmol., 90, 367–371

Donshik, P. C. and Ballow, M. (1983) Tear immunoglobulins in giant papillary conjunctivitis induced by contact lenses. Am. J. Ophthalmol., 96, 460–466

Donshik, P., Weinstock, F. J., Weschler, S. et al. (1988) Disposable hydrogel contact lenses for extended wear. Contact Lens Assoc. Ophthalmol. J., 14, 191–194

Douglas, J. P., Lowder, C. Y., Lazorik, R. et al. (1988) Giant papillary conjunctivitis associated with rigid gas permeable contact lenses. Contact Lens Assoc. Ophthalmol. J., 14, 143–147

Drubaix, I., Legeais, J. M., Robert, L. et al. (1997) Corneal hyaluronan content during post-ablation healing: evidence for a transient depth-dependent contralateral effect. Exp. Eye Res., 64, 301–304

du Toit, R., Papas, E., Stahl, U. et al. (2003) Initial comfort ratings of soft contact lenses [ARVO Abstract]. Invest. Ophthalmol. Vis. Sci., 44, 3696

Dumbleton, K. A., Chalmers, R. L., Richter, D. B. et al. (1999) Changes in myopic refractive error in nine months' extended wear of hydrogel lenses with high and low oxygen permeability. Optom. Vis. Sci., 76, 845–849

Dumbleton, K., Jones, L., Chalmers, R. et al. (2000) Clinical characterization of spherical post-lens debris associated with

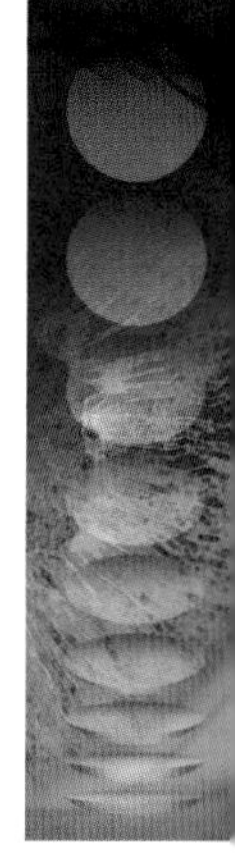

lotrafilcon high-Dk silicone lenses. Contact Lens Assoc. Ophthalmol. J., 26, 186–192

Dumbleton, K. A., Chalmers, R. L., Richter, D. B. et al. (2001) Vascular response to extended wear of hydrogel lenses with high and low oxygen permeability. Optom. Vis. Sci., 78, 147–151

Dumbleton, K. A., Chalmers, R. L., McNally, J. et al. (2002) Effect of lens base curve on subjective comfort and assessment of fit with silicone hydrogel continuous wear contact lenses. Optom. Vis. Sci., 79, 633–637

Dunn, J. P. Jr, Mondino, B. J., Weissman, B. A. et al. (1989) Corneal ulcers associated with disposable hydrogel contact lenses. Am. J. Ophthalmol., 108, 113–117

Edwards, K., Brian, G., Stretton, S. et al. (2004) Microbial keratitis and silicone hydrogels. Contact Lens Spectrum, 19, 38–43

Efron, N. and Carney, L. G. (1979) Oxygen levels beneath the closed eyelid. Invest. Ophthalmol. Vis. Sci., 18, 93–95

Efron, N., Wohl, A., Toma, N. et al. (1991) Pseudomonas corneal ulcers associated with daily wear of disposable hydrogel contact lenses. Int. Contact Lens Clin., 18, 46–51

Efron, N., Perez-Gomez, I. and Morgan, P. B. (2002) Confocal microscopic observations of stromal keratocytes during extended contact lens wear. Clin. Exp. Optom., 85, 156–160

Eichebaum, J. W., Feldstein, M. and Podos, S. M. (1982) Extended wear aphakic soft contact lenses and corneal ulcers. Br. J. Ophthalmol., 66, 663–666

Eliason, J. A. (1978) Leukocytes and experimental corneal vascularisation. Invest. Ophthalmol. Vis. Sci., 17, 1087–1095

Erickson, P., Comstock, T. L., Doughty, M. J. et al. (1999) The cornea swells in the posterior direction under hydrogel contact lenses. Ophthal. Physiol. Opt., 19, 475–480

Estil, S., Primo, E. J. and Wilson, G. (2000) Apoptosis in shed human corneal cells. Invest. Ophthalmol. Vis. Sci., 41, 3360–3364

Fanti, P. (1980) Gas permeable lenses in Germany. Contact Lens Forum, 5, 29–41

Fanti, P. and Holly, F. J. (1980) Silicone contact lens wear III. Physiology of poor tolerance. Contact Intraocul. Lens Med. J., 6, 111–119

Fatt, I. (1969) Oxygen tension under a contact lens during blinking. Am. J. Optom., 46, 654–661

Fatt, I. (1979) Negative pressure under silicone rubber contact lenses. Contacto, 23, 6–9

Fatt, I. (1996) New physiological paradigms to assess the effect of lens oxygen transmissibility on corneal health. Contact Lens Assoc. Ophthalmol. J., 22, 25–29

Fatt, I. and Bieber, M. T. (1968) The steady-state distribution of oxygen and carbon dioxide in the in vivo cornea. I. The open eye in air and the closed eye. Exp. Eye Res., 7, 103–112

Fatt, I. and Chaston, J. (1980) Temperature of a contact lens on eye. Int. Contact Lens Clin., 7, 195–198

Fatt, I. and Hill, R. M. (1970) Oxygen tension under a contact lens – a comparison of theory and experimental observations. Am. J. Optom., 47, 50–55

Fatt, I. and St Helen, R. (1971) Oxygen tension under an oxygen-permeable contact lens. Am. J. Optom., 48, 545–555

Fatt, I. and Wiessman, B. A. (1992) Physiology of the eye: and introduction to the vegetative functions. Boston: Butterworth-Heinemann

Fatt, I., Bieber, M. T. and Pye, S. D. (1969) Steady state distribution of oxygen and carbon dioxide in the in vivo cornea of an eye covered by a gas-permeable contact lens. Am. J. Optom., 46, 3–14

Ficker, L., Hunter, P., Seal, D. and Wright, P. (1990) Acanthamoeba keratitis occurring with disposable contact lens wear. Am. J. Ophthalmol., 108, 453

Fink, B. A., Hill, R. M. and Carney, L. G. (1990) Corneal oxygenation: blink frequency as a variable in rigid contact lens wear. Br. J. Ophthalmol., 74, 168–171

Fischer, F. H., Schmitz, L., Hoff, W. et al. (1978) Sodium and chloride transport in the isolated human cornea. Pflugers Arch., 373, 179–188

Fonn, D. and Dumbleton, K. A. (2003) Dryness and discomfort with silicone hydrogel contact lenses. Eye Contact Lens, 29(IS), S101–204

Fonn, D. and Holden, B. A. (1986) Extended wear of hard gas permeable contact lenses can induce ptosis. Contact Lens Assoc. Ophthalmol. J., 12, 93–94

Fonn, D. and Holden, B. A. (1988) Rigid gas-permeable vs. hydrogel contact lenses for extended wear. Am. J. Optom., 65, 536–544

Fonn, D., Holden, B. A., Roth, P. et al. (1984) Comparative physiological performance of polymethyl methacrylate and gas-permeable contact lenses. Arch. Ophthalmol., 102, 760–764

Fonn, D., Pritchard, N., Garnett, B. et al. (1996) Palpebral aperture of rigid and soft contact lens wearers compared with nonwearers. Optom. Vis. Sci., 73, 211–214

Fonn, D., du Toit, R., Simpson, T. L. et al. (1999) Sympathetic swelling response of the control eye to soft lenses in the other eye. Invest. Ophthalmol. Vis. Sci., 40, 3116–3121

Fonn, D., MacDonald, K. E., Richter, D. et al. (2002) The ocular response to extended wear of high Dk silicone hydrogel contact lenses. Clin. Exp. Optom., 85, 176–182

Fowler, S. A., Greiner, J. V. and Allansmith, M. R. (1979) Soft contact lenses from patients with giant papillary conjunctivitis. Am. J. Ophthalmol., 88, 1056–1061

Freeman, R. D. and Fatt, I. (1973) Environmental influences on ocular temperature. Invest. Ophthalmol., 12, 596–602

Fromer, C. H. and Klintworth, G. K. (1976) An evaluation of the role of leukocytes in the pathogenesis of experimentally induced corneal vascularisation. III. Studies related to the vasoproliferative capability of polymorphonuclear leukocytes and lymphocytes. Am. J. Pathol., 82, 157–167

Galentine, P. G., Cohen, E. J., Laibson, P. R. et al. (1984) Corneal ulcers associated with contact lens wear. Arch. Ophthalmol., 102, 891–894

Garcia, G. E. (1976) Continuous wear of gas-permeable lenses in aphakia. Contact Intraocul. Lens Med. J., 16, 29–34

Garcia, G. E., Aucoin, J. and Gladstone, G. (1990) Extended wear rigid gas permeable lenses used for correction of aphakia. Contact Lens Assoc. Ophthalmol. J., 16, 195–199

Gasset, A. R. and Kaufman, H. E. (1970) Therapeutic uses of hydrophilic contact lenses. Am. J. Ophthalmol., 69, 252–259

Gauthier, C., Holden, B. A. and Terry, R. (1992) Can contact lens wearers be correctly identified from their 'appearance'? [ARVO Abstract]. Invest. Ophthalmol. Vis. Sci., 33, S1294

Gerry, P. (1995) Bilateral superior epithelial arcuate lesions: a case report. Clin. Exp. Optom., 78, 194–195

Gleason, W., Tanaka, H., Albright, R. A. et al. (2003) A 1-year prospective clinical trial of Menicon Z (tisilfocon A) rigid gas-permeable contact lenses worn on a 30-day continuous wear schedule. Eye Contact Lens, 29, 2–9

Grant, T. (1991) Clinical aspects of planned replacement and disposable lenses. In The Contact Lens Year Book, pp. 7–11, ed. C. Kerr. Hythe, Kent: Medical and Scientific Publishing

Grant, T. and Holden, B. A. (1988) Clinical performance of disposable (58%) extended wear lenses. Trans. BCLA Conference, 63–64

Grosvenor, T. (1975) Changes in corneal curvature and subjective refraction of soft contact lens wearers. Am. J. Optom. Physiol. Opt., 52, 405–413

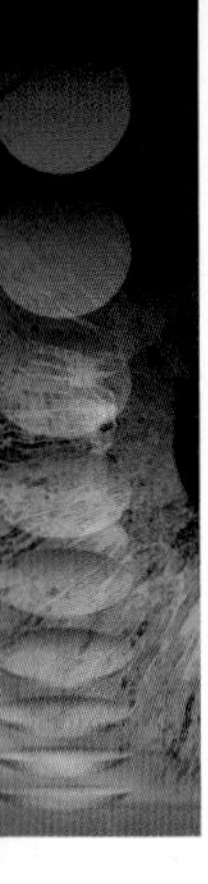

Guillon, J. P. and Guillon, M. (1993) Tear film examination of the contact lens patient. Optician, 206, 21–29
Guzey, M., Satici, A., Kilic, A. et al. (2002) Oedematous corneal response of the fellow control eye to Lotrafilcon A and Vifilcon A hydrogel contact lenses in the rabbit. Ophthalmolgica, 216, 139–143
Hamano, H. (1978) Fundamental researches on the effect of contact lenses on the eye. In Soft Contact Lenses – Clinical and Applied Technology, pp. 121–141, ed. M. Ruben. London: Baillière Tindall
Hamano, H., Hori, M., Hamano, T. et al. (1983) Effects of contact lens wear on mitosis of corneal epithelium and lactate content of aqueous humor of rabbits. Jpn J. Ophthalmol., 27, 451–458
Hamano, H., Jacob, J. T., Senft, C. et al. (2002) Differences in contact lens-induced responses in the corneas of Asian and non-Asian subjects. Contact Lens Assoc. Ophthalmol. J., 28, 101–104
Harris, M. G. and Mandell, R. B. (1969) Contact lens adaptation: osmotic theory. Am. J. Optom., 46, 196–202
Harvitt, D. M. and Bonanno, J. A. (1999) Re-evaluation of the oxygen diffusion model for predicting minimum contact lens Dk/t values needed to avoid corneal anoxia. Optom. Vis. Sci., 76, 712–719
Henry, V. A., Bennett, E. S. and Forrest, J. F. (1987) Clinical investigation of the Paraperm EW rigid gas-permeable contact lens. Am. J. Optom., 64, 313–320
Hickson, S. and Papas, E. (1997) Prevalence of idiopathic corneal anomalies in a non contact lens-wearing population. Optom. Vis. Sci., 74, 293–297
Hill, J. F. (1975) A comparison of refractive and keratometric changes during adaptation to flexible and non-flexible contact lenses. J. Am. Optom. Assoc., 46, 290–294
Hill, R. M. (1965) Oxygen uptake of the cornea following contact lens removal. J. Am. Optom. Assoc., 36, 913–915
Hill, R. M. and Fatt, I. (1964a) How dependent is the cornea on the atmosphere? J. Am. Optom. Assoc., 35, 873–875
Hill, R. M. and Fatt, I. (1964b) Oxygen measurements under a contact lens. Am. J. Optom., 41, 382–387
Hine, N., Back, A. and Holden, B. A. (1987) Aetiology of arcuate epithelial lesions induced by hydrogels. Trans. BCLA Conference, 48–50
Hirst, L. W., Auer, C., Cohn, J. et al. (1984) Specular microscopy of hard contact lens wearers. Ophthalmology, 91, 1147–1153
Hodd, N. F. B. (1975) Some observations on 62 permanent wear soft lens cases. Ophthalmic Optician, 15, 2–8
Holden, B. A. (1977) High magnification examination and photography with the slit-lamp. In Clinical Slit-lamp Biomicroscopy, p. 335, ed. R. H. Brandreth. San Leandro, CA: Blaco
Holden, B. A. and Mertz, G. W. (1984) Critical oxygen levels to avoid corneal oedema for daily and extended wear contact lenses. Invest. Ophthalmol. Vis. Sci., 25, 1161–1167
Holden, B. A. and Sweeney, D. F. (1985) The oxygen tension and temperature of the superior palpebral conjunctiva. Acta Ophthalmol., 63, 100–103
Holden, B. A. and Sweeney, D. F. (1991) The significance of the microcyst response: a review. Optom. Vis. Sci., 68, 703–707
Holden, B. A. and Zantos, S. G. (1981) Corneal endothelium: transient changes in atmospheric anoxia. In The Cornea in Health and Disease (Sixth Congress of the European Society of Ophthalmology). Royal Society of Medicine International Congress and Symposium Series No 40. pp. 79–83. London: Academic Press and Royal Society of Medicine
Holden, B. A., Mertz, G. W. and McNally, J. J. (1983) Corneal swelling response to contact lenses worn under extended wear conditions. Invest. Ophthalmol. Vis. Sci., 24, 218–226
Holden, B. A., Sweeney, D. F. and Sanderson, G. (1984) The minimum precorneal oxygen tension to avoid corneal oedema. Invest. Ophthalmol. Vis. Sci., 25, 476–480
Holden, B. A., Williams, L. and Zantos, S. G. (1985a) The etiology of transient endothelial changes in the human cornea. Invest. Ophthalmol. Vis. Sci., 26, 1354–1359
Holden, B. A., Sweeney, D. F., Vannas, A. et al. (1985b) Effects of long-term extended contact lens wear on the human cornea. Invest. Ophthalmol. Vis. Sci., 26, 1489–1501
Holden, B. A., Vannas, A., Nilsson, K. et al. (1985c) Epithelial and endothelial effects from the extended wear of contact lenses. Curr. Eye Res., 4, 739–742
Holden, B. A., Mcnally, J. J., Mertz, G. W. et al. (1985d) Topographical corneal oedema. Acta Ophthalmol., 63, 684–691
Holden, B. A., Sweeney, D. F. and Seger, R. G. (1986a) Epithelial erosions caused by thin high water content lenses. Clin. Exp. Optom., 69, 103–107
Holden, B. A., Sweeney, D. F., Swarbick, H. A. et al. (1986b) The vascular response to long-term extended contact lens wear. Clin. Exp. Optom., 69, 112–119
Holden, B. A., Ross, R. and Jenkins, J. (1987a) Hydrogel contact lenses impede carbon dioxide efflux from the human cornea. Curr. Eye Res., 6, 1283–1290
Holden, B. A., Grant, T., Kotow, M. et al. (1987b) Epithelial microcysts with daily and extended wear of hydrogel and rigid gas permeable contact lenses [ARVO Abstract]. Invest. Ophthalmol. Vis. Sci., 28, S372
Holden, B. A., Sweeney, D. F., La Hood, D. et al. (1988) Corneal deswelling following overnight wear of rigid and hydrogel contact lenses. Curr. Eye Res., 7, 49–53
Holden, B. A., La Hood, D., Grant, T. et al. (1996) Gram-negative bacteria can induce contact lens related acute red eye (CLARE) responses. Contact Lens Assoc. Ophthalmol. J., 22, 47–52
Holden, B. A., Stephenson, A., Stretton, S. et al. (2001) Superior epithelial arcuate lesions with soft contact lens wear. Optom. Vis. Sci., 78, 9–12
Horowitz, G. S., Lin, J. and Chew, H. C. (1985) An unusual corneal complication of soft contact lenses. Am. J. Ophthalmol., 100, 794–797
Høvding, G. (1983a) Variations of refractive error during the first year of contact lens wear. Acta Ophthalmol., 61, 129–140
Høvding, G. (1983b) Variations of central corneal curvature during the first year of contact lens wear. Acta Ophthalmol., 61, 117–128
Imayasu, M., Petroll, W. M., Jester, J. V. et al. (1994) The relation between contact lens transmissibility and binding of Pseudomonas aeruginosa to the cornea after overnight wear. Ophthalmology, 101, 371–388
Imre, G. (1972) Neovascularisation of the eye. In Contemporary Ophthalmology, pp. 88–91, ed. J. Bellows. Baltimore: Williams and Wilkins
Inagaki, Y., Akahori, A., Sugimoto, K. et al. (2003) Comparison of corneal endothelial bleb formation and disappearance processes between rigid gas-permeable and soft contact lenses in three classes of Dk/L. Eye Contact Lens, 29, 234–237
Iruzubieta, J. M., Ripoll, J. R. N., Chiva, J. et al. (2001) Practical experience with a high Dk lotrafilcon A fluorosilicone hydrogel extended wear contact lens in Spain. Contact Lens Assoc. Ophthalmol. J., 27, 41–46
Jalbert, I. (2004) The effects of soft contact lens wear on the corneal stroma. University of New South Wales, Sydney, Australia

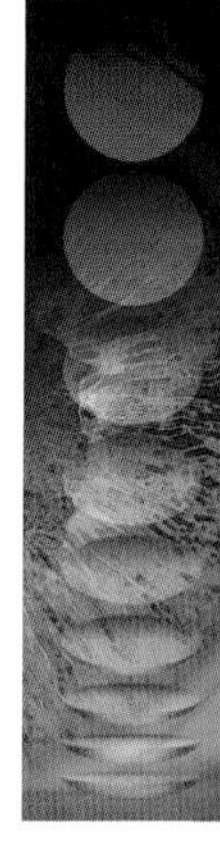

Jalbert, I. and Stapleton, F. (1999) Effect of lens wear on corneal stroma: preliminary findings. Aust. N. Z. J. Ophthalmol., 27, 211–213

Jalbert, I., Stapleton, F., Papas, E. et al. (2003) In vivo confocal microscopy of the human cornea. Br. J. Ophthalmol., 87, 225–236

Jalbert, I., Stretton, S., Naduvilath, T. J. et al. (2004) Changes in myopia with low Dk hydrogel and high Dk silicone hydrogel extended wear. Optom. Vis. Sci., 81, 591–596

Jalbert, I., Augusteyn, R. and Stapleton, F. (2005) The effect of atmospheric composition and hydrostatic pressure on keratocyte viability: preliminary experiments [ARVO Abstract]. Invest. Ophthalmol. Vis. Sci., 46, Abstract no. 2190

Jones, L., Senchyna, M., Glasier, M.-A. et al. (2003) Lysozyme and lipid deposition on silicone hydrogel contact lens materials. Eye Contact Lens, 29, S75

Josephson, J. E. (1978a) Comments on: Pitting stain with soft Hydrocurve lenses (L. Kline & T. Deluca). J. Am. Optom. Assoc., 49, 445

Josephson, J. E. (1978b) A corneal irritation uniquely produced by hydrogel lathed lenses and its resolution. J. Am. Optom. Assoc., 49, 869–870

Josephson, J. E. and Caffery, B. E. (1979) Infiltrative keratitis in hydrogel lens wearers. Int. Contact Lens Clin., 6, 223–241

Josephson, J. E. and Caffery, B. E. (1980) Clinical experiences with the Tesicon™ silicone lens. Int. Contact Lens Clin., 7, 235–245

Kallinikos, P. and Efron, N. (2004) On the etiology of keratocyte loss during contact lens wear. Invest. Ophthalmol. Vis. Sci., 45, 3011–3020

Kamiya, C. (1980) Temporary changes in corneal endothelial mosaic observed soon after wearing contact lenses. J. Jpn Contact Lens Soc., 22, 269–277

Kastl, P. R. and Johnson, W. C. (1989) FluoroPerm extended wear RGP contact lenses for myopia, hyperopia, aphakia, astigmatism and keratoconus. Contact Lens Assoc. Ophthalmol. J., 15, 61–63

Keay, L., Sweeney, D. F., Jalbert, I. et al. (2000) Microcyst response to high Dk/t silicone hydrogel contact lenses. Optom. Vis. Sci., 77, 582–585

Kent, H. D., Cohen, E. J., Laibson, P. R. and Arentsen, J. J. (1990) Microbial keratitis and corneal ulceration associated with therapeutic soft contact lenses. Contact Lens Assoc. Ophthalmol. J., 16, 49–52

Kenyon, E., Polse, K. A. and O'Neal, M. R. (1985) Ocular response to extended wear of hard gas-permeable lenses. Contact Lens Assoc. Ophthalmol. J., 11, 119–123

Kenyon, E., Polse, K. A. and Mandell, R. B. (1988) Rigid contact lens adherence: incidence, severity, and recovery. J. Am. Optom. Assoc., 59, 168–174

Kenyon, E., Mandell, R. B. and Polse, K. A. (1989) Lens design effects on rigid lens adherence. J. Br. Contact Lens Assoc., 12, 32–36

Key, J. E. and Mobley, C. L. (1989) Paraperm EW lens for extended wear. Contact Lens Assoc. Ophthalmol. J., 15, 134–137

Khodadoust, A. A. and Hirst, L. W. (1984) Diurnal variation in corneal endothelial morphology. Ophthalmology, 91, 1125–1128

Kline, L. N. and De Luca, T. J. (1977) Pitting stain with soft contact lenses – Hydrocurve® thin series. J. Am. Optom. Assoc., 48, 372–376

Klintworth, G. K. and Burger, P. C. (1983) Neovascularisation of the cornea: current concepts of its pathogenesis. Int. Ophthalmol. Clin., 23, 27–39

Klyce, S. D. (1981) Stromal lactate accumulation can account for corneal oedema osmotically following epithelial hypoxia in the rabbit. J. Physiol., 321, 49–64

Knighton, D. R., Hunt, T. K., Scheuenstuhl, H. et al. (1983) Oxygen tension regulates the expression of angiogenesis factor by macrophages. Science, 221, 1283–1284

Koers, D. (1982) Overnight corneal swelling. Am. J. Optom. Physiol. Opt., 59, 45

Kotow, M., Holden, B. A. and Grant, T. (1987a) The value of regular replacement of low water content contact lenses for extended wear. J. Am. Optom. Assoc., 58, 461–464

Kotow, M., Grant, T. and Holden, B. A. (1987b) Avoiding ocular complications during hydrogel extended wear. Int. Contact Lens Clin., 14, 95–99

Kruse, F. E. (1994) Stem cells and corneal epithelial regeneration. Eye, 8, 170–183

La Hood, D. (1988) Edge shape and comfort of rigid lenses. Am. J. Optom., 65, 613–618

La Hood, D. and Grant, T. (1990) Striae and folds as indicators of corneal oedema. Optom. Vis. Sci., 67(Suppl), 196

La Hood, D., Sweeney, D. F. and Holden, B. A. (1988) Overnight corneal oedema with hydrogel, rigid gas permeable and silicone elastomer lenses. Int. Contact Lens Clin., 15, 149–154

Ladage, P. M., Yamamoto, K., Ren, D. H. et al. (2001a) Effects of rigid and soft contact lens daily wear on corneal epithelium, tear lactate dehydrogenase, and bacterial binding to exfoliated epithelial cells. Ophthalmology, 108, 1279–1288

Ladage, P. M., Yamamoto, K., Ren, D. H. et al. (2001b) Proliferation rate of rabbit corneal epithelium during overnight rigid contact lens wear. Invest. Ophthalmol. Vis. Sci., 42, 2804–2812

Ladage, P. M., Jester, J. V., Petroll, W. M. et al. (2003a) Role of oxygen in corneal epithelial homeostasis during extended contact lens wear. Eye Contact Lens, 29, S2–5

Ladage, P. M., Jester, J. V., Petroll, W. M. et al. (2003b) Vertical movement of epithelial basal cells toward the corneal surface during use of extended-wear contact lenses. Invest. Ophthalmol. Vis. Sci., 44, 1056–1063

Ladage, P. M., Ren, D. H., Petroll, W. M. et al. (2003c) Effects of eyelid closure and disposable and silicone hydrogel extended contact lens wear on rabbit corneal epithelial proliferation. Invest. Ophthalmol. Vis. Sci., 44, 1843–1849

Lam, D. S., Houang, E., Fan, D. S. et al. (2002) Incidence and risk factors for microbial keratitis in Hong Kong: comparison with Europe and North America. Eye, 16, 608–618

Lee, J. S., Park, W. S., Lee, S. H. et al. (2001) A comparative study of corneal endothelial changes induced by different durations of soft contact lens wear. Graefes Arch. Clin. Exp. Ophthalmol., 239, 1–4

Lemp, M. A. and Gold, J. B. (1986) The effects of extended-wear hydrophilic contact lenses on the human corneal epithelium. Am. J. Ophthalmol., 101, 274–277

Lemp, M. A., Blackman, H. J., Wilson, L. A. et al. (1984) Gram-negative corneal ulcers in elderly aphakic eyes with extended-wear lenses. Ophthalmology, 91, 60–63

Levy, B. (1983) The use of a gas permeable hard lens for extended wear. Am. J. Optom. Physiol. Opt., 60, 408–409

Levy, B. (1985) Rigid gas-permeable lenses for extended wear – a 1 year clinical evaluation. Am. J. Optom., 62, 889–894

Levy, B. (1991) Complications of rigid gas permeable lenses for extended wear. Am. J. Optom., 68, 624–628

Levy, B., McNamara, N., Corzine, J. et al. (1997) Prospective trial of daily and extended wear disposable contact lenses. Cornea, 16, 274–276

Liesegang, T. J. and Forster, R. K. (1980) Spectrum of microbial keratitis in South Florida. Am. J. Ophthalmol., 90, 38–47

Lim, L., Loughnan, M. S. and Sullivan, L. J. (2002) Microbial keratitis associated with wear of silicone hydrogel contact lenses. Br. J. Ophthalmol., 86, 355–357

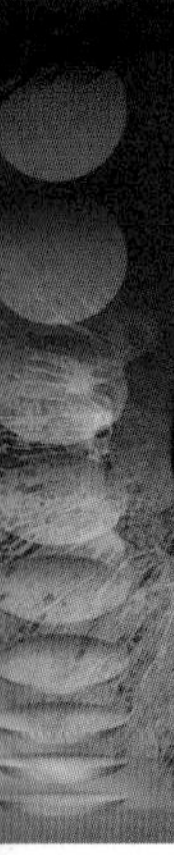

Liu, Z. and Pflugfelder, S. C. (2000) The effects of long-term contact lens wear on corneal thickness, curvature, and surface regularity. Ophthalmology, 107, 105–111

Long, B., Robird, S. and Grant, T. (2000) Six months of in-practice experience with a high Dk lotrafilcon A soft contact lens. Cont. Lens Anterior Eye, 23, 112–118

MacRae, S. M., Matsuda, M., Shellans, S. et al. (1986) The effects of hard and soft contact lenses on the corneal endothelium. Am. J. Ophthalmol., 102, 50–57

MacRae, S. M., Matsuda, M. and Phillips, D. S. (1994) The long-term effects of polymethyl methacrylate contact lens wear on the corneal endothelium. Ophthalmology, 101, 365–370

Madigan, M. C. (1989) Cat and monkey as models for extended hydrogel contact lens wear in humans. PhD Thesis. University of New South Wales, Sydney, Australia

Madigan, M. C., Holden, B. A. and Kwok, L. S. (1987) Extended wear of contact lenses can compromise corneal epithelial adhesion. Curr. Eye Res., 6, 1257–1259

Malinovsky, V., Pole, J. J., Pence, N. A. et al. (1989) Epithelial splits of the superior cornea in hydrogel contact lens patients. Int. Contact Lens Clin., 16, 252–255

Mandell, R. M. (1975) Corneal oedema and curvature changes from gel lenses. Int. Contact Lens Clin., 2, 88–98

Mandell, R. M. and Farrell, R. (1980) Corneal swelling at low atmospheric oxygen pressures. Invest. Ophthalmol. Vis. Sci., 19, 697–702

Mandell, R. B. and Fatt, I. (1965) Thinning of the human cornea on awakening. Nature, 208, 292–293

Mannarino, R. B., Belin, M. W. and Weiner, B. M. (1985) Clinical fitting characteristics of extended wear silicone (Silsight) lenses. Contact Lens Assoc. Ophthalmol. J., 11, 339–342

Martin, D. K. and Fatt, I. (1986) The presence of a contact lens induces a very small increase in the anterior corneal surface temperature. Acta Ophthalmol., 64, 512–518

Martin, D. K. and Holden, B. A. (1983) Variations in tear osmolarity, chord diameter and movement during wear of high water content hydrogel contact lenses. Int. Contact Lens Clin., 10, 323–342

Mauger, T. F. and Hill, R. M. (1992) Corneal epithelial healing under contact lenses: quantitative analysis in the rabbit. Acta Ophthalmol., 70, 361–365

McKenney, C., Becker, N., Thomas, S. et al. (1998) Lens deposits with a high Dk hydrophilic soft lens [AAO Abstract]. Optom. Vis. Sci., 75, S276

McMonnies, C. W. (1983) Contact lens-induced corneal vascularisation. Int. Contact Lens Clin., 10, 12–21

McMonnies, C. W., Chapman-Davies, A. and Holden, B. A. (1982) The vascular response to contact-lens wear. Am. J. Optom. Physiol. Opt., 59, 795–799

Mertz, G. W. (1980) Overnight swelling of the living human cornea. J. Am. Optom. Assoc., 51, 211–214

Millar, T. J., Papas, E. B., Ozkan, J. et al. (2003) Clinical appearance and microscopic analysis of mucin balls associated with contact lens wear. Cornea, 22, 740–745

Miller, J. P., Coon, L. J. and Meier, R. F. (1980) Extended wear of Hydrocurve II soft contact lenses. J. Am. Optom. Assoc., 51, 225–230, 232–233

Millodot, M. (1974) Effect of soft lenses on corneal sensitivity. Acta Ophthalmol., 52, 603–608

Millodot, M. and O'Leary, D. J. (1980) Effect of oxygen deprivation on corneal sensitivity. Acta Ophthalmol., 58, 434–439

Mishima, S. and Maurice, D. M. (1961) The oily layer of the tear film and evaporation from the corneal surface. Exp. Eye Res., 1, 39–45

Mizutani, Y., Matsunaka, H., Takemoto, N. and Mizutani, Y. (1983) [The effect of anoxia on the human cornea.] Jpn Ophthalmol. Soc. Acta, 87, 644–649

Molinari, J. F. (1983) Review: giant papillary conjunctivitis. Aust. J. Optom., 66, 59–67

Morgan, B. W. and Bennett, E. S. (1989) How to prevent RGP lens adherence. Contact Lens Update, 8, 17, 31–32

Morgan, P. B., Maldonado-Codina, C. and Efron, N. (2003) Comfort response to rigid and soft hyper-transmissible contact lenses used for continuous wear. Eye Contact Lens, 29(IS), S127–130

Morgan, P. B., Efron, N., Woods, C. A. et al. (2004) International contact lens prescribing in 2003. Contact Lens Spectrum, 19, 34–37

Morgan, P. B., Efron, N., Hiu, E. A. et al. (2005a) Incidence of keratitis of varying severity among contact lens wearers. Br. J. Ophthalmol., 89, 430–436

Morgan, P. B., Efron, N., Brennan, N. A. et al. (2005b) Risk factors for the development of corneal infiltrative events associated with contact lens wear. Invest. Ophthalmol. Vis. Sci., 46, 3136–3143

Morgan, P. B., Efron, N., Woods, C. A. et al. (2005c) International contact lens prescribing 2004. Contact Lens Spectrum. Online. Available: www.clspectrum.com

Mueller, N., Caroline, P., Smythe, J. et al. (2001) A comparison of overnight swelling response with two high Dk silicone hydrogels [AAO Abstract no. 126]. Optom. Vis. Sci., 78, S199

Nelson, L. B., Cutler, S. I., Calhoun, J. H. et al. (1985) Silsoft extended wear contact lenses in pediatric aphakia. Ophthalmology, 92, 1529–1531

Nilsson, K. T. (1983) Preventing extended wear problems, the Swedish way. Contact Lens Forum, 8, 21–29

Nilsson, S. E. G. (2001) Seven-day extended wear and 30-day continuous wear of high oxygen transmissibility soft silicone hydrogel contact lenses: a randomized 1-year study of 504 patients. Contact Lens Assoc. Ophthalmol. J., 27, 125–136

Nilsson, S. E. and Montan, P. G. (1994) The annualized incidence of contact lens induced keratitis in Sweden and its relation to lens type and wear schedule: results of a 3-month prospective study. Contact Lens Assoc. Ophthalmol. J., 20, 225–230

Nilsson, S. E. G. and Persson, G. (1986) Low complication rate in extended wear of contact lenses: a prospective two-year study of non-medical high water content lens wearers. Acta Ophthalmol., 64, 88–92

O'Donnell, C. and Maldonado-Codina, C. (2004) A hyper-Dk piggyback contact lens system for keratoconus. Eye Contact Lens, 30, 44–48

O'Hare, N. A., Naduvilath, T. J., Jalbert, I. et al. (2000) Superior epithelial arcuate lesions (SEALs): a case control study [ARVO Abstract]. Invest. Ophthalmol. Vis. Sci., 41, S74

O'Hare, N., Stapleton, F., Naduvilath, T. et al. (2002) Interaction between the contact lens and the ocular surface in superior epithelial arcuate lesions. Adv. Exp. Med. Biol., 506(Part B), 973–980

O'Leary, D. J. and Millodot, M. (1981) Abnormal epithelial fragility in diabetes and in contact lens wear. Acta Ophthalmol., 59, 827–833

O'Leary, D. J., Madgewick, R., Wallace, J. et al. (1998) Size and number of epithelial cells washed from the cornea after contact lens wear. Optom. Vis. Sci., 75, 692–693

O'Neal, M. R. and Polse, K. A. (1985) In vivo assessment of mechanisms controlling corneal hydration. Invest. Ophthalmol. Vis. Sci., 26, 849–856

Orsborn, G. N. and Schoessler, J. P. (1988) Corneal endothelial polymegethism after the extended wear of rigid gas-permeable contact lenses. Am. J. Optom., 65, 84–90

Orsborn, G. N. and Zantos, S. G. (1988) Corneal desiccation staining with thin high water content contact lenses. Contact Lens Assoc. Ophthalmol. J., 14, 81–85

Papas, E. (1998) On the relationship between soft contact lens oxygen transmissibility and induced limbal hyperaemia. Exp. Eye Res., 67, 125–131

Papas, E. (2003) The role of hypoxia in the limbal vascular response to soft contact lens wear. Eye Contact Lens, 29, 72–74

Papas, E. B., Vajdic, C. M., Austen, R. et al. (1997) High-oxygen-transmissibility soft contact lenses do not induce limbal hyperaemia. Curr. Eye Res., 16, 942–948

Patel, S. V., McLaren, J. W., Hodge, D. O. et al. (2002) Confocal microscopy in vivo on corneas of long-term contact lens wearers. Invest. Ophthalmol. Vis. Sci., 43, 995–1003

Pérez, J. G., Méijome, J. M. G., Jalbert, I. et al. (2003) Corneal epithelial thinning profile induced by long term wear of hydrogel lenses. Cornea, 22, 304–307

Poggio, E. C. and Abelson, M. (1993) Complications and symptoms in disposable extended wear lenses compared with soft daily wear and soft extended wear lenses. Contact Lens Assoc. Ophthalmol. J., 19, 31–39

Poggio, E. C., Glynn, R. J., Schein, O. D. et al. (1989) The incidence of ulcerative keratitis among users of daily-wear and extended-wear soft contact lenses. N. Engl. J. Med., 321, 779–783

Polse, K. A. (1979) Tear flow under hydrogel contact lenses. Invest. Ophthalmol. Vis. Sci., 18, 409–413

Polse, K. A. and Mandell, R. M. (1970) Critical oxygen tension at the corneal surface. Arch. Ophthalmol., 84, 505–508

Polse, K. A. and Mandell, R. B. (1976) Etiology of corneal striae accompanying hydrogel lens wear. Invest. Ophthalmol., 15, 553–556

Polse, K. A., Sarver, M. D., Kenyon, E. et al. (1987) Gas permeable hard contact lens extended wear: ocular and visual responses. Contact Lens Assoc. Ophthalmol. J., 13, 31–38

Polse, K. A., Rivera, R. K. and Bonanno, J. (1988) Ocular effects of hard gas-permeable-lens extended wear. Am. J. Optom., 65, 358–364

Polse, K. A., Graham, A. D., Fusaro, R. E. et al. (2001) The Berkeley Contact Lens Extended Wear Study: Part II. Ophthalmology, 108, 1389–1399

Quin, T. G. (1990) Manipulation of edge design to resolved RGP lens adherence. Contact Lens Forum, 15, 23–29

Rao, G. N., Aquavella, J. V., Goldberg, S. H. et al. (1984) Pseudophakic bullous keratopathy: relationship to preoperative corneal endothelial status. Ophthalmology, 91, 1135–1140

Ren, D. H., Petroll, W. M., Jester, J. V. et al. (1999a) The effects of rigid gas permeable contact lens wear on proliferation of rabbit corneal and conjunctival epithelial cells. Contact Lens Assoc. Ophthalmol. J., 25, 136–141

Ren, D. H., Petroll, W. M., Jester, J. V. et al. (1999b) The relationship between contact lens oxygen permeability and binding of Pseudomonas aeruginosa to human corneal epithelial cells after overnight and extended wear. Contact Lens Assoc. Ophthalmol. J., 25, 80–100

Ren, D. H., Yamamoto, K., Ladage, P. M. et al. (2002) Adaptive effects of 30-night wear of hyper-O_2 transmissible contact lenses on bacterial binding and corneal epithelium: a 1-year clinical trial. Ophthalmology, 109, 27–40

Ren, H. and Wilson, G. (1996) Apoptosis in the corneal epithelium. Invest. Ophthalmol. Vis. Sci., 37, 1017–1025

Reynolds, R. M. P. (1978) Giant papillary conjunctivitis: a mechanical aetiology. Aust. J. Optom., 61, 320–323

Rivera, R. K. and Polse, K. A. (1991) Corneal response to different oxygen levels during extended wear. Contact Lens Assoc. Ophthalmol. J., 17, 96–101

Rom, M. E., Keller, W. B., Meyer, C. J. et al. (1995) Relationship between corneal oedema and topography. Contact Lens Assoc. Ophthalmol. J., 21, 191–194

Roszkowska, A. M., Tringali, C. G., Colosi, P. et al. (1999) Corneal endothelium evaluation in type I and type II diabetes mellitus. Ophthalmologica, 213, 258–261

Ruben, M. (1976) Acute eye disease secondary to contact-lens wear. Lancet, 1, 138–140

Ruben, M. (1977) Constant wear vs daily wear. Optician, August, 5, 7, 9, 11–14

Ruben, M. and Guillon, M. (1979) Silicone rubber lenses in aphakia. Br. J. Ophthalmol., 63, 471–474

Sack, R. A., Tan, K. O. and Tan, A. (1992) Diurnal tear cycle: evidence for a nocturnal inflammatory constitutive tear fluid. Invest. Ophthalmol. Vis. Sci., 33, 626–640

Salz, J. J. and Slanger, J. L. (1983) Complications of aphakic extended wear lenses encountered during a seven-year period in 100 eyes. Contact Lens Assoc. Ophthalmol. J., 9, 241–244

Sankaridurg, P. R., Vuppala, N., Sreedharan, A. et al. (1996) Gram negative bacteria and contact lens induced red eye. Ind. J. Ophthalmol., 44, 29–32

Sankaridurg, P. R., Sweeney, D. S., Sharma, S. et al. (1999) Adverse events with extended wear of disposable hydrogels: results for the first 13 months of lens wear. Ophthalmology, 106, 1671–1680

Sankaridurg, P. R., Sharma, S., Willcox, M. et al. (2000) Bacterial colonization of disposable soft contact lenses is greater during corneal infiltrative events than during asymptomatic extended lens wear. J. Clin. Microbiol., 38, 4420–4424

Sankaridurg, P. R., Skotnitsky, C., Pearce, D. et al. (2001a) Contact lens papillary conjunctivitis: a review. Optom. Pract., 2, 19–28

Sankaridurg, P. R., Sweeney, D., Naduvilath, T. et al. (2001b) Papillary response in contact lens papillary conjunctivitis is either general or localised [ARVO Abstract no. 3205]. Invest. Ophthalmol. Vis. Sci., 42, S596

Sarver, M. D. (1971) Striae corneal lines among patients wearing hydrophilic contact lenses. Am. J. Optom., 48, 762–763

Schein, O. D., Glynn, R. J., Seddon, J. M. et al. (1989) The relative risk of ulcerative keratitis among users of daily-wear and extended-wear soft contact lenses. N. Engl. J. Med., 321, 773–778

Schein, O. D., McNally, J. J., Katz, J. et al. (2005) The incidence of microbial keratitis among wearers of a 30-day silicone hydrogel extended wear contact lens. Ophthalmology, 112, 2172–2179

Schnider, C. M., Zabiewicz, K. and Holden, B. A. (1988) Unusual complications associated with extended wear. Int. Contact Lens Clin., 15, 124–128

Schnider, C. M., Terry, R. L. and Holden, B. A. (1996) Effect of patient and lens performance characteristics on peripheral corneal desiccation. J. Am. Optom. Assoc., 67, 144–150

Schoessler, J. P. (1983) Corneal endothelial polymegethism associated with extended wear. Int. Contact Lens Clin., 10, 148–155

Schoessler, J. P., Woloschak, M. J. and Mauger, T. F. (1982) Transient endothelial changes produced by hydrophilic contact lenses. Am. J. Optom., 59, 764–765

Schoessler, J. P., Barr, J. T. and Freson, D. R. (1984) Corneal endothelial observations of silicone elastomer contact lens wearers. Int. Contact Lens Clin., 11, 337–340

Schulz, R. O., Matsuda, M., Yee, R. W. et al. (1984) Corneal endothelial changes in type I and II diabetes mellitus. Am. J. Ophthalmol., 98, 401–410

Seger, R. G. and Mutti, D. O. (1986) Corneal swelling and epithelial compromise with hard gas permeable contact lenses. Trans. BCLA Conference, 92–94

Sholley, M. M., Gimbrone, M. A. and Cotran, R. S. (1978) The effects of leukocyte depletion on corneal neovascularisation. Lab. Invest., 38, 32–40

Sibug, M. E., Datiles, M. B. I., Kashima, K. et al. (1991) Specular microscopy studies on the corneal endothelium after cessation of contact lens wear. Cornea, 10, 395–401

Sigband, D. J. and Bridgewater, B. A. (1994) FluoroPerm 151 extended wear: a clinical study. Contact Lens Assoc. Ophthalmol. J., 20, 37–40

Sjöstrand, J., Linner, E., Nygren, B. et al. (1981) Severe corneal infection in a contact lens wearer. Lancet, 1, 149–150

Skotnitsky, C., Sweeney, D. F., Keay, L. et al. (1999) Patient responses and attitudes to 30 night continuous wear of high Dk silicone hydrogel lenses and attitudes to refractive surgery [AAO Abstract]. Optom. Vis. Sci., 76, S214

Skotnitsky, C., Sankaridurg, P. R., Sweeney, D. F. et al. (2002a) General and local contact lens induced papillary conjunctivitis (CLPC). Clin. Exp. Optom., 85, 193–197

Skotnitsky, C., Naduvilath, T., Sweeney, D. F. et al. (2000b) Contact lens papillary conjunctivitis (CLPC): a case control study [AAO Abstract]. Optom. Vis. Sci., 77, S257

Smelser, G. K. and Ozanics, V. (1952) Importance of atmospheric oxygen for maintenance of the optical properties of the human cornea. Science, 115, 140

Snyder, C. (1995) Infiltrative keratitis with contact lens wear – a review. J. Am. Optom. Assoc., 66, 160–177

Spoor, T. C., Hartel, W. C., Wynn, P. et al. (1984) Complications of continuous-wear soft contact lenses in a nonreferral population. Arch. Ophthalmol., 102, 1312–1313

Stapleton, F., Dart, J. K. G. and Minassian, D. (1993) Risk factors with contact lens related suppurative keratitis. Contact Lens Assoc. Ophthalmol. J., 19, 204–210

Stapleton, F., Kasses, S., Bolis, S. et al. (2001) Short term wear of high Dk soft contact lenses does not alter corneal epithelial cell size or viability. Br. J. Ophthalmol., 85, 143–146

Stein, R. M., Clinch, T. E., Cohen, E. J. et al. (1988) Infected vs sterile corneal infiltrates in contact lens wearers. Am. J. Ophthalmol., 105, 632–636

Stern, J., Wong, R., Naduvilath, T. J. et al. (2004) Comparison of the performance of 6- or 30-night extended wear schedules with silicone hydrogel lenses over 3 years. Optom. Vis. Sci., 81, 398–406

Stocker, E. G. and Schoessler, J. P. (1985) Corneal endothelial polymegethism induced by PMMA contact lens wear. Invest. Ophthalmol. Vis. Sci., 26, 857–863

Swarbrick, H. A. (1988) A possible etiology for RGP lens binding (adherence). Int. Contact Lens Clin., 15, 13–19

Swarbrick, H. A. (1991) Rigid gas-permeable contact lens adherence: frequency, features and etiology. PhD Thesis. University of New South Wales, Sydney, Australia

Swarbrick, H. and Holden, B. A. (1987) Rigid gas permeable lens binding: significance and contributing factors. Am. J. Optom. Physiol. Opt., 64, 815–823

Swarbrick, H. A. and Holden, B. A. (1989) Rigid gas-permeable lens adherence: a patient dependent phenomenon. Optom. Vis. Sci., 66, 269–275

Swarbrick, H. A. and Holden, B. A. (1993) Complications of hydrogel extended wear lenses. In Anterior Segment Complications of Contact Lens Wear, pp. 289–316, ed. J. A. Silbert. New York: Churchill Livingstone

Swarbrick, H. A. and Holden, B. A. (1996) Effects of lens parameter variation on rigid gas-permeable lens adherence. Optom. Vis. Sci., 73, 144–155

Sweeney, D. F. (1991) Factors contributing to the human corneal oedema response. PhD Thesis. University of New South Wales, Sydney, Australia

Sweeney, D. F. (1992) Corneal exhaustion syndrome with long-term wear of contact lenses. Optom. Vis. Sci., 69, 601–608

Sweeney, D. F. and Holden, B. A. (1983) The closed-eye swelling response of the cornea to Polycon and Menicon O_2 gas-permeable hard lenses. Aust. J. Optom., 66, 186–189

Sweeney, D. F. and Holden, B. A. (1987) Silicone elastomer lens wear induces less overnight corneal oedema than sleep without lens wear. Curr. Eye Res., 6, 1391–1394

Sweeney, D. F., Madigan, M. C. and Holden, B. A. (1987) The effects of silicone elastomer lenses on the corneal epithelium [ARVO Abstract no. 45]. Invest. Ophthalmol. Vis. Sci., 28, 163

Sweeney, D. F., Grant, T., Chong, M. S. et al. (1993) Recurrence and acute inflammatory conditions with hydrogel extended wear [ARVO Abstract]. Invest. Ophthalmol. Vis. Sci., 34, S1008

Sweeney, D. F., Terry, R. L., Papas, E. et al. (1996) The prevalence of 'infiltrates' in a non-contact lens wearing population [ARVO Abstract]. Invest. Ophthalmol. Vis. Sci., 37, S71

Sweeney, D. F., Sankaridurg, P. R., Holden, B. A. et al. (2000) Atypical presentation of contact lens induced peripheral ulcers – multiple focal corneal infiltrates [AAO Abstract no. 146]. Optom. Vis. Sci., 77, S164

Sweeney, D. F., Stern, J., Naduvilath, T. et al. (2002a) Inflammatory adverse event rates over 3 years with silicone hydrogel lenses [ARVO Abstract no. 976]. The Association for Research in Vision and Ophthalmology Annual Meeting, Florida, USA. Online. Available: www.arvo.org

Sweeney, D. F., Keay, L., Carnt, N. et al. (2002b) Practitioner guidelines for continuous wear with high Dk silicone hydrogel contact lenses. Clin. Exp. Optom., 85, 161–167

Sweeney, D. F., Jalbert, I., Covey, M. et al. (2003) Clinical characterisation of corneal infiltrative events observed with soft contact lens wear. Cornea, 22, 435–442

Sweeney, D. F., du Toit, R., Keay, L. et al. (2004) Clinical performance of silicone hydrogel lenses. In Silicone Hydrogels: Continuous-wear Contact Lenses, pp. 164–216, ed. D. F. Sweeney. Edinburgh: Butterworth-Heinemann

Sweeney, D. F., Carnt, N. A., Du Toit, R. et al. (2005) Silicone hydrogel lenses for continuous wear. In Clinical Contact Lens Practice, pp. 693–717, eds. E. S. Bennett and B. A. Weismann. Philadelphia: Lippincott Williams and Wilkins

Szaflik, J. P., Ambroziak, A. M. and Szaflik, J. (2004) Therapeutic use of a lotrafilcon A silicone hydrogel soft contact lens as a bandage after LASEK surgery. Eye Contact Lens, 30, 59–62

Tan, K. O., Sack, R. A., Holden, B. A. et al. (1993) Temporal sequence of changes in tear film composition during sleep. Curr. Eye Res., 12, 1001–1007

Tan, J., Keay, L., Sweeney, D. F. et al. (2000) Mucin balls and high Dk soft lenses. Contact Lens Spectrum, July, 42–44

Tan, J., Keay, L., Jalbert, I. et al. (2003) Mucin balls with wear of conventional and silicone hydrogel contact lenses. Optom. Vis. Sci., 80, 291–297

Terry, J. E. and Hill, R. M. (1978) Human tear osmotic pressure: diurnal variation and the closed lid. Arch. Ophthalmol., 96, 120–122

Terry, R., La Hood, D., Schnider, C. et al. (1986) Continuous wear of a high Dk gas permeable lens. Am. J. Optom., 63, 6P

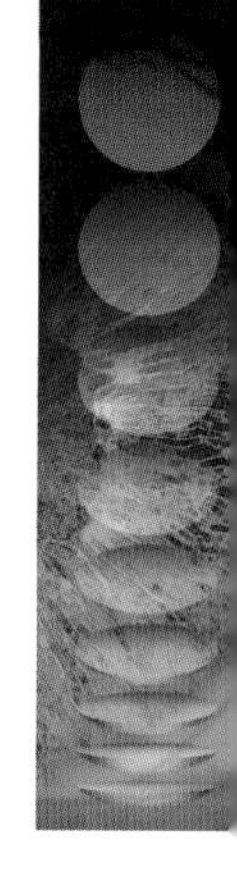

Terry, R. L., Schnider, C. M., Holden, B. A. et al. (1993) CCLRU standard for success of daily and extended wear contact lenses. Optom. Vis. Sci., 70, 234–243

Thakur, A. and Willcox, M. D. P. (1998) Cytokine and lipid inflammatory mediator profile of human tears during contact lens associated inflammatory diseases. Exp. Eye Res., 67, 9–19

Thakur, A. and Willcox, M. D. P. (2000) Contact lens wear alters the production of certain inflammatory mediators in tears. Exp. Eye Res., 70, 255–259

Tighe, B. J., Jones, L., Evans, K. et al. (2000) Patient-dependent and material dependent factors in contact lens deposition processes. Adv. Exp. Med. Biol., 438, 745–751

Tomlinson, A. and Haas, D. D. (1980) Changes in corneal thickness and circumcorneal vascularisation with contact lens wear. Int. Contact Lens Clin., 7, 26–37

Tripathi, R. C. and Bron, A. J. (1972) Ultrastructural study of non-traumatic recurrent corneal erosion. Br. J. Ophthalmol., 56, 73–85

van Setten, G. B., Tervo, T., Andersson, R. et al. (1990) Plasmin and epidermal growth factor in the tear fluid of contact-lens wearers: effect of wearing different types of contact lenses and association with clinical findings. Ophthalmic Res., 22, 233–240

Vannas, A., Makitie, J., Sulonen, J. et al. (1981) Contact lens induced transient changes in corneal endothelium. Acta Ophthalmol., 59, 552–559

Vannas, A., Sweeney, D. F., Holden, B. A. et al. (1992) Tear plasmin activity with contact lens wear. Curr. Eye Res., 11, 243–251

Weston, B. C., Bourne, W. M., Polse, K. A. et al. (1995) Corneal hydration control in diabetes mellitus. Invest. Ophthalmol. Vis. Sci., 36, 586–595

Wichterle, O. and Lim, D. (1960) Hydrophilic gels for biological use. Nature, 185, 117–118

Willcox, M., Sankaridurg, P. R., Zhu, H. et al. (2004) Inflammation and infection and the effects of the closed eye. In Silicone Hydrogels: Continuous Wear Contact Lenses, pp. 90–125, ed. D. F. Sweeney. Edinburgh: Butterworth-Heinemann

Williams, L. (1986) Transient endothelial changes in the in vivo human cornea. PhD Thesis. University of New South Wales, Sydney, Australia

Williams, L. and Holden, B. A. (1986) The bleb response of the endothelium decreases with extended wear of contact lenses. Clin. Exp. Optom., 69, 90–92

Wilson, G., O'Leary, D. J. and Holden, B. A. (1989) Cell content of tears following overnight wear of a contact lens. Curr. Eye Res., 8, 329–335

Wu, P. Z., Thakur, A., Stapleton, F. et al. (2000) Staphylococcus aureus causes acute inflammatory episodes in the cornea during contact lens wear. Clin. Exp. Ophthalmol., 28, 194–196

Yamamoto, K., Ladage, P. M., Ren, D. H. et al. (2002) Effect of eyelid closure and overnight contact lens wear on viability of surface epithelial cells in rabbit cornea. Cornea, 21, 85–90

Yamauchi, K., Hirst, L. W., Enger, C. et al. (1989) Specular microscopy of hard contact lens wearers II. Ophthalmology, 96, 1176–1179

Young, G. and Mirejovsky, D. (1993) A hypothesis for the aetiology of soft contact lens-induced superior arcuate keratopathy. Int. Contact Lens Clin., 20, 177–180

Young, G. and Port, M. (1992) Rigid gas-permeable extended wear: a comparative clinical study. Am. J. Optom., 69, 214–226

Young, G., Holden, B. A. and Cooke, G. (1993) Influence of soft contact lens design on clinical performance. Optom. Vis. Sci., 70, 394–403

Zabkiewicz, K., Swarbrick, H. A. and Holden, B. A. (1986) Clinical experiences with low to moderate Dk hard gas-permeable lenses for extended wear. Trans. BCLA Conference, 101–102

Zantos, S. G. (1981) The ocular response to continuous wear of contact lenses. PhD Thesis. University of New South Wales, Sydney, Australia

Zantos, S. G. (1983) Cystic formations in the corneal epithelium during extended wear of contact lenses. Int. Contact Lens Clin., 10, 128–146

Zantos, S. G. and Holden, B. A. (1977a) Transient endothelial changes soon after wearing soft contact lenses. Am. J. Optom., 54, 856–858

Zantos, S. G. and Holden, B. A. (1977b) Research techniques and materials for continuous wear of contact lenses. Aust. J. Optom., 60, 86–95

Zantos, S. G. and Holden, B. A. (1978) Ocular changes associated with continuous wear of contact lenses. Aust. J. Optom., 61, 418–426

Zantos, S. G. and Zantos, P. O. (1985) Extended wear feasibility of gas-permeable hard lenses for myopia. Int. Eyecare, 1, 66–75

Zieske, J. D. (1994) Perpetuation of stem cells in the eye. Eye, 8, 163–169

Chapter 14

Bifocal and multifocal contact lenses

Edward S. Bennett

CHAPTER CONTENTS

INTRODUCTION

Presbyopia, resulting from a gradual decrement in visual function at near, is one of the most prevalent ocular conditions resulting in patient complaints and dissatisfaction in the 40 years and older age group. Nevertheless, it also represents an outstanding opportunity for potential contact lens wearers. The presbyopic patient represents the largest growing segment of the population and the largest untapped segment of the contact lens market (Bennett & Jurkus 2005).

- There were 78 million 'baby boomers' born in the United States between 1946 and 1964 (Schwartz 1999).
- Only 3% of presbyopes currently wear some form of presbyopic contact lens correction (Wooley 1998, Rigel & Castellano 1999).
- In the United Kingdom, the presbyopic market has greater potential than the younger contact lens market (Edwards 1999, Meyler & Veys 1999).

Presbyopic contact lens options include:

- Single-vision contact lenses worn in combination with reading glasses.
- Monovision – one eye is corrected optimally for distance vision and the other eye for near vision.
- Bifocal rigid gas-permeable (RGP) or hydrogel lenses having separate corrections for near and distance.
- Multifocal RGP and hydrogel lenses having corrections for greater than two distances (i.e. typically distance, near and intermediate corrections).

It has been predicted that the contact lens multifocal market will increase rapidly in the next 10–20 years (Schwartz 1999, Pujol et al. 2003) as many baby boomers who have never worn corrective eyewear may choose contact lenses over spectacles simply because of vanity. Current emerging presbyopes are more active than their predecessors and appear to be more determined to maintain their youthful appearance. The increase in multifocal contact lens use will accompany the popularity of progressive addition spectacles as this generation pursues alternative treatments to standard bifocal/trifocal spectacles, which includes monovision contact lenses and refractive surgery.

Multifocal contact lenses have numerous benefits compared to spectacles (Fisher et al. 1999):

- Multifocal spectacles require numerous head movements to find the optimum position for tasks such as computer use or

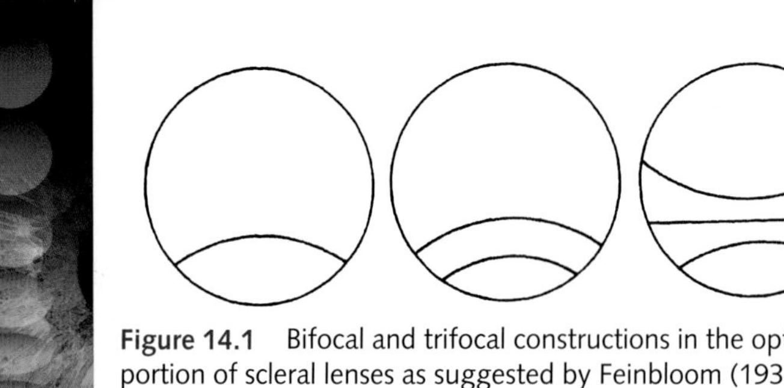

Figure 14.1 Bifocal and trifocal constructions in the optic portion of scleral lenses as suggested by Feinbloom (1938)

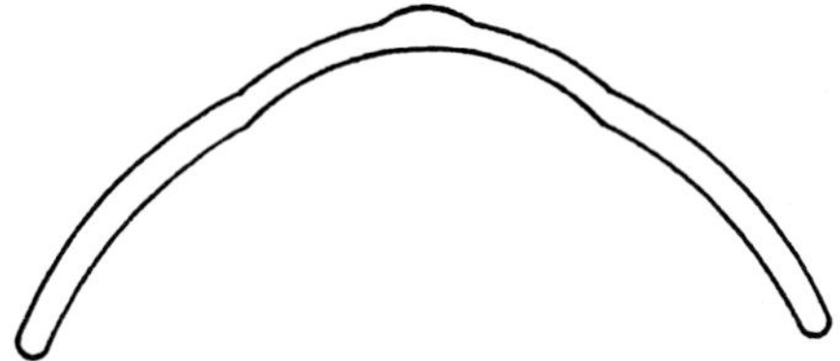

Figure 14.2 Bifocal scleral lenses suggested by Williamson-Noble (1951) with a small convex central near portion on the front surface

Figure 14.3 Diagrammatic representation of the Bicon translating bifocal design with the distance vision zone located centrally

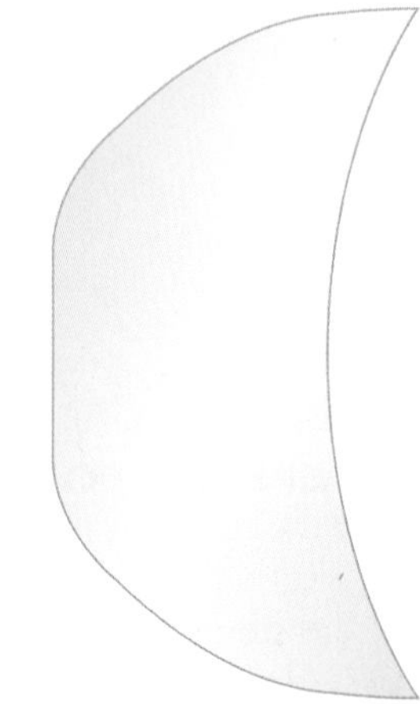

shelf stacking (Vassilieff & Dain 1986, Martin & Dain 1988) due to the varying corrective powers during any eye movement (Afanador et al. 1986). Multifocal contact lenses move with the eye and minimize these possible problems.

- Progressive addition spectacles can result in distortions in the size and shape of objects whose images extend beyond the limited intermediate and near zones (Diepes & Tameling 1988).

The low usage of presbyopic contact lenses is probably because:

- These lenses are perceived by practitioners as being complicated or challenging to fit, which leads to an easier option being chosen for the patient such as monovision, single-vision contact lenses in combination with reading glasses, and multifocal spectacles (Hansen et al. 2003).
- It is not uncommon for patients to be told that bifocal contact lenses either do not exist or they are not a successful option (Bennett & Hansen 2004).
- Multifocal lenses are often not presented as an option.

Contact lens practitioners can successfully build their practice by offering soft and RGP presbyopic contact lenses, and patients fitted with these lenses can be among the most satisfied patients. They also represent the high end of earnings potential; therefore practice income generated from these patients – and their referrals – can build a contact lens practice.

HISTORY

Bifocal contact lenses date back to 1938 when William Feinbloom filed the first contact lens patent application (Moss 1962). He showed diagrams of bifocal and trifocal segments in the optic zone of scleral polymethylmethacrylate (PMMA) contact lenses (de Carle 1997) (Fig. 14.1).

The Williamson-Noble design (Fig. 14.2), introduced in 1951, was also a scleral design, which had the reading zone positioned in the centre and the distance zone surrounding it (Caffery & Josephson 1991). The central near section was made 2.00 D more convex than the remainder of the front surface.

The next generation of lenses comprised concentric or annular corneal designs, the first of which was the translating Bicon lens (Fig. 14.3). This design had a central distance optical zone of 4.0–6.0 mm surrounded by a single annular near zone (Caffery & Josephson 1991).

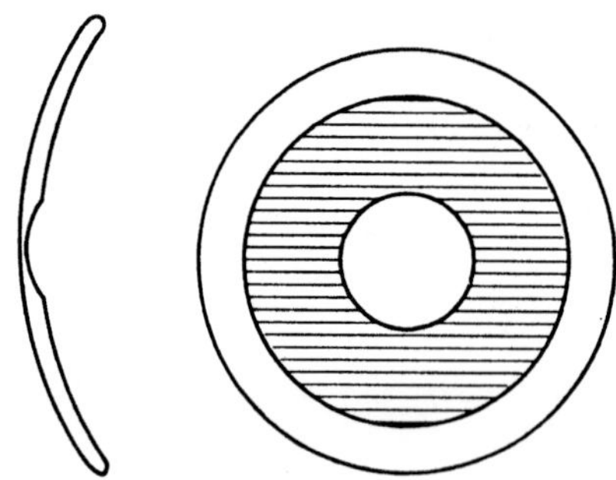

Figure 14.4 The De Carle concentric back surface bifocal (1957) with a 2.0–4.0 mm central distance portion surrounded by the near portion used as a bearing surface

There are two ways to achieve bifocal vision:

- Translation or shifting upward of the lens during near gaze to allow the wearer to view through the near optics during downward gaze.
- Simultaneous vision where multiple powers (i.e. near, distance and possibly intermediate) are in front of the eye at the same time.

The pioneer of concentric or annular lens designs was John de Carle. He placed the bifocal surface on the back of the lens so that the partial neutralization of the tears would be constant (de Carle 1959, 1997). The centre of the de Carle concentric back surface bifocal had a 2.0–4.0 mm central distance portion surrounded by the annular near section (Fig. 14.4).

These were lenses with the central distance zone sufficiently small in diameter to cover only part of the pupil and allow both

Figure 14.5 The Black bifocal design

partial distance and partial near coverage at all times. De Carle described this as 'bi-vision' with the premise that, while the patient looks at a distant object, the light entering the pupil from the near zone forms a blurred image. The near image blur circle covers a large area of the retina and is essentially ignored.

The Wesley–Jessen bifocal, introduced shortly afterwards, was a concentric design with the bifocal on the front surface and a larger central distance zone (i.e. 5–6 mm) (Jessen 1960a,b). This was essentially a translating alternating design.

From about 1960, a number of different bifocal contact lens designs were introduced that were similar to bifocal spectacles. Almost all of these were prism ballasted to prevent excessive rotation and maintain visual quality at distance and near. They were translating designs that would shift up into the near zone with downward gaze during reading. The early designs – by Hodd and others – had a front surface correction with separate powers, but the optical quality was slightly compromised and image jump was a problem.

These disadvantages were overcome by fused bifocals:

- The Camp lens could incorporate a front surface cylinder if necessary (Caffery & Josephson 1991).
- The Black bifocal was a prism-ballasted D-shaped design (Fig. 14.5).
- The Mandell 'No-Jump' monocentric bifocal (Mandell 1967) was a major breakthrough as image jump was eliminated by having the centre of the distance and near sections in the same focal plane. The near portion was cut into the front surface, creating a slight ledge between the distance and near portions (Fig. 14.6).

Monocentric fused bifocals in PMMA lens materials were quite popular in the 1970s and 1980s but difficulty was experienced in fusing RGP lens materials.

- Paragon Vision Sciences successfully introduced the first fused RGP bifocal (FluoroPerm St) in the early 1990s but the small D-shaped segment limited the area provided for near viewing and this bifocal was later discontinued.
- The Tangent Streak Bifocal (Fused Kontacts) was the first one-piece segmented RGP lens to have monocentric optics with the near and distance optical centres at a tangent at the top of the executive-style segment.

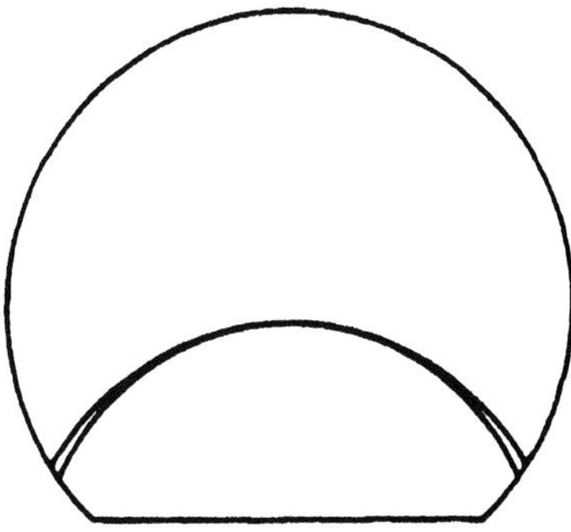

Figure 14.6 The Mandell 'No-Jump' front surface bifocal design

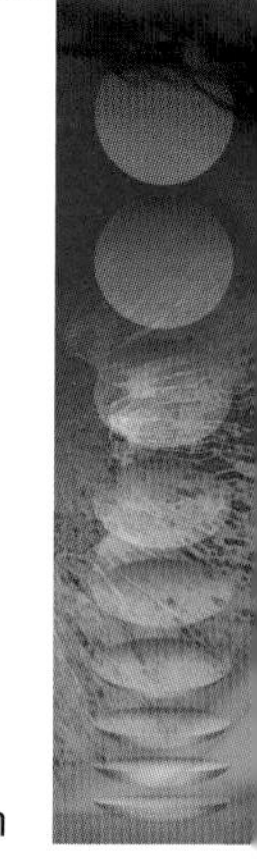

Recent advances in translating designs include the introduction of intermediate corrections in several of the new designs (see below).

The first aspheric multifocal lens was produced in the early 1960s. With these designs, the back surface flattened at a particular rate, generating a gradual increase in plus power away from the centre of the lens. Feinbloom developed an elliptical posterior surface lens in 1961, followed by innovative multifocal pioneer Joe Goldberg who introduced several aspheric designs (e.g. Ellip-See-Con, VFL), manufactured under a Volk patent (de Carle 1997). Back surface aspheric multifocal RGP lenses are popular today due to advancements in manufacturing technology which have resulted in better optical quality and the ability to incorporate higher add powers.

Hydrogel bifocal lenses were introduced in the early 1980s. The early designs differed dramatically:

- CIBA Vision BiSoft had a centre-distance concentric zone with a blended bifocal zone junction and three optional add powers (Josephson & Caffery 1991).
- Bausch & Lomb PA-1 was a back surface aspheric design.
- Wesley–Jessen developed the first segmented translating soft bifocal.

All these early designs had low success rates due to a variety of problems including:

- Poor optical quality.
- Limited add powers.
- For translating designs, difficulty in achieving adequate translation.
- Visual compromise in the case of soft bifocal and multifocal lens designs.

In recent years, several innovations have resulted in a higher success rate including:

- Better optical quality.
- Variable add powers.
- Disposability.

The last has:

- Reduced costs to the patient.
- Allowed for replacement lenses.

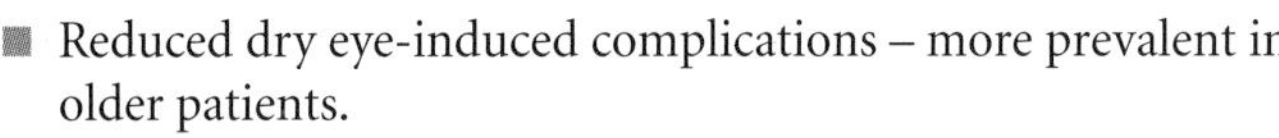

- Reduced dry eye-induced complications – more prevalent in older patients.
- Allowed the practitioner to try different lenses on a trial basis.

PRELIMINARY EVALUATION AND PATIENT SELECTION

Normal physiological changes

- The most important change for the presbyopic patient is reduction in tear volume, which can result in dry eye symptoms. A progressive reduction in tear production results from a reduction in both the goblet cells of the conjunctiva and the mass of the lacrimal glands (Weale 1982). Extended wear is not usually advisable, due both to the tear physiology and to thicker presbyopic lens designs.
- Tear film quality and quantity is likely to be reduced (Gromacki 2004) and assessment should be carried out before deciding on lens material and replacement schedule. RGP or disposable and frequent-replacement soft lenses are recommended (Veys & Davies 1995).
- Reduced tear flow results in
  - increased lens surface deposition.
  - blurred vision.
  - discomfort.
  - possible papillary hypertrophy.

  It is important, therefore, to rule out clinical signs of dry eye (Bennett & Jurkus 2005).
- A reduction in eyelid tone is common, which can make translating rigid bifocal lenses more challenging as these designs depend upon lid tone to shift the lens upward with downward gaze.
- Natural changes in the crystalline lens may affect acuity. Where this occurs, the contact lenses must not further compromise the vision, especially for distance.
- There is an increased likelihood for pingueculae and pterygia formation, which can result in decreased lens comfort.
- Handling of lenses must be considered since presbyopes find near tasks such as checking whether the lens is inside out more difficult. Handling tints and lenses that are less 'floppy' help with lens insertion.

Examination procedures

PATIENT REQUIREMENTS

The primary goals of presbyopic contact lens patients differ from those of pre-presbyopes in various aspects:

- What they expect from contact lens wear.
- What distance(s) are most important to them.
- What their occupational/avocational vision requirements are.

Various extra details and measurements are needed prior to fitting bifocal lenses.

History

A history of eye surgery, in particular cosmetic lid surgery, can affect RGP translating and aspheric multifocal lens success by causing excessive lifting and superior decentration with blinking.

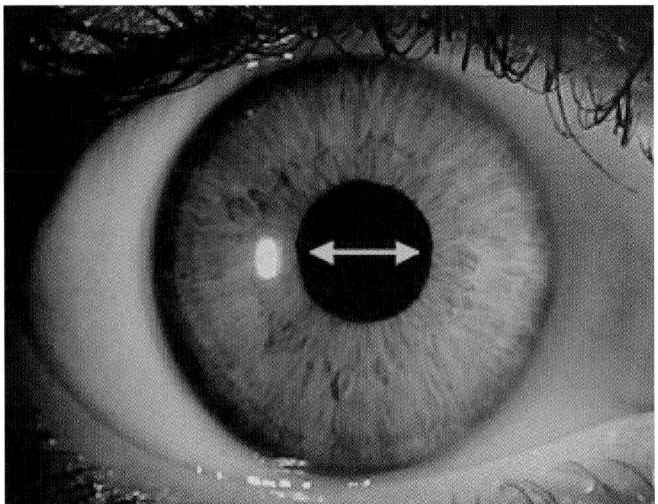

Figure 14.7 Pupil size determination in photopic and scotopic illumination is critical to lens selection. (Courtesy of Dr Peter Kollbaum)

Medication, especially if it reduces tear volume, will affect comfort and lens tolerance. This can include ibuprofen, oestrogen, antihypertensives, tricyclic antidepressants, anticholinergics and the scopolamine patch (du Toit et al. 2001).

Tears (see also Chapter 5)
Tear volume decreases with age and can help to determine whether the patient is a good candidate for contact lenses in general. A tear break-up-time (tear BUT) of less than 10 seconds suggests potential difficulties with lens wear (Andres et al. 1987). Between 6 and 9 seconds should limit the patient to a daily wear schedule, and 5 seconds or less typically contraindicates contact lens wear, especially if the measurement is repeatable (Bennett 2004a).

Blepharitis or meibomian gland dysfunction indicates poor tear quality and needs to be managed prior to reassessing tear quality for possible contact lens wear.

Tear volume can be assessed either with the Schirmer tear test or with a phenol red thread test (Zone-Quick from Menicon/Allergan). In the latter test a value of less than 9 mm of wetting in a 15-second time period should contraindicate contact lens wear (Hamano et al. 1983, Sakamoto et al. 1993).

Pupil size

This should be measured both in normal room illumination (Fig. 14.7) and with the room lights dimmed such that the millimetre rule readings are barely visible.

The presence of a large pupil in normal room illumination (i.e. more than 5 mm), although not common in the presbyopic population, would contraindicate an aspheric rigid multifocal lens design because of the ghost images and glare that the patient would experience in low illumination.

The lid-to-limbus relationship should be observed; in particular, the position of the lower lid. Individuals with a

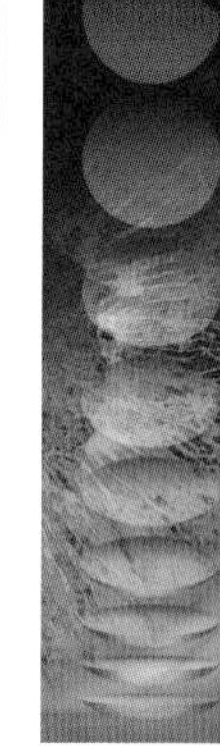

Table 14.1: Recommended examination procedures for the potential presbyopic contact lens patient

- Case history
  - medications
  - surgical history
  - primary visual requirements and goals
  - occupational requirements
- Anatomical/external measurements
  - pupil size (room illumination/dim illumination)
  - lid position and tonicity
  - vertical fissure size
  - blink rate and quality
- Tear quality and volume
- Corneal integrity
- Keratometry/corneal topography
- Manifest refraction/best corrected visual acuity

low-positioned lower lid (i.e. more than 1 mm below the inferior limbus) will not be good candidates for translating RGP lens designs.

Corneal topography

Keratometry provides an estimate of the paracentral curvature and assists in the initial back optic zone radius (BOZR) selection; however, videokeratography (VKG) provides several benefits including determining:

- The location of the corneal apex – a centrally located apex lends itself better to aspheric multifocal lens designs, whereas an inferior-positioned apex is preferable in translating designs (Hansen 1998).
- Irregular corneas (i.e. keratoconus, trauma, postsurgical) – these patients are typically poor candidates for bifocal, multifocal, or monovision contact lens correction.

Refraction

The best candidates for bifocal/multifocal contact lenses have more than 1.25 D of myopia or 1 D of hyperopia (Josephson & Caffery 1991). Emmetropes or near emmetropic patients should not be dismissed, however, if they are motivated to avoid spectacle lens wear. Fitting amblyopic patients is not advisable, due to the potential for further compromise in distance vision.

Table 14.1 summarizes the extra examination procedures required by a potential presbyopic contact lens wearer.

PATIENT CONSULTATION

The best time to discuss the presbyopic options is actually before a patient becomes presbyopic. They will therefore be expecting reading difficulties and know that contact lens options are available (Hansen et al. 2003). The pre-presbyopic high myope will experience an increase in accommodation demand when changing to contact lenses (see Chapter 6) and should be advised accordingly.

Discuss the patient's expectations and goals and the various options available to them, i.e. spectacles or bifocal/multifocal soft and RGP lenses.

Table 14.2: Good and challenging candidates for presbyopic contact lens correction

Good candidates	Challenging candidates
Patients with distance vision correction	Emmetropes
Realistic visual expectations	Unrealistic expectations
Spectacles interfere with lifestyle	Satisfied with spectacle wear
Current contact lens wearer	Satisfied with spectacle wear
Good tear volume and quality	Tear BUT ≤5 s; ≤9 mm Zone-Quick (phenol red thread)

Occupational and recreational information required includes:

- The patient's goal with these lenses.
- The distance(s) they want to see most clearly – for example:
  - If they use a computer 30% or more in a normal day, then a multifocal lens design would be indicated to help optimize the intermediate vision. Sit the patient in front of a computer to determine their working distance.
  - If critical distance vision is expected, a translating RGP lens should be considered.
  - Perfect vision is not possible at all distances and some compromise is necessary. Patients not prepared to accept this are not good candidates.
- A description of the work environment. Excessive wind or dust, poor air quality or prolonged computer use lead to dryness necessitating frequent application of rewetting drops.
- Do they play sport? A soft or aspheric RGP multifocal should be fitted 'tight' enough to minimize decentration or loss while allowing satisfactory vision.

Explain that these lenses differ from spectacles and the stability of correction is not like multifocal spectacles. Patients may experience transient blur in certain directions of gaze but if they feel that spectacles interfere with their lifestyle, they are often willing to accept compromise.

The goal of presbyopic contact lens wear should be to satisfy 'most of the visual needs, most of the time, or essentially to reduce, rather than eliminate the need for supplemental near correction' (Schwallie 2000, Bennett 2004b). Table 14.2 summarizes good candidates for presbyopic contact lens correction and those less likely to succeed.

Be realistic about the time needed to achieve the ideal fit. With multifocal designs, one or more lens exchanges may be necessary and the patient should be informed of this.

PRESBYOPIC CONTACT LENS OPTIONS

Single-vision contact lens wear and reading glasses

Single-vision lenses in combination with reading glasses provide the following benefits:

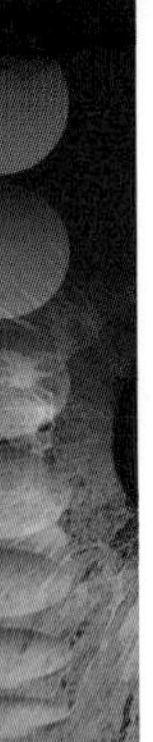

- Good bilateral vision at both distance and near.
- Simplicity of fit.
- Low cost.

The over-spectacles are typically single-vision or bifocal lenses but may be progressive addition lenses (PALs) to assist with intermediate correction. However, patients with varied near and distance tasks complain of the inconvenience of frequent application and/or removal of spectacles (Bennett & Jurkus 2005). Also, many patients desire contact lenses with the intent of cosmetically eliminating spectacles. Nevertheless, it is important for this option to be presented. Some patients prefer to begin with this option and change to a presbyopic contact lens system later.

Monovision

In monovision, one eye is optimally corrected for distance vision and the other eye for near, either with contact lenses or after refractive surgery (Jain et al. 2001). Both distances can therefore be seen, as long as both eyes are open.

The origin of monovision is unclear although the use of the monocle in the 1800s was an early method of monovision correction. Use of a contact lens in this fashion was first attributed to Westsmith in 1966 (Fonda 1996). The advantages of monovision include (Gasson & Morris 2003, Bennett & Jurkus 2005):

- Use of conventional lenses so that special lens designs are rarely necessary.
- Decreased professional time.
- Less expense.
- Thin, non-prism-ballasted lenses.
- Only one lens is changed for current contact lens wearers.
- The patient is usually able to determine whether they are likely to be successful soon after initiating lens wear.
- Avoidance of many of the symptoms/compromises associated with bifocal contact lenses including ghost images, reduced contrast sensitivity, and fluctuating vision related to pupil size changes.

However, the primary limitation of monovision is the lack of balanced binocular vision. A literature review by Johannsdottir and Stelmach (2001) indicates that monovision may:

- Stress the visual system.
- Impair stereoscopic depth perception.
- Affect performance on complex spatial–motor tasks such as driving.

PATIENT SELECTION

Good and poor candidates for monovision are shown in Table 14.3. Other considerations include:

- The patient's lifestyle and visual needs.
- Motivation.
- Visual needs equally distributed between far and near distances (Schwartz 1999).
- Personality – various studies have evaluated personality and psychological factors predictive of successful monovision wear (Josephson et al. 1990, MacAlister & Woods 1991, and others). Du Toit et al. (1998) found that patients with realistic expectations and the willingness to persevere were more successful.
- Age – younger presbyopes with lower adds are more successful than older presbyopes (Erickson & McGill 1992, Jain et al. 2001, and others).

Table 14.3: Good and poor candidates for monovision

Good monovision candidates
■ Early presbyopes who have a significant refractive error are generally better candidates than emmetropes or previously uncorrected hyperopes and low myopes ■ Individuals who read in positions other than the standard downward gaze such as office workers, executives, auto mechanics, pharmacists, etc., as well as individuals who have divided near and distance visual demands ■ Current contact lens patients ■ Highly motivated patients; individuals who have realistic expectations and willingness to persevere
Poor monovision candidates
■ Individuals with concentrated, specific visual needs ■ Individuals with dry eye symptoms or clinical signs ■ Individuals with high visual demands and expectations

Modified from Bennett & Jurkus (2004).

Schwartz (1996) recommends monovision screening criteria that evaluate:

- Age.
- Reading add.
- Distance prescription.
- Prior use of contact lenses.
- Motivation.
- Pupil size.
- Occupational and avocational needs.
- Apprehension of handling lenses.

Once the initial screening has been completed, the best predictor of success is a trial period with appropriately selected lens powers.

LENS SELECTION AND TYPE

The input from the two eyes does not produce identical input in the cerebral cortex; one eye generates a dominant response, which creates ocular dominance (Michaels 1974, Pearlman 1987). Jain et al. (1996) reviewed a series of papers on monovision and found that 95% corrected the dominant eye for distance.

Ocular dominance

It cannot be assumed which eye is dominant and if the wrong eye is thought dominant and monovision prescribed, the patient may ultimately fail with this mode of correction (Pointer 2001):

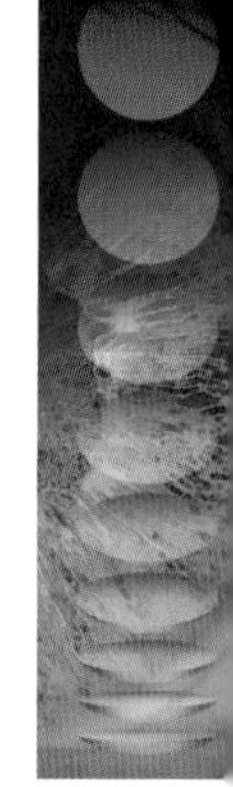

- Right handedness does not prove right eye dominance.
- The apparently better-sighted eye may not be the dominant eye.
- Keeping both eyes open, the patient should hold their arms straight and centre an object, such as a letter on the Snellen chart, through an opening formed by their hands (Quinn 1997). The eye that aligns the target is the dominant eye. If one eye instinctively closes, it is most likely the non-dominant eye.
- Alternatively, introducing a plus lens over the best corrected distance correction for near will determine which eye most readily accepts extra plus with minimal disruption of vision (Woods et al. 1998).

Once ocular dominance is established, the plus correction should be increased over the non-dominant eye with both eyes open. When transferring to distance vision, little or no visual disruption should be noticed. If the distance vision blurs, monovision is unlikely to be successful.

The full distance and near powers are prescribed as 'cutting the power' to minimize the dioptric span may alter the suppression pattern. Patients with little or no sighting preference may be better candidates than those with strong sighting preferences, as the latter have reduced interocular blur suppression and decreased binocular depth of focus, making it difficult to ignore the out of focus monovision image (Schor & Landsman 1987).

FITTING THE LENSES

The concept of monovision may be difficult for the patient to understand and it is often easier to actually demonstrate the system.

- Insert the lenses with appropriate powers into each eye.
- Ask the patient to read the distance chart with both eyes open. With a Snellen projection chart, having 6/7.5 (20/25) as the 'bottom line' gives the patient confidence that their distance vision is good.
- Have the patient read their usual reading material to provide a real-world view of their near vision.
- Ask about the visual comfort as well as measuring it. If the patient complains of feeling off-balance or that a headache is starting, monovision should be reconsidered. Try switching the eye powers before abandoning monovision altogether.
- Full adaptation to monovision can take as long as 8 weeks, although most subjects adapt in 2–3 weeks and about one-half in 1 week (Collins et al. 1994, Jain et al. 1996, Westin et al. 2000).

A benefit of monovision is the ability to modify the system. The initial powers can be altered to provide more comfortable vision. For example, if a patient reports that distance vision is not comfortable and becomes better when the near eye is covered, the plus power on the near eye can be reduced. After determining the lenses for the patient, always show the new monovision wearer what monocular and binocular acuity is like (see 'Modified monovision' or the modified bifocal approach, p. 328). Fitting and prescribing guidelines for monovision are provided in Table 14.4 (Bennett & Jurkus 2005).

Table 14.4: Fitting and prescribing considerations in monovision

1. Fit patients who do not require long periods of critical distance vision.
2. Perform binocular function testing to determine the effect of monovision on stereopsis.
3. Demonstrate the add power effect to the patient. Subjective reaction to providing the indicated plus power over one eye at times helps determine the preferred distance-corrected eye.
4. Select the appropriate eye for near. As it is more important for distance vision to be less impaired, the near eye typically represents the non-dominant eye and/or the eye in which vision is reduced relative to the other eye. If the patient is anisometropic, the more highly myopic eye should be considered for near, all other factors being equal.
5. Prescribe the full amount of correction. It is tempting to underplus the near eye and overplus the distance eye to lessen the anisometropia. However, for optimum near and distance vision, it is preferable to prescribe the full add amount.
6. Strongly encourage – if not require – monovision patients to purchase either a pair of 'driving' spectacles (i.e. minus power over near eye) or a second distance contact lens for use while driving. The patient should also be encouraged to first be a passenger in the car to experience the monovision effect prior to driving.
7. An informed consent that discusses the benefits and limitations of monovision in addition to discussing alternative forms of presbyopic correction (contact lens and spectacle) should be reviewed and signed by the patient.
8. Although most patients adapt to monovision within 2–3 weeks, they nevertheless should be told it could take up to several weeks for complete adaptation. If they experience difficulty in adapting, consider changing lenses (i.e. 'distance' lens on previous 'near' eye and vice versa or abandoning monovision altogether).

Modified from Bennett & Jurkus (2005).

PROBLEMS WITH MONOVISION

Monovision may present some visual challenges including a small reduction in high-contrast visual acuity such as reading or viewing the vision chart, and loss of contrast sensitivity function (CSF) that is proportional to the amount of add (Bennett & Jurkus 2005).

Monocular and binocular clues are used to judge depth and distance. Monocular clues include:

- Object interposition hiding parts of an object.
- Judging the customary object size.
- Colour and clarity of objects.
- Lines converging to a vanishing point.
- Shadows.

These remain unchanged but monovision can reduce stereo-acuity. With age, the mean angle of stereopsis reduces from 20 to 58 seconds of arc and monovision reduces this further from

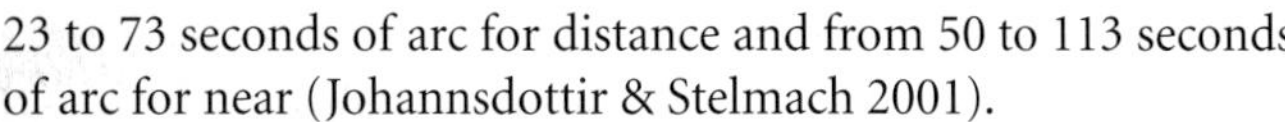

23 to 73 seconds of arc for distance and from 50 to 113 seconds of arc for near (Johannsdottir & Stelmach 2001).

There is generally no significant effect on peripheral field but low-contrast binocular distance acuity may be reduced, which may affect distance judgement when driving at night (Loshin et al. 1982, Rajagopalan et al. 2003).

Woods et al. (1998) found no difference in driving performance when the adapted monovision lens wearer was compared to a binocular spectacle wearer. However, they noted that night driving conditions may offer different challenges. It is wise, therefore, to advise caution to the new monovision wearer, regarding distance perception, until they feel confident in viewing distances as a passenger.

Some monocular suppression of blur occurs in monovision, which is useful; however, the blurred eye will still contribute to binocular summation (Westendorf et al. 1982). Collins et al. (1993) found that suppression increased as the add increased, and observed that residual astigmatism caused a significantly greater reduction of binocular visual acuity in monovision than in normal binocular conditions. This effect appeared to be related to meridional interocular suppression.

PATIENT EDUCATION

It is possible that a practitioner could be held liable if monovision lenses are found to be a contributory factor in injury (see also Chapter 32). Nakagawara and Veronneau (2000) reported on an aviation accident with a pilot wearing monovision lenses. All monovision patients should be made aware of potential problems and presented with alternative forms of correction.

SUCCESS WITH MONOVISION

Despite the compromises of this modality, monovision gives high patient satisfaction and success rates of up to 76% (Jain et al. 1996). Visual performance of patients wearing less than +2.50 D add is comparable to that of patients with balanced binocular corrections with suprathreshold stimuli in photopic conditions (Jain et al. 2001) although success rates vary when compared to bifocal and multifocal contact lenses (Back et al. 1984, du Toit et al. 2000, and others).

BIFOCAL/MULTIFOCAL CONTACT LENS DESIGNS

Some 'clinical pearls' to assist in achieving success with presbyopic patients are summarized in Table 14.5.

Numerous advancements have been made in recent years to improve the success of both RGP and soft bifocals. The large number of designs can be divided into *simultaneous* or *alternating* vision types, although the two are becoming more alike.

Definition: Simultaneous or bivision – having multiple powers positioned within the pupil at the same time (available in both RGP and soft lens designs).

Definition: Translating or alternating designs, which shift upward or translate, resulting in only one corrective power being in front of the pupil at any one time (almost exclusively RGP lens designs).

Table 14.5: Contact lens multifocal and bifocal fitting pearls

1. When fitting these designs it is important to begin by fitting patients who have great potential for success. This includes highly motivated individuals, existing single-vision contact lens wearers who are entering presbyopia, and monovision failures.
2. If possible, provide lenses that are to the correct prescription to optimize the initial experience. This is easier to accomplish with soft lens bifocals and aspheric RGPs which can often be empirically ordered. Alternating/translating RGP patients typically require fitting with diagnostic lenses.
3. When over-refracting, use loose trial lenses or ± 0.25–0.50 D flip lenses as opposed to the phoropter to provide a more natural environment.
4. Likewise, check vision binocularly to simulate a real-world environment.
5. When the patient is first dispensed their lenses, let them settle for 15–20 minutes prior to evaluating the lens-to-cornea fitting relationship.
6. Have the patient walk around the office and simulate tasks that they perform on a daily basis (i.e. look at a magazine or newspaper, view a computer screen, look outside, etc.) and determine their level of satisfaction with their vision for the various tasks and possible areas of improvement.
7. Be willing to try different multifocal/bifocal options including two different designs on the same patient.
8. Do not hesitate to prescribe unequal adds or a 'modified bifocal' approach in which one eye is slightly overplused at distance to optimize near vision.

Simultaneous vision ('bivision')

Light rays from both distance and near targets are imaged on the retina at the same time. The patient will selectively suppress the most blurred images that are not desired for a given visual task.

This concept functions on the basis of blur interpretation and/or blur tolerance of superimposed multiple images on the retina, which are formed by the various powers of the lens (Benjamin & Borish 1991). For true simultaneous vision, the two primary segments must remain within the pupillary boundary in all positions of gaze and, in order to give equally bright images, should cover nearly equal areas of the pupil. The lenses must therefore centre well.

Three designs using the simultaneous vision concept are aspheric, concentric/annular (or target) and diffractive.

- *Aspheric lenses* have a gradual change of curvature along one of their surfaces based on the geometry of conic sections. This rate of flattening (or eccentricity) is much greater than with aspheric single-vision lenses and creates a plus add power effect.
  - In centre-distance aspheric lenses, the eccentricity is located on the posterior surface and causes an increase in plus power from the centre to periphery.

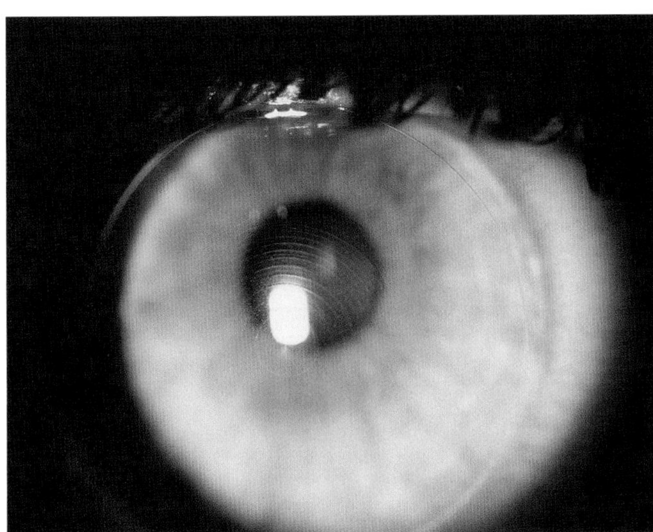

Figure 14.8 A rigid diffractive lens design

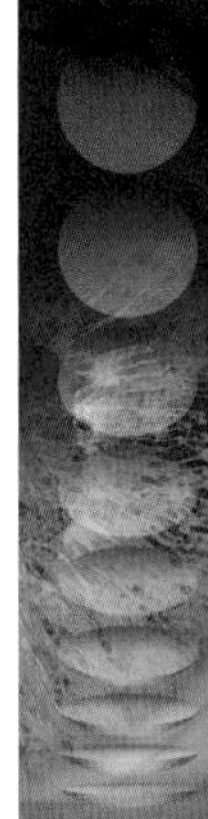

– Centre-near aspherics have their maximum plus power at the centre, which then gradually decreases away from the geometrical centre.

- *Concentric/annular* (or target) lenses are structured with a small annular zone, which is typically two-thirds to three-quarters the size of the pupil in normal room illumination. In most designs, this provides the distance vision correction; the near correction is ground on the annulus that surrounds the distance zone.

Both aspheric and concentric near zone lenses do gain some additional near power via slight shifting or translating of the lens upward with downward gaze for reading.

- *Diffractive* (or holographic) bifocal lenses have true equality of near and distance powers. They function through a central diffractive zone plate that focuses images at distance by refraction of light, and near through diffraction principles created by the zone eschelettes* (Churms et al. 1987) (Fig. 14.8). This design has the advantage of being pupil independent as equal amounts of light pass though both the distance and near-power elements of the lens for all normal pupil diameters, making the resolution of the in-focus image better than with pupil-sharing designs.
- In *alternating vision*, lenses move vertically or translate, such that only one power zone is in front of the pupil (or visual axis) at any one time (the superior zone for distance and the inferior zone for near).

* Eschelettes are grooves on the back surface of the lens which constitute the diffractive central zone. The add power is determined by the diameter and number of eschelettes and the depth determines the percentage of light that is transmitted (de Carle 1997). The original diffracting lens was the (now discontinued) Pilkington Diffrax™ RGP lens (Bennett et al. 1990, Eggink et al. 1990) and currently only the Echelon (Ocular Sciences) soft lens is available.

Typically, these designs incorporate prism ballast, sometimes in combination with inferior truncation, to stabilize the lens and allow a smooth translation when lowering the gaze to read. They are most commonly rigid, as translation is attained much more easily with rigid lenses than with hydrogels.

Several types have been developed over the years, including:

- Decentred concentric.
- One-piece segmented.
- Fused crescent and segmented.

General fitting considerations

There are several factors important to fitting bifocal/multifocal lens designs regardless of whether soft or rigid lenses are fitted and it is recommended to initially fit less complex designs (i.e. soft multifocals, aspheric RGP multifocals) prior to fitting alternating designs.

Lens designs

Two different lens designs and adds can be prescribed for the same patient, especially with soft bifocal lens wearers or patients experiencing blur at near but who desire little compromise of their distance vision.

A 'modified bifocal' approach in which one eye is slightly overplused is also a viable option for the moderate or advanced presbyope who desires better vision for near tasks.

INITIAL EXPERIENCE

Try to provide the patient with lenses in the correct prescription to make their initial experience more positive and increase the likelihood of success. This can be done with soft lens designs or with empirical ordering of some RGP designs (notably aspheric multifocal).

Diagnostic fitting of RGP designs – notably alternating lenses – is recommended although after some experience is gained, empirically fitting aspheric multifocals often results in success (Ames 2001). It can help to insert the first lenses after instilling a local anaesthetic and to allow at least 20 minutes before evaluating the fit.

PRESCRIPTION

In order to provide a more natural environment, over-refract binocularly, using ± 0.25–0.50 D flip lenses or lenses in a trial frame as opposed to a phoropter.

VISUAL COMFORT

After inserting the correct lenses, ask the patient to determine their level of satisfaction and possible areas of improvement, particularly for those tasks that they perform most frequently.

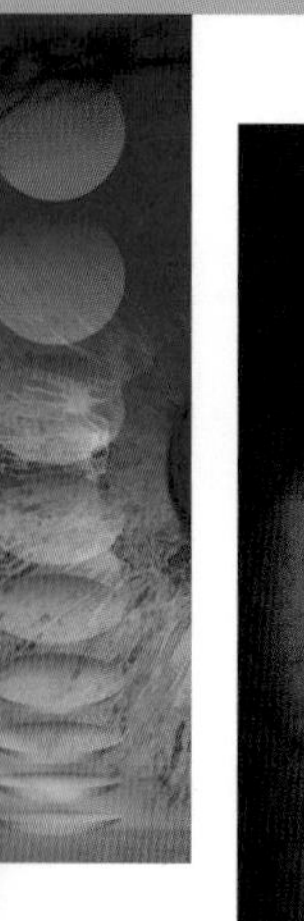

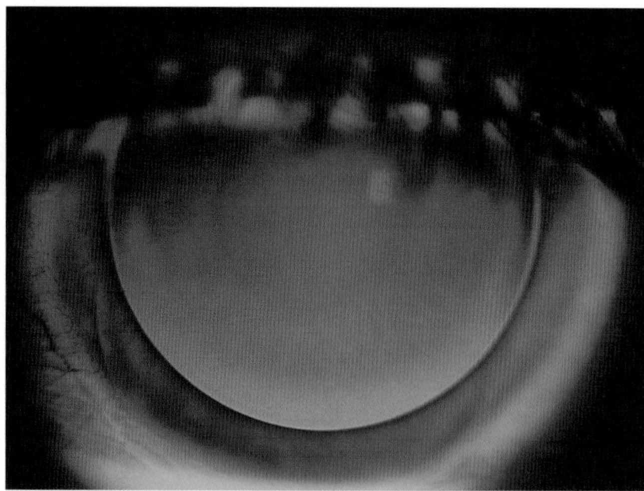

Figure 14.9 A high eccentricity value aspheric multifocal lens

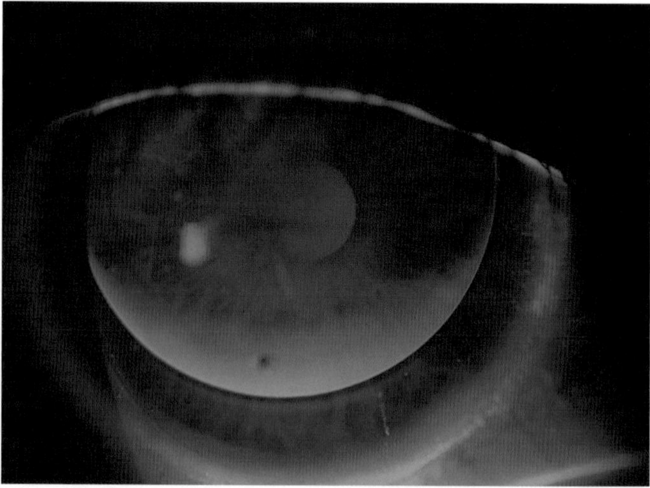

Figure 14.10 A low eccentricity value aspheric multifocal lens

RIGID BIFOCAL AND MULTIFOCAL LENS DESIGNS

Due to advances in manufacturing technology, various new designs of rigid bifocals have become available including:

- Aspheric multifocal designs.
- Monocentric optics with alternating designs.
- Alternating designs with an intermediate aspheric correction.

As a result, a trend toward RGP multifocal and bifocal lenses and away from monovision was demonstrated in the results of a survey from the American Academy of Optometry (Bergenske 2001) and online (Shovlin & Eisenberg 2003).

Simultaneous vision

Although some RGP concentric designs are in use today, as a result of numerous design and manufacturing improvements the most common forms of simultaneous vision correction are aspheric multifocals (see above). However, these designs are not strictly simultaneous vision. To be successful, they must exhibit some upward shift or translation on downward gaze.

Aspheric lens designs

There are numerous presbyopic designs having an entirely (i.e. not only peripheral) aspheric back surface geometry. The peripheral flattening of the back surface provides a continuously variable near addition. To provide the maximum near addition, a high degree of peripheral curvature flattening or asphericity must be used. This departure from spherical shape is known as eccentricity or '*e*' factor (see also Chapter 9). The first designs that were introduced were fitted as much as 0.6 mm (3 D) steeper than '*K*' and had a very high *e* value. Some of these designs are still in common use. Because of the back surface geometry, only slight apical clearance is noticed with fluorescein application (Fig. 14.9).

More recent designs have a lower eccentricity and are commonly fitted approximately 0.20–0.30 mm (1–1.5 D) steeper than *K*. They show alignment or slight central clearance because of the aspheric geometry and rate of flattening (Fig. 14.10).

The best candidates for aspheric lenses are individuals who are not good candidates for translating designs. With aspheric RGPs, it is difficult to generate the necessary add power within the pupillary zone without inducing disturbing aberration effects on distance vision. Early or emerging presbyopes are the best candidates as it is difficult to incorporate more than +2.00 D effective add power. Several lens designs now incorporate higher add powers, often via a smaller effective distance optical zone and/or a modification of the front surface, resulting in increased plus power. Other good candidates include any one of the following anatomical characteristics:

- Lower lid margin well above the limbus (below the limbus will prevent good centration).
- Small-to-average pupil size – a larger than normal pupil size is a contraindication due to the aberrations induced, particularly at night.
- Loose lids that will not support any necessary prism ballast.
- Steep corneal curvatures.

The benefits of aspheric designs include:

- Absence of prism and truncation.
- Thickness profile similar or better than conventional single-vision lenses.
- Lenses exhibiting little movement that rarely decentre or dislodge even when playing sport.
- Good intermediate vision. This design has been recommended for any motivated presbyopic contact lens candidate who spends at least 35% of their time at a computer (Hansen 1999) or who requires 'arm's length' vision, including accountants, electricians, and those involved in mechanics or plumbing.

This design is not recommended for patients who have:

- Very critical distance vision demands.
- Large pupils.
- Poor motivation.

As these are thin lenses, the material chosen should be similar to a single-vision lens. The author recommends a low-Dk (i.e. 25–50 ISO/Fatt units) lens material for myopic patients and a higher Dk for hyperopic patients. The lenses should centre well and display minimal movement with blinking.

FITTING PROBLEMS

- Excessive decentration and/or excessive movement will result in variable and generally unsatisfactory vision at all distances.
- Lenses tend to decentre laterally in against-the-rule eyes.

Both these problems can be eliminated by steepening the BOZR by at least 0.05–0.10 mm (0.25–0.50 D) and/or increasing the TD.

- Insufficient add power
  - if the lens design is available in multiple add powers (see below), incorporate a higher add, typically on the non-dominant eye.
  - using a 'modified bifocal' (see p. 328) approach with the non-dominant eye slightly overplused (i.e. 0.25–0.50 D) still provides satisfactory vision at all distances.

If these lens changes do not eliminate the problem, another lens design would be indicated.

ASPHERIC LENSES WITH MULTIPLE POWERS

Numerous aspheric lens designs have been reviewed in the literature (Hansen 2002, Loveridge 2003, Norman 2004, and others). Two representative designs, available in multiple adds, are discussed here.

VFL-3 (Conforma contact lenses)

This is a high-eccentricity back-surface surface aspheric design. It is fitted approximately 0.4–0.6 mm (2–3 D) steeper than *K*. The TD typically ranges from 9.0 to 9.4 mm. It is also available in a 'SuperAdd' design which incorporates the traditional VFL posterior surface with an annular progressive front zone (Davis 2003). The aim is to create a fitting relationship that exhibits mild central clearance accompanied by alignment in the intermediate and peripheral zones.

Essentials multifocal (Blanchard)

This is a low-eccentricity back-surface aspheric lens design. It utilizes the S-curve technology which creates a power gradient over the entire optical area and minimizes spherical aberration effects (Gasson & Morris 2003). It is available in Series I (low add), Series II (medium add) and Series III (high add) lens designs. As the add power increases, the near section of the lens encroaches further into the central area of the lens to improve near acuity. This lens is fitted approximately 0.2 mm (1 D) steeper than *K*; however, as a result of the back surface geometry, an alignment lens-to-cornea fitting relationship should be achieved.

Interpalpebral and lid attachment fitting relationships are both acceptable with this design. Nevertheless, particularly for advanced presbyopes and those exhibiting a smaller than average pupil size, it is often difficult to achieve a sufficiently effective add for near work. Therefore, Blanchard have introduced their 'CSA' design which allows more add power in a paracentral ring on the front surface of all three series of lenses (Fig. 14.11).

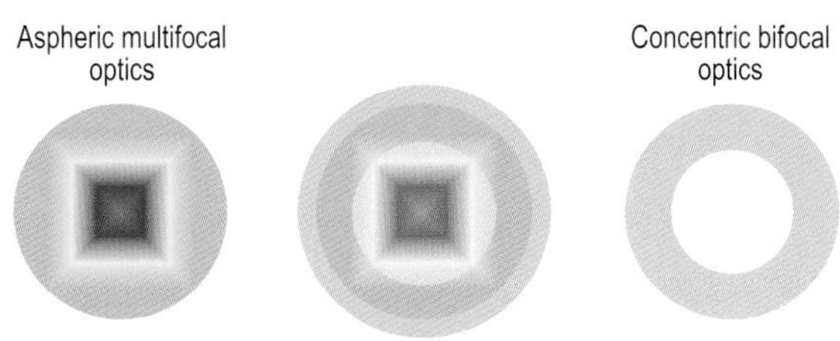

Figure 14.11 The Essentials CSA Enhancement Multifocal design (Blanchard)

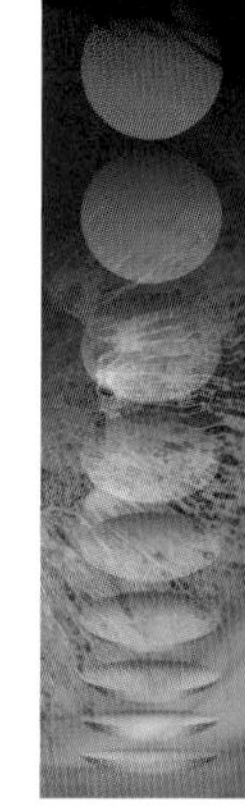

Concentric (annular)

Concentric designs that are used for simultaneous vision purposes are not in common use today as their translating counterparts are more popular. Most designs are centre-distance with a near surround. The pupil diameter is critical for these lenses and should be measured in dim illumination. The centre-distance annular zone is made 0.75–1.5 mm smaller than the pupil diameter (Caffery & Josephson 1991, de Carle 1997) (Table 14.6).

A diagnostic fitting set is recommended for optimum fitting and the ideal lens should show:

- Good centration or slight superior decentration.
- Limited movement – approximately 1 mm with the blink.
- The central zone covering approximately 50% of the pupil when looking straight ahead. Using the 'zone-check technique' (Caffery & Josephson 1991), a +4.00 D hand-held trial lens is held in front of the patient's eye and the red reflex viewed with an ophthalmoscope held at approximately 50 cm. The central zone can be clearly observed and its position and amount of pupil coverage noted. The lens should be able to move up to 1 mm and still have the distance zone in front of the pupil (Fig. 14.12).
- Slight shift or translation when the patient views inferiorly.

Centre-near lenses typically favour near vision due to the decrease in pupil size in bright illumination but, conversely, can result in blur at distance during daylight conditions. They are less commonly used.

Alternating vision

There are two types of alternating (translating) bifocal rigid design:

- Segmented.
- Concentric/annular (or target) lens designs.

SEGMENTED

History

Segmented bifocal lenses are more complex in design but provide the best vision. From 1960 to 1980, PMMA bifocal

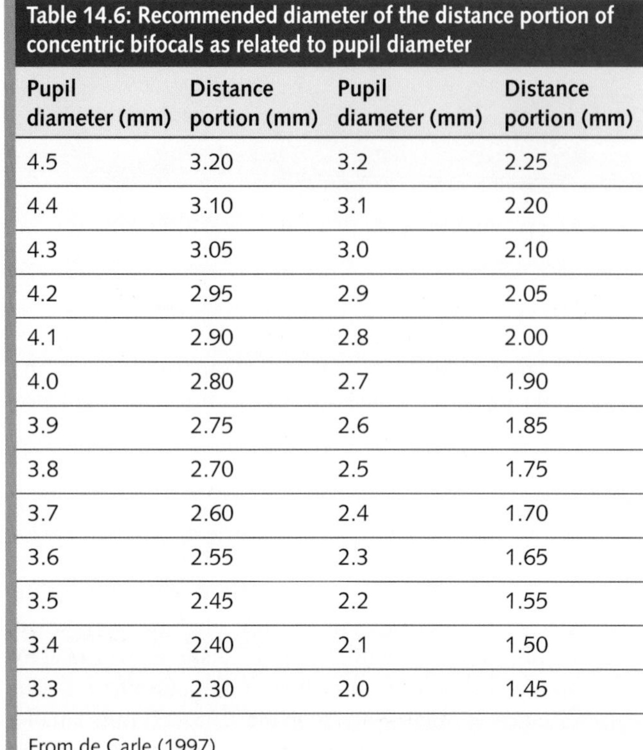

Table 14.6: Recommended diameter of the distance portion of concentric bifocals as related to pupil diameter

Pupil diameter (mm)	Distance portion (mm)	Pupil diameter (mm)	Distance portion (mm)
4.5	3.20	3.2	2.25
4.4	3.10	3.1	2.20
4.3	3.05	3.0	2.10
4.2	2.95	2.9	2.05
4.1	2.90	2.8	2.00
4.0	2.80	2.7	1.90
3.9	2.75	2.6	1.85
3.8	2.70	2.5	1.75
3.7	2.60	2.4	1.70
3.6	2.55	2.3	1.65
3.5	2.45	2.2	1.55
3.4	2.40	2.1	1.50
3.3	2.30	2.0	1.45

From de Carle (1997).

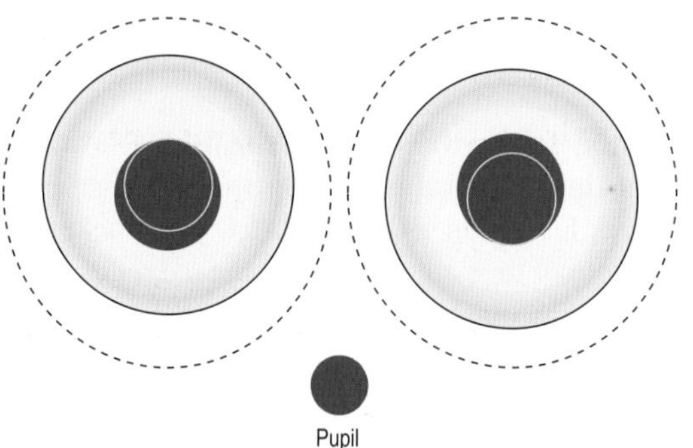

Figure 14.12 A well-fitting concentric bifocal can move up to 1.0 mm and still have all of the distance portion in front of the pupil (shaded)

lenses were manufactured in a wide range of shapes similar to spectacle bifocals, including executive, D-shaped and crescent. Typically, the segment was fused into the distance carrier, thus eliminating the optical problem of 'image jump'. However, the inability to fuse the softer RGP materials often resulted in patient symptoms of image displacement when changing focus. Segmented one-piece RGP bifocals were then introduced, utilizing monocentric optics by George Tsuetaki of Fused Kontacts (see below), having near and distance optical centres coincident at a tangent at the segment line.

Representative designs

There are a large number of segmented bifocals available today: two representative designs are discussed here.

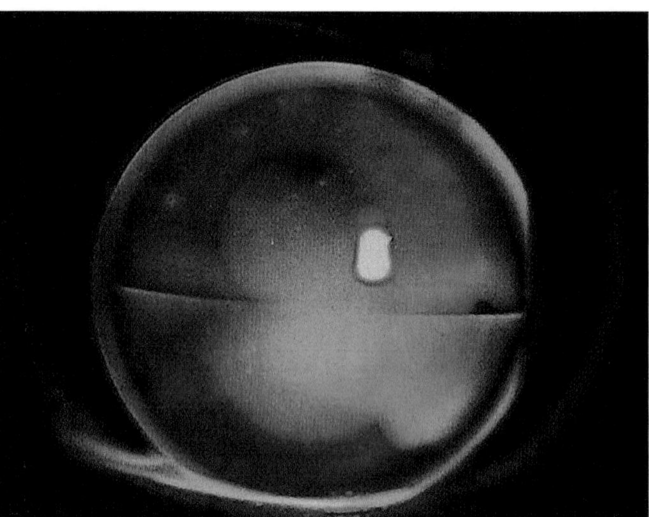

Figure 14.13 The Tangent Streak bifocal lens (Fused Kontacts)

Tangent Streak (Firestone Optics)

This custom-designed lens is heavily prism ballasted (between 1.75 and 3.00 Δ) and truncated. It can be up to 0.8 mm thick in moderate plus powers and is therefore made in high-Dk materials. The segment shape is similar to an 'executive' bifocal and can be ordered at any height, although it is recommended that it is made 1.3 mm less than the distance from the centre of the pupil to the lower lid (Davis 2003) (Fig. 14.13).

The following diagnostic lens specifications are recommended (20 lenses) by the manufacturer:

BOZR	7.50–8.40 mm (41.00–45.50 D)
Segment height	4.2 mm
Power	±2.00 D
Add	+2.00 D
TD	9.4 × 9.0 mm
Prism	2 Δ

These lenses – like all alternating designs – are fitted 0.05–0.1 mm (0.25–0.5 D) flatter than *K*, such that the lens rests on or near the lower lid during distance gaze. The segment line should be positioned at or slightly below the lower pupil margin with the superior edge of the lens overlapping the pupil in dim illumination. The lens must translate 2 mm or more on down-gaze to position enough of the segment in front of the pupil for near tasks. With the patient fixating straight ahead, the lens should move 1–2 mm upwards on blink and rapidly drop back to the lower position.

Solutions Bifocal (X-Cel)

This lens aims to be easy to fit. It is a crescent segment design that is fitted similarly to the Tangent Streak in terms of BOZR and segment position (Fig. 14.14) and has five segment heights, each separated by 0.5 mm, and a choice of three prisms (low, medium and high).

The standard design is not truncated and the diagnostic set has medium prism, intermediate segment height, 9.6 mm TD and similar distance and near powers to the Tangent Streak diagnostic set.

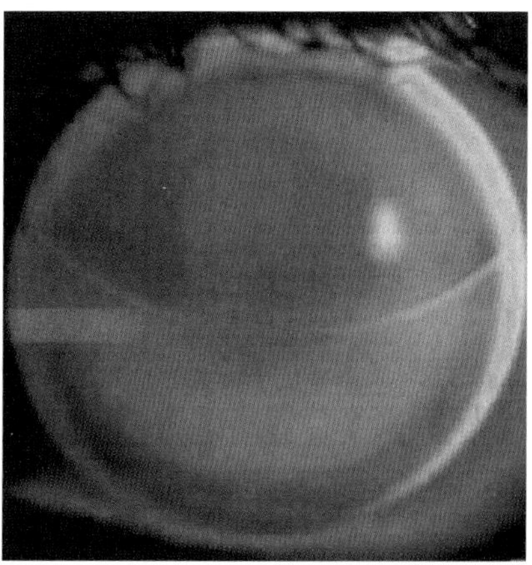

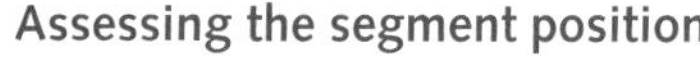

Figure 14.14 The Solutions Bifocal (X-Cel)

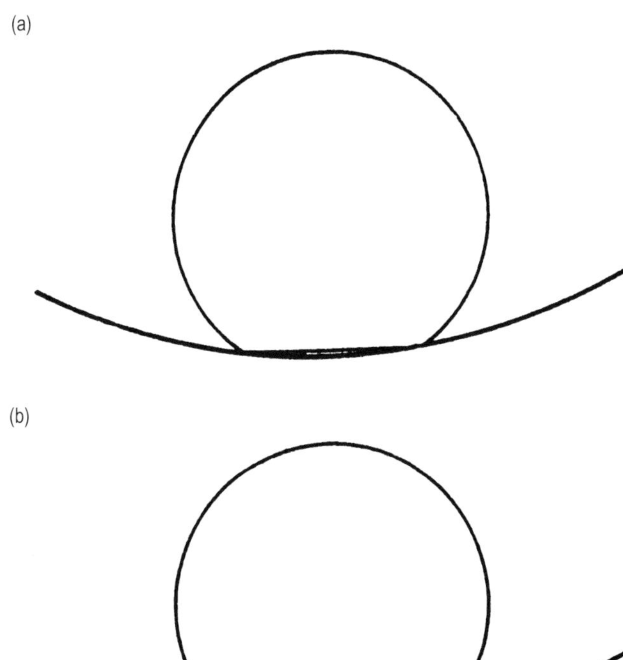

Figure 14.15 The lower edge of a truncated prism-ballasted lens should not be straight as shown in (a) but curved to match the line of the lower lid as shown in (b)

Assessing the segment position

- Use diagnostic lenses to accurately assess the segment position and translation. These lenses position inferiorly, so it is important to ensure that the superior edge overlaps the pupil in dim illumination (Yager 2002).
- Evaluate the lower lid-to-limbus relationship using a biomicroscope for accuracy. Patients whose lower lids are 1 mm or more below the lower limbus are not good candidates for translating designs, as the lens does not translate sufficiently to allow the near zone to cover the pupil. If the lower lid is less than 1 mm below the lower limbus, a larger than average TD and segment height are indicated to provide sufficient pupil coverage during distance gaze and satisfactory near vision with downward gaze.
- Assess the position of the segment line either visually or photographically (de Carle 1997) with the patient looking straight ahead. Ideally, the segment line should be positioned at or slightly below the lower pupil margin such that the movement of the lens with the blink will not move the segment more than 1 mm into the pupillary zone. Patients should be advised that even the simple act of smiling can occasionally interfere with their distance vision, an important consideration when driving.
- Ask the patient to look down and lift their upper lid in order to evaluate the lens translation. Assess the upward shift of the lens through the biomicroscope. The segment line should sit in front of the pupil or, at least, bisect the pupil.

Alternative methods of assessing segment position

- View the pupil in dim light with a direct ophthalmoscope held at arm's length from the patient (Quinn 2001). With the patient looking straight ahead, increase the plus power in the ophthalmoscope until the edge of the pupil is focused in the red reflex and then ask the patient to blink. The segment should rise into the pupil zone immediately and then drop quickly. If it remains in the pupil zone for a prolonged period, the patient is likely to complain of distance blur.
- Ask the patient to look at a reading card held straight in front of them then gradually lower the reading material until it becomes clear. If it does not become clear in their normal reading position and distance, a higher segment height will be necessary (Edwards 1999).

Both lids affect lens translation during down gaze.

- The upper lid pulls the lens upward during down gaze (Borish & Perrigin 1985, Borish 1986).
- The lower lid pushes the lens up and this movement is enhanced by incorporating prism and truncation into the lens. Any truncation should not be straight but should contour the lower lid (de Carle 1997) (Fig. 14.15).

If the lower lid is upswept or the lens rotates excessively in one direction, the segment can be offset relative to the prism base to correct for it. The lens position is assessed using a graticule in the biomicroscope (see Chapter 12). The RALS acronym (right add, left subtract) can be used to order the lens so that the truncation or segment aligns with the lower lid (Davis 2003). When the lens rotates to the practitioner's right, the amount is added; it is subtracted if it rotates to the left. For example, if the right lens rotates nasally by 15°, the lens is ordered with the prism at 105°.

Problem solving

Problems with translating lens designs can be one of the following (Gasson & Morris 2003) (Table 14.7).

- Insufficient or absence of translation (Fig. 14.16) may be resolved by increasing the amount of edge clearance to allow the lens edge to increase the contact with the lower lid. This can be accomplished by selecting a flatter BOZR or, alternatively, flattening the peripheral curve radii (Fig. 14.17).

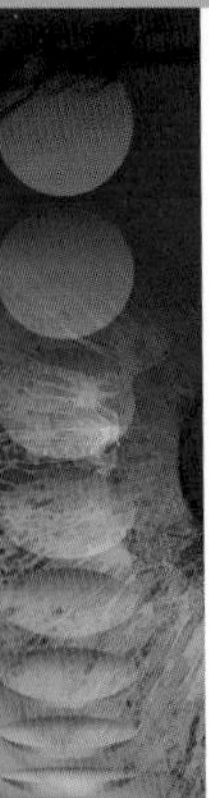

Table 14.7: Troubleshooting rigid gas-permeable (RGP) translating bifocal lens designs

Problem	Management options
Excessive rotation (see Fig. 14.18)	1. Flatten BOZR 0.10 mm (0.50 D) if with-the-rule cylinder; steepen 0.10 mm (0.50 D) if against-the-rule cylinder 2. Offset prism if upswept lower lid; order prism at 105° OD and 75° OS
Superior decentration (see Figs 14.16, 14.17)	1. Increase prism by 0.50 Δ 2. Flatten BOZR by 0.10 mm (0.50 D) 3. Thin the apex of the lens edge
Poor translation (see Fig. 14.19)	1. Flatten BOZR 0.10 mm (0.50 D) or flatten peripheral curve 2. Thin upper edge (see text) 3. Increase prism or truncation 4. Change to another lens design due to flaccid lower lid
Poor distance vision	1. Superior decentration: increase prism by 0.50 Δ 2. Inadequate pupil coverage: increase TD ≥0.5 mm 3. If segment height into pupil: reduce segment height
Poor near vision	1. Poor lens translation: manage as indicated above 2. Excessive rotation: manage as indicated above 3. Too low segment height: increase segment height 4. Patient is dropping head, not eyes, to read: educate patient appropriately
Poor intermediate vision	1. Over-spectacles for intermediate distance 2. Select an RGP translating lens design with an intermediate correction

BOZR, back optic zone radius; TD, total diameter.

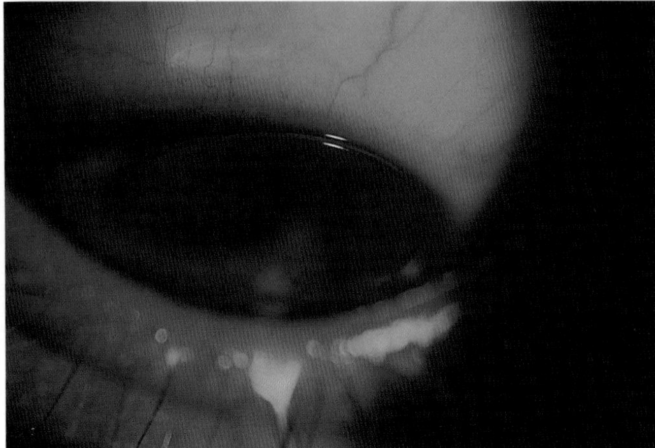

Figure 14.16 A segmented translating lens exhibiting poor translation

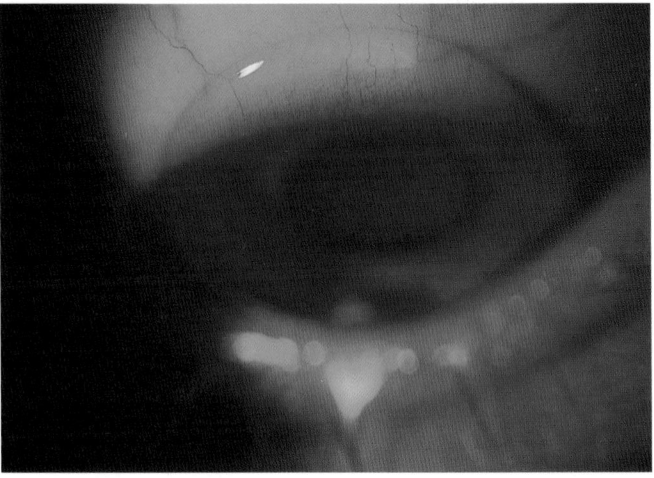

Figure 14.17 Same patient as in Figure 14.16 with a flatter lens design which exhibits good lens translation with downward gaze

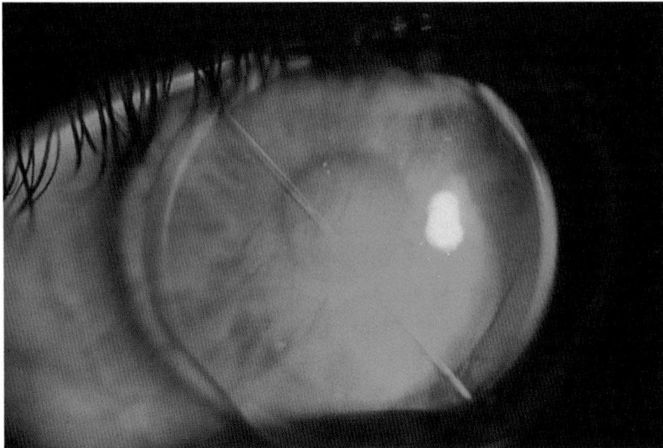

Figure 14.18 Excessive rotation of a segmented translating lens design fitted steeper than *K*

The former change is typically the easiest to perform in-office (see Chapter 28). If this is no better and the lens is still not translating, it is most likely because of a flaccid lower lid. Increasing the amount of prism ballast may help.

- Excessive rotation with the blink. This can occur with a steep BOZR (Fig. 14.18). While this can assist in promoting centration, it also has a greater upper lid torquing effect. Flattening the BOZR by 0.10 mm (0.50 D) should allow the lens to fall more quickly to the lower lid and be less prone to the rotational effects of the upper lid (Bennett & Luk 2001).
- Excessive movement on blinking (Fig. 14.19). If the lens is lifted too high on blinking, increasing the prism should result in less upward displacement (Bennett & Luk 2001, Yager 2002). Likewise, either flattening the BOZR or thinning the upper edge may minimize or eliminate this problem. The latter can be accomplished by placing tape around the circumference of the lens edge, leaving the apex exposed and then performing a standard edge polish procedure limited to that area (see Chapter 28).
- Poor vision at distance can have several of the above causes or result from excessive superior decentration. If the upper

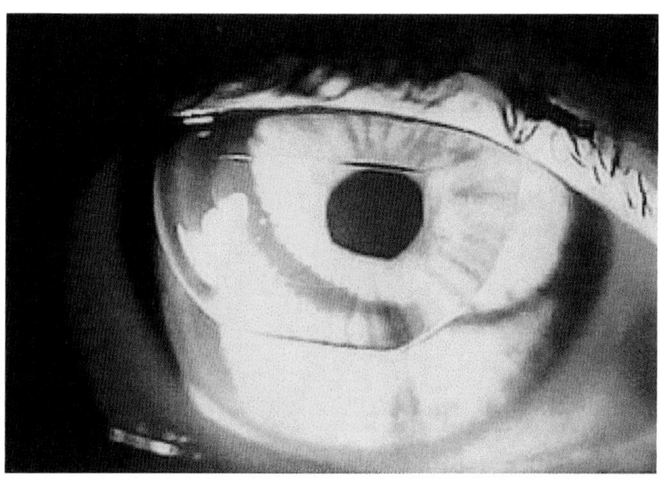

Figure 14.19 A segmented translating lens design which is picked up too superiorly with the blink

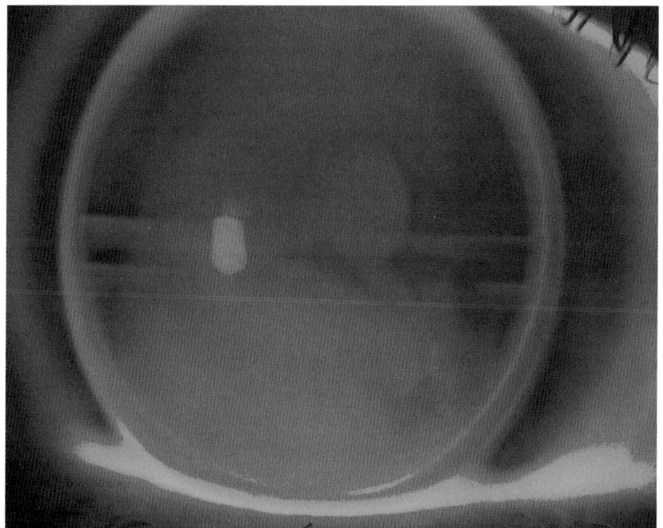

Figure 14.20 The Llevations trifocal design (Tru-Form)

lens edge is not providing sufficient pupil coverage, a larger TD is indicated. Also, if the segment line is well within the pupil, a lower height would be indicated.

- Poor vision at near could be caused by either poor lens translation or excessive rotation and managed as described previously. The segment height may also need to be increased if it is too low. Always check that the patient is dropping their eyes, not their head, when reading, otherwise, they are likely to be looking at near through the distance zone.
- To overcome the problem of poor intermediate vision, some segmented bifocal lens designs are also available as a trifocal – for example, Tangent Streak Trifocal (Firestone Optics) and Llevations (Tru-Form Optics) (Fig. 14.20).

Presbylite (Lens Dynamics)

This non-truncated lens design has spherical distance and near zones, a unique triangle-shaped aspheric intermediate zone and 1.5 Δ prism (Fig. 14.21) (www.lensdynamics.com). The large distance zone allows up to 30° of nasal rotation with minimal

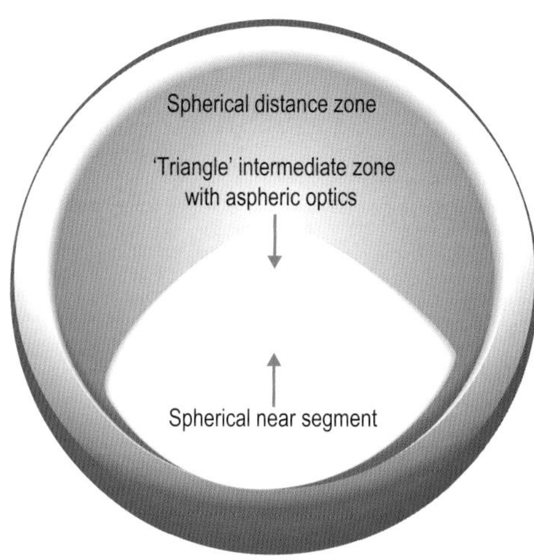

Figure 14.21 Presbylite (Courtesy of Lens Dynamics)

effect on vision. The standard TD is 9.3 mm, although 9.0 mm and 9.6 mm are available. The lens is fitted 0.05–0.1 mm (0.25–0.5 D) flatter than *K*.

X-Cel ESSential-Solution (X-Cel and Blanchard)

The posterior geometry of this lens generates about 1.00 D of add power using the S-form technology (www.blanchardlab.com). The front surface is similar to the X-Cel Solutions Bifocal (see above) with a crescent-shaped segment configuration incorporating a prismatic correction. Because of its aspheric posterior surface, the lens is fitted about 0.10 mm (0.5 D) steeper than the Solutions bifocal.

Patient selection

Translating bifocal lenses include concentric/annular lenses (see below).

- Good candidates
  - early and advanced presbyopes.
  - lower lid above, tangent to, or no more than 1 mm below the limbus.
  - myopic and low hyperopic powers.
  - normal-to-large palpebral fissure sizes.
  - normal-to-tight lid tension.
- Poor candidates
  - high hyperopes because of the increased thickness of the lenses.
  - individuals with loose lower lids as the lenses will not translate on down gaze.

Advantages:
- the ability to achieve precise correction and good vision.
- any amount of presbyopic adds can be corrected successfully.

Disadvantages:
- lenses are thicker.
- sufficient translation is essential with down gaze.

CONCENTRIC/ANNULAR (OR TARGET) LENSES

'Target' bifocals are front surface concentric designs. They are constructed with a larger centre-distance zone than

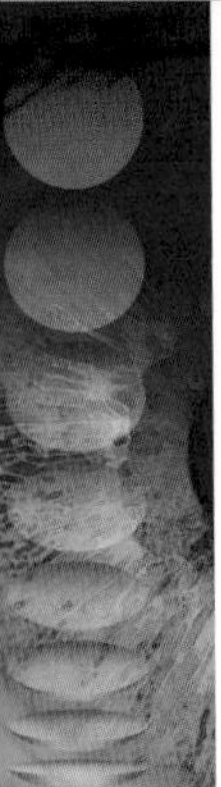

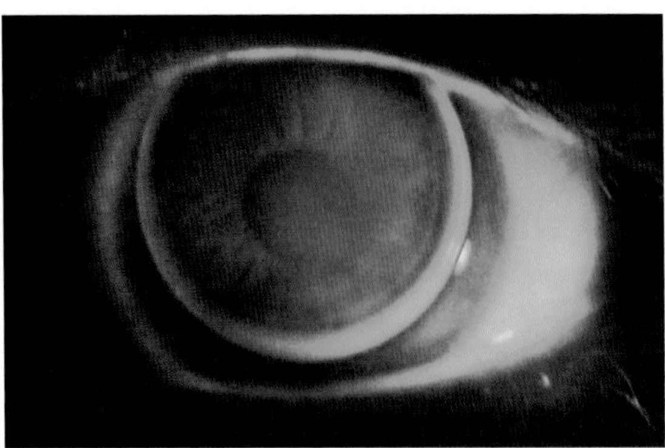

Figure 14.22 The Mandell Seamless lens design (Con-Cise)

simultaneous vision designs, and translate with near gaze to shift the concentric near zone in front of the pupil. Lenses typically have a 3–5 mm central distance zone, which is decentred 1–2 mm upwards, and incorporate 1–1.5 Δ prism and truncation to facilitate translation.

As with segmented designs, the use a diagnostic fitting set is recommended. The lenses are fitted 0.05–0.10 mm (0.25–0.5 D) flatter than *K*.

Designs

Mandell Seamless Bifocal (Con-Cise)

This bifocal lens has an aspheric transition zone between the distance and near annular zones. It is a front surface concentric design with central distance zone diameters ranging from 3.0 to 3.8 mm and an average TD of 9.8 mm (Mandell 2002, Davis 2003, Bennett 2004c). The lens is actually only slightly thicker than single-vision lens designs and should be fitted to centre well (Fig. 14.22).

Menifocal Z (Menicon)

This concentric design has a centre-distance area, a transition zone and a peripheral reading zone (www.menicon.com) and provides potentially good vision at all distances. It is made in a hyper Dk material and fitted like a single-vision lens with an alignment fluorescein pattern (Fig. 14.23).

Lens fitting

Translating RGP lenses yield the highest success rate of any contact lens bifocals available today. However, their fitting requires:

- Precise measurements.
- Familiarity with the translating concept.
- Use of a reliable diagnostic lens.
- Willingness to consult with the manufacturer.

Patient selection and benefits are the same as for segmented translating lenses (see above) although the lenses are the thinnest of the prism ballast bifocals and better for hypermetropes than segmented lenses. However, the distance zone must be large enough to minimize distance flare. Image jump, due to prismatic effects of the bicentric construction of these lenses, may result in patient problems during gaze shift.

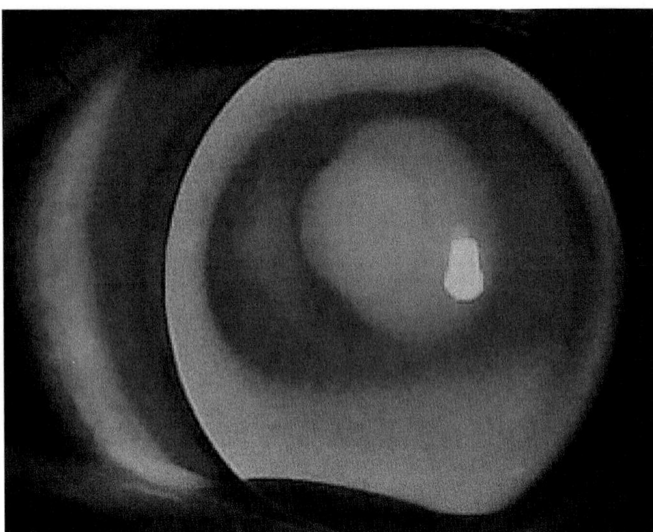

Figure 14.23 The Menicon Z Bifocal (Menicon)

SOFT BIFOCAL AND MULTIFOCAL LENS DESIGNS

The initial hydrogel multifocal and bifocal lens designs were developed in the 1970s, typically emulating PMMA lens designs (Josephson & Caffery 1991). The early results were not encouraging as little research had been performed and they were expensive to manufacture.

Soft bifocal and multifocal lens designs still have certain limitations compared to their RGP counterparts. The quality of vision is compromised as a result of both the water content and the dependence upon the simultaneous vision concept (Gispets et al. 2002, Pujol et al. 2003) with one exception (see 'Translating bifocal', below). However, presbyopes are so motivated not to wear spectacles they are often satisfied with reduced vision, although this can become an ethical issue for the practitioner.

Perhaps the most important change in soft lens usage has been the availability of disposable and frequent replacement modalities. As tear volume decreases with age, it is important to minimize the impact of deposits, both on ocular health and quality of vision.

Although these designs utilize the simultaneous vision principle, the design in each eye can be altered in order to optimize vision at various distances. Patients can trial the lenses while the practitioner adjusts the design to optimize both the fitting relationship and vision at all distances.

PATIENT SELECTION

Good candidates for soft bifocal lenses are shown in Table 14.8.

FITTING CONSIDERATIONS

Many of the fitting considerations mentioned with RGP designs also pertain to soft presbyopic lenses. The practitioner should have available several different soft multifocal lens designs as diagnostic fitting is important to determine the recommended lens design(s) and parameters. Lenses can be fitted from stock,

Table 14.8: Soft multifocals and bifocals – patient selection

Good candidates

- Existing soft lens wearers who are emerging presbyopes
- Soft lens monovision wearers who are dissatisfied with their vision
- Individuals with moderate intermediate vision requirements (i.e. computer users)
- Spherical or near-spherical refractive correction
- Individuals willing to accept some compromise in distance vision

Poor candidates

- Individuals who do not desire any compromise of their distance vision
- Individuals with moderate hyperopic refractive correction
- Individuals with emmetropic or near-emmetropic distance refractive error
- Individuals who best benefit from a toric correction
- Individuals with small pupil size (i.e. ≤3 mm)

making it easier for the patient to decide how closely the lenses meet their primary visual goals. Issue the optimum lenses for a 1-week trial period and then alter accordingly.

Design of soft multifocals

CENTRE-DISTANCE

Like RGP multifocal lenses, centre-distance lens designs can be either aspheric or concentric, although most are concentric with a central annular distance zone surrounded by an annular near zone. The benefit of these designs is the quality of distance vision when the pupil constricts in high illumination, although near vision may be compromised (Josephson & Caffery 1991).

Acuvue Bifocal (Johnson & Johnson)

This centre-distance concentric design has five alternating distance and near zones (www.acuvue.co.uk) (Fig. 14.24). This multizone design enhances distance and near vision as the pupil dilates or constricts.

Rigel (1998) found that 51% of patients were successful with the 'full binocular' approach to fitting Acuvue Bifocals, 32% with a 'modified bifocal' approach (adding plus power to the distance Rx of the non-dominant eye to enhance near vision) and 17% with the 'enhanced monovision' approach (fitting the non-dominant eye with a single-vision lens for near and the dominant eye with a reduced add).

Guidelines for problem-solving reduced vision with the Acuvue Bifocal are provided in Table 14.9 (Vehige 1992).

CENTRE-NEAR

The reading zone of these lenses is central and distance vision is optimized in mesopic or scotopic conditions. Conversely, under high illumination such as reading, the pupil constricts as a response to light and convergence; therefore, reading is optimized. However, this design is limited in bright daylight when the pupil constricts and good distance vision is required.

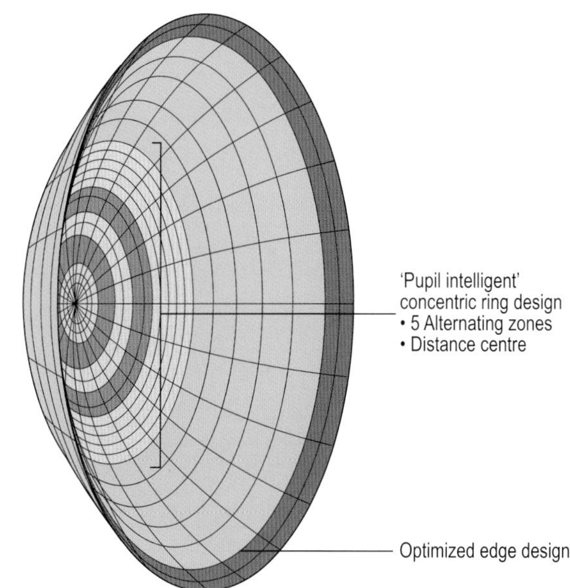

Figure 14.24 The Acuvue Bifocal (Vistakon)

Table 14.9: Acuvue Bifocal problem solving

1. Distance single-vision Acuvue on the dominant eye and Acuvue Bifocal on the non-dominant eye for patients with critical distance vision demands
2. Acuvue Bifocal on the dominant eye and Acuvue single-vision on the non-dominant eye for patients with extremely fine near work
3. Both eyes wearing Acuvue Bifocals with less add on the dominant eye to provide greater intermediate correction if needed
4. Fit Acuvue Bifocals on both eyes but increase the distance plus power on the non-dominant eye (i.e. 'modified monovision') to increase the effective add
5. Use a single Acuvue Bifocal on the dominant eye of low myopes or on the non-dominant eye of low hyperopes

From Lee (1999).

There are several aspheric or progressive centre-near designs.

Focus Progressive (CIBA Vision)

This 2-week or 1-month replacement lens has two BOZR (Fig. 14.25) (www.cibavision.co.uk).

It is reported to have a nominal add that can provide up to 3 D addition, although advanced presbyopes usually need extra plus in the non-dominant eye (Quinn 2002). The lens is approved for up to 6 nights extended wear.

Focus DAILIES Progressive lenses (CIBA Vision) are available in one BOZR and discarded daily.

SofLens Multi-focal (Bausch & Lomb)

This cast-moulded lens is available in two BOZR. A comparison of the lens design and problem solving of the SofLens Multi-Focal, Focus DAILIES Progressive and the Acuvue Bifocal is provided by Schofield et al. (2003).

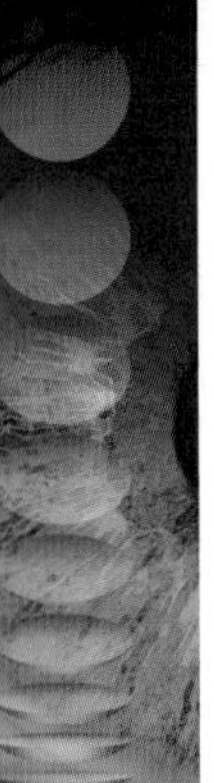

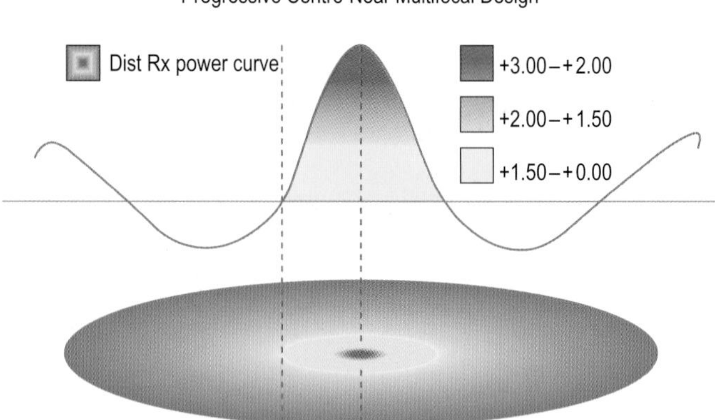

Figure 14.25 The Focus Progressive lens design (Courtesy of CooperVision)

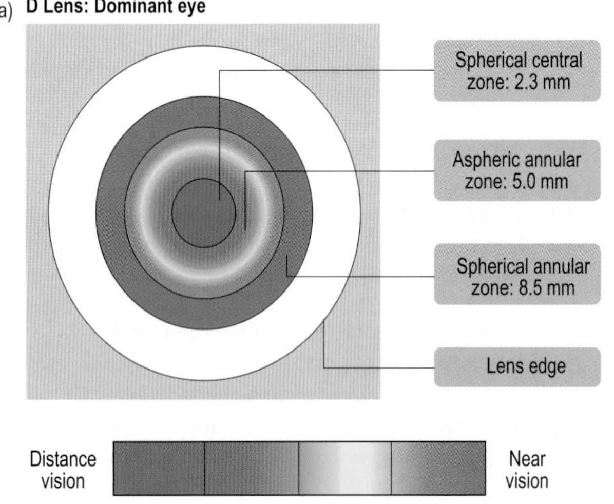

Figure 14.26 The Frequency 55 Multifocal lenses (CooperVision)

Simulvue lens (Unilens)

This lens is available in two centre-near diameters, 2.35 and 2.55 mm, and two BOZR (www.unilens.com). As with many of the soft multifocal and bifocal lens designs, the near add should be, at minimum, +0.50 D greater than the spectacle reading addition.

MODIFIED MONOVISION

Frequency 55 Multifocal (CooperVision)

This lens originated from the UltraVue lens design from Acuity One and combines multifocal optics with monovision. It has a combination of spherical and aspheric surfaces with little-compromised visual acuity of all distances present with binocular vision corrections (Shovlin & Eisenberg 2003, www.coopervision.co.uk) A centre-distance (D) lens, which transitions through an aspheric intermediate to an outer near zone, is placed on the dominant eye. A centre-near (N) lens, which transitions through an aspheric intermediate to a spherical peripheral distance zone is placed on the non-dominant eye (Wan 2003) (Fig. 14.26). It is hoped that binocular summation will occur, providing acceptable vision at all distances under binocular conditions. The central zone sizes are different between the D lens (2.3 mm) and N lens (1.7 mm) to enhance visual performance at each distance.

It is available in one total diameter and BOZR with +1.50, +2.00 and +2.50 D adds, and is recommended for monthly replacement. Patients may experience possible shadowing and ghost images initially.

Daniels and Cottam (2002) found that 20–40% of patients needed a different lens design in each eye and approximately half of their successful patients benefited from using uneven adds. In addition, patients with reduced distance vision were more comfortable with a single-vision aspheric design (e.g. Frequency 55 Aspheric) on the distance eye and the 'N lens' on the other eye.

The Frequency 55 Multifocal lens is also available in omafilcon material, as the Proclear Multifocal, which is useful for marginal dry eye patients.

DIFFRACTIVE BIFOCALS

The only diffractive bifocal lens available today is the Echelon (Ocular Sciences). This design uses a diffraction zone plate to separate light rays equally to distance and near. The distance power is refracted but the near power is achieved by diffraction. The major advantage is that it is independent of pupil size.

The near diffractive power is achieved through the circular annular grooves (echelettes) on the back surface of the lens and the refractive index of the tear layer that pools in the grooves.

The radii and spacing of the annular grooves determine the add power of the lens.

The diffractive zone is approximately 4.0–4.5 mm in diameter and the entire lens contains the distance power. This zone, particularly in higher adds, can be problematic for patients with large pupils although patients with small pupils typically report good vision at both distance and near (de Carle 1997).

Approximately 20% of the illumination is lost to higher orders of diffraction (40% of light goes to the distant image, 40% to the near image), thereby reducing contrast sensitivity; illumination should therefore be high when performing near tasks. Soni et al. (2003) described two experimental diffractive/refractive soft multifocal lens designs from Austria which produced no compromise in contrast sensitivity.

Fitting the lens

Insert a trial lens and check the overall fit then assess the position of the central zone against the dark background of the pupil with biomicroscopy. If only slight decentration is present, the patient can still be successful but extra add power may be required.

TRANSLATING BIFOCAL

The Triton Translating Soft Bifocal Lens (Gelflex) is the only translating soft lens currently available. Vision is excellent but there is potential for lid awareness as a result of the lens bulk and truncation (Gasson & Morris 2003). The lens consists of:

- Back surface design with truncation and a bi-prism to allow for lens stability and location (Ezekiel 2002, Ezekiel & Ezekiel 2002).
- TD in the horizontal meridian – 14.5 or 15.0 mm (14.5 mm most common). The larger lens is recommended for low-positioned lower lids (i.e. 2 mm below the lower limbus).
- Vertical sizes 11.4–13.9 mm in 0.5 mm steps.
- Two location dots engraved at the 3 and 9 o'clock positions at the periphery of the lens, which are on line with the geometrical centre of the lens.
- The near power segment positioned 1 mm below the geometrical centre.

Fitting information is available at www.gelflex.com.

TORIC BIFOCAL DESIGNS

Some of the aforementioned bifocal lenses are not yet available with toric prescriptions but lens designs are constantly changing with more toric bifocals becoming available all the time. Manufacturers' websites provide information about the latest developments.

Bifocal and multifocal success rates

RGP success rates are high (Woods et al. 1999, Lieblein 2000, Van Meter et al. 1990, and others). Previous soft bifocal studies resulted in only a 40–50% success rate (Hanks 1984, Edwards & Haig-Brown 1987, and others), although with the introduction of innovative designs and frequent replacement modalities, the success rate is increasing (Odineal 2001).

Rajagopalan et al. (2003) found RGP multifocal wearers had a higher contrast sensitivity function than any other presbyopic lens wearers.

PATIENT EDUCATION AND FOLLOW-UP CARE

Presbyopic patients need to be monitored more closely than younger patients as complications may arise from the aforementioned physiologic changes of the ageing eye.

Care and handling (see Chapter 11)

Older individuals – especially novices – may be apprehensive and lack confidence, and require patience during instruction. It is important that the patient leaves the office feeling confident in the handling of their lenses.

As a result of their predisposition for dryness-related problems, follow-up should be at least 6-monthly. Because bifocal lens designs are often thicker than their single-vision counterparts and the number of corneal endothelial cells is lower, the cornea should be evaluated for signs of hypoxia. If there is evidence of any such signs, a thinner design and higher oxygen transmissible material are indicated. Likewise, there may be changes in keratometry, corneal topography or refraction as a result of the thicker bifocal designs.

SUMMARY

Fitting the presbyopic patient can be challenging but, as this chapter hopefully shows, not nearly as complicated as perceived. Be realistic; let the patient know that visual compromise may be necessary compared to single-vision lenses and spectacles and that fees and potential chair time will be greater. If the patient has been adequately informed, and demonstrates sufficient motivation, then success will usually follow.

References

Afanador, A. J., Aitsemaomo, P. and Gertzman, D. R. (1986) Eye and head contribution to gaze at near through multifocals: the usable field of view. Am. J. Optom. Physiol. Opt., 63, 187–192

Ames, K. (2001) Fitting the presbyope with gas permeable contact lenses. Contact Lens Spectrum, 16(10), 42–45

Andres, S., Henriques, A., Garcia, M. L. et al. (1987) Factors of the precorneal fluid break-up time (BUT) and tolerance of contact lenses. Int. Contact Lens Clin., 4, 81–120

Back, A. P., Woods, R. and Holden, B. A. (1984) The comparative performance of monovision and various concentric bifocals. Trans. BCLA Conference, 46–47

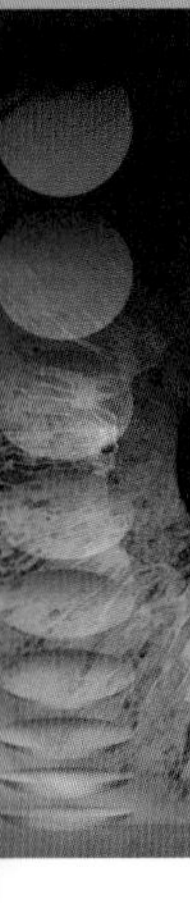

Benjamin, W. J. and Borish, I. M. (1991) Physiology of aging and its influence on the contact lens prescription. J. Am. Optom. Assoc., 62(10), 743–752

Bennett, E. S. (2004a) Patient selection, evaluation, and consultation. In Manual of Gas Permeable Contact Lenses, 2nd edn, pp. 58–85, eds. E. S. Bennett and M. M. Hom. St Louis, MO: Elsevier Science

Bennett, E. S. (2004b) Guide to fitting RGP multifocals and bifocals: Part 1. Rev. Contact Lenses, May 15, 14

Bennett, E. S. (2004c) Guide to fitting RGP multifocals and bifocals: Part 4. Rev. Contact Lenses, October, 14

Bennett, E. S. and Hansen, D. (2004) Presbyopia: gas-permeable bifocal fitting and problem-solving. In Manual of Gas Permeable Contact Lenses, 2nd edn, pp. 324–356, eds. E. S. Bennett and M. M. Hom. St Louis, MO: Elsevier Science

Bennett, E. S. and Jurkus, J. M. (2005) Presbyopic correction. In Clinical Contact Lens Practice, 2nd edn, pp. 27-1 to 27-18, eds. E. S. Bennett, and B. A. Weissman. Philadelphia, PA: Lippincott Williams and Wilkins

Bennett, E. S. and Luk, B. (2001) Rigid gas permeable bifocal contact lenses: an update. Optom. Today, June 15, 34–36

Bennett, E. S., Henry, V. A., Morgan, B. W. (1990) The Diffrax™ bifocal. What the practitioner needs to know. Contact Lens Forum, 15(3), 31–35

Bergenske, P. D. (2001) The presbyopic fitting process. Contact Lens Spectrum, 16, 34–41

Borish, I. M. (1986) Presbyopia. In Rigid Gas-Permeable Contact Lenses, pp. 385–414, eds. E. S. Bennett and R. M. Grohe. New York: Professional Press

Borish, I. M. and Perrigin, D. M. (1985) Observations of bifocal contact lenses. Int. Eyecare, 1(3), 241–248

Caffery, B. E. and Josephson, J. E. (1991) Rigid bifocal lens correction. In Clinical Contact Lens Practice, pp. 42-1 to 42-12, eds. E. S. Bennett and B. A. Weissman. Philadelphia, PA: Lippincott

Churms, P. W., Freeman, M. H., Melling, J. et al. (1987) The development and clinical performance of a new diffractive bifocal contact lens. Optom. Today, 27(22), 721–724

Collins, M. J., Goode, A. and Brown, B. (1993) Distance visual acuity and monovision. Optom. Vis. Sci., 70(9), 723–728

Collins, M., Bruce, A. and Thompson, B. (1994) Adaptation to monovision. Int. Contact Lens Clin., 21, 218–224

Daniels, K. and Cottam, L. (2002) Independent clinical evaluation of inverse geometry multifocal for presbyopic correction. Presented at the Annual Meeting of the American Academy of Optometry, San Diego, CA, December 2002

Davis, R. (2003) Pinpoint success with RGP multifocal lenses. Contact Lens Spectrum, 18(10), 25–38

de Carle, J. (1959) The de Carle bifocal contact lens. Contacto, 3, 5, 6, 8, 9

de Carle, J. T. (1997) Bifocal and multifocal contact lenses. In Contact Lens Practice, 4th edn, pp. 540–565 eds. A. J. Phillips and L. Speedwell. Oxford: Butterworth-Heinemann

Diepes, H. and Tameling, A. (1988) Comparative investigations of progressive lenses. Am. J. Optom. Physiol. Opt., 65, 571–579

du Toit, R., Ferreira, J. T. and Nel, Z. J. (1998) Visual and nonvisual variables implicated in monovision wear. Optom. Vis. Sci. 75, 119–125

du Toit, R., Situ, P., Simpson, T. and Fonn, D. (2000) Factors that discriminate between monovision and bifocal contact lens preference. Presented at the Annual Meeting of the American Academy of Optometry, December 2000

du Toit, R., Situ, P., Simpson, T. and Fonn, D. (2001) The effects of six months of contact lens wear on the tear film, ocular surfaces, and symptoms of presbyopes. Optom. Vis. Sci., 78, 455–462

Edwards, K. (1999) Contact lens problem-solving: bifocal contact lenses. Optician, 218, 26–32

Edwards, K. and Haig-Brown, G. (1987) An evaluation of bifocal contact lens performance and the design of a new fitting protocol. Trans. BCLA Conference, 30–34

Eggink, F. A. G. J., Pinkers, A. J. L. G. and DeGraaf, R. (1990) Visual acuity and contrast sensitivity with Diffrax contact lenses. Contact Lens J., 18(2), 37–39

Erickson, P. and McGill, E. C. (1992) Role of visual acuity, stereoacuity, and ocular dominance in monovision patient success. Optom. Vis. Sci. 69, 761–764

Ezekiel, D. F. (2002) A 'genuinely' new bifocal lens design. Optom. Today, May 17, 34–35

Ezekiel, D. F. and Ezekiel, D. J. (2002) A soft bifocal lens that does not compromise vision. Contact Lens Spectrum, 17(5), 40

Feinbloom, W. (1938) United States Patent 2, 129, 305. Application 21 August, patented 6 September, 1938

Fisher, K., Bauman, E. and Schwallie, J. (1999) Evaluation of two new soft contact lenses for correction of presbyopia: the Focus Progressives Multifocal and the Acuvue Bifocal. Int. Contact Lens Clin., 26, 92–103

Fonda, G. (1996) Presbyopia corrected with single vision spectacles or corneal lenses in preference to bifocal corneal lenses. Trans. Ophthalmol. Soc. Aust. XXV, 46–50

Gasson, A. and Morris, J. (2003) Lenses for presbyopia. In The Contact Lens Manual: A Practical Fitting Guide, 3rd edn, pp. 298–317, eds. A. Gasson and J. Morris. London: Butterworth-Heinemann

Gispets, J., Arjona, M. and Pujol, J. (2002) Image quality in wearers of a centre distance concentric design bifocal contact lens. Ophthalmic Physiol. Opt., 22, 221–223

Gromacki, S. J. (2004) Preventing contact lens challenges for presbyopes. Contact Lens Spectrum, 19(8), S2–S7

Hamano, H., Hori, M., Hamano, T. et al. (1983) A new method of measuring tears. CLAO J., 9, 281–289

Hanks, A. (1984) Contact lenses for presbyopia. Eye Contact, 9–14

Hansen, D. W. (1998) Mapping the way to successful bifocal RGP selection. Contact Lens Spectrum, 13(3), 14

Hansen, D. W. (1999) Advanced multifocal fitting and management. Contact Lens Spectrum, 14(8), 25–33

Hansen, D. W. (2002) Multifocal contact lenses – the next generation. Contact Lens Spectrum, 17(11), 42–47

Hansen, D., Baker, R. and Bennett, E. S. (2003) Why today's RGP designs are easier to fit. Rev. Optom., 140, 43–46

Jain, S., Arora, I. and Azar, D. T. (1996) Success of monovision in presbyopes: review of the literature and potential applications to refractive surgery. Surv. Ophthalmol., 40, 491–499

Jain, S., Ou, R. and Azar, D. T. (2001) Monovision outcomes in presbyopic individuals after refractive surgery. Am. Acad. Ophthalmol., 108, 1430–1433

Jessen, G. N. (1960a) Recent developments in bifocal contact lenses. Am. J. Optom. Arch. Am. Acad. Optom., 37, 379–387

Jessen, G. N. (1960b) Bifocal contact lenses. Br. J. Physiol. Opt., 17, 217–221

Johannsdottir, K. R. and Stelmach, L. B. (2001) Monovision: a review of the scientific literature. Optom. Vis. Sci., 78, 646–651

Josephson, J. E. and Caffery, B. E. (1991) Bifocal hydrogel contact lenses. In Clinical Contact Lens Practice, pp. 43-1 to 43-20, eds. E. S. Bennett and B. A. Weissman. Philadelphia, PA: Lippincott

Josephson, J. E., Erickson, P., Back. A. et al. (1990) Monovision. J. Am. Optom. Assoc., 61, 820–826

Lee, W. C. (1999) Factors for fitting success. Contact Lens Spectrum, 14(3), 7a

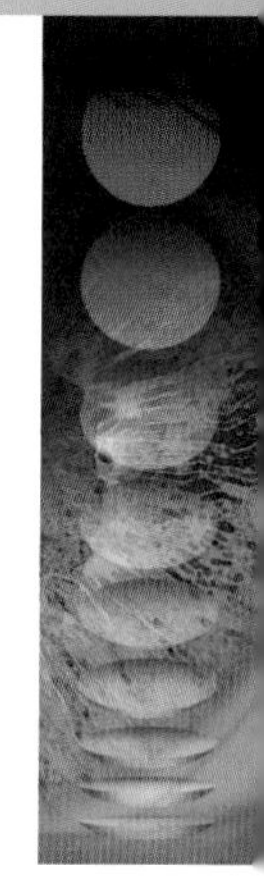

Lieblein, J. S. (2000) Fitting success with multifocal contact lenses. Contact Lens Spectrum, 14(3), 50–51
Loshin, D. S., Loshin, M. S. and Comer G. (1982) Binocular summation with monovision contact lens correction for presbyopia. Int. Contact Lens Clin., 9, 161–165
Loveridge, R. (2003) In practice assessment of an RGP multifocal contact lens. Optician, 226(5926), 28–30
MacAlister, G. O. and Woods, C. A. (1991) Monovision versus RGP translating bifocals. J. Br. Contact Lens Assoc., 14, 173–178
Mandell, R. B. (1967) A no jump bifocal contact lens. Optom. Weekly, 58, 19–21
Mandell, R. B. (2002) A new concept in RGP bifocal contact lenses. Contact Lens Spectrum, 17(10), 34–40
Martin, D. K. and Dain, S. J. (1988) Postural modifications of VDU operators wearing bifocal spectacles. Appl. Ergonom., 19, 293–300
Meyler, J. and Veys, J. (1999) A new pupil-intelligent design for presbyopic correction. Optician, 217, 18–23
Michaels, D. D. (1974) Ocular dominance. Surv. Ophthalmol., 17, 151–163
Moss, H. I. (1962) Bifocal contact lenses – a review. Am. J. Optom. Arch. Am. Acad. Optom. 39, 653–668
Nakagawara, V. B. and Veronneau, S. J. H. (2000) Monovision contact lens use in the aviation environment: a report of a contact lens-related aircraft accident. Optometry, 71(6), 390–395
Norman, C. W. (2004) Cut down on fitting and chair time with a new RGP multifocal. Contact Lens Spectrum, 19(5), 15
Odineal, C. (2001) Fitting a soft disposable bifocal contact lens. Contact Lens Spectrum, 16(4), 44–46
Pearlman, A. (1987) The central visual pathways. In Adler's Physiology of the Eye: Clinical Application, pp. 583–618, eds. R. A. Moses and W. M. Hart. St Louis, MO: Mosby
Pointer, J. S. (2001) Sighting dominance, handedness, and visual acuity preference: three mutually exclusive modalities? Ophthalmic Physiol. Opt., 21, 117–126
Pujol, J., Gispets. J. and Arjona, M. (2003) Optical performance in eyes wearing two multifocal contact lens designs. Ophthalmic Physiol. Opt., 23, 347–360
Quinn, T. G. (1997) Identifying the presbyopic contact lens candidate. Contact Lens Spectrum, 12(9), 3s–6s
Quinn, T. G. (2001) Translating bifocals into success. Contact Lens Spectrum, 16(3), 16
Quinn, T. G. (2002) Making sense of frequent replacement soft multifocals. Contact Lens Spectrum, 17(3), 17
Rajagopalan, A. S., Bennett, E. S., Lakshminarayanan, V. and Henry, V. A. (2003) Performance of presbyopic contact lenses under mesopic conditions. Presented at ARVO, Fort Lauderdale, FL, April 2003
Rigel, L. E. (1998) What to expect from the Acuvue Bifocal. Optom. Today, 6(6), 26–27
Rigel, L. E. and Castellano, C. F. (1999) How to fit today's soft bifocal contact lenses. Optom. Today, 7 (Suppl), 45–51
Sakamoto, R., Bennett, E. S., Henry, V. A. et al. (1993) The phenol red thread test: a cross-cultural study. Invest. Ophthalmol. Vis. Sci., 34, 3510–3514
Schofield, J., Richmond, M. and Evans, V. (2003) Over-refraction with multifocal soft lenses. Optom. Today, September 19, 42–44
Schor, C. and Landsman, L. (1987) Ocular dominance and the interocular suppression of blur in monovision. Am. J. Optom. Physiol. Opt., 64, 723–730
Schwallie, J. (2000) Multifocal contact lenses: a valuable alternative for your presbyopic patient. Contact Lens Spectrum, 15(12), 29–32
Schwartz, C. A. (1996) Presbyopia: monovision. In: Specialty Contact Lenses: A Fitter's Guide, 1st edn, pp. 85–93, ed. C. A. Schwartz. Philadelphia, PA: W. B. Saunders
Schwartz, C. A. (1999) Portrait of a presbyope in 1999. Optom. Today, (Suppl), 5–7
Shovlin, J. P. and Eisenberg, J. S. (2003) Monovision vs. multifocal: which would you choose? Rev. Optom., 140, 36–38
Soni, P. S., Patel, R. and Carlson, R. S. (2003) Is binocular contrast sensitivity at distance compromised with multifocal soft contact lenses used to correct presbyopia? Optom. Vis. Sci., 80(7), 505–514
Van Meter, W. S., Gussler, J. R. and Litteral, G. (1990) Clinical evaluation of three bifocal contact lenses. CLAO J., 16(3), 203–207
Vassilieff, A. and Dain, S. (1986) Bifocal wearing and VDU operation: a review and graphical analysis. Appl. Ergonom., 17, 82–86
Vehige, J. G. (1992) Hydron Echelon lens fitting guide Part III: fitting factors for success. Contact Lens Spectrum, 7(2), 39–46
Veys, J. and Davies, I. (1995) Basic contact lens practice – part eight: managing the presbyope. Optician, 210, 30–35
Wan, L. (2003) Take some frustration out of multifocal fitting. Contact Lens Spectrum, 18(9), 42–44
Weale, R. A. (1982) A biography of the eye: development, age, and growth. London: H. K. Lewis
Westendorf, D. H., Blake, R., Sloane, M. and Chambers, D. (1982) Binocular summation occurs during interocular suppressions. J. Exp. Psych., 8, 81–90
Westin, E., Wick, B. and Harrist, R. B. (2000) Factors influencing success of monovision contact lens fitting: survey of contact lens diplomats. Optometry, 71, 757–763
Woods, C., Ruston, D., Hough, T. and Efron N. (1999) Clinical performance of an innovative back surface multifocal contact lens in correcting presbyopia. CLAO J., 25(3), 176–181
Woods, J. M., Wick, K., Shuley, V. et al. (1998) The effect of monovision contact lens wear on driving performance. Clin. Exp. Optom., 81(3), 100–103
Wooley, S. (1998) 'Doctor, do I need to give up my contact lenses just because I need bifocals?' Optom. Today, 6, 40–42
Yager, J. (2002) Pearls for fitting the presbyopic patient. Rev. Contact Lenses, September, 28–32

Further information/useful websites

The GP Lens Institute (www.gpli.info)
The International Association of Contact Lens Educators (IACLE) – module on contact lens multifocals (www.iacle.org)

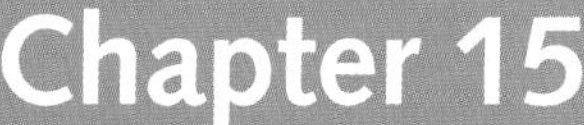

Chapter 15

Scleral contact lenses

Ken Pullum

CHAPTER CONTENTS

INTRODUCTION

Scleral contact lenses have retained a uniquely valuable role in contact lens practice, even though they predated all other lens forms by about six decades. Rigid gas-permeable (RGP) materials have enabled straightforward, predictable and effective fitting methods, often when a successful visual outcome is most needed. However, even in countries where scleral lens practice has remained relatively strong, teaching has virtually ceased to exist, so there is a poor recognition of their attributes and indications.

Following the development of corneal and hydrogel lenses in the 1950s and 1960s, the use of scleral lenses rapidly declined. They became considered only useful as a last resort, i.e. before transplantation in keratoconus or when all other contact lens options failed, and were perceived as generally cumbersome. The reality is that there are opportunities for effective, non-surgical visual rehabilitation at all levels of pathology whenever there is a sound indication for contact lens management.

Advantages of scleral lenses

Contrary to popular belief, rather than disadvantages, the large size and bearing surface provide positive benefits:

- Virtually any corneal topography can be fitted because close alignment between the corneal surface and the lens is not necessary.
- An extensive power range is possible.
- Retention of the precorneal tear reservoir allows some highly effective therapeutic applications.
- The endpoint to the fitting process is well defined and usually reached quickly.
- There is no eyelid/lens edge interaction.
- Foreign bodies behind lenses are not a problem.
- There is no localized exposure due to disrupted blinking.
- Inserting may be easier for less dextrous patients, because the lens is held between the thumb and a finger rather than balanced on one finger.
- Maintenance is straightforward
  - dry storage is generally satisfactory, even with RGP materials.
  - polishing or resurfacing is possible.

Disadvantages of scleral lenses

However, there are also disadvantages with scleral lenses:

- Even if skilfully fitted, the oxygen available to the cornea is reduced.

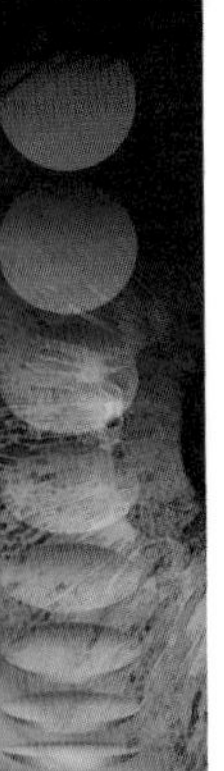

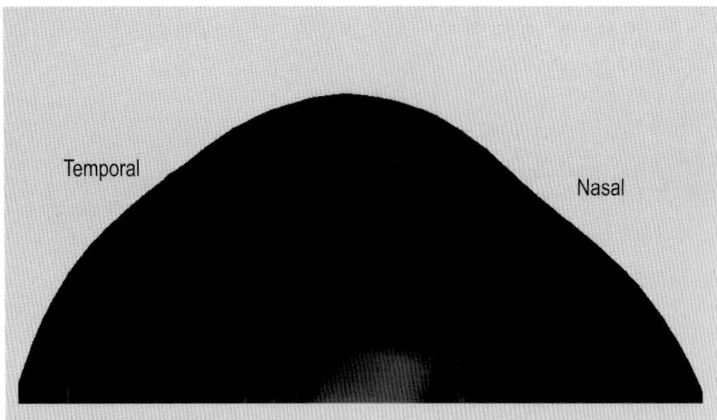

Figure 15.1 Cross-section of the author's eye cast in the horizontal meridian. The nasal scleral radius of curvature is flatter and with a more pronounced topographical change between the cornea and the sclera than at the temporal limbus

Figure 15.2 Vertical meridian cross-section of the same eye as in Figure 15.1 showing a greater similarity between the superior and inferior sclera compared to the clear asymmetry along the horizontal. The contour is virtually conical, with a barely discernible distinction between the cornea and the sclera at the limbus. In spite of the asymmetry about the geometric axis, many eyes remain fittable with coaxially designed scleral lenses

- Production is labour intensive.
- The large size can be intimidating.
- Some patients are conscious of the feeling and appearance of bulk.
- Visual performance is not always as good as corneal lenses.
- There are significant prismatic effects, especially in the vertical meridian.
- Some apparently successful fittings are not well tolerated.

Corneal and scleral topography relevant to scleral lens fitting

The normal cornea flattens towards the periphery, affecting the choice of back optic zone radius (BOZR). The limbus is a not a well-defined junction, but a continuous aspheric curve linking the cornea and the sclera. The normal scleral contour is not spherical or symmetrical about the visual axis (Marriott 1966); typically the centre of curvature of the temporal sclera is contralaterally offset, giving a less pronounced limbal sulcus, while the nasal sclera is most often the flattest sector, accentuating the limbus. Figure 15.1 is the horizontal and Figure 15.2 the vertical cross-section of a normal eye cast. Many scleras tend to be toroidal, more often flatter in the horizontal meridian, but retaining the difference between the nasal and temporal sectors.

Impression and preformed PMMA scleral lenses

Polymethylmethacrylate (PMMA) scleral lenses are lathe-cut according to the appearance of diagnostic preformed fitting set lenses or individually fabricated from the basis of an eye impression. Although preformed lenses have limitations if the scleral topography is excessively toroidal or irregular, they prove satisfactory for many topographically normal eyes. The greater versatility of impression lenses allows their use with virtually any ocular topography.

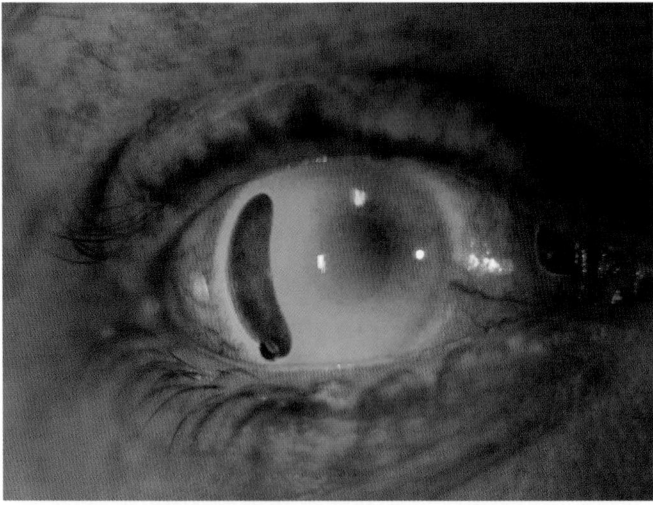

Figure 15.3 Fenestrated scleral lens in situ, illustrating full clearance extending just beyond the limbus in all meridians but with a crescent-shaped air bubble on the temporal side at the site of the fenestration

Ventilating PMMA scleral lenses

Addressing the problem of hypoxia is crucial for a successful outcome. A means of ventilation to allow some fresh oxygenated tears exchange, usually a fenestration at the temporal limbus, is necessary with PMMA. However, an air bubble is nearly always admitted behind the lens, its shape and size traditionally used to qualify the fitting characteristics of the lens. Figure 15.3 shows a fenestrated lens with a just acceptable crescent-shaped bubble at the temporal limbus. In addition, the lens settles back on the globe as the hydrostatic pressure of the precorneal fluid reservoir is brought into equilibrium with atmospheric pressure.

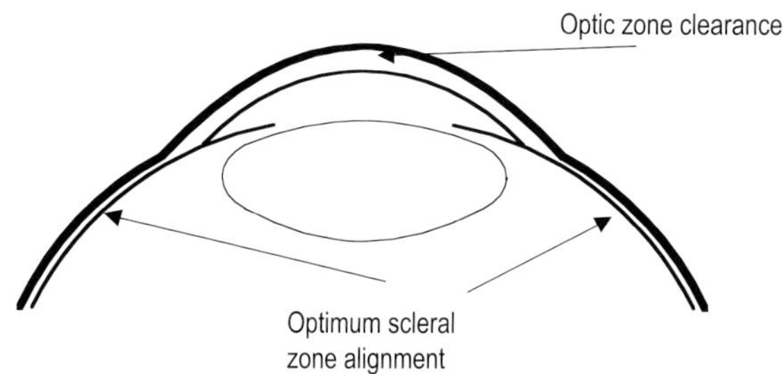

Figure 15.4 Optimum scleral fit

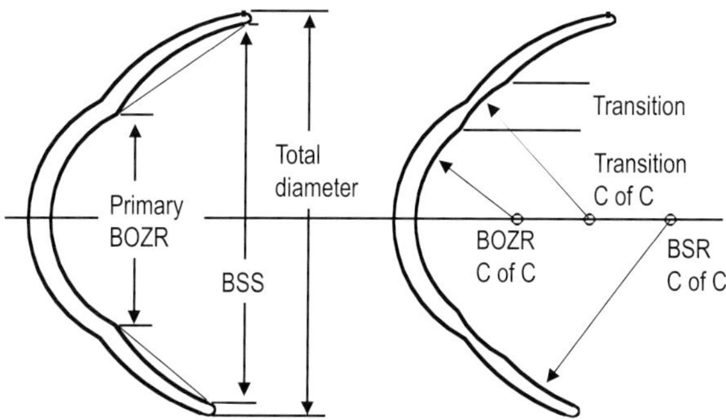

Figure 15.5 Diagrammatic preformed scleral lens

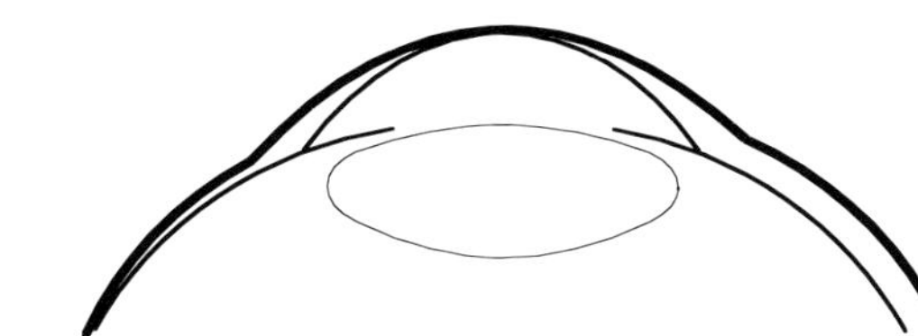

Figure 15.6 Lens displacement and lifting off from the sclera due to apical contact during scleral zone fitting gives an incorrect appearance of a flat-fitting scleral zone

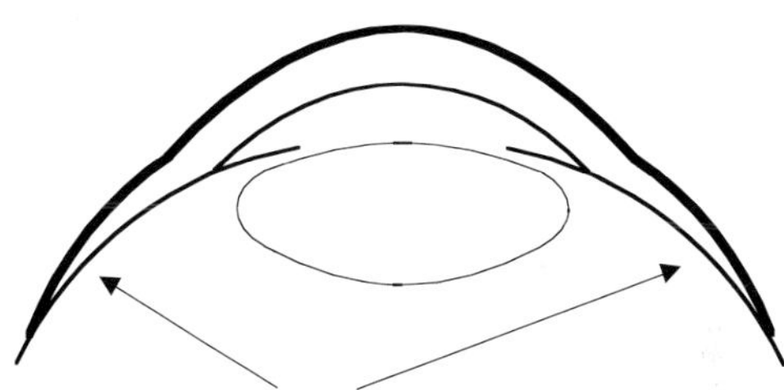

Figure 15.7 Vaulting from peripheral contact only with steep scleral zone fitting

Rigid gas-permeable scleral lenses

RGP materials have transformed scleral lens practice, shifting the emphasis from impression lenses to preformed. Blanks are lathe-cut or the material is individually cast polymerized to produce a range of preformed designs. The substance required for scleral lenses is greater than for corneal lenses, so there was initially some doubt that RGP materials would have sufficient transmissibility. However, there are encouraging results in corneal swelling studies (Ruben & Benjamin 1985, Bleshoy & Pullum 1988, Pullum et al. 1990, 1991, Mountford et al. 1994, Pullum & Stapleton 1997, Smith et al. 2004) and also in clinical reports where scleral lenses have been fitted for a variety of visual and therapeutic conditions (Ezekiel 1983, 1991, Pullum et al. 1989, 2005, Schein et al. 1990, Visser 1990, Kok & Visser 1992, Tan et al. 1995, Pullum & Buckley 1997, Cotter & Rosenthal 1998, Swann & Mountford 1999, Ramero-Rangel et al. 2000, Rosenthal et al. 2000, Tappin et al. 2001, Segal et al. 2003).

The materials are not thermoplastic, but when impression lenses are needed, they can be made by drilling out the centre of a PMMA shell and cementing an RGP optic in its place, or by duplicating a PMMA lens in an RGP material (Lyons et al. 1989). Early manufacturing techniques favoured the former; however, more recently, duplication has become the more satisfactory method.

PREFORMED SCLERAL LENS FITTING

The objective is that of corneal clearance extending far enough into the scleral zone to avoid compression of the limbus, with optimum scleral alignment over the broadest possible area (Fig. 15.4).

General principles of scleral zone fitting

The principles are the same for all preformed scleral lenses, but there are notable differences for fenestrated and non-ventilated systems. Figure 15.5 shows a diagram of a preformed lens using BSI terminology (UK Vocabulary Standards 1988).

BACK SCLERAL RADIUS (BSR)

Two or three lenses should establish the optimum scleral zone fit, or show that preformed lenses are not suitable. A glove fit is not a prerequisite, but there should be only minimal occlusion of the conjunctival blood vessels. Provided there is no compressive optic zone contact, which could lift the whole lens off the globe (Fig. 15.6), the scleral zone fit may be assessed in isolation from the optic zone. However, it is not possible to make a final evaluation without taking both into consideration at the same time.

If the BSR is too steep, the lens may vault the whole anterior eye from its periphery (Fig. 15.7). Fluorescein in the precorneal fluid reservoir spreads too far into the scleral zone, and the peripheral conjunctival vessels are occluded (Fig. 15.8). Vaulting from a localized flat scleral region causes tilting or decentration (Fig. 15.9). If too flat, the scleral zone stands off the globe, allowing fluorescein under the periphery, and may occlude the mid-peripheral conjunctival vessels (Figs 15.10, 15.11). There may be more settling back because of the narrow bearing surface (Fig. 15.12).

The range of back scleral zone radii traditionally included in a PMMA scleral fitting set is from 12.5 to 15.0 mm with increments of 0.25 mm. Increments of 0.5 mm may be more appropriate as the difference between the steepest and flattest sections of a normal sclera is greater than 0.25 mm. The

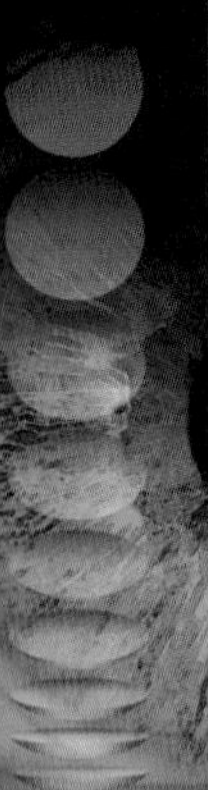

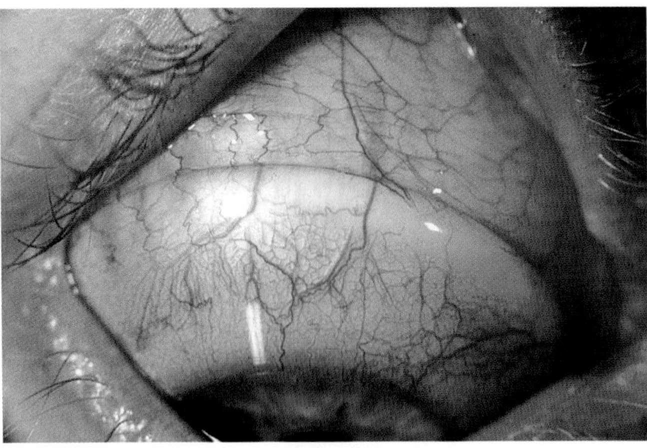

Figure 15.8 Steep-fitting scleral zone. The lens vaults from the periphery, and may occlude the peripheral conjunctival vessels

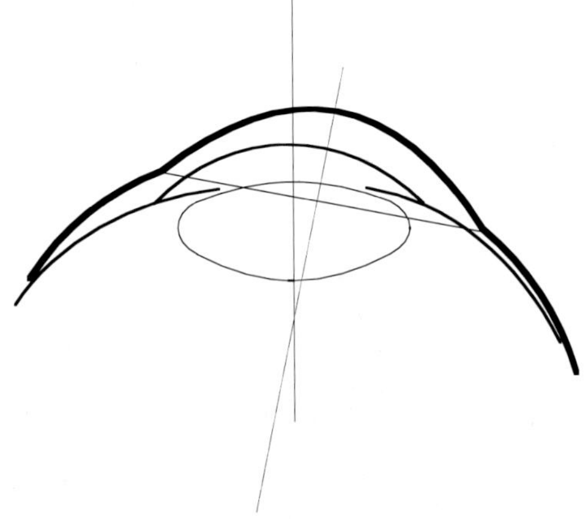

Figure 15.9 Partial vaulting and decentration from a single flat sector of the sclera

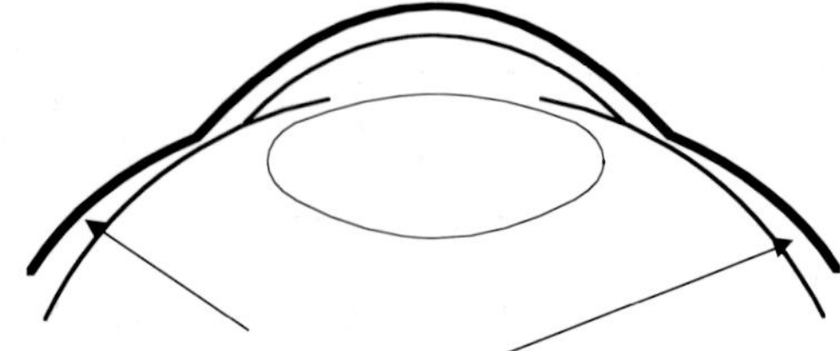

Figure 15.10 Flat scleral zone standing off the globe at the periphery

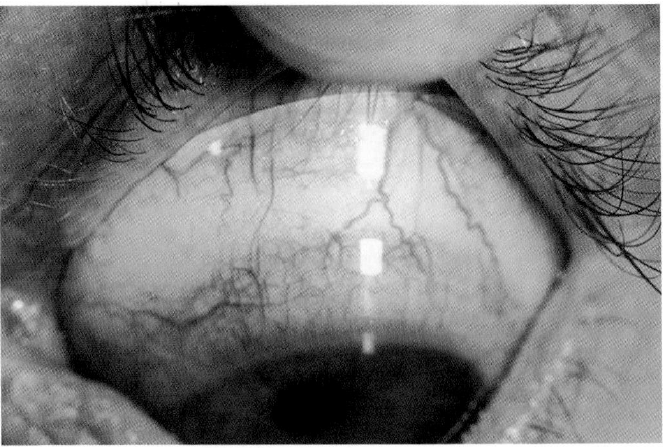

Figure 15.11 Flat-fitting scleral zone. The lens stands off the globe from just outside the limbus, and may occlude the mid-peripheral conjunctival vessels

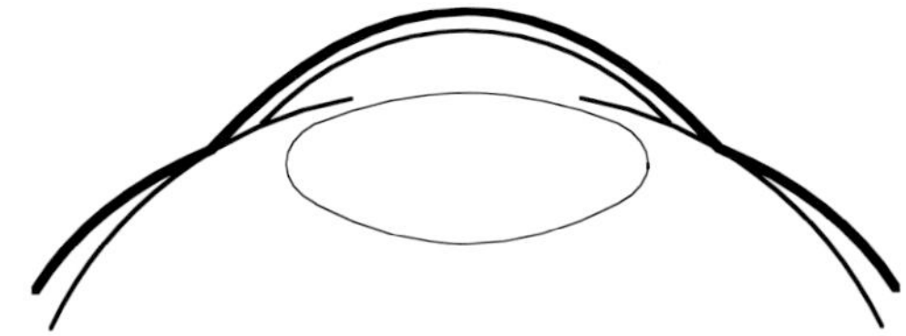

Figure 15.12 There may be more settling back on the globe compared to a steep scleral zone because of the narrow bearing surface. This leads to reduction of the apical clearance

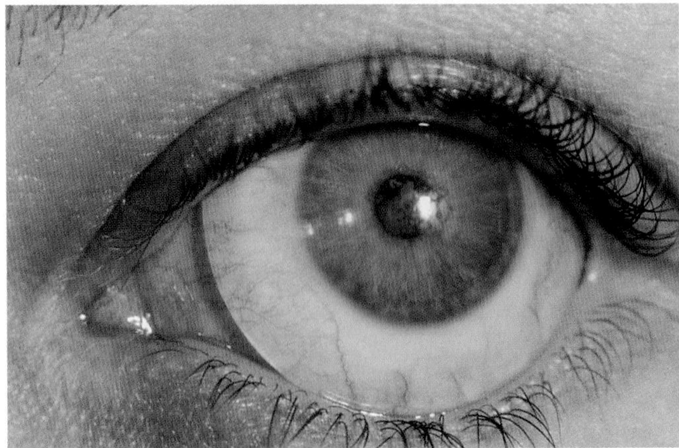

Figure 15.13 Small-diameter (20 mm) scleral lens snagging on the lower lid

precorneal fluid reservoir retained by a non-ventilated RGP scleral lens has a distinct cushioning effect, allowing more extension of the optic zone clearance into the scleral zone, increasing the latitude for optimal scleral zone fitting as well as for the optic zone. A 1.0 mm increment is only just discernible on some eyes.

TOTAL DIAMETER

The lens diameter may vary from just larger than perilimbal, but enough to have a scleral bearing surface, up to 25 mm. If too small, the edge is more noticeable, and may catch on the lower lid (Fig. 15.13). If too large, the lens impinges on the inner canthus or the lower fornix with nasal or downward eye movements. The diameter of the first trial lens should be approximately 23 mm as the distance between the medial and lateral recti muscle insertion points in an adult is usually slightly greater than that.

A small alteration in the diameter gives a relatively large change in the area of the bearing surface (Fig. 15.14). As the sclera does not flatten towards the equator (unlike the cornea, which flattens towards the periphery), increasing the diameter does not necessarily have a great effect. However, a larger lens may impinge on a single flatter scleral sector, or on irregular areas such as the recti muscle insertion points.

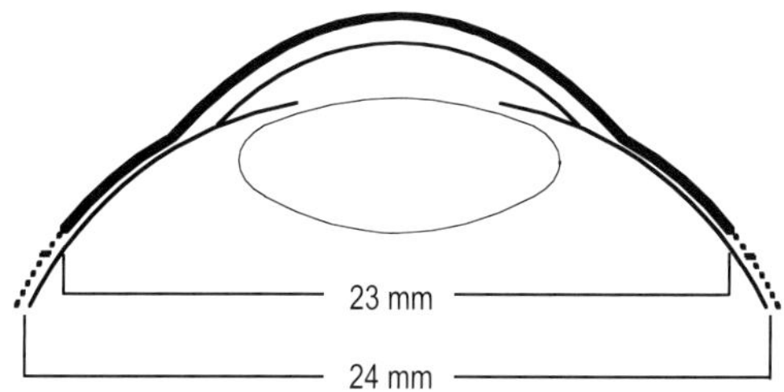

Figure 15.14 A small alteration in the diameter gives a relatively large change in the area of the bearing surface

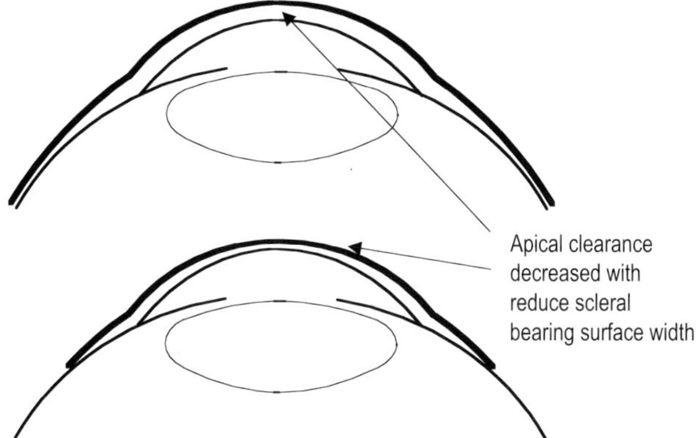

Figure 15.15 If the diameter is reduced by a critical amount (e.g. from 23 mm to 19 mm or 18 mm), the original bearing surface may be completely removed, leading to a reduction in the optic zone clearance

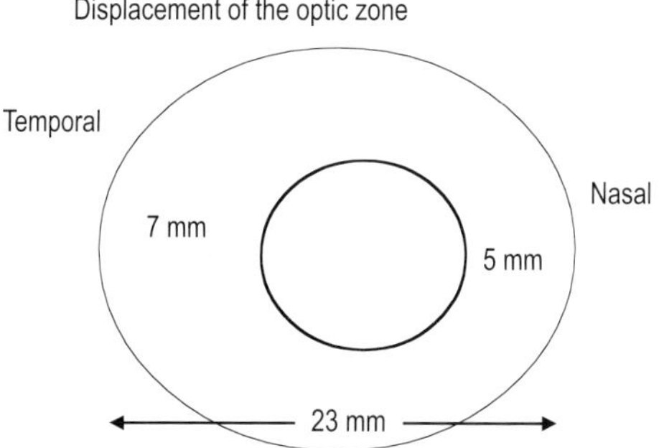

Figure 15.16 The optic is normally displaced 1–1.5 mm towards the nasal side so the temporal scleral zone is 2 mm wider

Similarly, if the diameter is reduced by a small amount, there may not be much difference in appearance but if reduced to the size of the area of perilimbal clearance, the original bearing surface may be completely removed, leading to a reduction in the optic zone clearance (Fig. 15.15). As a rule, reducing the 23 mm diameter by more than 2–3 mm should be undertaken with caution, and a special trial lens should be made to test the effect of diameter changes. If the diameter is to be reduced by more than 3 mm, the lens should be redesigned to allow for the predicted change.

DISPLACEMENT OF OPTIC

The optic should be displaced 1–1.5 mm towards the nasal side (Fig. 15.16). Reducing the width of the nasal scleral zone helps prevent the edge impinging on the inner canthus on adduction.

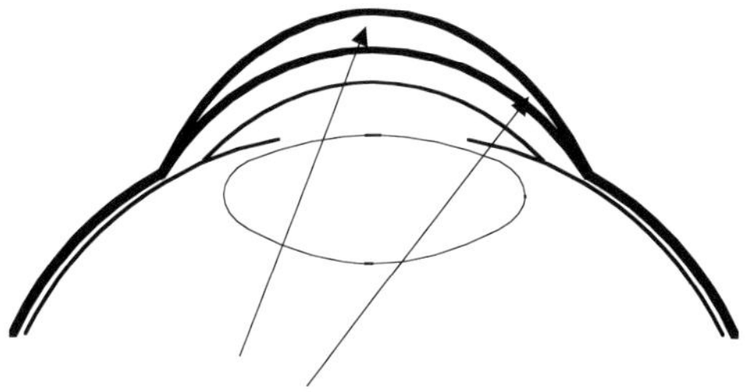

Figure 15.17 The apical clearance increased with a steeper BOZR and an unchanged BOZD, but there is only a minimal change to the limbal clearance

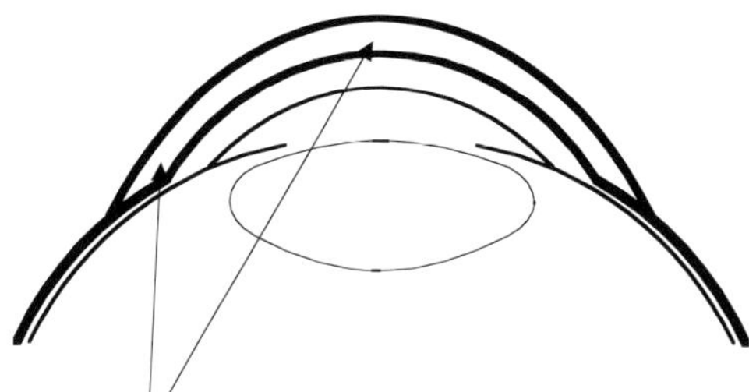

Figure 15.18 Both apical and limbal clearance are increased with a larger BOZD if the BOZR is unchanged

The optic zone in preformed RGP scleral lenses

SAGITTAL DEPTH (SAG)

Having established the optimum scleral zone alignment, the optic zone sag – and hence the corneal clearance – is determined by varying the BOZR and the back optic zone diameter (BOZD) in combination (Figs 15.17, 15.18). Modern designs blend the junction between the optic and scleral zones, or include an aspheric transition zone. The primary BOZD is measured at the junction between the continuation of the BOZR and BSR.

CONTROLLED CLEARANCE USING OPTIC ZONE PROJECTION (OZP)

An alternative method is to use progressive increments in the projection of the optic zone (OZP) from the extrapolation of the BSR, but without reference to the BOZR or BOZD (Pullum 1997) (Figs 15.19, 15.20).

Part of the design process of these lenses analysed the parameter changes, so that the differences between lenses are clinically significant: 0.25 mm is a suitable apical increment for non-ventilated lenses. That way fitting sets are not too cumbersome and need not include rarely used lenses. Most normal corneas are 1–2 mm in the OZP scale, while a rare, highly globic corneal profile may be up to 5.0 mm.

Interaction with OZP and BSR

Reflecting the more forgiving nature of non-ventilated lens fitting, the BSR options have been simplified to steep or flat –

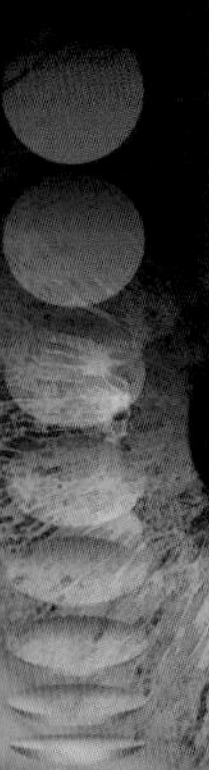

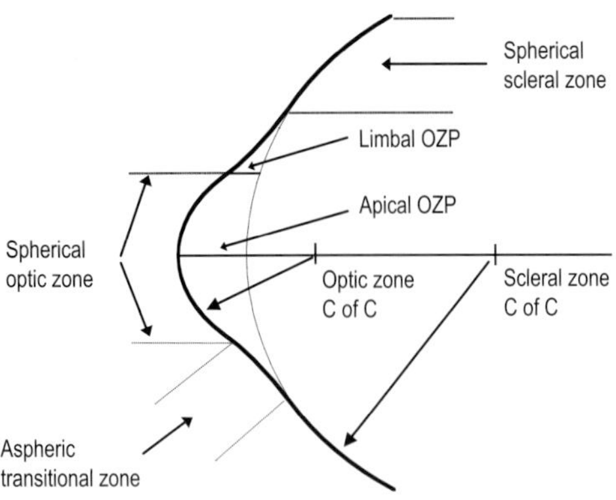

Figure 15.19 Definition of scleral lens parameters according to the optic zone projection (OZP) from the extrapolation of the (BSR)

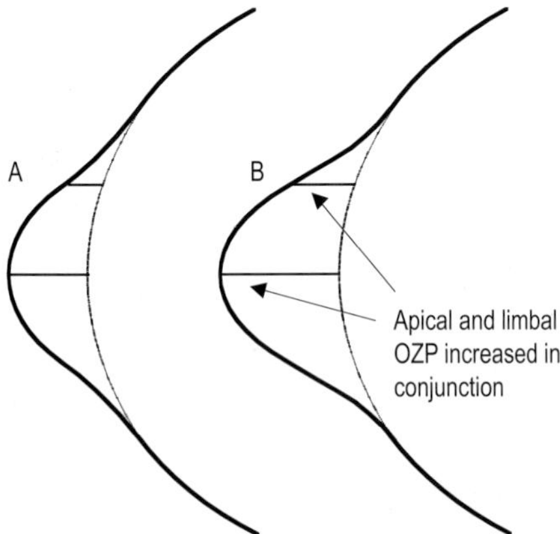

Figure 15.20 Lens B is designed with an increment to the projection of the optic zone (OZP) from the extrapolation of the back scleral radius, but without reference to the BOZR or BOZD

13.50 or 14.50 mm – from which the majority of eyes can be fitted. In the absence of a reliable measure of scleral radius or topography, the steeper BSR is a more appropriate first choice because some partial vaulting from the mid-periphery may help to increase the limbal clearance. The final choice is determined by the appearance of the underlying conjunctival blood vessels and the clearance beyond the limbus. Spherical lenses fitted to a moderately toroidal sclera may stand off in the steep meridian, or vault in the flat meridian, but may provide some tear exchange and still retain a bubble-free precorneal fluid reservoir.

SELECTION OF OPTIC ZONE PARAMETERS FOR NON-VENTILATED SCLERAL LENSES

Normal flat corneas have less corneal projection than steep corneas. Keratometry and topographical mapping do not provide sufficient information about the corneal projection or the limbal topography. Where the topography is irregular, instrumentation is of even less use. A more appropriate indicator is a simple assessment of the corneal profile, as illustrated in Figures 15.21, 15.22 and 15.23, showing the variation in corneal projection from the scleral plane and eccentricity of the corneal apex.

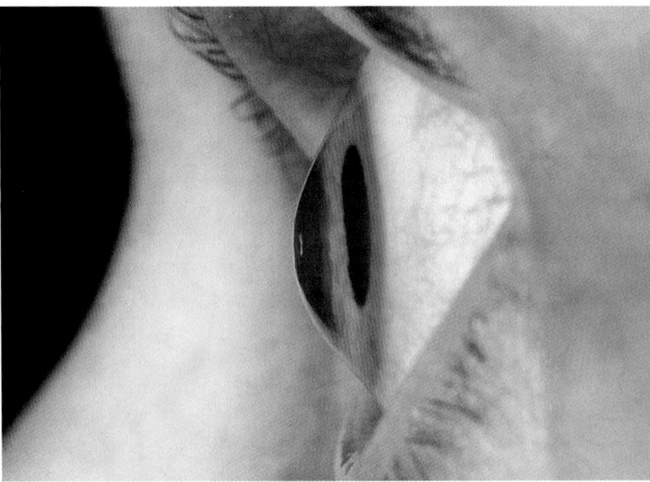

Figure 15.21 Corneal profile: keratoconus with moderate distension and a central apex

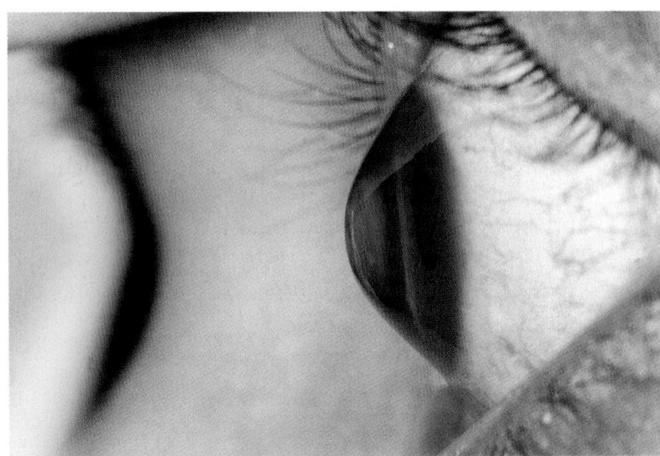

Figure 15.22 Corneal profile: keratoconus with medium distension and a central apex

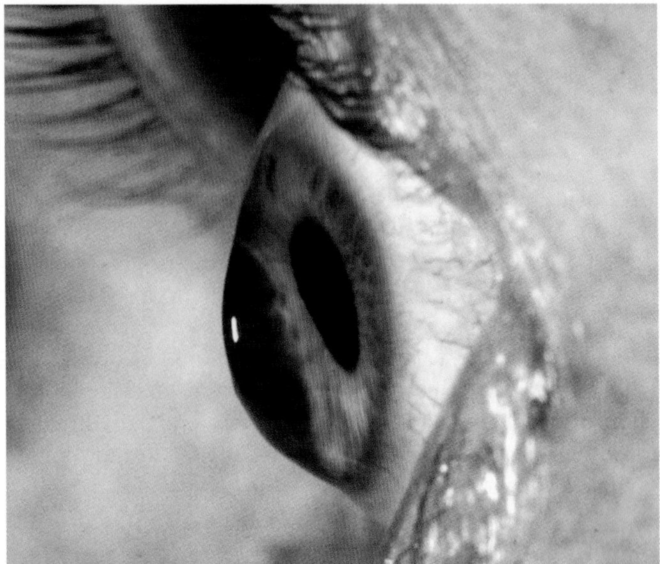

Figure 15.23 Corneal profile: keratoconus with moderate distension and a downwardly decentred apex

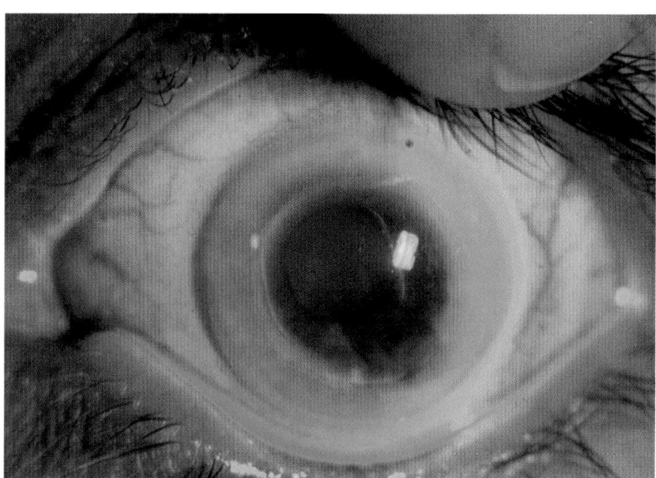

Figure 15.24 Non-ventilated RGP scleral lens in situ with a compressive central corneal contact zone

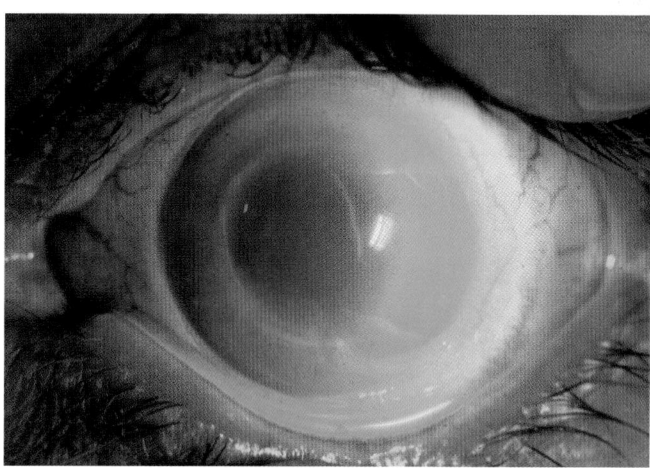

Figure 15.26 Same eye as seen in Figures 15.24 and 15.25 wearing a non-ventilated RGP scleral lens in situ with full corneal clearance

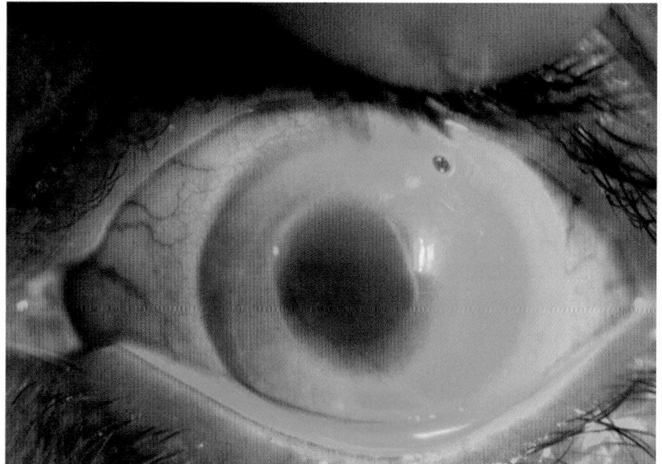

Figure 15.25 Same eye as seen in Figure 15.24 wearing a non-ventilated RGP scleral lens in situ with a glancing central corneal contact zone

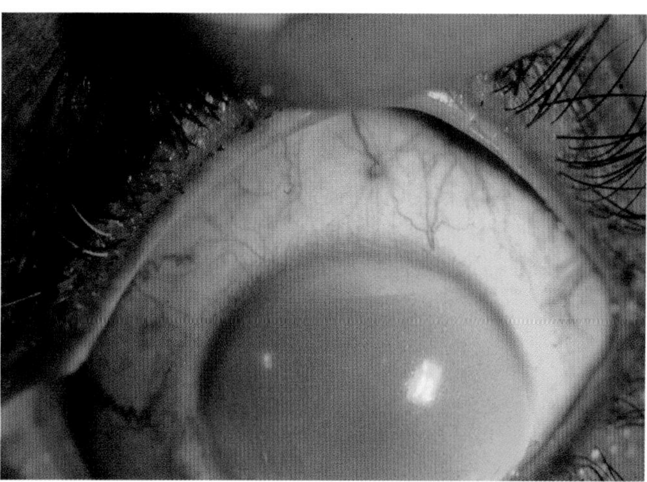

Figure 15.27 Non-ventilated RGP scleral lens in situ with a circumferential limbal contact zone

ASSESSMENT OF CORNEAL CONTACT AND CLEARANCE

Contact zones are designated:

- Compressive if the cornea conforms significantly to the shape of the lens for the duration of lens wear.
- Glancing if there is no or minimal change to corneal topography.

Figures 15.24, 15.25 and 15.26 illustrate the difference between optic zone clearance increments of 0.24 and 0.48 mm, where the latter provides corneal clearance. The depth of the precorneal reservoir can be estimated by comparing it to corneal thickness, using an optical section on a slit-lamp. It is more difficult to assess by how much the OZP or sag should be increased to give clearance if the first trial lens is in contact with the cornea.

VARYING LIMBAL CLEARANCE

It may be necessary to increase the limbal clearance independently – for example, if there is a circumferential limbal contact as in Figure 15.27. Figure 15.28 shows a lens with 0.25 mm increase in the limbal OZP but an unchanged apical OZP, diagrammatically represented in Figure 15.29. Increasing the limbal clearance removes some substance from the scleral zone, so may lead to more settling, with a possible small reduction in apical clearance.

ENDPOINT TO THE FITTING PROCESS

Between 0.20 and 0.30 mm apical corneal clearance with the scleral zone optimally aligned usually allows an air-free precorneal reservoir with non-ventilated lenses. By comparison, 0.10 mm is the maximum that would retain fluid coverage with fenestrated lenses. Pachometry is not necessary as the depth of the precorneal fluid reservoir is sufficiently estimated in comparison to the corneal thickness. Figure 15.30 illustrates a precorneal fluid reservoir with an RGP scleral lens in situ. It is possible that corneal contact over the visual axis may regularize the corneal surface and improve the acuity, but corneal

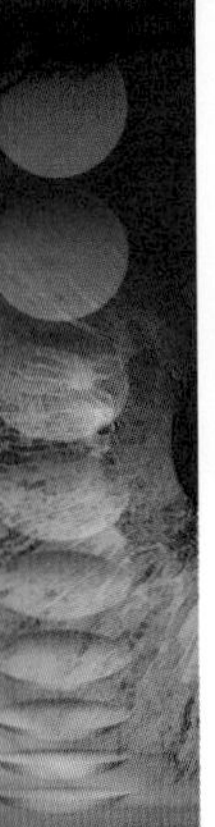

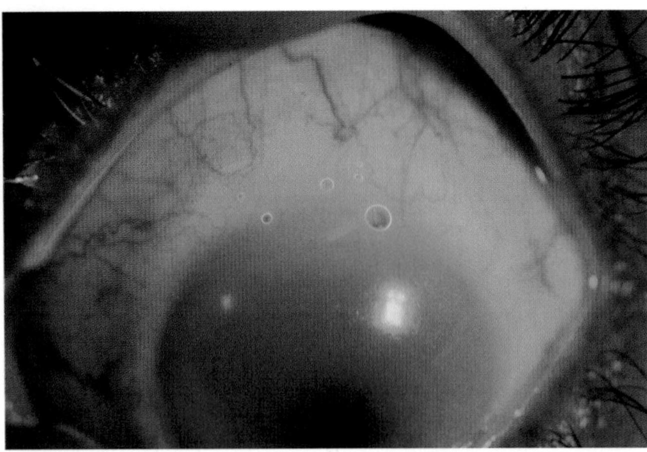

Figure 15.28 Same eye as seen in Figure 15.27 showing a lens designed to give a 0.25 mm increase in the limbal optic zone projection (OZP) but an unchanged apical OZP. The small glancing apical contact zone is due to some settling back because the limbal bearing surface has been eased, but the increase in the limbal clearance is a greater amount

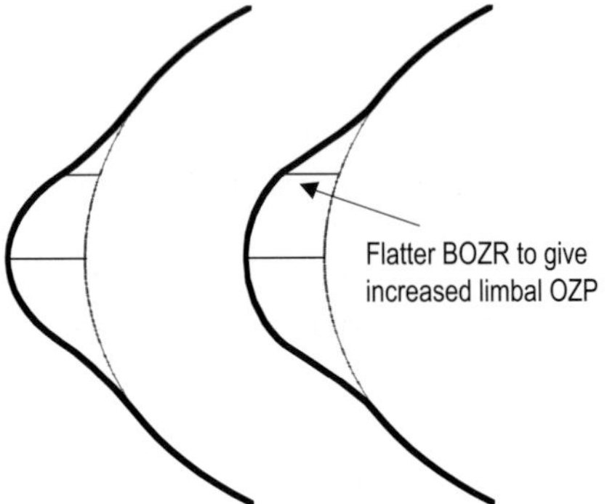

Figure 15.29 A redesigned lens giving an increased limbal optic zone projection (OZP) but an unchanged apical OZP

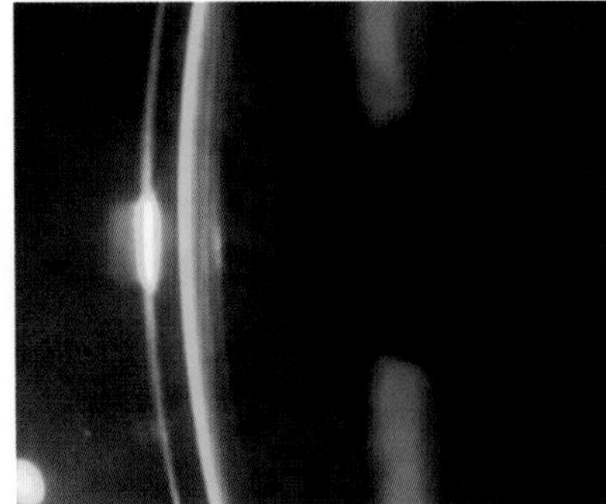

Figure 15.30 Scleral lens in situ. Optical section showing the front surface of the lens, the fluoresceinated precorneal fluid reservoir and the cornea. The precorneal fluid reservoir is about the same thickness as the cornea; ideally, it should be more like half the thickness of the cornea, i.e. approximately 0.25 mm. (Courtesy of Paolo Formichella)

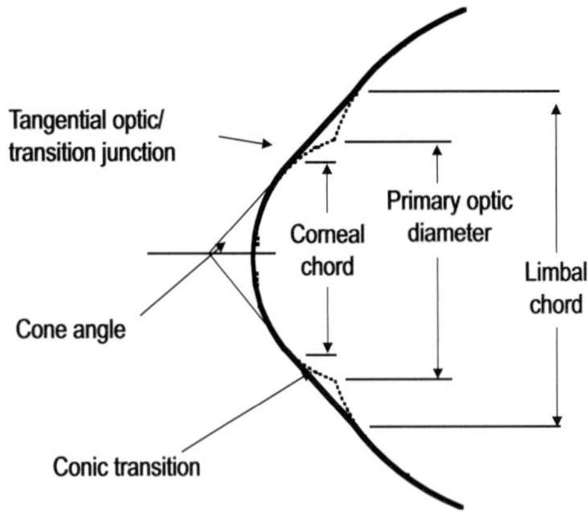

Figure 15.31 Principle of the wide-angle design illustrating the spherical optic and scleral zones with a conic transition and a tangential optic zone/transition zone junction

clearance is usually better tolerated. At a later stage, it may be appropriate to reduce the clearance to improve vision.

Traditional fenestrated preformed scleral lenses

There are some occasions when traditional fenestrated PMMA lenses are necessary but, as previously discussed, there is much less latitude for corneal clearance. The BOZR, BOZD and BSR all influence the fitting processes and, if these are assessed simultaneously, large numbers of lenses would be required to cover all the permutations. The scleral and optic zones can be assessed separately but the outcome is more predictable with simultaneous fitting.

SIMULTANEOUS FITTING WITH WIDE-ANGLE LENSES

Wide-angle lenses (Cowan 1948) are a successful way to simplify simultaneous preformed fitting and are suitable for many normal topographies. The system is straightforward and quick to fit and has been used for over 50 years.

The terms corneal and limbal chords are used rather than BOZD, referring to the optic/transition junction and the transition/scleral junction. The transition is a conic section, designed to be tangential at the corneal chord. Figure 15.31 illustrates the principle of the wide-angle design. The BOZR range from 7.50 to 9.00 mm, with 8.25–8.75 mm the most commonly used. The diameter can vary but the standard fitting diameter is 23 mm round with some 23 × 21 mm oval lenses. Table 15.1 lists the parameters for a comprehensive wide angle set (those in bold showing a scaled-down set).

Selection of first wide-angle lens

- A mid-range BOZR of 8.50 mm is chosen, or 8.75 mm for flatter corneas.
- The initial BSR is 13.50 mm.
- When assessing the scleral zone, the back optic surface should be clear of the cornea.
- The apical clearance is increased or decreased by steepening or flattening the BOZR.

Table 15.1: A comprehensive wide-angle fitting set with 30 lenses

BSR (mm)			BOZR (mm)		
12.50	8.00	8.25	8.50		
12.75	8.00	8.25	8.50		
13.00	8.00	8.25	8.50	8.75	
13.25	8.00	8.25	8.50	8.75	9.00
13.50	**8.00**	**8.25**	**8.50**	**8.75**	**9.00**
13.75		8.25	8.50	8.75	9.00
14.00			8.50	8.75	9.00
14.25			**8.50**	**8.75**	**9.00**

- If a lens from the fitting set does not provide the final parameters, intermediate variants can be made.
- If altering parameters is still unsuccessful, preformed fitting is probably not possible, and an impression may be preferable.

SEPARATE OPTIC AND SCLERAL ZONE FITTING

Although a major section in previous texts, the author's view is that separating the scleral and optic zones is too complex and unpredictable for a mainstream technique. However, a brief outline follows.

Fenestrated lenses for optic measurement (FLOMs)

The optimum BSR is determined by inspection of scleral shells with a range of radii, designed with the optic well clear to eliminate corneal contact. FLOMs (Bier 1948) are not intended for issue and may be quite uncomfortable, so a topical anaesthetic may be necessary.

These lenses are made up of:

- A narrow 2 mm scleral zone to exclude vaulting.
- An intentionally unblended transition to give a precise BOZD.
- A fenestration at the limbus.
- A BOZR range of 8.00–9.50 mm and BOZD of 13.0–14.75 mm, both in 0.25 mm increments, usually omitting the flat radii with small diameters and steep radii with large diameters.

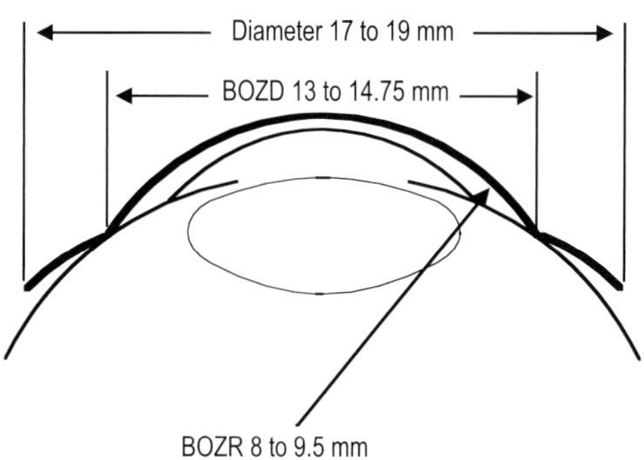

Figure 15.32 A FLOM in situ. The scleral zone is narrow and flat to avoid any excessive optic zone clearance due to scleral zone vaulting

Figure 15.32 illustrates a FLOM in situ, and Table 15.2 shows the parameter range of a FLOM fitting set.

The first trial FLOM

- Choose a middle of the range lens – for example, 8.50 mm BOZR/13.75 mm BOZD (8.50/13.75) or 0.25 mm steeper or flatter, depending on corneal curvature.
- BOZD should be approximately 2.0 mm larger than the horizontal visible iris diameter (HVID).
- Insert the lens and instil fluorescein to observe the depth and extent of the precorneal reservoir.
- The ideal appearance is fluid coverage over the whole cornea, not exceeding 0.10 mm in depth, extending 2 or 3 mm beyond the HVID with a mobile crescent-shaped bubble.
  - too much apical clearance traps a spherical air bubble behind the lens.
  - correct apical clearance with excessive limbal clearance gives a bubble extending too far around the limbus.
  - insufficient limbal clearance may give an annular contact at the limbus.

Alteration of BOZR and BOZD independently

- A steeper BOZR increases the apical clearance by approximately twice as much as if the BOZD is increased by the same amount.
- Steepening the BOZR with a constant BOZD increases apical clearance, but the limbal clearance is unaffected.

Table 15.2: Specifications for a FLOM fitting set

BOZR (mm)				BOZD (mm)				
8.00	13.00	13.25						
8.25	13.00	13.25	13.50	13.75	14.00			
8.50	13.00	13.25	13.50	13.75	14.00	14.25		
8.75	13.00	13.25	13.50	13.75	14.00	14.25	14.50	
9.00		13.25	13.50	13.75	14.00	14.25	14.50	14.75
9.25			13.50	13.75	14.00	14.25	14.50	14.75
9.50							14.50	14.75

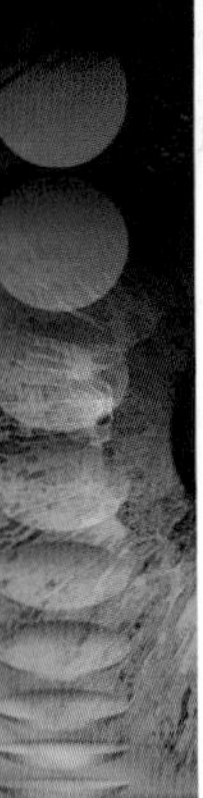

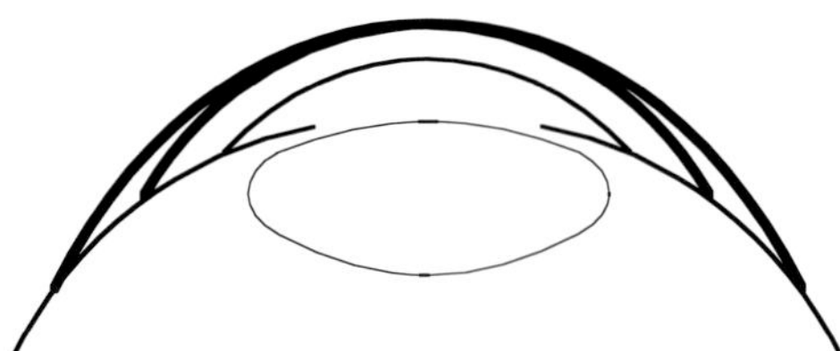

Figure 15.33 Clinically equivalent FLOMs (optic zones only) with equal apical but an increased limbal clearance when the BOZR is flattened

- Increasing the BOZD with a constant BOZR increases both apical clearance and depth and extent of the limbal clearance.

Alteration of BOZR and BOZD simultaneously

- Changing the BOZR and BOZD together may be additive or subtractive.
- A steeper BOZR with a larger BOZD gives a large increase in clearance.

Clinical equivalents (e.g. 8.50/13.50 and 8.75/14.00) give an unchanged apical clearance, but the limbal clearance is greater with the lens having the larger diameter. Figure 15.33 shows two clinical equivalent FLOMs.

Limitations of FLOM fitting

- Changing the BOZR alone gives a precisely calculable change to the clearance.
- BOZD changes, including clinical equivalents, are dependent on a poorly measurable scleral curvature.
- The settling and decentration characteristics with a FLOM and a finished lens are different as the bearing surfaces are dissimilar and any scleral vaulting of the finished lens cannot be estimated by the appearance of a FLOM.

Unless the practitioner has sufficient experience to estimate the final parameters prior to inspection of the trial lenses in situ, the chances of successfully combining the optic and scleral zones in the finished lens are not high.

EYE IMPRESSIONS

Eye impressions enable fabrication of the optic zone according to the individual corneal topography and are not subject to influence from the fit of the scleral zone, which is aligned whatever the scleral contour.

Impression materials

Polyvinyl siloxanes (PVS), such as Panasil Contact Plus, and dental alginates, such as Orthoprint (Zhermack), separate easily from moist surfaces, so can be used for eye impressions.

The base compound of PVS is mixed with a hardener to initiate the gelling process. There is little deterioration during storage, and no effect with humidity. The impression retains its shape indefinitely, so can be cast in stone at a later time, or can be re-cast. Products are presented in kit form with tubes of the two

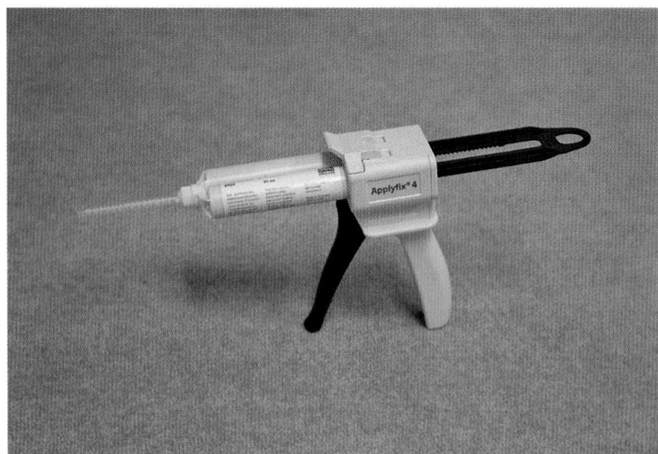

Figure 15.34 Polyvinyl siloxane (Panasil) mixing equipment. (Courtesy of Panadent Ltd)

components forming a single cartridge which fits into a mixing device (Fig. 15.34) to produce a perfectly homogeneous paste.

Alginate is less commonly used, mainly because once a packet is opened, it begins to degrade, slowing down the gelling process and reducing the quality of the final impression. Gelling is accelerated by high ambient humidity, sometimes reaching completion before the material has covered the eye. Once removed from the eye, casting with dental stone is required immediately because an alginate impression begins to dehydrate in a few minutes.

The alginate powder is mixed with the appropriate amount of distilled water and spatulated until it forms a paste which gels after 30–40 seconds. Some alginates are unsuitable because of additives such as peppermint.

Taking the impression

- The impression of the cornea must be reasonably well centred, but with a wider scleral portion superiorly and temporally.
- The patient should be seated, with a straight back and head upright.
- Two or three drops of topical anaesthetic are instilled into the conjunctival sac.
- To ensure correct positioning during moulding, just before the impression material is applied, the patient establishes fixation with the fellow eye, so that the eye to be moulded is looking slightly in and down from the primary position.
- The largest impression tray (Fig. 15.35) that can be inserted easily is selected, marked at the top with R or L and cleaned.
- The tray is charged with mixed PVS material, inserted under the upper lid and the lower lid is everted over the edge of the tray.
- Once under both lids, rotating the tray spreads the impression material which gels after approximately 30–40 seconds.

Gelling alginate has a less sticky texture than PVS so can be transferred to a 10 ml syringe and injected continuously through the tubular handle of the tray. The extremities of the

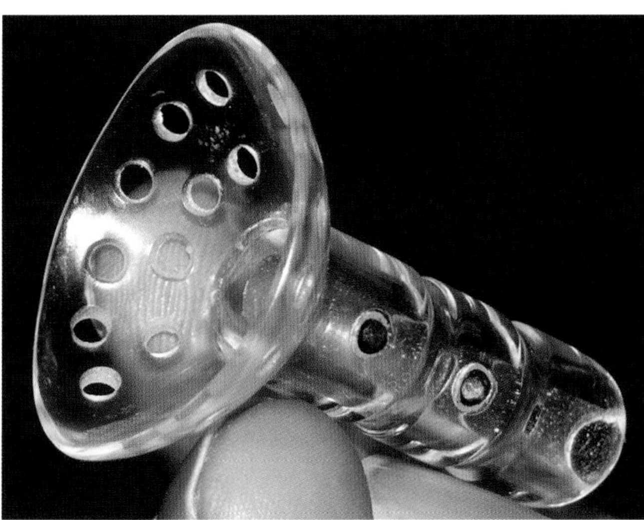

Figure 15.35 Impression tray

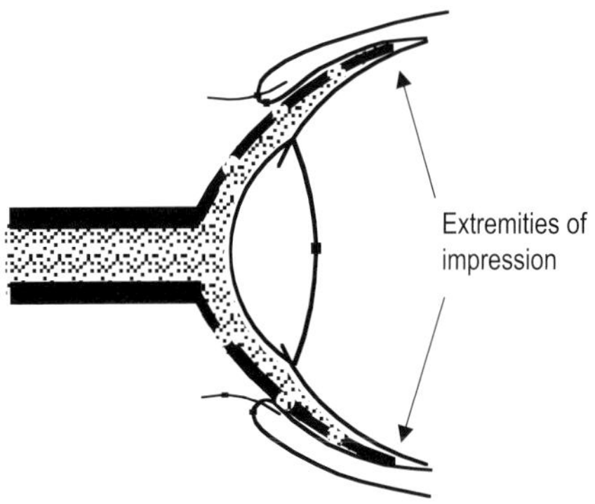

Figure 15.36 The extremities of the tray rest on the sclera, allowing maximum coverage of the ocular surface. The impression material extrudes through the holes in the tray to lock it in position

tray rest on the sclera, allowing maximum coverage of the ocular surface, as in Figure 15.36. Holding the tray slightly away from the globe and moving it up, down, left and right as the plunger is pressed helps spreading over the ocular surface. Gelling is accelerated by high ambient humidity, sometimes reaching completion before the material has covered the eye.

Before removing the tray, the top should be re-marked and excess material removed from the lids. The lower lid is pulled down below the impression and gently pressed underneath the cast to relieve the suction, allowing the impression to slide out.

Inspection of the cornea using the slit-lamp and fluorescein reveals any abrasions or punctate epithelial stain. If significant, a prophylactic antibiotic may be indicated. The conjunctival sac should be examined for any residual particles of impression material which can be flushed out with irrigation.

Casting

A ratio of approximately 1:5 of cold water and dental stone powder are mixed together in a flexible bowl to give a homogeneous cream from which a cast of the impression is made. Agitating helps to eliminate air bubbles. A PVS impression retains its shape indefinitely, so can be cast in dental stone at leisure, but alginate dehydrates after a few minutes so must be cast immediately. The stone is set after about 1 hour when it can be separated from the impression, identified with the patient's name, and the top marked R or L. Surplus material and conjunctival folds or vessels recorded on the cast are removed by scraping lightly with a plaster knife. A plaster of Paris base is added to the base of the cast afterwards to provide a solid foundation.

Production of impression lenses

In the past, it was preferable for as much handwork as possible to be carried out on impression shells by practitioners or under their immediate supervision so that the effect of any modification could be seen immediately. While this is still ideal, it is not practical. Few practitioners have the necessary skills or equipment, and it is more appropriate to preserve the technical skills in the manufacturing sector. However, for practitioners who wish to modify their own lenses, this is described in Chapter 28. Practitioner modification saves multiple appointments and can be done in small steps to assess the effect of each modification.

Impression scleral lenses can be PMMA or RGP materials. Ventilation must be provided, by means of a fenestration, a channel or a slot in PMMA lenses, otherwise hypoxia can occur within a few minutes of wear.

RGP lenses can be either ventilated or non-ventilated, although non-ventilated is the more straight forward option. Both require a well-fitting PMMA lens for duplication as the first stage in the process.

NON-VENTILATED IMPRESSION RGP SCLERAL LENSES

A PMMA trial shell with a well-aligned scleral zone provides a bubble-free fluid reservoir. Substance is removed as evenly as possible over the optic zone to give clearance of approximately 0.20–0.30 mm. This may be the final shape for duplication in an RGP material, but further optic zone substance can easily be removed if necessary.

FENESTRATED IMPRESSION RGP SCLERAL LENSES

Elderly or disabled patients may find it impossible to insert an air-free non-ventilated RGP lens. Fenestrated lenses can be inserted with the head upright. Impression fitting is more likely to provide a good outcome because the starting point is nearly the exact corneal contour rather than an approximation, making the exclusion of air bubbles behind the lens more likely. Fabrication is a skilled process and varies according to the topography of the individual eye.

For a topographically normal eye, a PMMA shell is made with 0.15 mm removed uniformly from the optic zone. If the lens is being made for an irregular cornea, the trial shell should be ground to remove substance as evenly as possible over the optic zone, removing just the bare minimum

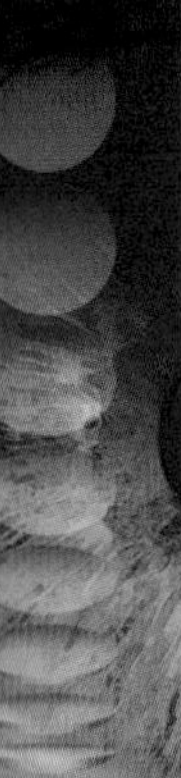

substance from the very centre. After assessing the fit of the shell, further substance can be ground out to give the optimum clearance.

If the apical clearance is excessive with a fenestrated impression lens, the space fills with air. An optimally fitting non-ventilated lens has greater clearance, so the chances of a satisfactory result simply from fenestrating are not great.

ORDERING SCLERAL LENSES

Preformed lens

For a preformed scleral lens of 'traditional' style, the practitioner should specify the following:

- BOZR.
- Primary BOZD.
- BSR.
- Optic zone displacement (D).
- Back scleral size (BSS), which is independent of the thickness.
- BVP.
- A transition curve to soften the optic/scleral junction – the practitioner should allow the manufacturer to select the optimum design.
- Size and position of fenestration.

Wide-angle lenses are manufactured to a predetermined design, so require just the BOZR, BSR, BSS, D and BVP.

RGP scleral lens ordering post-dates the latest BSI terminology document. It has become more usual for manufacturers to have their own ordering system which should be followed to avoid errors. Usually, this includes:

- Optimum lens used from the set, the specifications of which are known to the manufacturer.
- Power formula details, in most cases obtained following a refraction over the trial lens.
- Any variations from the trial set parameters.

Impression shells

- A cast of an impression, or a shell pressed over the cast, can be sent to a competent laboratory from which a moulded lens can be made. The manufacturer should be given full freedom to produce the back surface.
- The BSS is indicated by drawing a line on the cast.
- The back surface is fabricated by lightly grinding, with diamond-coated spherical stones, onto the back surface of the shell. The optimum is reached by a skilled trial and error process, after which the shell should be inspected in situ. The practitioner is not necessarily in a position to decide on the correct tools, or combination, to be used.
- A power formula should be provided, i.e. the result of a refraction over a scleral lens or a large-diameter corneal lens of known BOZR and BVP. The manufacturer can then make the appropriate power allowance for the difference between the calculated BOZR and that of the final lens.

SOLUTIONS AND MAINTENANCE OF SCLERAL LENSES

Storage

Both PMMA and RGP scleral lenses can be stored dry. Where enhanced surface wetting is necessary, lenses can be soaked in soft lens multipurpose solutions (MPS). These are better than the more viscous rigid lens soaking solutions.

Cleaning and conditioning

Rigid lens conditioning solutions can be used but if the lenses are non-ventilated, there is little tear exchange, so viscous solutions remain in contact with the cornea for much longer than when corneal lenses are worn. This may lead to an accumulative sensitivity to the preservatives. Many scleral lens wearers prefer a non-preserved cleaner rather than a conditioning solution, and rinse with non-preserved saline prior to insertion. Cleaners containing isopropyl alcohol appear to be significantly more effective.

Filling solutions for RGP non-ventilated scleral lenses

Non-preserved saline is necessary for filling non-ventilated RGP lenses prior to insertion. Because the solution is retained in contact with the cornea for the duration of wear, some wearers are sensitive to the buffer in preservative-free multidose saline, so unit dose preparations are preferable. Aerosol saline tends to be too gassy and appears to sting more than unit dose saline.

Rewetting

If lenses need refreshing during the day, soft lens MPS may be beneficial. The cleaning action is not as powerful as dedicated cleaners, but they are more eye compatible and easier to rinse off before reinsertion.

SCLERAL LENSES IN PATHOLOGICAL CONDITIONS

Scleral lenses have a particularly important place in the management of some pathological conditions with irregular corneal topography, for high refractive errors and in the management of ocular surface disease (OSD). Figure 15.37 shows the breakdown of recent indications for scleral lens assessment at a scleral lens clinic at Moorfields Eye Hospital, London.

Keratoconus and other primary corneal ectasia (PCE)

Keratoconus provides over 50% of the total referrals for scleral lens fitting (see Fig. 15.37). Primary corneal ectasia (PCE) describes conditions where there has been a dystrophic corneal thinning and distension.

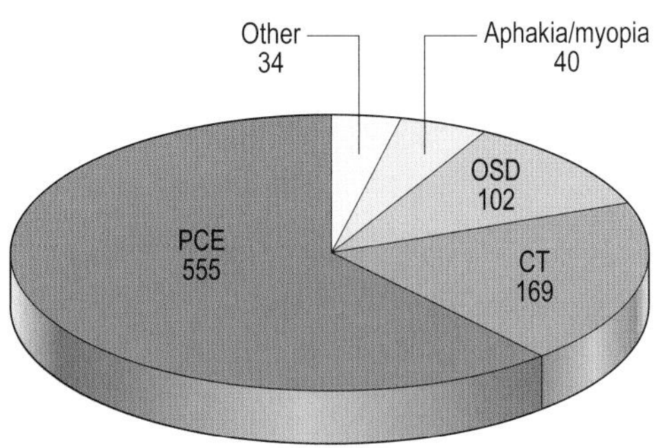

Figure 15.37 A breakdown of the indications for 570 patients (900 eyes) continuing scleral lens wear seen at after-care consultations between 1999 and 2004

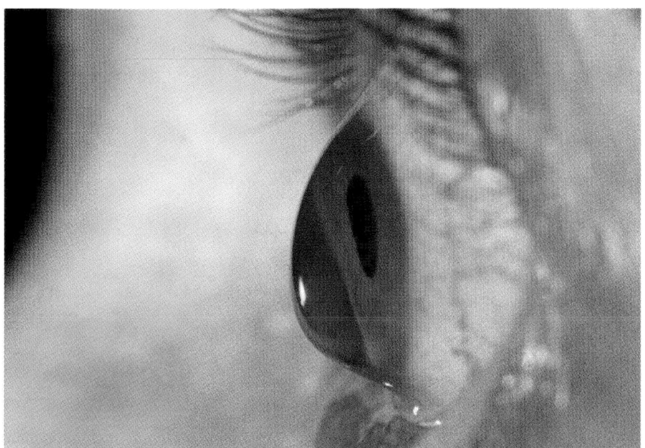

Figure 15.38 Primary ectasia with downwardly decentred apex, otherwise referred to as pellucid marginal degeneration

TOPOGRAPHICAL CLASSIFICATION BY EXAMINATION OF THE CORNEAL PROFILE

An appreciation of the corneal profile is essential for scleral lens practice. The projection of the cornea from the scleral plane and any displacement of the apex can be seen by retracting the eyelids.

- An area of thinning in the central third of the cornea gives rise to a relatively symmetrical protrusion of the affected cornea with a central apex (see Figs 15.21, 15.22).
- Figure 15.23 illustrates the topography when the ectasia is mid-peripheral and displaced downwards.
- Pellucid marginal dystrophy is an ectasia affecting the periphery of the cornea (Fig. 15.38, and Fig. 15.39 with a non-ventilated RGP scleral lens in situ) with flat central curvature.
- Keratoglobus is consequent to a larger area of thinning in the central region; advanced cases may be almost hemispherical (Fig. 15.40). In spite of the massive corneal distension, keratoglobus can be the simplest to fit with scleral lenses because it is usually symmetrical (Fig. 15.41).

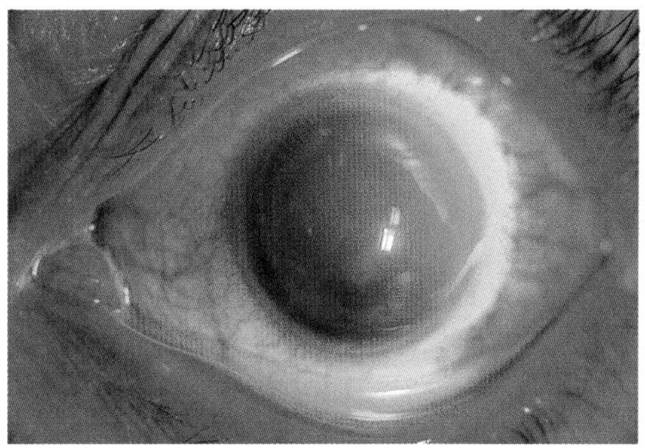

Figure 15.39 Same eye as seen in Figure 15.38 with a non-ventilated RGP scleral lens in situ. The optic zone is clear of the central cornea, and extending beyond the limbus, but with a glancing contact zone corresponding to the most prominent part of the cornea

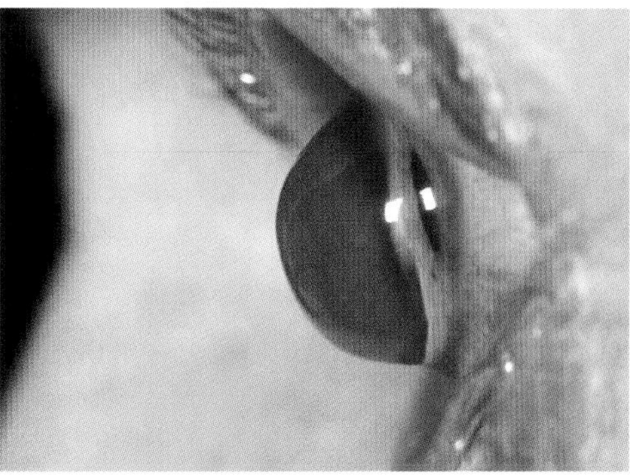

Figure 15.40 Keratoglobus corneal profile. The corneal profile is extremely protrusive, but almost hemispherical

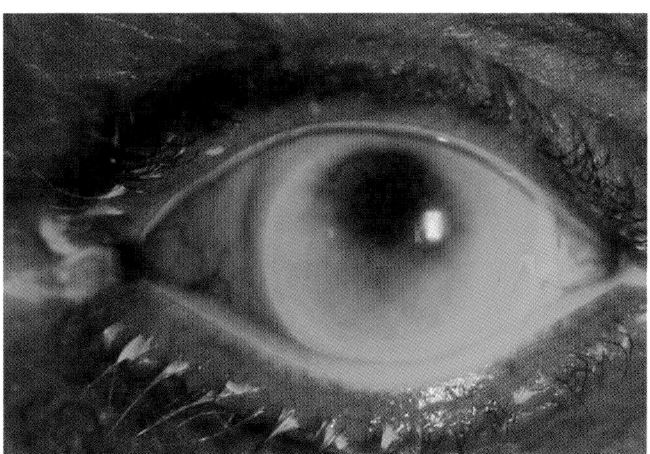

Figure 15.41 Same eye as seen in Figure 15.40 with a non-ventilated RGP scleral lens in situ. Note the contact zone corresponding to the central apex. This could be alleviated with an increased apical optic zone projection if considered necessary

Topographical mapping (see Chapter 7) is not of particular relevance in scleral lens practice. However, a view from the top and from the side of a keratoconic cornea cast in dental stone (Figs 15.42, 15.43) gives a striking illustration of the asymmetry sometimes encountered.

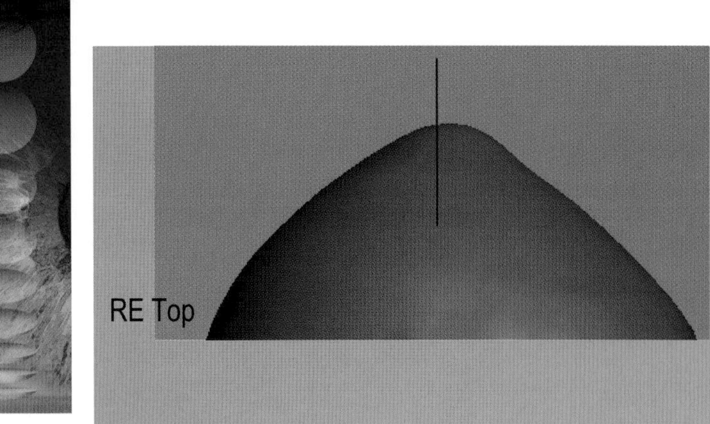

Figure 15.42 Cross-section of keratoconic cast, vertical meridian. The geometric centre of the cornea is indicated; note the downward displacement of the cone apex

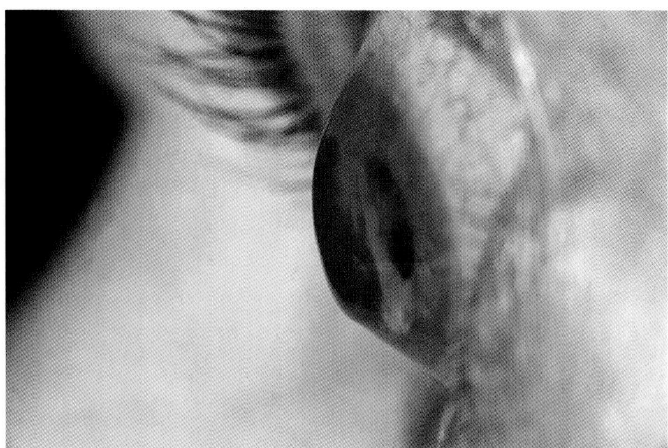

Figure 15.44 Post corneal transplant corneal profile. Donor survival over 20 years, but astigmatism over 20.00 DC

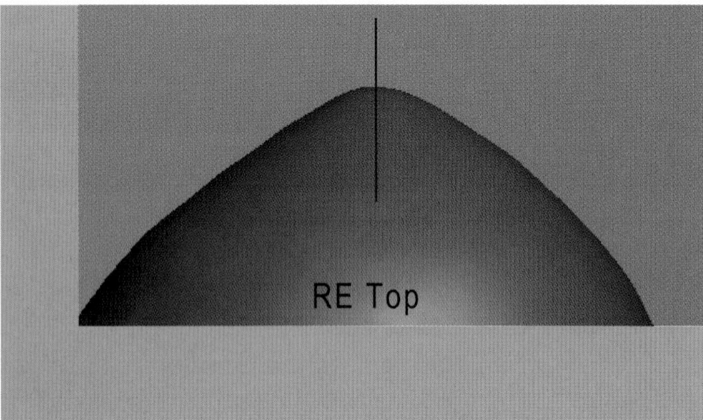

Figure 15.43 Cross-section of keratoconic cast, horizontal meridian. The cone apex is nearer the geometric centre of the cornea along the horizontal

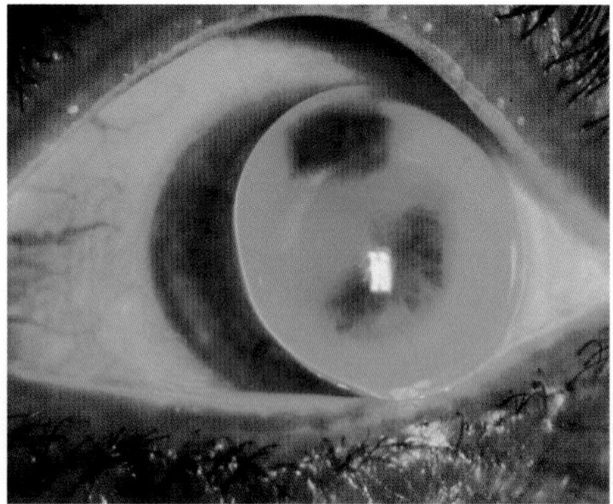

Figure 15.45 Same eye as seen in Figure 15.44 with an RGP corneal lens in situ. The astigmatism is corrected, but alignment with the cornea and centration is poor, giving rise to variable vision

INDICATIONS FOR SCLERAL LENSES IN PRIMARY CORNEAL ECTASIA

The alternative to corneal transplant

The prognosis of keratoplasty for advanced PCE is favourable, with studies indicating survival rates (i.e. a clear donor cornea) of over 95% for 5 years and 92% for 10 years (Williams et al. 1991, Thompson et al. 2003). However, for those with transplant rejections, the only option is repeat surgery with a higher risk of rejection. Furthermore, in the cases that survive, the level of success varies. The visual outcome may not be regarded as satisfactory if there is a high refractive error or uncorrectable astigmatism. It is crucial, therefore, that all contact lens management options, including scleral lenses, are available and fully investigated prior to surgery.

Vision should be measured with both eyes open. If the ectasia is bilateral, with poor acuity in the worse eye, it still may be worthwhile to correct that eye if there is some improvement in stereopsis or visual field gain (Sherafat et al. 2001).

Poor tolerance to corneal lenses

Scleral lenses should be considered before corneal lenses become unwearable, as RGP materials permit their use with less pathology than before. Tolerance of corneal lenses may be poor due to the extra mobility and greater peripheral clearance in keratoconus fitting. Alternating between scleral and corneal lenses can maximize wearing time.

Scleral lenses after corneal transplant

Continually improving surgical techniques, including post-transplant refractive surgery, have reduced the incidence of high corneal astigmatism, high refractive errors and protrusive corneal profiles. However, there can still be a considerable variation in the postoperative corneal topography. The donor cornea may shift forward at the time of removal of the sutures, even if they are left in place for over a year. Postoperative astigmatism in excess of 20 D still occurs occasionally and may not be sufficiently improved with refractive surgery. Corneal lenses fitted to transplanted corneas (e.g. on a 'plateau' type of topography), or if excessively toroidal, can be very mobile (Figs 15.44, 15.45).

In such cases, scleral lenses offer a good prospect of a satisfactory outcome. There is usually a greater symmetry about the visual axis compared to keratoconus, and even very high

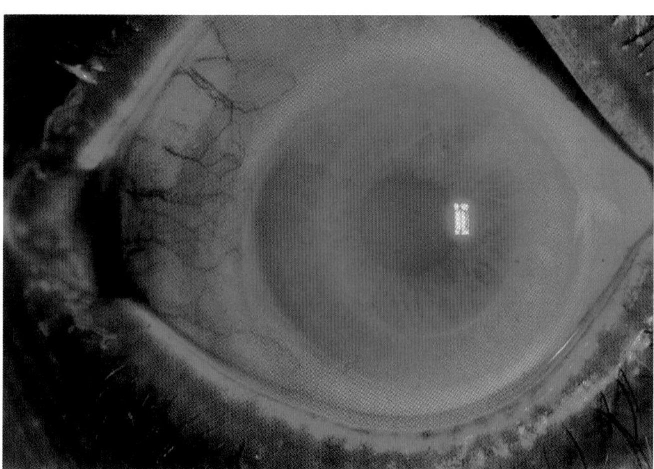

Figure 15.46 Same eye as seen in Figure 15.44 with a non-ventilated scleral lens in situ. Visual acuity is 6/9 with full corneal clearance

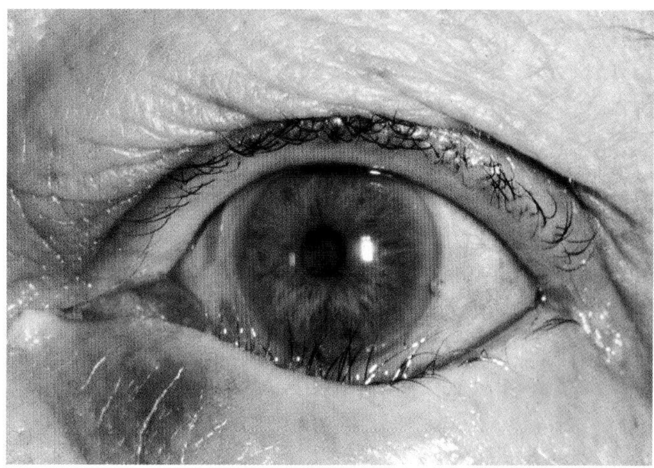

Figure 15.47 Age-related entropion and trichiasis with intermittent low-grade symptoms fitted with a fenestrated preformed PMMA scleral lens, worn as and when necessary to relieve the discomfort

postoperative astigmatism is often almost fully corrected with the precorneal fluid reservoir (Fig. 15.46).

Reduced levels of corneal oxygen may be a factor contributing to rejection after transplant surgery due to the reduction in endothelial cell density. Reduced postoperative corneal sensation may allow early subjective indications of oedema (i.e. discomfort) to pass unnoticed by the patient. Misty vision is an early symptom of rejection as well as being a symptom of contact lens hypoxia, so careful follow-up is necessary.

Management of aphakia and high myopia with scleral lenses

High myopia is usually well managed with corneal or hydrogel lenses. Aphakia is still an occasional contact lens indication when intraocular lenses are not implanted, especially after trauma (see Chapter 21). Extended-wear hydrogels are convenient but there is a well-documented risk of sight-threatening infection (see Chapter 13). Where problems occur with other lens types, the improved stability, simple maintenance and relative ease of handling of scleral lenses can be advantageous.

Established scleral lens wearers may not like the increased mobility and lid sensation of corneal lenses, or the more complex maintenance of hydrogel lenses, so continued supervision of scleral lens wear is necessary. From a clinical standpoint, there is no reason to change if there are no sight-threatening sequelae.

Elderly patients

- Many patients were successful with PMMA scleral lenses prior to the introduction of RGP materials.
- RGP non-ventilated scleral lenses are not without problems and, as discussed earlier, PMMA may be a satisfactory or even a better option for elderly aphakes and myopes.
- Spectacles are often satisfactory for sedentary activities, but scleral lenses may be useful when mobility is important, requiring short wearing spells only.
- Long-term contact lens-induced ocular changes are less of a problem as there is a shorter life expectancy.
- If the anterior ocular topography is regular, a preformed PMMA fenestrated lens may be a simple option and preferable to non-ventilated RGP scleral lenses for ease of handling.
- An impression may give a better result for aphakia because high positive powers may require precise positioning of the front optic over the visual axis.

Therapeutic and protective applications of scleral lenses

Scleral lenses play a unique therapeutic role for certain conditions because they cover the whole cornea while retaining a precorneal fluid reservoir (see also Chapter 26).

TRICHIASIS

A therapeutic soft lens used as a protective barrier may alleviate the problems from trichiasis but the lashes sometimes erode the surface or are forced under the lens. Scleral lenses provide effective protection without these drawbacks (Fig. 15.47), even after treatment with cryotherapy or electrolysis when scar tissue may still be uncomfortable.

SEVERE DRY EYE AND MUCOSAL DISEASE

In serious dry eye conditions, the tear quality may be so poor that the surface spoilation negates any beneficial effect from conventional therapeutic lenses. Retention of a precorneal fluid reservoir behind a scleral lens may be a more effective way to maintain corneal hydration. Such conditions include:

- Stevens–Johnson syndrome.
- Ocular cicatricizing pemphigoid.
- Chemical burns.

Patients with these conditions may all suffer from:

- Conjunctival dysfunction.
- Entropion.

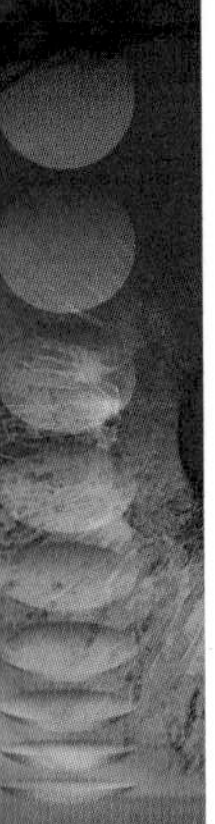

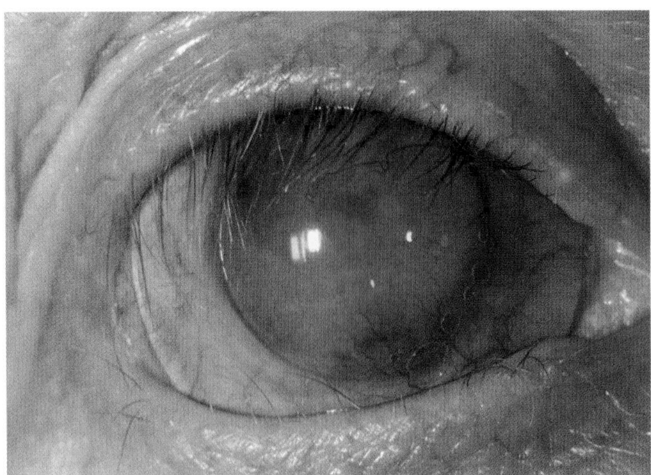

Figure 15.48 Aftermath of Stevens–Johnson syndrome. Non-ventilated scleral lens fitted to retain a precorneal fluid reservoir for corneal hydration and protection from misdirected and metastatic lashes

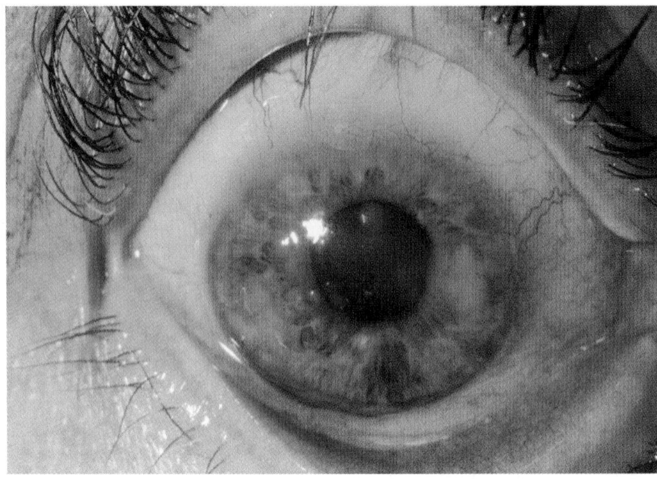

Figure 15.49 Salzmann's nodular dystrophy. The corneal surface is irregular with some nodules within the pupillary area giving rise to discomfort and impaired vision

- Trichiasis.
- Symblepharon.

Figure 15.48 shows the eye of a patient with Stevens–Johnson syndrome fitted with a scleral lens giving full corneal fluid coverage.

Other advantages of scleral lenses for therapeutic use

- The surface of an RGP lens is also subject to deterioration, but the lens can be cleaned or polished as necessary.
- A scleral lens also offers complete protection from the action of ingrowing or metastatic lashes emergent from the meibomian glands, and from keratinized lid margins, all of which are features of mucosal disorders.
- Shells or scleral rings may help prevent symblepharon reforming after surgical separation.

SUPERFICIAL CORNEAL DYSTROPHIES

Superficial corneal disorders – such as in Salzmann's nodular or lattice dystrophies – can be painful and visually debilitating. A scleral lens provides protection and neutralization of the ocular surface by means of the precorneal fluid reservoir behind the lens. Figure 15.49 shows an example of Salzmann's dystrophy and Figure 15.50 a non-ventilated scleral lens in situ.

CORNEAL EXPOSURE

Impaired lid closure disrupts the precorneal tear film and results in exposure keratitis. Scleral lenses may be the only way to provide fluid coverage and prevent evaporation.

The aetiology may be:

- Ectropion.
- Coloboma of the lid.
- Loss of lid tissue.
- Exophthalmos.
- Lid retraction after surgery.
- Neurological (e.g. VIIth nerve lesions).

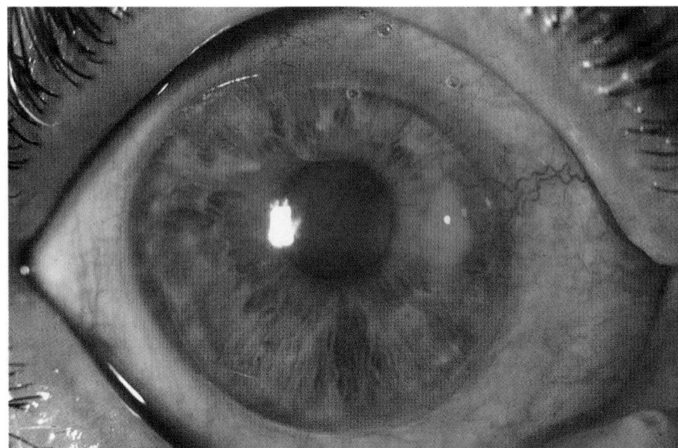

Figure 15.50 Same eye as seen in Figure 15.49 fitted with a non-ventilated scleral lens giving full corneal clearance. Ocular comfort and vision both significantly improved

NEUROTROPHIC KERATITIS

Loss of epithelium may occur as a consequence of degeneration of the nerve supply to the cornea (e.g. in diabetes). The precorneal fluid reservoir retained behind an RGP scleral lens may assist reformation in some cases. Figures 15.51 and 15.52 give an example of epithelial healing with a non-ventilated RGP lens.

An anaesthetic cornea is at risk of injury from foreign bodies lodging in the epithelium or tarsal plate. Scleral lenses give excellent protection but the patient will not report symptoms of discomfort and problems may arise without their knowledge.

OVERNIGHT WEAR OF THERAPEUTIC SCLERAL LENSES

Therapeutic soft lenses are often worn overnight for remedial purposes. Scleral lenses are usually advised for day wear only, with nocturnal application of ointment or lid taping. Patients are reluctant to follow this course of treatment, as the ointment is sticky and may clog the lens for much of the following day.

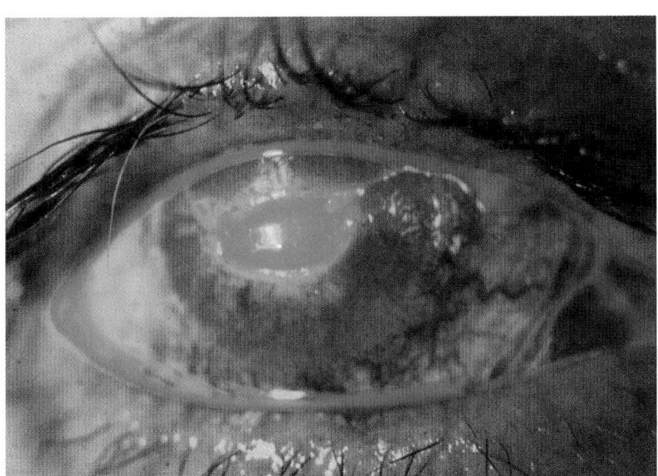

Figure 15.51 Neurotrophic corneal ulcer secondary to exposure in the aftermath of acoustic neuroma

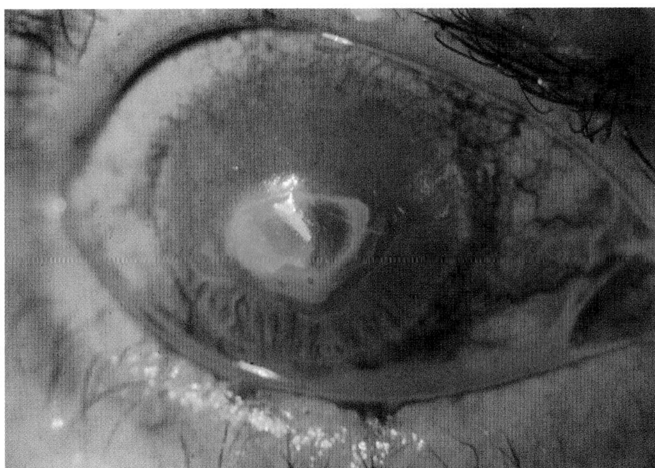

Figure 15.52 Neurotrophic ulcer seen in Figure 15.51 epithelializing following night and daytime non-ventilated RGP scleral lens wear

Overnight use of RGP scleral lenses may be indicated on occasions (Pullum & Buckley 1997, Cotter & Rosenthal 1998, Ramero-Rangel et al. 2000, Rosenthal et al. 2000, Tappin et al. 2001) but has been shown to generate more hypoxic response than for day wear (Smith et al. 2004). There must therefore be a justifiable reason for overnight protection or corneal hydration. However, if there is poor nocturnal lid closure, the hypoxia threat from a scleral lens worn overnight is considerably less since it is effectively an open eye situation. Some patients have normal lid closure during sleep and can be fitted with scleral lenses for daytime wear only.

It is necessary to remove a scleral lens for regular cleaning, so it is important that overnight wear is not confused with extended uninterrupted continuous wear.

PTOSIS

Ptosis may be present

- Following lid trauma.
- As a result of third nerve palsy.
- As part of general myasthenia gravis or in ocular myopathy when the condition is specific to the levator muscle.

A ledge can be cemented onto the front of a scleral lens or made by cutting through a thick shell to hold the upper lid open. Sometimes a second shelf may be added to rest on the lower lid to prevent lens depression (Fig. 15.53). A description of ptosis prop manufacture can be found in the fourth edition.

COSMETIC SHELLS

Cosmetic shells are time consuming to fit compared to cosmetic hydrogel lenses (see Chapter 25) but they last for many years and have virtually no maintenance costs. The whole anterior eye is covered and any iris and scleral features, such as conjunctival blood vessels, can be included for the best possible match with the fellow eye. The appearance of unsightly, phthisical eyes can be improved by building up the thickness of a cosmetic shell.

The exception to the general rule that shells are the best cosmetic option is if the eye is proptosed when the extra bulk may be unfavourable.

(a)

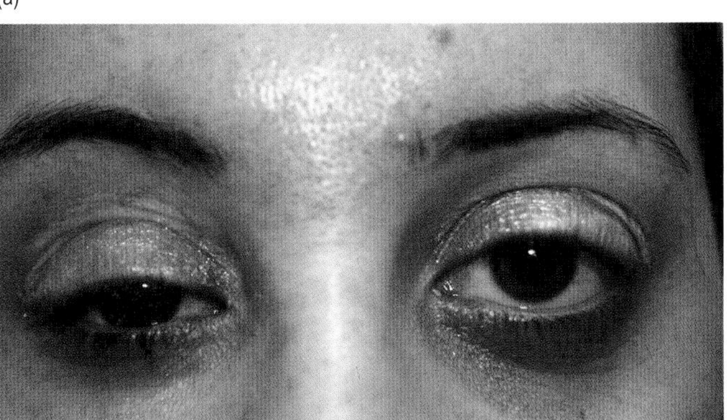

(b)

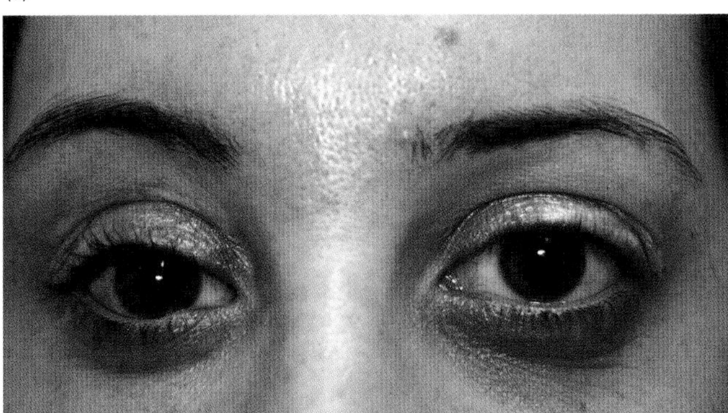

Figure 15.53 Young female adult with a right ptosis (a) fitted with a 1.5 mm thick RGP non-ventilated scleral lens providing a nearly 3 mm ptosis-propping effect (b). The normal thickness for a 23 mm diameter scleral lens is more like 0.8 mm

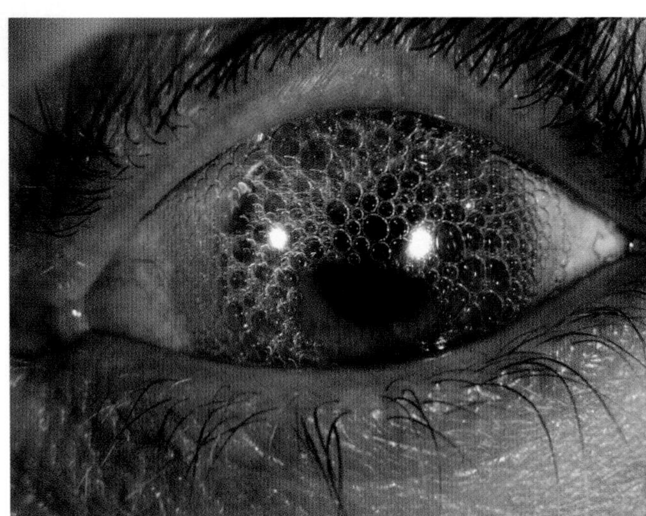

Figure 15.54 Frothy bubbles behind a non-ventilated RGP scleral lens. The indication was advanced keratoconus associated with learning difficulties. Surprisingly, the wearer was not particularly troubled by the bubbles, presumably because there was a significant visual gain

MINOR PROBLEMS WITH SCLERAL LENS WEAR

Bubbles

Elimination of air bubbles from behind the lens is not always possible, especially when the depth of the precorneal reservoir is not uniform. They may enter via non-aligned scleral zone sectors but rarely disappear without removing and reinserting the lens. Peripheral air bubbles cause reflections, but small frothy bubbles disrupt vision when they cross the visual axis (Fig. 15.54). If static, they lead to dimpling and localized corneal dehydration. In addition, clicking sounds can result from air bubbles entering the space behind the lens through fenestrations and can be very annoying.

A non-preserved viscous eye drop, such as Celluvisc (Allergan), used for filling prior to inserting, helps to reduce bubbles. If the lens is fenestrated, instilling the drop into the eye, just at the site of the fenestration, may solve the problem temporarily.

If the problem becomes so great that satisfactory wear is not possible, refitting is required. The following changes are necessary:

For a preformed lens

- Reducing corneal clearance, if there is scope, pushes the bubble towards the periphery.
- A flatter BSR improves the scleral zone seal by shifting the bearing surface onto the more symmetrical sclera closer to the limbus.
- Reducing the diameter may have the same effect.
- An eye impression may be necessary to improve alignment on the sclera.

For an impression lens

- If the lens is already fenestrated, another drilled into an area retaining a permanent bubble may reduce its size.

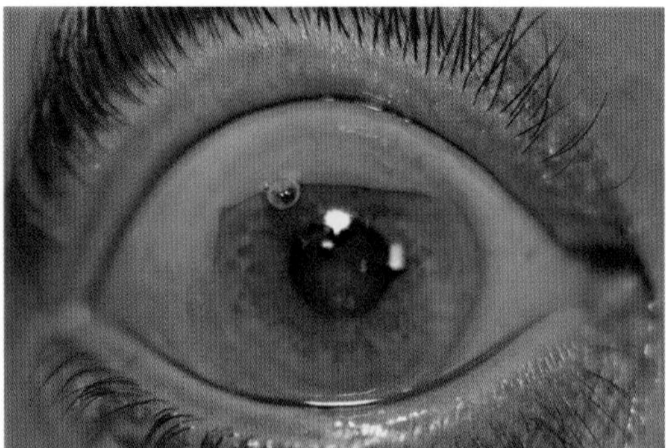

Figure 15.55 The conjunctiva is often displaced over the limbus during scleral lens wear. This does not constitute a serious complication as return to normality is immediate after removal of the lens

- Removal of substance from the whole of the scleral zone reduces the corneal clearance, but is only feasible if there is sufficient scleral zone substance.
- Remaking the lens with reduced optic zone clearance may be preferable.

Like many scleral lens modifications, the results are far from predictable.

Accumulation of mucus

Scleral lenses sometimes generate oversecretion of mucus which is trapped in the precorneal space. This is more of a problem with non-ventilated RGP lenses as there is some flushing action through a fenestration. Removal and reinsertion with fresh saline is necessary, and filling with Celluvisc (Allergan) appears to give an improvement in some cases. Instillation of mucolytic drops such as acetylcysteine before reinsertion may be an option, but consideration must always be given to the long corneal contact time.

Conjunctival hyperaemia

On lens removal, localized conjunctival hyperaemia may indicate an area of tight scleral zone fitting. The limbus should be watched carefully for early signs of limbal vessel engorgement, which may be the precursor of corneal neovascularization. However, some hyperaemia is not a threat and may be impossible to alleviate.

Conjunctival displacement over the limbus

Displacement of conjunctiva over the limbus and peripheral cornea can occur with scleral lenses, in particular non-ventilated RGP lenses, if there is insufficient limbal clearance (Fig. 15.55). It does not cause a serious problem but patients notice it when looking in a mirror.

Discomfort

Discomfort cannot always be completely eliminated from all types of contact lens. With scleral lenses it can be a consequence of:

- Apical corneal contact zones.
- Limbal occlusion.
- An ill-fitting scleral zone.
- An early symptom of corneal hypoxia in PMMA scleral lenses.

Settling back

Scleral lens fitting should be assessed both immediately after insertion and after a period of settling back. Use of non-ventilated RGP lenses reduces settling back, or makes the effect more manageable in comparison to PMMA fenestrated lenses.

COMPLICATIONS

Abrasions or corneal staining

Abrasions can be caused by clumsy insertion or central touch on a fragile corneal apex, especially with central contact in PCE. Unusual discomfort after a period of wear is an early symptom. The author's observations suggest there is more discomfort and corneal staining from contact zones with RGP materials than PMMA, probably due to greater friction between the lens and the corneal surface with no precorneal fluid reservoir. However, apical clearance can be achieved even in the most advanced cases with non-ventilated controlled clearance lenses but is more difficult to achieve with fenestrated lenses.

Corneal dehydration

Localized dehydration caused by static bubbles behind the lens can lead to epithelial desiccation. In some advanced cases there may be corneal neovascularization.

Exacerbation of corneal scarring

Corneal scarring may be exacerbated by corneal contact zones, but this is unproven as it is also an established part of the disease process of keratoconus (Krachmer et al. 1984, Zadnik et al. 1996). There is no reason why avascular scarring should jeopardize a future corneal transplant and in any case poor unaided vision precludes withdrawal of lenses in such cases.

Giant papillary conjunctivitis

Giant papillary conjunctivitis (GPC) does not often appear to cause the typical discomfort described by soft lens wearers, presumably because there is no tarsal plate/lens edge interaction and deposits are easily cleaned from rigid lens surfaces.

Hypoxic changes

Corneal neovascularization is the most serious complication of scleral lens wear. Discomfort due to corneal oedema may reduce the wearing time but the onset may be retarded after a period of adaptation. Misty vision is not necessarily obvious if there is concurrent pathology (e.g. from corneal or lenticular opacities).

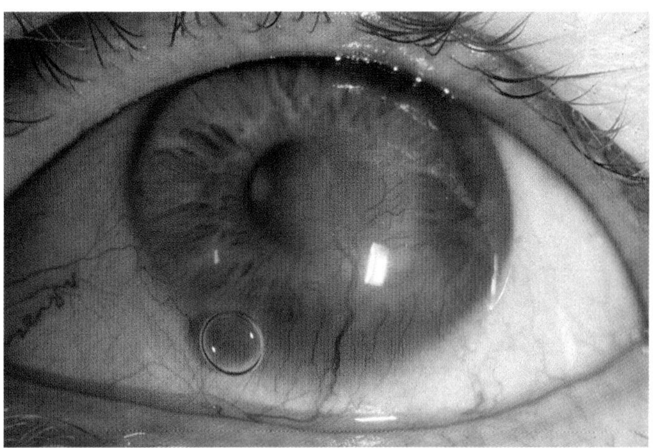

Figure 15.56 Corneal neovascularization following 40 years of a PMMA channelled scleral lens. The onset was very rapid, the patient reporting hazy vision in between after-care consultations, occurring in both eyes simultaneously. Although sight threatening, it must be remembered that prior to this event there had been 40 years of fully functional vision with no feasible alternative to a scleral lens

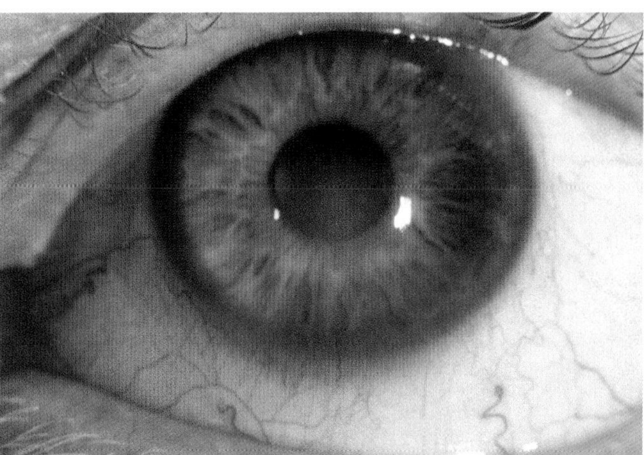

Figure 15.57 The eye in Figure 15.56 had been refitted with a non-ventilated RGP scleral lens as a matter of some urgency, and after 3 months the vascularization had regressed, leaving ghost vessels only. Some corneal haze remained, but the visual acuity recovered to 6/9, and has been retained at that level for 9 years with full daytime lens wear

Neovascularization

The long-term effect of chronic corneal oedema is corneal neovascularization, but a small amount may be an acceptable complication if there is no alternative management option. Neovascularization may be self-limiting or very slowly progressive and any changes may not be sight threatening for many years.

Hypoxia and consequent corneal neovascularization was a major problem with PMMA scleral lenses, but it has been significantly reduced with the introduction of RGP materials. In some cases, neovascularization caused by PMMA lenses can be reversed when refitted with RGP materials, leaving only ghost vessels (Figs 15.56, 15.57).

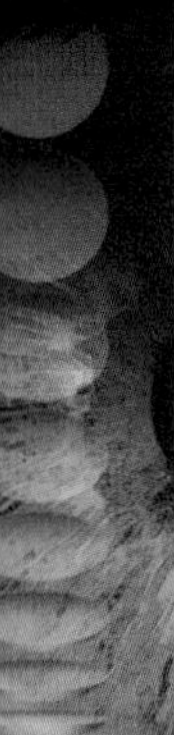

Neovascularization in PCE

The possible complications of contact lenses are insignificant compared to the possible consequence of the surgical alternatives, but neovascularization may increase the risk of any future corneal transplant rejection. This is particularly the case when the apex is eccentric, requiring a larger donor cornea which is in closer proximity to the limbal arcades. Most cones are decentred downwards and a common origin of major new vessels is from the inferior sector of the cornea. Careful monitoring is clearly essential.

Lipid keratopathy

New vessels *per se* do not necessarily cause visual loss but the vessels have a tendency to leak lipid, and can cause a dense opacity. Sudden-onset visual loss can occur even if the vessels are apparently quite fine in calibre. Some absorption is possible after a time, but the rate is slower for older patients.

CONCLUSION

Scleral lens application constitutes a very small percentage of all lens fittings, but they are often invaluable when other contact lenses are unsuccessful or when the patient faces potentially hazardous ocular surgery. It is vital to preserve the clinical skills in order to avoid discredit due to too many unsatisfactory results. A relatively small number of practitioners need to be actively involved but those who may not wish to undertake the work personally should still be familiar with the application of scleral lenses so that suitable patients can referred to a specialist.

References

Bier, N. (1948) The practice of ventilated contact lenses. Optician, 116, 497–501

Bleshoy, H. and Pullum, K. W. (1988) Corneal response to gas permeable impression scleral lenses. J. Br. Contact Lens Assoc., 11(2), 31–34

Cotter, J. and Rosenthal, P. (1998) Scleral contact lenses. J. Am. Optom. Assoc., 69, 33–40

Cowan, J. M. (1948) The wide angle contact lens. Optician, 115, 359

Ezekiel, D. (1983) Gas permeable haptic lenses. J. Br. Contact Lens Assoc., 6(4), 158–161

Ezekiel, D. F. (1991) Gas permeable scleral lenses. Spectrum, July, 19–24

Kok, J. H. C. and Visser, R. (1992) Treatment of ocular surface disorders and dry eyes with high gas-permeable scleral lenses. Cornea, 11, 518–522

Krachmer, J. H., Feder, R. S. and Benin, M. W. (1984) Keratoconus and related noninflammatory corneal thinning disorders. Surv. Ophthalmol., 28, 293–322

Lyons, C. J., Buckley, R. J., Pullum, K. W. and Sapp, N. (1989) Development of the gas-permeable impression-moulded scleral contact lens. A preliminary report. Acta Ophthalmol., 67(Suppl 192), 162–164

Marriott, P. J. (1966) An analysis of the global contours and haptic lens fitting. Br. J. Physiol. Opt., 23, 3–40

Mountford, J., Carkeet, N. and Carney, L. (1994) Corneal thickness changes during scleral lens wear: effect of gas permeability. ICLC , 21, 19–21

Pullum, K. W. (1997) The role of scleral lenses in modern contact lens practice. In Contact Lenses, 4th edn, pp. 566–608, eds. A. J. Phillips and L. Speedwell. Edinburgh: Butterworth-Heinemann

Pullum, K. W. and Buckley, R. J. (1997) A study of 530 patients referred for rigid gas permeable scleral contact lens assessment. Cornea, 16(6), 612–622

Pullum, K. W. and Stapleton, F. J. (1997) Scleral lens induced corneal swelling: what is the effect of varying Dk and lens thickness? CLAO J., 23(4), 259–263

Pullum, K. W., Parker, J. H. and Hobley, A. J. (1989) Development of gas permeable impression scleral lenses. The Josef Dallos Award Lecture, part one. Trans. BCLA Conference, 77–81

Pullum, K. W., Hobley, A. J. and Parker, J. H. (1990) Hypoxic corneal changes following sealed gas permeable impression scleral lens wear. The Josef Dallos Award Lecture, part two. J. Br. Contact Lens Assoc., 13(1), 83–87

Pullum, K. W., Hobley, A. J. and Davison, C. (1991) 100 + Dk: Does thickness make much difference? J. Br. Contact Lens Assoc., 6, 158–161

Pullum, K. W., Whiting, M. A. and Buckley, R. J. (2005) Scleral contact lenses: the expanding role. Cornea, 24(3), 269–277

Ramero-Rangel, T., Stavrou, P., Cotter, J. M., Rosenthal, P., Baltatzis, S. and Foster, C. S. (2000) Gas-permeable scleral contact lens therapy in ocular surface disease. Am. J. Ophthalmol., 130, 25–32

Rosenthal, P., Cotter, J. M. and Baum, J. (2000) Treatment of persistent corneal epithelial defect with extended wear of a fluid-ventilated gas-permeable scleral contact lens. Am. J. Ophthalmol., 130, 33–41

Ruben, C. M. and Benjamin, W. J. (1985) Scleral contact lenses: preliminary report on oxygen-permeable materials. Contact Lens, 13(2), 5–10

Schein, O. D., Rosenthal, P. and Ducharme, C. (1990) A gas-permeable scleral contact lens for visual rehabilitation. Am. J. Ophthalmol., 109, 318–322

Segal, O., Barkana, Y., Hourovitz, D. et al. (2003) Scleral contact lenses may help where other modalities fail. Cornea, 22(4), 308–310

Sherafat, H., White, J. E. S., Pullum, K. W., Adams, G. G. W. and Sloper, J. S. (2001) Anomalies of binocular function in patients with longstanding asymmetric keratoconus. Br. J. Ophthalmol., 85, 1057–1060

Smith, G. T. H., Mireskandari, K. and Pullum, K. W. (2004) Corneal swelling with overnight wear of scleral contact lenses. Cornea, 23(1), 29–34

Swann, P. G. and Mountford, J. (1999) Facial nerve palsy and scleral contact lenses. Br. J. Optom. Dispensing, 7, 85–87

Tan, D. T. H., Pullum, K. W. and Buckley, R. J. (1995) Medical applications of scleral contact lenses: 2. Gas-permeable scleral contact lenses. Cornea, 14(2), 130–137

Tappin, M. J., Pullum, K. W. and Buckley, R. J. (2001) Scleral contact lenses for overnight wear in the management of ocular surface disorders. Eye, 15, 168–172

Thompson, R. W. Jr, Price, M. O., Bowers, P. J. and Price, R. W. Jr. (2003) Long-term graft survival after penetrating keratoplasty. Ophthalmology, 110(7), 1396–1402

UK Vocabulary Standards (1988) Terms relating to ophthalmic lenses and spectacle frames. Part 3: Glossary of terms and symbols relating to contact lenses. BS 3521, Part 3. ISO 8320-1986

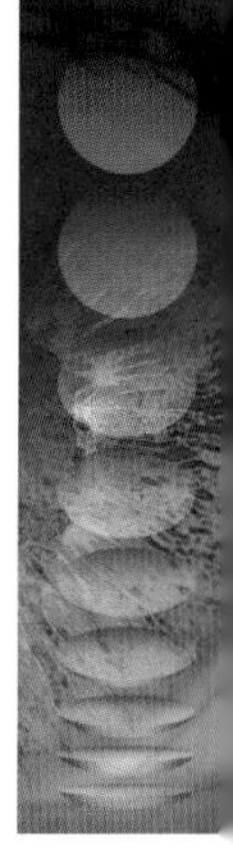

Visser R. (1990) Een nieuwe toekomst hoogzuurtofdoorlatende scleralenzen bij verschillende pathologie. Ned. Tijdschr. Optom. Contactol., 3, 10–14

Williams, K. A., Roder, D., Estermann, A., Muehlberg, S. M. and Coster, D. J. (1991) Factors predictive of corneal graft survival. Report from the Australian Corneal Graft Registry. Ophthalmology, 99, 403–414

Zadnik, K., Gordon, M. O., Barr, J. T. et al. (1996) Biomicroscopic signs and disease severity in keratoconus. Cornea, 15, 139–146

Chapter 16

Lens checking: soft and rigid

Wolfgang Cagnolati

CHAPTER CONTENTS

INTRODUCTION

Successful contact lens fitting requires the manufacture of high-precision contact lenses and the establishment of meaningful tolerances. Such tolerances are established by national and international standards organizations including the British Standards Institute (BSI), the American National Standards Institute (ANSI), Deutsches Institut für Normung (DIN), Comité Europeén de Normalisation (CEN) and the International Organization for Standardization (ISO).

Contact lens standards are drafted exclusively by ISO working groups before national working groups review them. Once an ISO standard has been passed, it will go through a predetermined process before being adopted as a CEN standard in Europe (Höfer 1999). Figure 16.1 outlines the relevant ISO/CEN standards development scheme.

The national and international standardization committees are made up of optometrists, ophthalmologists and other experts with a clinical background or experience in training and research.

Contact lens parameters must fall within individual tolerances, especially with the huge number of frequent-replacement lenses now available. Efron et al. (1999) investigated the accuracy and reproducibility of 1-day disposable lenses and found that 14 of the 15 parameters measured (five parameters of each of five makes of lens) proved to be within ISO tolerances. Accurate dispensing, however, remains the responsibility of the clinician, although it is not viable to verify each individual disposable lens.

Depending on the classification, contact lens type and design, the inspection and verification of a lens may include any of the parameters listed in Tables 16.1 and 16.2. Tolerances for dimensional and optical parameters of rigid lenses are given in Tables 16.3 and 16.4 (International Standard 2004b).

Soft lenses are more difficult to verify than rigid lenses because of greater flexibility and dehydration effects. The dimensional properties are influenced by dehydration but also by factors such as pH and tonicity of the storage solution (Masnik & Holden 1972, Patel 1983, Gundel & Cohen 1986, Fonn et al. 1999, Young & Benjamin 2003). Table 16.5 outlines the dimensional and optical tolerances for soft contact lenses (International Standard 2004b).

TERMINOLOGY

Unification of terms and definitions in the field of contact lenses is important in a globalized world. ISO/DIS 18369-1

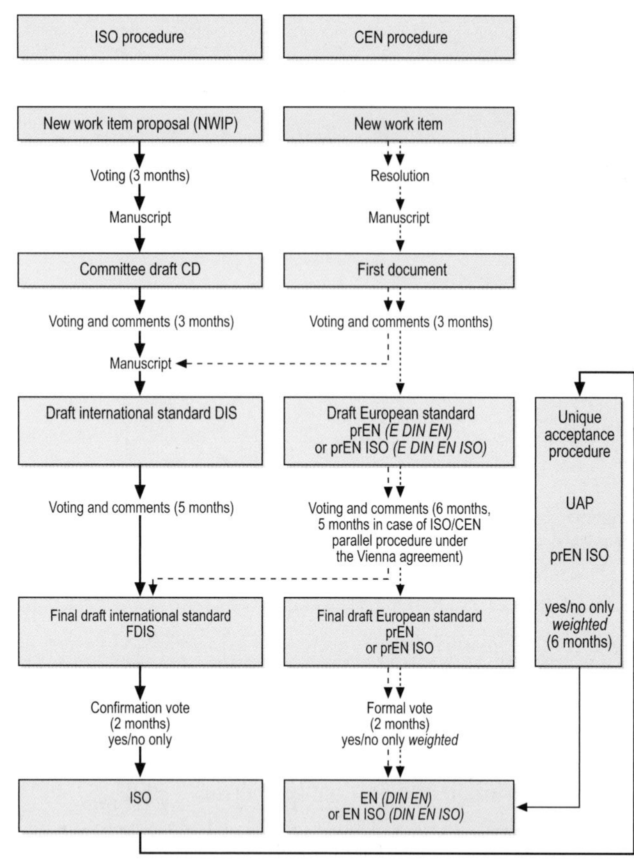

Figure 16.1 ISO/CEN standards development scheme. (From Höfer 1999, with permission of DOZ Verlag)

(International Standard 2004a) identifies and defines the terms applicable to the physical, chemical and optical properties of contact lenses, their manufacture and uses. It also contains an alphabetical list of terms with the relevant international symbols and abbreviations. The terms relating to contact lens care products and the classification and specification of soft and rigid contact lenses are also listed.

INSTRUMENT CALIBRATION

When a measurement is made, the resultant reading may or may not represent the true value. The error in a system is represented by the difference between the true and the measured value. In taking measurements, a learning curve is involved for both the operator and the instrument. With experience, repetitive learning or practice, the spread or standard deviation of multiple measurements is normally reduced and the reliability of the system improved. Ideally, measurements should be calibrated, independent, multiple, masked and randomized.

The calibration procedure requires validation in the form of test plates. These should be of confirmed and known accuracy, which have been certified by an independent, acceptable and traceable source. ISO/DIS 18369-3 (International Standard 2004c) describes the calibration of most relevant instruments for the measurement and evaluation of contact lenses.

LENS SPECIFICATION

The recommendation of the ISO/DIS 18369-1 (International Standard 2004a) is that all linear dimensions are made in millimetres (mm) and all additional specific requirements – edge form, material tint or power and orientation of specified prism – may be included as 'Additional notes'.

Examples

Tri-curve corneal contact lens

$r_0:\varnothing_0/r_1:\varnothing_1/r_2:\varnothing_T/F'_v/t_c$

7.60:7.00/8.30:8.80/12.25:9.60/–5.00/0.10

where:

r_0 = back optic zone radius
$\varnothing_0$ = back optic zone diameter
r_1 = first back peripheral radius
$\varnothing_1$ = first back peripheral diameter
r_2 = second back peripheral radius
$\varnothing_t$ = total diameter
F'_v = back vertex power in air
t_c = specified value of centre thickness

Bicurve hydrogel contact lens

$r_0:\varnothing_0/r_1:\varnothing_T/F'_v$

8.80:12.00/9.50:14.50/–2.00

where:

r_0 = back optic zone radius
$\varnothing_0$ = back optic zone diameter
r_1 = first back peripheral radius
$\varnothing_T$ = total diameter
F'_v = back vertex power in air

RADII, ECCENTRICITY AND EDGE LIFT

There are different methods available for measuring rigid and soft contact lenses but they are not all suitable for checking both types of lens.

Keratometers

In clinical practice, keratometers are used primarily to measure the central curvature of the cornea but they can also be used to verify front and back surface radii of contact lenses. A convex surface, such as the anterior cornea, produces a reduced, virtual and upright image of the keratometer mires whilst the concave back surface produces a reduced, real and inverted image.

RIGID CONTACT LENSES

The keratometer is used with a special contact lens holder (Fig. 16.2). In order to view the mires reflected from the back

Table 16.1: Contact lens parameters which may need verifying

Group	Corneal lenses	Scleral lenses
Radii (spherical and/or toroidal)	Back optic zone radius Back central optic zone radius Back peripheral optic zone radius/radii* Back peripheral zone radius/radii* Front optic zone radius Front central optic zone radius Front peripheral optic zone radius/radii* Front peripheral zone radius/radii*	As for corneal lenses
	Effective or equivalent back optic zone radius	Back scleral zone radius/radii* Back transition zone radius/radii*
Diameters and linear parameters (maximum and minimum dimensions if not circular)	Back optic zone diameter Back central optic zone diameter Back peripheral optic zone diameter(s)* Back peripheral zone diameter(s)* Front optic zone diameter Front central optic zone diameter Front peripheral optic zone diameter(s)* Front peripheral zone diameter(s)* Total diameter Displacement of optic Bifocal segment size and position	As for corneal lenses
	Back diffractive zone diameter Axial and/or radial edge lift	Primary optic diameter Back scleral size Transition width(s)
Thickness	Central (optic and/or geometric) Edge Lenticular junction At any other specified point	Central optic Average scleral Edge Transition At any other specified point
Optic – lens prescription	Back vertex power Front vertex power Near addition Prism and base direction Cylinder power and axis Aberration	As for corneal lenses
Quality etc.	Finish and quality Polish Edge form Transitions Tint Material	As for corneal lenses

* Where there is more than one such zone.

surface and suppress the reflections from the front surface, the lens rests on saline in a small depression on a horizontal support. A mirror is set at 45° to the optical axis of the instrument and reflects light from the instrument onto the surface being measured.

In a different type of holder the lens is attached to a depression in the vertical plane using double-sided sticky tape or plasticine, making sure that there is no tension on the lens being measured.

In some keratometers, the mires are reflected from regions outside the paraxial zone, and an allowance is made during calibration for the aberrations thus introduced.

Aberrations from concave and convex surfaces are different. Keratometers are calibrated for convex surfaces and so errors occur when they are used to measure concave back optic zone radii (BOZR). Some manufacturers have produced tables for converting convex radii to concave. The radii for concave surfaces are greater than for convex surfaces and range from 0.02 mm for steep radii to 0.04 mm for flat. Thus, for lenses used in practice, it is sufficient to add 0.03 to the radius reading given by the keratometer. The Zeiss 30 SL/M and the Rodenstock CMES keratometer do not need a conversion factor added.

An autorefractor/keratometer with a rigid contact lens holder can be used to determine BOZR (Fig. 16.3). Computer-

Table 16.2: Possible methods of test for rigid contact lenses

Back central optic zone radius	(1) Optical radiuscope microspherometer (2) Keratometer (calibrated for concave surfaces) (3) Interferometry techniques
Back (central) optic zone diameter	× 10 measuring magnifier
Back scleral zone radius (of preformed lenses)	(1) Radiuscope (2) Keratometer (calibrated for concave surfaces)
Basic or primary optic diameter	Sagitta method
Back peripheral (optic) radius	(1) Radiuscope (2) Topographical keratometer (3) Interferometry techniques
Back peripheral (optic) diameter	× 10 measuring magnifier
Axial edge lift, radial edge lift	(1) Radiuscope (2) Sagitta method
Total diameter	(1) V-channel gauge (2) × 10 measuring magnifier (3) Projection magnifier with scale
Front (central) and/or peripheral optic zone diameter	× 10 measuring magnifier
Bifocal segment height	× 10 measuring magnifier
Centre thickness	(1) Measuring dial gauge (2) Radiuscope (3) Projection magnifier with scale
Edge thickness	Measuring dial gauge
Scleral vertex clearance (from cast)	Measuring dial gauge
Back vertex power, prism, optical centration	Focimeter with contact lens support
Surface quality, edge form	(1) Binocular microscope (2) Projection magnifier (3) Measuring magnifier

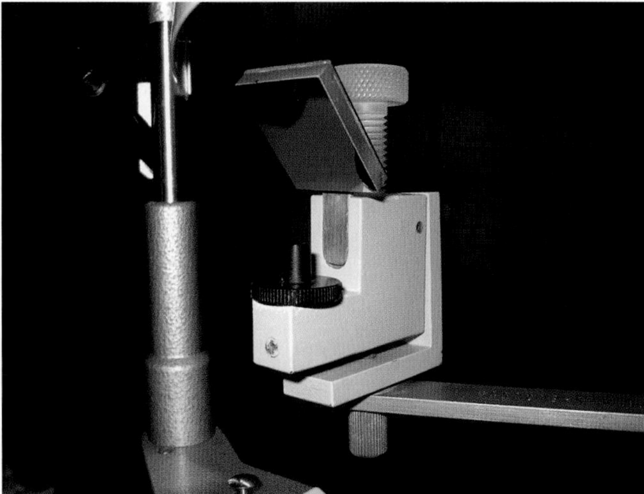

Figure 16.2 Contact lens holder for use with a keratometer

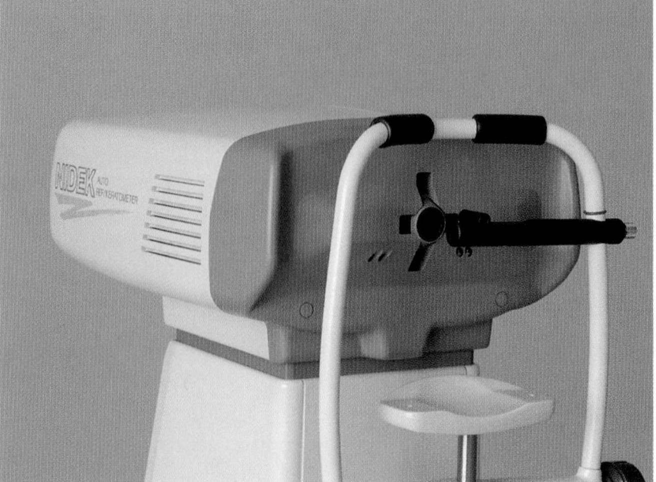

Figure 16.3 Nidek contact lens holder for use with an autokeratometer. (Courtesy of Nidek Co., Ltd)

assisted videokeratography equipment, such as the EyeSys, can also be used, although not with the same degree of accuracy, by mounting the lens on double-sided sticky tape or plasticine in the plane of the eye.

A correction factor must also be added when verifying radii of aspheric lenses, as the mire images of the keratometer are reflected from a zone significantly flatter than the contact lens centre. The correction factor is the difference between the

Table 16.3: Dimensional tolerances for rigid contact lenses

Property	Tolerance limit: Corneal contact lens, *PMMA (mm)*	*Gas permeable (mm)*	Scleral contact lens (mm)	Relevant method
Back optic zone radius	±0.025	±0.05	±0.10	ISO 18369-3, Clause 4.1
Back optic zone radii of toroidal surfaces[a, b]				ISO 18369-3, Clause 4.1
where 0 < Δr ≤0.2	± 0.025	± 0.05	±0.12	
where 0.2 < Δr ≤0.4	±0.035	±0.06	±0.13	
where 0.4 < Δr ≤0.6	±0.055	±0.07	± 0.15	
where Δr >0.6	±0.075	±0.09	±0.17	
Back optic zone diameter[c]	±0.20	±0.20	±0.20	ISO 18369-3, Clause 4.4
Back scleral radius (of preformed lens)	–	–	±0.10	ISO 18369-3, Clause 4.1
Basic or primary optic diameter	–	–	±0.20	ISO 18369-3, Clause 4.4
Back or front peripheral radius (where measurable)[c]	±0.10	±0.10	±0.10	ISO 18369-3, Clause 4.1
Back peripheral diameter[c]	±0.20	±0.20	±0.20 (for preformed lenses)	ISO 18369-3, Clause 4.4
Total diameter[b]	±0.10	±0.10	±0.25	ISO 18369-3, Clause 4.4
Front optic zone diameter[c]	±0.20	±0.20	±0.20	ISO 18369-3, Clause 4.4
Bifocal segment height	–0.10 to +0.20	–0.10 to +0.20	–0.10 to +0.20	ISO 18369-3, Clause 4.4
Centre thickness	±0.02	±0.02	±0.10	ISO 18369-3, Clause 4.5
Vertex clearance from cast (for impression scleral lenses)	–	–	±0.02	ISO 18369-3, Clause 4.1

[a] Δr is the difference between the radii of the two principal meridians.
[b] The tolerance applies to each meridian.
[c] These tolerances apply only to contact lenses with spherical surfaces and distinct curves; they are for a finished contact lens and any blending may make measurement difficult.
Permission to reproduce extracts of International Standard Draft ISO/DIS 18369-2 (2004a) Table 1 is granted by BSI (see Glossary).

nominal vertex radius and the nominal sagittal radius at a semi-chord that is half the keratometer mire image separation on the surface (Dietze et al. 2003).

When measuring the eccentricity of aspheric contact lenses, a special lens holder is used. This needs to pivot around its vertical axis (Wilms 1972) so that the central vertical radius and the sagittal radius at 30° can be measured (Fig. 16.4). The eccentricity of the contact lens can be quantified with the equation

$$e = \sqrt{\frac{r_s^2 - r_0^2}{\sin^2 \varphi \times r_s^2}}$$

where e is the eccentricity, r_s is the sagittal radius, r_0 is the vertex radius and φ is the angle at which the sagittal radius is measured (Dietze et al. 2003).

STEEP AND FLAT RADII

The range of the keratometer needs to be extended when measuring back scleral radii. This is done by recalibrating the keratometer using a –1.00 or –2.00 D trial case lens taped in front of the objective. Three steel balls, of known radii (e.g. 9.00, 12.00 and 15.00 mm) are used for recalibration and entered onto a graph with measured radius on the x-axis and actual radius on the y-axis. Provided the same trial case lens is always used, the same graph can determine longer radii than the keratometer was designed to measure.

Steep radii can be determined (useful in keratoconic corneas) by taping a positive trial case lens of about +1.50 D in front of the keratometer objective and recalibrating with steep steel balls.

SOFT CONTACT LENSES

Measuring radii of soft lenses with a keratometer is complicated by lens flexibility and dehydration effects. The lens must be placed in a wet cell containing normal saline ($n = 1.336$) and the wet cell separated from the keratometer by air. The contact lens–liquid lens–air system acts as an equivalent mirror (Chaston 1973) so that the vertices of the mirror are displaced towards

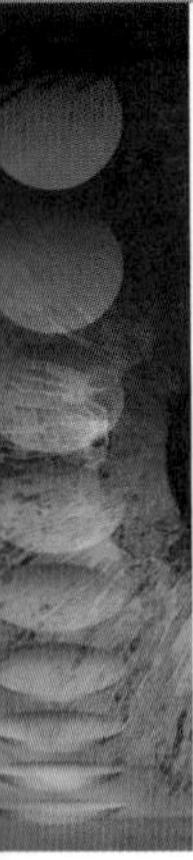

Table 16.4: Optical tolerances for rigid contact lenses

Dimension	Tolerance limit	Relevant method
Back vertex power in the weaker meridian		ISO 18369-3, Clause 4.2
0 to ±5.00 D	±0.12 D	
over ±5.00 D to ±10.0 D	±0.18 D	
over ±10.00 D to ±15.0 D	±0.25 D	
over ±15.00 D to ±20.0 D	±0.37 D	
over ±20.00 D	±0.50 D	
Prismatic error (measured at geometrical centre of the optic zone)		ISO 18369-3, Clause 4.3
Back vertex power 0 to 6 D	0.25 Δ	
Back vertex power over 6 D	0.50 Δ	
Specified prism	±0.25 Δ	ISO 18369-3, Clause 4.3
Optical centration for scleral lenses only (maximum error)	0.50 mm	ISO 18369-3, Clause 4.4
Cylinder power		ISO 18369-3, Clause 4.2
to 2.00 D	±0.25 D	
over 2.00 D to 4.00 D	±0.37 D	
over 4.00 D	±0.50 D	
Cylinder axis	±5°	ISO 18369-3, Clause 4.2

Permission to reproduce extracts of International Standard Draft ISO/DIS 18369-2 (2004b) Table 2 is granted by BSI (see Glossary).

each other. The wet cell is mounted on an inverting prism/mirror, which is in front of the keratometer (Fig. 16.5).

There are various difficulties that must be taken into account when measuring soft lenses in liquid using a keratometer.

- Keratometer mires appear smaller in solution (between 5.40 and 7.10 mm) than in air and the refractive index (RI) of the storage solution must be considered. Either measurements must be converted or compensating lenses must be used. The Rodenstock CMES keratometer incorporates an additional objective lens mounted on a turret on the telescope to directly measure the radii of soft contact lenses in saline.
- If reflected light is used to measure the radii of a submerged lens, then a double image is formed by reflections at the front and back surfaces. The surface proximal to the mires will produce a brighter image, which is smaller for negative and larger for positive lenses (Forst 1974). Figure 16.6 shows the classification of the Zeiss mires when measuring the radius of a soft lens. Less light is reflected from each surface in liquid than in air.

  Fresnel's Law for light of normal incidence is:

  $R = \left[\frac{n' - n}{n' + n}\right]^2 \times 100\%$ where R = percentage of light, n = RI of surrounding medium (1.336 for saline solution and 1.00 for air), n' = RI of the second medium (≈1.430 for hydrogel material). In air; therefore, $R = 3.13\%$, in saline $R = 0.115\%$.

Table 16.5: Dimensional and optical tolerances for soft contact lenses

Property	Tolerance limits	Relevant method
Back optic zone radius (see Notes 1 and 2)	±0.20 mm	ISO 18369-3, Clause 4.1
Sagitta at specified diameter (see Note 1)	±0.05 mm	ISO 18369-3, Clause 4.1
Total diameter	±0.20 mm	ISO 18369-3, Clause 4.4
Optic zone diameter	±0.20 mm	ISO 18369-3, Clause 4.4
Centre thickness	(see Note 3)	ISO 18369-3, Clause 4.5
≤0.10 mm	± [0.010 mm + 0.10 t_c]	
>0.10 mm	± [0.015 mm + 0.05 t_c]	
Back vertex power		ISO 18369-3, Clause 4.2
$\lvert F'v \rvert \le 10$ D	±0.25 D	
10 D < $\lvert F'v \rvert \le 20$ D	±0.50 D	
$\lvert F'v \rvert > 20$ D	±1.00 D	
Prismatic error	(see Note 4)	ISO 18369-3, Clause 4.3
$\lvert F'v \rvert \le 6$ D	0.25 cm/m	
$\lvert F'v \rvert > 6$ D	0.50 cm/m	
Prescribed optical prism	(see Note 5)	ISO 18369-3, Clause 4.3
$\lvert F'v \rvert \le 6$ D	±0.25 cm/m	
$\lvert F'v \rvert > 6$ D	±0.50 cm/m	
Prism axis	±5°	
Cylinder power		ISO 18369-3, Clause 4.2
$\lvert F'_c \rvert \le 2$ D	±0.25 D	
2 D < $\lvert F'c \rvert \le 4$ D	±0.37 D	
$\lvert F'_c \rvert > 4$ D	±0.50 D	
Cylinder axis	5°	ISO 18369-3, Clause 4.2

NOTE 1: Tolerance is applicable when this property is the one specified by the manufacturer as the expression of the back surface curvature.
NOTE 2: Tolerance is applicable when the step between successive back optic zone radii is 0.40 mm or greater. For smaller steps the tolerance is equal to half the design step (e.g. back optic zone radius design step 0.30 mm, tolerance ± 0.15 mm).
NOTE 3: Examples of tolerance calculations:

Nominal thickness	*Tolerance*
0.035 mm	± [0.010 + 0.004] = ±0.014 mm
0.070 mm	± [0.010 + 0.007] = ±0.017 mm
0.150 mm	± [0.015 + 0.008] = ±0.023 mm
0.300 mm	± [0.015 + 0.015] = ±0.03 mm

NOTE 4: Prismatic error is measured at the geometrical centre of the optical zone.
NOTE 5: The reference for the prismatic axis in toric lenses is the basic axis on apex.
Permission to reproduce extracts of International Standard Draft ISO/DIS 18369-2 (2004b) Table 3 is granted by BSI (see Glossary).

(a)

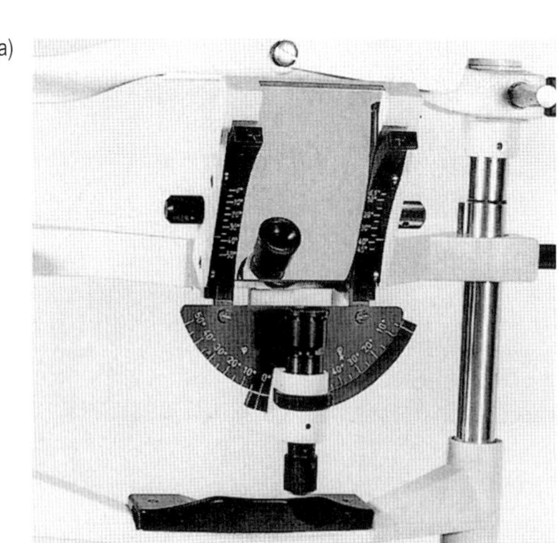

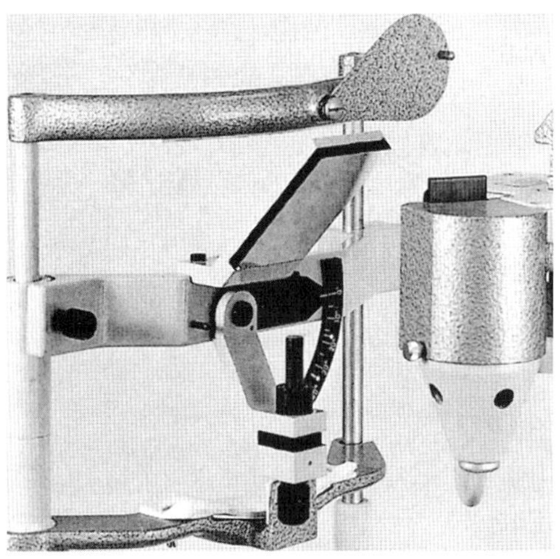

(b) **Figure 16.4** (a, b) Special contact lens holder for aspheric contact lens back surfaces. (From Baron 1991, with permission of DOZ Verlag)

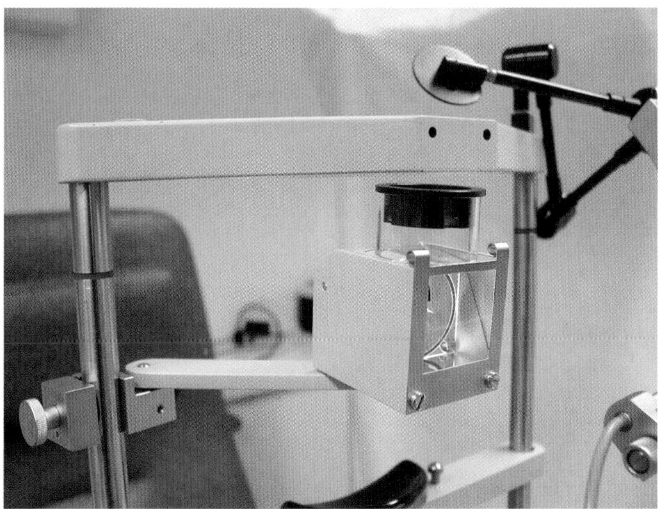

Figure 16.5 Contact lens holder for soft contact lenses for use with a keratometer. (Courtesy of A. Müller-Treiber)

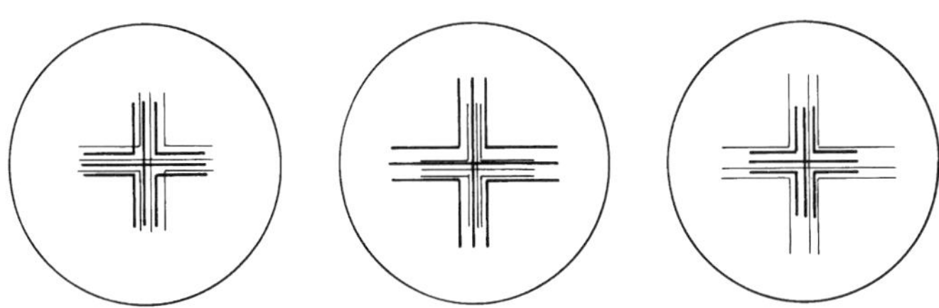

Figure 16.6 Classification of the mires when measuring the radius of a hydrogel contact lens. Coincidence position with a weak minus lens (left), strong plus lens (middle) and strong minus lens (right). (From Baron 1991, with permission of DOZ Verlag)

- The luminosity of the mires must be increased significantly to compensate for the reduction in intensity of reflected light when a contact lens is measured in a saline cell. Many modern keratometers are illuminated with brightness-controlled halogen bulbs and provide scale intervals of 0.01 mm, which read to radii of 5.00 mm or less.

As the water content of the contact lens increases, keratometer measurement becomes more difficult. Quesnel and Simonet (1994) studied the precision repeatability of keratometry in measuring BOZR of soft lenses. Thirty-two lenses (+5.00 to −5.00 D and 38% and 55% water content (WC)) were measured. For 38% WC, radii were ±0.058 to ±0.107 mm, and for 55% WC, radii were ±0.140 to ±0.198 mm.

SILICONE RUBBER CONTACT LENSES

Silicone rubber lenses should be floated on the surface of a liquid without tension (Baron 1991). As measurements are carried out in air, the values measured correspond to real radii.

AXIAL EDGE LIFT AND ECCENTRICITY

The pillar and collar technique

Axial edge lift of multicurve rigid lenses (Douthwaite & Hurst 1998) and flattening gradient (*p*-value or eccentricity) of aspheric rigid lenses (Dietze et al. 2003) can be derived from measurements of the sagittal depth across single or multiple chord diameters.

- A pillar, whose diameter is smaller than the total lens diameter, serves as a contact lens holder and the collar, whose diameter is slightly larger than the contact lens diameter (0.1–0.2 mm), ensures proper centration of the lens on the pillar (Fig. 16.7).
- A travelling microscope is focused on the front surface of the lens, the lens removed and the microscope refocused on the surface of the pillar.
- The distance the microscope has travelled between the two foci minus the central thickness of the lens gives the sagittal depth across a chord corresponding to the pillar diameter.
- Using the sag formula $s = r - \sqrt{(r^2 - y^2)}$, where r = radius of curvature and s = sagittal at semi-aperture y, the required sag of the lens under test (b) at the total diameter can be calculated. The axial edge lift (e) then is given by the formula $e = b - s$.

For determining the axial edge lift of multicurve rigid lenses, this method is accurate and reproducible (Douthwaite & Hurst 1998).

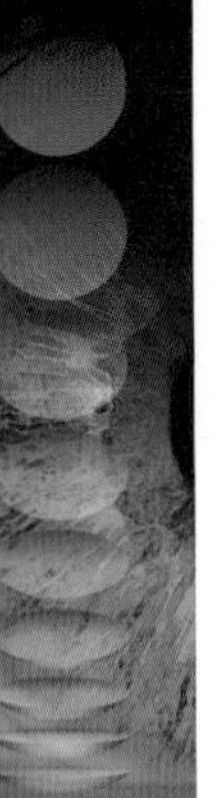

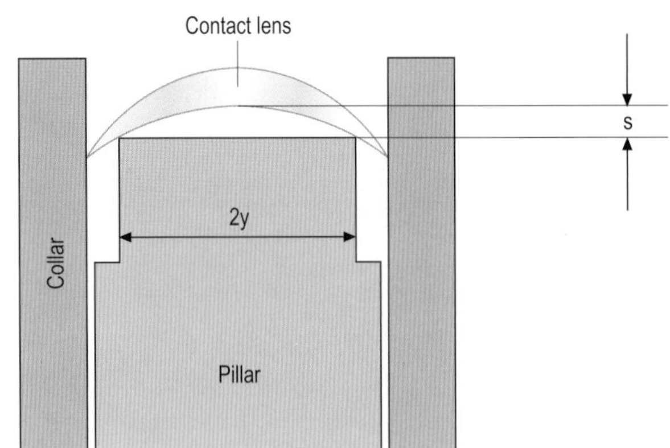

Figure 16.7 Pillar and collar method. (Courtesy of H. H. Dietze)

- Rearranging Baker's equation for ellipsoids as $p = \dfrac{2r_0s - y^2}{s^2}$ gives the *p*-value, *p*, of an elliptical lens surface, where r_0 is the vertex radius and *y* is half the pillar diameter over which the sagitta, *s*, has been measured. The *p*-value and the eccentricity, *e*, of a surface are related by $e = \sqrt{1 - p}$.
- Deriving the eccentricity or the *p*-value of aspherical lenses with increasing eccentricity is far more complex and requires the mathematical description of the surface to be known.

  For determining the eccentricity of an aspheric lens, this method is less precise than a keratometer-based method using central and peripheral radii (Dietze et al. 2003).

Optical microspherometers (radiuscopes)

The optical microspherometer is commonly known as a radiuscope (the trade name of an American Optical instrument).

The measurement of small radii with a radiuscope was originally described by Drysdale (1900) and is based on the principle that, for a curved mirror, an image is formed in the same plane as the object when the object is at the centre of the curvature because reflected light returns along its incident path. An image is also formed on the surface and the distance between the two images is equal to the radius of the surface (Fig. 16.8).

- A radiuscope essentially consists of a microscope with a linear scale (calibrated to 0.01 mm), which reads the position of the microscope body or microscope stage.
- Light from an illuminated target (consisting of a ring of dots or radial lines) attached to the microscope is imaged by the microscope objective after being reflected through a right angle by a semi-transparent mirror.
- The radius is determined by shifting the contact lens or the mire coupled with the microscope objective from one focus to the next.

The radiuscope can be used to measure the concave and convex surfaces of both rigid and soft lenses.

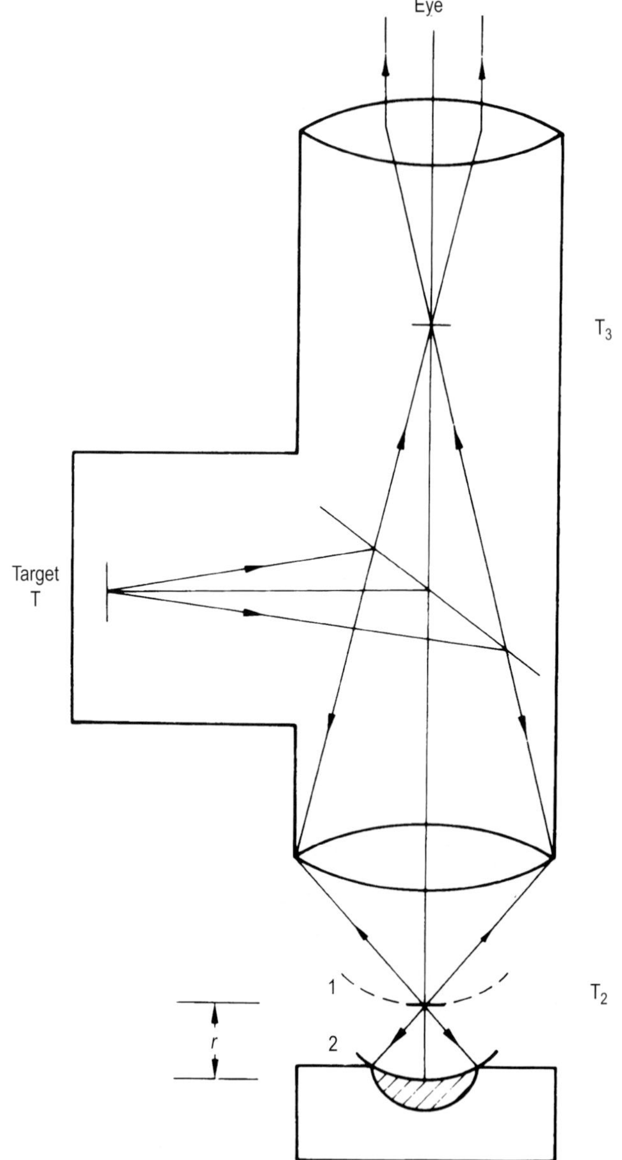

Figure 16.8 Diagram to show Drysdale's principle. (1) First position of lens, image focused on lens surface; (2) second position of lens, image is now at centre of curvature of surface. *r* = lens radius

Examples of radiuscopes are shown in Figure 16.9. The CG Auto Microspherometer MS/T by Neitz Instruments (Fig. 16.9b) eliminates the operator's subjective judgement by automatically focusing the mires using a microgrid. A number of horizontal and vertical points are focused and analysed by a computer (Meszaros 2003).

RIGID CONTACT LENSES

The BOZR of a rigid lens is determined as follows:

- A concave lens holder on the microscope stage is filled with saline or sterile water.
- The lens is centred on the holder convex side down; this prevents distortion of the contact lens and eliminates reflections from the front surface.

(a)

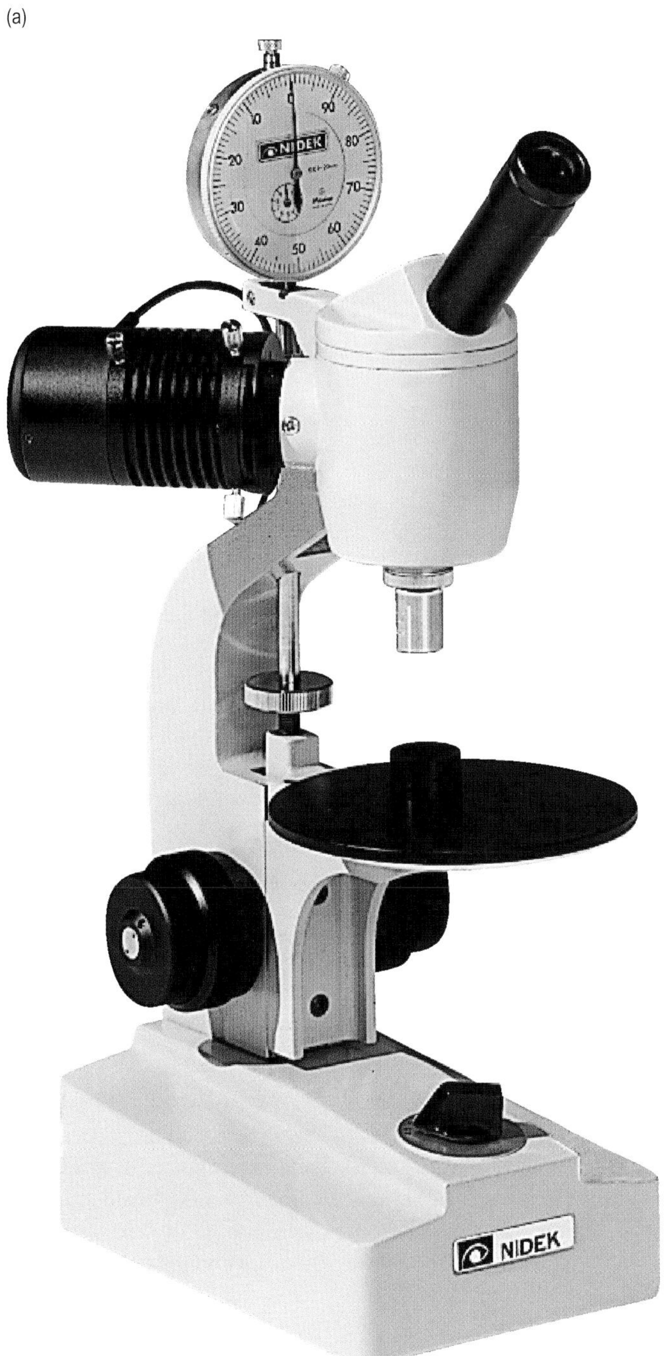

(b)

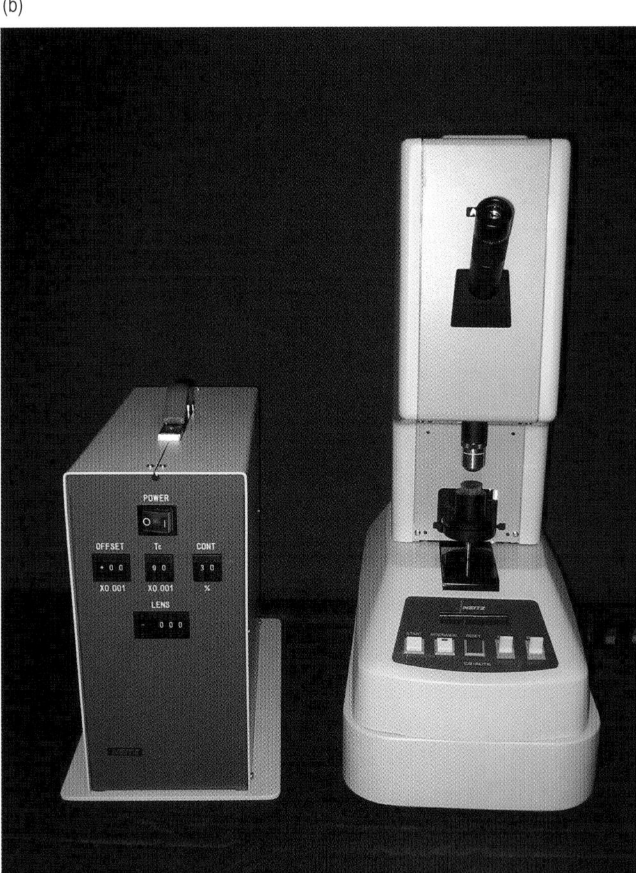

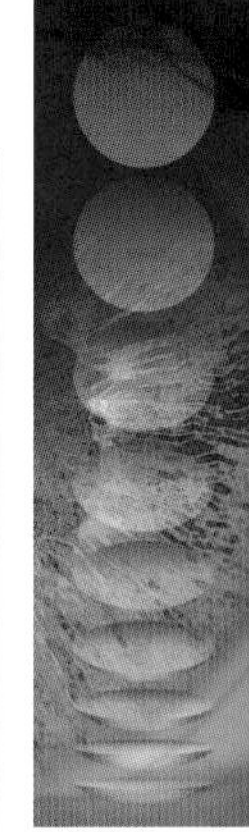

Figure 16.9 (a) Nidek Radiusgauge RG-200. (Courtesy of Nidek Co., Ltd) (b) CG Auto Microspherometer MS/T. (Courtesy of Neitz Instruments Co., Ltd)

- The microscope eyepiece is then focused on the target on the surface of the lens by moving either the microscope and target or the microscope stage.
- The measurement is recorded or the gauge set to zero.
- A second focus, at the centre of curvature of the surface, is obtained by racking the microscope stage up or down.
- The difference between the two dial gauge readings gives the radius of curvature of the surface.

To measure back peripheral radii, the holder must be tilted and the microscope stage moved across so that the target is focused in the peripheral band of the contact lens. Provided that the band is 1 mm wide and incident light is still normal to the surface being measured, it is possible to measure its radius. Where the peripheral curve is too narrow, the image at the centre of curvature is similar to that of a toroidal surface. A line image, formed by the surface along the circumference of the band, is closest to the correct radius and can be focused parallel to the direction of the tilt.

Stone (1975) described a method to measure axial edge lift of rigid lenses:

- The lens is placed on the radiuscope holder in the usual manner, and a microscope cover slide placed on the top.
- Central readings are taken successively on the underside of the cover slide and then the back surface of the lens.

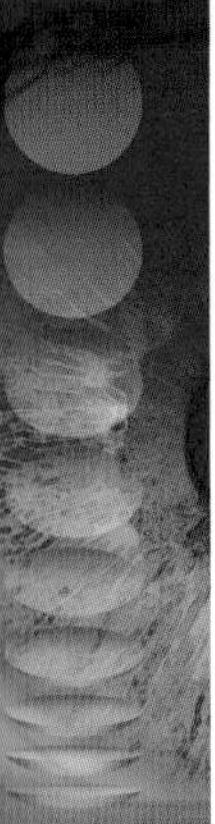

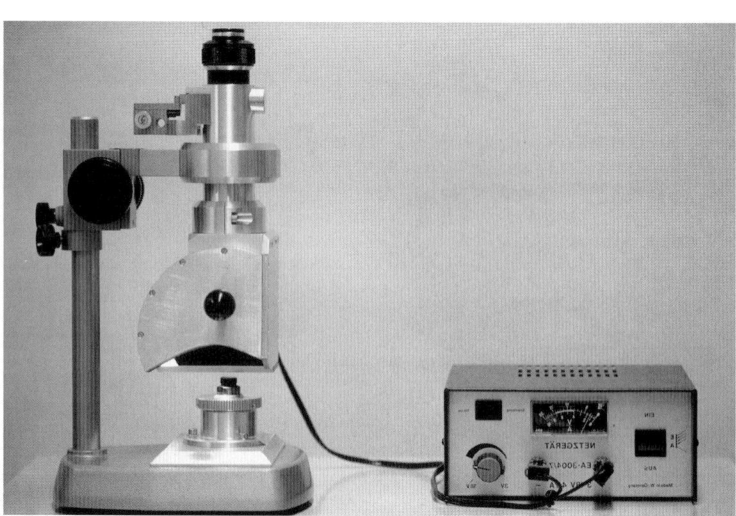

Figure 16.10 Toposcope. (Courtesy of H. Bussacker)

- The difference between these readings gives the lens primary sag, i.e. from the sag formula $s = r - \sqrt{r^2 - y^2}$, where r = radius of curvature, s = sagitta at a semi-aperture y.
- The sag b, corresponding to the BOZR of the lens under test at a diameter corresponding to the total diameter of the lens, is found. The axial edge lift $e = b - s$.

Newlove (1974) and Stone (1975) also described a method to determine radial edge lift using a radiuscope.

DeFazio and Lowther (1979) investigated two methods of clinically checking and verifying the aspherical back surfaces of rigid contact lenses. In the first method, a radiuscope was modified with a tilting table. By measuring radii at off-axis points, the eccentricity was calculated for each aspherical surface tested. The conformity of the surface to a true conicoid could then be evaluated.

Rabbetts (1995) published correction factors for aspheric contact lenses to be subtracted from the radiuscope reading for various lens designs and diameters.

SOFT CONTACT LENSES

There are different methods available for measuring the BOZR of soft contact lenses with a radiuscope. The method used for rigid lenses is not usually effective as capillary attraction between the lens and the holder distorts the lens.

Soft lenses are usually measured in a wet cell, designed so that there is no layer of air between the liquid and the cover. The radius of the lens measured in air is calculated from the radius of the lens measured in liquid, taking the refractive index of the liquid in the wet cell into account: $r = r' \times n$, where r = radius of curvature in air, r' = radius of curvature in liquid and n = RI of saline solution (1.336).

The reflected mires produce a poor image in the wet cell (Baron 1991).

Spherometers (mechanical and electronic)

The radii of spherical surfaces can be determined using a mechanical or electronic spherometer. The radius is calculated from the sagittal depth.

The contact lens is placed on a support ring with a fixed chord diameter and the thumbscrew turned until contact is made between the spherometer stylus and the contact lens apex.

In an electronic device, the vertical stylus is moved by a small motor, which produces electrical contact, and the radius measured digitally, directly from the scale.

With either type, in order to maintain the shape and avoid dehydration, the lens is placed in a wet cell with normal saline solution and illuminated by an external light source.

Toposcopes

Moiré interference fringes are the basis of many lens-testing techniques. They are utilized in the toposcope (Fig. 16.10) to measure the following lens parameters:

- Radii and diameters.
- Back vertex power (Keren et al. 1992) and quality assessment (e.g. in the Rotlex ConTest). The Rotlex ConTest uses Moiré deflectometry to measure the back vertex power of a soft lens immersed in saline. Spherical, toric and multifocal lenses can be checked and the instrument can also be used for checking rigid lenses in air. The Moiré fringes are imaged on a computer screen and the optical quality assessed at the same time. An accuracy of 0.06 D is claimed for 38% water contact lenses.
- Contact lens peripheries.
- Quality assessment of aspheric lens geometries (Bussacker 1983).

With the toposcope, the shape and orientation of the fringes are a function of the relationship between the two sets of lines:

- Straight parallel fringes indicate a spherical surface.
- Curved fringes indicate an aspheric surface.
- Irregularly shaped fringes indicate warpage or dimples in the surface.

Ultrasound

The sagittal depth, and thus the BOZR, can also be determined using ultrasound (Port 1975, 1976, Patella et al. 1982).

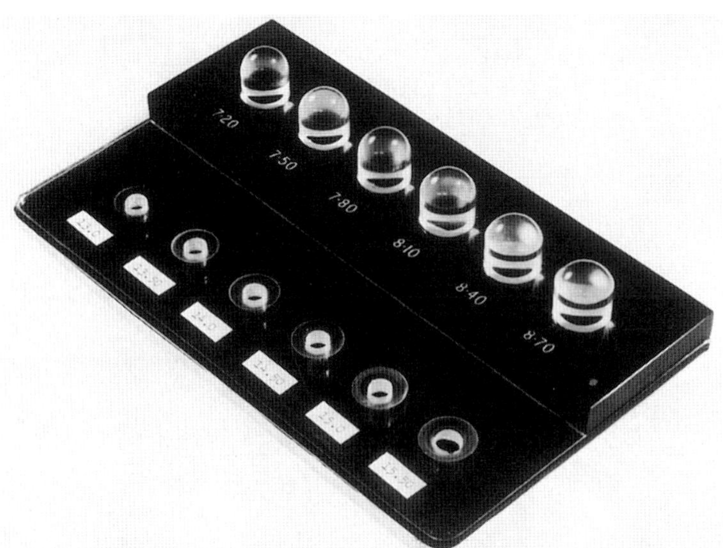

Figure 16.11 The Lensmaster, formerly produced by Contactalens Ltd, which uses optical gauging to determine the approximate back optic zone radius in air, using the hemispheres at the back and determining total diameter, using the circles engraved at the front. Known as a comparator

Ultrasound pulses, emitted from a transducer, are reflected onto the back of the contact lens and electronically analysed.

Interferometry

El-Nasher and Larke (1980) and Dörbrand (1985) found interferometry to be an accurate and reproducible method to measure the contact lens radii. Incident monochromatic light is shone on the surface of a contact lens suspended in normal saline. The interference patterns thus produced are measured with a microdensitometer and mathematically converted into radii. Rottenkolber and Podbielska (1996) described a method for measuring the front surface of rigid contact lenses with a Twyman-Green interferometer.

Optical gauging

MASTER SPHERES

One of the simplest and oldest methods of obtaining an approximate value for the radius of a soft lens is optical gauging using master spheres (Fig. 16.11). The system is inexpensive, rapid and simple, and can measure lenses in air but it is of little use with current ultrathin disposable lenses.

- The hydrated contact lens is placed, convex face up, onto one of a series of accurately made acrylic spheres of known radii.
- If the two surfaces are not aligned, a bubble forms, a central bubble indicating a BOZR steeper than the master sphere, and a peripheral bubble indicating a BOZR flatter than the master sphere.

PROJECTION METHODS

Projections methods were used widely in the 1970s and 1980s to measure:

- Optic zone radii.
- Centre thickness.
- Contact lens diameters.
- Edge profile.

An example is the Söhnges Optik (Fig. 16.12) (Söhnges Optik 1974, Lester & Lester 1979, Port 1981a).

- The contact lens is placed concave side up in a wet cell filled with liquid whose RI corresponds to that of the contact lens material.
- The profile of the lens is projected onto a screen engraved with horizontal and vertical millimetre scales and a series of annuli, graded from 7.2 to 9.5 mm in 0.10 mm steps. These are adjusted vertically until alignment is achieved.
- The screen is approximately 1 metre away.
- The projector incorporates a high luminosity halogen bulb and a cooling system.

The Optimec Soft Contact Lens Analyser is another projection system, available in two forms, both with temperature control of the wet cell and saline filtration (Port 1981a).

The Chiltern Analyser (Fig. 16.13) is a front projection system. It allows verification of total diameter at intervals of 0.25 mm and central thickness with an accuracy of 0.05 mm (Gisler 1993). For BOZR measurement:

- The lens is mounted and centred in saline, convex side up, on an 8.50 mm diameter cylinder containing a probe.
- The lens profile is viewed on a built-in screen at 15× magnification.
- The probe is manually advanced until the observer detects a barely perceptible edge lift confirming contact.
- It is then lowered by the same amount and the BOZR read directly in millimetres.

For contact lenses of 40% water content, the reported precision for the model without temperature control is ±0.03 mm and unexpectedly, it was ±0.05 mm with temperature control (Port 1981b).

ABERRATIONS OF RIGID AND SOFT CONTACT LENSES

The influence of contact lens-induced aberrations on the retinal image was first discussed by Westheimer in 1961 and more

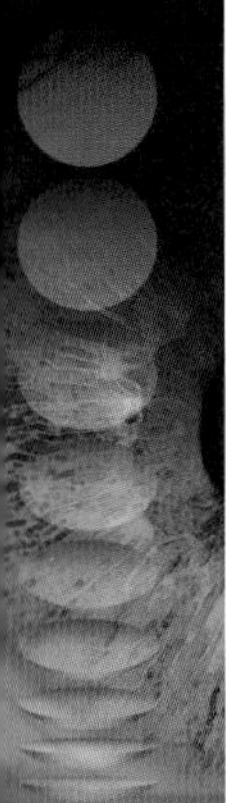

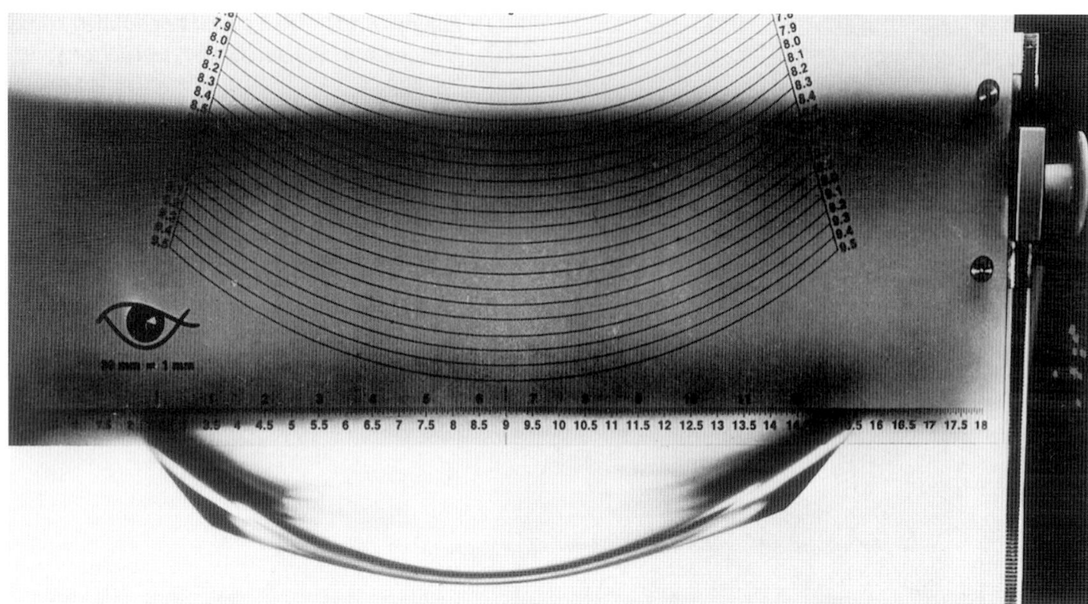

Figure 16.12 The image of the sagittal section of an immersed lens projected in the Söhnges system on to a screen containing annuli which may be adjusted vertically until alignment is achieved. (Courtesy of Söhnges Optik; reproduced by kind permission of the National Eye Research Foundation)

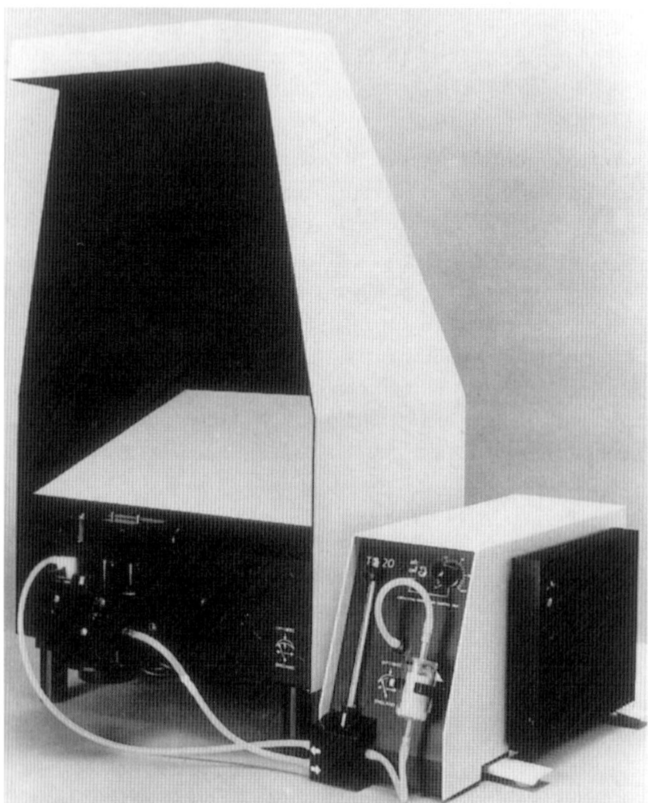

Figure 16.13 The Chiltern Optimec Soft Lens Analyser, Front Projection Model with temperature control and saline filtration. (Courtesy of Optimec Ltd)

recently by Thibos et al. (2002), Yoon and Williams (2002) and Dorronsoro et al. (2003).

Wavefront-guided contact lens design has been suggested by Lopez-Gil et al. (2002), Thibos (2003) and Dietze and Cox (2004).

Contact lens aberrations can be verified on-eye (Hong et al. 2001, Lopez-Gil et al. 2002, Dietze & Cox 2003, 2004, Dorronsoro et al. 2003) and off-eye (Bauer 1979, Dietze & Cox 2004).

One interesting method using modern instrumentation is to place the contact lens in the ray path of a Hartman Shack aberroscope (Dietze & Cox 2004).

Diameters and widths

Draft ISO/DIS 18369-2 (International Standard 2004b) gives a tolerance of ±0.20 mm for the back optic zone diameter (BOZD), ±0.10 mm for the total diameter of rigid contact lenses and ±0.20 mm for the BOZD and the total diameter of soft contact lenses.

Total diameter

RIGID CONTACT LENSES

It is easy to check the total diameter (TD) of rigid contact lenses and there are a number of simple-to-use instruments available to do so. With some methods, the problem of parallax occurs as the measuring scale is not in the same plane as the parameter being measured.

- V gauges (Fig. 16.14a) are probably the easiest to use. They are made of metal or plastic and have a V-shaped channel cut into the material. The channel ranges in width from 6.0 to 12.5 mm in 0.10 mm increments. A rigid lens is placed at the widest end of the channel, concave side down, and allowed to slide down the 'V' under gravity until it is stopped by the sides of the gauge. The TD is then read from a scale beside the channel.
- Hand-held scale magnifiers (Fig. 16.14b) are equally simple to use and have a reading accuracy of ±0.01 mm (Baron 1991).

(a)

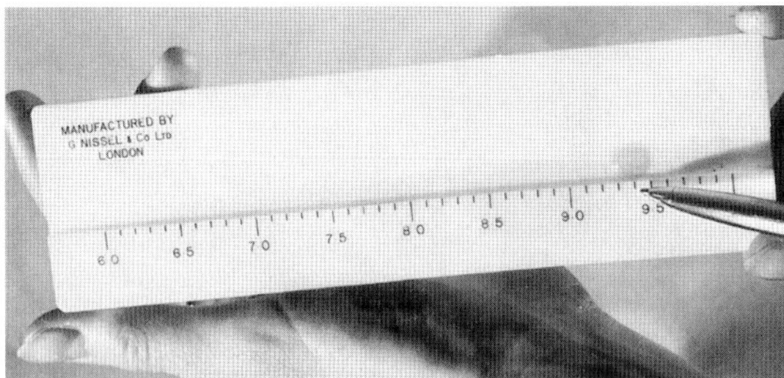

(b)

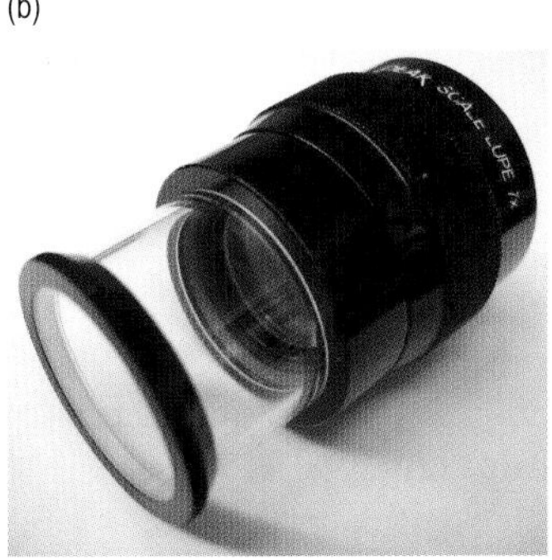

Figure 16.14 (a) V gauge in use. Pen indicates position to read lens total diameter of 9.40 mm to nearest 0.10 mm. (b) Hand-held scale magnifier

- A graticule in the eyepiece of a keratometer or a slit-lamp can also be used.

SOFT CONTACT LENSES

ISO guidelines for measuring the total diameter of soft lenses are more complicated than for rigid lenses.

Draft ISO/DIS Standard 18369-3 (International Standard 2004c) recommends the projection comparator method for this purpose with the contact lens in normal saline solution at a temperature of 20°C ±0.5°C.

Other projection methods include the Söhnges system and the Optimec Analyser described above.

The TD can also be measured with a slit-lamp. The soft lens is placed convex surface down in a wet cell with standard saline solution (Forst 1993). The wet cell is set on a deflecting prism with two scales on its undersurface in the shape of a cross. The TD is measured in the two meridians and the mean calculated.

Zone diameters and widths

Instruments used to measure optic zone diameters and secondary and peripheral diameters or widths include hand-held scale magnifiers, slit-lamps, projection comparators and toposcopes. As a rule, the measurement of optic zone diameters is carried out with soft lenses placed in a wet cell and the rigid lenses measured in air.

Depending on the quality of the blending of the edges of the different zones, it can be difficult to check these parameters in practice.

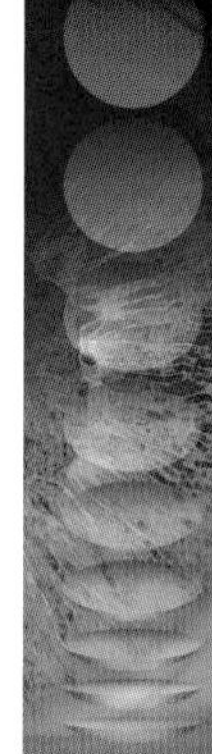

Thickness

Lens thickness affects:

- Oxygen transmissibility.
- Optical stability.
- Durability of a lens.

As with other parameters, thickness is easier to check in rigid lenses than soft.

Draft ISO/DIS Standard No. 18369-3 (International Standard 2004c) recommends a dial gauge be used for checking the thickness of rigid lenses and a low-force dial gauge for soft lenses.

Optical instruments such as microspherometers or projection comparators should only be used for comparative measurements of different contact lenses.

RIGID CONTACT LENSES

The easiest method to measure the central thickness of rigid lenses is with a mechanical or electronic stylus (Fig. 16.15).

No liquid is used in the lens holder when the thickness of a lens is being determined using a radiuscope. The target is focused on each lens surface in turn. The distance between the two foci multiplied by the refractive index of the material gives the lens thickness. A direct reading of the lens thickness is possible when a flat plate is placed on the radiuscope holder, and the radiuscope focused on this surface and then set to zero. The lens is then placed, convex side down, on the plate and the radiuscope focused at the centre of its back surface.

Guillon et al. (1986) described the use of a modified digital pachometer for the measurement of axial edge thickness of rigid lenses, giving an accuracy for single measurements of ±20 μm.

Franco et al. (2000) described a laboratory measurement of the central thickness of rigid lenses using video pachometry. A CCD camera (COU 2252) was mounted on the observation arm of a biomicroscope and the slit-lamp images digitized and sent to a computer for processing. The contact lenses were mounted in a support. The slit-lamp was placed perpendicular to the central corneal plane with an angular separation of 50° of the light source from the microscope and a magnification of 40×. After acquiring the image, a vertical edge enhancement algorithm was applied to the original image to enhance the contact lens borders.

Port (1987) evaluated a modified thickness gauge, which allowed radial edge thickness to be measured at a precisely determined distance from the edge of the lens.

SOFT CONTACT LENSES

Central thickness can be measured using:

- A radiuscope – as with rigid lenses.
- A wet cell in conjunction using a radiuscope and allowing for the RI of the liquid in which the contact lens is stored (multiply by 1.336 for saline).

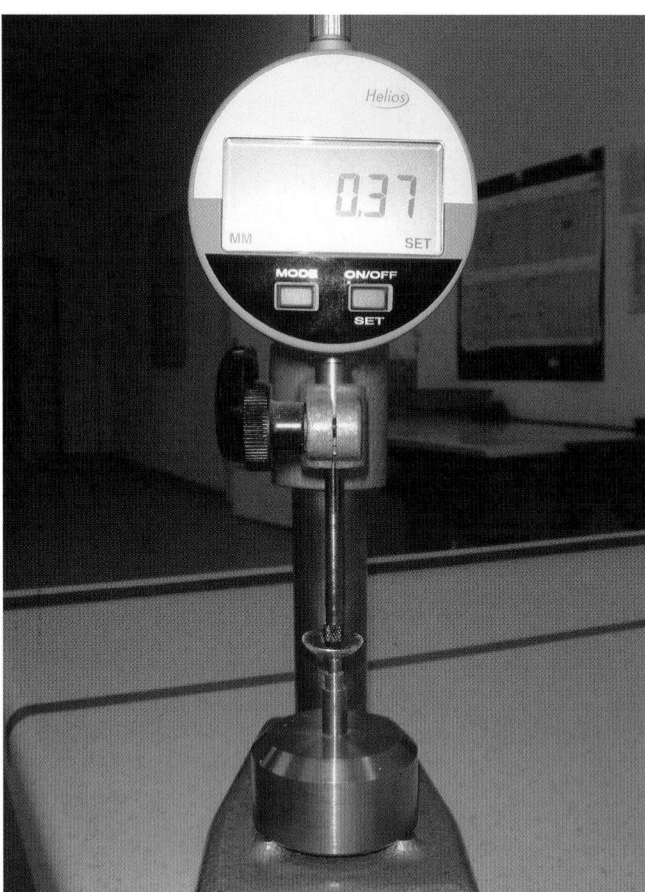

Figure 16.15 Measurement of the thickness of a rigid lens

- Projection methods, such as the Söhnges system or the Optimec Analyser (see above).
- Pachometry (Ruben 1974) with the lens in situ on the eye and viewed through a slit-lamp. With a modern ultrasonic pachometer, care must be taken not to indent the contact lens.

The Rehder Electronic Thickness Gauge is used by manufacturers to measure lens thickness accurately. It has a motorized sensor drive which automatically lowers the sensor to take a measurement. As it approaches the lens, the velocity of the sensor slows so that it is the same for every measurement. This avoids interoperator differences and improves the accuracy of the measurements.

Back vertex power

RIGID CONTACT LENSES

The back vertex power (BVP) of rigid contact lenses can be measured using a manual or automated focimeter but if the focimeter is used in the normal way, the measurement may be inaccurate. The back vertex focal length of a contact lens is measured from the plane of the stop to the target position. Because contact lenses have highly curved surfaces, the back surface is further away than the plane of the stop, resulting in a greater back vertex focal length. This error can be minimized either by using a smaller stop or removing the stop collar, if possible, so that the back surface of the contact lens is in approximately the correct position.

With scleral contact lenses, the scleral zone may prevent the back surface of the contact lens from lying in the correct plane. Special contact lens holders are available for many focimeters.

Adequate calibration of focimeters is important when measuring contact lenses as different calibration methods do influence results. Wang et al. (2002) found that when focimeters are calibrated as described in ISO 9337-1: (2001), a measurement error will exceed 0.50 D as a result of mainly spherical aberration when the ISO 9337-1: (2001) proposed spectacle lens support is used.

SOFT CONTACT LENSES

Draft ISO/DIS Standard 18369-3 (International Standard 2004c) recommends that the BVP of soft lenses with a focimeter is carried out in air as follows.

- Dry the lens on filter paper or lint-free absorbent cloth.
- Take five measurements.
- Calculate the mean of the readings.
- Ensure adequate lens support on a holder.
- Care is needed to avoid artefacts from, for example, incorrect surface liquid removal or dehydration of the contact lens.

A conventional vertometer (lensometer) is a device that measures the BVP of a lens. Where the BVP varies across the optic zone, the accurate measurement is relatively difficult with this instrument. Collins et al. (1997) used a standard projection vertometer, together with a wet cell, Scheiner discs, a shaft encoder and computer interface and software, to measure and produce a profile of the BVPs of soft and rigid lenses. The computer interface to the vertometer allows rapid acquisition of the readings. Software-based ray tracing derives in-air dioptric power readings across the optic zone at specific ray heights, which improves the accuracy over a conventional vertometer.

Water content

Water content affects:

- Flexibility.
- Comfort.
- Dehydration.
- Permeability.

Brennan (1983) described a method that determines the water content of soft lenses indirectly by measuring the RI. As the water content increases, the RI decreases and the two are closely correlated, especially in the 30–70% water content range (Fatt & Chaston 1980, Teuerle 1984).

Under controlled environmental conditions and for a given wavelength, RI = sine of angle of incidence/sine of angle of reflection.

The angle at which total internal reflection occurs can be measured using a hand-held Abbé Refractometer (Fig. 16.16) (Brennan 1983).

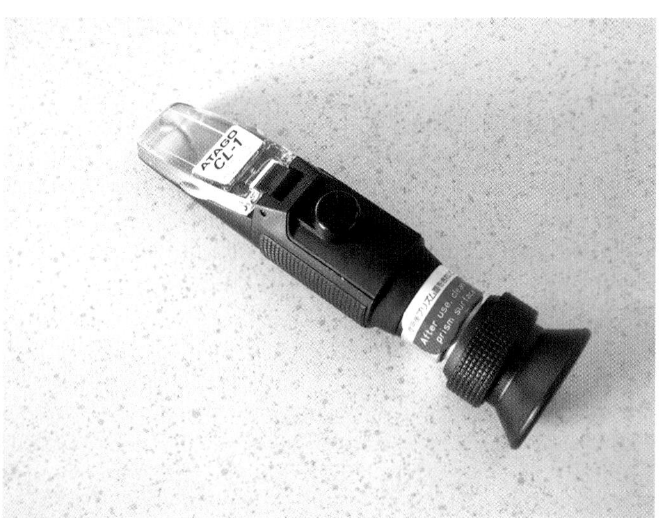

Figure 16.16 The Atago CL-1 soft lens refractometer

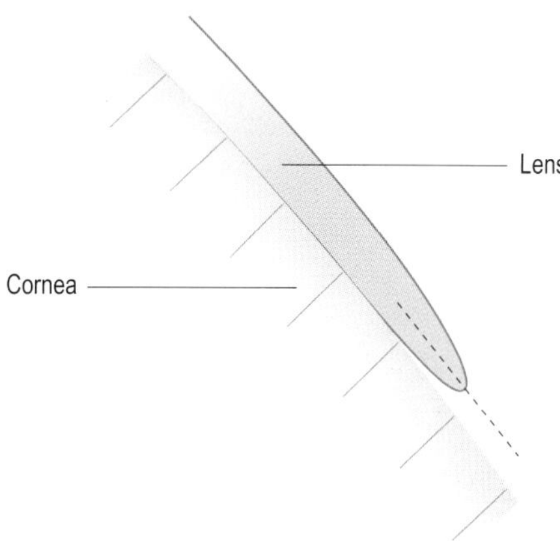

Figure 16.17 Theoretical ideal contact lens profile. The lens with an ideal edge profile will move parallel to the cornea as shown by the dotted line. (From Forst 1993, with permission of DOZ Verlag)

- The hydrated contact lens is blotted dry and applanated with a glass plate onto the fixed prism of the refractometer.
- The instrument is directed towards an external light source, and the border between the dark and light fields viewed in the eyepiece.
- The water content is then read directly from the internal scale.

The CLR 12-70 (Index Instruments, UK) is an automated refractometer with ten programmable water content scales to assess different polymer materials which have been found to give reliable readings (Nichols & Berntsen 2003).

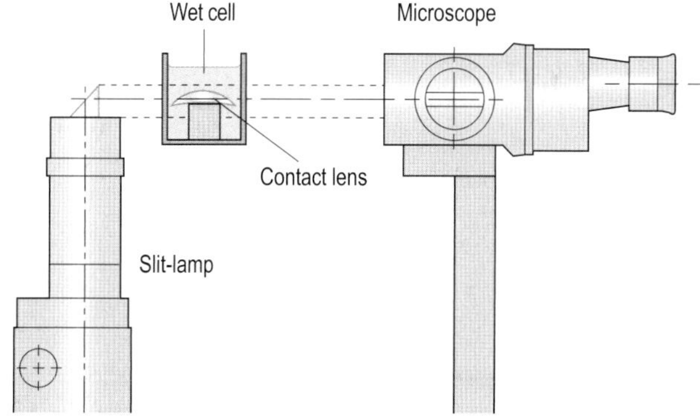

Figure 16.18 Slit-lamp technique for checking the edge profile of a soft lens. (From Forst 1993, with permission of DOZ Verlag)

Edge quality

The design of the edge profile affects the comfort of rigid lenses. An edge profile that is approximately symmetrical is most comfortable (Forst 1980). The ideal radial edge lift should be approximately 0.08–0.10 mm and the ideal rounding of the lens edge should have an approximate radius of 0.03–0.06 mm (Forst 1980, Adrasko 1991) (Fig. 16.17). Soft lenses have a larger diameter and drape over the eye onto the sclera. The edge profile requirements are therefore not as critical as in rigid lenses but must still be well rounded to aid comfort.

Various methods are available to check lens edge, including projection methods, slit-lamps, simple binocular microscopes or hand-held magnifiers. Rigid lenses are mounted on a rotating lens holder (a suction holder can be used) for examination. Forst (1993) described a special slit-lamp technique that uses a wet cell to assess the edge profile of a soft lens (Fig. 16.18).

Surface quality

Despite the high percentage of frequent replacement systems, checking the surface of rigid and soft contact lenses is still important. Surface deposits and spoilage of contact lenses are the main reasons for complications occurring with conventional lenses (Fleiszig et al. 1996).

The surface or the edge of a contact lens can be examined using a loupe, slit-lamp, scanning electron microscope, reflective light and transmission light microscope, as well as projection magnifiers.

According to Sickenberger (2001), there are three categories of contact lens deposit:

- Endogenous deposits (from the eye): lipids, proteins, mucins and salts. These deposits are made up of calcium, magnesium, sodium chloride and potassium.
- Exogenous deposits (external source): cosmetics, drug intake, nicotine, microorganisms, fungi and metallic oxides.
- Mixed deposits.

ENDOGENOUS DEPOSITS

Lipid

This can be observed on all lens materials but especially on rigid silicone or fluorosilicone lenses. Figure 16.19 shows lipid on a rigid contact lens.

Protein

Protein, seen as a whitish-grey coating, which appears crazed when observed through the microscope (Fig. 16.20a), makes

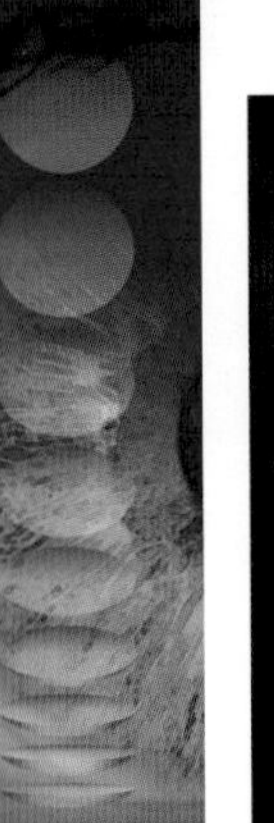

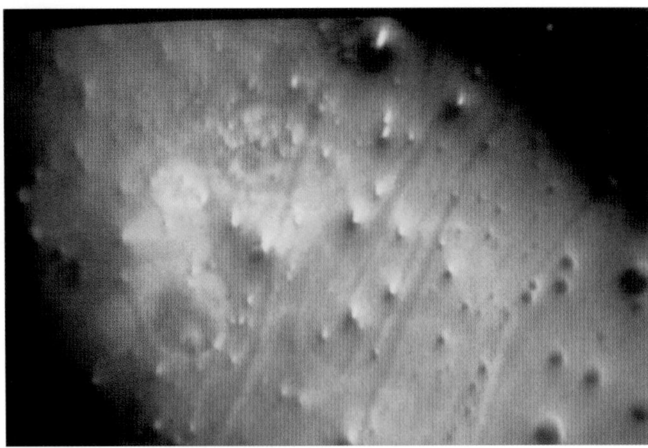

Figure 16.19 Lipid droplets in the tear film (magnification 200×). (Courtesy of W. Sickenberger)

surfaces hydrophobic. It can cause problems on rigid lenses but plays a greater role in the build-up of deposits on soft lenses.

Protein may result in allergic reactions (e.g. giant papillary conjunctivitis).

High-water-content materials bind to more proteins (mainly lysozymes) than low-water-content materials (Stone 1984); ionic materials bind to all proteins (Sack 1985).

Mucin

Mucin is a neutral mucopolysaccharide that contains amino sugars and monosugars (Berke & Blümle 1997). These deposits are less common and may be mistaken for lipid. They cause a reduction in lens wettability (Fig. 16.20b).

EXOGENOUS DEPOSITS

Nicotine and cosmetics

A large number of exogenous substances can adhere to the surface of rigid and soft contact lenses and reduce comfort in different ways. Exogenous substances include nicotine, dust and cosmetics (Fig. 16.21a) as well as drugs.

Discolouration

Discolouration is more commonly seen in soft lenses. There are many different causes of lens discolouration, one of which is drug intake (including prescription drugs). In general, discolouration is more common with conventional high-water-content lenses than low-water-content materials (Fig. 16.21b).

Fungi

Poor lens hygiene can result in fungal deposits although minimal contamination is required for fungi to grow (as opposed to bacteria which need contamination to adhere to the lens surface). They initially adhere to the lens surface with polysaccharides and ionic bonds before forming a fibrillary film, which protects them from contact lens cleaners (Berke & Cagnolati 2002). Fungal enzymes destroy high-water-content lenses more than low-water-content. *Aspergillus* (Fig. 16.22a), *Candida* (Fig. 16.22b) and *Penicillium* varieties have been observed on contact lenses.

There are two types of fungus associated with contact lenses:

- Yeast.
- Mould.

Metallic deposits

The environmental effects of air pollution or particles found in the workplace can result in metallic deposits, especially on soft lenses. Rust spots, which can be caused by metallic particles, are a classic type (Fig. 16.23a).

Scratches and edge spoilage

Scratches occur on all types of lens, but are most common on rigid lenses (Fig. 16.23b). They will:

(a)

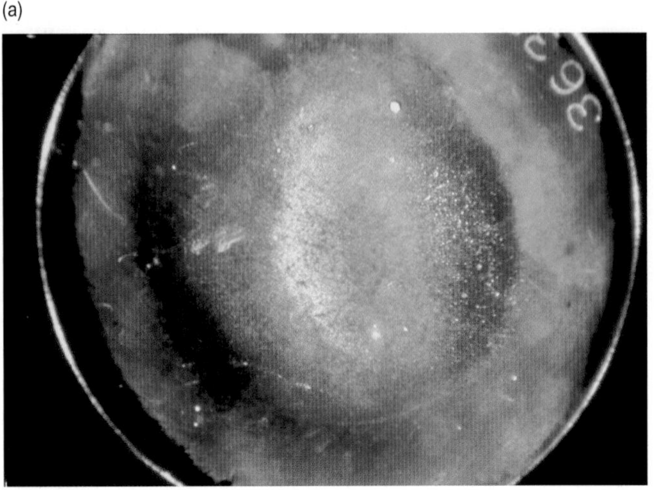

(b)

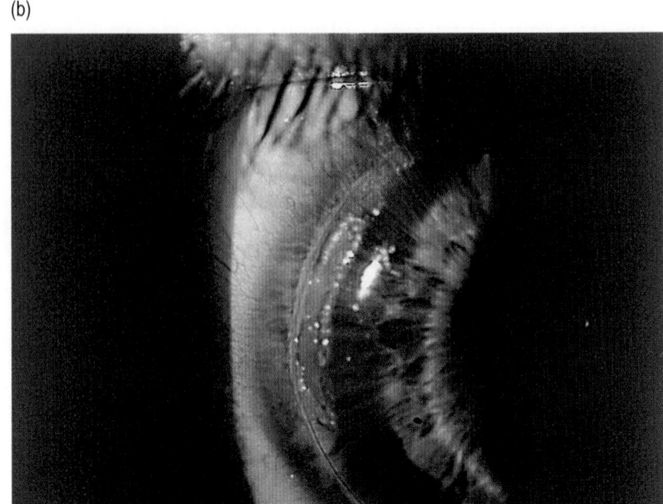

Figure 16.20 (a) Extensive protein deposits (magnification 6×); (b) 9 o'clock deposits on the lenticular zone of a rigid contact lens. (Courtesy of W. Sickenberger)

(a)

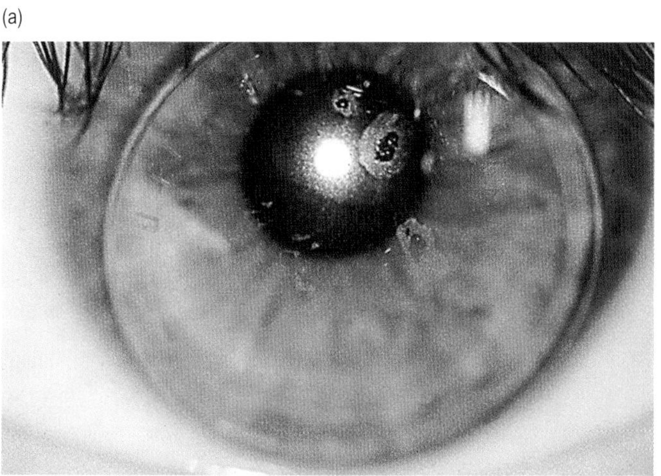

(b)

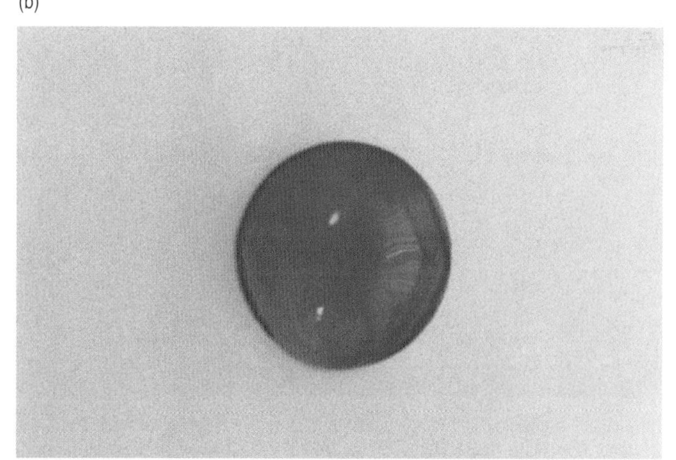

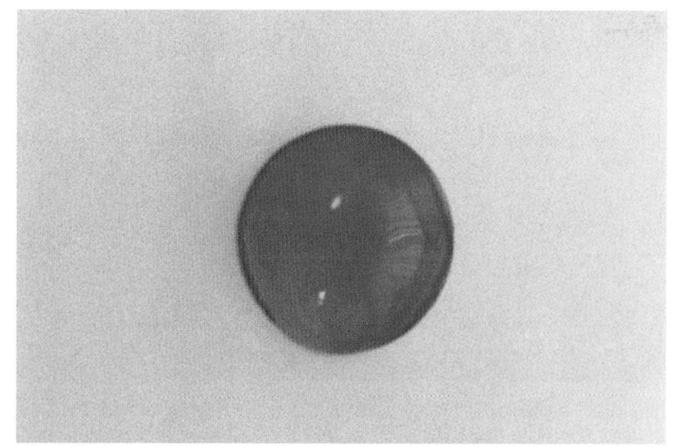

Figure 16.21 (a) Hydrophobic areas due to eyeliner residue on a rigid contact lens. (Courtesy of W. Sickenberger) (b) Discoloration by phenolphthalein (macroscopic). (From Berke & Blümle 1997, with permission of DOZ Verlag)

(a)

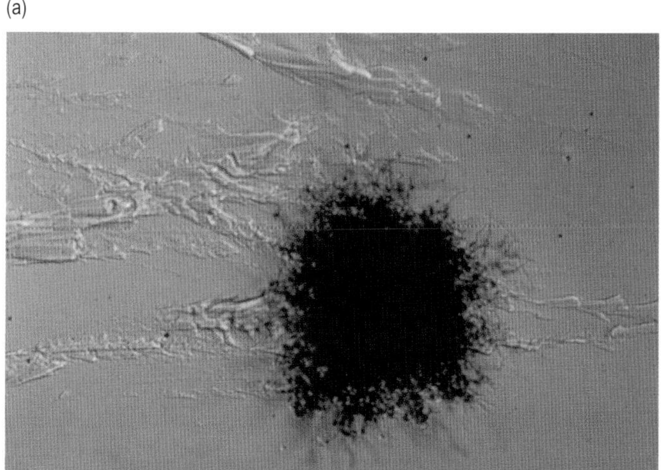

(b)

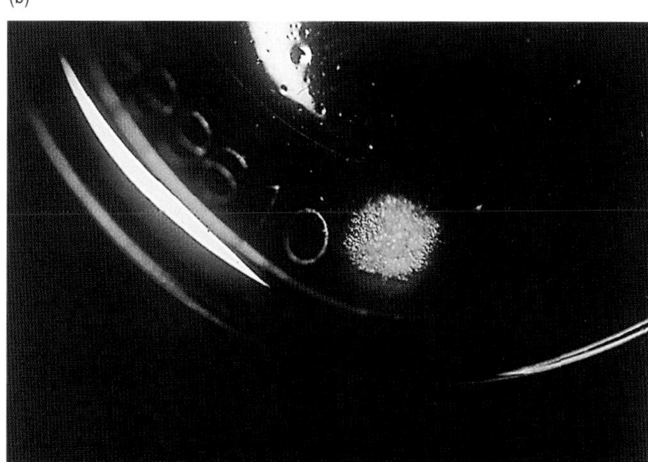

Figure 16.22 (a) *Aspergillus niger* (magnification 200×); (b) *Candida albicans* (magnification 12×). (Courtesy of W. Sickenberger)

- Affect comfort.
- Reduce wettability.
- Cause deposit build-up.

As mentioned previously, many instruments can be used to check contact lenses for scratches and edge spoilage. The slit-lamp will provide a general overview of the lens using diffuse illumination, followed by more detailed examination with direct illumination and a wide beam or an optic section and a narrow beam.

CONCLUSION

The contact lens curriculum taught today no longer corresponds with the contents of the first edition of this book, published in 1972, when the verification of contact lens parameters was so much more complex. Nevertheless, today's practitioners must have a basic knowledge of lens checking because they are still responsible for the health of their patients' eyes. Contact lens verification is still taught and is an examination subject in the European Diploma in Optometry (ECOO).

Knowledge develops continuously in the contact lens field, and at national and international levels we see a steady increase in publications relating to contact lenses. For this reason I have referred to some German publications which are not always available internationally.

Acknowledgements

When writing this chapter, I was able to base my research on the excellent work of Rita Watts and Don Loran from the fourth edition of this book which has been of great assistance. I have adopted many of their contributions that are still topical today.

(a)

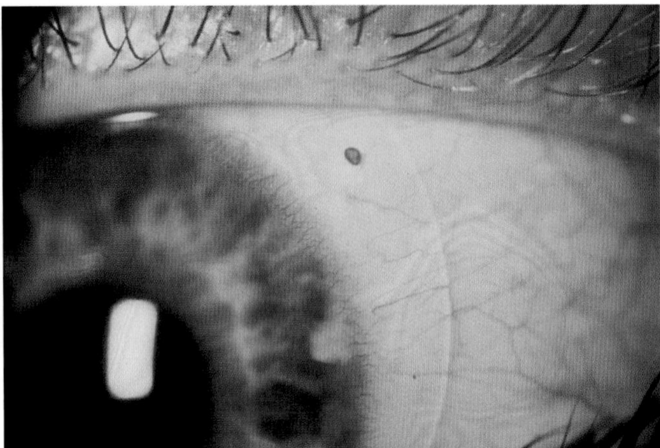

(b)

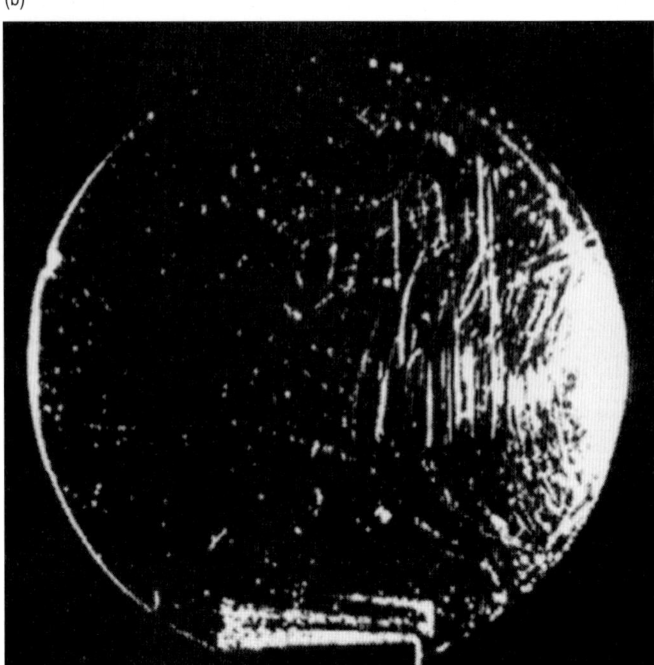

Figure 16.23 (a) Rust spot on a contact lens. (Courtesy of W. Sickenberger). (b) Scratches and edge damage of a rigid contact lens after use. (From Forst 1993, with permission of DOZ Verlag)

My sincere thanks go to Peter V. Moest, University of Applied Sciences (TFH), Berlin, Germany, and to Holger Dietze, formerly of the University of Bradford, UK, for the critical and constructive review of my manuscript. I am also indebted to all those who kindly provided many of the photographs and illustrations used in this chapter, in particular to Wolfgang Sickenberger, University of Applied Sciences (FH), Jena, Germany; Andrea Müller-Treiber, School of Optometry (HFA), Olten, Switzerland; Hilmar Bussacker, formerly Head School of Optometry (HFA), Olten, Switzerland; as well as to the DOZ Verlag, Heidelberg, Germany.

References

Adrasko, G. J. (1991) Keeping your eye on edge quality. Spectrum, 6(9), 37–39

Baron H. (1991) Kontaktlinsen, pp. 617–619. Heidelberg: Verlag Optische Fachveröffentlichung

Bauer, G. T. (1979) Longitudinal spherical aberration of soft contact lenses. Int. Contact Lens Clin., 6, 143–150

Berke, A. and Blümle, S. (1997) Kontaktlinsenhygiene. Pforzheim: Boden

Berke, A. and Cagnolati, W. (2002) Contact Lens Hygiene. In Antiseptic Prophylaxis and Therapy in Ocular Infections, pp. 328–342, eds. A. Kramer and W. Behrens-Baumann. Basel: Karger

Brennan, N. A. (1983) A simple instrument for measuring the water content of hydrogel lenses. Int. Contact Lens Clin., 10, 357–361

Bussacker, H. (1983) Toposkopische Beurteilung von asphärischen Kontaktlinsenrückflächen. Neues Optikerjournal, 25(1), 56–59

Chaston, J. (1973) A method of measuring the radius of curvature of a soft contact lens. Optician, 165(4271), 8–12

Collins, M., Goode, A., Davis, B. et al. (1997) A computer-interfaced vertometer system for contact lenses. Optom. Vis. Sci., 74(1), 59–65

DeFazio, A. J. and Lowther, G. E. (1979) Inspection of back surface aspheric contact lenses. Am. J. Optom. Physiol. Opt., 56(8), 471–479

Dietze, H. H. and Cox, M. J. (2003) On- and off-eye spherical aberration of soft contact lenses and consequent changes of effective lens power. Optom. Vis. Sci., 80(2), 126–134

Dietze, H. H. and Cox, M. J. (2004) Correcting ocular spherical aberration with soft contact lenses. J. Opt. Soc. Am. A, 21(4), 473–485

Dietze, H. H., Cox, M. J. and Douthwaite, W. A. (2003) Verification of aspheric contact lens back surfaces. Optom. Vis. Sci., 80(8), 596–605

Dörbrand, B. (1985) Interferometrische Meßtechnik zur Prüfung asphärischer Kontaktlinsen. die Kontaktlinse, 19(1), 14–31

Dorronsoro, C., Barbero, S., Llorente, L. et al. (2003) On-eye measurement of optical performance of rigid gas permeable contact lenses based on ocular and corneal aberrometry. Optom, Vis. Sci., 80(2), 115–125

Douthwaite, W. A. and Hurst, M. A. (1998) 'Pillar and collar' technique for measuring the axial edge lift of multicurve rigid lenses. Optom. Vis. Sci., 75(3), 217–220

Drysdale, C. V. (1900) On a simple direct method of measuring the curvature of small lenses. Trans. Opt. Soc., 2, 1–12

Efron, N., Morgan, P. and Morgan, S. (1999) Accuracy and reproducibility of one-day disposable contact lenses. Int. Contact Lens Clin., 26(6), 168–173

El-Nasher, N. and Larke, J. K. (1980) Interference measurements of soft lenses. J. Br. Contact Lens Assoc., 3, 64–70

Fatt, I. and Chaston, J. (1980) The effect of temperature on RI, water content and central thickness of hydrogel contact lenses. Int. Contact Lens Clin., 7, 250–255

Fleiszig, S. M., Evans, D. J., Mowrey-McKee, M. F. et al. (1996) Factors affecting Staphylococcus epidermidis adhesion to contact lenses. Optom. Vis. Sci., 73(9), 590–594

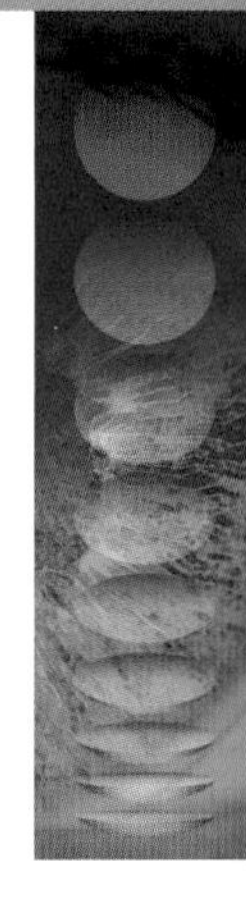

Fonn, D., Situ, P. and Simpson, T. (1999) Hydrogel lens dehydration and subjective comfort and dryness ratings in symptomatic and asymptomatic contact lens wearers. Optom. Vis. Sci., 76(10), 700–704

Forst, G. (1974) New methods of measurement for controlling soft lens quality. Contacto, 18(6), 6–9

Forst, G. (1980) Zur Gestaltung des Randprofils einer Kontaktlinse. Dtsch. Optikerztg., 35(9), 99–103

Forst, G. (1993) Grundlagen der Kontaktlinsenanpassung, p. 86. Heidelberg: Verlag Optische Fachveröffentlichung

Franco, S., Almeida, J. B. and Parafita, M. (2000) Measurement of corneal thickness by videopachymetry: preliminary results. J. Refract. Surg., 16(5), 661–663

Gisler, T. (1993) Praxis der Kontaktlinsenanpassung – Ein Handbuch für den Praktiker, p. 88. Mülheim: Gisler-Verlag

Guillon, M., Crosbie-Walsh, J. and Byrnes, D. (1986) Application of pachometry to the measurement of hard contact lens edge profile. Trans. BCLA Conference, pp. 56–59

Gundel, R. E. and Cohen, H. I. (1986) Dehydration induced parameter changes. Int. Eyecare, 2, 311–314

Höfer, P. (1999) Die Normung: Strukturen, Entstehung und Inhalte am Beispiel Kontaktlinse. Dtsch. Optikerztg., 54(10), 84–87

Hong, X., Himebaugh, N. and Thibos, L. N. (2001) On-eye evaluation of optical performance of rigid and soft contact lenses. Optom. Vis. Sci., 78, 872–880

International Standards: ISO 9337–1 (2001) Contact Lenses. Determination of back vertex power. Method using jocimeter with manual focusing. Geneva: International Organization for Standardization

International Standard Draft ISO/DIS 18369-1 (2004a) Ophthalmic Optics – Contact Lenses – Part 1: Terminology. Geneva: International Organization for Standardization

International Standard Draft ISO/DIS 18369-2 (2004b) Ophthalmic Optics – Contact Lenses – Part 2: Tolerances. Geneva: International Organization for Standardization

International Standard Draft ISO/DIS 18369-3 (2004c) Ophthalmic Optics – Contact Lenses – Part 3: Methods of measurement. Geneva: International Organization for Standardization

Keren, E., Kreske, K. and Livnat, A. (1992) Darstellung der optischen Wirkung und Qualitätsbeurteilung von weichen Kontaktlinsen in Flüssigkeit mit dem Moiré-Deflectometer. die Kontaktlinse, 26(9), 14–16

Lester, W. R. and Lester, S. F. (1979) The soft lens analyzer. Contact Lens Forum, 4(2), 85–91

Lopez-Gil, N., Castejon-Mochon, J. F., Benito, A. et al. (2002) Aberration generation by contact lenses with aspheric and asymmetric surfaces. J. Refract. Surg., 18, 603–609

Masnick, K. B. and Holden, B. A. (1972) Studies of water content and parametric variations of hydrophilic contact lenses. Aust. J. Optom., 55, 481–487

Meszaros, G. (2003) A new method to achieve better quality quickly. Online. Available: www.gclabsite.com

Newlove, D. B. (1974) Development of a new hard lens material. Optician, 169(4368), 16–23

Nichols, J. J. and Berntsen, D. A. (2003) The assessment of automated measures of hydrogel contact lens refractive index. Ophthalmic Physiol. Opt., 23(6), 517–525

Patel, S. (1983) Effects of lens dehydration on back vertex power, apical height, and lens mass off high water content hydrogel lenses. Int. Contact Lens Clin., 10, 38–42

Patella, V. M., Harris, M. G., Wong, V. A. et al. (1982) Ultrasonic measurement of soft contact lens base curves. Int. Contact Lens Clin., 9(1), 41–53

Port, M. J. A. (1975) The radius measurements of hydrophilic contact lenses using ultrasonics. MSc Thesis. Birmingham: University of Aston

Port, M. J. A. (1976) New methods of measuring hydrophilic lenses. Ophthalmic Opt., 16, 1079–1082

Port, M. J. A. (1981a) The Optimec Contact Lens Analyser. Optician, 181(4683), 11–14

Port, M. J. A. (1981b) The radius measurement of soft contact lenses in air. J. Br. Contact Lens Assoc., 5, 168–176

Port, M. J. A. (1987) A new method of edge thickness measurement for rigid lenses. J. Br. Contact Lens Assoc., 10, 16–20

Quesnel, N-M. and Simonet, P. (1994) Precision and reliability study of a modified keratometric technique for measuring the radius of curvature of soft contact lenses. Ophthalmic Physiol. Opt., 4, 320–326

Rabbetts, R. B. (1995) Radiuscope correction factors for aspheric lenses. Optician, 210(5513), 26–27

Rottenkolber, M. and Podbielska, H. (1996) High precision Twyman-Green interferometer for the measurement of ophthalmic surfaces. Acta Ophthalmol. Scand., 74(4), 348–353

Ruben, M. (1974) Soft lenses: the physico-chemical characteristics. Contacto, 18(5), 11–23

Sack, R. A. (1985) Specificity and biological activity of lens bound protein layer to hydrogel structure. Presentation, American Academy of Optometry Meeting, Atlanta

Sickenberger, W. (2001) Klassifikation von Spaltlampenbefunden – Ein praxisnahes Handbuch für Kontaktlinsenanpasser. Aschaffenburg: CIBA Vision

Söhnges Optik (1974) Information Deutsche Kontaktlinsen GmbH No. 9. Munich: Deutsche Kontaktlinsen GmbH

Stone, J. (1975) Corneal lenses with constant axial edge lift. Ophthalmic Optician, 15, 818–824

Stone, R. P. (1984) Protein: a source of lens discoloration. Contact Lens Forum, 9, 33–41

Teuerle, W. (1984) Refractive index calculation of hydrogel contact lenses. Int. Contact Lens Clin., 11, 625–628

Thibos, L. N. (2003) Wavefront-guided contact lens design – principles, techniques and limitations. Optom. Today, 2, 35–37

Thibos, L. N., Hong, X., Bradley, A. et al. (2002) Statistical variation of aberration structure and image quality in a normal population of healthy eyes. J. Opt. Soc. Am. A, 19(12), 2329–2348

Wang, L. R., Zhang, J. Y. and Ya, Z. (2002) Calibration error on the measurement of back vertex power for contact lenses with method using focimeter with manual focusing. Optom. Vis. Sci., 79(2), 126–133

Westheimer, G. (1961) Aberrations of contact lenses. Am. J. Ophthalmol., 38, 445–448

Wilms, K. H. (1972) Zur Vorgeschichte der Betrachtung des Kontaktlinsenprofils in Immersion. Neues Optikerjournal, 14(4), 329–331

Yoon, G. Y. and Williams, D. R. (2002) Visual performance after correcting the monochromatic and chromatic aberrations of the eye. J. Opt. Soc. Am. A, 19(2), 266–275

Young, M. D. and Benjamin, W. J. (2003) Calibrated oxygen permeability of 35 conventional hydrogel materials and correlation with water content. Eye Contact Lens, 29(2), 126–133

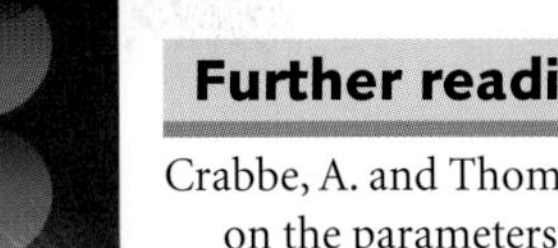

Further reading

Crabbe, A. and Thompson, P. (2001) Effects of microwave irradiation on the parameters of hydrogel contact lenses. Optom. Vis. Sci., 78(8), 610–615

Douthwaite, W. A. (2002) Application of linear regression to videokeratoscope data for tilted surfaces. Ophthalmic Physiol. Opt., 22(1), 46–54

Fatt, I. (1997) Comparative study of some physiologically important properties of six brands of disposable hydrogel contact lenses. CLAO J., 23(1), 49–54

Leitenberger, W., Wendrock, H., Bischoff, L. et al. (2004) Pinhole interferometry with coherent hard X-rays. J. Synchrotron Radiat., 11(2), 190–197

Merindano, M. D., Canals, M., Saona, C. et al. (1998) Rigid gas permeable contact lenses surface roughness examined by interferential shifting phase and scanning electron microscopies. Ophthalmic Physiol. Opt., 18(1), 75–82

Song, J. S., Lee, Y. H., Jo, J. H. et al. (1998) Moiré patterns of two different elongated circular gratings for the fine visual measurement of linear displacements. Opt. Commun., 154, 100–108

Woods, C. A. (2001) Measuring non-spherical optical surfaces. Cont. Lens Anterior Eye, 24, 9–15

Chapter 17

After-care

Charles McMonnies and Russell Lowe

CHAPTER CONTENTS

INTRODUCTION

Contact lens after-care is the key to developing good lens performance and sustaining ocular tissue health; successful contact lens practice depends on this. It provides an opportunity not only to modify lenses and maintenance methods, but also to solve problems of discomfort (the primary reason for discontinuation of contact lens wear; Vadjic et al. 1999) so that optimum results are achieved and maintained.

After-care may be time consuming and demanding of contact lens practitioners, and draws on all aspects of optometric and contact lens knowledge. Symptoms and signs require differential diagnosis from ocular pathology that is unrelated to contact lens wear and forethought is needed to predict problems so that appropriate steps can be taken.

An after-care examination should include the following:

- History of contact lens use, including:
  - hours worn per day.
  - days per week.
  - overall period of wear.
  - any limitations on wearing time.
- Prevalence, onset, duration of symptoms and when they occur.
- Evaluation of visual acuity and over-refraction using objective (retinoscopy, keratometry) and subjective methods.
- Examination of lens fitting:
  - centration.
  - movement.
  - tear circulation.
  - lens/cornea alignment.
- Examination at low magnification using a hand-held ultraviolet and white light, and at higher magnification using a slit-lamp biomicroscope. Contact lens and ocular tissue changes should be noted in white light before instilling staining agents to assist diagnosis.
- Further examination of lenses off the eye, including microscopic examination for signs of degradation and reassessment of lens parameters.
- Non-routine tests and measurements such as videokeratoscopy, tear film analysis, corneal sensitivity and a more thorough assessment of ocular health, including the posterior segments if indicated.

The above points are not intended to imply a rigid examination sequence. Usually symptoms are discussed throughout the examination in order to resolve any problems. Skilled interviewing and observation techniques are needed to build on information gained prior to fitting (if available). Abnormalities can only be recognized if the practitioner is aware of the normal variations in physiology and the pathological and physiological responses to contact lens wear. An observer who is unaware of

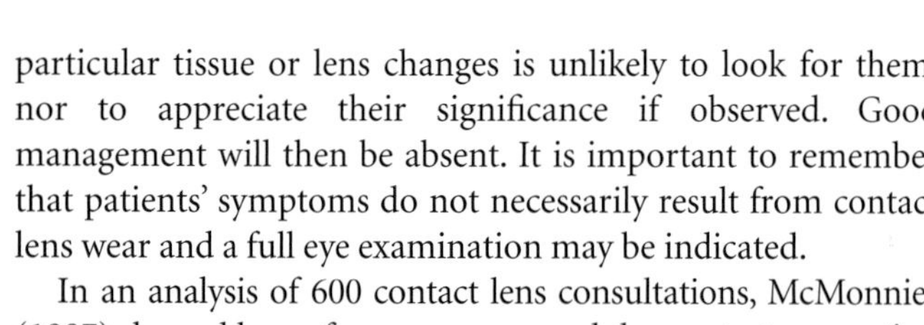

particular tissue or lens changes is unlikely to look for them, nor to appreciate their significance if observed. Good management will then be absent. It is important to remember that patients' symptoms do not necessarily result from contact lens wear and a full eye examination may be indicated.

In an analysis of 600 contact lens consultations, McMonnies (1987) showed how after-care consumed the greatest proportion of contact lens professional time. A second series of 600 after-care visits indicated 126 subtypes of problem requiring 64 subtypes of remedial strategy. Patients described no significant symptoms in 32% of after-care visits and yet 81% showed adverse signs which resulted in remedial action being taken, indicating that after-care is a time when potential problems are averted. Within the first year of prescribing, only 26% of remedial action was concerned with lens modification, increasing to 33% after the first year, indicating that the majority of after-care management was concerned with areas *other than* the technical aspects of lens and fit modification. Of the remaining two-thirds of patients, changing the lens fit did not improve their symptoms.

A systematic approach to the after-care examination provides the necessary information for correct identification of problems and their causes.

In the early stages of fitting, the concern is to determine how adaptation can be facilitated and tolerance improved. When problems develop, a systematic approach to analysis is helpful. For example: Is lost tolerance due to changes in:

- The eye's receptivity?
- The lens material or surface properties?
- The ambient conditions under which the lenses are worn?

Deductive analysis leads to remedial action, which in turn leads to remedial strategies.

INTERVIEWING AND HISTORY TAKING

Good patient interviewing is the key to effective after-care and derives in part from the trust, confidence and rapport developed between practitioner and patient (Enelow & Swisher 1972). Interview technique varies depending on whether the visit is prompted by an emergency, a particular problem, or a routine appointment with or without symptoms.

Open-ended questions are appropriate initially but questions should become more direct as specific details are sought. 'What kind of troubles have you been having?' is not open-ended enough to start, because it assumes that problems exist. A preferred start is 'How have you been getting on with your lenses?' followed by 'Do you wear your lenses every day?' and 'Are there any restrictions on wear?' If reduced or occasional wear is reported, the more direct 'Could you wear them longer or more often if you needed to?' may identify a reactive rather than preferential pattern of use.

The interviewer's tone should vary, depending on the patient's personality or mood. As clues lead to a solution, active authoritarian tone changes to a guiding and cooperative one and then one of mutual discussion between patient and practitioner. A patient's embarrassed attitude may correctly indicate problems in following instructions. Shared responsibility demonstrated by mutual participation in the discussion should elicit the reasons for non-compliance. Humour may help, combined with an acknowledgement that lack of strict discipline is a common failing, and the use of the euphemistic 'casual approach' rather than 'incorrect' may help expose the need for changes in the patient's attitude.

When change is essential, stronger terms such as 'dangerous procedures' may be required (e.g. if there is a high risk of infection). An authoritative tone risks an unproductive defensive patient attitude, whereas a passive tone may not solve the problem – the ideal tone is between the two.

Interviewing is time consuming but there is no completely satisfactory alternative. Questionnaires may be useful (McMonnies 1978, 1986, McMonnies & Ho 1987a,b), especially when they can be completed without supervision; however, a questionnaire limits the area of enquiry, and may be best suited to pre-fitting visits.

SYMPTOM ANALYSIS

Symptoms related to vision and comfort may occur together but should be considered separately.

Visual symptoms

Poor vision may result from the following although the list is not comprehensive.

- Blurred vision suggests an incorrect lens power; distortion suggests faulty optical quality, residual astigmatism or macular problems.
- A ghost image suggests incomplete pupil coverage, faulty optical quality or cataract.
- Near vision difficulties may result from presbyopia or from the nature of the near vision task, such as computer use which is associated with decreased blinking.
- Intermittent symptoms can be caused by lens flexure or rotation of an unstable toric lens.
- As surface deposits accumulate, difficulties may increase.
- Are symptoms relieved upon removing, cleaning and replacing the lenses?
- Lenses that are soiled or exhibit poor surface wetting characteristics will exhibit better vision with increased blinking.
- Does the difficulty only occur with reduced illumination because of a myopic shift under these conditions?

Reference to established findings may help identify the cause, for example:

- Patient's age, occupation and hobbies.
- Poor blinking.
- Poor lens optical quality or power when checked prior to delivery.
- Too thin a lens.
- Lens warpage from handling.

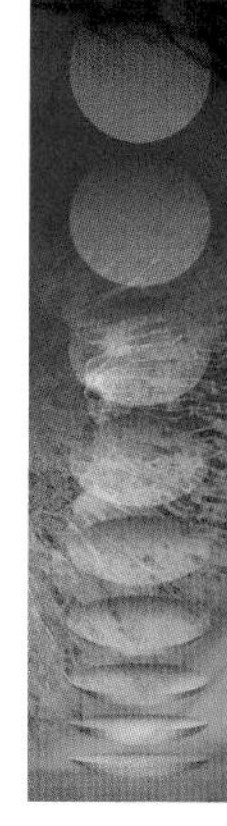

Tests such as retinoscopy or front surface keratometry can detect lens flexure. Ophthalmoscopy may indicate cataract development, retinal changes or other pathology. Further questions may be needed, such as:

- Does the problem become more apparent when reverting to spectacles after lens wear?
- Have there been systemic health changes and possible ocular side-effects of medications or general anaesthesia?
- Has there been an increase in near vision, possibly due to examinations or to a change in work practices such as more VDU use?

Simple explanations should be kept in mind; for example, if over-refraction indicates antimetropia, right and left lenses may have been inadvertently swapped.

Note any variations from expected acuity and the difference between quantitative and qualitative visual performance when acuity is good but complaints of poor vision persist; contrast sensitivity tests will help. Retinoscopy may indicate irregular astigmatism due to a distorted lens or one with poor optics, or possibly keratoconus. Biomicroscopy may reveal a soiled and/or non-wetting lens surface.

The parameters and condition of the lens should be checked before reordering or carrying out modifications. Even a copy of the lens prescription from a previous practitioner only tells what the lenses are supposed to be; the actual parameters are often different. Patients may also present wearing lenses from an earlier fitting.

Symptoms of discomfort

The cause of discomfort needs to be investigated. Pertinent questions include the following.

- Does discomfort occur immediately upon insertion?
- Does discomfort occur following lens removal?
- Discomfort disappearing on lens insertion suggests trichiasis, a retained foreign body or extruding concretion in the upper palpebral conjunctiva.
- Is the discomfort constant – only on application; only after several hours of wear; only when reading; only in glare situations?
- Was this lens previously comfortable?
- Is the discomfort a chemical sting or a gritty, foreign body sensation?
- Grade the intensity of discomfort (e.g. lens awareness = 1; irritation = 2; pain = 3).
- Does the eye itch (allergy)?
- Is the lens damaged or ill fitting?
- Are signs of localized limbal hyperaemia or corneal epitheliopathy present?
- Is the lens inside out or mixed (left with right or old with new)?
- Is there any corneal oedema?
- Are rigid lens back surface transitions smooth?
- Is the edge shape satisfactory?
- Is the lens too thick?
- Has a duplicate lens been incorrectly made?
- Are different lens care products being used?
- Are the lenses being over-worn?
- Are the lenses being worn in a harsh environment?
- Is the discomfort associated with the use of certain cosmetics?
- Does lens application require multiple attempts that cause irritation?
- Are there psychological reasons for the patient to exaggerate or fabricate discomfort symptoms?
- Is the patient unhappy with the choice of tint?
- Has the patient lost motivation for wearing contact lenses?
- Has the patient been subjected to adverse comments about their appearance without spectacles?
- Is this a case of an industrial compensation claim that is yet to be settled?

Good record keeping is the key to good after-care. A systematic examination should reveal the cause of any problem. Examine the anterior eye, tear film, lens fit and condition in diffuse illumination or with a hand-held lamp, then instil fluorescein and reassess.

If new symptoms arise with lenses that have previously been worn successfully, the following may give a clue as to the source.

- *The eye*: patient is less tolerant – medication side-effects, reduced tear function, allergy.
- *The lens*: lenses are less wearable – lens or case contamination, lens damage, surface deposits.
- *The environment*: wearing conditions have changed significantly – increased exposure to air conditioning or glare, work-related increase in visual demand.

After-care glossary

The entries in this glossary are chosen according to their relevance to after-care consultations rather than contact lens fitting in general, and reference to other chapters of this book is made where appropriate. The distinction between rigid gas-permeable (RGP) and polymethylmethacrylate (PMMA) lenses is only made when necessary and other references to rigid lenses include both types. Similarly, entries in this glossary refer to both rigid and soft lenses unless otherwise stated.

Variations in terminology used may cause difficulty in locating information. The reader should refer to the main index to search for particular entries.

Cross-references in **bold type** refer to other entries within the glossary.

Allergy

Atopy generally predisposes against contact lens wear (see also Chapter 8) and it is difficult and impractical to attempt to identify the precise allergen(s). Sensitivity to lens materials and solutions (see **Preservative reaction**) occurs, as do reactions to cosmetics (see **Cosmetics**), and it may be difficult to differentiate from sensitivity to lens surface deposits.

Signs

- Oedematous lids.
- Watery discharge.
- Conjunctival hyperaemia and oedema.

General corneal superficial punctate keratitis may be the sign of a material allergy, and grey stromal infiltrates the signs of a solution (especially thimerosal) allergy (see **Fit evaluation**; **Vascularization**; Fig. 17.28).

Symptoms

- Burning.
- Itching.
- Irritation.

Management

- Challenge and rechallenge tests to identify and eliminate suspected antigenic factors.
- Reduce exposure to seasonal antigens.
- Consider allergenic potential of household pets, indoor plants, dust mites.
- Prescribe topical therapeutic agents such as mast cell stabilizers, corticosteroids and antihistamines. Contact lens wear may be contraindicated when using drops, although if daily disposable lenses are worn the risk of any adverse reaction is minimal.

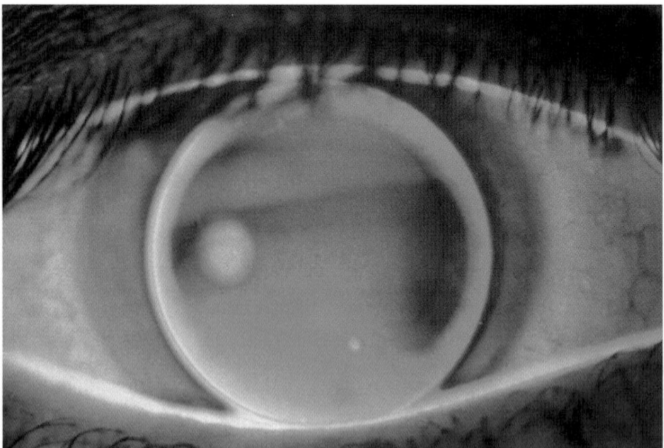

Figure 17.1 An interrupted tear layer (prowline) across the lens front surface indicating that the blink prior to the photograph was partial or incomplete

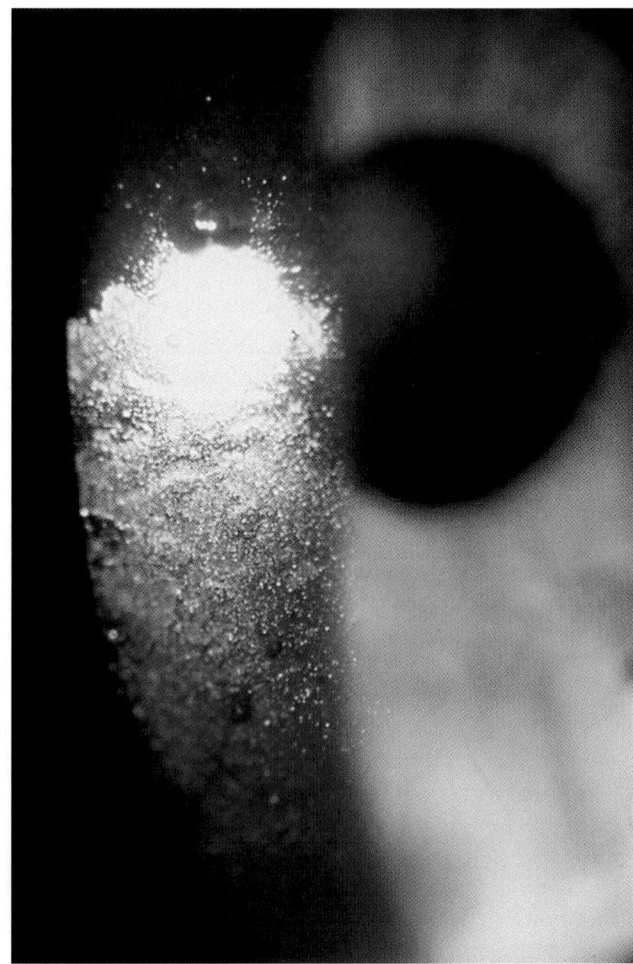

Figure 17.2 A partial blink allows the inferior portion of the lens to dry, increasing the deposition of tear residues

Blepharitis (see **Dermatological conditions; Lid hygiene;** Fig. 17.17 and Chapter 18)

Blink efficiency

Efficient, complete blinks help to position lenses correctly, promote tear circulation, eliminate debris from under lenses and prevent deposits from forming. A combination of partial and complete blinks is normal, but an excess of partial blinks compared with full, complete blinks is commonly found with new contact lens wearers (Korb 1974). It is likely that contact lenses increase the blink frequency during adaptation or when discomfort is present but, when lenses are worn comfortably by adapted patients, the frequency of blinks is determined by factors such as the patient's personality, mood, fatigue level, visual task, state of alertness and ambient atmosphere conditions, etc.

Helping the patient understand these various blink functions and the nature of their problem will motivate them to make the effort required to develop more efficient blinks. They need to be made aware of their blink action and when they make a relaxed, full or complete blink (when the top lid lightly touches the bottom lid) and does not involve facial muscles. Facial muscles can either increase the force of closure (blepharospasm) and/or increase the widening of the palpebral aperture but should be avoided as they appear unnatural.

Signs

- Interrupted tear layer (prowline) across the front surface in the pupil region of the lens (Fig. 17.1).
- Excess tear debris under lenses.
- Excess drying and deposits on the inferior, exposed area of lenses, which are particularly noticeable on lenses that do not rotate (toric and/or prism ballast, etc.) (Fig. 17.2; see also Figs 17.21 and 17.22).
- Superficial punctate epitheliopathy on the inferior area of the cornea exposed by partial blinks in some soft lens wearers.

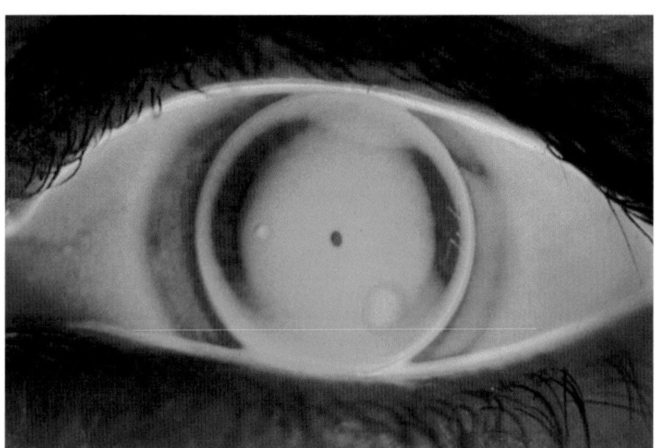

Figure 17.3 Excess apical clearance can permit bubble formation

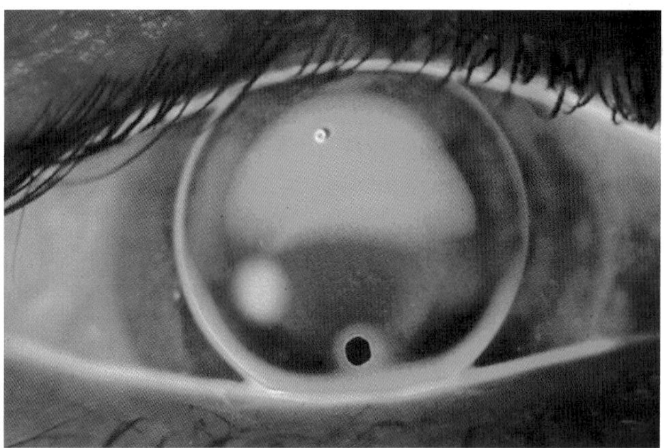

Figure 17.4 In keratoconus, bubble formation can easily occur

Management

- Improve contact lens comfort.
- Remove contact lenses for extended reading periods, especially in air conditioning/central heating.
- Use tear supplements.
- Prescribe blink efficiency exercises (see **Tear deficiency**).
- Advise patients to practise relaxed complete blinks that do not involve the facial muscles.
- Warn against slow blinks, as these look unnatural and reduce efficiency.
- The ratio of full blinks to incomplete blinks can be increased with practice. Sessions of 20 blinks, 20 times per day for a week should be sufficient, but the patient needs to be motivated. The matter may be crucial as inefficient blinking may be the only barrier to contact lens success (see also Chapter 8).

Bubbles of air

A steep lens may trap a bubble of air at the time of application (Fig. 17.3) or during eye movements. Successive blinks cause the bubble to break up into froth. Rigid lenses require a flatter fitting but in some keratoconus fittings, flattening the fit will not help (Fig. 17.4). Fenestration may relieve the problem but may cause more bubbles to form.

Bubbles appear under the edge, and possibly into the back optic portion, of a lens with excessive edge clearance. With soft lenses, bubbles or fine froth can form under an immobile lens (Fig. 17.5), often observed together with stationary tear debris.

Centrally located froth will reduce vision only slightly but can cause increased flare due to light scattering. Froth or bubbles cause epithelial indentation or 'dimpling' that generally disappears within an hour of lens removal. These fill with fluorescein (Fig. 17.6) but do not actually stain unless the epithelial cells are damaged. The areas of fluorescence are typically larger, brighter and have sharply defined edges compared to punctate keratitis staining. Staining lasts no more than a few minutes as normal blink action (or irrigation) will remove the fluorescein from the hollow since true staining has not occurred. Even with no staining the dimples may be seen by indirect slit-lamp illumination both against the dark pupil and the light iris background (retroillumination). The long-term effects of dimpling on epithelial integrity have not been recorded but do not appear to harm the cornea and may be acceptable in advanced cases of keratoconus if attempts to modify the lens do not eliminate the froth (Fig. 17.7) (see also Chapters 9, 10 and 20).

(a)

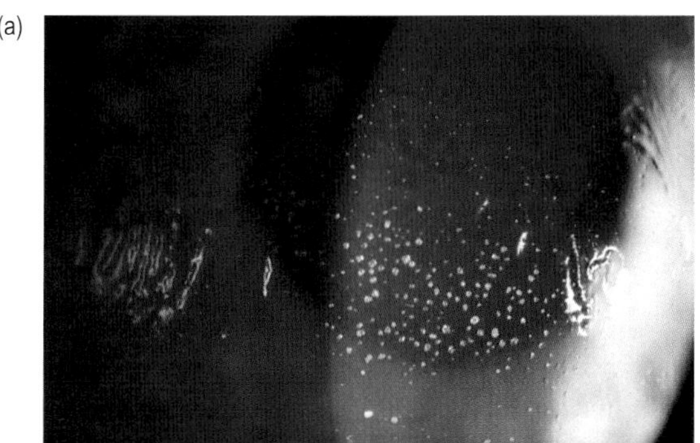

(b)

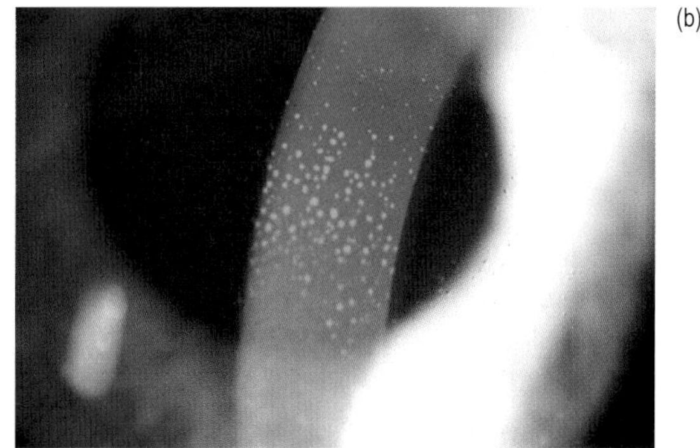

Figure 17.5 Dimple staining can occur with both rigid (see Fig. 17.6) and soft lenses. (a) Lipid droplets shown beneath a soft lens. (b) Dimpling can be recognized by its bright staining and sharply defined edges. (Courtesy of A. J. Phillips)

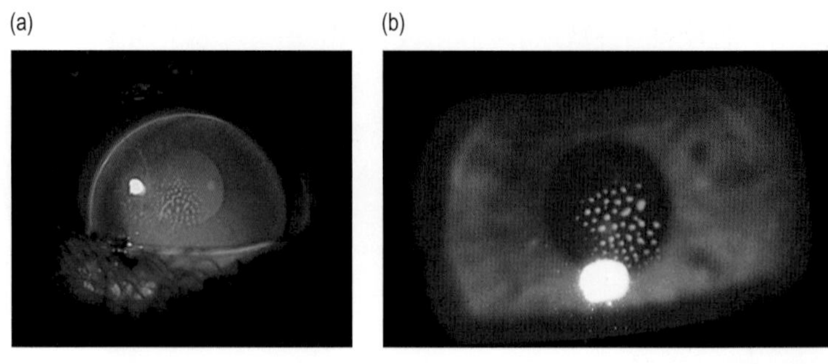

Figure 17.6 (a) Small bubbles trapped under a corneal lens have caused furrows and dimples in the epithelium during lens movement; (b) fluorescein has collected in these furrows and dimples. The resultant deterioration in vision is known as dimple veil (see also Fig. 17.5). (Courtesy of A. J. Phillips)

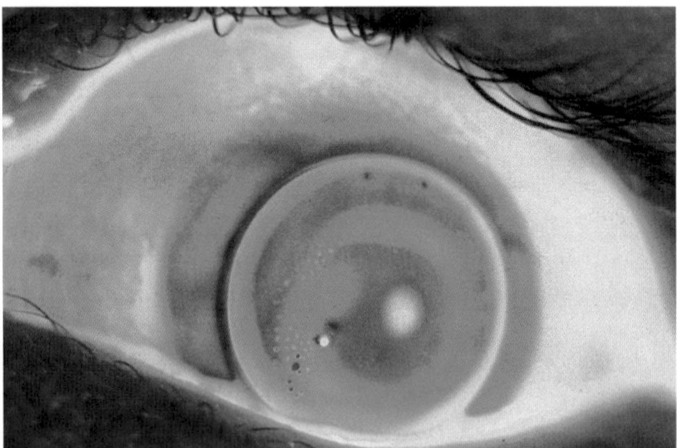

Figure 17.7 In some cases of keratoconus, minor frothing can be regarded as acceptable

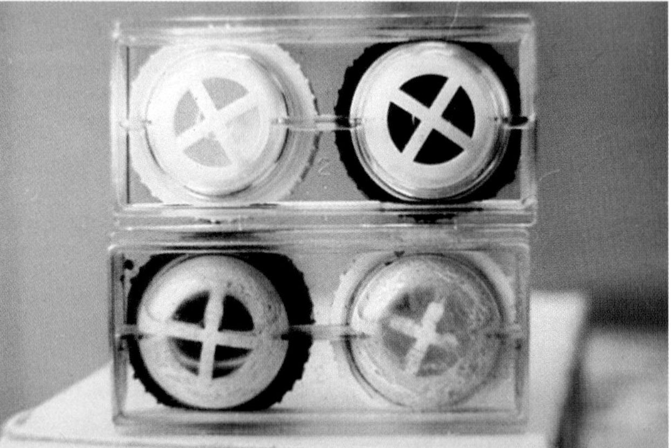

Figure 17.8 The soiled case (below) contrasts with the new case (above). Dark-coloured cases are not ideal because they conceal dirt and biofilm

Symptoms

- Deteriorating vision.
- Increased flare/glare later in the wearing day (dimple veil).

Management

- Fit RGP lenses flatter or with less edge clearance.
- Fit looser soft lenses.
- In keratoconus, a steeper fitting with a smaller back optic zone diameter (BOZD) may be indicated or a steeper and/or toroidal back peripheral radius (BPR_1) or differential edge clearance (see also Chapter 20).

Burton lamp (hand UV lamp)

Evaluation of lens fittings with white and ultraviolet light has several advantages not available with the slit-lamp.

- Rapid evaluation of eyes and lenses, which is useful if the patient is very uncomfortable or uncooperative (e.g. small children).
- Both eyes are visible within the field of the magnifier so the lens position on the two eyes can be compared.
- Rapid assessment of lens fit.
- The patient can sit with their head held naturally.

The biomicroscope can then be used for more detailed examination. The hand UV lamp is also ideal for low magnification with white light (see also Chapters 8 and 9).

Case contamination (see **Infection** and Chapters 4 and 8)

- Light-coloured cases show accumulated biofilm and other contamination (Fig. 17.8).
- Soiled cases provide nutrients for microorganisms that cause infection or irritation.
- Patients frequently need re-instruction on cleaning their lens case.
- A clear plastic pouch is useful to store the case in their pocket or handbag to stop dust and dirt soiling the case exterior.
- Case contamination should be suspected when infection occurs.

Management

- Advise patient of association between case contamination and infection.
- Improve maintenance compliance.
- Replace case more frequently.

Chronic hyperaemia

This may be evident at after-care visits (McMonnies et al. 1982, McMonnies & Chapman-Davies 1987a) although some patients have chronically hyperaemic eyes without lenses and contact lens wear exacerbates the problem (see **Reactive eye** and Figs 17.9, 17.10).

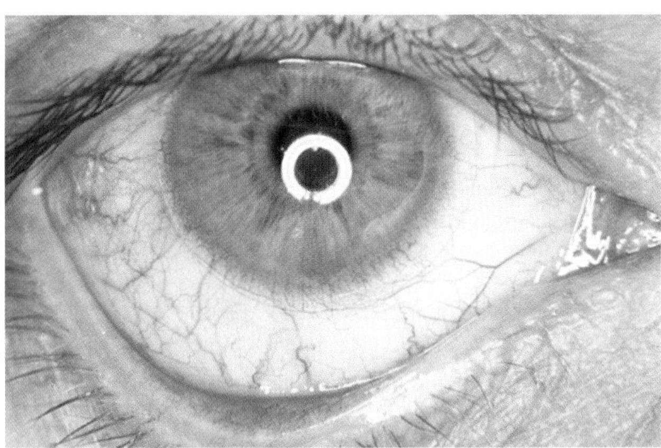

Figure 17.9 Conjunctival hyperaemia may be due to lack of sleep, eye rubbing, exposure to dust or any other occasional cause. Alternatively, conjunctival hyperaemia may be caused by contact lenses and become chronic

The cause may relate to:

- Lens wear in smoke, smog, wind, dust or glare.
- Hay fever or other allergy.
- Poor tears (see **Tear deficiency** and Chapter 5).
- Poor fitting.
- Solution toxicity.
- Over-wear.
- Soiled or damaged lenses.
- Excess reading/VDU work.
- Chronic low-grade infection.
- Lack of sleep.
- Swimming with or without lenses.
- Poor lens maintenance compliance.

(See **Reactive eye; Three and nine o'clock peripheral stain** and Chapter 11.)

Management

- Remove, treat or reduce risk factors where possible.
- Stress lens hygiene.
- Improve lens fit.
- Reduce wear.
- Differentiate from general ocular pathology.

Compliance

It is useful to ask the patient to go through their hygiene routine at every after-care appointment. Despite good initial instruction (see Chapter 11), departures from recommended techniques are common (Collins & Carney 1986), sometimes because of laziness but sometimes because of misunderstanding or incorrect advice from other sources. Patients need a responsible attitude towards lens hygiene and soiled lenses act as a prompt for discussing infection risks and consequences. The risk of increased hyperaemia and discomfort, reduced vision and the inability to wear lenses should be stressed as the consequences of poor compliance. Repeated or additional literature may be helpful but it may have to be read and discussed with the patient for it to have the desired effect (see also Chapters 8 and 11).

Computer vision syndrome (CVS)

The combination of air conditioning or central heating together with intense visual tasks tends to reduce blink efficiency and increase symptoms when doing prolonged computer work, particularly in contact lens wearers (Patel & Port 1991). Symptoms of dryness, irritation and ocular fatigue lead to a condition that is becoming known as computer vision syndrome (CVS).

Management

- 'Ocular gymnastics' should be carried out intermittently throughout the day. This involves looking away from the screen, preferably into the far distance, while blinking vigorously and making exaggerated versional eye movements. This helps clean and rewet lenses and encourages lens movement.
- Instil rewetting drops or ocular lubricants.
- Refit with lenses that are less prone to dehydration.
- Limit wear to part time as required for social and recreational activities.

Concretions

These develop from retention cysts in goblet cells or accessory lacrimal glands in the palpebral conjunctiva, resulting in the formation of discrete white aggregates of sebaceous material and crystals (Fig. 17.11). The formation stage is characterized by a clear vesicle that traps the gland production and the accumulated secretions form a hardened core that is gradually extruded on to the conjunctival surface.

Concretions are benign and associated with chronic hyperaemia, but at the stage of extrusion they may cause symptoms of a foreign body sensation (see **Foreign body sensation**) although lenses often act as a barrier to discomfort and discomfort is only noticed when the lens is removed. This also applies if a foreign body is retained under the upper lid or there is irritation from a misaligned eyelash (Fig. 17.12).

Management

Counsel the patient to expect symptoms to disappear as concretion naturally extrudes.

Conjunctivitis (see **Infection**)

Contact lens-induced papillary conjunctivitis (CLPC) (see **Giant papillary conjunctivitis**)

Corneal exhaustion syndrome (CES)

CES or 'corneal fatigue' is a term used to describe the loss of tolerance to contact lens wear. The reason may not be evident, especially when the patient is examined without their lenses, but may be caused by chronic corneal hypoxia and acidosis

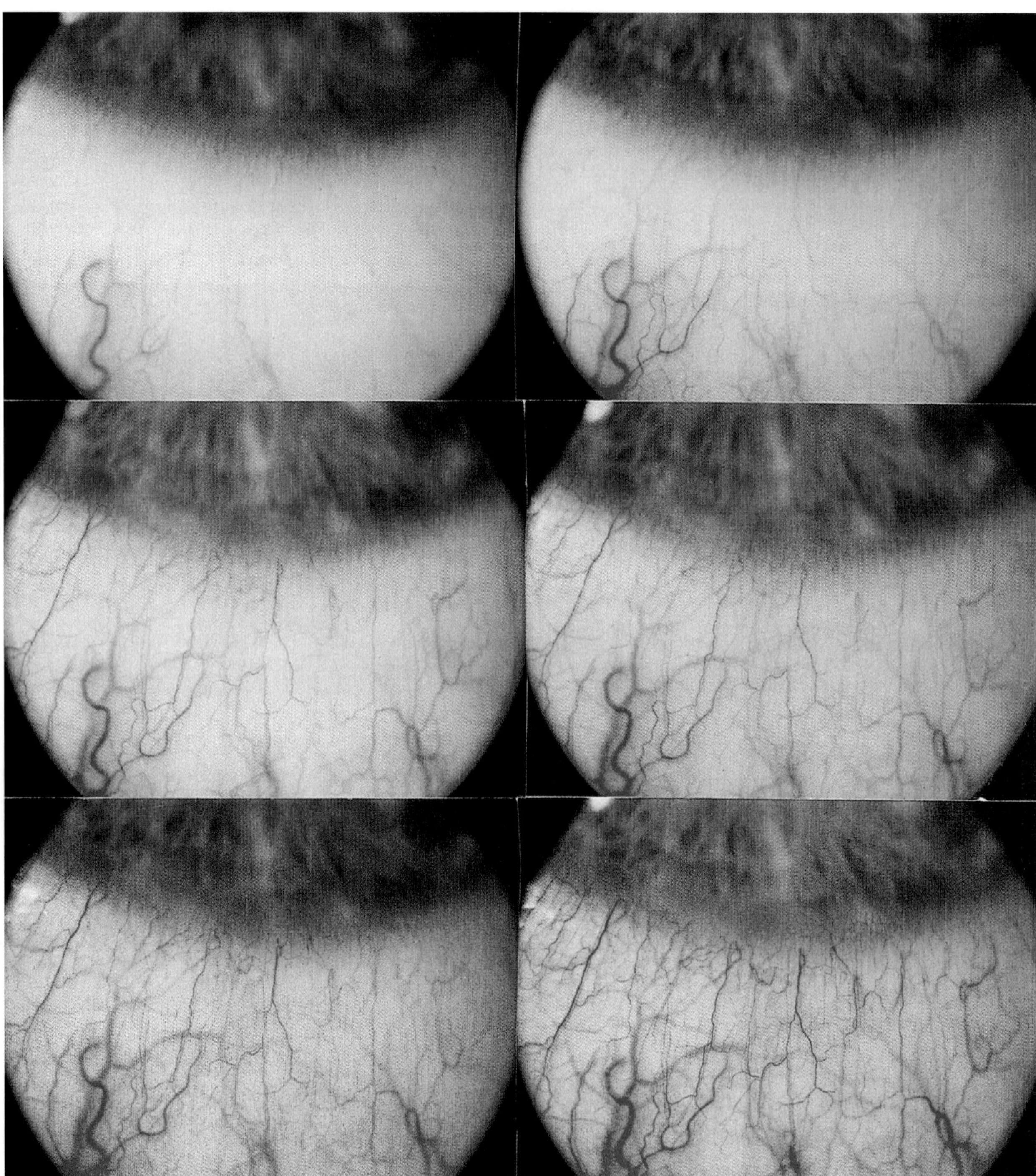

Figure 17.10 A photographic reference scale can be used to assess hyperaemia associated with contact lenses, reactive eyes, over-wear, infection, allergy irritation, cosmetics, preservatives, tear deficiency, etc. These may be graded from H0 (top left) to H5 (bottom right). (From McMonnies & Chapman-Davies 1987b, with permission of the American Journal of Optometry and Physiological Optics). (See also Appendix B)

together with endothelial dysfunction (Sweeney 1992). The lenses cannot then be worn without discomfort. The patient is frustrated because of the previous record of satisfactory tolerance, and the practitioner finds attempts to relieve symptoms, at best, only moderately successful.

Systemic factors are associated with corneal fatigue, such as chronic fluid retention and hormonal imbalance, or emotional or physical stress (see also **Hormonal factors**).

Signs

- History of chronic over-wear, tight lens fit or low-Dk materials.
- History of conjunctivitis where careful biomicroscopy reveals residual infiltrates in the cornea suggestive of a viral infection (see **Infiltrates**).
- Endothelial bedewing (Fig. 17.13), epithelial basement membrane dystrophy, endothelial guttata and polymegethism (see Figs 13.18 and 13.19).

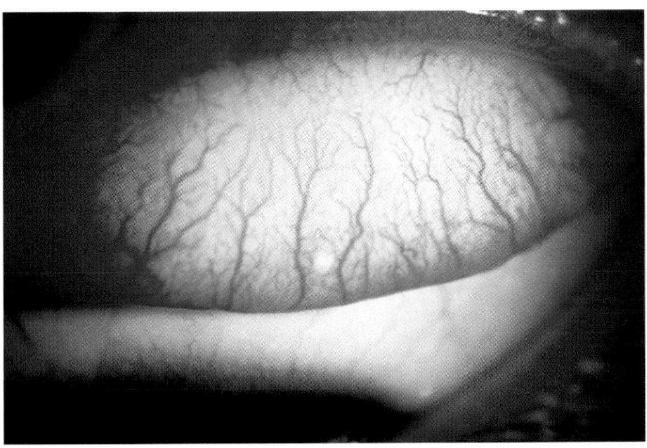

Figure 17.11 Retention cysts in goblet cells or accessory lacrimal glands in the palpebral conjunctiva may result in the formation of discrete white aggregates of mucus, sebaceous material and crystals. These concretions may cause irritation when they extrude to the surface

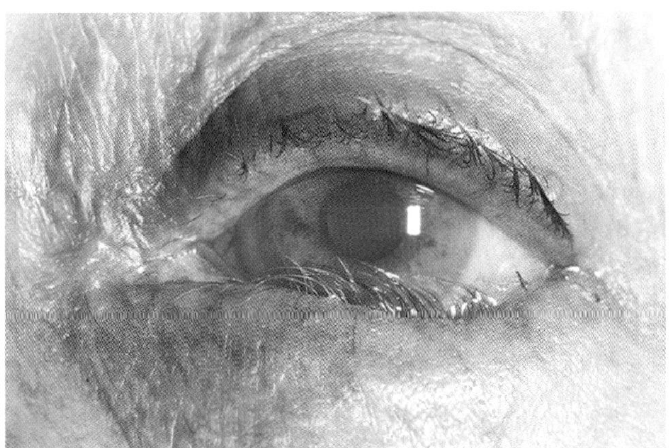

Figure 17.12 Severe entropion and trichiasis associated with blepharitis. The use of a bandage soft lens allowed regeneration of damaged corneal epithelium and prevented further disturbance prior to surgery. (Courtesy of D. Westerhout)

- Tear deficiency may be evident.
- The eyes are comfortable until the lenses are re-worn when signs include:
  - Hyperaemia.
  - Photophobia.
  - Lacrimation.
  - Stinging and discomfort.

Management

- Discontinue lens wear.
- Refit with very high-Dk gas-permeable material when corneal integrity is fully recovered, including regularity and stability of keratometric readings and corneal topography.
- Build up wearing time very slowly from as little as half an hour a day.

Corneal oedema (see also Chapter 13)

Low levels of corneal oedema are not uncommon with contact lens wear although it occurs much less often than with older materials (see **Over-wear**). For some patients, low levels of corneal oedema are a normal response to sleep and need to be considered when evaluating contact lens oedema symptoms in the first hours of waking, especially for extended-wear patients (see Chapter 13).

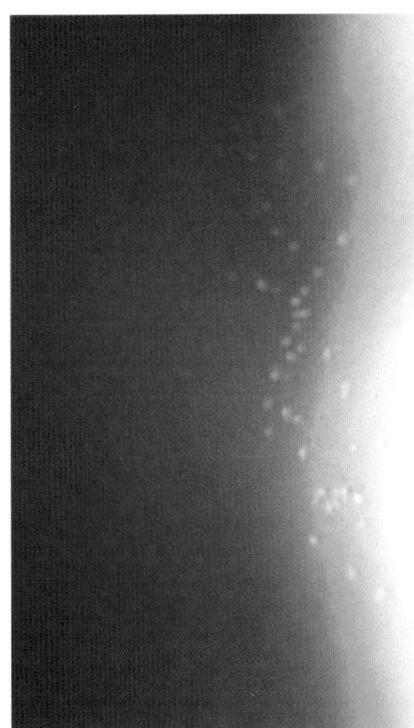

Figure 17.13 Endothelial bedewing observed in the region of the inferior pupil margin 3 days after the intense oedema from an over-wear episode had cleared. Bedewing is thought to represent inflammatory cells adhering to the endothelium

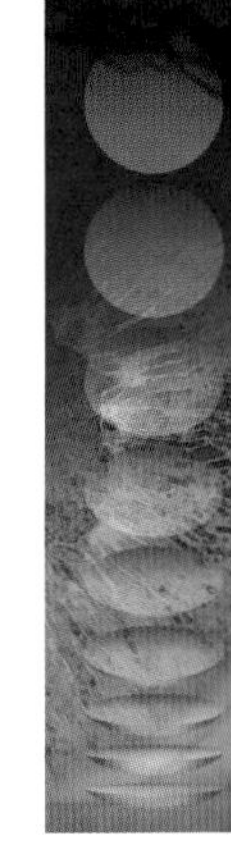

Epithelial oedema may be observed when a foreign body causes excess tearing (see **Foreign body sensation**), especially in the early stages of adaptation to rigid lenses or by prolonged emotional tearing or exposure to hypotonic water during swimming. Stromal oedema is a common response to contact lens-induced hypoxia and increased corneal thickness is evident using a pachometer.

Early oedema is seen, using a parallelepiped slit-lamp beam, as vertical striae (see Chapter 7, Fig. 13.13 and Appendix B). These wispy white lines lie in the posterior stroma and do not have the discrete appearance of lines of Vogt seen in keratoconus, or more anterior nerve fibres observed in normal corneas. Higher levels of stromal oedema cause folds in Descemet's membrane to appear as dark lines that traverse the specular reflection from the endothelium (see Fig. 13.14 and Appendix B). Very high levels of oedema result in loss of corneal transparency and some limbal and conjunctival hyperaemia.

Symptoms

- Photophobia.
- Haloes.
- Spectacle blur.
- Stinging, burning and pain.

Management

- Refit silicone hydrogel soft or more gas-permeable materials.
- Reduce wearing times.
- Consider cyclical influence of menstrual factors or pregnancy (see **Hormonal factors**).
- Consider other factors such as glaucoma.

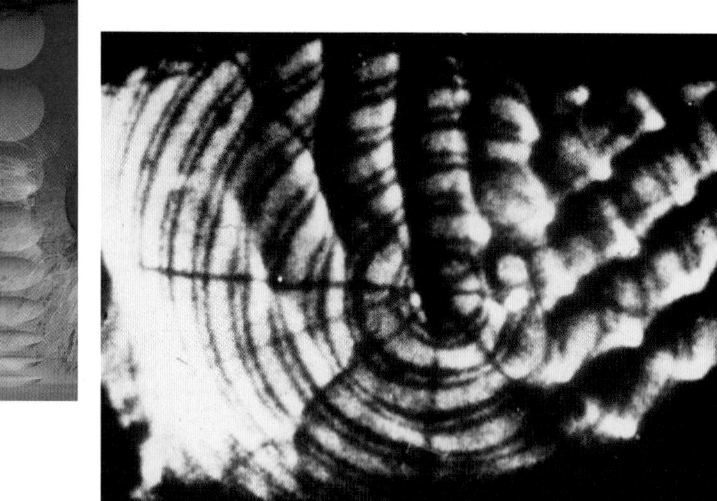

Figure 17.14 Reflection of keratoscope rings showing corneal wrinkling caused by a thin soft lens. (Reprinted from Lowe & Brennan 1987, with permission from the British Contact Lens Association)

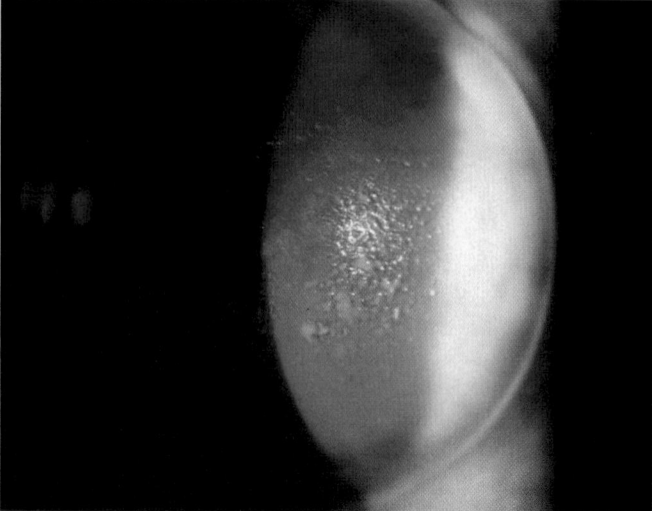

Figure 17.15 Poor surface wetting of an RGP lens due to residual hand cream, following failure to wash hands adequately. A similar appearance is seen on lenses coated with excess lipid secretion

Corneal wrinkling

Wrinkling (Fig. 17.14) is an uncommon, non-inflammatory, reversible wave-like alteration to corneal shape associated with thin, high water content soft lenses (Lowe & Brennan 1987). The condition may present as an unexplained reduction in visual acuity that varies in severity from one or two lines to less than 6/60. Wrinkling results from deformation of low-modulus lenses during the blink action. Careful observation of the retinoscope reflex may reveal small localized shadows that appear to change in shape and orientation with blinking. The diagnosis is confirmed with videokeratoscopy. Management requires refitting with a higher-modulus lens.

Cosmetics

Cosmetics need not cause problems for contact lens wearers but advice may be required if problems arise. The main difficulties are accidental soiling of lens surfaces (Fig. 17.15) and cosmetic contamination of lashes, lid margins and tears, leading to a chronically infected and irritated eye.

- Eye make-up should be applied after lens insertion.
- Special spectacles with hinged lenses may be necessary to ensure accurate cosmetic application for presbyopes.
- Mascara that releases particles onto the conjunctiva and water-based ones should be avoided, so that dust under a rigid lens, for example, does not become an embarrassment.
- Grease-based cosmetics can increase the oil in the tear film and tinting the lashes may be a safer option for some.
- A cream eye shadow that smudges easily should be avoided if lid manipulation is required, but powders can also cause problems.
- Hypoallergenic make-up is preferred, especially for atopic patients.
- Sensitivities can develop, particularly because cosmetics and their containers become increasingly contaminated with use.
- Eye-liner applied to the lid margin can block or irritate the meibomian glands.

Problems also arise from make-up-removing agents and from false eyelash glue, skin conditioners and soaps. Eliminating each agent separately may lead to the irritant. Over-frequent application of suntan lotions and anti-wrinkle creams to the lids and adnexa may be associated with excessive and/or contaminated tear lipid (see also Chapters 5, 8 and 11).

Dellen (See **Pseudopterygia**)

Dermatological conditions

These can be associated with irritation, dryness and contact lens intolerance. Signs of these conditions include erythema and pustules of acne rosacea, oiliness, scales or crusts of seborrhoea, erythema and various localized eruptions, including exudative lesions associated with eczema and dermatitis (Figs 17.16, 17.17). If possible, contact lenses should not be worn during treatment for these conditions (see also Chapter 8).

Diabetes

Diabetics may be predisposed to lens intolerance, although published studies provide conflicting evidence (see also Chapter 8). The corneal endothelium in diabetes has been found to be both normal (Pardos & Krachmer 1980) and morphologically abnormal (Schultz et al. 1984). Healing rates for the epithelium were found to be the same for diabetics and non-diabetics (Snip et al. 1980), although the same study found a tendency towards recurrent epithelial defects in diabetics and O'Leary and Millodot (1981) showed that diabetic corneas have increased epithelial fragility and reduced touch sensitivity. Variation in sampling criteria in these studies may explain the different results found (Snip et al. 1980). Some diabetics show good tolerance to contact lenses and individual response to contact lens trauma may depend

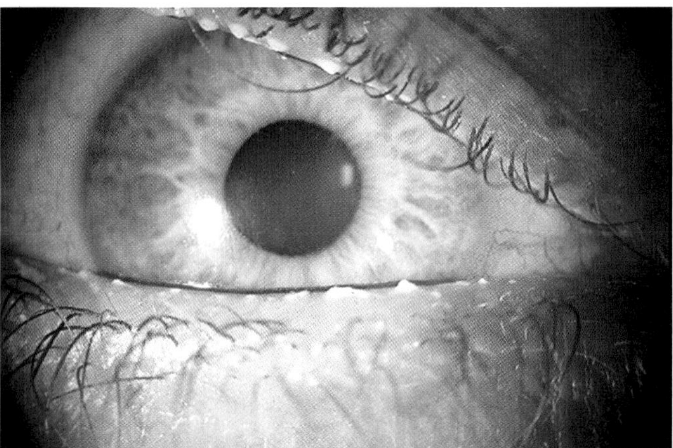

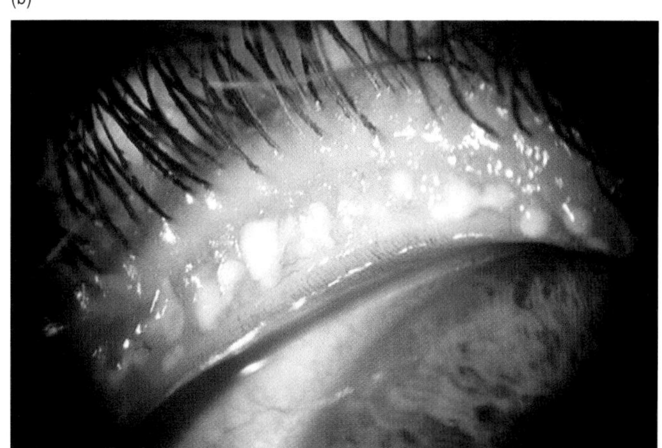

Figure 17.16 Severe meibomian hypersecretion: (a) the excess cloudy secretion contrasts with normal clear gland products; (b) the upper lid margin shown in more detail

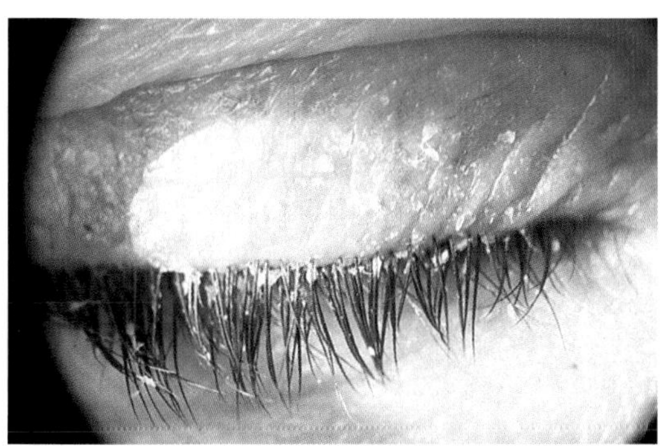

Figure 17.17 Blepharitis indicating the need for treatment and sustained lid hygiene to improve the chances of good contact lens tolerance. Dead epithelial tissue accumulates around the base of the lashes. This material is a nidus for infection and is irritating in the tear film

on age of onset of diabetes, whether there is insulin dependency and whether the diabetes is well controlled. If epithelial fragility or contact lens intolerance is evident at after-care, diabetes should be considered as a possible cause in a patient who has not been previously diagnosed with diabetes.

Dimple veil (see **Bubbles of air**)

Diplopia

This may present as a symptom of unstable binocular vision during adaptation in a patient with intermittent strabismus or it may be monocular, for example in bifocal lenses (see **Ghost images**). Vision training may help in cases of binocular diplopia. However, a patient who has been able to maintain single vision with decentred spectacles may not be able to achieve single vision with contact lenses (see also Chapters 6 and 14).

Discoloration

This occurs as conventional soft lenses degrade with use, although the reasons for these changes are not completely understood. Possible reasons include:

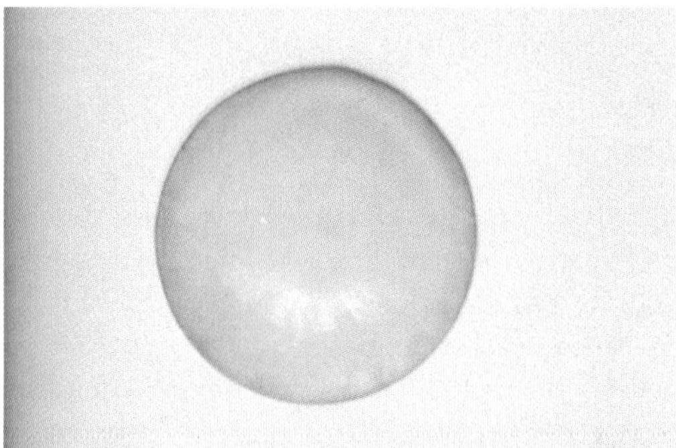

Figure 17.18 Soft lens discoloration of unknown aetiology. (Courtesy of A. P. Gasson)

- Selective adsorption of amino acids or other by-products of the protein-denaturing process on the lens surface, leading to gradual loss of transparency (Wardlaw & Sarver 1986).
- Adsorption of substances from the skin of the hands during surfactant use.
- Tear chemistry.
- Systemic medication (see Chapter 4).
- Heat disinfection and certain preservatives, such as sorbic acid, in higher-water-content lenses (Wardlaw & Sarver 1986).

Mild to moderate degrees of discoloration do not seem to have clinical consequences; however, some patients demonstrate rapid lens discoloration which is cosmetically unacceptable (Fig. 17.18) (see also Chapter 10).

Management

- Mild discoloration can be ignored.
- Hydrogen peroxide disinfection or intermittent sodium perborate cleaning (see Chapter 4).
- Change to disposable or frequent-replacement lenses.

Disposable lenses

Many after-care problems can be prevented or reduced by the use of disposable or frequent-replacement lenses – in particular, surface deposits and giant papillary conjunctivitis. A short-term

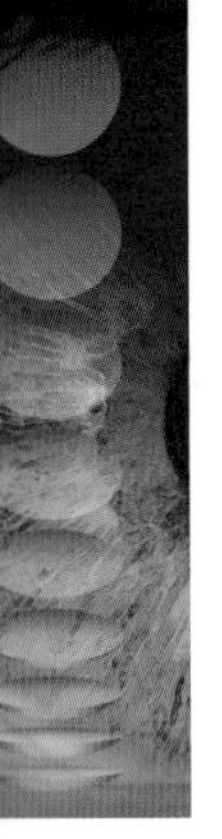

(a)

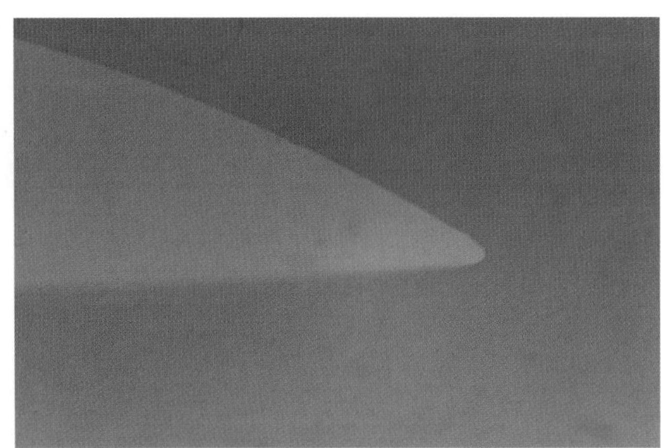

(b)

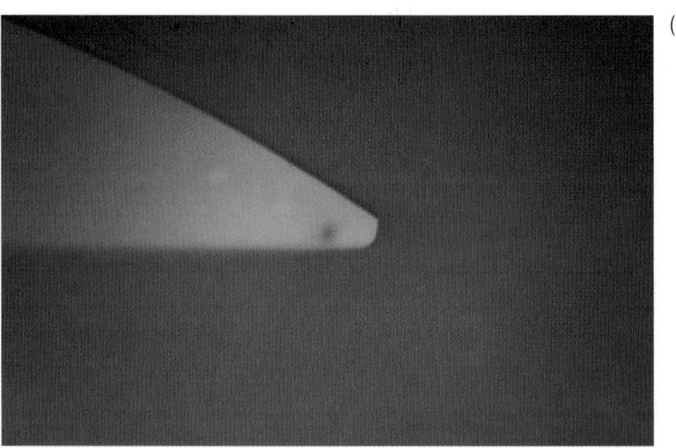

Figure 17.19 (a) Example of a desirable edge shape showing good taper, rounding and thickness. (b) Poor rounding on the anterior edge may cause increased awareness of the lid margin

trial with a disposable lens can be an inexpensive and simple way of deciding whether a patient can tolerate lenses.

Distortion

Distortion or warpage of rigid lenses occurs due to lens ageing or accidental stress in handling and affects lens performance and alters the refraction. Lens parameters should always be checked before re-prescribing.

Distorted soft lenses will show irregular edge contours when placed on a fingertip and focimeter readings are unclear. Retinoscopy is a good method of examining for lens distortion and/or poor optical quality that is not detectable by any other objective means (clinical or laboratory) (see also Chapters 11 and 16).

Dry eyes (see **Tear deficiency; Three and nine o'clock peripheral stain**)

Duplicate lenses

Duplicate lenses may be significantly different from the ones they replace, especially if a different laboratory is used. Even if the parameters measure the same, other aspects of the lens may differ (e.g. front optic zone diameter, edge shape, etc.). The older the prescription, the greater the chance of problems arising with a duplicate, especially if the original lens was modified to improve performance, or has undergone age-related changes. The potential for problems with duplicate soft lenses is not as great.

Edge shape (see also Chapter 16)

RGP lenses will be uncomfortable if there is an unsatisfactory edge shape (Fig. 17.19b). Adapted patients may be able to wear lenses with poor edges without discomfort but for a new wearer these can cause problems. The edge can be examined using a slit-lamp or with a loupe. Modifications can be done by the practitioner or by the laboratory (see Chapter 28). Edge shape should balance between the thickness, roundness and taper (Fig. 17.19a). Variations from this model may be indicated when matching the shape of a patient's previous lens which has proved to be comfortable.

Emergency examinations

The urgency of an appointment may depend on a patient's personality; for example, a lost lens can be a greater crisis for a low ametrope than for one with a high refractive error. Some patients may worry that a lens is stuck under the lid and may 'lodge in the brain'.

True emergencies are usually caused by infection. Severe over-wear oedema from PMMA lenses (see **Over-wear**) is seldom encountered with gas-permeable materials. Patients should be instructed to remove lenses immediately if the eyes are:

- Painful.
- Red.
- Sticky.
- Photophobic.

The earliest re-examination should be arranged and medical treatment given when appropriate.

Pathology may not be contact lens-related and the signs and symptoms must be differentiated from those of other ocular emergencies, such as acute glaucoma or retinal detachment (see **Out of hours emergencies** and Chapter 11). For these reasons, after-care appointments should always be performed by an optometrist or ophthalmologist and not by ancillary staff.

Endothelial bedewing

This is now rare with modern materials. It appears as a cluster of drop-like particles on the endothelial surface, usually located near to the inferior pupil margin, and is normally only visible using marginal retro-illumination (see Chapter 7) and high magnification. It appears after contact lens-induced corneal oedema has subsided and represents cellular keratic precipitates without obvious exudates. McMonnies and Zantos (1979) reported that chronic contact lens intolerance can be associated with endothelial bedewing in a cornea that otherwise appears to be normal (see also **Over-wear** and Fig. 17.13). In the absence of adverse lens performance, endothelial bedewing can be regarded as non-diagnostic.

Management

Use a higher-Dk material.

Endothelial guttata

Some endothelial guttata are a normal observation in the corneas of middle-to-older age groups but may occasionally be seen in younger patients. They are wart-like excrescences on Descemet's membrane, sometimes referred to as Hassall-Henle bodies, seen as dark spots in specular reflection. When located in the central cornea in sufficient numbers, endothelial function may be compromised. Stromal oedema develops, followed by epithelial oedema and bullous keratopathy as found in Fuchs' endothelial dystrophy (Grayson 1979).

The significance of corneal guttata in contact lens wearers is greater when seen in the central cornea (usually older female patients) as lens tolerance may be limited, with oedema developing after a short time. Corneal guttata need to be distinguished from the transient endothelial bleb response to contact lens wear (see **Endothelial response** and Chapter 13).

Management

- Limit contact lens use.
- Prescribe silicone hydrogel lenses.
- Change from soft to RGP lenses.

Endothelial response

A normal response to contact lens wear consists of dark areas of non-reflecting individual cells (blebs) observed by specular reflection (see Fig. 13.17). This peaks approximately 30 minutes after application and then slowly disappears. If these are observed more than an hour after lens insertion, they are likely to be endothelial guttata (see above). However, in the adapting stage of conventional extended-wear lenses, bleb responses show peaks at eye opening and 6 hours later. These responses are not detected after about 5 days of extended wear (Williams & Holden 1986) (see also Chapter 13).

Epithelial dimpling (see **Bubbles of air**)

Epithelial staining (see **Superficial punctate epitheliopathy**)

Fenestrations

Fenestrations are seldom used with RGP lenses but where necessary they should have polished bevels to avoid epithelial abrasion. If they become plugged with a solid core of mucus and tear debris, a sharpened wooden matchstick or a fine nylon bristle from a hairbrush, together with polishing fluid, can be used to clear the blockage. Where possible, care should be taken not to position a fenestration over the pupil area as this can lead to visual interference.

Fenestrations facilitate tear circulation, which improves oxygen levels, reduces oedema and possibly helps eliminate metabolic waste products. Red eye reactions in extended wear may be reduced if fenestrations increase tear circulation.

Fenestrations are unnecessary in most current-generation RGP and soft lenses (see also Chapters 9 and 28).

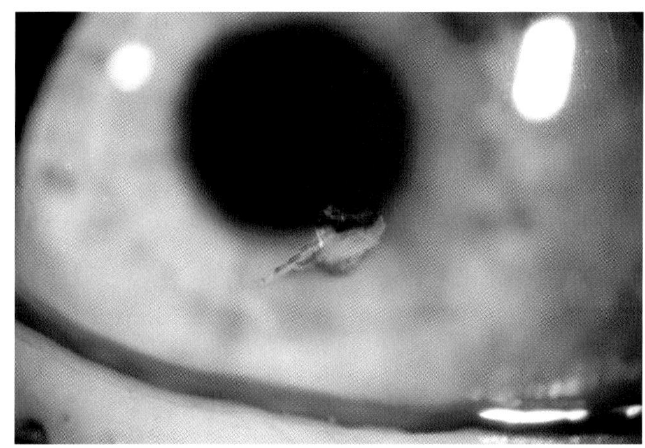

Figure 17.20 Damaged soft lens, with central nick possibly caused by a foreign body or fingernail, or due to folding a partially dehydrated lens. (Courtesy of A. J. Phillips)

Fingernails

Long nails can damage both the eyes and soft lenses. Jagged nicks and gouge marks should be suspected of being caused by accidental fingernail contact (Fig. 17.20). If possible, advise the patient to cut or file the nails of one index finger and thumb. Alternatively, teach a technique that avoids possible lens or eye damage.

Fit evaluation (see also Chapters 9, 10 and 12–15)

Patients should try to wear their lenses for after-care examinations, even in the presence of symptoms, because useful evaluations depend on seeing lenses in situ.

Flare

Inadequate pupil coverage by the optic zone of the lens causes flare and is most apparent when light sources are seen against a dark field and at night with dilated pupils. This occurs mostly with rigid lenses from:

- Large pupils.
- Small optic zone diameters on either the front or back surface.
- Lenses that decentre.
- Bifocal designs with small central optic zones.

The problem may be insurmountable with bifocal lenses but patients usually adapt to small amounts of flare as lacrimation reduces and blink efficiency improves (see also Chapters 6, 9 and 14). Flare can also be caused by mucus in the tear film in both rigid and soft lens wear.

Management

For new RGP wearers, flare should subside during the first month of wear. If it persists, refit with:

- Larger front and/or back surface central optic zone diameters.
- Better lens centration.
- Soft lenses.
- If flare is caused by mucus in the tear film, consider the causes:
  - infection.
  - irritation.
  - allergy.

Flexure (see also Chapters 6 and 9)

This is seldom a problem with soft lenses that wrap around the cornea but thin rigid lenses can flex with lid pressure during blinks, depending on corneal astigmatism and the material used (see Chapter 9). The cornea/back optic zone radius (BOZR) fitting relationship also affects flexure: steep lenses flex more than flat lenses, and lenses fitted in alignment (0.08 mm flatter than the flattest corneal meridian) flex least (Herman 1983). The critical centre thickness for PMMA lenses is about 0.12 mm. Most RGP materials need to be thicker to reduce flexure. Changes in residual astigmatism due to lens flexure should be considered as a possible cause of altered acuity noted at after-care visits.

Lens flexure caused by blinking affects keratometry mire images when taken over a rigid lens. To improve image quality, measurements should be taken immediately after a blink. Blinking increases lens flexure and the shape returns to normal between blinks; this causes the vision to improve just before a blink and be worst just after a blink.

Very thin lenses may become permanently flexed into a toric shape that aligns with corneal astigmatism. Although distorted from their manufactured shape, such lenses may give satisfactory performance if they exhibit meridian stability on the eye.

Management

- Ignore flexure that does not cause significant fluctuation or deterioration in vision.
- Change to a thicker design if necessary, preferably using a material with more stable characteristics, but be aware of reduced oxygen permeability.
- Flatten the fit slightly (see Chapter 9).

Fluorescein

Sodium fluorescein (NaFl) is commonly used to evaluate the fit of RGP lenses. For RGP materials that absorb ultraviolet light, a cobalt blue filter on a biomicroscope or appropriate filters over a white hand-UV or Burton lamp can be used instead (Pearson 1986) (see Chapter 9). Fluorescein also stains damaged epithelium and should be used to examine the cornea after rigid or soft lens removal. The eyes should be irrigated with physiological saline or a tear supplement prior to reapplication of soft lenses. Residual discoloration of soft lenses is not usually permanent and if necessary can be removed with hydrogen peroxide or sodium perborate. (See also **Tear deficiency**.)

Flying

Reduced oxygen levels or dehumidified cabin air both cause contact lens intolerance, especially when systemic oedema develops during a long flight. Window glare exacerbates the discomfort. Tear supplements help but, for long flights, lenses should be removed before boarding, even with highly gas-permeable materials.

Foreign body sensation

This may be otherwise described as a gritty or 'lash in the eye' sensation. A real foreign body sensation occurs when solid matter is trapped under a lens and causes epithelial abrasion. Instantaneous lacrimation should wash the foreign matter away in the case of rigid lenses but a soft lens needs to be deliberately moved onto the sclera with an index finger to allow the foreign body to be displaced from under the lens (see Chapters 8 and 11). Discomfort in the early stages of RGP wear causes a foreign body sensation which gradually reduces. If discomfort persists, lenses should be checked for faults.

A foreign body sensation that occurs with a previously comfortable lens may be due to a lens split, chip or other form of damage or deposit (see Figs 17.20, 17.35) or by conditions such as concretions or tear deficiencies.

Edge shape and other qualitative features should be checked with a hand-magnifier or slit-lamp, especially if a well-fitting lens is uncomfortable.

Management

- Consider possible causes.
- Check whether switching lenses (right and left or new and old) helps, especially if the problem is monocular. This assumes that the lens fit is similar.

(See **Concretions; Edge shape; Irritation; Tear deficiency** and Chapters 8 and 9.)

Frequent replacement lenses (see **Disposable lenses**)

Front surface keratometry

This assesses the image-forming properties of the contact lens front surface. However, with some lens powers, supplementary lenses are needed to extend the effective range of the keratometer (see Chapters 7 and 16). Surface deposits may degrade the mire image quality as does excessive lens movement. Mire image quality and reliability improves with blinks but readings derived from repeated blinks measure maximum lens flexure (see **Flexure**). Information yielded by front surface keratometry can be derived with other methods of assessment, such as retinoscopy, videotopography or biomicroscopy.

Front surface lens deposits (localized)

These typically form on non-rotating lenses in the area of lens exposed by inefficient blinking and/or lagophthalmos, either in the inferior area or 3 and 9 o'clock positions (Figs 17.21, 17.22).

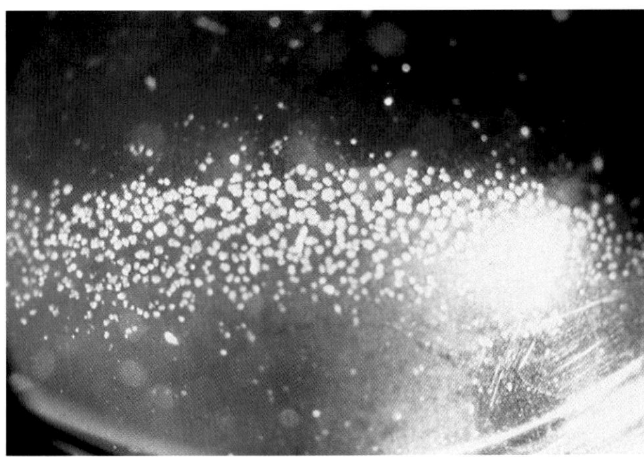

Figure 17.21 Non-rotating RGP lens with inferior deposits on the exposed area of the lens

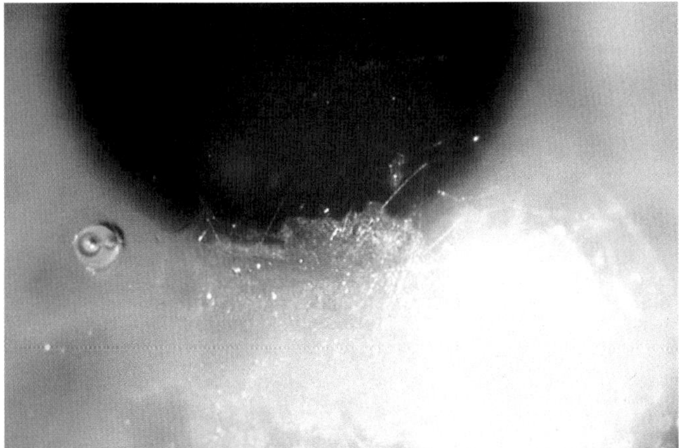

Figure 17.22 Non-rotating hydrogel lens with inferior deposits apparently due to habitual incomplete blinks

Management

- Improve blink efficiency.
- Improve maintenance, with particular emphasis on surfactant cleaning of the front surface (see Fig. 17.22).
- Consider changing to frequent replacement lenses if possible.

(See **Blink efficiency; Surface deposits.**)

Ghost images

These are secondary images that appear briefly adjacent to the primary image. They are due to tears, poor lens wetting and lens displacement but are more consistent when due to incomplete pupil coverage, a distorted lens or one with faulty optics. Ghosting is a monocular symptom, although it can occur simultaneously in both eyes and will be most obvious when a bright image is viewed in a relatively dark field. It is a common symptom with bifocal contact lenses (see also **Diplopia; Flare** and Chapters 14 and 16).

Management

- Images may disappear with adaptation.
- For poor optical quality, replace the lens.
- If due to poor pupil coverage, change design to increase lens centration and/or increase central optic diameter(s).
- In bifocals, try an alternative design; for example, an alternating design instead of a simultaneous vision design.
- If due to surface deposits, recondition or replace the lens.

Giant papillary conjunctivitis (GPC) or contact lens-induced papillary conjunctivitis (CLPC) (see also Chapter 18)

GPC is an extreme form of palpebral conjunctival response in contact lens wear (Allansmith et al. 1977) or other mechanical irritants such as protruding nylon suture ends following cataract surgery (Spring 1974). CLPC is a response specific to contact lens wear and presents less in wearers of disposable lenses than conventional soft and RGP lenses. Two distinct categories of CLPC may be defined depending on whether they are distributed across the entire palpebral conjunctiva (general CLPC) or confined to one or two areas (local CLPC). Local CLPC may result from mechanical trauma between the lens and the superior palpebral conjunctiva and is typically associated with less developed symptoms than the generalized condition (Skotnitsky et al. 2002).

Symptoms

- First (preclinical) stage:
  - a mild increase in mucus that accumulates at the inner canthus during sleep (morning mucus).
  - mild symptoms of itchiness on lens removal.
  - ***Signs***: none.
- Second stage:
  - moderate increase in mucous discharge.
  - mild blurring.
  - increased lens awareness.
  - mild itch late in the day that increases on lens removal.
  - ***Signs***: normal papillae show some elevation and the thickened conjunctiva has a hyperaemic appearance.
- Third stage:
  - moderate to severe mucous discharge and accumulation on lens surfaces.
  - increased lens awareness and movement on blinking.
  - lens wearing time decreases.
  - mild to moderate itch during wear.
  - moderate to severe itch on lens removal.
  - ***Signs***: loss of translucency of the conjunctiva; giant papillae begin to form from confluent smaller papillae, producing a clover-like appearance.
- Fourth (or terminal) stage:
  - morning mucous discharge causes the lids to stick together.
  - lenses are uncomfortable and mobile.
  - surface deposits are excessive, with mucus accumulating at the inner canthus.
  - wearing times are very restricted.
  - itch is mild to severe.
  - ***Signs:*** giant papillae of increased size and elevation with flattening of the top surfaces that show fluorescein staining during active development. At later stages, scar

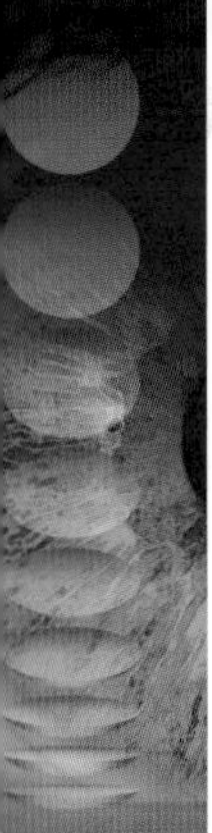

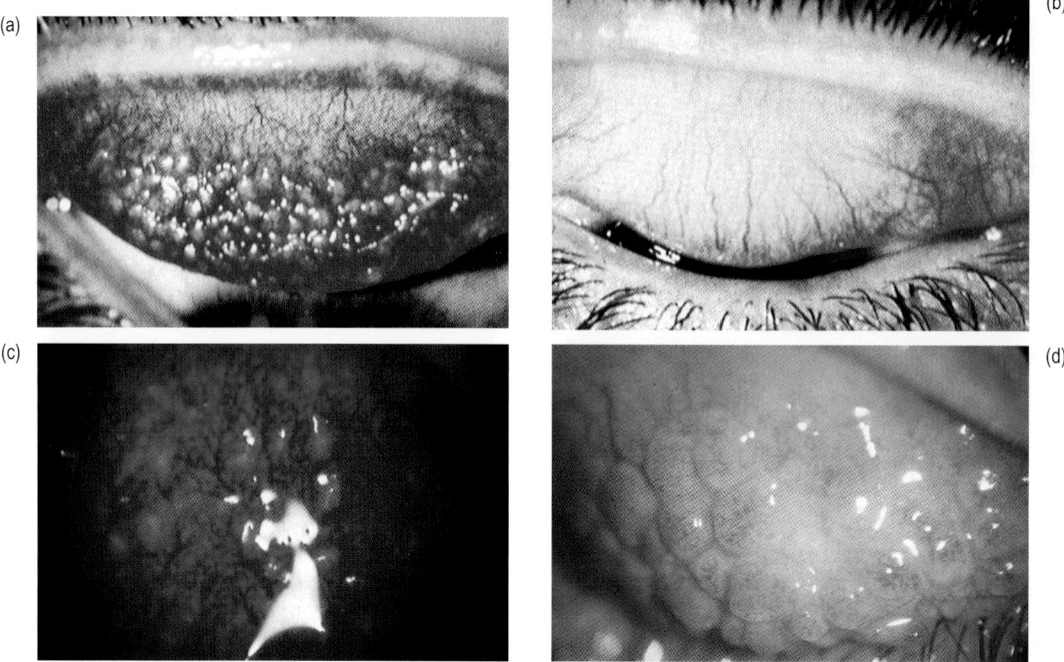

Figure 17.23 Giant (GPC) or contact lens-induced papillary conjunctivitis (CLPC) of the upper palpebral conjunctiva due to contact lens wear shown in (a) and compared to the normal conjunctiva in (b). Shown in (c) is the early 'tapioca' granule appearance of early GPC compared to the more advanced papillary formations shown in (d). ((a, b) Courtesy of M. R. Allansmith and (c, d) courtesy of D. J. Coster)

tissue at the top of papillae obscures the characteristic papillary blood vessel stalk (glomerulus).

Signs of papillary conjunctivitis may exist without significant symptoms. The observation of papillae on the non-tarsal palpebral conjunctiva is not relevant to contact lens-induced changes that are restricted to the tarsal area (Allansmith et al. 1977).

Aetiologies such as vernal conjunctivitis or chlamydial infection should be considered in cases of giant papillary conjunctivitis, especially when no progress is made with contact lens management methods (see Fig. 17.23 and Appendix B).

Management

- Improve lens maintenance.
- Change to disposable lenses if parameters permit.
- Change to daily disposable lenses, either temporarily or permanently.
- Change to a material with lower modulus of elasticity.
- Change maintenance products and include protein removal.
- Reduce wear (hours per day or from extended wear to daily wear).
- Change from soft to RGP lenses with well-rounded edges.
- Prescribe sodium cromoglycate and/or a weak, short-term topical steroid.
- In severe cases, cease lens wear until symptoms and acute signs subside (1–3 months).

(See also **Surface deposits** and Chapter 18.)

Glare or photophobia

Glare and photophobia used to result from early oedema in PMMA lenses. With RGP materials, this is much less common. However, in some patients, photophobia is caused by the discomfort of rigid lenses.

The problem is exacerbated if the patient wore tinted prescription spectacles prior to starting with contact lenses. Glare is worse in the mornings and evenings when higher levels of oedema may be present and when sunlight is oblique to the Earth's surface. Symptoms in adapted patients may signal loss of tolerance, corneal pathology associated with ciliary injection or cataract development, or other changes in the transparency of ocular media (see also Chapters 10 and 11).

Management

- If glare is caused by corneal oedema, change the lens material to one with a higher Dk and check the lens fit.
- During periods of adaptation, sunglasses may be beneficial.
- Good-quality sunglasses can include a correction for residual astigmatism if indicated.
- Increasing the contact lens tint is not indicated as reduced transmission is a disadvantage at night.

Glaucoma treatment

This can usually continue without interruption of contact lens wear. Morning and evening drops should be instilled before and after lens wear so that soft lenses cannot absorb the drug or any preservative. If a mid-day instillation is required, the lens may need to be removed; however, if disposable lenses are worn, the risk of a build-up causing a problem is unlikely. Daily disposables are ideal.

Soft lenses can be used as a means of achieving greater anterior segment penetration for protracted periods (see Chapter 26).

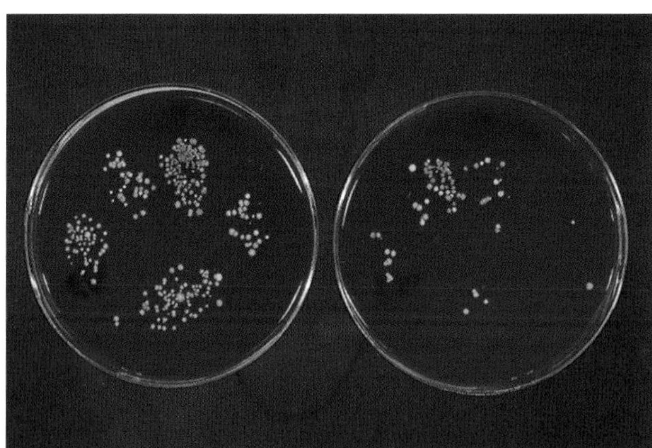

Figure 17.24 Hygiene and hand-washing. Two agar plates are shown with a practitioner's fingers and thumbprint before (left) and after (right) hand-washing. The reduction but not complete elimination of bacterial colonies is clearly visible. (Courtesy of C. Copley)

Hand-washing

Hygiene should be stressed when a negligent attitude is noted at after-care. If previous advice regarding hygiene has been disregarded, compliance can be improved by discussing the risks caused by non-compliance and by providing information on the prevalence of contact lens-related infection (Lippman 1986) (Fig. 17.24; see also **Infection**). Patients whose hands become soiled at work (e.g. car mechanics) need to wash their hands two or three times (lather/rinse cycles) before lenses can be handled safely.

Natural skin secretions or hand creams affect lens surfaces and hands should be rinsed thoroughly after washing to avoid irritation. Always wash your hands in front of the patient to show that you take hand-washing seriously (see Figs 17.15, 17.24; see also Chapters 8 and 11).

Hormonal factors

Many women experience significant systemic oedema as part of their menstrual cycle. Systemic fluid retention increases the risk of contact lens-induced corneal oedema (see also **Over-wear**) and causes intermittent symptoms of discomfort. An association with menstruation may be confirmed during subsequent cycles, together with other systemic signs of fluid retention (e.g. weight gain, ring tightness, etc.). Reduced contact lens use may be necessary during these phases (Serrander & Peek 1993, Guttridge 1994).

Tear volume and corneal sensitivity reduce during pregnancy and corneal curvature steepens. Corneal thickness also increases, which can lead to oedema developing earlier than usual when contact lenses are worn (Imafidon & Imafidon 1991) (see also **Oral contraceptives**).

Infection (see also Chapter 18)

Poor hygiene is a common cause of infection in contact lens wear. After resolution, hygiene should be completely reassessed. Cases must be disinfected (see **Case contamination**) or replaced and patients encouraged to comply with hygiene instructions. Extended-wear patients are at greater risk than daily wear patients (Dart 1993) (see also Chapter 13).

Management

- Discontinue lens wear and discard lenses after culturing.
- Treat the infection.
- Resumption of lens wear must be undertaken with caution.
- Many soft lens wearers need to be refitted with RGP lenses, especially if there is corneal scarring.
- Review lens maintenance and hygiene.

(See also **Hand-washing; Infection; Infiltrates; Microbial keratitis.**)

Infiltrates (see also Chapter 18)

Infiltration of the cornea with inflammatory cells occurs in response to solution preservatives or an immune stimulus associated with contact lenses. These are sterile infiltrates and should dissipate on lens removal. They do not stain and some are only visible with careful marginal retro-illumination or sclerotic scatter.

Stromal infiltrates may occur in association with a variety of adverse reactions to lens wear, such as the acute red eye reaction, contact lens-induced superior limbic keratoconjunctivitis, stromal vascularization and corneal ulceration. They typically occur near the limbus and the adjacent conjunctiva is often hyperaemic. Infiltrates are most probably leucocytes or monocytes lying between collagen fibres in the stroma.

Infiltrates associated with the chronic phase of an infection do not clear easily (Fig. 17.25) after lens removal and a history of red eye may indicate a staphylococcal or viral infection. These infiltrates may require many weeks without lenses and may then recur within a few days of resuming lens wear.

Infiltrates in nummular keratitis cause corneal scarring and stain better with Rose Bengal than fluorescein. They do not stain at all when superficial healing has taken place as the infiltrates become subepithelial.

Management

- Abandon lens wear until the cornea is clear.
- Consider improvement in lid hygiene and other treatment for blepharitis.
- Suspect contaminated lenses and solution toxicity.
- Refit with RGPs or a higher-Dk material.

Informed patients

Poor compliance with lens maintenance is common (Collins & Carney 1986), partly because of the large amount of information given initially (see **Compliance**; **Re-instruction**). Priluck et al. (1979) found that, although 97% of patients presenting for retinal detachment surgery acknowledged the thorough preoperative discussion that they were given, overall retention of disclosures was only 57%. When patients failed to remember particular aspects, more than half denied having discussed that aspect previously.

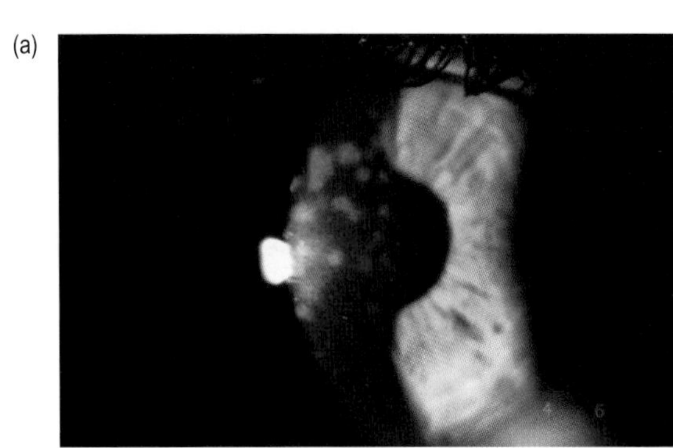

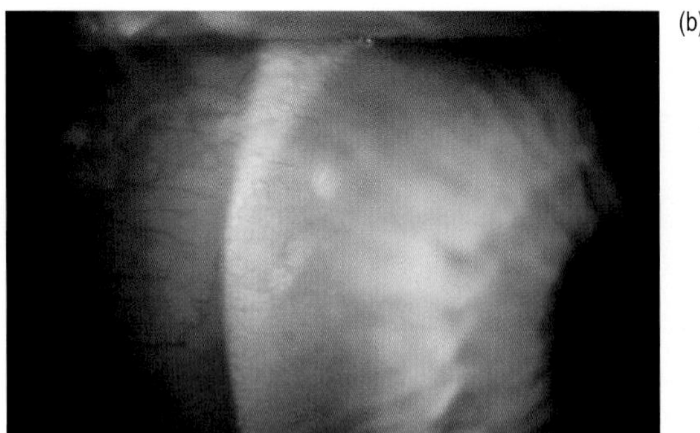

Figure 17.25 Infiltrates appear as hazy, grey areas which (a) may be focal, or (b) diffuse. ((a) Courtesy of T. Grant; (b) courtesy of A. J. Phillips)

A patient's signature on written information will not necessarily improve compliance, so important points should be repeated at each after-care appointment (see also Chapters 8 and 32). Spacing the instructions throughout the after-care period is helpful. For example, instruction regarding the use of protein-removing tablets can be left until a subsequent examination when lens deposition can be assessed.

Irritation

This is a general term used for symptoms from a range of problems. Ask the patient to distinguish between a chemical sting and a foreign body sensation and also when the irritation occurs; for example, immediately following lens application, or end of day. The former may be due to clumsy application, lens contamination or an adverse reaction to care solutions. An irritation later in the day may be due to oedema, an increase in surface deposition during wear or progressive drying of the lenses.

Intermittent irritation may be due to a damaged lens that only causes abrasion in one position.

Management

- Check the lens (damage, soiling, manufacturing faults, etc.).
- Check the eyes (epithelial lesions, tear deficiency, etc.).
- Consider sensitivity to the lens material or solutions and change as necessary.

(See **Foreign body sensation; Stinging.**)

Itching

This may be associated with allergy although not necessarily from contact lenses or solutions. A day without lenses will determine if the itch occurs independently of lens wear.

Symptoms may be mild but instigate vigorous eye rubbing. Patients should be encouraged to avoid eye rubbing, especially those with keratoconus. Giving an alternative is helpful; for example, hot and/or cold compresses after lens removal which also helps clear allergens from the lids and lashes at the same time (see **Lid hygiene**). Itching can indicate giant papillary conjunctivitis (see **Giant papillary conjunctivitis**).

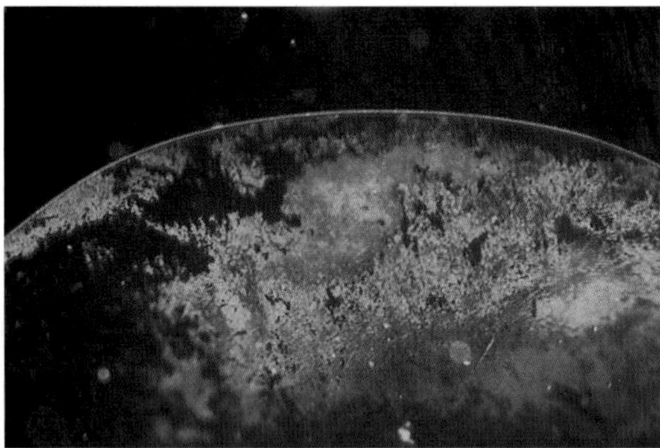

Figure 17.26 Protein deposits with superimposed calcium deposits centrally and lower right shown by dark-field microscopy. (Courtesy of R. Payor)

Management

- If possible, identify and remove/avoid any allergic stimulus (change lens maintenance, replace soiled lenses, change cosmetics, etc.).
- Fit daily disposable lenses.
- Prescribe an antihistamine or mast cell stabilizing drops.

(See **Allergy** and Chapter 18.)

Lens condition

This should first be assessed with the lens on the eye using the slit-lamp. Any nicks or deposits should be noted as they may correspond to an area of epithelial stain after lens removal. Deposits are more apparent off the eye after the lens surface has dried using an external spotlight.

Lens surface deposits and scratches may not always be visible with routine biomicroscopy. Transillumination of the lens off the eye with the microscope mirror rotated and ×10–×40 magnification provides a dark-field effect that improves the visibility of various refractile changes (Figs 17.18, 17.20, 17.26; see also Fig. 17.31).

Lens eversion (inside out lenses)

Everted soft lenses are usually uncomfortable, although hyperthin lenses cause few problems if they are inside out (see

Chapter 10). Mild symptoms in a previously comfortable low-power lens warrant suspicion that the lens is inside out.

Although this is rare, very thin rigid lenses can invert and this results in irreversible changes in parameters.

Management

Control the orientation of lenses during removal and place correctly in the storage case.

Lens insertion (see Chapter 11)

Common problems associated with lens insertion are poor fixation control, inaccurate lens positioning (aim) and failure to maintain a wide palpebral aperture due to lack of lid control. Re-instruction can help. Try to ensure that the contralateral eye remains open to reduce muscle tonus and blepharospasm, and holds the lashes of the upper lid against the supraorbital margin.

Lens parameters

Rigid lens parameters should be rechecked if there is any suspicion of change and before reordering spare lenses. Soft lenses rarely require inspection for parameter changes because significant loss of shape or optical quality can be detected on the eye from the fit or retinoscopy findings. Predelivery findings should be recorded on the record card.

(See **Irritation; Transition quality in rigid lenses**; see also Chapter 16.)

Lenses lost in the eye

Lenses may unknowingly be retained in the eye with minimal symptoms, sometimes for many months. Rigid lenses and ultrathin soft lenses that have folded can be displaced and retained in the superior fornix. Large eyes and lids with loose tonus make finding and retrieving the lenses more difficult.

Management

- Evert the upper lid and ask the patient to look as far down and laterally as possible.
- Instil fluorescein to look for a whole or broken soft lens.

(See **Emergency examinations**; see also Chapter 11.)

Lid hygiene (see also Chapters 8 and 18)

Patients with chronic blepharitis, meibomian gland dysfunction or palpebral conjunctivitis require lid hygiene prior to, or together with, antibiotic treatment (see **Reactive eye**; **Tear deficiency**). Hot compresses on waking and before retiring can improve lid condition and mild meibomian gland dysfunction. Clean lids are less conducive to the proliferation of *Staphylococcus* spp. (Catania 1987) and hordeola will resolve more rapidly and are less likely to recur (see Figs 17.16, 17.17).

Management

- Hot compresses on waking and before going to bed
  - hold a clean, steaming hot face cloth, as hot as the eyes can accept, against closed lids for 5 minutes, renewing the heat every minute.
  - gently massage the lids and lashes to remove the discharge and dust particles from the lid margin, lashes and canthi.
- Lid scrubs Lid Care (CIBA Vision) or Adapettes (Alcon) to thoroughly clean around the base of the lashes. Alternatively, dilute a teaspoon of bicarbonate of soda or baby shampoo in 1 pint (568 cc) of boiled cooled water and use a cotton wool bud to clean the lashes.
- Express the meibomian glands
  - after the hot compress, press downwards on the upper lid, and upwards on the lower lid, using either a clean finger or a cotton wool ball wetted with one of the above solutions.
  - wipe along the lid margin with a solution-soaked cotton wool bud.
- Treat with antibiotics or weak steroids.
- A course of systemic tetracycline may be necessary in recalcitrant cases. This both eliminates any staphylococcal infection and lowers the melting temperature of the meibomian mucus.

(See also **Tear deficiency [management]**.)

Lid twitch sensation

This is caused by the nerve fibres to the lid muscle (of Riolan) discharging haphazardly, resulting in minor flexing of the surrounding tissue. This may be related to low calcium levels in the diet, leading to a lowered concentration of calcium ions at myoneural junctions (Hall & Cusack 1972).

Under conditions of fatigue, stress and/or debility, haphazard discharge causes a nuisance symptom which is unlikely to be related to contact lens wear.

Limbal indentation (see **Fit evaluation; Vascularization**)

Medication

Ocular side-effects of medication can interfere with contact lens performance or be mistaken for contact lens symptoms; for example, tear production may be reduced by antihistamines, diuretics, sleeping tablets, tranquillizers, oral contraceptives (see **Oral contraceptives**) or medication for duodenal ulcer, digestive problems and high blood pressure.

Medication for many conditions may affect accommodation including psychiatric disorders, depression, insomnia, anxiety, tension headaches, hypertension, cardiac and vascular conditions, malaria, rheumatic disorders, epilepsy, diabetes, fluid retention, painful muscular conditions, cramps, torticollis and infections (O'Connor Davies 1972) and some patients experience delayed recovery of accommodation after general anaesthesia.

Unusual changes in refraction or accommodation or increased myopia should suggest medication side-effects as a contributing cause.

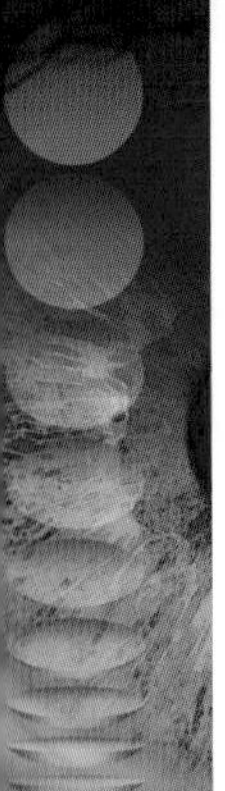

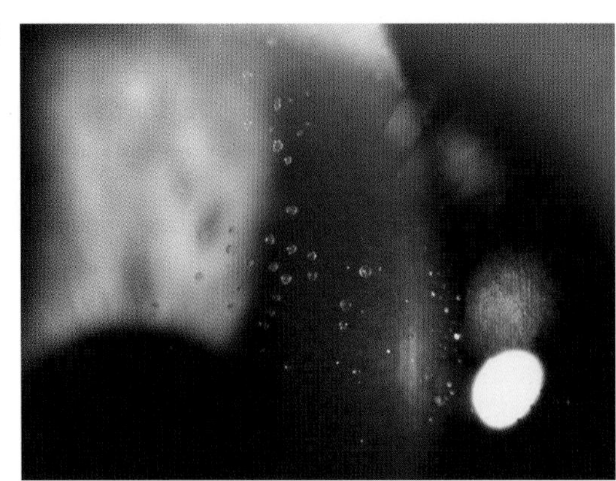

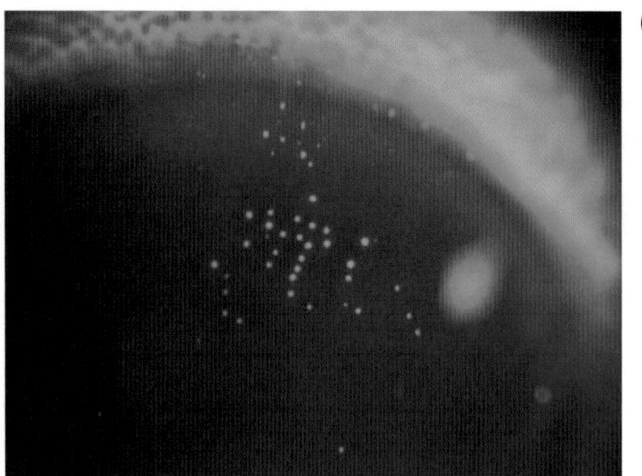

Figure 17.27 (a) Mucin balls shown in direct and indirect illumination; (b) fluorescein has collected in the resultant dimples upon lens removal (compare Fig. 17.6b)

Soft lenses may discolour in response to systemic medication (see Chapter 4).

Meibomian gland dysfunction (see **Lid hygiene**; **Tear deficiency**; Fig. 17.16)

Microbial keratitis (corneal ulcer, ulcerative keratitis) (see Chapter 18)

Mixed lenses

Lenses are frequently swapped, left to right or old with new. Lens prescriptions may be similar and wearing them on the wrong eyes is of little or no consequence. Where prescriptions differ significantly, an induced antimetropia, where one eye accepts plus and the other minus, or one lens fitting steep and the other flat, indicates that lenses are probably switched. It is easier to make differentiations between rigid lenses than soft.

Management

- Engrave rigid lenses R and L or with one and two dots (see Chapter 9).
- For patients with darker irides, prescribe different handling tints for each eye.

Modifications (see Chapter 28)

Simple modifications of rigid lenses such as polishing surfaces, reshaping edges, adding posterior edge curves, or making small power changes can be carried out in practice with suitable equipment.

Sending lenses to a laboratory inconveniences the patient. Modifications cannot easily be carried out in small increments and reassessed at each stage.

RGP materials require ammonia-free polishing compounds and very wet conditions to minimize overheating and distortion.

Soft lens modification is difficult and unreliable.

Monovision

Over-refraction may reveal that a presbyopic patient is corrected for distance in one eye and for near in the other. This may also be caused by a monocular increase in myopia. In this case the patient may be unaware of one eye being superior for distance and the other for near and is likely to be disappointed if both eyes are then corrected for distance as they will experience near vision difficulties (see also **Supplementary spectacles** and Chapter 14).

Mucin balls (see also Chapter 13)

Mucin balls are commonly found with extended wear of silicone hydrogel lenses and to a lesser extent in other lens types and modalities (Dumbleton et al. 2000). Mucin balls are small (20–200 μm), spherical, opalescent bodies that may occur singly or in clusters (Figs 17.27a and Fig. 13.30). They lie trapped between the posterior lens surface and the corneal epithelium, and are easily blinked away upon lens removal, whereupon fluorescein pools in the imprint, resembling dimple staining (Fig. 17.27b). They are of little clinical significance but need to be differentiated from epithelial microcysts and vacuoles (see **Corneal oedema** and Chapter 13).

Management

- Small numbers of mucin balls cause no symptoms and require no treatment.
- Where there are several mucin balls, use lens lubricant drops and/or remove and clean the lenses more frequently.

Neovascularization (see **Vascularization**)

No symptoms

The asymptomatic patient still needs careful examination for early signs of problems. Findings such as hyperaemia, surface deposits, oedema, etc. may be symptomless in early stages, but improvement in lens fitting and advice regarding better lens care can prevent problems from occurring.

Oral contraceptives

Older versions of these drugs, with higher dosages, were reported to be associated with contact lens intolerance but the

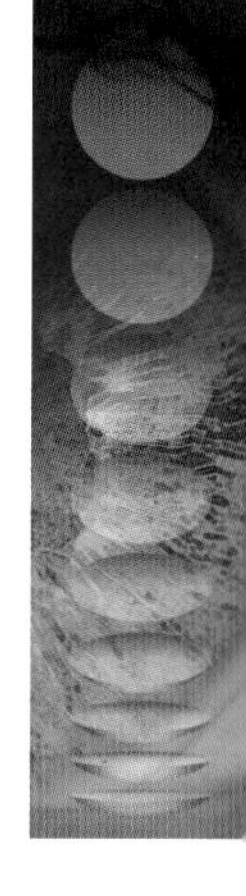

evidence for a causal relationship is circumstantial (Ruben et al. 1976, de Vries Reilingh et al. 1978). It is still possible that individual adverse reactions could occur (see **Hormonal factors** and Chapter 8).

Out of hours emergencies

Emergencies, such as red eye, loss of vision or failure to neutralize a lens soaked in hydrogen peroxide, all indicate the importance of an out of hours contact number. In some countries, such as the UK, practitioners are required to provide patients with such a number.

Over-refraction

This is performed with contact lenses on the eyes. If the expected visual acuity and binocular balance are achieved, then the only point of interest may be to determine whether any additional plus will be accepted for distance in an early presbyope.

A hand-held spectacle trial set lens provides adequate over-refraction in most cases and confirms that the contact lens power is correct. If the expected acuity is not achieved, retinoscopy should be carried out, which may reveal residual astigmatism, deposits, poor wetting and/or poor lens optical quality.

It is always important to consider that ocular pathology may be the cause of reduced acuity (see also Chapters 9 and 10).

Over-spectacles (see **Supplementary spectacles**)

Over-wear

The over-wear syndrome, involving significant oedema and pain a few hours after PMMA lens removal, is rare nowadays with most rigid lenses being gas permeable. This syndrome is known as the '3 a.m. syndrome' because symptoms often occur around that time in the morning after the patient has been sleeping for a few hours.

Symptoms

Symptoms include intense pain and photophobia, depending on the degree of oedema and epithelial disturbance.

Examination is difficult because of photophobia, but symptoms and the history of lens use, together with the obvious gross signs, permit the syndrome to be diagnosed without detailed biomicroscopic examination. Usage of a topical anaesthetic will assist this examination. Usually PMMA lenses have been over-worn, or worn all day; for example, when a patient has worn a spare non-gas-permeable lens.

There may be systemic factors, such as fluid retention, that predispose the patient towards the over-wear syndrome. The presumed mechanism is greater than usual corneal swelling due to increased oxygen deprivation associated with over-wear. The thickened cornea then becomes mechanically abraded. Sufficient corneal anaesthesia develops for symptoms to be minimal at the time of lens removal. However, as the corneal sensitivity returns, the rapid eye movement phase of sleep results in intense irritation through lid movements over a swollen cornea.

Once the cornea has cleared, endothelial bedewing may be detected, indicating that an anterior uveal response occurred in association with the corneal insult (see **Endothelial bedewing** and Fig. 17.13).

Management

- The patient requires maximum reassurance that vision is not permanently impaired and that the symptoms will dissipate slowly during the course of the following day.
- Advise oral analgesics and dark glasses.
- Prescribe prophylactic antibiotic drops to minimize the risk of secondary infection.
- Refit lenses with good oxygen permeability after complete resolution.

(See also **Hormonal factors** and Chapter 9.)

Photophobia (see **Glare**)

Polishing

Convex lens surfaces attract deposits and scratches. RGP lenses can be polished unless scratches are deep, in which case the lens must be replaced. However, polishing the concave surface may alter the radius and cause discomfort.

Polished lenses are easier to clean and stay cleaner for longer. High-Dk RGP materials are difficult to polish and, if possible, should be replaced every 6–9 months (Woods & Efron 1996).

Surface-treated materials, such as 'Menicon Z', cannot be polished (see also Chapters 9 and 28).

Pregnancy (see **Hormonal factors**)

Presbyopia (see Chapter 14)

Contact lens wearers returning for after-care may complain of presbyopic symptoms. The simplest solution is an over-correction for near work and, with some patients, this may be the most appropriate approach rather than fitting bifocal contact lenses. However, with modern multifocal designs being much more straightforward to fit, alternatives should be considered and discussed with the patient (see **Monovision; Reading difficulties**).

Preservative reaction

Adverse reactions to preservatives may present with delayed and insidious, or immediate and acute, responses. Symptoms of stinging and burning occur on lens application (see Chapter 4) although in chronic responses, symptoms may be mild with only increased lens awareness reported.

Signs

These include:

- Hyperaemia of the limbal, bulbar and palpebral conjunctiva.
- Conjunctival oedema.

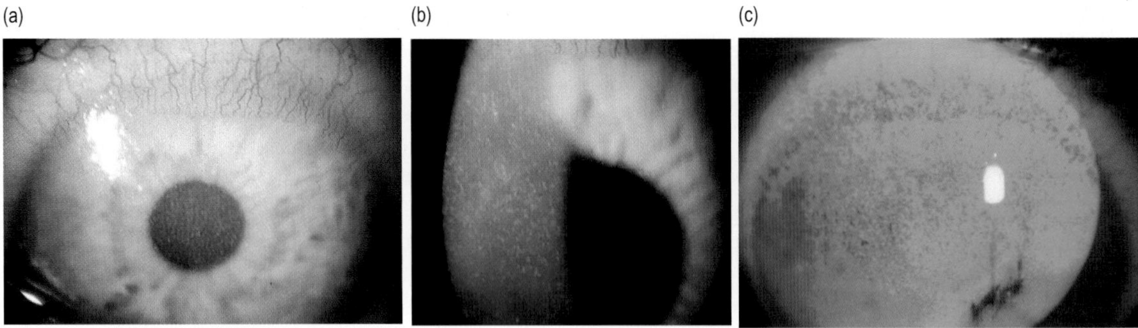

Figure 17.28 Toxic keratitis may arise from several sources but is commonly due to a hypersensitivity or toxic reaction to the preservative in a lens storage solution which leaches onto the cornea when the lens is inserted. The pattern is that of a diffuse to heavy punctate keratitis over a large area or the whole area of the cornea. The limbal area is also commonly injected. (a, b) Low- and high-magnification white light photographs, respectively; (c) low-magnification blue light photograph showing long-term thimerosal toxicity with diffuse fluorescein staining of the epithelium and a pronounced dark dry spot. (Courtesy of T. Grant)

- Punctate epithelial staining.
- Corneal infiltration with inflammatory cells.

Evidence of hypersensitivity may be obtained from a positive ocular reaction to a provocative test with a suspected preservative or from a skin patch test, or if cytology results show eosinophils. However, management can proceed on the basis of a presumed diagnosis by a trial elimination of suspected preservative care solutions.

Before resuming lens wear, corneal infiltrates should be given time to disperse because early resumption may cause symptoms to recur (see **Infiltrates**).

Soft lenses are more likely to bind with preservatives and therefore adverse preservative responses are more common than with rigid lenses (see Figs 17.9, 17.28).

Management

- Replace or purge lenses (see **Purging**).
- Change lens care system to one that has a different preservative or is preservative free.

Pseudopterygia (or Dellen)

These appear as a sequel to chronic epithelial erosion (see **Three and nine o'clock peripheral stain**) in rigid lens wearers (Stainer et al. 1981). The temporal and/or nasal limbal cornea becomes scarred and vascularized superficially, leading to subepithelial opacities which appear similar to pterygia but with a diffuse leading edge.

Initially, there are no symptoms but increased lens awareness, burning and stinging occur.

Predisposing factors include:

- Over-wear.
- Inferiorly locating lenses.
- Superiorly locating lenses with low lower lids.
- Tear deficiency.
- Lenses with excess peripheral clearance.
- Lenses with thick edges.
- Inefficient blinking.

(See Fig. 17.29.)

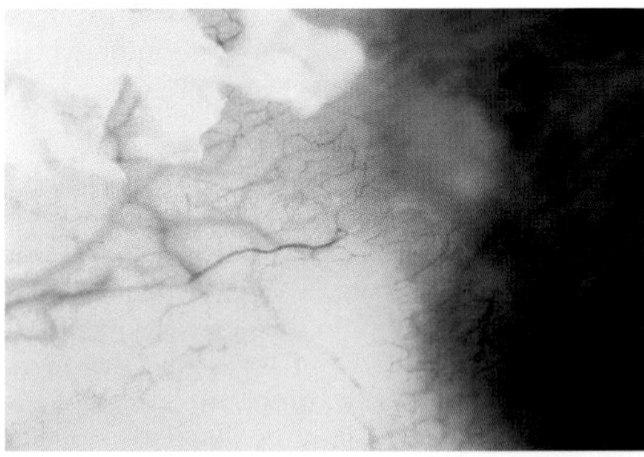

Figure 17.29 A case of pseudopterygium in an RGP lens wearer. This is the sequel to chronic 9 o'clock epithelial desiccation, staining and erosion

Management

- Refit thinner, better-centred RGP lenses with reduced edge clearance and smaller TD.
- Improve blink efficiency.
- Treat any tear deficiency.
- Reduce concentrated close work in contact lenses.
- Prescribe in-eye rewetting drops.
- Change to soft lenses.

(See **Blink efficiency** and **Tear deficiency**.)

Pterygia and pingueculae

Because these lesions are highly vascularized, any stimulus to conjunctival injection will result in a greater hyperaemic response (Fig. 17.30). Well-fitted and -maintained contact lenses do not appear to cause significant problems but may be incorrectly regarded as the cause of pterygium growth.

Soft lenses, especially with a UV inhibitor, may act as a bandage for the head of a pterygium and prevent the epithelial drying associated with increased growth. An advancing pterygium can alter corneal astigmatism (see Chapters 8 and 10).

Management

- Refit unstable RGP lenses as they may mechanically irritate vascularized scar tissue.
- Refit with soft lenses incorporating a UV inhibitor.

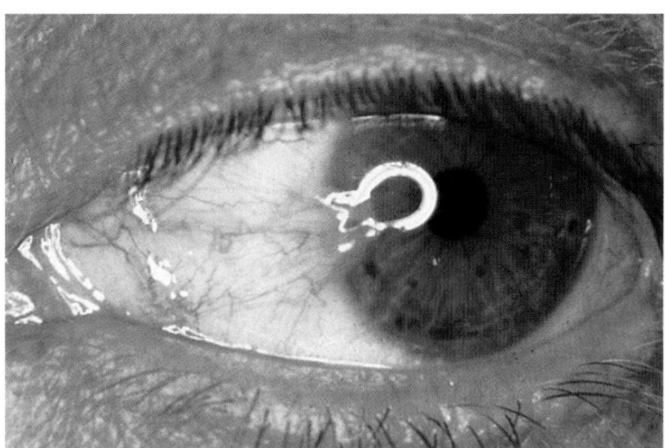

Figure 17.30 Pterygium

- Monitor corneal astigmatism and refer for surgery if the pterygium is advancing towards the pupil.
- Prescribe sunglasses with a good UV inhibitor (see **Ultraviolet protection**).

Purging

Purging lenses is rarely carried out nowadays as there are extensive ranges of relatively cheap disposable lenses. However, should a problem arise with a complicated conventional lens, for example absorbing irritant substances from storage solutions or toxic gases, vapours and sprays (see **Toxic fumes**), the lens should be purged prior to reuse.

In order to carry out purging:

- Soak the lens in a large volume of unpreserved saline in a lens vial or specimen bottle for 12 hours.
- Agitate the bottle to circulate the fluid.
- Repeat three or four times.
- If the lens can tolerate it, sterilize or autoclave.
- Cautiously resume lens wear.

(See also Chapter 4.)

Quality control

Laboratories must maintain quality control and satisfactory tolerances for all lens parameters.

Practitioners should check the parameters of rigid lenses prior to collection but soft lenses are rarely checked. If errors are noted, the rigid lens can be rejected, which should reduce after-care problems. Small inaccuracies, while not rejected, should be noted on the record card so that if a problem is noticed later, the reason for it will be apparent (see also **Edge shape**; **Transition quality in rigid lenses**, and Chapters 16 and 27).

Reactive eye

These eyes react more readily than normal to any stimulus (McMonnies 1978). They are chronically hyperaemic and signs include:

- Pterygia or pingueculae.
- Lid conditions such as blepharitis.
- Tear deficiency.
- Chronic follicular or papillary changes in the palpebral conjunctiva.
- Meibomian gland dysfunction.

There may be a history of:

- Skin conditions such as acne rosacea.
- Atopic conditions such as hay fever.
- An adverse response to wind, dust, glare, smoke, smog, lack of sleep, eye strain and food allergies.

Figures 17.16, 17.17 and 17.30 illustrate some of these conditions.

Management

- Reiterate strict lens care and lid hygiene.
- Moderate lens wear to minimize adverse responses.
- Refit with disposable or frequent-replacement lenses.
- Avoid solution preservatives.
- Control meibomian gland dysfunction and blepharitis.

(See **Chronic hyperaemia; Lid hygiene.**)

Reading difficulties

Some myopic patients, especially early presbyopes, will report difficulty reading with their lenses because they need to accommodate more in contact lenses than in spectacles (see Chapter 6). This problem is greater for higher degrees of myopia. Younger myopes who usually read unaided may experience difficulties with contact lenses.

Conversely, hypermetropic patients accommodate less with contact lenses than with spectacles.

Management

- Discuss potential problems before fitting lenses.
- Consider blink efficiency and associated lens drying as contributing factors (see **Monovision**; **Presbyopia**).

Reconditioning

Rigid lenses that are scratched can be polished. Lenses coated in protein can be reconditioned by rigorously rubbing with a tissue soaked in abrasive cleaner, liquid enzyme or chemical cleaner such as Progent (Menicon), and soft lenses can be purged. However, it is advisable to replace any lenses that need these procedures. Where reconditioning is necessary, always advise about the risk of lens breakage for which the practitioner cannot be held responsible (see also **Polishing; Purging**.)

Record keeping

There is a balance between filling cards with unnecessary details and not recording sufficient information. For example, poor compliance with hygiene should be noted so that this can be rechecked at a subsequent visit. However, if no note is made, it

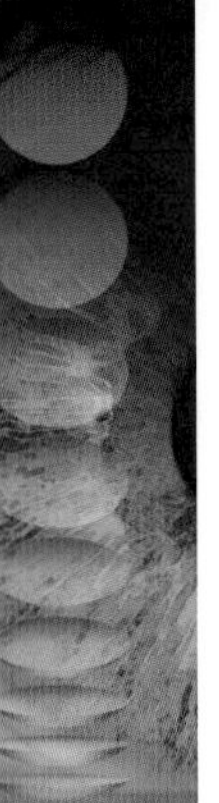

does not necessarily mean that the patient showed good compliance.

Abbreviations can be used, for example:

WT 12, No S, R&L 6/6, No O/R, R&L (o, o) M1, B-ve Rep 12/12

indicating a wearing time of 12 hours a day, no symptoms, each eye reads 6/6 with no significant over-refraction, both lenses centre and move 1 mm on upward gaze blink, biomicroscopy results are unremarkable, and the patient is to report for the next after-care visit in 12 months. It is important that shorthand terms are readily understood by those who need to see the record cards (see Chapter 32).

Many observations are readily rated on nominal or ordinal scales that can be described economically. For example, rigid lens/corneal curvature relationships can be described by the following shorthand system (A. J. Phillips, 1987, personal communication):

Borderline flat = AL–
Alignment = AL
Slight clearance = AL+
Definite clearance = AL++.

The recording of conjunctival hyperaemia is another example, where a photographic reference scale allows six grades of hyperaemia to be determined (McMonnies & Chapman-Davies 1987b) and these can be recorded as H0 through to H5 so that time and record card space is conserved (see Fig. 17.10).

The CCLRU/IER grading scale of commonly observed conditions is shown in Appendix B and on the CD-ROM.

An illustration of right and left eyes on the record card allows any abnormalities to be drawn in. This provides a diagrammatic representation of the location and intensity of any findings. A digital photograph is even better (see Chapter 7).

Refitting contact lenses

Contact lenses should be refitted to an existing wearer when changes in refraction and/or a degraded lens indicate it or where a new lens material or design has been produced that would be better for the patient.

Degraded rigid lenses show accumulated surface scratches and/or changes to the BOZR, including warpage (see Fig. 17.31). Degraded soft lenses can also show surface scratches (see Figs 7.2, 7.22), as well as loss of shape, deposits and discoloration. A gradual loss of lens performance (comfort and vision) may not be appreciated until the change is made.

Refractive changes after wearing contact lenses

Ideally patients should be able to alternate between contact lenses and spectacles, both having a similar visual performance. If corneal shape is altered by lens wear, or there is any corneal oedema, this is not possible.

There are differences of opinion as to when refraction should be carried out in order to prescribe a pair of spectacles with the optimum prescription. With current materials, it should be possible to refract a few minutes after lens removal, especially as this is the time when spectacles are most likely to be worn.

Patients with higher levels of ametropia are likely to experience difficulty with spatial orientation and other perceptual problems (see Chapter 21) when changing from contact lenses to spectacles.

Problems are compounded when lens design, material or lens location induce corneal shape changes, especially when the same lens design is worn for many years. Long-term PMMA wearers may have great difficulty with spectacles (see **Spectacles**) and may take many months after refitting with RGP lenses to be able to alternate spectacles and contact lenses comfortably.

Corneal shape changes may occasionally be beneficial and an orthokeratology effect may occur which reduces the refractive error (see Chapter 19).

Management

- Counsel patients about potential problems when changing to spectacles.
- Try to establish realistic expectations for variation in performance of spectacles depending on how recently contact lenses have been worn (on removal, on waking, etc.) (see **Spectacles**).

Re-instruction

Re-instruction of lens handling and maintenance is sometimes needed at after-care when patients have forgotten techniques or developed bad habits. Additional instruction may be needed that cannot be anticipated earlier; for example, after-care patients may require instruction regarding blink efficiency, lid hygiene, cleaning the inferior portion of non-rotating lenses, tear supplement use, etc. Written hand-outs can be issued for home reference to reinforce consulting room discussion (see **Blink efficiency**, **Lid hygiene** and Chapter 11).

Reports

These should be written for patients who require after-care from another practice when travelling or moving house. They should include:

- A copy of the latest keratometry findings.
- Spectacle and contact lens prescriptions, including recommended maintenance products.
- Other significant details which will facilitate the transfer of after-care responsibility.

(See also Chapter 32.)

Residual astigmatism

Suspect residual astigmatism when acuity is worse than expected with spherical over-refraction. This can be confirmed by retinoscopy, which allows the assessment of varying lid position and lens movement. A decentred lens, especially one with high power, will induce an astigmatic effect and variations in RGP flexure may be induced with changes in palpebral aperture and lid tonus.

The degree and axis of residual astigmatism is checked by subjective refraction but variations do occur between blinks in lenses that are scratched or deposited as the surface wetness alters. Allow longer viewing time of the alternatives during subjective refraction so that blinking can clear vision and stabilize the lens position.

Where residual astigmatism is found in toric lenses, especially soft, check the axis of the lens.

Sometimes lens flexure in rigid lenses fortuitously compensates for residual astigmatism that would occur if a non-flexing lens were fitted. This phenomenon may explain some of the differences in visual performance found with lenses of the same prescription made with different centre thickness or in a different material. For either rigid or soft lenses, front and/or back toroidal surfaces can be used to compensate for residual astigmatism, or supplementary spectacles can be prescribed for occasional use (see also Chapters 6, 9, 10 and 12).

Management

- Refit with toric lenses.
- Overcorrect with spectacles which can be photochromic to expand their usefulness.
- Increase centre thickness and improve lens/cornea fitting relationship (see **Flexure**).

Rigid lens verification (see **Lens parameters**; **Quality control**; see also Chapter 16)

Scratches

Scratches that develop earlier than expected can be due to faulty case design, rough skin on hands, from a ring on a finger, the lens dropping onto a hard surface or difficulty in retrieving a lens that has fallen.

Sliding a lens from a smooth or basket-type case can cause scratches from dust or degraded plastic surfaces. Soft lens case wells should be ribbed and/or flat bottomed to minimize this problem. Some RGP lens cases suspend the lens in solution in soft plastic holders, free from flexure stress. However, a large-diameter lens may flex and become warped and these cases are difficult to clean.

Polishing RGP lenses does cause a small reduction in thickness.

The appearance of deep scratches may in fact be surface crazing (Fig. 17.31) in which case the lens will need to be replaced (see also Chapters 9, 16 and 28).

Management

- Ignore minor scratches.
- Polish or replace RGP lenses yearly.
- Replace very scratched lenses or lenses manufactured from materials that cannot be polished.
- Avoid storage case designs that increase scratch damage.
- If rough skin is the problem, suggest the use of a clean, lint-free tissue or a mechanical cleaner.

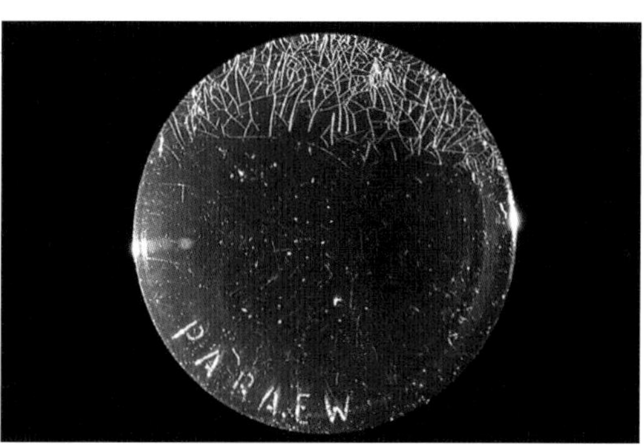

Figure 17.31 Surface crazing and cracking of high-oxygen-permeable silicone-acrylate lenses is now rarely seen as the lenses age. Symptoms can range from slight loss of vision if occurring centrally, to some loss of comfort. Removal of the cracks is not possible and lens replacement is the only answer, but in the early stages of surface crazing it may be possible to repolish the surface. (Courtesy of A. J. Phillips)

Sequential stain

This occurs with multiple instillations of fluorescein over a period of several minutes and is associated with contact lens intolerance. It may be observed in mild form in successful wearers (Korb & Herman 1979). Several instillations of 2% liquid fluorescein at 5-minute intervals will identify at-risk patients. Absence of fluorescein stain upon sequential instillation suggests normal epithelial integrity.

Silicone rubber lenses

These may be found to adhere tightly to the ocular surface because of pervaporation, i.e. the tears vaporize and the vapour passes through the silicone rubber material, reducing the volume of liquid beneath the lens causing lens adherence to the cornea (Refojo & Leong 1981). The lens can usually be safely removed after instilling a local anaesthetic and using the edge of a rubber suction holder to lift the edge of the lens away from the eye. If lenses still prove resistant, removal can be effected with round-ended forceps.

Slit-lamp biomicroscopy

During after-care, careful slit-lamp examination should be undertaken of lens condition and fit, and any changes in appearance of ocular tissue. These can be compared with a baseline record of pre-fitting observations (see also Chapters 7 and 8).

Corneal integrity should be assessed before and after lens removal, as removal affords an opportunity to use stains in the case of soft lens wear.

'Smile' stain

An arcuate stain (Fig. 17.32), usually in the lower third of the cornea, caused by dehydration. This can result from poor blinking or because of rapid dehydration of the soft lens. Refitting with a material less prone to dehydration (e.g. Proclear [CooperVision]) or with a looser lens usually solves the problem.

Spectacles (see also **Refractive changes after wearing contact lenses**)

Spectacle prescriptions are unlikely to be reliable if keratometry readings are unclear after lenses have been removed. If spectacle blur is apparent, lenses need to be left out for several hours or overnight before refracting. PMMA lens wearers, who have no spectacles, may require a compromise spectacle prescription while they reduce their wearing time in order to be refitted with a gas-permeable material (see also **Supplementary spectacles** and Chapter 9).

Stinging

Possible causes of stinging after lens insertion include:

- An adverse reaction to the pH, buffering, tonicity or preservative in a storage or rinsing solution.
- Hydrogen peroxide that has not been effectively neutralized.
- Cleaning solution that has not been rinsed off.
- Contamination from unwashed hands.
- Misapplied cosmetics.

If the sensation is mild, it should settle after a minute or two, otherwise the lens should be removed, rinsed or immersed in saline and reapplied.

New lenses may sting if not completely leached of toxic substances introduced during manufacture (see also Chapter 4).

Striae (see **Corneal oedema**)

Suction holders

Suction holders intended for contact lens removal are not usually advisable. Patients with loose lids that do not dislodge a rigid lens, or who have long fingernails that inhibit soft lens removal, should have further instruction before suggesting a suction holder. These devices can become contaminated and are potential sources of corneal abrasion if an attempt is made to remove a dislodged lens. However, patients should have a suction holder available for emergencies. A suction holder may provide a feeling of security for a patient who lacks confidence even if it is never used. Suction holders may help to remove silicone rubber and large RGP or scleral lenses (see also Chapters 11 and 15).

Superficial epithelial arcuate lesions (SEALs)

SEALs are horizontal splits, usually adjacent to the superior limbus in soft lens wearers, especially those wearing thick periphery high-water-content or first-generation silicone hydrogel lenses (Figs 17.32, 17.33; see also Chapters 10 and 13). They show diffuse stain into the surrounding cornea.

The cause of SEALs is not known but is thought to result from a mechanical chaffing secondary to inward pressure from the upper lid, in combination with predisposing lens design, increased lens rigidity and susceptible corneal topography (Holden et al. 2001). Precipitating factors may include tightening of lens fittings through tear hypotonicity, localized drying associated with the upper lid tear meniscus or overall lens dehydration.

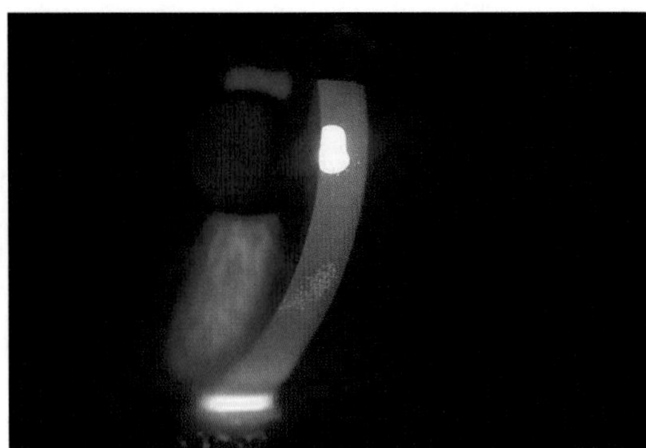

Figure 17.32 Smile stain. (Courtesy of J. Morris)

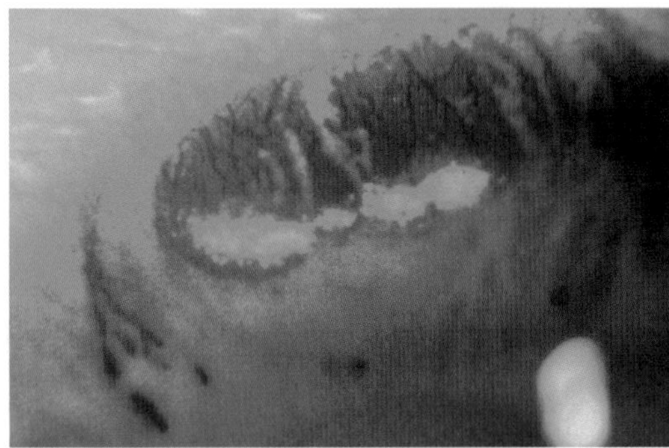

Figure 17.33 Superior limbal epithelial split found in a hydrogel lens wearer causing pain, dense staining and diffusion of the stain into the underlying stroma, with increased vascularization.

The split may occur during the following:

- Blinking.
- Lens removal.
- Prolonged periods of reading.
- When lid shear forces are increased by
  - surface deposits.
  - palpebral conjunctival thickening.
  - tear deficiency.
- Any combination of these factors.

SEALs may be symptomless but are usually associated with irritation leading to intolerance. In mild cases, superficial healing can occur overnight.

Management

- If possible, abandon lens wear until the epithelium heals. The basal cell layer takes much longer than superficial healing (indicated when staining has disappeared).
- Resume lens wear cautiously with the existing fitting.
- Preferably, refit lenses with improved movement or different water content.

- Refit with RGP lenses.
- Be conscious of the risk of secondary infection.

(See **Superficial punctate epitheliopathy**.)

Superficial punctate epitheliopathy (SPE)

Mild SPE is not uncommon in the normal eye and is a common finding in contact lens wearers. It is caused by many factors including:

- Abrasion from surface deposits or damaged lenses.
- Incomplete tear distribution.
- Tear deficiency.
- Toxic or sensitivity reactions to solution preservatives.

In addition, most corneal pathologies exhibit SPE (see Chapters 9, 10 and 18). Epithelial erosions may occur when soft lenses dehydrate on the eye. Figure 17.34 shows multiple confluent erosions following short-term wear of a very thin high-water-content hydrogel lens. Holden et al. (1986) postulated that small areas of epithelial tissue become attached to the lens and are torn away when the lens is removed. They may also occur when mild degrees of punctate stain remain untreated for long periods, in cases of sterile ulceration, and when debris builds up under a lens or adheres to its back surface.

Increased visibility of punctate epithelial lesions suggests associated infiltration with inflammatory cells that reduce transparency, rendering them visible with direct focal illumination. Deeper lesions, especially if necrotic with greyish stromal infiltrates, may be observed in the bed of an epithelial injury that appears to be ulcerating. This type of change is rare but is an indication for immediate action.

Table 17.1 shows the most likely cause of various locations of SPE staining.

Prolonged soft contact lens-induced hypoxia can significantly reduce epithelial adhesion. This may provide an explanation for the SLACH syndrome (soft lens-associated corneal hypoxia syndrome) where there is spontaneous loss of up to 40% of the epithelial surface during lens wear (Fig. 17.36).

(See also Fig. 17.43.)

Table 17.1: Probable causes of superficial punctate epitheliopathy staining

Type of stain	Cause
Deep, appearing translucent, with marginal retro-illumination	Abrasions and corneal desiccation
Haphazard linear distribution	Foreign body abrasion (Fig. 17.35)
Localized or arcuate lesion	A damaged lens, especially a non-rotating one
Circular localized lesion	A damaged lens that rotates
Lower corneal stain	Inefficient blinking and tear deficiency or poor eyelid closure during sleep
Generalized stain	Sensitivity and toxic reactions
Superiorly located stain	Superior limbic keratitis

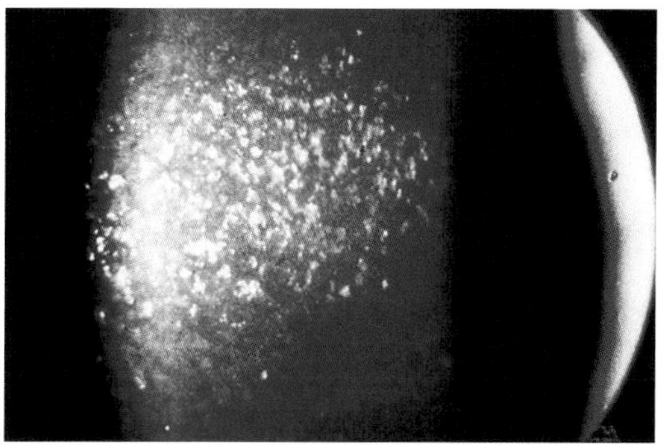

Figure 17.34 Epithelial erosions. (From Holden et al. 1986, with permission)

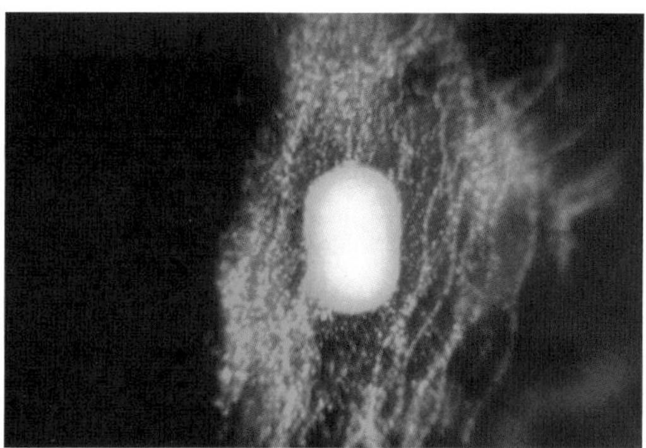

Figure 17.35 Multitrack foreign body corneal abrasion and staining seen under high magnification

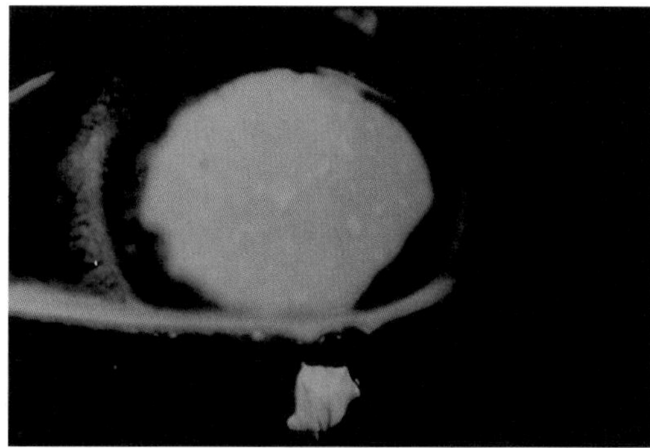

Figure 17.36 Spontaneous loss of epithelium. (Courtesy of B. Holden and D. Sweeney)

Management

- Remove lenses and allow SPE to heal.
- Refit with a different material or lens modality.
- Deeper lesions must be carefully monitored and treated with antibiotic drops as a precaution.

Superior limbic keratitis (SLK)

SLK resulting from contact lenses should not be confused with SLK of Theodore. The latter is a sectoral inflammation and injection of the superior bulbar conjunctiva and limbal cornea, often associated with a filamentary keratitis. The tarsal

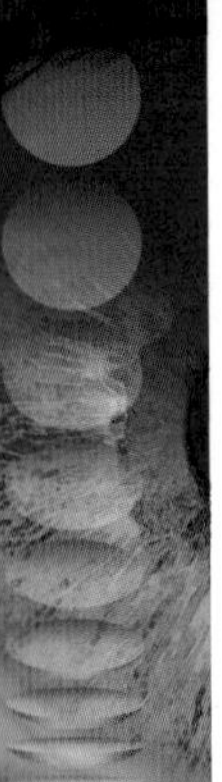

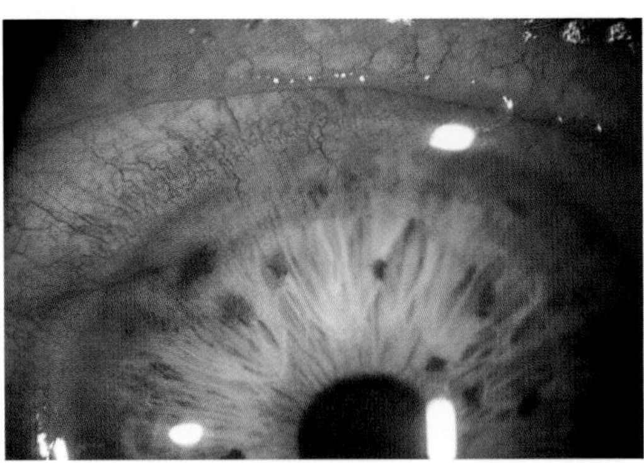

Figure 17.37 Contact lens-induced superior limbic keratitis shows hyperaemia of the superior limbus and adjacent conjunctiva, stromal infiltrates, a fibrovascular micropannus, epithelial haziness and corneal and conjunctival staining to fluorescein (see also Figs 17.32 and 17.33). (Courtesy of A. J. Phillips)

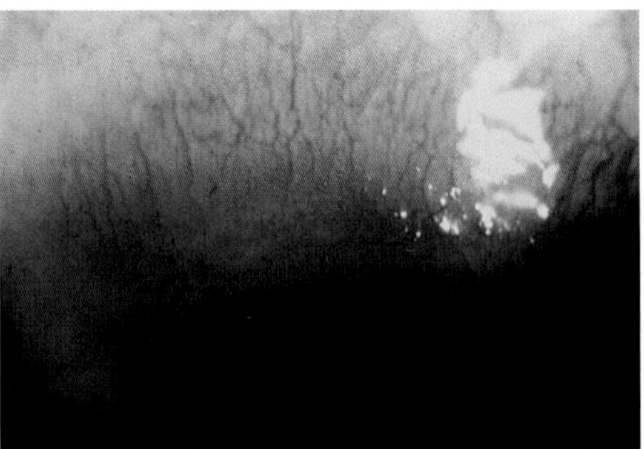

Figure 17.38 The same type of contact lens-induced superior limbal keratitis as in Figures 17.33 and 17.37, showing Rose Bengal staining of the damaged epithelium. This should be differentiated from that in Figure 17.39. (Courtesy of A. J. Phillips)

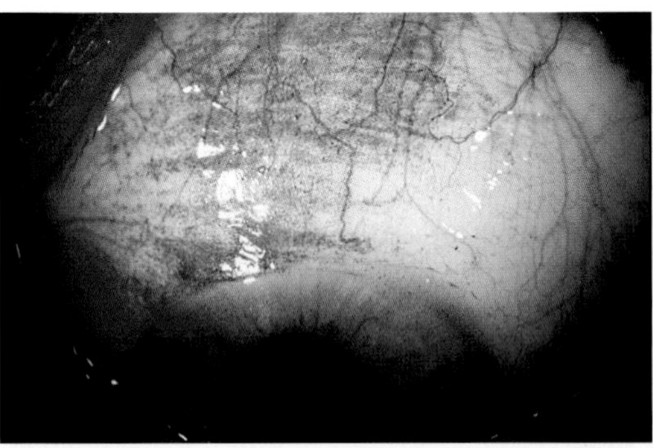

Figure 17.39 Superior limbic keratitis (SLK) or Theodore's SLK occurs when there is abnormal frictional force between lid and globe. The condition is commonly associated with thyrotoxicosis. Epithelial staining to Rose Bengal can be seen in the area above the globe and a fold of loose or stretched conjunctiva hangs over the upper limbal area. The condition often responds to the use of an extended-wear bandage lens, ocular lubricants and, of course, the treatment of any underlying condition. True SLK should be differentiated from contact lens-induced SLK (see Figs 17.33, 17.37, 17.38) which also stains similarly with Rose Bengal. (Courtesy of A. J. Phillips)

conjunctiva reveals small uniform papillae. Theodore's SLK occurs when there is abnormal friction between lid and globe. It is associated with thyroid eye disease and autoimmune disease, and affects females more than males. Soft therapeutic lenses are used as treatment to prevent shearing of the conjunctiva, as well as mast cell stabilizer drops and cautery of the filaments.

SLK from contact lens wear affects young healthy contact lens wearers. It is associated with prolonged hypoxia and mechanical irritation from the lens edge and were formerly seen with thimerosal preserved solutions (Sendele et al. 1983). Patients become increasingly intolerant of their lenses and examination reveals localized superior bulbar conjunctival injection, corneal stromal haze and infiltrates, and hyperaemia and staining of the palpebral conjunctiva (Figs 17.37–17.39). Resolution can take many months.

Management

- Cease contact lens wear.
- Unpreserved ocular lubricants.
- Resume lens wear with new lenses once the condition has resolved.
- If soft lens intolerance recurs, refit with RGP lenses.

Supplementary spectacles

Spectacles may be required in conjunction with contact lenses for reading (see **Presbyopia**) or when toric lenses cannot easily be fitted to correct residual astigmatism (e.g. in keratoconus). Photochromic lenses increase the usefulness.

Monovision patients may require supplementary spectacles for optimum binocular vision, especially when driving (see **Monovision** and Chapter 14).

Surface deposits

Some lens types and some patients are especially prone to developing surface deposits (see Chapters 9 and 10).

Management

- Change to daily disposable or frequent-replacement lenses where possible.
- Polish RGP lenses more frequently.
- Change the material to one which is more deposit resistant (e.g. avoid high-water-content ionic materials) (see Chapters 3, 9 and 10).
- Stress hygiene compliance.
- Increase surfactant lens cleaning time.
- Advise use of surfactant night and morning.
- Change surfactant to one containing abrasives (emulsion cleaners).
- Increase frequency of enzyme tablets (see Chapter 4) or, for RGP lenses, use a chemical cleaner such as Menicon's Progent.
- Use a different type of enzyme (e.g. animal- or vegetable-derived).

- Stress surfactant cleaning before and after enzyme tablets. This exposes the bound (older) deposits to a greater concentration of enzyme and removes broken-down protein deposits.
- Improve blink efficiency.
- Improve tear function with hot compresses and lid hygiene (see **Lid hygiene** and **Tear deficiency**).
- Prescribe tear supplements.

Swimming

Swimming in lenses carries a risk of infection. Goggles can be worn over lenses but are seldom effective enough to be completely safe. In the event of contamination with water, lenses should be disinfected by a method considered active against possible *Acanthamoeba* contamination (see Chapter 4).

Tear circulation

Tear circulation should be assessed at after-care when lenses have fully settled as poor tear circulation leads to discomfort and oedema.

Indications of poor circulation include:

- Static lenses that do not move with blinking.
- Accumulation of stationary tear debris under lenses.
- Delayed movement of fluorescein under a rigid lens.

Management

- Increase RGP edge lift.
- Loosen hydrogel lenses.
- Avoid matching toric RGP back optic radii to corneal curvature too exactly.
- If the lens fits well but tears are poor, prescribe rewetting drops.
- Consider fenestrating RGP lenses (see **Fenestration**).

(See also Chapters 9 and 15.)

Tear deficiency (see Chapter 5)

Older patients are more prone to tear deficiency than younger patients and patients with marginal dry eye conditions are more likely to be susceptible to problems when contact lenses are worn. A dry eye questionnaire (McMonnies & Ho 1987a,b), slit-lamp examination and the Tearscope (Guillon & Guillon 1993, McPherson 1993) (see Chapter 5) can be used to identify these patients.

Signs

- Contact lens surface drying and associated surface deposits.
- Conjunctival hyperaemia.
- Reduced height, irregular or excessively viscous marginal tear prism.
- Excessive precorneal tear debris.
- Dull specular reflection from a desiccated bulbar conjunctiva.
- Excessive meibomian gland secretion.
- Oil in the tear film from skin emollients (see Fig. 17.15).
- Staining at 3 and 9 o'clock with rigid lenses (see **Three and nine o'clock peripheral stain**).
- Superficial punctate epitheliopathy in the exposed area of the cornea with soft lenses (especially torics).

(See Figs 17.40–17.43.)

Symptoms

Dryness and grittiness for rigid lens wearers, and dryness and soreness for soft lens wearers (Bron & Quinlan 1993).

Management

- Preservative-free tear supplements.
- Treat any blepharitis and meibomitis (see **Lid hygiene**).
- Advise against using face cream around eyes and on eyelids.
- Blink exercises (see **Blink efficiency**).
- Reduce wearing time, especially in air-conditioned or centrally heated rooms or for computer use (see **Computer vision syndrome**).
- Consider punctual occlusion (Bockin 1993, Anon 1994).
- Use a soft lens material less susceptible to dryness or switch to an RGP, scleral or semi-scleral lens.

Three and nine o'clock peripheral stain
(see also Chapter 9)

This localized staining occurs in rigid lens wearers when areas of the cornea are not wetted adequately during blinking. It is more common with RGP materials than with PMMA (Bennett & Egan 1986). It presents as a chronic condition and may progress to scarring and vascularization of the cornea (see **Pseudopterygia**).

The lids are unable to evenly resurface the cornea with mucin due to lid-bridging over the contact lens edge and a possible abrasive effect from the lens. These factors combine with predisposing conditions such as a hot dry climate, tear deficiency and inefficient blinking (Sarver et al. 1969) (see Fig. 17.43).

Management

- Refit lenses with reduced edge clearance and/or smaller or larger total diameters.
- Ensure edge is not too thick and is well polished.
- Improve blink efficiency and treat tear deficiency.
- Ensure rigorous surfactant lens cleaning.
- Reduce lens wear for prolonged periods of reading or high vision demand.
- Refit with soft lenses.

Toric lenses (see **Residual astigmatism** and Chapter 12)

These may not give expected visual results because of incorrect prescribing of power or axis, inaccurate manufacture, poor fit, or meridional mislocation that is either constant or variable.

Toric soft lenses can be rotated in 2.5° steps to find the axis of maximum acuity using a cotton bud to move the lens. If this does not give satisfactory acuity, the lens power is likely to be incorrect or the quality poor.

(a)

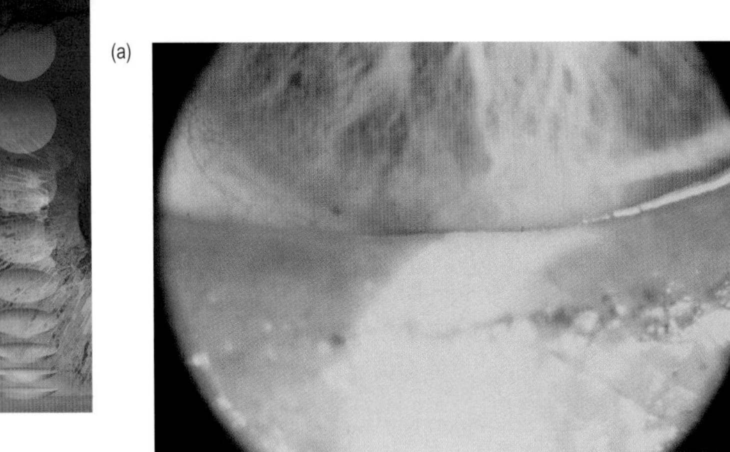

(b)

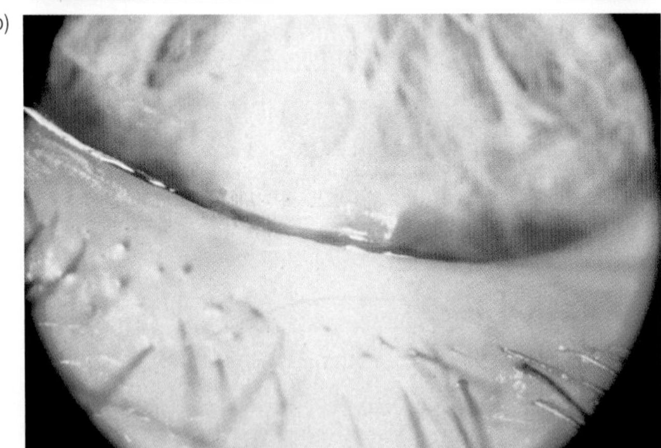

(c)

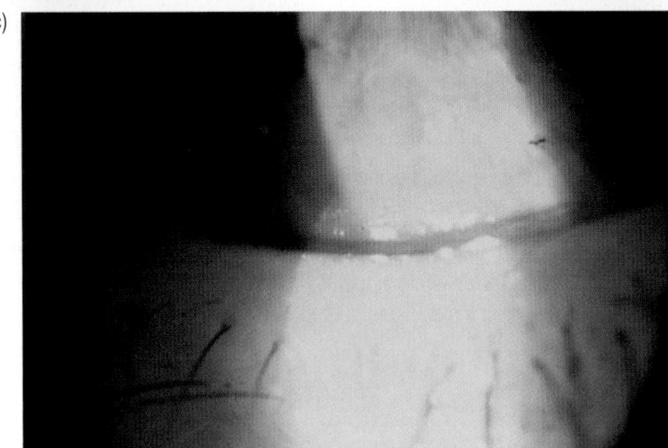

Figure 17.40 Tear prism height is one method of estimating tear volume: (a) deficient; (b) normal; (c) excess. Ectropion may significantly invalidate this type of observation

A lens that gives good acuity when rotated to the correct axis needs a change in axis. If the acuity varies, the lens fit is likely to be incorrect.

Management

- Check over-refraction.
- If the lens is stable, reorder a lens with the correct power.
- If the lens is unstable, refit the lens.
- In the case of soft lenses, a larger TD (e.g. 0.5–1.00 mm) often helps stabilization.

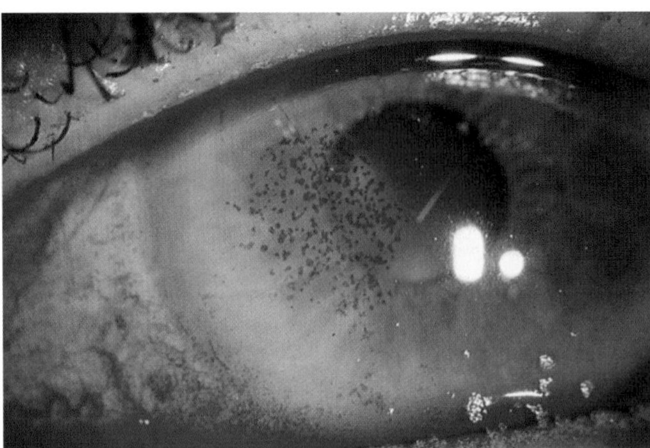

Figure 17.41 Rose Bengal staining of a dry eye: note tear debris. (Courtesy of A. J. Phillips)

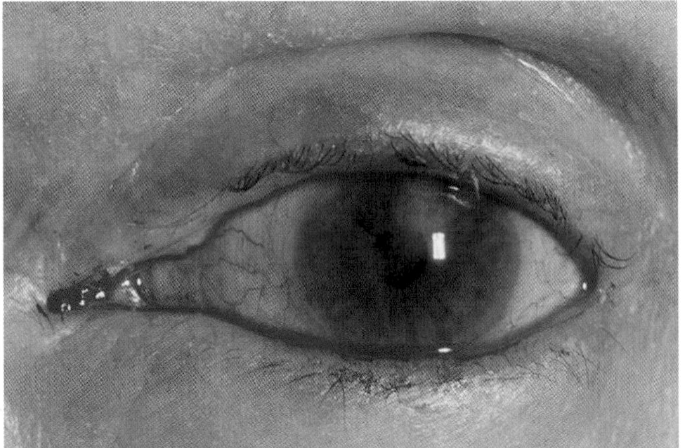

Figure 17.42 Keratoconjunctivitis sicca associated with chronic blepharitis where both aqueous and lipid layers of the precorneal tear film are affected. (Courtesy of D. Westerhout)

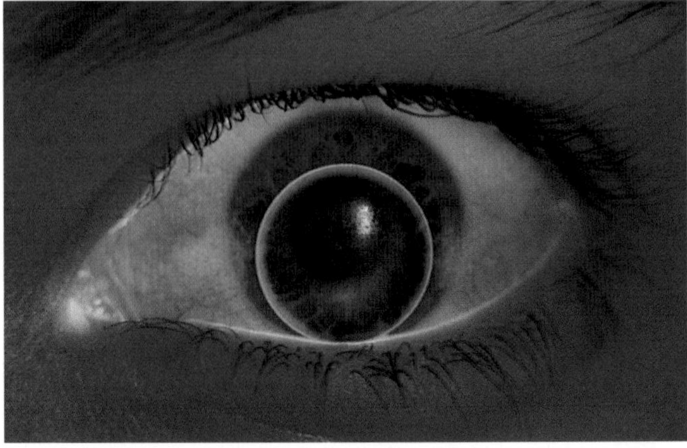

Figure 17.43 Three and 9 o'clock corneal staining here shown associated with a dry and lipid-coated rigid lens. This type of staining only occurs in those areas exposed to the atmosphere between blinks. If the lower lid is very low then similar staining may also occur in the 6 o'clock position. (Courtesy of D. Westerhout)

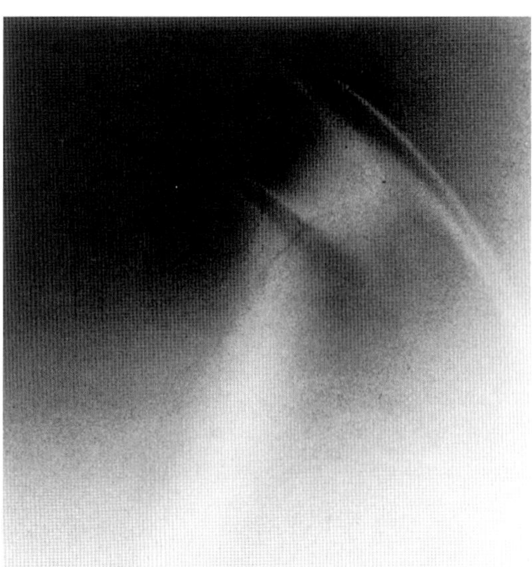

Figure 17.44 Lack of continuity in a fluorescent tube image followed by reflection from the back surface of a rigid lens indicates a poor transition between optic zone and periphery. Additionally, the non-paraboloidal shape of image towards the edge indicates unsatisfactory formation of the most peripheral curve and its transition to the posterior edge. This image can be viewed using a ×7 to ×10 hand-held magnifier (see Fig. 17.45)

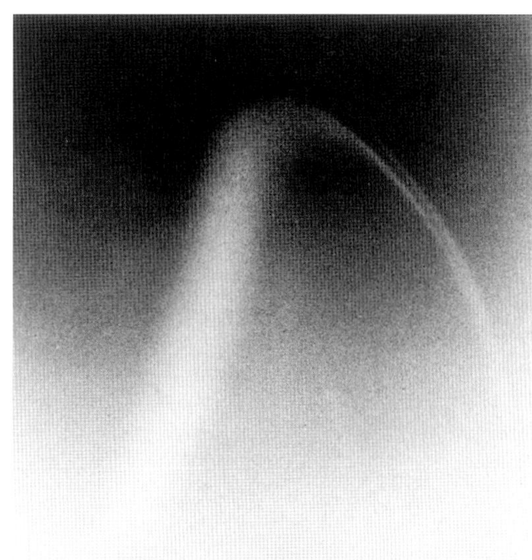

Figure 17.45 The fluorescent tube image from the back surface of this rigid lens has a satisfactory shape. Smooth transition between optic zone and periphery is evident. In addition, the paraboloidal shape of the peripheral part of the image indicates a well-formed transition between flattening peripheral curves and posterior edge (see Fig. 17.44)

Toxic fumes

These are likely to be absorbed into soft lens materials resulting in pain, lacrimation and epitheliopathy. Lenses should, if possible, be discarded or, if that is not possible, they must be purged (see **Purging**).

Anti-splash protective goggles worn when toxic liquids are handled are not enough protection against adsorption from the air. Goggles need to be airtight for adequate protection.

Apart from vocational risk, hobbyists (e.g. model makers) and home renovators may also be exposed to toxic fumes intermittently.

Transition quality in rigid lenses

Lack of continuity in an elongated fluorescent tube image, formed by reflection from the back surface of a rigid lens, indicates a poor transition between optic zone and periphery (Figs 17.44, 17.45) that may require modification or remaking (see Chapters 16 and 28).

Travelling

Restriction on baggage allowance with air travel limits the quantity of lens solutions that can be carried. Small-quantity containers are preferred. Frequent travellers may find daily disposable lenses more convenient.

Hygiene problems are common, depending on water supply. If in doubt, spectacles should be worn. (See **Flying** and Chapter 8.)

Ultraviolet protection

Conjunctival injection may be associated with exposure to excess levels of ultraviolet radiation (e.g. when skiing). Ultraviolet-absorbing materials help protect the cornea and internal eye but protective sunglasses are still necessary to protect the peripheral cornea (in corneal lenses) and the conjunctiva (see **Pterygia and pingueculae**).

Vascularization

Contact lens wear causes both acute and chronic injection of limbal vessels of the cornea and is more common in soft lens wearers (McMonnies 1984).

Causes include:

- Over-wear.
- Adverse reactions to preservatives.
- Hypoxia.
- Loss of epithelial integrity, such as 3 and 9 o'clock staining.
- Tight lenses which trap debris and metabolic waste and which cause passive hyperaemia by restriction of limbal blood flow.
- Poorly finished edges.
- Environmental causes of ocular irritation and injection.

Terminal limbal capillaries lying in the translucent peripheral corneal tissue should be at least partly empty. They should extend no more than 1 mm into the visible iris (2 mm superiorly where the transitional conjunctiva encroaches over the transparent stroma). These are measured using the scale on a biomicroscope.

Normal vessels should loop back; spikes indicate new vessels (Figs 17.46, 17.47). Once established, spikes can be seen to consist of arterial and venous portions when viewed under high

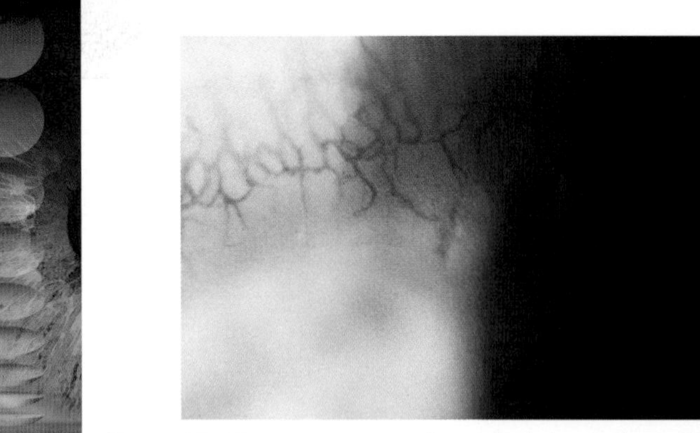

Figure 17.46 Active stage of new limbal vessel growth showing a new spike projecting from an existing arcade and surrounded by exudate

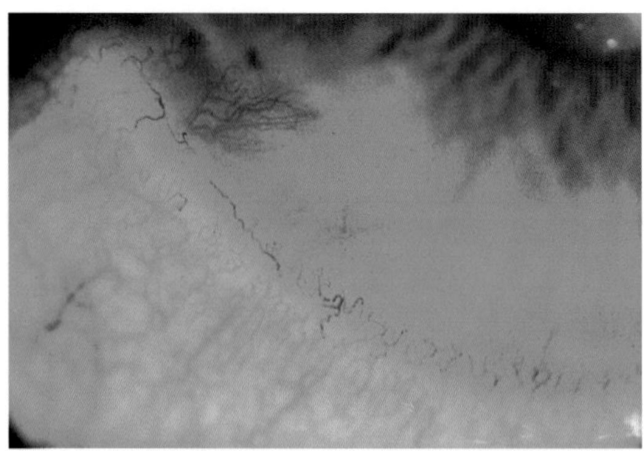

Figure 17.47 Red-free illumination may help detect stromal vessels (seen around 8 o'clock) that are partly obscured by inflammatory lipid exudate when examined with white light

magnification. Adjacent spikes join to form a new arcade. Stromal vessels are not continuous with the conjunctival vessels; their growth is more serious and indicates a deeper pathology.

New vessels can leak lipid (see Fig. 18.8), which, if extensive, can affect vision. They are also more common and extensive if there is existing scar tissue.

(See Figs 17.37–17.39; see also Figs 13.11 and 18.9, Chapters 7 and 13, and Appendix B.)

Management

- Avoid tight lenses and conditions that promote chronic hyperaemia.
- Refit soft lens wearers with silicone hydrogel or higher-water-content materials.
- Refit soft lens wearers with RGP lenses.
- Refit RGP wearers with higher-Dk materials or smaller lenses.
- If neovascularization becomes too advanced, abandon lens wear.

Vasoconstrictors

The cause of hyperaemia should be considered and, if possible, treated. Vasoconstrictors should be used only occasionally as they mask the problem and frequent use can lead to rebound hyperaemia.

CONCLUSION

Ocular tissue responses should be monitored during after-care to reduce the risk of complications. Improvements in lens materials, design and care systems are under constant development as the search for a greater understanding of contact lens adaptation goes on.

References

Allansmith, M. R., Korb, D. R., Greiner, J. V. et al. (1977) Giant papillary conjunctivitis in contact lens wearers. Am. J. Ophthalmol., 83, 697–708

Anon. (1994) Dry eye. Int. Ophthalmol. Clin., 34(1), 27–36

Bennett, E. S. and Egan, D. J. (1986) Rigid gas permeable lens problem solving. J. Am. Optom. Assoc., 57, 504–511

Bockin, D. (1993) How to perform punctal occlusion. Contact Lens Spectrum, 8(11), 30–32

Bron, A. J. and Quinlan, M. (1993) Causes and treatment of dry eyes. Optometry Today, 28, 22–24

Catania, L. J. (1987) Contact lenses, staphylococcus and 'crocodile O. D.'. Int. Contact Lens Clin., 14, 113–115

Collins, M. J. and Carney, L. G. (1986) Compliance with care and maintenance procedures amongst contact lens wearers. Clin. Exp. Optom., 69, 174–177

Dart, J. K. G. (1993) Disease and risks associated with contact lenses. Br. J. Ophthalmol., 77, 49–53

de Vries Reilingh, A., Reiners, H. and Van Bijsterveld, D. P. (1978) Contact lens tolerance and oral contraceptives. Am. J. Ophthalmol., 10, 947–952

Dumbleton, K., Jones, L., Chalmers, R. et al. (2000) Clinical characterization of spherical post-lens debris associated with lotrafilcon high-Dk silicone lenses. Contact Lens Assoc. Ophthalmol. J., 26, 186–192

Enelow, A. J. and Swisher, S. N. (1972) The problem-oriented medical record. In Interviewing and Patient Care, pp. 66–101. London: Oxford University Press

Grayson, M. (1979) Diseases of the Cornea, pp. 240–248. St Louis, MO: Mosby

Guillon, J. and Guillon, M. (1993) Tear film examination of the contact lens patient. Optician, 206(5421), 21–29

Guttridge, N. (1994) Changes in ocular and visual variables during the menstrual cycle. Ophthalmol. Physiol. Opt., 14(1), 38–48

Hall, R. J. and Cusack, B. L. (1972) The measurement of eye behaviour: critical and selected reviews of voluntary eye movements and blinking. Technical Memorandum 18–72, pp. 67–69. Human Engineering Laboratory, US Army Aberdeen Research & Development Center, Maryland, AMCMS code 501B.11.84100

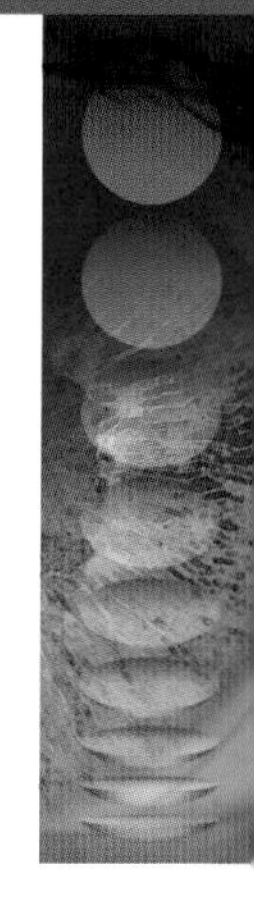

Herman, J. P. (1983) Flexure of rigid contact lenses on toric corneas as a function of base curve fitting relationship. J. Am. Optom. Assoc., 54, 209–214

Holden, B. A., Sweeney, D. F. and Seger, R. G. (1986) Epithelial erosions caused by thin high water content lenses. Clin. Exp. Optom., 69(3), 103–107

Holden, B. A., Stephenson, A., Stretton, S. et al. (2001) Superior epithelial arcuate lesions with soft contact lens wear. Optom. Vis. Sci., 78(1), 9–12

Imafidon C. O. and Imafidon, J. E. (1991) Contact lens wear in pregnancy. J. Br. Contact Lens Assoc., 14(2), 75–78

Korb, D. (1974) The role of blinking in successful contact lens wear. Int. Contact Lens Clin., 1, 59–71

Korb, D. R. and Herman, J. P. (1979) Corneal staining subsequent to sequential fluorescein instillation. J. Am. Optom. Assoc., 50, 361–367

Lippman, R. E. (1986) FDA awaits results of acanthamoeba extended wear studies. Contact Lens Forum, 11, 32–33

Lowe, R. and Brennan, N. A. (1987) Corneal wrinkling caused by a thin medium water content lens. Int. Contact Lens Clin., 14, 403–406

McMonnies, C. W. (1978) Allergic complications in contact lens wear. Int. Contact Lens Clin., 5, 182–189

McMonnies, C. W. (1984) Risk factors in the aetiology of contact lens-induced corneal vascularisation. Int. Contact Lens Clin., 11, 286–293

McMonnies, C. W. (1986) Key questions in a dry eye history. J. Am. Optom. Assoc., 57, 512–517

McMonnies, C. W. (1987) Contact lens after-care: a detailed analysis. Clin. Exp. Optom., 70, 121–127

McMonnies, C. W. and Chapman-Davies, A. (1987a) Assessment of conjunctival hyperaemia in contact lens wearers: Part II. Preserved versus unpreserved storage of soft lenses. Am. J. Optom. Physiol. Opt., 64, 251–255

McMonnies, C. W. and Chapman-Davies, A. (1987b) Assessment of conjunctival hyperaemia in contact lens wearers: Part I. Am. J. Optom. Physiol. Opt., 64, 246–250

McMonnies, C. W. and Ho, A. (1987a) Patient history in screening for dry eye conditions. J. Am. Optom. Assoc., 58, 296–301

McMonnies, C. W. and Ho, A. (1987b) Responses to a dry eye questionnaire from a normal population. J. Am. Optom. Assoc., 58, 588–591

McMonnies, C. W. and Zantos, S. (1979) Endothelial bedewing of the cornea in association with contact lens wear. Br. J. Ophthalmol., 63, 478–481

McMonnies, C. W., Chapman-Davies, A. and Holden, B. A. (1982) Vascular response to contact lens wear. Am. J. Optom. Physiol. Optics, 59, 795–799

McPherson, S. (1993) The Tearscope in practice. Optician, 206(5421), 30

O'Connor Davies, P. H. (1972) The Actions and Uses of Ophthalmic Drugs, pp. 237–262. London: Barrie and Jenkins

O'Leary, D. J. and Millodot, M (1981) Abnormal epithelial fragility in diabetes and in contact lens wear. Acta Ophthalmol., 59, 827–833

Pardos, G. J. and Krachmer, J. H. (1980) Comparison on endothelial cell density in diabetes and a control population. Am. J. Ophthalmol., 90, 172–174

Patel, S. and Port, M. J. A. (1991) Tear characteristics of the VDU operator. Optom. Vis. Sci., 68(10), 798–800

Pearson, R. M. (1986) The mystery of missing fluorescein – a postscript. J. Br. Contact Lens Assoc., 9, 36–37

Priluck, I. A., Robertson, D. M. and Buettner, H. (1979) What patients recall of the preoperative discussion after retinal detachment surgery. Am. J. Ophthalmol., 87, 620–623

Refojo, M. F. and Leong, F. (1981) Water pervaporation through silicone rubber contact lenses: a possible cause of complications. Contact Intraoc. Lens Med. J., 7, 226–233

Ruben, M., Brown, N., Lobascher, D., Chaston, J. and Morris, J. (1976) Clinical manifestations secondary to soft contact lens wear. Br. J. Ophthalmol., 60, 529–531

Sarver, M. D., Nelson, J. L. and Polse, K. A. (1969) Peripheral corneal staining accompanying contact lens wear. J. Am. Optom. Assoc., 40, 310–315

Schultz, R. O., Matsuda, M., Yee, R. W., Edelhauser, H. F. and Schultz, K. J. (1984) Corneal endothelial changes in type I and type II diabetes mellitus. Am. J. Ophthalmol., 98, 401–410

Sendele, D. D., Kenyon, K. R., Mobilia, E. F., Rosenthal, P., Steinert, R. and Hanninen, L. A. (1983) Superior limbic keratoconjunctivitis in contact lens wearers. Ophthalmology, 90(6), 616–622

Serrander, A. and Peek, K. F. (1993) Changes in contact lens comfort related to the menstrual cycle and menopause. J. Am. Optom. Assoc., 64(3), 162–166

Skotnitsky, C., Sankaridurg, P. R., Sweeney, D. F. et al. (2002) General and local contact lens induced papillary conjunctivitis (CLPC). Clin. Exp. Optom., 85, 193–197

Snip, R. C., Thoft, R. A. and Tolentino, F. L. (1980) Similar epithelial healing rates of the corneas of diabetic and non-diabetic patients. Am. J. Ophthalmol., 90, 463–468

Spring, T. F. (1974) Reaction to hydrophilic lenses. Med. J. Aust., 1, 449–450

Stainer, G. A., Brightbill, F. S., Holm, P. and Laux, D. (1981) The development of pseudo-pterygia in hard contact lens wearers. Contact Intraoc. Lens Med. J., 7, 1–4

Sweeney, D. F. (1992) Corneal exhaustion syndrome with long-term wear of contact lenses. Optom. Vis. Sci., 69(8), 601–608

Vadjic, C., Holden, B. A., Sweeney, D. F. et al. (1999) The frequency of ocular symptoms during spectacle and daily soft and rigid contact lens wear. Optom. Vis. Sci., 76(10), 705–711

Wardlaw, J. L. and Sarver, M. D. (1986) Discolouration of hydrogel contact lenses under standard care regimens. Am. J. Optom. Physiol. Opt., 63, 403–408

Williams, L. and Holden, B. A. (1986) The bleb response of the endothelium decreases with extended wear of contact lenses. Clin. Exp. Optom., 69, 90–92

Woods, C. A. and Efron, N. (1996) Regular replacement of daily-wear rigid gas-permeable contact lenses. J. Br. Contact Lens Assoc., 19, 83–90

Chapter 18

Medical aspects of contact lenses, diagnosis and treatment

Lalitha C. M. Moodaley

CHAPTER CONTENTS

INTRODUCTION

Contact lens-related disease accounts for between 3 and 10% of all new ophthalmic Accident and Emergency patients in London (Dart 1993). However, since the 1990s, the spectrum of contact lens-related complications has changed significantly due to:

- Improvements in the physiological performance of new-generation contact lens materials.
- Improved manufacturing techniques.
- The withdrawal of thimerosal from contact lens care products.
- The complete elimination of care products and cases for some patients, with the advent of daily disposable lenses and the greater use of disposable cases.
- Better patient education.

As a result, many complications, such as thimerosal keratopathy (Wilson-Holt & Dart 1989), corneal warpage syndrome, deep stromal opacification (Remeijer et al. 1990) and tight lens syndrome are now rarely seen. However, microbial keratitis remains the main sight-threatening complication of contact lens wear and its incidence remains unchanged. The Addendum on pp. 419–422 (adapted from Dart 1993) summarizes the spectrum of complications seen before 1993.

This chapter reviews the serious, together with the most prevalent, medical complications of contact lens wear.

EFFECTS OF CONTACT LENS WEAR

Contact lens wear has physiological, metabolic and anatomical effects on the eye.

Liesegang (2002) described the main physiological effects from hypoxia and hypercapnia as:

- Decreased metabolic rate.
- Reduced sensation.
- Altered epithelial morphology, fragility and integrity.
- Neovascularization and pannus formation.
- Corneal thinning.
- Endothelial polymegethism and bleb formation.

The high oxygen permeability of silicone hydrogel lens materials should significantly reduce some of these effects.

Anatomical effects include altered blinking and tear resurfacing, which in turn can lead to increased evaporation of tears and alteration of the lipid layer. The accumulation of deposits on the contact lens surface makes it biologically active and can

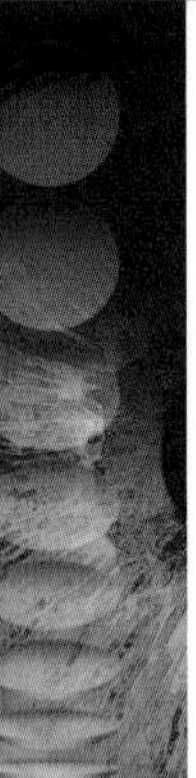

provoke an immunological response in the tarsal conjunctiva; for example, contact lens-induced papillary conjunctivitis (CLPC), similar to that seen in ocular allergic conditions such as vernal keratoconjunctivitis (VKC), perennial allergic conjunctivitis (PAC) and atopic keratoconjunctivitis (AKC) (Henriquez et al. 1981).

Contact lens wear can unmask underlying asymptomatic external disease (e.g. blepharitis and poor tear film) or be confused with, and delay the diagnosis of, active external eye disease such as marginal keratitis, conjunctivitis and Thygeson's keratitis. It is important, therefore, to be able to distinguish the two since contact lens-related disease and external disease may co-exist.

Many contact lens-related problems are reversible and symptoms should resolve soon after discontinuing lens wear, although signs may remain for weeks. Drops and contact lens solutions can cause physiological effects and toxic and allergic reactions. They can occasionally have metabolic effects but do not have anatomical effects.

HISTORY AND EXAMINATION

Establishing a diagnosis requires a detailed history and careful examination (see also Chapter 17). History taking should include:

- A brief medical history.
- Details of any systemic medication and allergies.
- A detailed contact lens history including
  - total duration of lens wear.
  - types of contact lens used.
  - average daily wearing time.
  - lens age.
  - daily hygiene routine.
  - care system used.
  - any topical medications, including over-the-counter preparations.

Examination should include:

- Observation of the skin, adnexae and ocular environment.
- Slit-lamp examination of the eye.
- Examination of the contact lens, lens case and care products, if available.

MICROBIAL KERATITIS

Between 80 and 100 million people worldwide wear contact lenses. There are approximately 30 million contact lens wearers in the USA and 3–4 million in the UK. Incidence figures suggest there are 1500–1800 cases of contact lens-related keratitis in the UK per year. Of these, 10% will lose vision (Poggio et al. 1989, Dart 1999). This makes contact lens wear the major cause of corneal infection in otherwise healthy eyes in developed populations with a high penetrance of contact lens wear (Bourcier et al. 2003).

Various studies (Schein et al. 1989a, Cheng et al. 1999) have calculated the relative risk of different types of contact lens use, and have shown that:

- Daily wear rigid gas-permeable (RGP) lenses carry the least risk.
- Daily wear soft lenses increase the risk nearly four-fold.
- Conventional soft lens extended-wear increases the risk 20-fold.

Fifty percent of cases of contact lens-related keratitis used to occur in conventional soft lens extended wear, although extended wear represented only 10% of total contact lens use. Extended wear, therefore, came to be regarded as unsafe.

Daily disposable lenses eliminate the need for care products and storage cases (and hence biofilm (see Chapter 4)) and silicone hydrogel lenses provide increased oxygen. Little relative or absolute risk data are currently available to show if these developments have reduced the incidence and relative risk of microbial keratitis (MK) for these modes of contact lens wear, although studies are underway. Pilot epidemiological estimates predict a decrease in risk rates for silicone hydrogels (Edmunds et al. 2001). The Silicone Hydrogels website (www.siliconehydrogels.org) gives ongoing global data on reported cases of microbial keratitis with these lenses.

MECHANISM

The mechanism by which corneal infection develops is complex; it requires both the presence of microbes and the increased susceptibility of the cornea to infection as a result of contact lens wear (Fleiszig & Evans 2003).

Microbes are present in the biofilm, which builds up in contact lens storage cases, and on the contact lens itself with wear (McLaughlin-Borlace et al. 1998). Microbes are present in contaminated environments including:

- Patients' skin and hands (e.g. *Staphylococcus*).
- Water supplies and pool water (e.g. *Acanthamoeba*).
- Used care products and contact lens cases (e.g. *Pseudomonas, Acanthamoeba*).

Contact lens disinfection systems are not as effective against organisms protected in biofilm as with free-living organisms against which care systems are tested. Contact lens wear probably reduces the resistance of the cornea to infection through microtrauma and hypoxia, compromising corneal epithelial integrity. Microbes adherent to the contact lens prolong their exposure to the cornea and reduce their clearance with blinking, giving organisms more time to invade the compromised cornea.

SYMPTOMS AND SIGNS

MK should be suspected in a contact lens wearer complaining of:

- Rapid-onset pain.
- Redness.
- Discharge.
- Photophobia.

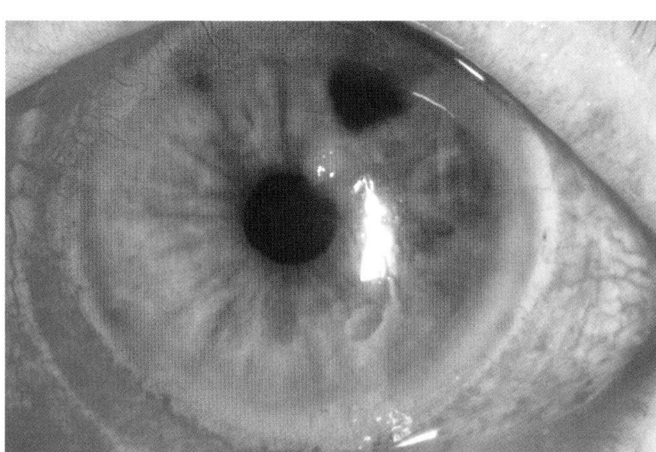

Figure 18.1 Early microbial keratitis

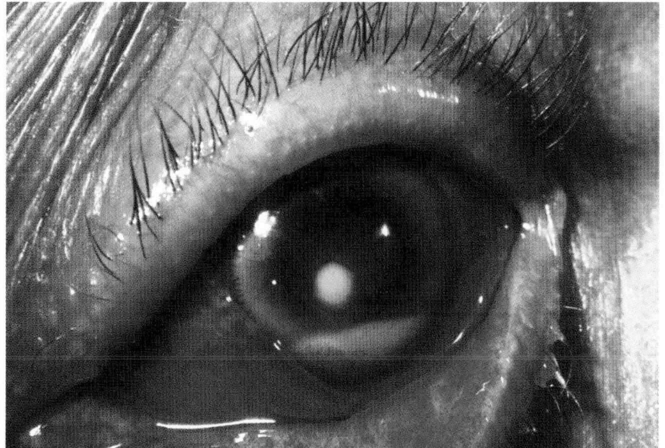

Figure 18.2 Hypopyon ulcer

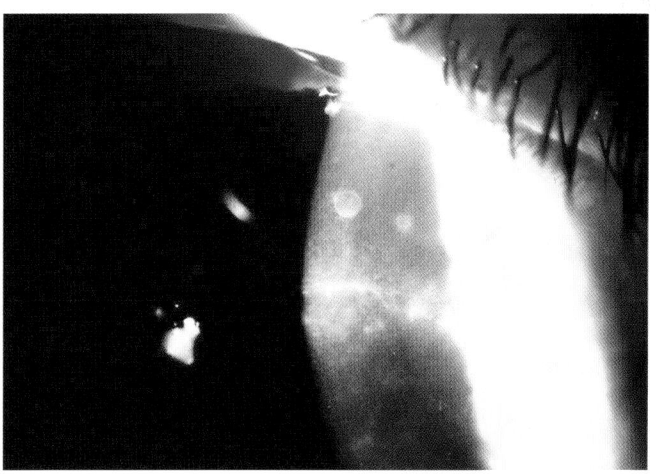

Figure 18.3 *Acanthamoeba* keratitis mimicking herpes simplex keratitis

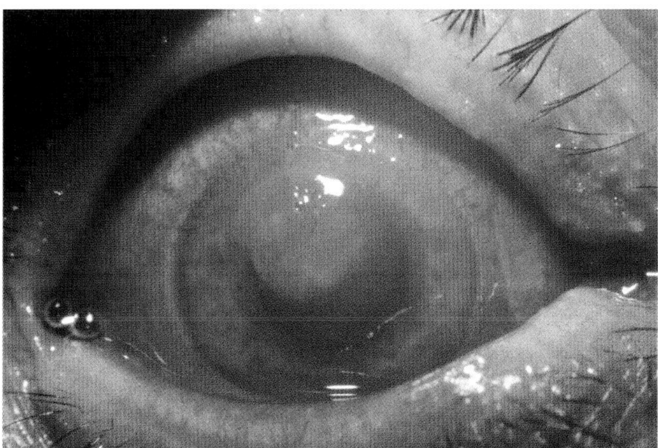

Figure 18.4 *Pseudomonas* ulcer

Slit-lamp examination reveals:

- An epithelial defect or ulcer – usually central but possibly peripheral (Bennett et al. 1998).
- Stromal infiltrates.
- Ciliary injection (Fig. 18.1).

This can rapidly progress to a hypopyon ulcer with virulent organisms such as *Pseudomonas aeruginosa* (Fig. 18.2).

Atypical keratitis (often mimicking herpes simplex keratitis) and the presence of perineural infiltrates (radial keratoneuritis) suggest *Acanthamoeba* infection (Fig. 18.3).

MANAGEMENT

The patient should be referred urgently for corneal scrapes and cultures before commencing broad-spectrum antimicrobial treatment selected on the basis of history and clinical features while awaiting the laboratory results. Treatment can then be modified accordingly. The contact lens and case should also be cultured (Martins et al. 2002) and patients informed that their lenses and case cannot then be returned. Some centres take an epithelial biopsy, which is sent for culture and histology.

ORGANISMS (see also Chapter 4)

Contact lens-related keratitis is usually caused by the following in order of incidence:

- *Pseudomonas aeruginosa*, a ubiquitous Gram-negative organism (Fig. 18.4).
- *Staphylococcus* spp. (Gram-positive).
- Other Gram-negative organisms (*Serratia* spp., *Proteus* spp., *Pseudomonas* spp.).
- *Acanthamoeba* (Galentine et al. 1984, Schein et al. 1989b).
- Fungi.

Organisms may also co-exist (e.g. *Acanthamoeba* with bacteria). It is not yet clear whether the spectrum of causative organisms will alter with the new lens types.

TREATMENT

Once samples have been taken, treatment should be commenced with a broad-spectrum topical antimicrobial active against Gram-negative organisms as this is the most likely pathogen. Broad-spectrum quinolones are:

- Ofloxacin.
- Ciprofloxacin.

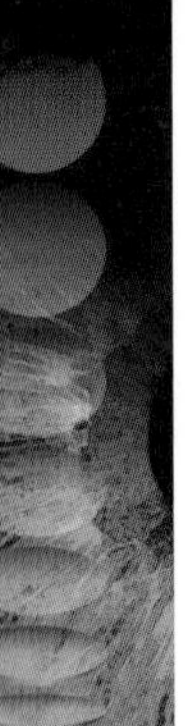

These are less toxic than gentamicin. It is important to achieve adequate dosage by treating intensively (1–2 hourly day and night) at the onset. Treatment can then be modified according to microbiological sensitivities. Topical steroids may also be required to control the inflammatory response and limit tissue damage (Allan & Dart 1995).

Acanthamoeba keratitis

Acanthamoeba keratitis is more common in the UK than elsewhere, with an incidence of 17.5 cases per million contact lens wearers; in the USA it is only 2 per million contact lens wearers. This is thought to be due to the use of stored water in UK household plumbing systems, leading to the contamination of the water supply to the bathroom (Seal et al. 1992, Radford et al. 2002, Kilvington et al. 2004) and a high rate of *Acanthamoeba* in tap cultures. Studies of the 1993 UK epidemic showed that poor contact lens hygiene and the use of ineffective chlorine-based contact lens disinfection systems played a major role in this outbreak (Radford et al. 1995).

Acanthamoeba is a family of cyst-forming protozoans that are free-living in air, soil and water. In its cystic form it is very resistant to contact lens disinfection solutions and Silvany et al. (1990) recommended that lenses be soaked in hydrogen peroxide 3% for at least 3 hours for effective disinfection against amoebae.

Contamination of lens cases is present in up to 10% of asymptomatic users (Larkin et al. 1990). Other risk factors include swimming in lenses, the use of homemade saline and poor hygiene with disposable contact lenses (Butler et al. 2005).

CLINICAL FEATURES

Acanthamoeba keratitis is often characterized by severe pain and photophobia. Early features of the disease include:

- Punctate keratitis.
- Pseudodendrites (often mimicking herpes simplex keratitis).
- Epithelial and subepithelial infiltrates.
- Perineural infiltrates which are pathognomonic for the condition (Bacon et al. 1993).

Late disease is characterized by:

- Ring-shaped infiltrates (Fig. 18.5).
- Corneal ulceration.
- Possible scleritis and rarely choreoretinitis.

TREATMENT

Early diagnosis is important as these cases respond well to medical therapy (Radford et al. 1998). Late disease is much more difficult to treat (Perez-Santonja et al. 2003) and may ultimately require a corneal transplant. Appropriate treatment is often delayed because the condition is misdiagnosed as herpes simplex keratitis or fungal keratitis (Auran et al. 1987).

To be effective against *Acanthamoeba*, drugs should have cysticidal activity as this is the form the organism adopts in chronic disease. Commonly used topical antiamoebic drugs include:

- Propramidine (Brolene).
- Hexamidine (Desomedine).

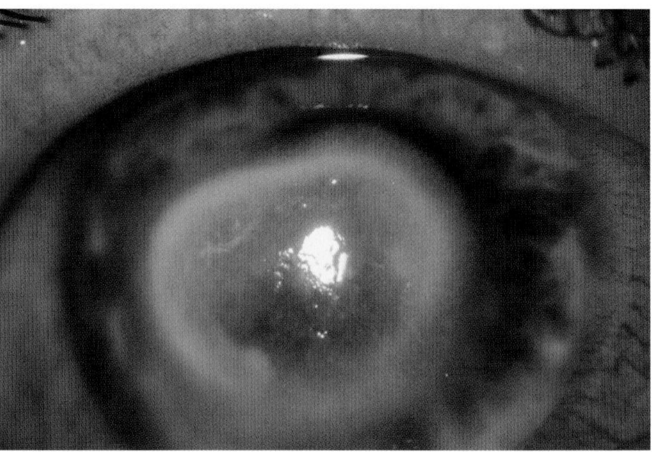

Figure 18.5 Ring-shaped infiltrate seen in late-stage *Acanthamoeba.* (Courtesy of S. Tuft)

- Polyhexamethyl biguanide (PHMB) – limited availability.
- Chlorhexidine.
- Neomycin.

Propamidine- and hexamidine-resistant strains are reported and neomycin has no effect on cysts. Resistance can develop during treatment but PHMB and chlorhexidine are currently the drugs of choice as they show almost no resistance. Propamidine and neomycin are toxic and may cause corneal ulceration with prolonged use.

Topical steroids may be required to control the inflammatory response; however, their use should be delayed until adequate antiamoebic treatment has been given (1–2 weeks). Although pain often responds well to oral non-steroidal anti-inflammatories (e.g. flurbiprofen), oral steroids and cyclosporin may be needed to control scleritis.

Overall, this is a difficult condition to treat. Treatment for months to years may be required and, if medical treatment fails, all affected tissue should be excised.

Fungal keratitis

Fungal keratitis is a major cause of blinding disease in tropical and subtropical climates. In temperate climates such as the UK and North America the incidence is low. However, contact lens wearers may travel to countries where it is common and where conditions for good contact lens hygiene are less than optimal.

Although trauma is the major risk factor (Srinivasan 2004), contact lens wear has also been identified as a risk and it must be considered in the differential diagnosis of fungal keratitis, particularly in those returning from high-risk areas.

Minimizing the risks of microbial keratitis

From the evidence discussed, it is clear that in order to reduce the risk of MK, patients should be advised to:

- Wash hands before handling contact lenses.
- Never use untreated or stored tap water or home-made saline solutions.

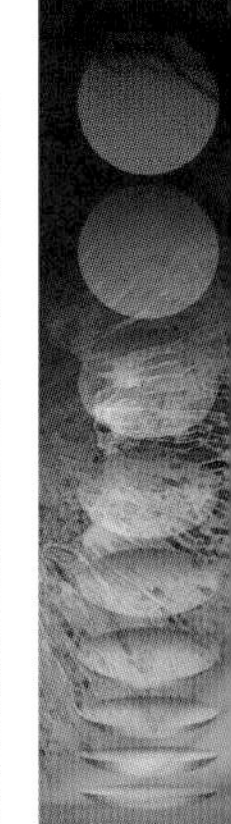

- Clean the lens case and change it regularly.
- Check that care products are in date and discarded after the recommended time after opening.
- Never swim in contact lenses.
- Avoid unplanned overnight wear and over-wear.
- Always disinfect lenses before re-wearing.

Wearers should be advised that even if they comply with all recommendations, there is still an increased risk of contact lens-related infection with continued lens wear.

RESUMING LENS WEAR

An obvious precipitating event resulting in keratitis – such as trauma, poor hygiene or unplanned overnight wear – can be avoided. However, in the absence of any obvious precipitating cause, the relative risk of a new infection remains the same. The risk can be reduced by switching to a mode of lens wear with less relative risk (e.g. soft-lens wear to RGP lens wear).

CONTACT LENS-INDUCED PERIPHERAL ULCER OR STERILE KERATITIS

Incidence figures for contact lens-induced peripheral ulcer (CLPU) vary greatly, ranging from zero to 41% of study populations (Robboy et al. 2003). CLPU is most often seen in soft contact lens wearers. It is non-progressive and usually spontaneously resolves on discontinuing contact lens wear.

Patients may be asymptomatic but more commonly experience:

- Slight discomfort.
- Mild focal hyperaemia.
- Photophobia and minimal discharge.

Slit-lamp signs include:

- Peripheral nummular or linear infiltrates, usually without epithelial ulceration although this may occur in late lesions.
- The lesions are usually small (<1 mm) and may be multiple.
- Old, quiet lesions may be evident.
- Anterior chamber activity is rare.

It is uncommon to culture organisms from these lesions, hence the term 'sterile'; however, inflammatory cells are present. These lesions probably represent an inflammatory hypersensitivity response to a variety of stimuli including:

- Preservatives.
- Bacteria (usually staphylococci).
- Bacterial products.
- Contact lens deposits.

Histologically, Bowman's layer remains intact whereas it is breached in MK (Holden et al. 1997).

DIFFERENTIAL DIAGNOSIS

Distinguishing between early MK and CLPU can be difficult as they may present with similar symptoms. In MK, symptoms are more acute, and lesions are more likely to be central and larger with associated anterior chamber activity, but this is by no means always the case (Fig. 18.6). Scoring systems have been proposed to aid differentiation (Aasuri et al. 2003).

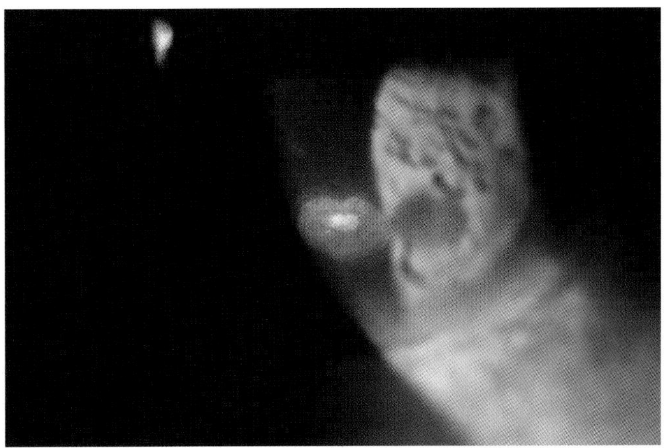

Figure 18.6 Microbial keratitis or contact lens-induced peripheral ulcer? Nocardia keratitis (culture positive)

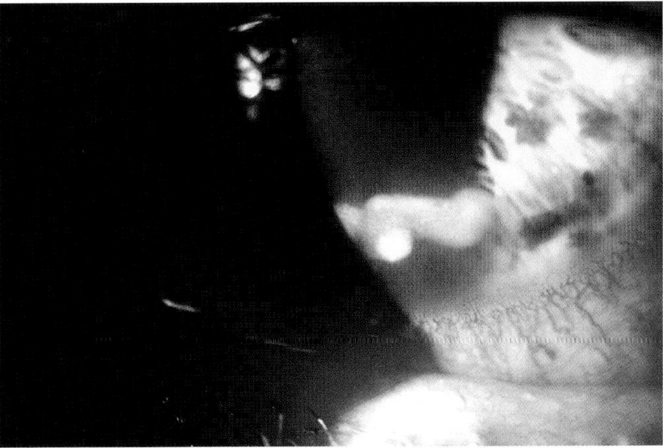

Figure 18.7 Marginal keratitis (culture negative)

Similar lesions may be seen in marginal keratitis (Fig. 18.7), herpes simplex keratitis, viral keratoconjunctivitis, chlamydial conjunctivitis and Thygeson's keratitis.

NEOVASCULARIZATION

Contact lens-induced corneal neovascularization is significant because it can lead to lipid keratopathy (see p. 414) and haemorrhage, which can cause loss of vision. In addition, the presence of corneal vessels may compromise the success of corneal surgery (e.g. corneal transplantation) by increasing the risk of rejection, suture loosening and infection.

AETIOLOGY

The stimulus for neovascularization is hypoxia resulting in the release of vasogenic mediators, which in turn stimulate the growth of superficial and deep vessels into the cornea to provide it with oxygen (Chang et al. 2001). These new vessels

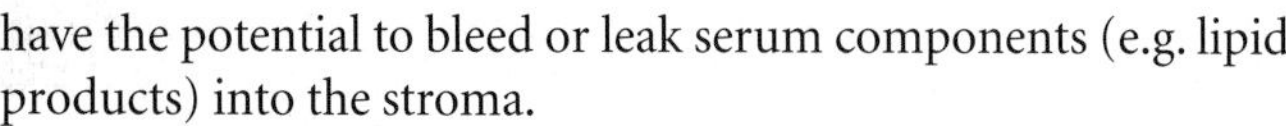

have the potential to bleed or leak serum components (e.g. lipid products) into the stroma.

CLINICAL FEATURES

Neovascularization is more commonly seen in soft contact lens wearers, particularly in extended wear with conventional hydrogel lenses, but can also occur in RGP wearers where the contact lens fit is occlusive. It is asymptomatic unless there is lipid keratopathy, haemorrhage or oedema affecting the visual axis, and highlights the need for regular after-care visits.

It is common to see up to 1 mm of limbal neovascularization in long-term soft contact lens wearers. These vessels are looped and self-limiting, i.e. they do not extend over time and require no change of management.

In contrast, active new vessels are branched and extend over time. They may leak serum components or blood into the stroma. Active neovascularization can arise and extend rapidly, even between 6-monthly after-care visits, or creep in gradually, depending on the degree of hypoxic stimulus.

TREATMENT

Treatment is aimed at improving corneal oxygenation causing the vessels to empty and become ghost vessels, which remain visible under slit-lamp examination. This can be achieved in a number of ways.

- Discontinue contact lens wear.
- Reduce contact lens wearing time.
- Refit hydrogel lenses with silicone hydrogel.
- Refit RGP instead of soft lens.
- Improve the fit of RGP lenses to improve tear exchange.

It should be noted that ghost vessels can easily refill in the presence of hypoxia.

LIPID KERATOPATHY

Lipid keratopathy should be considered irreversible. However, once the cause of neovascularization has been addressed and corneal oxygenation improved, the stromal oedema surrounding the vessels resolves, often giving the impression that the extent of lipid keratopathy has reduced.

Monitored use of topical corticosteroids such as fluorometholone (FML) and prednisolone 0.5% (Predsol) will aid in shutting down feeder vessels. Feeder vessels can also be treated with limbal argon laser treatment (Mendelsohn et al. 1986, Marsh 1988) or photodynamic therapy (Epstein et al. 1991, Primbs et al. 1998), providing the vessels are not too numerous. As a precaution, patients should have their serum, lipid and cholesterol levels checked to exclude hypercholesterolaemia. If visual acuity is significantly reduced, patients may require corneal surgery.

Case report 1

Lipid keratopathy in a patient with a 4-year history of daily wear soft lens use with extended wearing time and failed after-care visits. Figure 18.8 shows the corneal appearance 6 months after discontinuing contact lens wear: visual acuity 6/9 with spectacles and normal blood lipid profile.

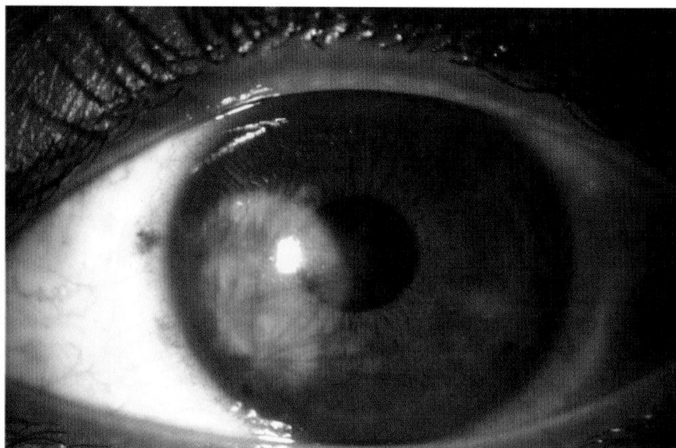

Figure 18.8 Lipid keratopathy in soft contact lens wear

Case report 2

Lipid keratopathy in a patient with keratoconus wearing RGP lenses with long daily wearing time and poor after-care attendance (Fig. 18.9).

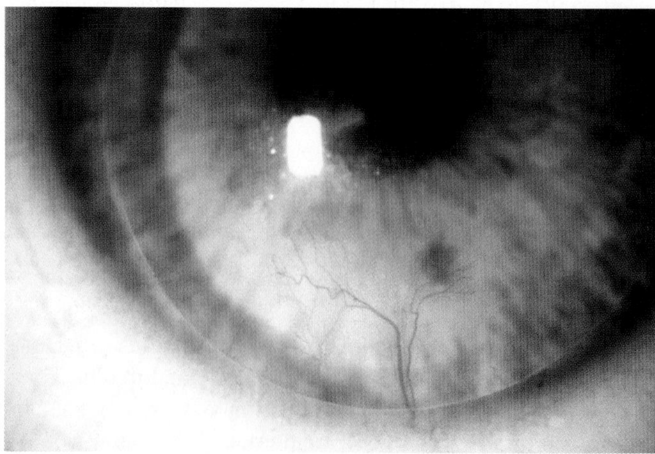

Figure 18.9 Lipid keratopathy in RGP lens wear

The patient presented with blurred vision (6/18) due to stromal oedema and lipid in the visual axis. The contact lens fit was immobile with a stagnant tear pool over the inferior cornea. As the patient was unable to discontinue lens wear, the lens was refitted with increased tear exchange, the Dk and wear time remaining the same. The oedema resolved and vessels regressed leaving the lipid. The visual acuity returned to 6/9. The blood lipid profile was normal.

CONTACT LENS-INDUCED PAPILLARY CONJUNCTIVITIS

Contact lens-induced papillary conjunctivitis (CLPC) or giant papillary conjunctivitis (GPC), first described as a contact lens-related complication by Spring (1974), is found with all lens types including silicone hydrogels (Yeniad et al. 2004). It is commonest in reusable soft contact lens wear (85%), with 15% in RGP wear (Donshik 2003). CLPC may develop after years of successful contact lens wear and is often markedly asymmetric (10%) (Donshik 2003). Symptoms usually precede signs and there is a poor correlation between the two.

SYMPTOMS

These include:

- Excess mucus production (white, stringy, elastic mucus).
- Itching, often worse after contact lens removal.
- Reduced contact lens tolerance due to increased contact lens movement, the deposited lens being dragged around by the lid.
- Blurred vision due to mucus deposition on the lens.

SIGNS

The bulbar conjunctiva usually remains white and the cornea clear, with the signs only apparent on everting the upper lid. The stages of CLPC are:

- Upper tarsal hyperaemia, with a fine papillary response.
- Macropapillae (0.3–1 mm diameter).
- Giant papillae (>1 mm diameter) with oedema and excess mucus building up in the papillary crypts (Fig. 18.10; see also Appendix B).
- Fibrosis at the papillary tips.

Even once the reaction is subsiding or inactive, evidence of the papillae and fibrosis persist; however, the hyperaemia, oedema and mucus production resolve. Eventually the papillae may flatten out.

AETIOLOGY

This is multifactorial, being a combination of an immune response (immediate Type 1 hypersensitivity and delayed Type 4 hypersensitivity) to antigenic proteins on the contact lens surface and mechanical effects of the lens edge and surface, causing trauma to the conjunctiva (Donshik 1994).

Bearing in mind the aetiology, the incidence of GPC is increased in atopic lens wearers. It is useful to diagnose any pre-existing allergic eye disease in patients before they embark on contact lens wear to clarify the aetiology.

Giant papillae are also seen in vernal keratoconjunctivitis (VKC) in the absence of contact lens wear, in ocular prosthetic wear, and resulting from protruding sutures.

TREATMENT

Treatment is aimed at eliminating the allergen and controlling the host response. The reaction will subside on discontinuing contact lens wear; however, in order that successful contact lens wear may continue, most cases will respond well to improved contact lens hygiene and lens condition (Donshik 2003) without the need for topical medication.

General treatment options are:

- Improve contact lens hygiene with more vigorous daily cleaning and regular enzymatic protein removal.
- Replace/polish damaged or scratched lenses.
- Improve RGP design (e.g. less edge clearance).
- Change to a more deposit-resistant material.
- Change from soft to RGP lenses (decreases deposition).
- Change from soft reusable to daily disposable lenses (decreases antigenic load).
- Reduce contact lens wear time (decreases contact time).

If the reaction persists and contact lens wear cannot be discontinued (e.g. in atopic keratoconus patients) then topical treatment is indicated.

Topical treatment options include:

- Mast cell stabilizers (e.g. sodium cromoglicate, nedocromil sodium, lodoxamide).
- Antihistamine and mast cell stabilizers (e.g. olopatadine, ketotifen).
- Mucolytic agents (e.g. acetylcysteine).
- Non-steroidal anti-inflammatory agents (e.g. diclofenac sodium, ketorolac, trometamol).
- Corticosteroids – the use of which must be monitored (e.g. prednisolone, fluorometholone).

It is also important to treat any associated lid margin disease (see below).

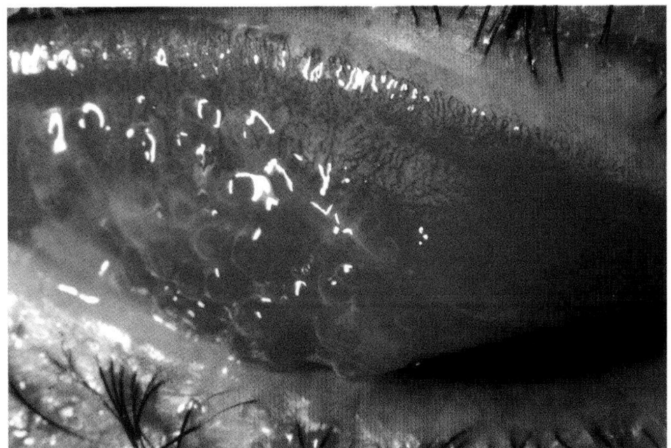

Figure 18.10 Active contact lens-associated papillary conjunctivitis

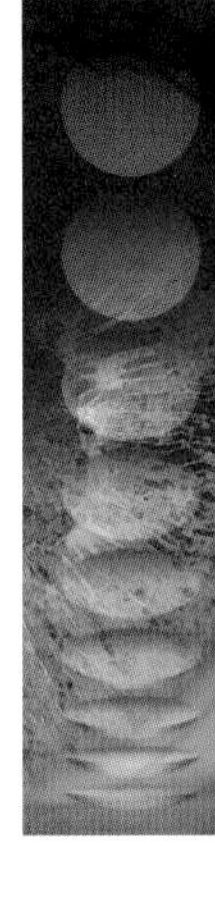

DIFFERENTIAL DIAGNOSIS

This includes:

- Superior limbic keratitis.
- Seasonal and perennial allergic conjunctivitis.
- Vernal keratoconjunctivitis.
- Atopic keratoconjunctivitis.

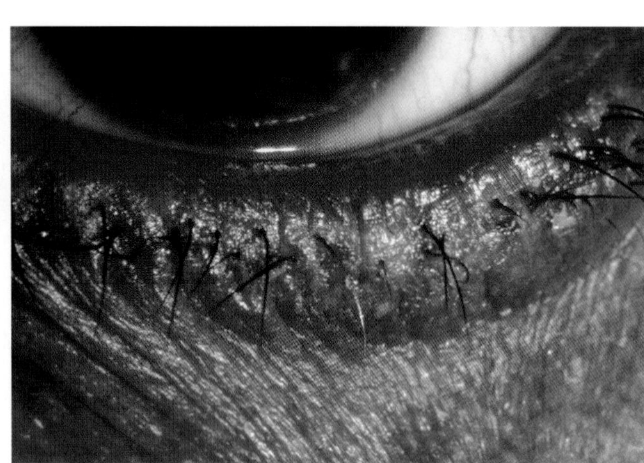

Figure 18.11 Blepharitis or lid margin disease with peripheral corneal opacification

LID MARGIN DISEASE (BLEPHARITIS) AND THE DRY EYE

Blepharitis

Blepharitis is a blanket term for inflammation affecting the lid margin. Associated skin and eye diseases include:

- Atopic eczema.
- Atopic keratoconjunctivitis.
- Conjunctivitis.
- Impetigo.
- Seborrhoea and acne rosacea. Ocular rosacea may occur in the absence of skin disease.

Blepharitis or lid margin disease (Fig. 18.11) is common in both general and ophthalmic practice, accounting for 1–5% of all consultations in general medical practice. It is the most common (approximately one-third) presenting complaint to ophthalmic Accident and Emergency Departments. It is also a common cause of contact lens intolerance due to its effect on the lid margin and tear film.

Contact lens wear often exacerbates symptoms and may unmask underlying asymptomatic blepharitis. It is not a contraindication to contact lens wear, although it should be controlled before contact lens wear is initiated, and lens wear should be halted temporarily if blepharitis becomes symptomatic. It usually responds well to treatment, allowing successful resumption of contact lens wear.

CLINICAL FEATURES

The main symptoms are itchy, burning eyes with foreign body sensation and photophobia. Patients may complain that the lids feel stuck together in the mornings and lens wearers also complain of:

- Loss of tolerance due to discomfort.
- Unstable visual acuity.
- Increased lens deposition due to effects on the tear film and corneal surface.

Chronic blepharitis can be classified into anterior lid margin disease (affecting lash-bearing skin) and posterior lid margin disease (affecting the mucocutaneous junction and meibomian glands) (McCulley et al. 1982). The two often coexist.

Features of lid margin disease are:

- Anterior (all or part of the lid margin may be involved)
  - brittle, fibrinous scales around lash bases forming collarettes.
  - dilated vessels.
  - styes, poliosis and madarosis.
- Posterior
  - distortion and notching of the lid margins.
  - distorted meibomian orifices.
  - meibomitis.
  - thick, 'toothpasty' meibomian secretions.
  - chalazia.
  - lid margin telangiectasia.

The conjunctiva may exhibit a mixed follicular and papillary response, with hyperaemia.

The cornea may exhibit:

- Coarse punctate staining, particularly of the lower third.
- Peripheral corneal ulceration with infiltrate (as in marginal keratitis).
- Scattered epithelial and subepithelial opacities (as in staphylococcal hypersensitivity) (see Fig. 18.11).
- Neovascularization.

Severe and chronic cases can lead to cicatrization.

Effects on the tear film include:

- Rapid break-up time.
- Reduction in the tear meniscus.
- Foam and debris.

AETIOLOGY

Anterior lid margin disease is usually caused by staphylococcal colonization. The associated keratitis is thought to be due to a combination of transient infection and hypersensitivity.

Posterior lid margin disease, or meibomian gland disease, is due to abnormalities in the production of meibum, the effects of bacterial lipases on the meibomian secretion at the lid margin and keratinization of meibomian ductules (Driver & Lemp 1996). The interaction between bacteria, the various lipid components in the tear film, the aqueous layer and the presence of a contact lens is complex (McCulley & Shine 2003).

MANAGEMENT

Investigations are of limited value in this condition.

TREATMENT

Anterior lid margin disease

- Regular lid hygiene to remove debris and scales from the lash bases.
- Staphylococcal colonization is treated with topical antibiotic (e.g. chloramphenicol, fusidic acid) applied to the lid margin and, in more severe cases, systemic antibiotic for 2 weeks.

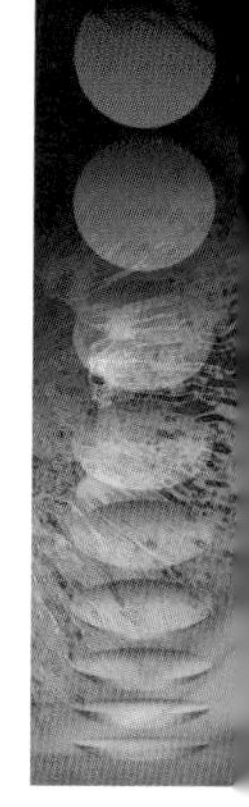

- Ulcerative blepharitis may require topical steroid (e.g. hydrocortisone) to the lid margins.

Posterior lid margin disease (Romero et al. 2004)

- Hot compress treatment to the lids for 5 minutes each day using a clean hot flannel in order to liquefy meibomian secretions (Olson et al. 2003), followed by
- Lid massage along the tarsal plate (upwards on the lower lid and downwards on the upper lid) to express the meibomian glands.
- Artificial tear supplements for symptomatic relief, particularly in contact lens wearers.
- Low-dose, long-term systemic antibiotic treatment (e.g. doxycycline, minocycline) will improve meibomian gland function and also the nature of the secretions, making them more fluid.

These treatments work slowly and may take 4–6 weeks to show an effect. Treatment should be continued for at least 2 months and often longer to achieve improvement in the tear film.

Marginal ulceration and staphylococcal hypersensitivity reactions respond well to treatment with a combination of topical corticosteroid (e.g. prednisolone 0.5%) and topical antibiotic (e.g. chloramphenicol, ofloxacin).

Dry eye

The diagnosis of 'dry eye' (see also Chapter 5) as a cause of contact lens intolerance is common. It is well recognized that an adequate, good-quality, stable tear film is important for successful contact lens wear and that lens wear increases tear evaporation (Foulks 2003). Primary dry eye from intrinsic tear pathology is rare. It is far more common for there to be a generally poor-quality tear film secondary to underlying external disease (e.g. blepharitis or allergic eye disease) or lagophthalmos (Bielory 2004). In a few contact lens-wearing patients 'dry eye' may be due to aqueous tear deficiency or indicate underlying systemic autoimmune disease such as diabetes, thyroid disease, Sjögren's syndrome, systemic lupus erythematosus and rheumatoid disease.

Once the underlying condition is diagnosed and treated, there is often improvement in the tear film, although this is not always the case and additional treatment may be required. Appropriate management requires an understanding of the nature of the tear deficiency.

DEFINITION AND CLASSIFICATION

'Dry eye' is defined as a disorder of the tear film caused either by tear deficiency or excessive tear evaporation that causes damage to the interpalpebral ocular surface. It is associated with symptoms of discomfort (Lemp 1995, Bron 2001).

- Aqueous tear deficiency is subdivided into:
  - Sjögren's syndrome-related.
  - Non-Sjögren's syndrome.
- Evaporative dry eye is subdivided into:
  - Lipid deficiency.
  - Pathologic eyelid and blinking conditions.
  - Contact lens wear.
  - Ocular surface abnormalities.

The aqueous-deficient dry eye is most often associated with reduced tear production and the evaporative dry eye with meibomian gland disease, the two types often occurring together.

Normal ocular surface sensation is important for the neural control of lacrimal secretion and the integrity of the ocular surface. Long-term contact lens wear can reduce corneal sensitivity.

Inflammation of the lacrimal tissue, ocular surface or lid margin, and the presence of inflammatory mediators in the tear film will suppress the secretion of certain components of the tear film, often leading to ocular surface damage. Control of inflammation is therefore essential in the management of dry eye. A poor tear film increases the risk of infection due to the reduction in bacteriostatic and protective proteins found in tears.

MANAGEMENT

Identify and treat the underlying cause! In contact lens wear, this is frequently a poor tear film due to meibomian gland disease (Korb & Henriquez 1980).

If symptoms persist after treatment, a number of options are available including:

- Artificial tear supplements (unpreserved if applied more than four times per day).
- Mucolytic agents.
- Topical anti-inflammatory agents (steroidal and non-steroidal).
- Tear conservation (protective spectacles; in severe cases, temporary or permanent punctal occlusion – see Chapters 5 and 17).
- Change to a less tear-dependent lens (i.e. reduce water content, change from soft to RGP).

Improving tear *quantity* may not improve symptoms if tear *quality* remains poor or if there is untreated inflammation or infection.

Acknowledgement

I would like to thank to Mr John Dart and Dr Elizabeth Millis for their help in the preparation of this chapter.

References

Aasuri, M. K., Venkata, N. and Kumar, V. M. (2003) Differential diagnosis of microbial keratitis and contact lens-induced peripheral ulcer. Eye Contact Lens, 29(1S), S60–S62

Allan, B. D. and Dart, J. K. (1995) Strategies for the management of microbial keratitis. Br. J. Ophthalmol., 79(8), 777–786

Auran, J. D., Starr, M. B. and Jakobiec, F. A. (1987) Acanthamoeba keratitis: a review of the literature. Cornea, 6, 2–26

Bacon, A. S., Dart, J. K. G., Ficker, L. A. et al. (1993) Acanthamoeba keratitis: the value of early diagnosis. Ophthalmology, 100(8), 1238–1243

Bennett, H. G. B., Hay, J., Kirkness, C. M. et al. (1998) Antimicrobial management of presumed microbial keratitis: guidelines for treatment of central and peripheral ulcers. Br. J. Ophthalmol., 82(2), 137–145

Bielory, L. (2004) Ocular allergy and dry eye syndrome. Curr. Opin. Allergy Clin. Immunol., 4(5), 421–424

Bourcier, T., Thomas, F., Borderie, V. et al. (2003) Bacterial keratitis: predisposing factors, clinical and microbiological review of 300 cases. Br. J. Ophthalmol., 87(7), 834–838

Bron, A. J. (2001) Diagnosis of dry eye. Surv. Ophthalmol., 45, S221–S226

Butler, T. K. H., Males, J. J., Robinson, L. P. et al. (2005) Six-year review of Acanthamoeba keratitis in New South Wales, Australia: 1997–2002. Clin. Exp. Ophthalmol., 33, 41–46

Chang, J-H., Gabison, E. E., Kato, K. et al. (2001) Corneal neovascularization. Curr. Opin. Ophthalmol., 12(4), 242–249

Cheng, K. H., Leung, S. L., Hoekman, H. W. et al. (1999) Incidence of contact-lens-associated microbial keratitis and its related morbidity. Lancet 254(9174), 181–185

Dart, J. (1993) The epidemiology of contact lens related disease in the United Kingdom: a review. J. Contact Lens Assoc. Ophthalmol., 19(4), 241–246

Dart, J. (1999) Extended-wear contact lenses, microbial keratitis, and public health. Lancet 254(9174), 174–175

Donshik, P. C. (1994) Giant papillary conjunctivitis. Trans. Am. Ophthalmol. Soc., 92, 687–744

Donshik, P. C. (2003) Contact lens chemistry and giant papillary conjunctivitis. Eye Contact Lens: Sci. Clin. Pract., 29(1)(Suppl 1), S37–S39

Driver, P. J. and Lemp, M. A. (1996) Meibomian gland dysfunction. Surv. Ophthalmol., 40, 343–367

Edmunds, F., Comstock, T., Crescuillo, T. et al. (2001) Cumulative experience of extended wear clinical trials of a silicone hydrogel contact lens. Optom. Vis. Sci., 78, S202

Epstein, R. J., Hendricks, R. L. and Harris, D. M. (1991) Photodynamic therapy for corneal neovascularisation. Cornea, 10, 424–432

Fleiszig, S. M. J. and Evans, D. J. (2003) Contact lens infections: can they ever be eradicated? Eye Contact Lens, 29(1S), S67–S71

Foulks, G. N. (2003) What is dry eye and what does it mean to the contact lens wearer? Eye Contact Lens: Sci. Clin. Pract., 29(1)(Suppl 1), S96–S100

Galentine, P. G., Cohen, E. J., Laibson, P. R. et al. (1984) Corneal ulcers associated with contact lens wear. Arch. Ophthalmol., 102, 891–894

Henriquez, A. S., Kenyon, K. R. and Allansmith, M. R. (1981) Mast cell ultrastructure. Comparison in contact lens associated giant papillary conjunctivitis and vernal conjunctivitis. Arch. Ophthalmol., 99(7), 1266–1272

Holden, B. A., Reddy, M. K., Sankaridurg, P. R. et al. (1997) The histopathology of contact lens induced peripheral corneal ulcer. Invest. Ophthalmol. Vis. Sci., 38, S201

Kilvington, S., Gray, T., Dart, J. et al. (2004) Acanthamoeba keratitis: the role of domestic tap water contamination in the United Kingdom. Invest. Ophthalmol. Vis. Sci., 45(1), 165–169

Korb, D. R. and Henriquez, A. S. (1980) Meibomian gland dysfunction and contact lens intolerance. J. Am. Optom. Assoc., 51, 243–251

Larkin, D. F. P., Kilvington, S. and Easty, D. L. (1990) Contamination of contact lens storage cases by Acanthamoeba and bacteria. Br. J. Ophthalmol., 74, 133–135

Lemp, M. A. (1995) Report of the National Eye Institute/Industry workshop on Clinical Trials in Dry Eyes. J. Contact Lens Assoc. Ophthalmol., 21, 221–232

Liesegang, T. J. (2002) Physiologic changes of the cornea with contact lens wear. J. Contact Lens Assoc. Ophthalmol., 28(1), 12–27

Marsh, R. J. (1988) Argon laser treatment of lipid keratopathy. Br. J. Ophthalmol., 72, 900–904

Martins, E. N., Farah, M. E., Alvarenga, L. S. et al. (2002) Infectious keratitis: correlation between corneal and contact lens cultures. J. Contact Lens Assoc. Ophthalmol., 28(3), 146–148

McCulley, J. P. and Shine, W. E. (2003) Eyelid disorders: the meibomian gland, blepharitis and contact lenses. Eye Contact Lens: Sci. Clin. Pract., 29(1), S93–S95

McCulley, J. P., Dougherty, J. M. and Deneau, D. G. (1982) Classification of chronic blepharitis. Ophthalmology, 89, 1173–1180

McLaughlin-Borlace, L., Stapleton, F., Matheson, M. et al. (1998) Bacterial biofilm on contact lenses and lens storage cases in wearers with microbial keratitis. J. Appl. Microbiol., 84(5), 827–838

Mendelsohn, A. D., Stock, E. L., Lo, G. G. et al. (1986) Laser photocoagulation of feeder vessels in lipid keratopathy. Ophthalmic Surg., 17, 502–508

Olson, M. C., Korb, D. R. and Greiner, J. V. (2003) Increase in tear film lipid layer thickness following treatment with warm compresses in patients with meibomian gland dysfunction. Eye Contact Lens: Sci. Clin. Prac., 29(2), 96–99

Perez-Santonja, J. J., Kilvington, S., Hughes, R. et al. (2003) Persistently culture positive Acanthamoeba keratitis: in vivo resistance and in vitro sensitivity. Ophthalmology, 110(8), 1593–1600

Poggio, E. C., Glynn, R. J., Schein, O. D. et al. (1989) The incidence of ulcerative keratitis among users of daily wear and extended wear soft contact lenses. N. Engl. J. Med., 321(12), 779–783

Primbs, G. B., Casey, R., Wamser, K. et al. (1998) Photodynamic therapy for corneal neovascularisation. Ophthalmic Surg. Lasers, 29, 832–838

Radford, C. F., Bacon, A. S., Dart, J. K. G. and Minassian, D. C. (1995) Risk factors for Acanthamoeba keratitis in contact lens users: a case control study. Br. Med. J., 310(6994), 1567–1570

Radford, C. F., Lehmann, O. J., Dart, J. K. G. for the National Acanthamoeba Keratitis Study Group (1998) Acanthamoeba keratitis: multicentre survey in England 1992–6. Br. J. Ophthalmol., 82(12), 1387–1392

Radford, C. F., Minassian, D. C. and Dart, J. K. (2002) Acanthamoeba keratitis in England and Wales: incidence, outcome and risk factors. Br. J. Ophthalmol., 86(5), 536–542

Remeijer, L., Van Rij, G., Beekhuis, H., Polak, B. and Van Nes, J. (1990) Deep corneal stromal opacities in long term contact lens wear. Ophthalmology, 97, 281–285

Robboy, M. W., Comstock, T. L. and Kalsow, C. M. (2003) Contact lens-associated corneal infiltrates. Eye Contact Lens: Sci. Clin. Pract., 29(3), 146–154

Romero, J. M., Biser, S. A., Perry, H. D. et al. (2004) Conservative treatment of meibomian gland dysfunction. Eye Contact Lens: Sci. Clin. Pract., 30(1), 14–19

Schein, O. D., Glynn, R. J., Poggio, E. C. et al. (1989a) The relative risk of ulcerative keratitis among users of daily wear and extended wear soft contact lenses. N. Engl. J. Med., 321(12), 773–779

Schein, O. D., Ormerod, L. D., Barraquer, E. et al. (1989b) Microbiology of contact lens-related keratitis. Cornea, 8, 281–285

Seal, D., Stapleton, F. and Dart, J. (1992) Possible environmental sources of Acanthamoeba spp. in contact lens wearers. Br. J. Ophthalmol., 76, 424–427

Silvany, R. E., Dougherty, J. M., McCulley, J. P. et al. (1990) The effect of currently available contact lens disinfection systems on Acanthamoeba castellani and Acanthamoeba polyphagia. Ophthalmology, 97, 286–290

Spring, T. F. (1974) Reaction to hydrophilic lenses. Med. J. Aust., 1, 449–450

Srinivasan, M. (2004) Fungal keratitis. Curr. Opin. Ophthalmol., 15(4), 321–327

Wilson-Holt, N. J. and Dart, J. K. (1989) Thiomersal keratoconjunctivitis: frequency, clinical spectrum and diagnosis. Eye, 3, 581–587

Yeniad, B., Seidu Adam, Y., Koser Bilgin, L. et al. (2004) Effect of 30-day continuous wear of silicone hydrogel contact lenses on corneal thickness. Eye Contact Lens: Sci. Clin. Prac., 30(1), 6–9

Further reading

Dart, J. D. (2003) Contact Lens and Prosthesis Infections. Duane's Foundations of Clinical Ophthalmology. Philadelphia, PA: Lippincott Wilkins and Williams

Mackie, I. A. (1993) Medical Contact Lens Practice: A Systematic Approach. Oxford: Butterworth-Heinemann

Millis, E. (2005) Medical Contact Lens Practice. London: Elsevier

Addendum

Classification of contact lens-related disorders

Classification	Disease (synonyms)	Probable aetiology	Symptoms	Corneal signs	Conjunctival signs	Associated lens
Metabolic (hypoxia, hypercapnia & related effects)						
Epithelial	Acute epithelial necrosis (over-wear syndrome)	Epithelial cell necrosis; separation of cells due to hypoxia	Blurred vision due to corneal oedema Delayed pain and epiphora from necrosis Resolves in hours or days if severe	Central punctate epithelial erosions may coalesce into an ulcer Involved area larger in SCL Stromal oedema in severe cases	Ciliary injection	PMMA-RCL and SCL
	Microcystic epitheliopathy	Impaired epithelial metabolic activity	Asymptomatic or minor discomfort	Small erosions during symptomatic episodes Clear or opaque epithelial cysts and punctate keratitis	None	All types
	Superior epithelial arcuate lesions (SEALs)	Multifactorial aetiology, including metabolic and mechanical effects	Often none	Superior arcuate epithelial staining	None	SCL
	Corneal warpage	Metabolic and mechanical factors	Irregular astigmatism: vision good with lenses and poor with spectacles	Irregular keratometry and topography	None	PMMA-RCL commonest
	Epithelial oedema (Sattler's veil)	Hypoxia and tear hypotonicity	Blurred vision after some hours of wear May progress to acute epithelial necrosis	Dull corneal reflex due to epithelial oedema	None	All lens types but more common with PMMA and low-Dk soft and RCL

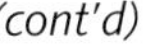
(cont'd)

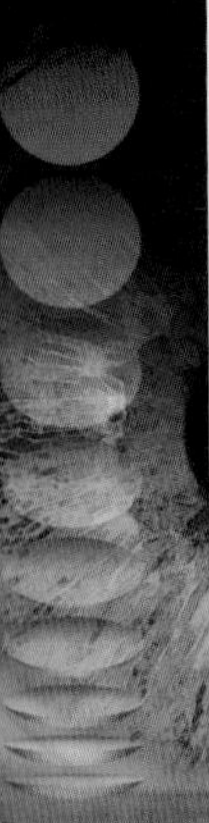

Classification of contact lens-related disorders (*cont'd*)

Classification	Disease (synonyms)	Probable aetiology	Symptoms	Corneal signs	Conjunctival signs	Associated lens
Stromal	Stromal oedema (striate keratopathy)	Stromal lactate accumulation, tear hypotonicity causing swelling	Blurring of vision in some cases only	Striae and stromal folds Folds from corneal oedema, seen in severe acute epithelial necrosis	None except when associated with acute epithelial necrosis	Usually EW-SCL
	Neovascularization (superficial and deep)	Hypoxia causes stromal oedema and release of vasogenic mediators	None unless lipid keratopathy or haemorrhage from deep vessels, causing loss of vision	Superficial/deep stromal vessels Lipid keratopathy associated with deep vessels	None	Rare with RCL; common with SCL
	Deep stromal opacity	Probably due to prolonged hypoxia and hypercapnia	Asymptomatic or reduced acuity	Pre-Descemet's opacity in central cornea	None	Rare with RCL
Epithelial and stromal	Tight lens syndrome	Lens tightening precipitated by hypoxia and reduced pH; also other factors	Starting during or after overnight wear Vision usually affected	As above, but stromal oedema and an epithelial defect common	Ciliary injection and limbal indentation from the tight lens	EW-SCL
Endothelial	Polymegethism and pleomorphism	Prolonged hypoxia and hypercapnia	None Evidence of functional changes and slower de-swell rates in polymegethism	Variations in endothelial cell size and shape	None	All
Mechanical/traumatic						
	Corneal abrasion	Trauma during lens handling or from trapped foreign bodies behind lens, deposits on lens or poor lens fitting	Sudden onset of pain and epiphora Resolves in hours	Linear/sharply circumscribed epithelial defect	Hyperaemia	Commoner with RCL

(cont'd)

Classification of contact lens-related disorders (*cont'd*)						
Classification	**Disease (synonyms)**	**Probable aetiology**	**Symptoms**	**Corneal signs**	**Conjunctival signs**	**Associated lens**
Toxic or allergic disorders						
	Toxic keratopathy	Exposure to compounds adsorbed onto or absorbed by lens	Pain arising after inserting lens soaked in proteolytic enzyme/ chemically preserved soaking solution	Widespread punctate stain	Ciliary injection	SCL
	Thimerosal keratopathy (thimerosal keratoconjunctivitis or soft lens-related superior limbic keratoconjunctivitis)	Preservatives act as haptens, causing a delayed hypersensitivity response	Irritation and redness soon after inserting lenses; symptoms increasing over 1–2 weeks Rapid relief of symptoms after lens removal in early disease; recur within hours of restarting lens wear Vision affected in severe cases	Keratopathy affecting superior quadrant and extending to visual axis in severe cases Changes include epithelial infiltrates, microcysts and anterior stromal opacity	Superior limbal hyperaemia, oedema and neovascularization of limbus and superior cornea Intense hyperaemia with lens in situ Follicular changes remain when lens removed	SCL; rare with RCL
	Contact lens-associated papillary conjunctivitis (giant papillary conjunctivitis)	Multifactorial aetiology; immune response to antigenic proteins on lenses, mechanical effects of lens edge May be compounded by use of preserved solutions	Subacute onset Increased discharge and greasing of lenses Itching on lens removal in early stages, later severe irritation and lens intolerance Acuity normal	None	Upper tarsal hyperaemia and fine papillary response 'Giant' (compound) papillae >1 mm in advanced disease with apical fibrosis Clear mucus discharge	All lens types Commoner with EW-SCLs and with prosthetic shells Associated with spoiled lenses, poor lens hygiene and a history of allergy
	Contact lens intolerance	Due to lens spoilation, chronic hypoxia, loss of adaptation	Chronic redness and/or discomfort and loss in tolerance Vision may be blurred	Punctate stain common	Hyperaemia, papillae and follicles common	All types

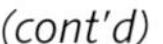

(cont'd)

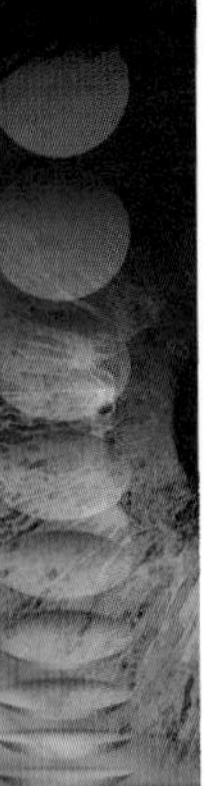

Classification of contact lens-related disorders (*cont'd*)

Suppurative keratitis					
Contact lens-related peripheral ulcer (sterile keratitis, aseptic keratitis, sterile corneal infiltrates)	Inflammatory response in the absence of infecting organism Hypersensitivity to preservatives, bacteria or bacterial products, and tight lens fitting implicated	Discomfort, redness and discharge minimal Symptoms non-progressive	Appearance similar to marginal keratitis Usually peripheral infiltrates with/without ulceration Peripheral lesions, occasionally central, may be multiple Lesions usually <1 mm, sometimes arcuate Intact epithelium in early lesions, ulcerated in late	Hyperaemia	Common with reusable soft lenses, EW-SCLs and some disposable soft lenses
Microbial keratitis	Multiple factors including increased ocular susceptibility and exposure to pathogens	Rapid onset, progressive pain, hyperaemia and discharge in bacterial disease *Acanthamoeba* slower onset but pain often a principal feature of early disease when signs are minimal	Epithelial ulcer with underlying stromal infiltrate *Pseudomonas, Staphylococcus* and *Acanthamoeba* implicated Lesions often central but may be in any location Anterior chamber reaction in bacterial disease but not in early *Acanthamoeba*, for which radial keratoneuritis is pathognomonic	Ciliary injection in bacterial disease, especially adjacent to affected corneal quadrant Anterior scleritis common in *Acanthamoeba* keratitis	Bacterial keratitis most common in EW-SCL, rare in rigid lens use *Acanthamoeba* commoner in daily wear soft lens users either using chlorine disinfection compared to other cold systems, or in those failing to use any disinfection system
Tear resurfacing disorders					
3 and 9 o'clock stain	Drying of corneal surface adjacent to lens edge and abnormal blink	Interpalpebral redness Rarely discomfort	Punctate keratopathy at 3 and 9 o'clock Severe cases = dellen formation and vascularized opacities	Interpalpebral hyperaemia	HCL
Inferior corneal stain	Incomplete blinking Localized lens dehydration	Inferior limbal redness and discomfort	Inferior/interpalpebral punctate stain	Inferior limbal hyperaemia	SCL
Dimple veil	Static air bubbles under lens	Asymptomatic or blurred vision	Fluorescein pooling in epithelial depressions	None	HCL

EW-SCL, extended-wear soft contact lenses; HCL, hard contact lenses; PMMA-RCL, polymethylmethacrylate rigid contact lenses; RCL, PMMA and rigid gas-permeable contact lenses; SCL, soft contact lenses.
Adapted from Dart (1993) Disease and risks associated with contact lenses, a review. Br. J. Ophthalmol., 77, 49–53. Reproduced with permission from the BMJ Publishing Group

Chapter 19

Orthokeratology

John Mountford

CHAPTER CONTENTS

INTRODUCTION

Due to the rapid changes occurring in the field since the fourth edition of this book, total revision of this subject has been necessary. This chapter outlines the changes in lens design and the results of controlled research into the field of orthokeratology, as well as the expanding fields of astigmatic and hypermetropic correction.

In academic circles, it is now common to see papers where the statement 'orthokeratology works' is made; however, such statements are usually followed by the proviso that more work needs to be done as the exact mechanisms of action and the corneal responses are not fully understood. This is as it should be. For low (3.00 D and less) myopia, orthokeratology has become a simple, straightforward clinical process that is highly predictable. The same cannot be said for myopia over 4.00 D or astigmatism of greater than 1.00 D with-the-rule or against-the-rule and oblique astigmatism. In addition, the correction of hypermetropia is undergoing renewed interest, with some novel designs and approaches (see p. 440).

HISTORY

Historically, orthokeratology consisted of a series of progressively flatter lenses that were used to 'gently' reshape the cornea by flattening the corneal radius with a concomitant change in refraction. The lenses were worn on a daily wear schedule until 'stabilization' or the maximum refractive change was achieved (usually 6–9 months), followed by a slowly reducing wear schedule to the minimum required to maintain the changes for the balance of the wakening hours. Unfortunately, this minimal wearing time was approximately 8 hours per day.

The results of the controlled studies (Kerns 1976, Polse et al. 1983, Coon 1984) were largely negative for the procedure using polymethylmethacrylate (PMMA) lenses with variable back optic zone radius (BOZR)/cornea fitting relationships. Outcome was largely unpredictable and poorly maintained.

The advent of reverse geometry lenses, CNC lathes, relatively high-Dk materials that allowed for overnight wear, and corneal topography led to a revolution in orthokeratology.

All orthokeratology lenses are now worn on an overnight-wear basis with removal in the morning. 'Night therapy' was first described by Grant (1995), who reasoned that since orthokeratology lenses took 8 hours to effect the required changes as well as maintain them, the treatment period should occur while the patient was asleep. This became possible with the introduction of high-Dk rigid gas-permeable (RGP) materials. The benefits include:

- Increased efficacy of the procedure.
- Little or no adaptation.
- No environmental problems (e.g. wind, dust and dryness).
- Less risk of loss.
- Freedom from corrective lenses during the day.

However, the overnight wear of contact lenses is associated with a higher risk of corneal complications (see p. 448).

LENS DESIGNS

The orthokeratology chapter in the fourth edition was restricted to a discussion on the Contex OK series of 3-zone lenses as they were the only commonly available lenses at that time. Since then, the designs have become more advanced, with 4- and 5-zone lenses being the norm. A 3-zone lens is typically:

- Central back optic zone diameter (BOZD) of 6.00 mm.
- 'Reverse curve', where the back peripheral radius (BPR_1) is *steeper* than the BOZR.
- Edge lift curve that provides the required edge lift (Fig. 19.1).

However, 4- and 5-zone lenses have a different construction with:

- Central BOZD of between 5.20 and 7.00 mm.
- Reverse curve(s) that are steeper than the BOZR.
- First alignment curve that is slightly steeper than the peripheral cornea.
- Second alignment curve that aligns the peripheral cornea but is flatter than the first alignment curve.

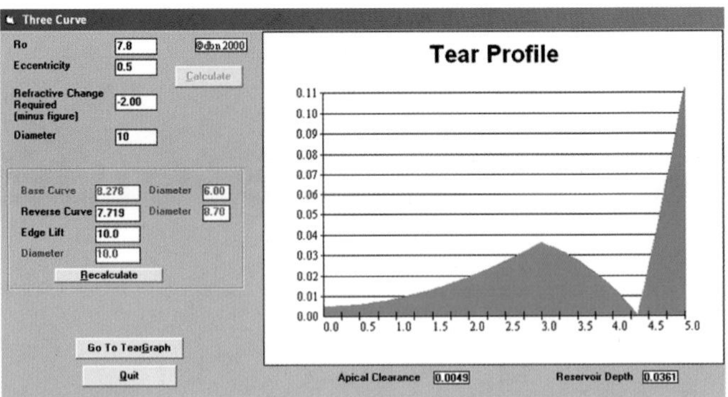

Figure 19.1 A 3-zone lens tear layer profile. Note the abrupt junction between the reverse curve and the edge lift, which resulted in poor centration

- 'Flat' or tangent curve as an alternative to the alignment curve(s).
- Peripheral curve that provides the required axial edge lift (Fig. 19.2).

Wlodyga and Stoyan (Joe et al. 1996) designed and developed the original 3-zone lenses. The 4-zone lens, which incorporated a wide alignment zone, was developed by Reim (Dreamlens), whilst El Hage and colleagues (1999) were the first to base the lens design on corneal topography and named the lens and fitting system 'controlled keratoreformation' (CKR). Mountford and Noack (Capricornia BE) incorporated the concept of a tangential periphery on the lens as a means of controlling centration and also introduced the concept of sag philosophy to the fitting of reverse geometry lenses. Day (Fargo) extended the 4-zone concept of Reim by splitting the alignment curve into two sections and making it wider, thereby increasing the common lens diameter from 10.00 to 10.60 mm. Leggerton (G., personal communication, 2005; Paragon CRT) modified the reverse curve zone by using a sigmoid curve instead of a spherical curve. The sagittal relationship of the lens to the cornea could therefore be controlled by alterations to the sag of the sigmoid proximity curve. Tung (D., personal communication, 2005; Vipok) added a second peripheral reverse curve that was flatter

(a)

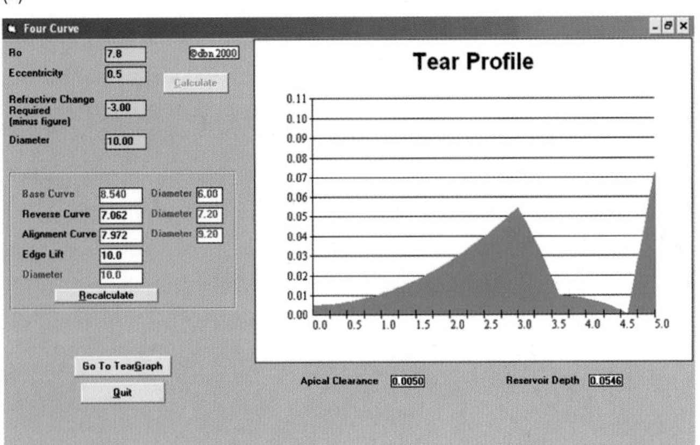

(b)

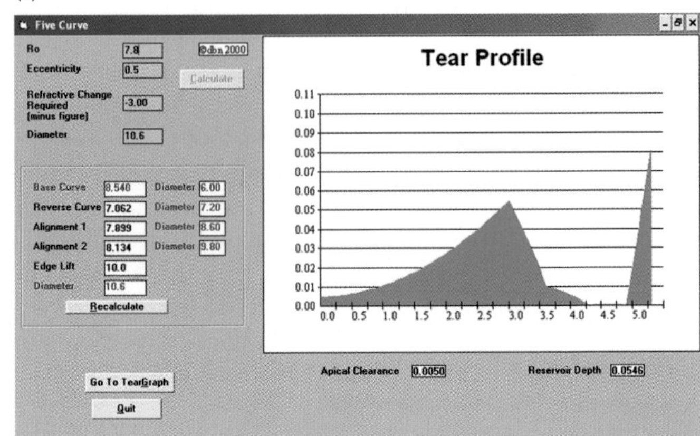

Figure 19.2 (a) A 4-zone lens. Note the steep and narrow reverse curve and the wide alignment curve. (b) A 5-zone lens, constructed by dividing the alignment curve into two sections, leading to an increase in total diameter and greater control of centration

than the first curve and reduced the BOZD to approximately 5.50 mm as a means of correcting higher myopic refractive errors. The European designers incorporate aspheric surfaces in their designs, particularly in the alignment zones.

The wide range of lens designs available for overnight orthokeratology (Table 19.1) all have the same basic construction. The differences in reverse zone designs and alignment curve/cornea relationships are minimal, much as tricurve RGP lenses may all have different peripheral curve values but similar clinical performance. There is no inherently superior orthokeratology lens design; the real differences are the underlying assumptions made with respect to corneal shape, the accuracy of lens manufacture and the standard of fitting.

These new designs have revolutionized orthokeratology, making it much more predictable.

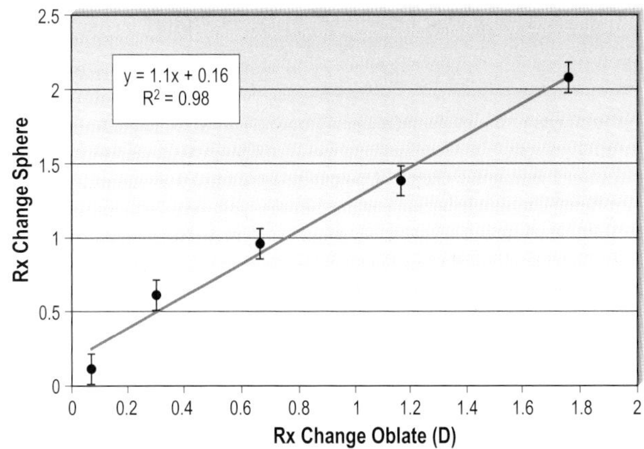

Figure 19.3 The relationship between refractive change, assuming the cornea is oblate following treatment, and the change possible if the corneal surface is spherical over discrete zones. There is no clinical difference between the two

PATIENT SELECTION

The selection criteria for patients undergoing orthokeratology are as follows:

Good candidates

- Low to moderate myopia (up to 4.50 D).
- With-the-rule astigmatism of 1.50 D or less.
- Pupil size less than 6.00 mm in dim illumination.
- Normal, healthy cornea, lids and conjunctiva.
- Normal tear break-up time.
- A corneal eccentricity that correlates with the refractive change required (see below).
- Non-habitual spectacle wearers.
- Soft lens wearers who complain of end-of-day dryness.
- Active sportspeople.

Poor candidates

- Any against-the-rule or oblique astigmatism of greater than 0.75 D.
- Lenticular astigmatism of greater than 0.50 D against-the-rule.
- Limbus to limbus astigmatism.
- Any active or recurrent ocular surface disease such as blepharitis, meibomianitis, dry eye and basement membrane dysfunction.
- Large pupils (>6.00 mm) in normal illumination.
- Low eccentricity corneas requiring high refractive change.
- Those with a prior history of poor compliance.
- Those with unrealistic expectations expecting a permanent 'cure'.

Other factors such as corneas flatter than 8.65 mm (39.00 D) or steeper than 7.50 mm (48.00 D) are also contraindications because flat corneas are associated with relatively low eccentricities, and some relatively high myopes (up to –10.00 D) have steeper corneas that are near spherical (Carney et al. 1997).

The important factor, however, is not the keratometry but whether the eccentricity value of the cornea is high enough to allow adequate refractive change.

Mountford (1997) showed that corneal eccentricity could be used to determine the refractive change possible for a particular eye. The relationship is:

$$e = 0.16x + 0.10$$

where e is the corneal eccentricity and x the refractive change required in dioptres. A 2.00 D refractive change would therefore require the corneal eccentricity to be 0.46.

El Hage et al. (1999) found a similar result when comparing refractive change to the corneal shape factor p (where $p = 1 - e^2$; see also Chapter 9).

The initial results suggested that the maximum refractive change was achieved when the cornea became spherical with an eccentricity of zero. However, the newer 4- and 5-zone lenses can achieve greater results either by making the cornea oblate or by producing smaller spherical surfaces over which the refractive change occurs (Mountford 2004c, Swarbrick 2004a).

Figure 19.3 shows the relationship between refractive change and Q (where $Q = -e^2$; see also Chapter 9), assuming the cornea becomes oblate following orthokeratology. This relationship indicates that the total refractive change possible may be twice the value expressed in the above formula. For example, the mean corneal shape of r_0 7.80 mm and Q –0.26 ($e = 0.50$) would have a maximum refractive change of 2.25 D assuming corneal sphericalization (Q and $e = 0$) as the endpoint of treatment. However, if the cornea became oblate to a Q value of +0.26, the total refractive change possible would become 4.50 D. The major difficulty in verifying this concept is that not all the currently available corneal topographers can reconstruct an oblate or bicurve surface accurately (Tang et al. 2000).

The final factor to consider is the treatment zone diameter with greater refractive change. As shown by Munnerlyn et al. (1988), the greater the refractive change required, the smaller the treatment zone (TxZ), and this has implications with respect to low-contrast vision. However, the correction of higher myopic refractive errors is possible and is discussed below.

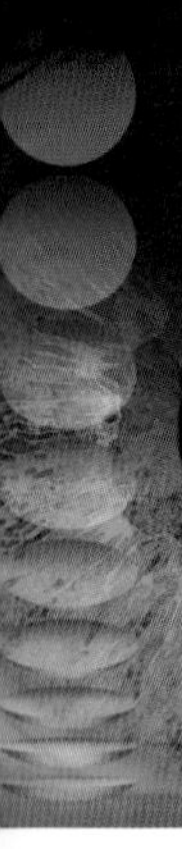

Table 19.1: Lens designs available for overnight orthokeratology

Lens name	Designer	Laboratory and material	Design	Fitting	Country
Contex OK	Nick Stoyan	Contex Boston XO and Equalens 2	4- and 5-zone	Empirical, trial lens	USA
Correctech	Breece/Herndon	Correctech Inc Boston XO and Equalens 2	4-zone	Empirical	USA
DK-4	Danny Fan	Custom Craft Boston XO and Equalens 2	4- and 5-zone	Trial lens/topography	Hong Kong
Dreamlens	Tom Reim	Correctech, Procornea, Hanita. No 7 Boston XO and Equalens 2	4- and 5-zone	Empirical, trial and topography	USA, Taiwan, Holland, Israel, UK
Emerald and Jade	George Glady	Euclid Systems Boston XO and Equalens 2	4- and 5-zone	Empirical, software based and topography	USA
EZM	Don Ezekiel	Gelflex Australia Boston XO and Equalens 2	3-zone/tangent	Software, trial lens and topography	Australia, USA Israel
BE	Mountford/Noack	Capricornia Contact Lens, Precision Technologies, Art Optical, NKL, Hanita B&L (UK) Boston XO and Equalens 2	4- and 5-zone with tangent Myopic, hypermetropic correction Astigmatic lens in development	Topography, software, trial lens fitting	Australia, Canada, USA, Holland Israel, UK
CRT	Jerry Leggerton	Paragon Vision Sciences Paragon HDS100	3-zone/tangent Sigmoid proximity reverse zone	Trial lens, topography, *K* readings	USA
Orthofocus	Al Blackburn	Metro Optics Boston XO and Equalens 2	4- and 5-zone	Empirical	USA
R&R	Rinehart/Reeves	Danker Laboratories, Nova (UK). Eyecon Boston XO and Equalens 2	4- and 5-zone	Trial lens and topography	USA, UK, Australia
Nightmove	Roger Tabb	Gelflex Australia Boston XO and Equalens 2	4- and 5-zone, hypermetropia, astigmatic lens	Empirical	USA, Australia
Luna	Christian Krusi	Galifa Contactlinsen AG, Switzerland Boston XO, other high-Dk materials	Double reverse zone 5 curve	Topography, trial lens	Switzerland
Seefree	Silke Lohrengel	HechtContactlinsen GmbH Boston XO	Aspheric 4-zone	Topography/software fitting	Germany
Sleep & See	Bruno Fantony	Techno-Lens SA Boston XO	4-zone, variable eccentricity alignment zone	Topography based	Switzerland
VIPOK	Tung Hiaso-Ching	E&E Boston XO	4-zone, hypermetropic and myopic designs	Trial lens and topography	Taiwan
Justsee	Tom Tao	Autekchina Boston XO	4-zone	Trial lens/empirical	China

Table 19.1: Lens designs available for overnight orthokeratology (*cont'd*)

Lens name	Designer	Laboratory and material	Design	Fitting	Country
Fokx	Michael Baertschi and Michael Wyss	Falco Laboratories, Switzerland Boston XO	4-zone, myopia, hypermetropia, astigmatism and mini-scleral designs	Topography and trial lens fitting	Switzerland
Wave	Jim Edwards	Custom Craft, Las Vegas Boston XO and Equalens 2	4- and 5-zone	Topography designed and fitted	USA
Quadra RG	Jim Day	Paragon Vision Science Paragon HDS 100	4- and 5-zone	Empirical	USA
CKR	Sammi El Hage	Progressive Vision Technologies, Texas Boston XO and Equalens 2	4-zone	Topography-based design and fitting	USA

FITTING REVERSE GEOMETRY LENSES

There are three ways to fit reverse geometry lenses for orthokeratology:

- Empirical.
- Trial lens fitting.
- Topography-based fitting.

Empirical fitting

This consists of supplying the laboratory with the patient's keratometry readings and refraction. The laboratory then designs the lens based on proprietary algorithms, manufactures it and sends it to the practitioner. The lens is issued and reviewed after the first overnight wear and then a week later. If the results are less than optimal (see below), the laboratory will send modifications of the original design until problems are resolved, or the patient deemed to be a failure.

In the majority of lens designs, changes to the lens fit are made by altering the reverse curve or the alignment curves. The BOZR is rarely altered, as it is used to effect the required refractive change.

The original 'orthofocus' technique as described by Jessen (1962) used the liquid lens as the basis of the lens fit. A 2.00 D refractive change was achieved by fitting the lens 2.00 D (0.40 mm) flatter than K_F. This has become the popular means of determining the BOZR in all reverse geometry lenses with the exception of 3-zone and BE lenses. The initial BOZR is selected such that the liquid lens is equal to the refractive change required. This is now commonly referred to as the Jessen factor. An additional 'compression factor' of between 0.50 and 1.00 D is incorporated into the final design to allow for regression. In other words, a slight over-correction is aimed for, such that the final lens BOZR for a 3.00 D refractive change would be 3.50 D (0.70 mm) flatter than K_F.

The first-fit success rate of empirically designed lenses is unknown as there are very few studies that have specifically set out to compare the different methods.

Tahhan et al. (2003) compared four different designs of reverse geometry lenses based on improvement in unaided visual acuity (VA), high- and low-contrast VA, refraction, glare and haloes, and patient acceptance. All lenses performed to the same level. However, the mean refractive change was only 2.00 D.

Maldonado-Codina et al. (2005) found the first-fit success rate of lenses designed from refraction and keratometry values was 66%, with two participants requiring one extra set of lenses and one requiring three (similar to the success rate achieved with conventional lenses; Bennett et al. 1989). Subjects fitted by topography data and an overnight trial achieved a 100% success rate with the first set of lenses. They concluded that the first-fit success rate of empirical lenses could be improved by supplying the laboratory with information on the topographical corneal shape. Further, the empirical method required approximately 50% more chair time to achieve a successful fit compared to the topography-based/overnight trial system. In addition, this does not allow for the cost in replacement lenses that usually occurs in practice.

When empirical fitting is used, the first lens simply becomes a 'trial lens' from which the correct lens specifications may be determined (Rinehart & Bennett 2004).

At the end of the first week of overnight wear, the effectiveness of a lens is usually determined by the results of VA and refractive change. However, these assessments can be somewhat influenced by practitioner bias. Post-wear topographical analysis is the preferred method of objective analysis as the outcome can be compared to the accepted optimal result and modifications made to the lens design (see 'Topography-based fitting', below).

The exact prescription of reverse geometry lenses is rarely given to the practitioner, as most manufacturers consider the designs to be proprietary information. However, as with conventional rigid lens fitting, there are 'rules' that can be used to modify the design in order to improve outcomes. These rules apply whether empirical, trial lens or topography-based fitting is used.

When a lens is prescribed empirically, based solely on refraction and keratometry values, a very large margin of error

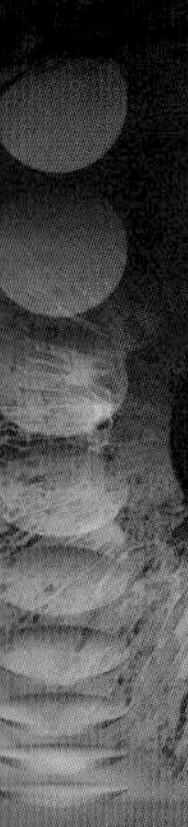

exists and studies to date indicate that it may not be the preferred method of fitting.

Trial lens fitting

The use of trial lenses in routine contact lens practice leads to a higher first-fit success rate than empirical fitting (Bennett et al. 1989). The ability to assess the fluorescein pattern, movement and centration is essential to achieve the correct design for the individual patient. Although most orthokeratology lens designs utilize trial lens fitting and the same fitting assessments, centration is of particular importance in determining the optimal lens design.

There is a certain inconsistency with this approach. Conventional lenses are fitted to be used in a dynamic state, with active blinking in the open-eye environment; factors such as lens recentration following a blink and peripheral tear exchange are the hallmarks of success or failure. The shape of the edge lift of a conventional lens determines the surface tension forces that maintain lens centration in conjunction with the post-lens squeeze film forces, which are determined by the BOZR/K_F relationship (Greber & Dybbs 1972, Hayashi & Fatt 1980, and others; see Chapter 9). Orthokeratology lenses, however, are used strictly in the static environment of the closed eye, with no movement, tear exchange or surface tension forces working around the lens edge to maintain centration. A lens that shows all the attributes of an 'ideal' fit in the open eye may decentre behind closed lids, leading to a poor outcome.

Another factor is the relative accuracy of fluorescein pattern assessment with reverse geometry lenses compared to that of conventional lenses. Brungart (1961) showed that, with training, the difference in fit of alignment lenses can be determined to a level of 0.05 mm in BOZR or approximately 10 μm in lens sag. Alternatively, the sensitivity with aspheric lenses is 0.10 mm in BOZR or 20 μm in tear layer thickness (TLT) (Osborne et al. 1989).

Mountford and Cho (2005) found that this level was not achievable with the static interpretation fluorescein patterns of orthokeratology lenses. Variations in lens fit using two designs of reverse geometry lenses (BE and Dreamlens) to a maximum variation of 40 μm were photographed and shown to two groups of practitioners: experienced orthokeratologists and non-orthokeratologists. Neither group could determine the correct, steeper or flatter lenses better than chance, and there was no statistically significant difference between the two groups, indicating that experience with orthokeratology lens fitting did not improve the practitioner's ability to determine the correct fit.

Beerten (2004) reported on the Dutch experience with orthokeratology over a 2-year period and concluded that fluorescein pattern analysis was of limited clinical value in predicting a successful outcome.

If orthokeratology lenses are to be fitted for overnight wear, the logical approach is to perform overnight trials in order to ascertain correctly the resting position of the lens during sleep.

Topography-based fitting

Corneal topography is an essential part of orthokeratology for two main reasons:

- The corneal data can be used to determine the closest matching sag between the lens and the cornea.
- The results of the trial lens wear period can be assessed objectively by comparing the difference between the pre- and post-wear topography, which is more sensitive and objective than measuring post-wear refraction and high or low contrast VA.

The major weakness of all published orthokeratology studies is that none gives an objective rating of the quality of the post-wear topography. The results all measure the reduction in myopia and increase in unaided VA. This is misleading: a lens that is not optimally centred can still give a good reduction in refraction and improvement in unaided VA.

The problems appear later as decentration increases with time, leading to symptoms of:

- Increased haloes and flare.
- Astigmatism.
- Poor retention of the effect, especially in low illumination.

Two papers have reported on cases where the results were compromised by poor post-wear topography outcomes. Maldonado-Codina et al. (2005) showed that a central island could produce reduced visual acuity even though the post-wear keratometry readings were normal, and Joslin et al. (2003) reported on a case of smiley face post-wear topography (see p. 431) causing a reduction in best-corrected VA and a large increase in higher-order aberrations.

Opponents of topography-based fitting point out that topography data are subject to variations due to:

- The capture method.
- The stability of the patient.
- The reconstruction algorithms used by the manufacturer.

Cho et al. (2002a,b) compared corneal data produced by four topographers and the lens parameters that each would have generated. The lenses were totally different, and none was interchangeable with the others. This only becomes a problem if an inherently inaccurate instrument is used. The majority of topographers have a repeatability of ±14 μm in the measurement of corneal sag over a 9.00 mm chord, and this degree of error is quite acceptable for designing the initial trial lens and then refining the fit. However, the Orbscan and PAR have poorer repeatability (approximately ±40 μm) and are not suitable for use with orthokeratology in their current design.

Trial lens sets for orthokeratology have two main curves: the alignment curve and, less importantly, the BOZR, which – unlike conventional lens fitting – has little or no influence in orthokeratology lens fitting.

The alignment curve or tangent is the critical curve that controls lens centration and from which trial lens sets are designed. Trial lenses are designed with a relatively constant difference in sag between successive lenses in the set, usually

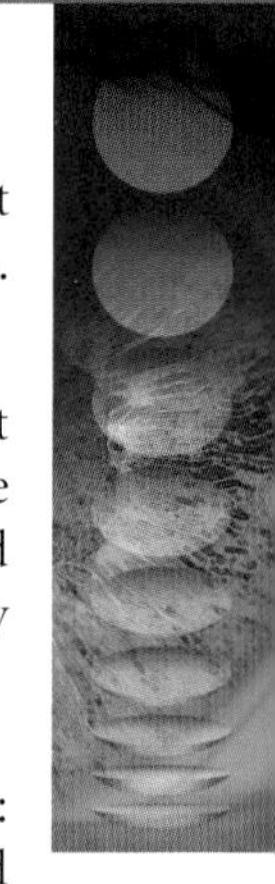

10 μm. The practitioner therefore must become conversant with alterations to lens sag by changing the alignment curve or tangent, rather than by alterations to the BOZR.

The routine for topography-based fitting is as follows:

- Take four repeated readings of the cornea and compare similarities in apical radius or power and either elevation or eccentricity (*e*) values. Delete any 'rogue reading' and replace it.
- Calculate the mean and standard deviation of error for apical radius, eccentricity and elevation. This is laborious and requires the use of an Excel spreadsheet (Mountford 2004c). Currently, only the Medmont E300 and Shin-Nippon CT incorporate a statistical analysis table of repeated readings.
- Enter the apical radius and eccentricity (or elevation) values into the manufacturer's software and the indicated trial lens determined (BE, Dreamlens, R&R, Euclid).
- Insert the trial lens and assess movement and centration.
- As stated previously, the dynamic appearance of the lens may be a poor indicator of the resting position behind the closed lid. A more accurate assessment of the closed lid resting position of the lens can be made by advising the patient to close their eyes for 10–20 seconds and then open them. Assess the position of the lens immediately on eye opening to decide whether the lens decentred during eye closure (P. Gerry, personal communication).
- If the lens decentres, increase the sag of the trial lens by one unit (steeper alignment curve) until the lens is centred behind the closed lid. Conversely, if the lens drops low, the alignment curve is considered to be too tight, and a lens with a lower sag (or flatter alignment curve/tangent) is used.
- Instruct the patient to insert the lens prior to sleep and to present the next morning with the lens in situ. Lens care is with the practitioner's preferred method.
- The following morning, examine with a slit-lamp and note any adverse signs such as striae and folds or corneal staining. Remove the lens and perform corneal topography.
- Use the difference or subtractive functions to assess the pre- and post-wear maps.
- Measure unaided VA and residual refractive error. Post-wear refraction is only valid if an ideal 'bull's-eye' response is achieved (see p. 430). If suboptimal outcomes such as 'smiley face' or 'central islands' occur, the refractive data are meaningless.

POST-WEAR TOPOGRAPHY OUTCOMES

The most complex and difficult aspect of orthokeratology is learning how to read topography maps, which are commonly misinterpreted. If the post-wear topography is misread, the final lens prescription will be incorrect, leading to a poor outcome. This is reflected in the re-make rate of lenses during the initial learning curve required for orthokeratology. The author reviewed the re-make rates for six different manufacturers on four continents, finding a re-make rate of approximately 30% for the first 15 cases, which then dropped rapidly to approximately 5% by case 20.

Practitioners tend to make some basic mistakes when first learning how to use the instrument and then read the maps. These include:

- *Poor patient alignment with the instrument*: The head must be turned to the left for the right eye, and to the right for the left, to reduce the effect of the lid, brow and nose and increase the area of cornea measured. This is particularly important if a large placido instrument is used.
- *Poor control of the focusing and alignment system.*
- *Capturing an image of an uneven or disrupted tear film*: Advise the patient to blink a few times until the reflected mires are crisp and even.
- *Dependence on a single reading*: Repeated readings are essential so that the relative repeatability of the data is assessable. Rogue readings can then be deleted and replaced.
- *Comparison between the two eyes*: It is rare to find significant differences in apical radius and eccentricity between the two eyes, assuming that the corneal shape is in the normal range (Keiley et al. 1984, Guillon et al. 1986).
- *Inability to learn how to change the scales*: A common source of misinterpretation of maps occurs when the scales are left at the manufacturer's default values. The absolute scale is only of value when different eyes are being compared. The general range of absolute maps is from 10 to 100 D and small changes will be totally missed if the maps are left on the absolute scale. However, most instruments will allow the practitioner to alter the scales manually to bring out more detail. This is done by increasing the low setting and decreasing the high setting. Alternatively, the 'normalized' scale can be used. When the normalized scale is selected, the software automatically finds the flattest and steepest values and sets these as the range. Practitioners must learn to manipulate scales in order to gain the maximum information from the instrument.
- *Inability to use and interpret other map presentations*: All topographers represent the cornea as axial, tangential or refractive, and these maps are either curvature or power. Power maps show the changes in dioptres, which are easier to understand and more intuitive than curvature maps.

  Practitioners often limit the display to only one of these, usually the axial power or tangential map. In Asia, for example, only the tangential power map is used as the majority of practitioners use the Keratron which reports tangential curvature and power as being 'true' curvature. This is not the case. It is simply a different mathematical method of looking at a surface.

Subtractive maps

There are six distinct subtractive map appearances following overnight trials. The accepted terminologies for the different outcomes are:

- Bull's-eye.
- Smiley face.
- Smiley face with a fake central island.

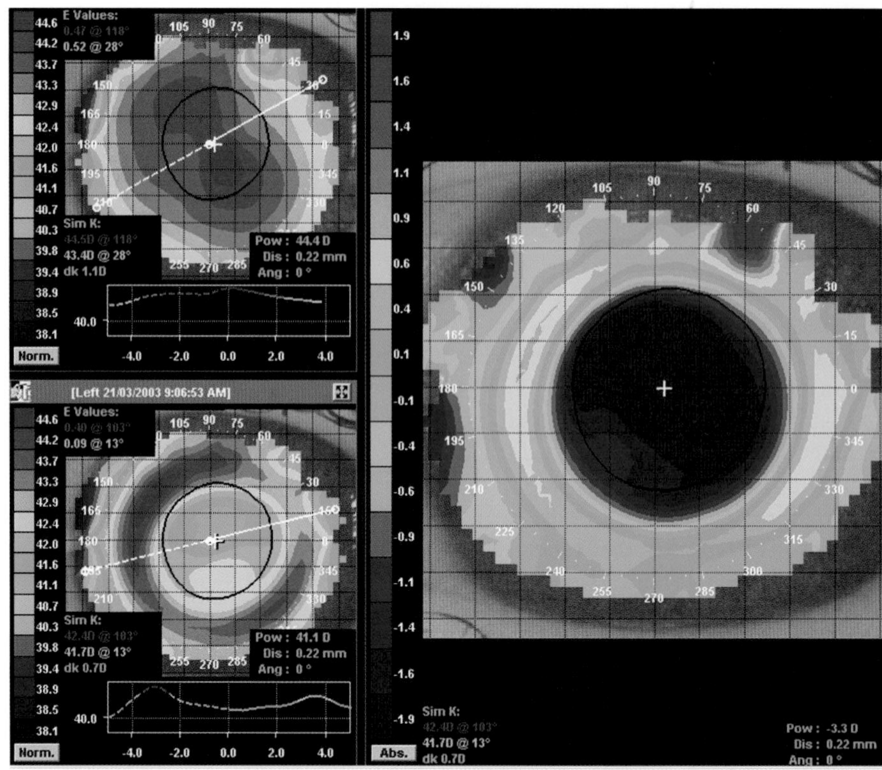

Figure 19.4 An axial power difference map of a bull's-eye. The cursor is set at the centre and shows the refractive change

- Central island.
- Frowny face.
- Lateral decentration.

Other than the bull's-eye, each is diagnostic of a less than optimal fit, and specific with regard to the method of lens correction. Each outcome has a different appearance depending on whether an axial, tangential or refractive power map is used. Note that *power* maps should be used, *not* curvature maps.

BULL'S-EYE

A bull's-eye results from perfect centration and fit of a reverse geometry lens. This is caused by an ideal balance between the post-lens squeeze film force and the lid force. The fluid pressure in the tear layer is negative, and tends to pull the lens towards the corneal surface somewhat like a suction cup. The lid force applies the compressive force that is required, but if it is greater than the negative force under the lens, the lens will decentre (Mountford 2004a).

When assessing the topographical maps, the following should be noted:

- There are two distinct bull's-eye maps: complete and incomplete.
- The axial power map shows the refractive change that has occurred when the cursor is placed at the corneal apex, which is usually designated as point zero at zero degrees (Fig. 19.4).
- The tangential power map shows the treatment centration and is the true diagnostic tool for a bull's-eye.
- The 'red ring' shows the rapid change of curvature that occurs with orthokeratology lenses at approximately 3 mm from centre. The hallmark of a bull's-eye is that the red ring should be perfectly centred on the pupil, although it can be inside the pupil zone (especially after only one night of wear) or outside (usually seen at the 1-week after-care appointment) (Fig. 19.5).
- The refractive power map shows the treatment zone diameter (TxZ), not the 'blue zone', which is commonly misinterpreted as the treatment zone. The real value of the TxZ is determined by moving the cursor from the centre of the cornea to that point on the nasal and temporal side where the difference between the pre- and post-treatment corneal refractive power is zero (Roberts & Wu 1998). Ideally, the TxZ should be greater in diameter than the pupil in dim illumination.

An 'incomplete' bull's-eye can occur following the first overnight trial and is commonly mistaken for a central island (Fig. 19.6). The difference map shows a well-centred treatment effect and red ring, but what appears to be a steeper centre than the surrounding area. There is often little refractive change at the corneal apex because *it is not steeper than the original cornea.* Figure 19.7 shows the same eye after another 2 nights' wear with the trial lens. The bull's-eye is now completely formed.

Incomplete bull's-eyes usually occur in high eccentricity corneas (the *e* value in this case is 0.78). The definitive diagnosis is that the apical corneal power is not steeper than the original cornea (which represents a true central island) and can be improved by allowing the patient an extra few nights of trial lens wear.

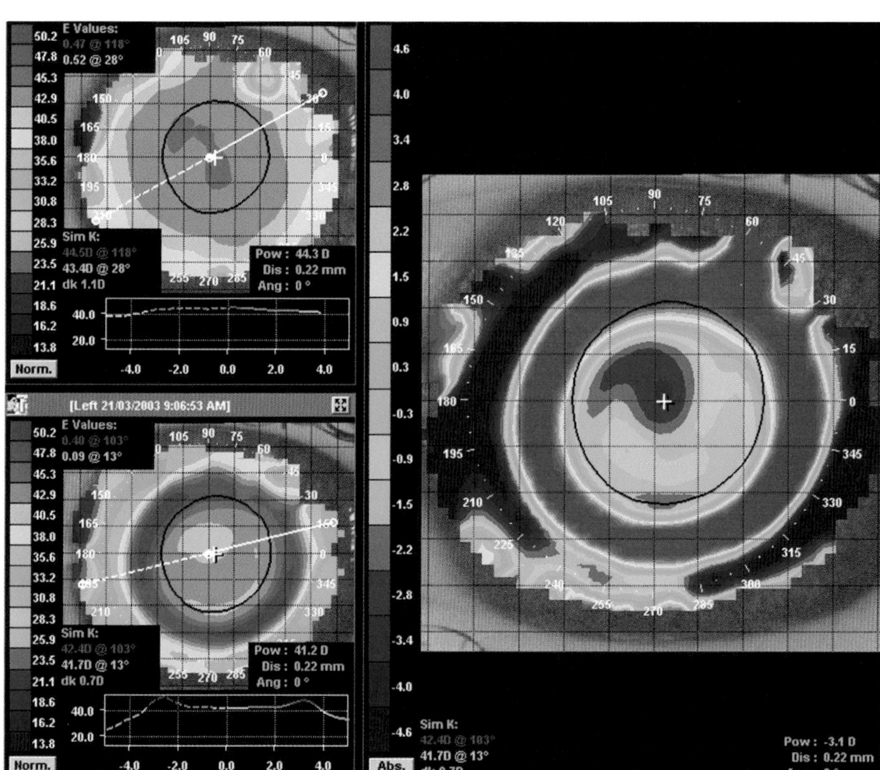

Figure 19.5 A tangential power difference map of a bull's-eye. Note the centration of the 'red ring' around the pupil zone

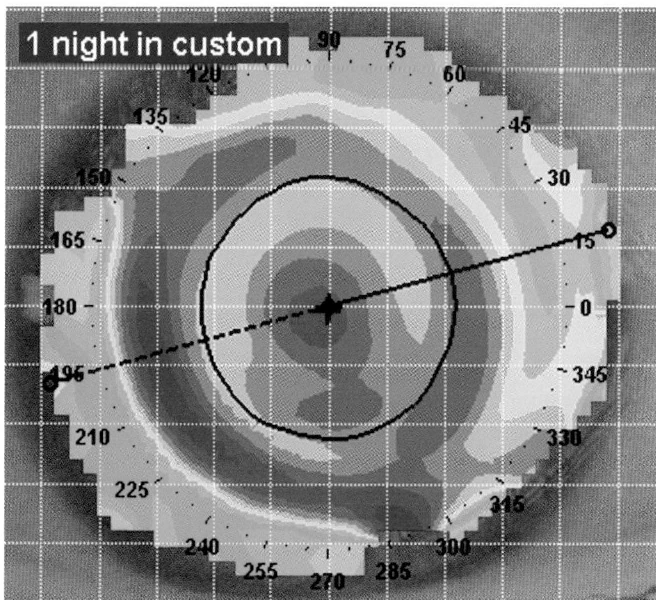

Figure 19.6 An 'incomplete' bull's-eye following the first night of lens wear. This can be common in cases of high corneal eccentricity. The difference map would show that the apex is marginally flatter (0.50 D) than the original cornea

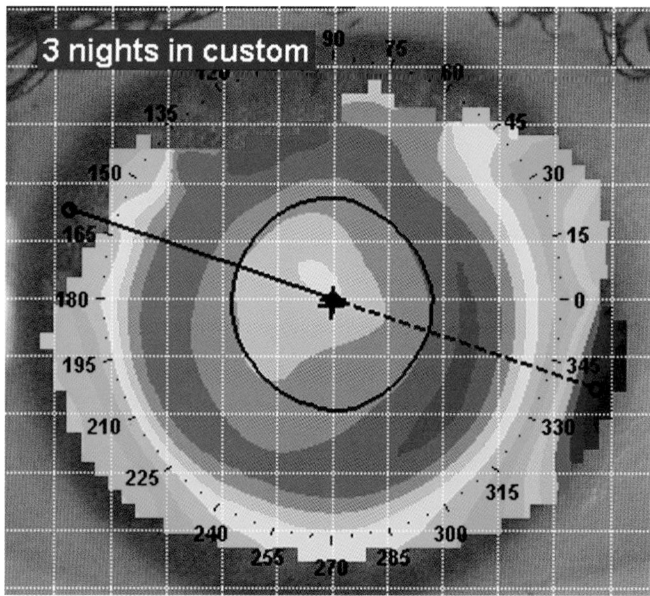

Figure 19.7 The same eye as in Figure 19.6 following 3 nights of lens wear. A fully formed bull's-eye is present

Small bull's-eyes usually occur on the first overnight trial and can lead to some concern with respect to the final treatment zone versus pupil size. Figure 19.8 shows a small bull's-eye with a small area of central flattening and the same eye after 7 nights' wear of the trial lens. Note the difference in TxZ.

SMILEY FACE

If the lens sag is less than the corneal sag, the lens comes into contact with the apical cornea. This does not allow for a squeeze film force to be generated in the post-lens tear layer (Hayashi & Fatt 1980), thereby allowing the lid force to decentre the lens. This commonly results in a high-riding lens that causes a smiley face topography plot. The diagnosis can be made with either the axial or tangential map, but the detail in the tangential map is

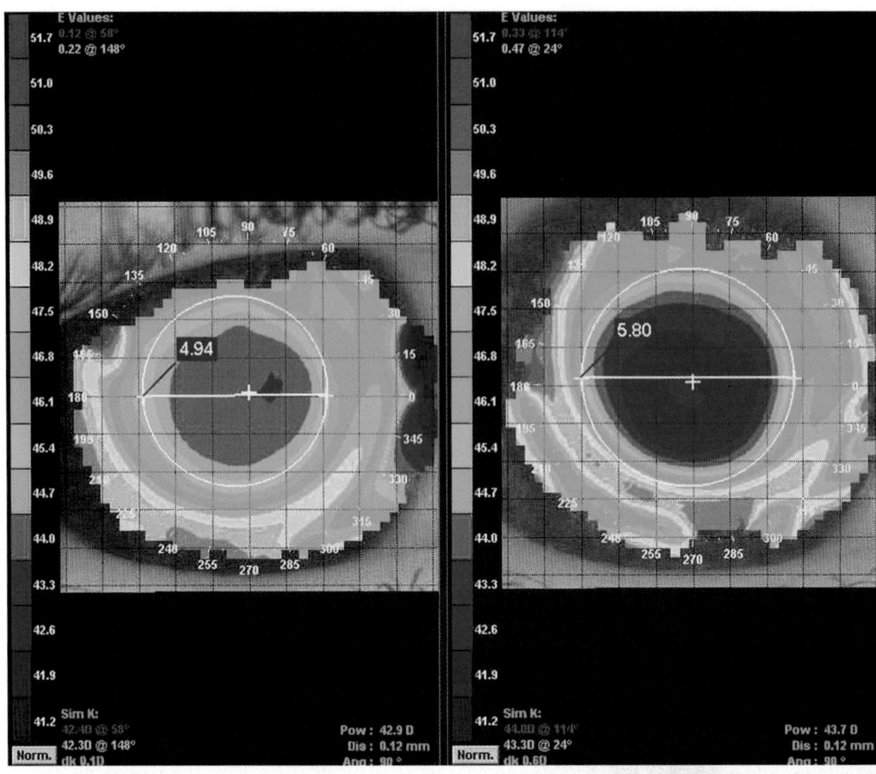

Figure 19.8 The change in TxZ following 1 week of wear. Note that the zone has increased by 1.00 mm between the first and seventh night of wear

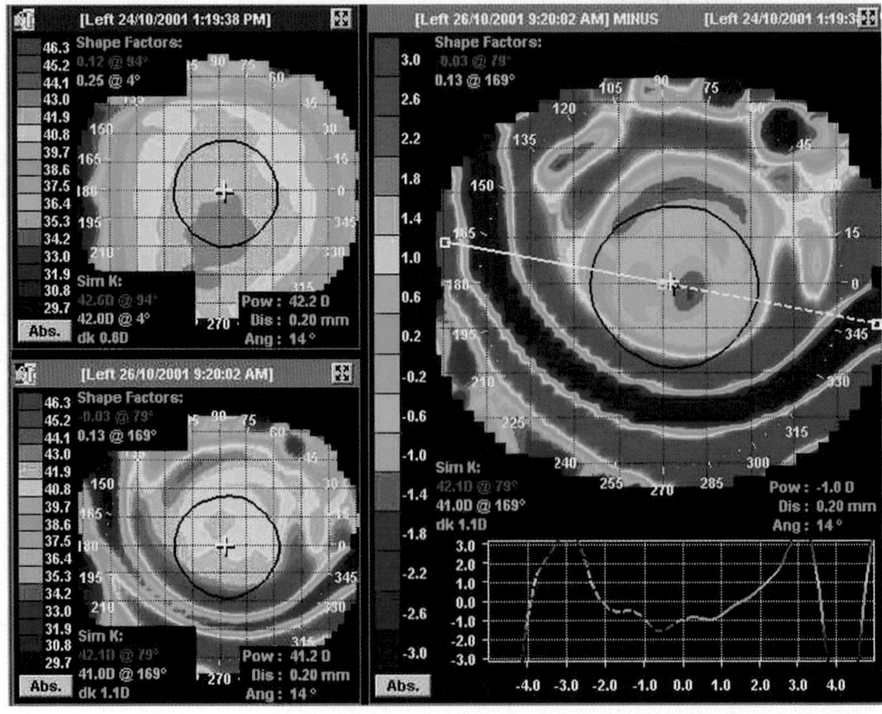

Figure 19.9 A tangential power difference map of a smiley face. Note the decentration of the 'red ring' towards the superior temporal area with respect to the pupil zone

much better as the complete red ring and its decentration are more evident.

Figure 19.9 shows a tangential map of a smiley face. The degree of decentration can be measured by drawing a circle around the red ring and then using the grid scale on the map to measure the displacement with respect to the pupil zone. This is an obvious smiley face. A mildly decentred smiley face is shown in Figure 19.10 with the decentration less than 1 mm. Unfortunately, smiley faces *always* get worse with time and decentration will increase following 1 week of wear (Fig. 19.11). This is commonly called 'creeping decentration'.

In all cases, the underlying cause is the same: the lens has insufficient sag.

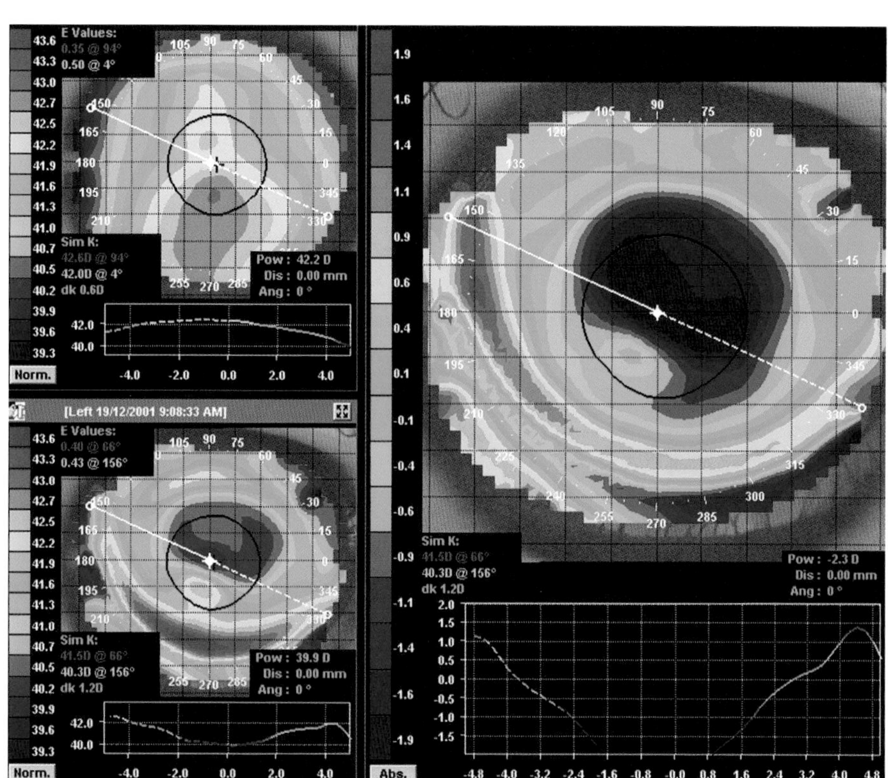

Figure 19.10 An axial power difference map of the same eye as in Figure 19.9. Note the flattened zone (blue) is not centred around the pupil. Even though the refractive change is 2.30 D, the patient would experience poor low-contrast vision and flare

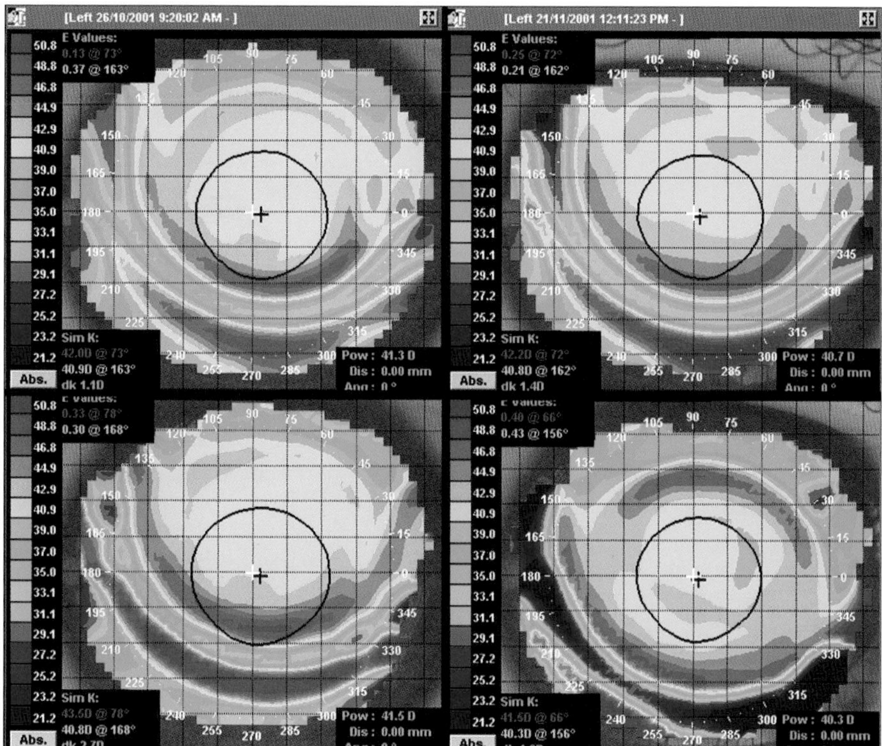

Figure 19.11 'Creeping decentration' from an initial smiley face. If the initial lens is decentred, the effect becomes worse with time

It cannot be assumed that the next steepest lens in the trial set will resolve the problem. The unknown quantity is how much lower the lens sag is compared to the corneal sag. Some degree of apical clearance is essential to avoid a smiley face, but this can change depending on the lid force. If the lids are tight, the lens may need to be appreciably steeper than expected in order to balance the forces. Figure 19.12 shows four repeated overnight trials with increasingly steeper trial lenses. The indicated lens was the 8.95 mm, but the lens that eventually caused the bull's-eye was the 8.80 mm.

Repeated overnight trials are therefore invaluable in making sure that the first lens ordered is the correct one, and that time and expense are not wasted in trying to correct for creeping decentration from an incorrect initial fit.

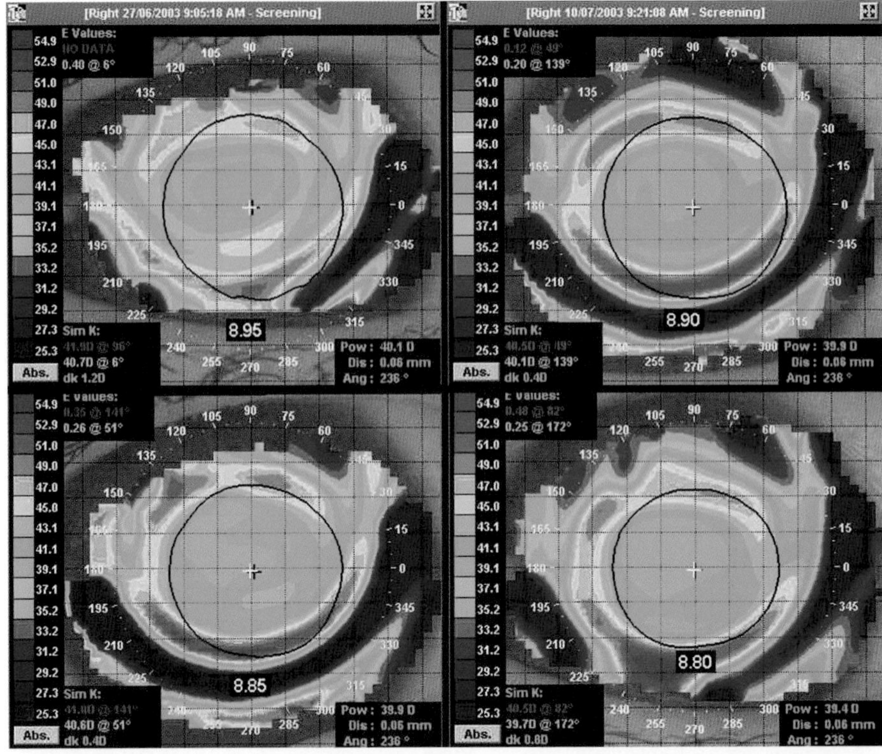

Figure 19.12 The results from four repeated overnight trials with progressively steeper lenses. The indicated lens was 8.95 mm, and caused a smiley face. The bull's-eye was achieved with an 8.80 mm BOZR lens

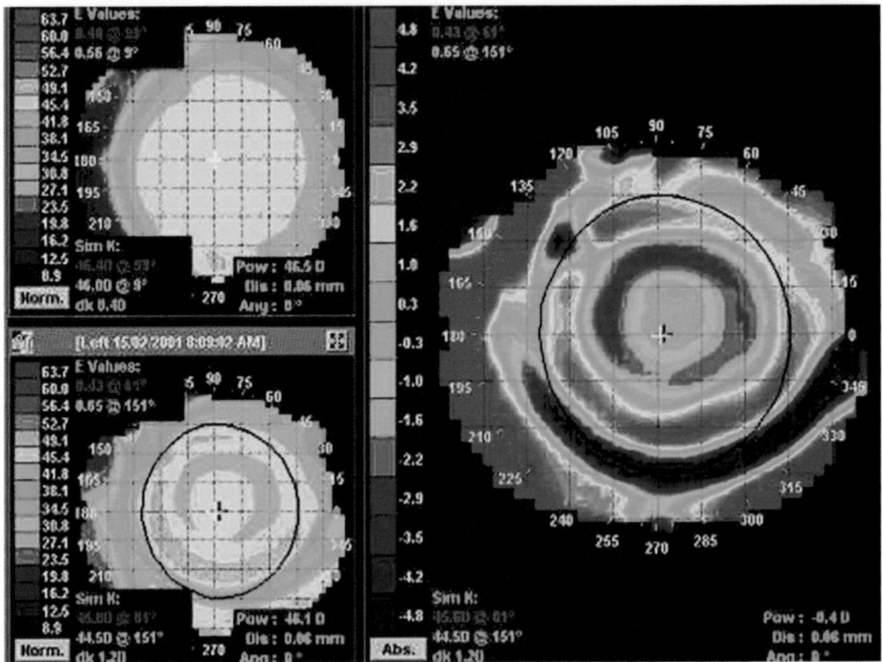

Figure 19.13 A tangential power difference map of the same eye as in Figure 19.12. The diagnosis is dependent on the 'red ring' and not the appearance of the island. Note the decentration of the red ring with respect to the pupil zone

SMILEY FACE WITH A FAKE CENTRAL ISLAND

There are three causes of a fake central island:

- *If an excessively flat lens comes into direct contact with the epithelium causing damage.* The resulting topography map will show what appears to be an island of central steepening with a decentred red ring. The distortion of the central mires due to the epithelial damage will cause inaccuracies in the reconstruction of the surface, resulting in the appearance of the steepened central zone.

It is easy to mistake a fake central island for a real central island. The practitioner orders a flatter lens (the correct treatment for a real central island) and it performs worse than the original lens. Once again, the diagnosis is made *not* by the presence of the island but by the *decentration of the red ring when compared to the pupil.* The tangential map (Fig. 19.13) shows this clearly.

- *When a lens binds on overnight wear and is poorly removed in the morning.* An island may be present but the red ring is perfectly centred. This is simply the distortion caused by

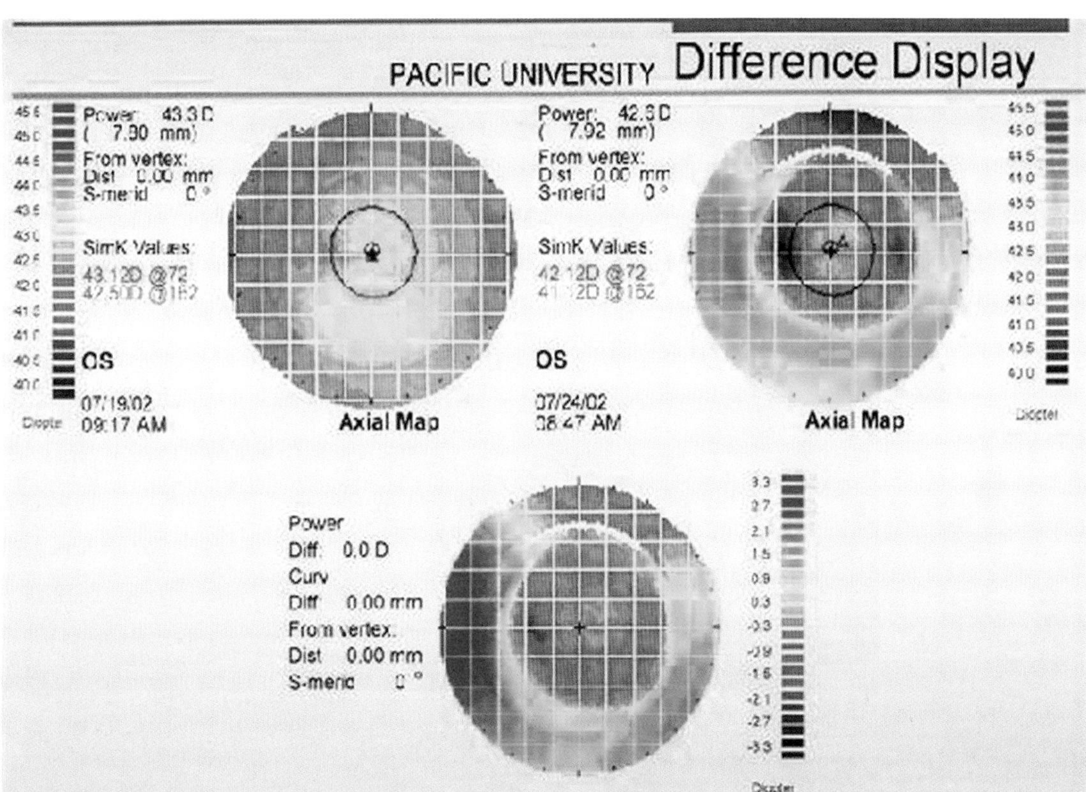

Figure 19.14 Another 'fake' central island due to the lack of smoothing as apex normal is reached. This is, in effect, a normal bull's-eye, but the result is clouded by the presence of 'noise' in the apical area. (Courtesy of Patrick Caroline)

epithelial disruption from lens binding. The patient should be taught the correct method of freeing up a bound lens and reviewed a few days later to confirm the diagnosis.

- *The actual reconstruction algorithm used by the instrument manufacturer*. The majority of topographers use an 'arc-step' method of surface reconstruction (see Chapter 7). However, as the corneal apex is approached, the tangent to the surface normally approaches 90° and the value of the apical radius approaches infinity. Some of the instruments overcome this contradiction by a process called 'smoothing' whereby the data from outside the central area are projected into the apex.

  Others (Humphrey, Keratron and Shin-Nippon), however, do not, and the resultant distortion of the apex appears as an island. An example of this is shown in Figure 19.14 where the associated fitting note diagnoses the problem as a central island. It is not. The island is basically a mathematical 'glitch' caused by the reconstruction algorithm and there is no valid reason why the algorithm cannot be smoothed to decrease confusion.

To rectify smiley faces with fake central islands, a steeper trial lens should be used until a bull's-eye appearance is achieved.

CENTRAL ISLAND

Central islands occur when the lens is:

- Too steep.
- Too large in total diameter (TD).
- Too tight in the alignment zone or tangent.

Central islands cause a reduction in refractive change and a drop in best-corrected visual acuity (BCVA). They are characterized by a 2.00 mm diameter area of central steepening where the apical power is actually steeper than the original cornea and surrounded by an annulus of corneal flattening (Fig. 19.15). The tangential difference map shows the red ring to be perfectly centred on the pupil. The difference between a real central island and an incomplete bull's-eye is that the apical corneal power is always steeper in the central island, whereas the incomplete bull's-eye will show either no change at the apex or a mild reduction of 0.50 D. Central islands do not improve with time whereas an incomplete bull's-eye will resolve with a few extra nights of trial wear.

Central islands are associated with topographers that underestimate corneal eccentricity because of:

- The reconstruction algorithm.
- The chord over which the eccentricity is measured.
- The use of a 'global' eccentricity instead of the eccentricity of the flat meridian.
- Topographers that utilize extrapolation to fill in missing areas.

Underestimation of the eccentricity leads to an overestimation of the lens sag such that the lens has excessive apical clearance and a tight periphery. If the alignment curves are designed from data that underestimate eccentricity, they will be too steep and raise the whole lens above the corneal surface. If the apical clearance is greater than the tear layer thickness in the steeper meridian, the squeeze film forces are reversed, resulting in a central island (Mountford 2004a).

FROWNY FACE

A frowny face (Fig. 19.16) occurs when:

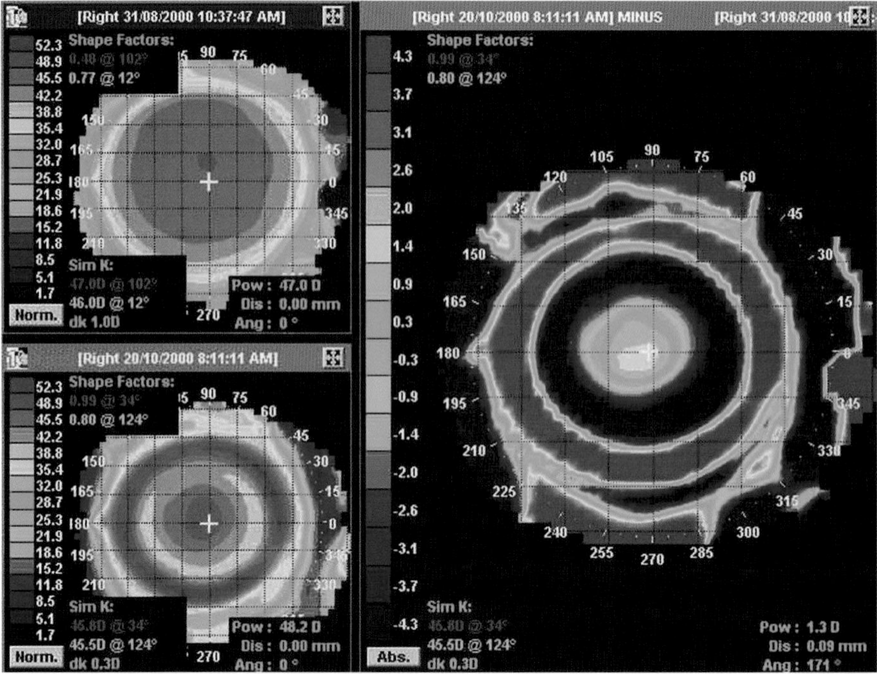

Figure 19.15 A tangential power difference map showing a central island. Note that the island is steeper than the original cornea, and that the 'red ring' is perfectly centred

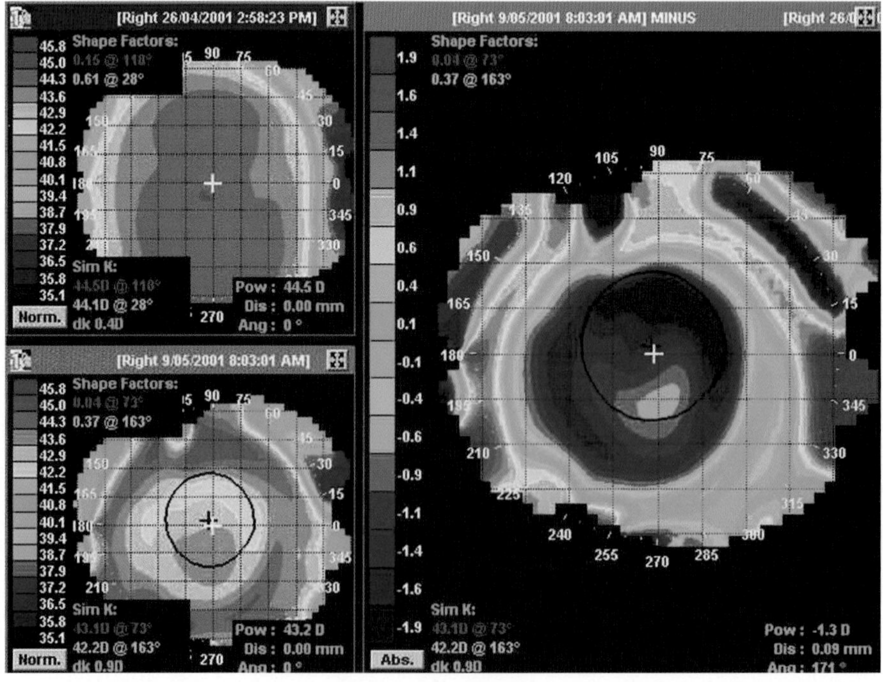

Figure 19.16 A frowny face difference map. Note that the treatment area is decentred inferiorly with respect to the pupil zone

- The lens is marginally tight, somewhere between a bull's-eye and a central island.
- The lens is too tight in the alignment curve.
- Lid tension is high.
- The TD too small.

In these cases the red ring is decentred inferiorly. If allowed to persist, a central island will occur (Fig. 19.17) and the decentration will increase. This leads to an increase in reports of flare and haloes at night and associated ghosting during the day. The quality of the unaided VA is also adversely affected.

LATERAL DECENTRATION

Lateral decentration is frustrating and intractable. It is more common in Asian eyes than Caucasian and reported causes are:

- TD too small.
- Tight or loose alignment curves.

A review of cases of lateral decentration shows that there are two common findings:

- Tight eyelids.
- A marked difference in curvature in the alignment zone between the nasal and temporal sides.

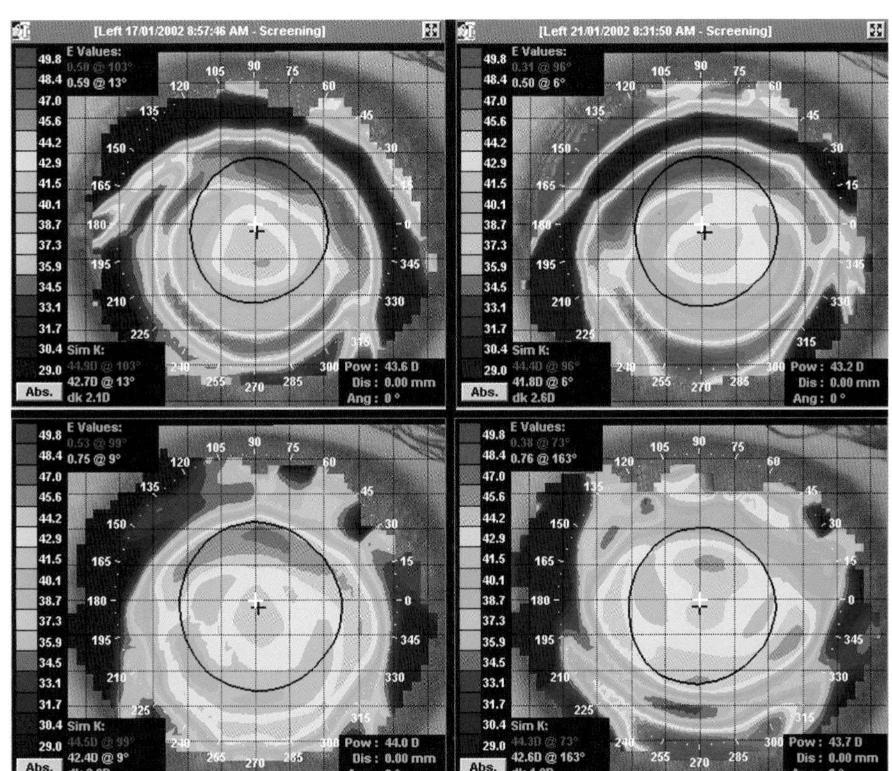

Figure 19.17 Sequential topography of a mild frowny face becoming worse with time and leading to island formation

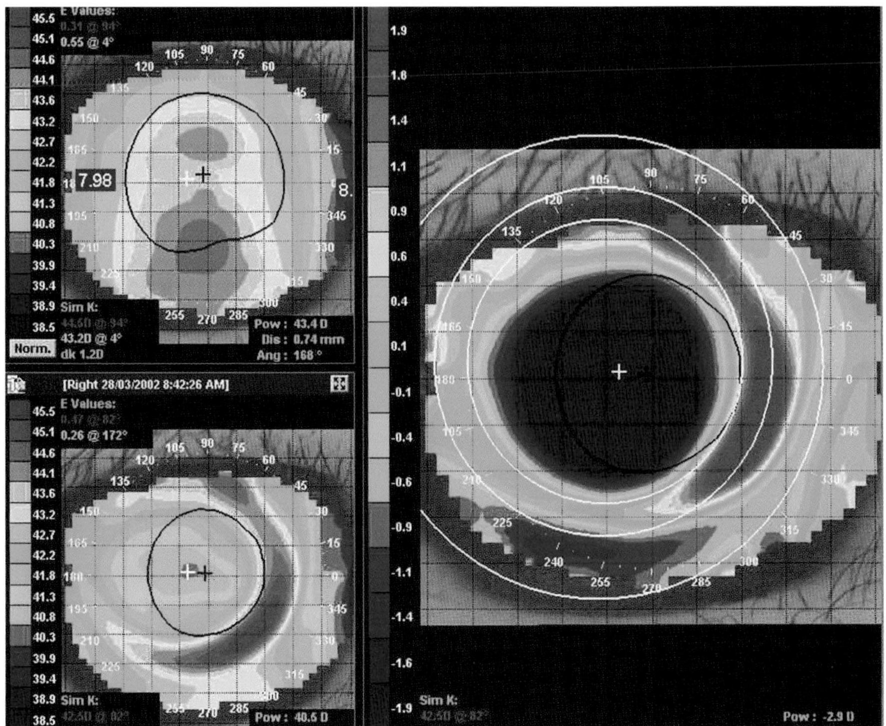

Figure 19.18 A case of lateral decentration. Note that the lens (with the BOZD, RC and AC drawn in white) is decentred temporally by approximately 1.50 mm. The presence of the red ring in the pupil zone will cause marked ghosting and flare

Figure 19.18 shows a subtractive map of lateral decentration. The treatment zone is decentred towards the nasal side with the red ring encroaching the pupil zone on the temporal side.

At present, there are no absolute or predictable rules for correcting lateral decentration. The author has attempted correction by increasing lens diameter, tightening or loosening the alignment curves or tangent, and even using a smaller TD. None appears to be effective with the exception of large-diameter lenses (12.00 mm). However, this is then compounded by inaccuracies in the measurement of the peripheral cornea, and the lens invariably ends up too tight, thus causing a central island. Where lateral decentration occurs on an overnight trial the practitioner is left with two choices:

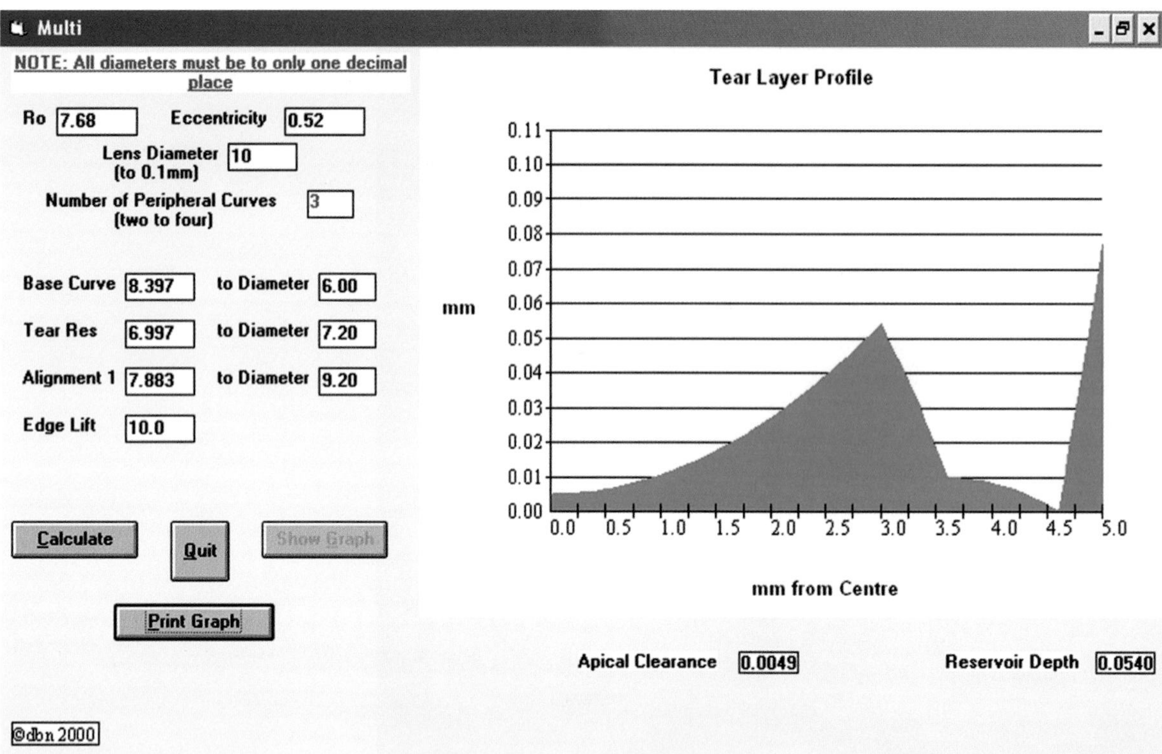

Figure 19.19 The tear layer profile of the original lens on the initial eye shape. If this lens decentres, then the probable cause is topography overestimation of eccentricity

- Advise that effective treatment is not possible.
- Be prepared for a time-consuming and expensive period of experimentation and lens re-makes.

Solving suboptimal outcomes

In routine rigid lens fitting, there are 'rules' that apply when a lens design needs to be altered to bring about an improvement in fit (see Chapter 9). The same rules apply to reverse geometry lenses except that the BOZD, BOZR and reverse curve (RC) zone width are not altered. Only the RC and alignment curve (AC) values can be altered to change the fit of the lens. The rules of thumb are:

- Flattening the AC by 0.05 mm (0.25 D) decreases the apical clearance by 5 µm.
- Steepening the AC by 0.05 mm (0.25 D) increases the apical clearance by 5 µm.
- Flattening the RC by 0.15 mm (0.75 D) decreases the apical clearance by 10 µm.
- Steepening the RC by 0.15 mm (0.75 D) increases the apical clearance by 10 µm.

If the trial wear period results in a bull's-eye then no changes need to be made to the final lens design.

SMILEY FACE OUTCOMES

If a smiley face occurs as a result of the trial, the lens sag is less than the corneal sag and must be increased to optimize the fit.

Figure 19.19 shows the tear layer profile of a lens based on the following data: r_0, 7.68; eccentricity, 0.52; standard deviation of eccentricity error from repeated readings, 0.10 or 15 µm; refractive change, 3.00 D.

The lens is worn overnight and a smiley face results. The degree of lens flatness can be assessed using the repeated readings and calculation of instrument error. The standard deviation of error in eccentricity values is typically ±0.10.

Smiley face outcomes are caused by the lens sag being less than the corneal sag. An *underestimation* of corneal sag occurs when the topographer *overestimates* eccentricity.

The same lens is now shown on a cornea where the eccentricity value has been changed to 0.42 (Fig. 19.20). If the eccentricity has been overestimated, then the standard deviation value is subtracted from the original data.

Note that the lens now shows apical touch. In order to correct the fit of the lens, the reverse curve and alignment curve must be steepened. In this case the reverse curve has been steepened by 0.15 mm (increasing the sag by 10 µm) and the alignment curve steepened by 0.10 mm (10 µm). The lens now has the ideal TLT of approximately 10 µm of apical clearance and 10 µm clearance at the RC/AC junction (Fig. 19.21). In total, the lens sag has been increased by 20 µm, so the patient should return for another overnight trial with a trial lens two steps 'steeper' (assuming a 10 µm difference in lens sag in the trial set).

If the trial wear period resulted in a smiley face with a fake central island, then the lens sag was appreciably less than the

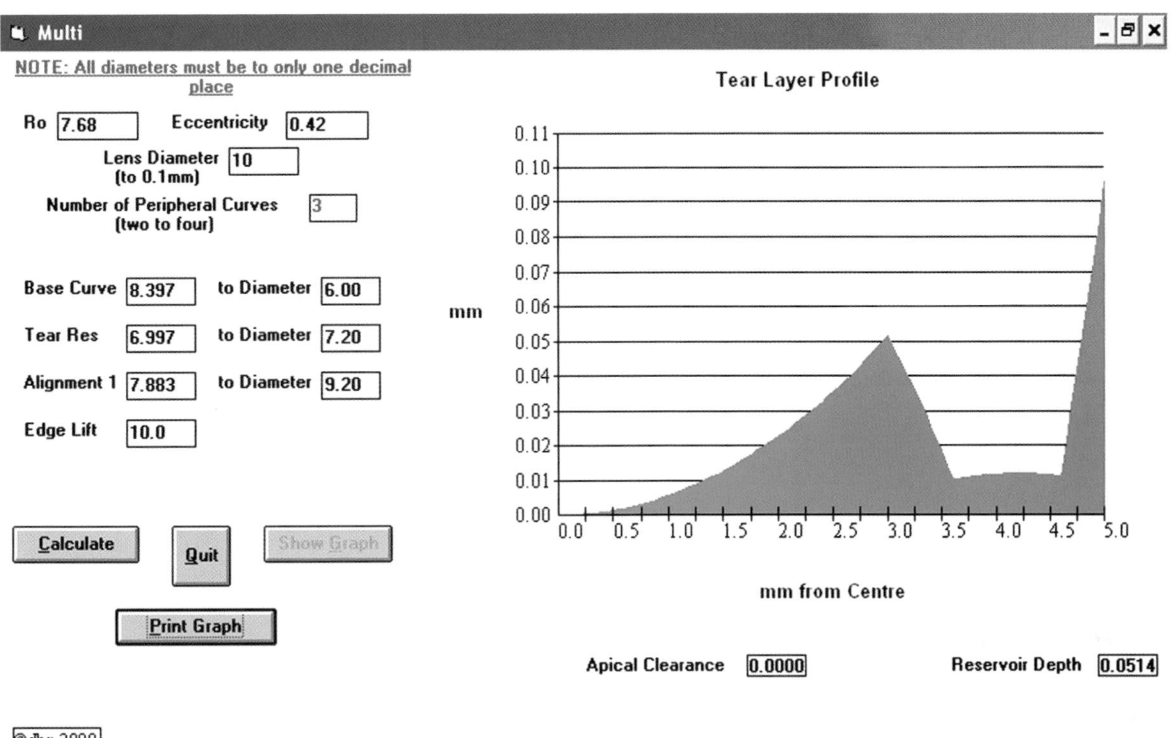

Figure 19.20 The same lens on the 'altered' corneal data with an eccentricity of 0.42. The lens is now effectively too flat, and will cause the smiley face

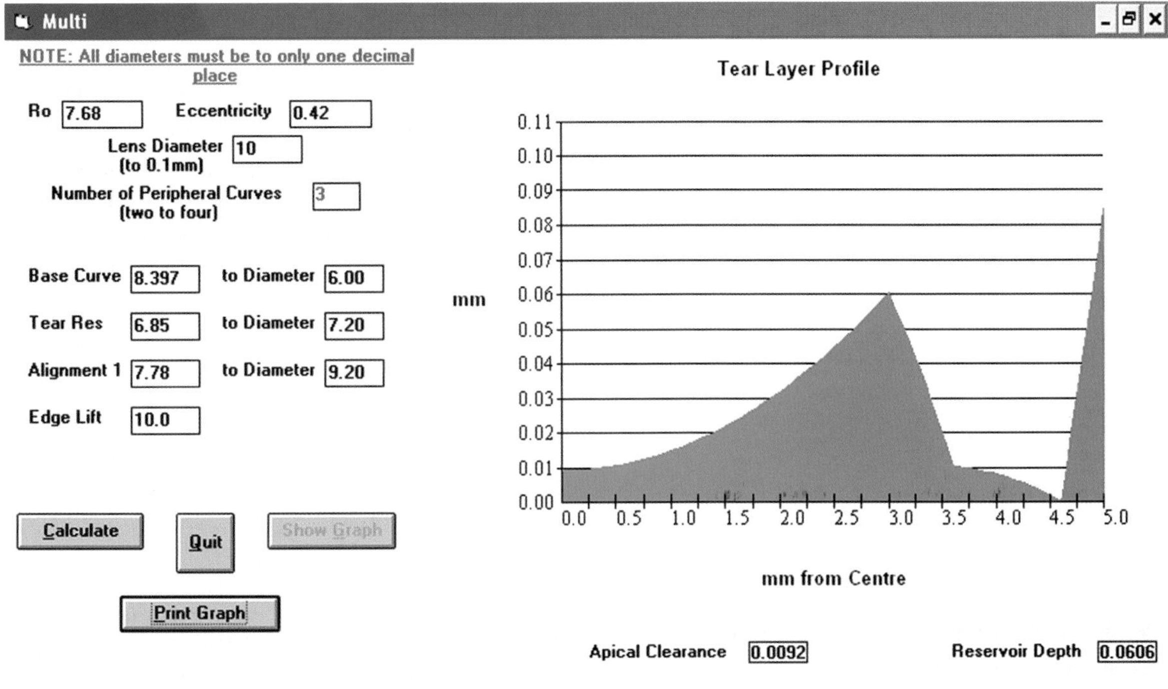

Figure 19.21 The reverse curve and alignment curve have been steepened and the lens now has the correct fitting relationship

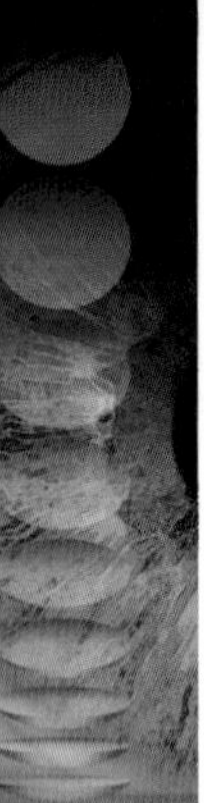

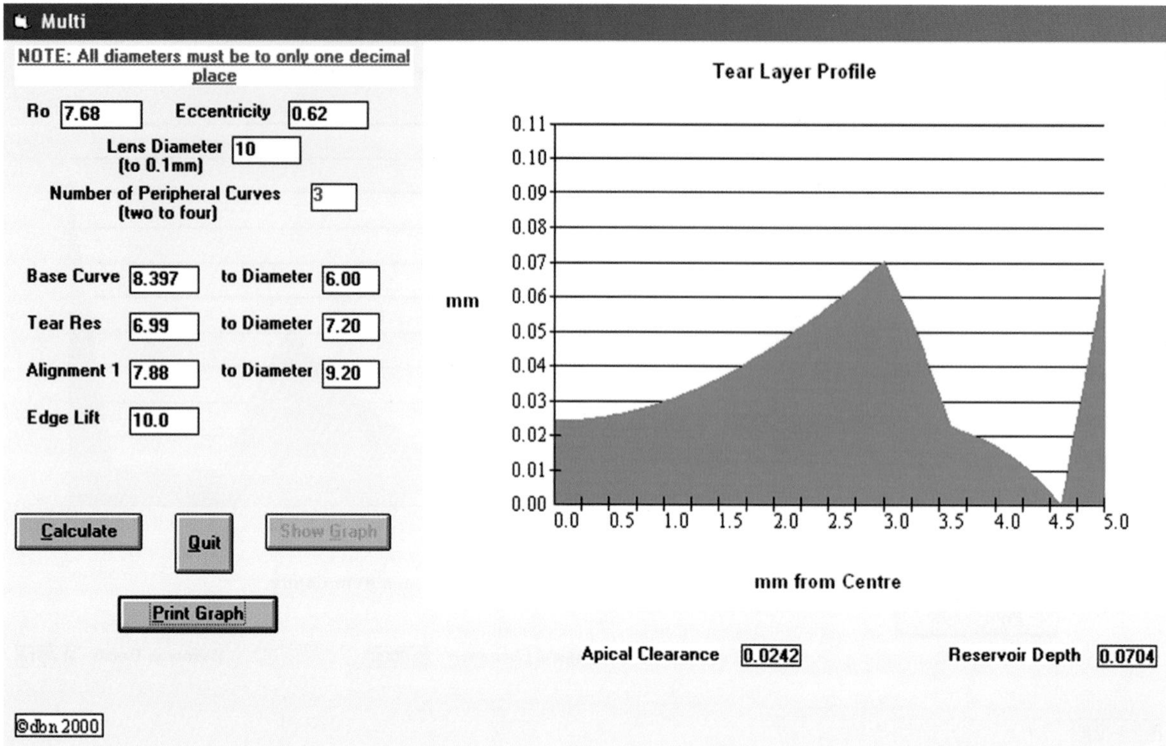

Figure 19.22 A case of central island formation due to topography underestimation of eccentricity. The lens is steep with a tight alignment curve

corneal sag due to an even greater overestimation of corneal eccentricity. In these cases it is wiser to assume that the error was closer to 0.20 in eccentricity. Once again, a re-trial with a lens of greater sag or steeper alignment curves will be necessary to arrive at the correct fit.

CENTRAL ISLANDS AND FROWNY FACE OUTCOMES

Central island and frowny face outcomes are due to the lens sag being appreciably greater then the corneal sag due to topographer underestimation of eccentricity. This will lead to a trial lens that has a tight alignment curve that will increase the apical clearance of the lens. Using the same data as above, the tear layer profile of a lens where the eccentricity has been underestimated by 0.10 ('real' eccentricity 0.62) is shown in Figure 19.22.

Note that the lens has a steep alignment and reverse curve leading to approximately 25 μm of apical clearance. In this case the reverse curve will be flattened by 0.15 mm and the alignment curve by 0.10 mm, leading to a decrease in lens sag of 20 μm. The 'final' lens design is shown in Figure 19.23.

In the case of a frowny face outcome, the changes are more subtle, and a simple flattening of the alignment curve by 0.10 mm may be all that is required.

If the basic design is known (the BOZD, RC and AC widths), the inputs can be altered to determine what RC was used. The errors in eccentricity can then be introduced and alterations to the design made. However, this programme uses the well-established sag philosophy approach and may need major alterations if the original lens design was based on keratometry values (i.e. assuming that the cornea is a sphere and not taking corneal eccentricity into account) instead of topography data.

HYPERMETROPIA CORRECTION

Interest in hypermetropia correction has increased since Tung presented his results at the 2004 Global Orthokeratology Symposium. Since then lens designs for hypermetropia correction have been developed by Tung (2004, Vipok-Dual Geometric Lens), Leggerton (CRT), Tabb (Nightmove) and Mountford and Noack (BE).

Historically, Jessen (1962) reported greater success in reducing hypermetropia than myopia due to the corneal moulding he was able to induce by using the de Carle bifocal design; however, he noted that central oedema may have influenced the outcome as all lenses were made from PMMA.

The use of highly aspheric lenses for hypermetropia reduction was reviewed by Goldberg (1996). He advocated the use of constant apical radii lenses with variations in eccentricity to correct varying levels of hypermetropia. The BOZR was based on the Jessen factor (see p. 427), but in reverse, and the application of mid-peripheral compression by altering the eccentricity, i.e. the higher the eccentricity of the lens back surface, the greater the control over the effect. This astute paper was ahead of its time as the basic tenets that he espoused are

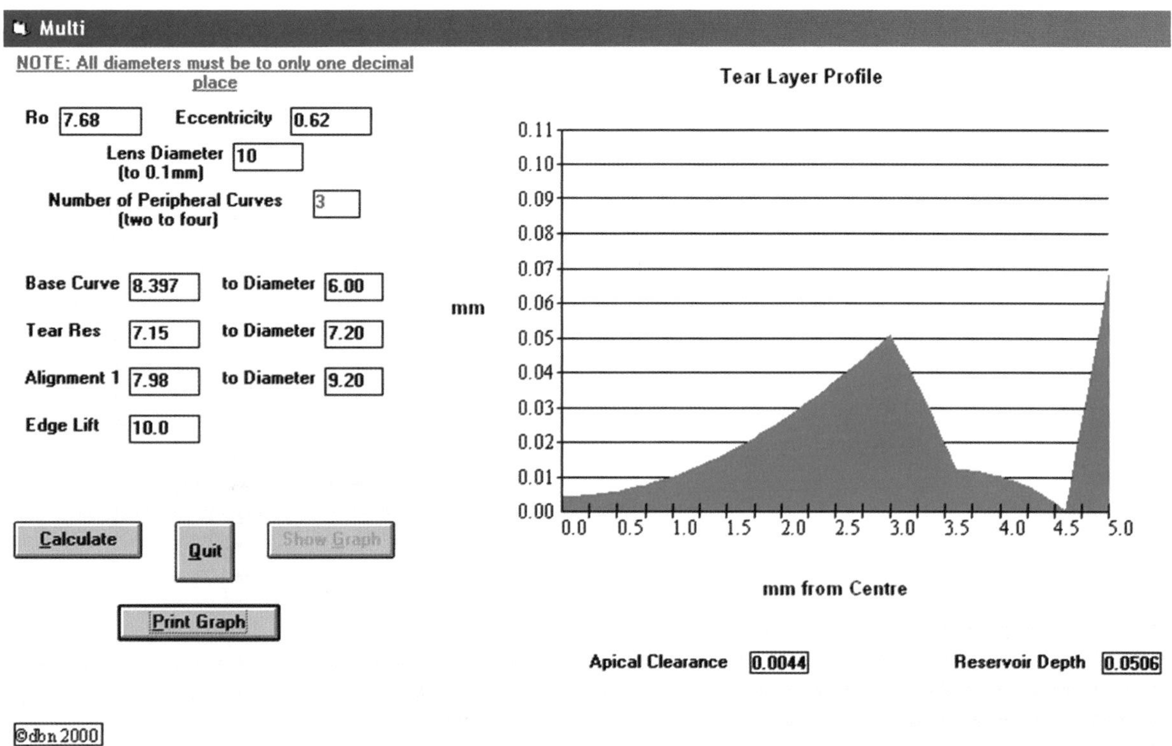

Figure 19.23 The fit of the lens has been corrected by flattening the reverse and alignment curves (see text)

currently being applied to the new generation of reverse geometry lenses.

It is well known that 'steep' lenses steepen the cornea although this has only recently been proven scientifically (Swarbrick 2004b). Orthokeratology 'works' the same for hypermetropia as myopia by applying a differential in pressure in the post-lens tear layer across the corneal surface (Mountford 2004a). The cornea alters shape in response to the pressure differential until some form of equalization of force occurs in the post-lens tear layer. In effect, the force is positive or compressive centrally and negative or tension at the BOZD/RC junction.

The correction of hypermetropia is effectively the application of the myopia theory in reverse: the compression is applied to the mid-peripheral cornea and the tension centrally.

Tung (2004) achieves this by using a steep central spherical curve with a wide, flat second curve and a peripheral reverse curve (Fig. 19.24).

Leggerton (CRT) alters the sigmoid proximity curve such that it makes contact along the curve with the peripheral zone being a tangent (Fig. 19.25). In both cases the Jessen factor is used to determine the BOZR such that a 3.00 D refractive change would require a BOZR 3.50 D (0.70 mm) *steeper* than K_F. The lenses are fitted with apical clearance.

The BE philosophy is to reverse the modelled squeeze film forces to the opposite of those used for myopic correction (Fig. 19.26). The central force for hypermetropia is now negative or tension, and that in the mid-periphery compressive or positive force. A fluorescein pattern is shown in Figure 19.27. Note that the fluorescein patterns between the designs are similar with apical clearance, mid-peripheral bearing followed by an area of steepening, and finally, a wide alignment zone.

A post-wear topography map of 1.50 D reduction of hypermetropia is shown in Figure 19.28. Note the central steepening and mid-peripheral flattening of the cornea. This is the exact opposite of what occurs with myopia, where the central cornea is flattened with an associated mid-peripheral steepening of the cornea.

Presbyopia

Leggerton (CRT) and Tung (2004, Vipok) are designing lenses that cause a multifocal effect on the cornea but research is still in its infancy (personal communication, 2005).

Astigmatism

Mountford and Pesudovs (2002) showed that the mean reduction in astigmatism with orthokeratology was approximately 50% and that it was unpredictable, with the major change occurring over the central 2.00 mm chord. With higher degrees of astigmatism, reverse geometry lenses may actually *increase* the astigmatism due to an inability to 'push' the astigmatism out of the pupil zone (Fig. 19.29). If the flat meridian is flattened, but the steep meridian is not flattened more, then astigmatism will increase. The problem, therefore, is to design a lens that will cause greater changes in the steeper than in the flatter meridian.

Baertschi and colleagues in Switzerland have designed a unique 'toric' reverse geometry lens design that effectively reduces

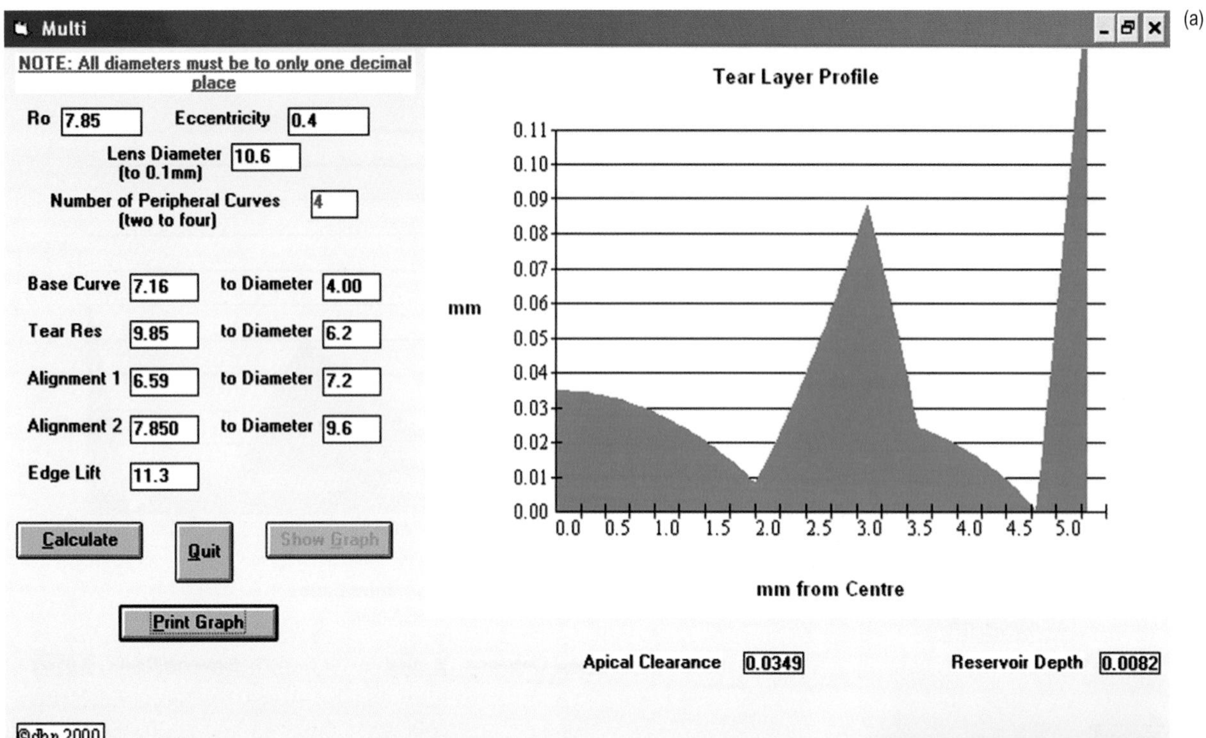

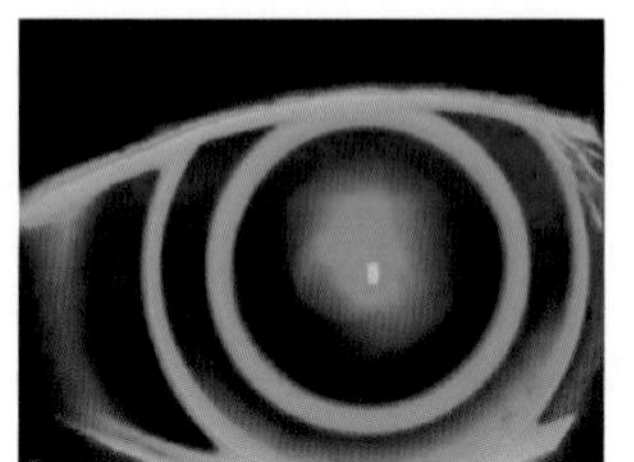

Figure 19.24 (a) Tear layer profile of the Vipok XC hypermetropia lens. Note the steep central curve, with a flatter secondary curve, a reverse curve and alignment zone. (b) Fluorescein pattern of the Vipok lens, showing apical clearance and mid-peripheral compression or touch. (Courtesy of Dr Hsiao-Ching Tung)

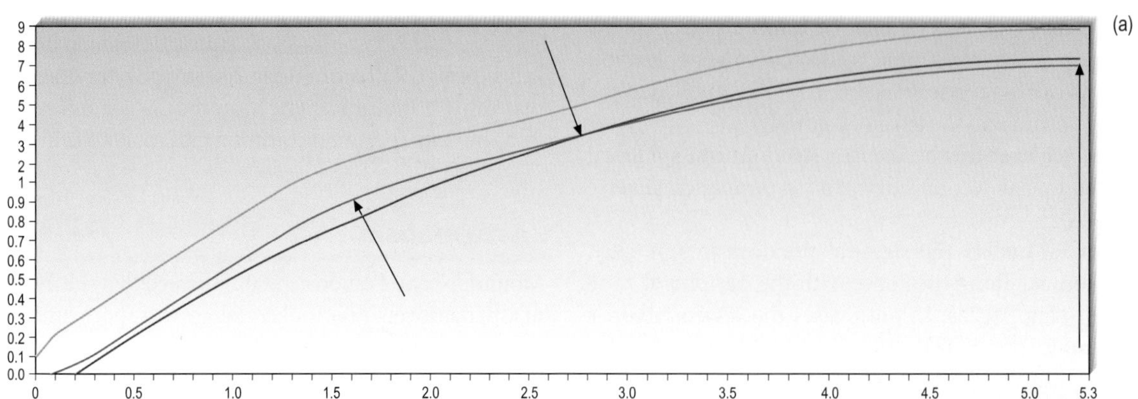

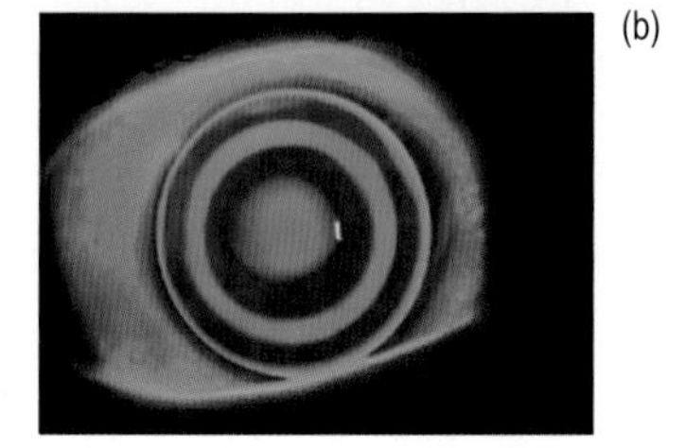

Figure 19.25 (a) A profile of the CRT hypermetropia lens showing the use of the sigmoid proximity curve to apply mid-peripheral compression at the edge of the BOZD (down arrow). The relief zone (up arrow) shows the sigmoid curve allowing clearance prior to meeting the tangent peripheral zone. (b) Fluorescein pattern of the CRT lens for hypermetropia. Note the central clearance, mid-peripheral touch, relief zone and tangent. (Courtesy of Jerry Leggerton)

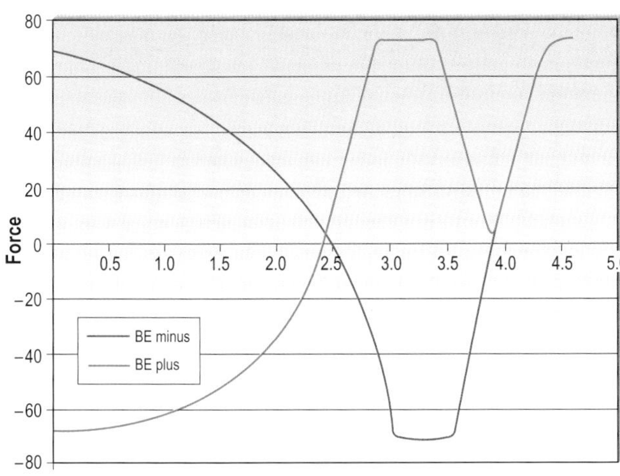

Figure 19.26 The squeeze film force graph of a standard myopia BE (purple line) and that of the hypermetropic BE (red line). Note that the forces generated over the central zones are opposites. The myopic BE shows central compression and peripheral tension, whereas the hyperopic design shows central tension and peripheral compression

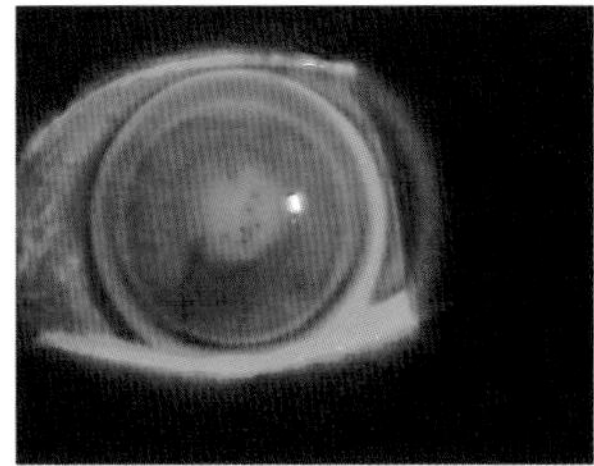

Figure 19.27 Fluorescein pattern of a hypermetropic BE. Note the similarities with all the hypermetropic designs

up to 3.00 D of corneal astigmatism (Mountford 2004b). In lower degrees of astigmatism (≤1.50 D), the BOZR is spherical but the reverse and alignment curves are toric in order to align the peripheral cornea and also manipulate the squeeze film force in the steep meridian. For higher astigmatism (>2.00 D) the BOZR, RC and AC are all toric. The fluorescein pattern of the lens is shown in Figure 19.30, and a topography map showing the correction of 2.50 D of astigmatism in Figure 19.31. The success of this design apparently lies in the ability to 'push' the astigmatism out past the pupil zone. The correction of astigmatism requires complex designs and high degrees of manufacturing tolerance. Once again, it is a fertile area for future controlled research.

High myopia correction

All the controlled studies on modern orthokeratology have involved the correction of up to 4.00 D of myopia as that has been considered to be the maximum change possible.

This is primarily due to two factors:

- Limitations of change due to the eccentricity model.
- The effect that larger refractive change may have on treatment zone diameter and corneal epithelial thickness.

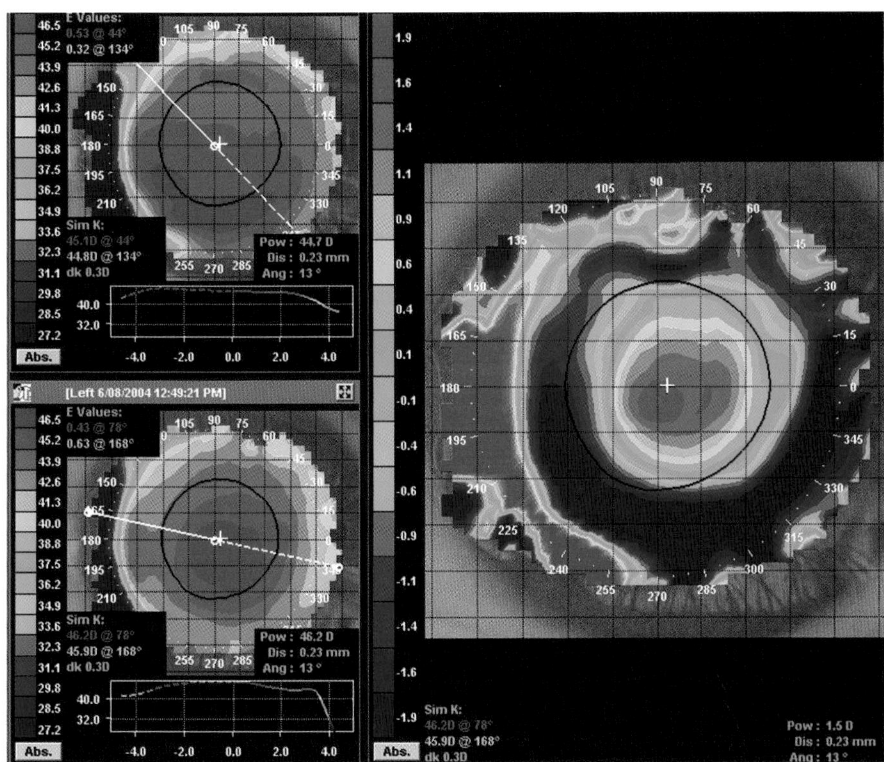

Figure 19.28 The result of one night's wear of a hypermetropic lens. The central cornea has steepened by 1.50 D. Note the flattening of the paracentral zone

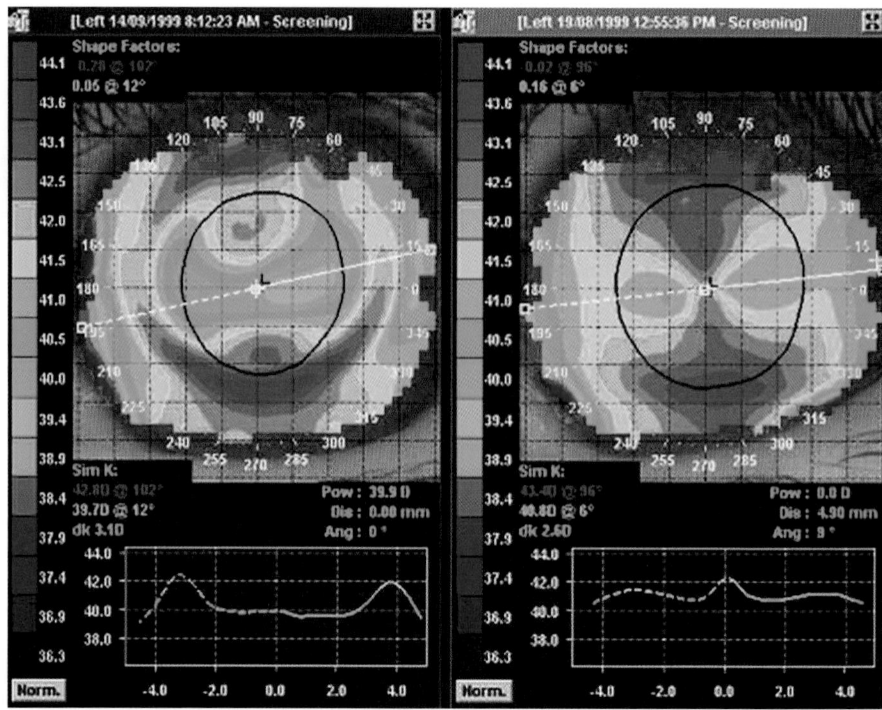

Figure 19.29 The map on the right is the pre-fit map and the one on the left the post-orthokeratography map. Although the horizontal meridian has flattened dramatically, the vertical meridian still has elements of the original astigmatism in the pupil zone, leading to an increase in post-treatment astigmatism

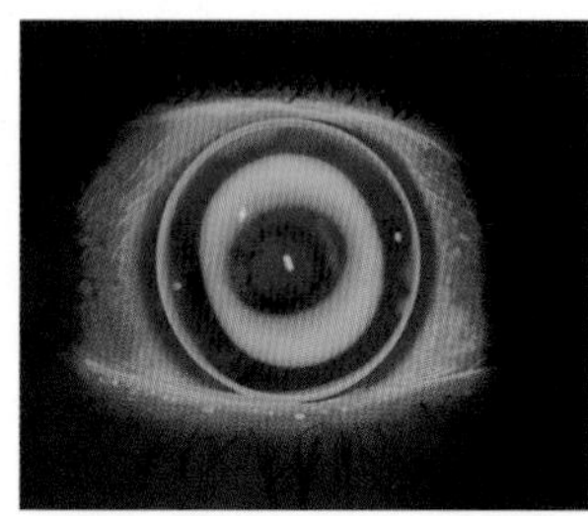

Figure 19.30 A fluorescein pattern of an astigmatic ortho-K lens. Note the difference in appearance of the reverse zone in the flat and steep meridians. (Courtesy of Michael Baertschi, and kind permission of Contact Lens Spectrum)

Alharbi and Swarbrick (2003) showed a correlation between epithelial thickness change and refractive change using Munnerlyn's formula for refractive surgery. The formula states:

Ablation depth = $RD^2/3$

where R is refractive change in dioptres, and D the diameter of the treatment zone.

A surgical refractive change of 3.00 D over a treatment zone diameter would therefore require an ablation depth of 25 µm. In the orthokeratology context, ablation depth is equivalent to central epithelial thinning which appears to be limited to a maximum of 20 µm (Alharbi & Swarbrick 2003). Therefore, the consensus has been that greater refractive change would automatically lead to the treatment zone being too small, resulting in flare and haloes in dim illumination. A 6.00 D change is shown in Figure 19.32. Note that the treatment zone is small and less than the pupil diameter in normal illumination.

The main impetus for greater refractive change is in Asia where myopia, in general, is higher in both incidence and severity than in western countries and is a major reason for parents to seek orthokeratology treatment for their children (Cho et al. 2005; see Chapter 30).

Tung (2004) has been involved in the correction of high (>6.00 D) myopia using the Vipok, Dk-4 and Contex designs. A 6.00 D refractive change is shown in Figure 19.33. Note the difference in treatment zone diameter between this case and that shown in Figure 19.32. In the first case, the BCVA was 6/12 and poorly maintained, but in the second case the unaided VA was 6/6 and maintained for all waking hours.

The difference between the two may be due to either the design or the fitting philosophy. The first example cited above was fitted with a single lens whereas the second case required refitting for greater refractive change with a second set of lenses. What these early results show is that it may indeed be possible to correct higher degrees of myopia without compromising both epithelial health and treatment zone diameter. This should be performed under controlled research.

CLINICAL RESEARCH RESULTS

As stated at the beginning of this chapter, there has been an explosion in academic interest in orthokeratology over the last 7 years. The following section briefly describes the results of the research.

Refractive change

Table 19.2 is a synopsis of the refractive changes achieved with the study groups. The mean change is approximately 2.00 D in

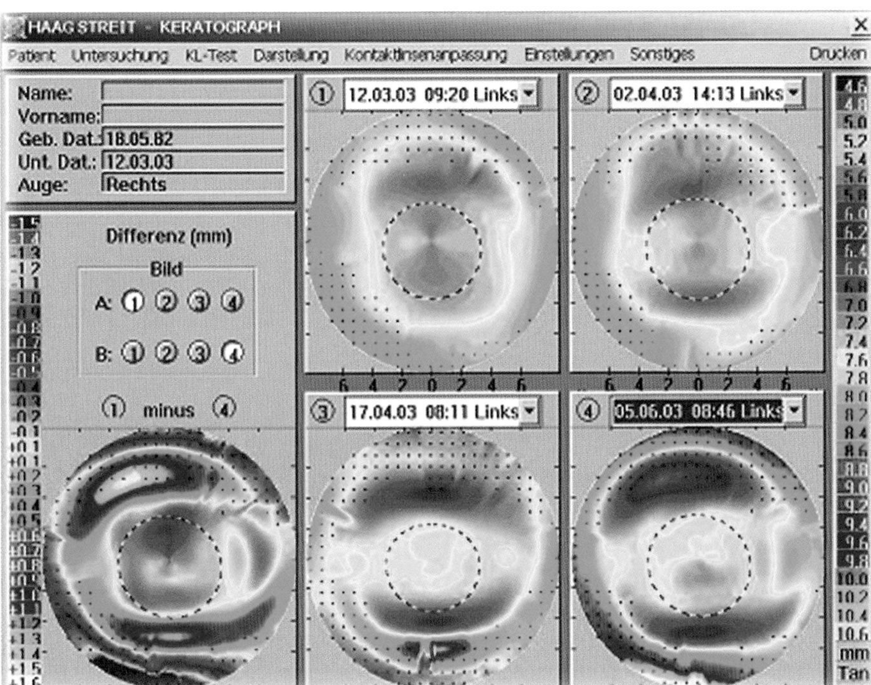

Figure 19.31 Sequential topography of a reduction of 2.50 D astigmatism. Note that the astigmatism has been 'pushed' out of the pupil zone. Initial Rx –2.25/–2.50 at 180°. Final Rx +0.25/–0.25 at 180°. (Courtesy of Michael Baertschi, and kind permission of Contact Lens Spectrum)

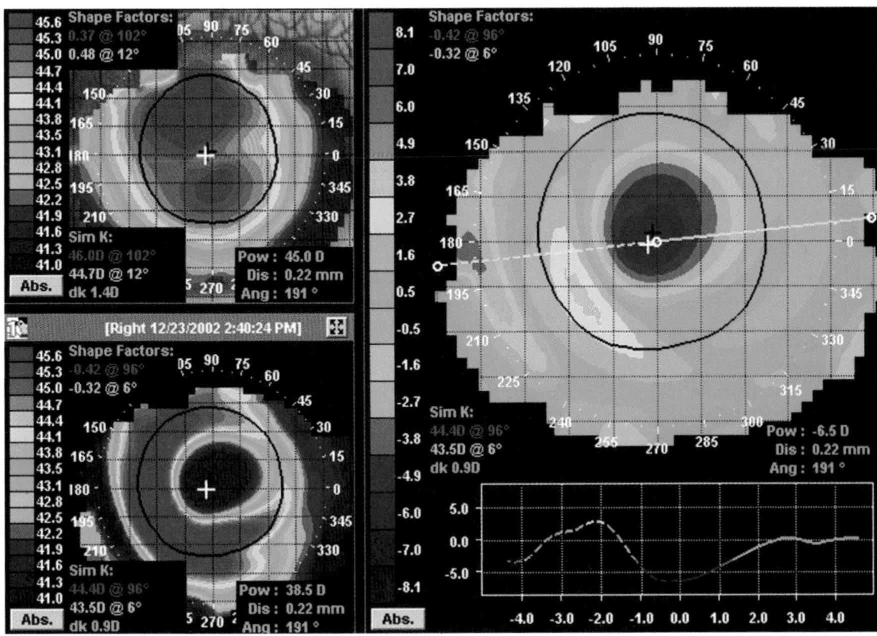

Figure 19.32 A 6.00 D refractive change associated with a small treatment zone, which is much smaller than the pupil diameter. The high-contrast VA was 6/12. (Courtesy of Shane Keddie)

the earlier studies but this could occur mainly due to the initial selection criteria that were used.

Tung (2004) presented the results of a retrospective study of attempting higher refractive changes using the Vipok XC lens. The results show an almost linear correlation between the attempted change and the achieved change. Larger studies would be useful to reassess this finding.

Myopia control (see also Chapter 30)

There has been a common belief amongst some orthokeratologists that the procedure can retard the progression of myopia. In Asia this is the most common reason why parents present their children for lens fitting (Cho et al. 2005).

Cho et al. (2005) studied myopia progression in a group of 43 Hong Kong Chinese children undergoing orthokeratology and compared the changes in axial length and vitreous chamber depth to an age-, sex- and refractive error-matched group of spectacle wearers. The data from the control group had come from a previous study on myopia increase in children. The participants were followed regularly over a 2-year period.

The spectacle group had a mean increase in myopia of 0.75 D per year associated with an annual increase in axial length of 0.27 mm. The orthokeratology group had an annual increase in

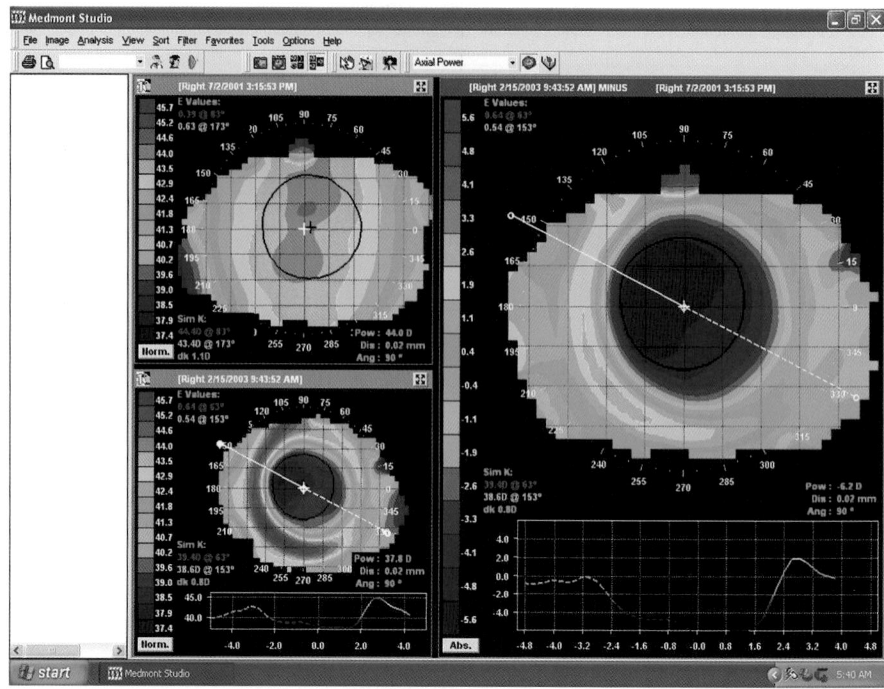

Figure 19.33 An ideal 6.00 D change with a large treatment zone. Unaided VA 6/6. (Courtesy of Stan Isaacs)

Table 19.2: The change in refractive error reported by different studies

Author(s)	Sample size	Lens design	Duration of lens wear	Mean Rx change (D)
Lui & Edwards (2000)	14	3-zone (Contex)	DW: 100 days	1.50 ± 0.49 D
Mountford (1997)	60	3-zone (Contex)	O/N wear: 90 days	2.19 ± 0.57 D
Nichols et al. (2000)	8	3-zone (Contex)	O/N wear: 60 days	1.83 ± 1.23 D
Rah et al. (2002)	60	4-zone (CRT, Fargo)	O/N wear: 90 days	2.08 ± 1.11 D
Soni et al. (2003)	8	4-zone (Contex)	O/N wear: 90 days	2.12 D
Tahhan et al. (2003)	60	All 4-zone: various designs	O/N wear: 30 days	2.00 D (approx.)
Alharbi & Swarbrick (2003)	18	BE design	O/N wear: 90 days	2.54 ± 0.63 D
Joslin et al. (2003)	9	CRT	O/N wear: 30 days	3.08 ± 0.93 D

DW, daily wear; O/N, overnight.

myopia of 0.39 D associated with an axial length increase of 0.14 mm. The differences were highly statistically significant.

The other interesting finding was that in the spectacle group the more myopic participants exhibited faster progression of their myopia whereas the more myopic participants in the orthokeratology group showed the greatest slowing in progression of the condition.

It would appear from the results of this pilot study that there is a positive role for orthokeratology in myopia control.

Corneal thickness changes

Alharbi and Swarbrick (2003) were the first to describe the corneal thickness changes occurring as a result of reverse geometry lens wear. They showed that the central epithelium thins and the mid-peripheral stroma thickens. The study was repeated with overnight wear of the lenses (Alharbi & Swarbrick 2003) with similar results (Fig. 19.34). The central epithelium thinned by approximately 16 μm, and the mid-peripheral stroma thickened by a similar amount. Interestingly, there was an apparent inhibition of the central stromal swelling response following overnight wear. The thickness changes were measured using the Holden-Payor optical pachometer.

Wang et al. (2003) used the Zeiss OCT2 ocular coherence tomographer to measure epithelial and total corneal thickness changes following overnight wear of the CRT lens. Their results, and those of Haque et al. (2004), agreed with those of Alharbi and Swarbrick (2003) that central epithelial thinning occurred, but differed in their findings that the stromal changes were apparent over the entire corneal surface and that stromal swelling returned to baseline after a few hours. However, their results showed both central epithelial thinning and also mid-peripheral

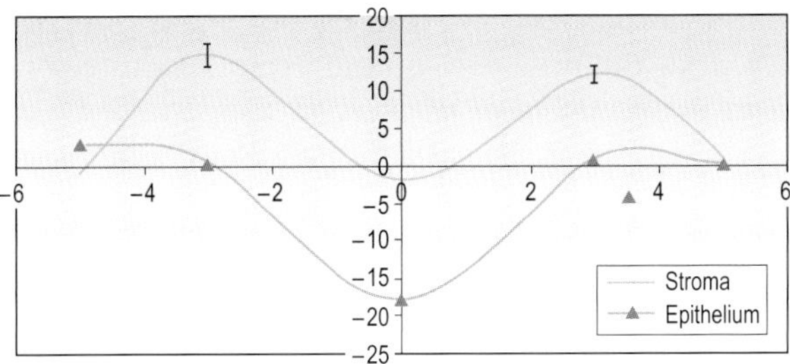

Figure 19.34 The change in epithelial and stromal thickness with overnight orthokeratology. The epithelium thins centrally, and the stroma thickens peripherally. (Courtesy of Helen Swarbrick and Ahmed Alharbi)

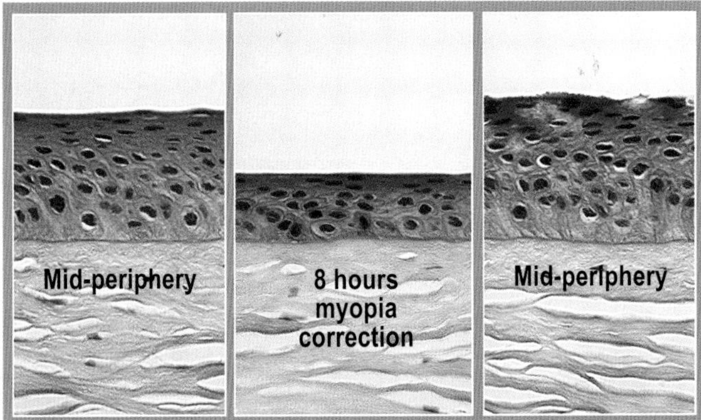

Figure 19.35 The change in epithelial thickness centrally and mid-peripherally (shown for each side) following 8 hours of CRT myopia control lens wear in cats. There is mild central thinning, and marked peripheral thickening. (Courtesy of Jennifer Choo and Patrick Caroline)

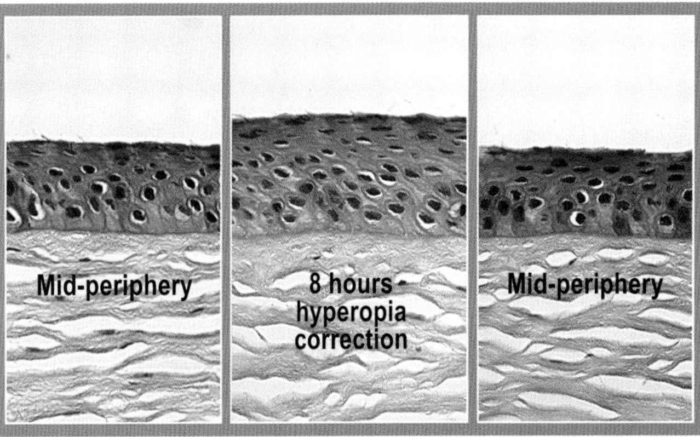

Figure 19.36 The epithelial changes occurring in cats corrected with the CRT hypermetropia lens following 8 hours of wear. The central epithelium is thickened and the periphery (shown for each side) thinned. (Courtesy of Jennifer Choo and Patrick Caroline)

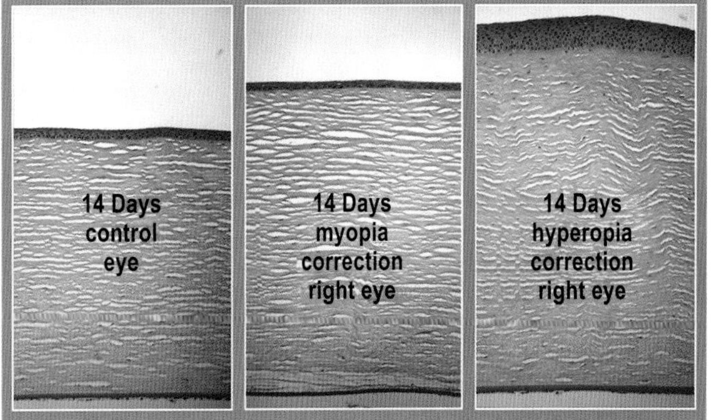

Figure 19.37 Stromal changes occurring after 14 days of continuous wear of CRT lenses for myopia and hypermetropia in cats. Note the difference between the control and treatment groups. This could be an artefact due to the prolonged continuous wear of the lenses. (Courtesy of Jennifer Choo and Patrick Caroline)

epithelial thickening. They did not demonstrate any prolonged mid-peripheral stromal thickening.

There appears to be a difference between the results obtained by Alharbi and Swarbrick (2003), which showed central epithelial thinning and mid-peripheral *stromal* thickening, and those of Wang et al. (2003) and Haque et al. (2004), which showed central epithelial thinning and mid-peripheral *epithelial* thickening, that is as yet unexplained.

Choo et al. (2004) fitted five cats with CRT lenses and examined the corneal changes following 4 and 8 hours of closed eye wear and 14 days of continuous wear. The nictating membrane was sewn into place over the lens to prevent lens loss. One eye was fitted to correct myopia and the other hypermetropia, while another cat simply had the membrane sewn closed and acted as a control.

The results for 8 hours of myopia correction are shown in Figure 19.35. The central epithelium thinned with no decrease in the number of cells, while the mid-periphery thickened with no increase in the number of cells. The thinning was thought to be due to cell compression and the thickening due to cell enlargement. The 8-hour change for hypermetropia correction is shown in Fig 19.36. It appears to be the exact opposite of the myopia changes in that the central epithelium thickens and the mid-periphery thins. These results appear to confirm the results of Wang et al. (2003) and Haque et al. (2004), but, as is shown in Figure 19.37, some stromal changes also occurred as found by Alharbi and Swarbrick (2003). In this group, however, the lenses were worn for 14 days of continuous wear and may not accurately reflect the changes that occur with only 8 hours of exposure to the lenses.

Matsubara (2004) also showed epithelial thinning centrally with rabbit eyes fitted with reverse geometry lenses.

Research may eventually help us to understand the underlying changes that occur with orthokeratology lens wear, but at present no clear answers are available.

Other epithelial, endothelial and stromal changes

Perez-Gomez et al. (2003) used confocal microscopy to study the changes in anterior and posterior keratocyte and endothelial cell density following 7 nights' wear of orthokeratology (OK) lenses and again 1-week post-lens removal. There was a statistically significant decrease in anterior keratocyte density following the 7 nights of lens wear which then returned rapidly towards baseline following the cessation of lens wear. They found no change in posterior keratocyte or endothelial cell density.

A similar result was found by Lin (2004) following a 6-month study of endothelial morphology in a group of 36 myopic children (mean age 9.9 years). He found no change in endothelial cell size or density in either the central or peripheral cornea.

Ladage et al. (2004) used in vivo confocal microscopy to study the effects of high-Dk RGP lenses and reverse geometry (CRT) lenses on rabbit epithelium. Both lenses caused central epithelial thinning following 24 hours of wear (RGP 9.8%, $p=0.001$; OK 6.4%, $p=0.03$) and epithelial thickening peripherally. Central epithelial cell size increased by 5.3% in the RGP group, and by 29% in the OK group.

Yamamoto et al. (2004) studied the binding of *Pseudomonas aeruginosa* to rabbit epithelial cells following 24 hours' wear of a high-Dk (Menicon Z) RGP and a CRT lens made of the same material. There was no statistically significant difference between the *P. aeruginosa* binding of the control and RGP group ($p=0.13$) but there was a significant difference between the control and OK group ($p=0.003$) and the RGP and OK group ($p=0.014$). Overnight wear of CRT lenses caused a significant increase in *P. aeruginosa* binding to rabbit epithelial cells but questions remain as to the accuracy of the fit of the lenses to the rabbit eyes.

Ocular aberrations and orthokeratology

Joslin et al. (2003) were the first to report on changes in corneal and ocular aberrations following overnight orthokeratology. Spherical aberrations increased by a factor of 1.79 for 3.00 mm pupils and 2.42 for 6.00 mm pupils as compared to four-fold (Moreno-Barriuso et al. 2001) and nine-fold increase (Oshika et al. 2002) with LASIK. One subject was found to have a large increase in horizontal coma due to lens decentration (smiley face post-wear topography).

Lu et al. (2004) found a correlation between treatment zone diameter and the change in higher-order aberrations (2.22 times greater than baseline), spherical aberration (4.02 times) and coma (2.27 times). The larger the treatment zone, the lower the total aberrations due to the correction of defocus, but concomitantly, the larger the treatment zone the greater the induction of higher-order aberrations.

Beerten (2004) also found an overall increase in higher-order aberrations over a 1-month period of CRT wear. However, the change in higher-order aberrations appeared to remain stable throughout the day and was not found to be responsible for subjective visual fluctuations.

Ocular infection and orthokeratology

Young et al. (2004) presented a case series study of orthokeratology-related corneal ulcers in China over a period of 2 years. Six children between the ages of 9 and 14 years were treated, with the male:female ratio being 1:5. All cases were monocular, with the onset of infection being between 3 and 36 months of lens wear. All participants suffered a loss of BCVA and five of the six cultured positively for *P. aeruginosa*. However, the patients' prior history was not recorded.

Swarbrick (2004b) reviewed the literature on orthokeratology-related corneal infections and found a total of 45 cases. Of these, 25 were due to *P. aeruginosa*, 14 to acanthamoeba, two to other bacteria, one to fungi and three unknown. There were 21 cases in China, 11 in Taiwan, seven in Hong Kong, one in Singapore, two in Australia and three in the USA/Canada.

Swarbrick pointed out that, in the majority of cases, the causative organism was related to a lack of lens maintenance compliance. *Acanthamoeba* is highly correlated to tap water storage, and *P. aeruginosa* to poor case maintenance. The materials used and practitioners' qualifications were unknown, especially in China.

Extended wear of contact lenses carries an increased risk of corneal infection, but at present the exact risks associated with orthokeratology lens wear are unknown. The prevalence of infection with orthokeratology lens wear can only be determined if the actual numbers of wearers is known and at present it is not. What is required is a method of reporting adverse outcomes and a means of tracking the actual number of wearers. Those who fit orthokeratology lenses must comply with the highest standards of practice and ensure that their patients are fully informed about the procedure.

Cho et al. (2005) studied the contamination of lenses, lens cases and suction holders in a group of 47 participants. Only 15 participants (32%) showed no contamination at all while wearing orthokeratology lenses. They concluded that regular case replacement and reinforcement of hygiene and lens care were vital in decreasing the rate of contamination.

CONCLUSIONS

Rapid changes have occurred in orthokeratology over the past 7 years. There has been a wealth of academic research and new designs for the correction of hypermetropia, presbyopia and astigmatism. The potential to correct higher degrees of myopia is also a possibility.

Nevertheless, any potential that orthokeratology may have is put at risk if the incidence of microbial keratitis increases. Good oxygen permeability of the materials used in lens manufacture is essential. At present, the majority of lenses are made from 100 ISO Dk materials, which, at a centre thickness of 0.20 mm, still fail to meet the Holden–Mertz criterion for overnight wear with no oedema. Paragon's CRT is now manufactured in Menicon Z material (Dk 300) and a high-Dk material is expected in the near future from Polymer Technology.

Another important area of research is the effect that epithelial thinning could have on the potential for infection and whether better lens design and fitting can reduce these risks.

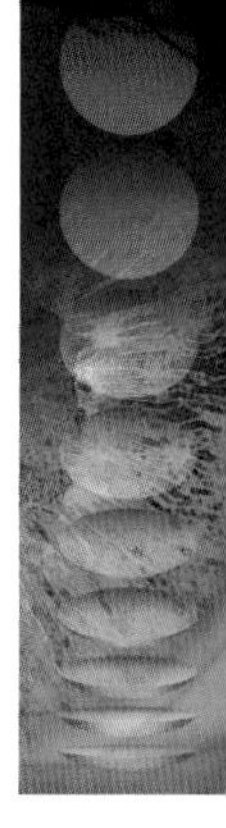

Practitioner interest (both optometric and ophthalmological) in orthokeratology is growing exponentially and this has been associated with a corresponding academic effort to answer some of the questions that provide a firm scientific foundation. Orthokeratology is unlikely to become part of routine practice but it certainly will become an important part of total contact lens practice.

References

Alharbi, A. and Swarbrick, H. A. (2003) The effects of overnight orthokeratology lens wear on corneal thickness. Invest. Ophthalmol. Vis. Sci., 44, 2518–2523

Beerten, R. (2004) Ortho-K: the Dutch experience. Paper presented at the Second Global Orthokeratology Symposium, Toronto, July 2004

Bennett, E. S., Henry, V. A., Davis, L. J. and Kirby, S. (1989) Comparing empirical and diagnostic fitting of daily wear fluoro-silicone acrylate contact lenses. Contact Lens Forum, 14, 38–44

Brungart, T. F. (1961) Fluorescein patterns: they are accurate and they can be mastered. J. Am. Optom. Assoc., 32, 973–974

Carney, L. G., Mainstone, J. C. and Henderson, B. A. (1997) Corneal topography and myopia. Invest. Ophthalmol. Vis. Sci., 38(2), 311–320

Cho, P., Lam, A., Mountford, J. and Ng, L. (2002a) The performance of four different corneal topographers on normal human corneas and its impact on orthokeratology lens fitting. Optom. Vis. Sci., 79, 175–183

Cho, P., Cheung, S. W. and Edwards, M. (2002b) Practice of orthokeratology by a group of contact lens practitioners in Hong Kong. Part 1. Clin. Exp. Optom., 85(6), 358–363

Cho, P., Cheung, S. W. and Edwards, M. H. (2005) The longitudinal orthokeratology research in children (LORIC) study in Hong Kong. A pilot study on refractive changes and myopic control. Curr. Eye Res., 30(1), 71–80

Choo, J., Caroline, P. J., Harlin, D. and Meyers, B. (2004) Morphologic changes in cat epithelium following overnight wear of Paragon CRT lenses for corneal reshaping. Paper presented at the Second Global Orthokeratology Symposium, Toronto, July 2004

Coon, L. J. (1984) Orthokeratology, part 2. Evaluating the Tabb method. J. Am. Optom. Assoc., 55, 409–418

El Hage, S. G., Leach, N. E. and Shahin, R. (1999) Controlled Kerato-Reformation (CKR): an alternative to refractive surgery. Pract. Optom., 10(6), 230–235

Goldberg, J. B. (1996) Ortho-K aspheric RGP corneal lenses. Contacto, March, 29–30

Grant, S. (1995) Orthokeratology night therapy and retention. Contacto, 35, 30–33

Greber, I. and Dybbs, A. (1972) Fluid dynamic analysis of contact lens motion. Cleveland, OH: Case Western Reserve University Report FTAS/TR-72-81

Guillon, M., Lyndon, D. P. and Wilson, C. (1986) Corneal topography: a clinical model. Ophthalmic Physiol. Opt., 6, 47–56

Haque, S., Fonn, D., Simpson, T. and Jones, L. (2004) Corneal and epithelial thickness changes after 4 weeks of overnight corneal refractive therapy lens wear, measured with optical coherence tomography. Eye Contact Lens 30(4), 189–193; discussion 205–206

Hayashi, T. and Fatt, I. (1980) Forces retaining a contact lens on the eye. Am. J. Optom. Physiol. Opt., 57(8), 485–507

Jessen, G. N. (1962) Orthofocus techniques. Contacto, 6, 200–204

Joe, J. J., Marsden, H. J. and Edrington, T. B. (1996) The relationship between corneal eccentricity and improvement in visual acuity with orthokeratology. J. Am. Optom. Assoc., 67, 87–97

Joslin, C. E., Wu, S. M., McMahon, T. T. and Shahidi, M. (2003) Higher-order wavefront aberrations in corneal refractive therapy. Optom. Vis. Sci., 80, 805–811

Keiley, P. M., Smith, G. and Carney, L. G. (1984) Meridional variations of corneal shape. Am. J. Optom. Physiol. Opt., 61(10), 619–626

Kerns, R. (1976–78) Research in orthokeratology, Part 7. J. Am. Optom. Assoc., 48, 1541–1553

Ladage, P. M., Yamamoto, N. and Cavanagh, H. D. (2004) Confocal microscopy of the rabbit corneal surface following orthokeratology lens wear. Invest. Ophthalmol. Vis. Sci. Online. Available: www.iovs.org

Lin, J-C. (2004) The effect of orthokeratology on the morphology of central and peripheral corneal endothelium. Paper presented at the Second Global Orthokeratology Symposium, Toronto, July 2004

Lu, F. (2004) The relationship between the treatment zone diameter and optical performance in CRT lens wearers. Paper presented to the Second Global Orthokeratology Symposium, Toronto, July 2004

Lui, W. O. and Edwards, M. H. (2000) Orthokeratology in low myopia. Part 2: corneal topographic changes and safety over 100 days. Cont. Lens Anterior Eye, 23, 90–99

Maldonado-Codina, C., Efron, S., Morgan, P., Hough, T. and Efron, N. (2005) Empirical versus trial set fitting systems for accelerated orthokeratology. Eye Contact Lens, 31(4), 137–147

Matsubara, M. (2004) Morphological findings of rabbit cornea produced by orthokeratology lens. Paper presented at the Second Global Orthokeratology Symposium, Toronto, July 2004

Moreno-Barriuso, E., Lloves, J. M., Marcos, S. et al. (2001) Ocular aberrations before and after myopic corneal refractive surgery: LASIK induced changes measured with laser ray tracing. Invest. Ophthalmol. Vis. Sci., 42, 1396–1403

Mountford, J. A. (1997) An analysis of the changes in corneal shape and refractive error induced by accelerated orthokeratology. ICLC, 24, 128–143

Mountford, J. A. (2004a) A model of forces acting in orthokeratology. In Orthokeratology Principles and Practice, pp. 269–302, eds. J. Mountford, D. Ruston and T. Dave. Edinburgh: Butterworth-Heinemann

Mountford, J. A. (2004b) Astigmatism and ortho-K. Contact Lens Spectrum, September, p. 8

Mountford, J. A. (2004c) Trial lens fitting. In Orthokeratology Principles and Practice, pp. 139–174, eds. J. Mountford, D. Ruston and T. Dave. Edinburgh: Butterworth-Heinemann

Mountford, J. A. (2004d) Computerized modelling of outcomes and lens fitting in orthokeratology. In Orthokeratology Principles and Practice, pp. 205–226, eds. J. Mountford, D. Ruston and T. Dave. Edinburgh: Butterworth-Heinemann

Mountford, J. A. and Cho, P. (2005) Is fluorescein pattern analysis a valid method of assessing the accuracy of reverse geometry lenses for orthokeratology? Clin. Exp. Optom. 88(1), 33–38

Mountford, J. and Pesudovs, K. (2002) An analysis of the astigmatic changes induced by accelerated orthokeratology. Clin. Exp. Optom., 85, 284–293

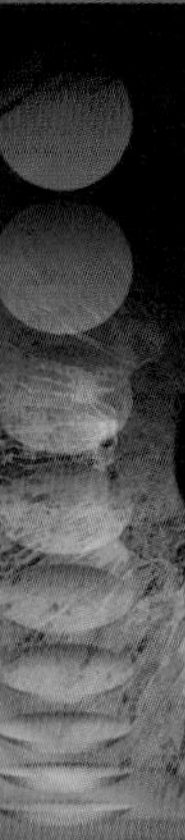

Munnerlyn, C. R., Koons, S. J. and Marshall, J. (1988) Photorefractive keratectomy: a technique for laser refractive surgery. J. Cataract Refract. Surg., 14, 46–51

Nichols, J. J., Marsich, M. M., Nguyen, M., Barr, J. T. and Bullimore, M. (2000) Overnight orthokeratology. Optom. Vis. Sci., 77(5), 252–259

Osborne, G. N., Zantos, S. G., Godio, L. B., Jones, W. F. and Barr, J. T. (1989). Aspheric rigid gas permeable contact lenses; practitioner discrimination of base curve increments using fluorescein pattern evaluation. Optom. Vis. Sci., 66(4), 209–213

Oshika, T., Miyata, K., Tokunaga, T. et al. (2002) Higher order wavefront aberrations of cornea and magnitude of refractive correction in laser in-situ keratomileusis. Ophthalmology, 109, 1154–1158

Perez-Gomez, I., Maldonado-Codina, C., Efron, S. et al. (2003) Confocal microscopic evaluation of corneal changes after orthokeratology. Optom. Vis. Sci., 80(12s), 190

Polse, K. A., Brand, R. J. and Schwalbe, J. S. (1983) The Berkeley orthokeratology study, Part 2: efficacy and duration. Am. J. Optom. Physiol. Opt., 60(3), 187–198

Rah, M. J., Jackson, J. M., Jones, L. A., Marsden, H. J., Bailey, M. D. and Barr, J. T. (2002) Overnight orthokeratology: preliminary results of the Lenses and Overnight Orthokeratology (LOOK) study. Optom. Vis. Sci., 79, 598–605

Rinehart, J. and Bennett, E. S. (2004) Orthokeratology. In Manual of Gas Permeable Contact Lenses, 2nd edn, Chapter 17, eds. E. S. Bennett and M. M. Hom. Edinburgh: Butterworth-Heinemann

Roberts, C. and Wu, Y. T. (1998) Topographical estimation of treatment zone size after refractive surgery using axial distance radius of curvature and refractive power algorithms. IVOS (Suppl), 39(4), 5131, 111.

Soni, P. S., Nguyen, T. T. and Bonanno, J. A. (2003) Overnight orthokeratology: visual and corneal changes. Eye Contact Lens, 29, 137–145

Swarbrick, H. (2004a) 'Mind your P's and Q's'. Paper presented at the Second Global Orthokeratology Symposium, Toronto, July 2004

Swarbrick, H. (2004b) Is Ok Okay? Paper presented at the Second Global Orthokeratology Symposium, Toronto, July 2004

Tahhan, N., Du Toit, R., Papas, E., Chung, H., La Hood, D. and Holden, A. B. (2003) Comparison of reverse-geometry lens designs for overnight orthokeratology. Optom. Vis. Sci., 80, 796–804

Tang, W., Collins, M., Carney, L. C. and Davis, B. (2000) The accuracy and precision performance of four videokeratoscopes in measuring test surfaces. Optom. Vis. Sci., 77(9), 483–491

Tung, H-C. (2004) Turning the fantasies into unequivocal innovations of ortho-K. Paper presented at the Second Global Orthokeratology Symposium, Toronto, July 2004

Wang, J., Fonn, D., Simpson, T. L., Sorbara, L., Kort, R. and Jones, L. (2003) Topographical thickness of the epithelium and total cornea after overnight wear of reverse-geometry rigid contact lenses for myopia reduction. Invest. Ophthalmol. Vis. Sci., 44, 4742–4746

Yamamoto, N., Ladage, P. M. and Cavanagh, H. D. (2004) Pseudomonas aeruginosa binding to the rabbit corneal surface following orthokeratology lens wear. Invest. Ophthalmol. Vis. Sci. Online. Available: www.iovs.org

Young, A. L., Leung, A. T., Cheng, L. L. et al. (2004) Orthokeratology lens-related corneal ulcers in children. Ophthalmology, 111, 590–595

Further reading

Canella, A. (2004) A Guide to Overnight Orthokeratology. Boston: Polymer Technology

Carney, L. (1994) Orthokeratology. In Contact Lens Practice, Chapter 37, eds. M. Rubin and M. Guillon. London: Chapman and Hall Medical

Institute for Eye Research/Polymer Technology. Overnight Orthokeratology: An Interactive Educational Programme (DVD). Institute for Eye Research (Sydney, Australia) and Polymer Technology, Boston

Mountford, J. (1997) Orthokeratology. In Contact Lenses, 4th edn, pp. 653–692, eds. A. J. Phillips and L. Speedwell. Oxford: Butterworth-Heinemann

Mountford, J. A., Ruston, D. and Dave, T. (eds) (2004) Orthokeratology: Principles and Practice. Oxford: Butterworth-Heinemann

Chapter 20

Keratoconus

E. Geoffrey Woodward and Martin P. Rubinstein

CHAPTER CONTENTS

Although keratoconus has been recognized as a clinical entity for more than two millennia, Nottingham (1854) was the first to appreciate that keratoconus is essentially a disease producing corneal thinning and subsequently ectasia, the initial corneal thinning rarely having been previously observed, or, if observed, not associated with the disease process. This is not surprising as the first in vivo measurement of corneal thickness was not carried out by Blix until 1880. Nottingham described the degradation of vision produced by the irregular keratoconic cornea and his management was mainly surgical. His techniques were designed to produce, in a controlled manner, scarring to strengthen the cornea – cauterization, using silver nitrate and mercury, and the passing of a seton (a fine thread or bristle) vertically through the cornea to produce scarring. However, he concluded that the most simple and least dangerous technique was a straightforward puncturing of the cornea. Nottingham also mentioned using glass shells filled with gelatine to improve vision, but the first report of a powered contact lens used in connection with keratoconus was by Fick (1888).

A number of keratoconus patients have a personal or family history of atopic disease (Cox 1984, Edwards et al. 2001). The advent of computerized photokeratoscopy has revealed many patients with a very mild form of the disease who have obtained a satisfactory level of vision with a spectacle correction (Fig. 20.1). Where patients retain a reasonable level of visual acuity in one or both eyes, either with spectacles or unaided, there is no indication to fit contact lenses. Such patients usually lack motivation and are notoriously unsuccessful with contact lenses; this is particularly the case where vision is affected in one eye but the contralateral eye retains normal vision. It is usually desirable to delay fitting until there is a significant difference between the best acuity achieved with spectacles and that achieved with contact lenses, thus increasing motivation.

INCIDENCE OF KERATOCONUS

Although keratoconus is described as rare, it is difficult to obtain consistent figures as to its prevalence.

The earliest reports by Jaensch (1929) gave an incidence of 1 in 3000 in Switzerland whereas Forrest (1929) found an incidence of 1 in 7000. Ruben (1978) found an incidence of 1 in 10,000 in England. His figures were based on the number of keratoconus patients treated at Moorfields Eye Hospital for a catchment area of approximately 5.5 million. However, more recent research would indicate that the incidence is much higher than previously thought, around 1 in 2000 (Rabinowitz & McDonnell 1999) and 1 in 1834 (Kennedy et al. 1986) for the reasons discussed below.

In studies on populations from different ethnic origins in the UK, Pearson et al. (2000) found that, compared with Caucasian

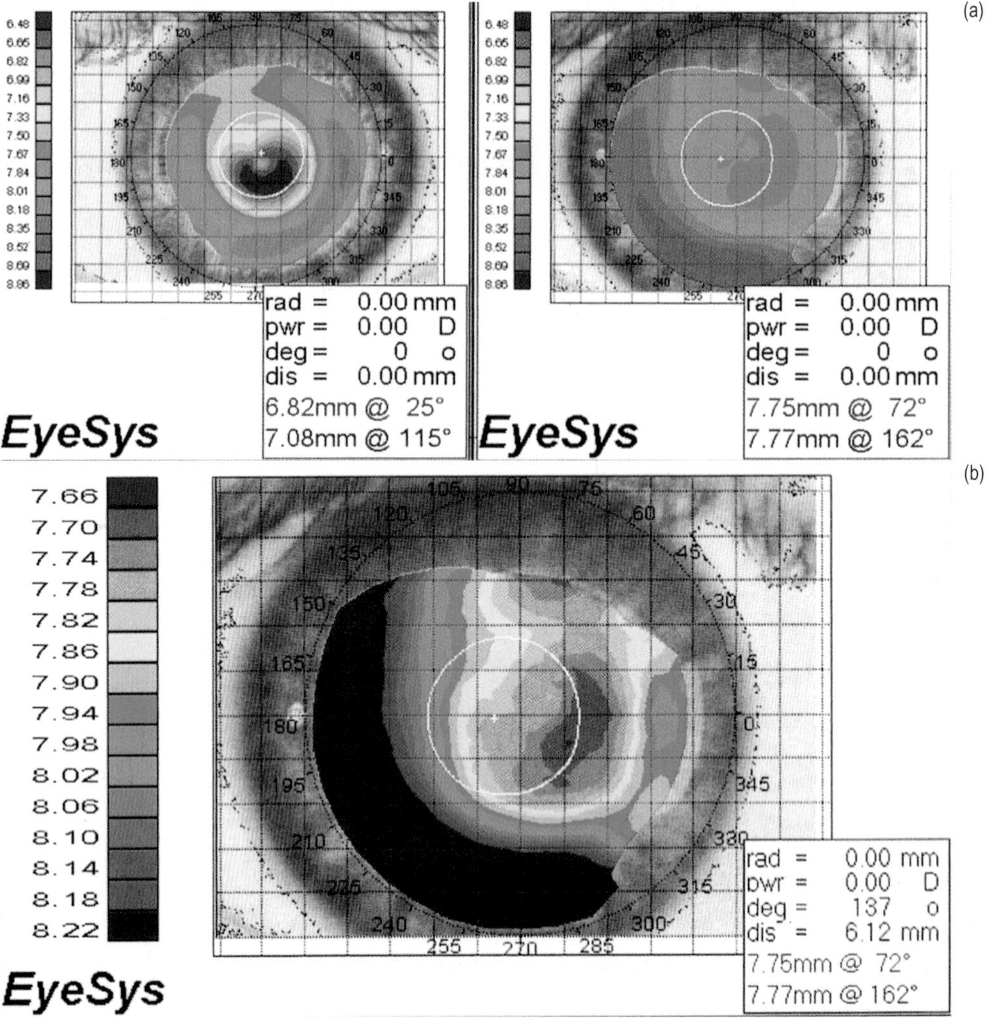

Figure 20.1 (a) A corneal topographical plot showing a monocular keratoconus. The right eye shows an obvious central cone requiring rigid lens correction. The left eye shows an apparently normal plot with 6/6 acuity wearing a spectacle correction only. (b) If the scale is now reduced from 1.00 D steps to 0.25 D steps the left eye can now be seen to show a mild early or 'forme fruste' keratoconus. (Courtesy of A. J. Phillips)

patients, Asians have a four-fold increase in incidence, are younger at presentation and require corneal grafting at an earlier age. Georgiou et al. (2004) found an incidence of 1 in 4000 per year for Asian patients, compared with 1 in 30,000 per year for Caucasian patients and postulated that the higher incidence in this population was suggestive of a genetic factor being significant in the aetiology.

The large variations in the quoted prevalence of the disease may be explained in two ways:

- The genetic nature of some manifestations of the condition, such that in some areas the condition is more common (Nottingham 1854, Woodward 1980a, Ihalainen 1986).
- Substantial variation in the diagnosis of the abortive forms of the condition. For example, Kornerup and Lodin (1959) showed that there is a significantly higher incidence of 'bi-oblique corneal astigmatism' among atopic dermatitis patients and some authors would classify these cases as keratoconus. Amsler (1961), using a classification based upon mire distortion, found that, of 600 cases, 52% were of the rudimentary type and might often not be diagnosed. Computer-assisted photokeratoscopy has also increased the number of reports of subclinical keratoconus (McDonnell 1991) because of its ability to detect mild forms of the disease without any overt clinical signs. Topographical abnormalities appear in family members of keratoconus patients, adding weight to the view that some keratoconus is inherited in an autosomal dominant manner with incomplete penetrance (Gonzalez & McDonnell 1992).

Kerr-Muir et al. (1987) showed that atopic patients with normal vision had an abnormal distribution of corneal thickness skewed to the thinner end of the range. It is thus possible that there is a continuum of corneal variation in thickness and topography whose extreme presentation is keratoconus.

Monocular keratoconus is sometimes described; however, in the vast majority of cases, if the eye with unaffected vision is carefully examined, signs of subclinical keratoconus such as corneal thinning or abnormal siting of the thinnest part of the cornea will be found (Fig. 20.1). True monocular keratoconus is extremely rare but has been described (Phillips 2003) (see p. 464).

Prior to 1958, it was suggested that there was a higher proportion of female sufferers (Nuel 1900, Barth 1948). More recently, an average ratio of 60:40 (male:female) has been found (Obrig & Salvatori 1958, Ihalainen 1986).

Most keratoconic patients fitted with contact lenses are of above average intelligence (Woodward 1981, Ihalainen 1986) and demand a clear explanation of the rationale of their treatment.

Some syndromes are associated with keratoconus. Figures for the incidence of keratoconus in people with Down's syndrome vary from 5.5% (Cullen & Butler 1963) to 15% (Walsh 1981).

Keratoconus as a localized dysfunction in collagen metabolism

There are reports supporting the theory that keratoconus is a localized manifestation of a mild connective tissue disorder causing corneal thinning and ectasia following a weakening of the corneal collagen. Keratoconus has been linked to connective tissue disorders such as Ehlers–Danlos syndrome, osteogenesis imperfecta (Maumenee 1975) and mitral valve prolapse (Beardsley & Foulks 1982, Sharif & Casey 1992). An increased hypermobility in the metacarpophalangeal and wrist joints has also been shown (Woodward & Morris 1990).

It has been suggested that patients with keratoconus have a shorter life expectancy due to underlying connective tissue-related disease; however, the largest cohort of patients investigated for this possibility at Moorfields Eye Hospital, London, did not show a shorter life expectation than the general population (Moodaley et al. 1992). The association of floppy eyelid syndrome with keratoconus was suggested as evidence of an underlying connective tissue disorder (Negris 1992).

SYMPTOMS AND SIGNS

The primary symptom of keratoconus is usually deteriorating vision, more marked in one eye than in the other. Occasionally patients first notice monocular diplopia in the form of a superior ghost image while retaining good vision. Refraction reveals an against-the-rule astigmatism becoming increasingly irregular. In the early stages, keratometry is not necessarily steep, but may appear irregular. Sometimes the mean keratometry readings are at the flatter end of the normal range, corneal thinning preceding ectasia by some considerable time (Woodward 1980a). In addition, if the ectasia is not central, the *K* readings can remain flat even with advanced cones, as the readings measure only the central 3 mm of the cornea.

Contact lens-induced warpage from rigid lens wear can be difficult to differentiate from early keratoconus, even with the aid of computer-assisted photokeratoscopes. In such cases, early keratoconus can best be diagnosed by topographical pachometry (see Chapter 7). A central or paracentral corneal thickness of less than 0.48 mm is almost certainly keratoconus, or where the thinnest part of the cornea can be shown to be off its visual axis.

As the condition progresses, the characteristic swirling retinoscopy reflex appears and the near visual acuity is found to be better than would be anticipated from the distance visual acuity. Pinhole acuity also shows a definite improvement.

An early sign of keratoconus is enhanced visibility of the corneal nerves and many corneas exhibit vertical striae (Fig. 20.2), first described by Elschnig (1894). These result from the buckling of the posterior cornea as the cone steepens. Pressure applied to the globe reduces the visibility of the striae.

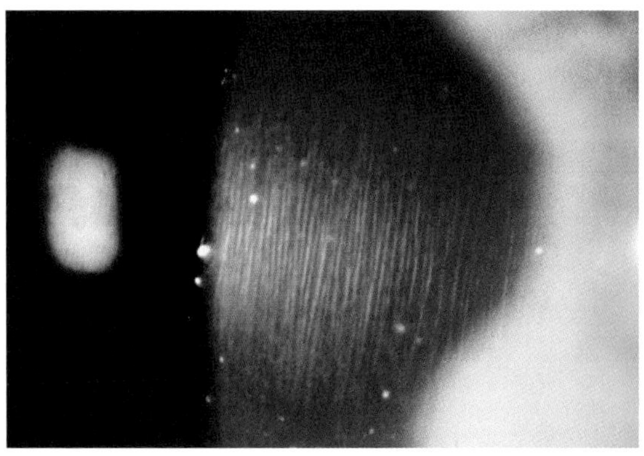

Figure 20.2 Striae form one of the diagnostic signs in keratoconus. They are almost invariably orientated vertically at the apex of the cone. They occur in the posterior stroma. (Courtesy of A. J. Phillips)

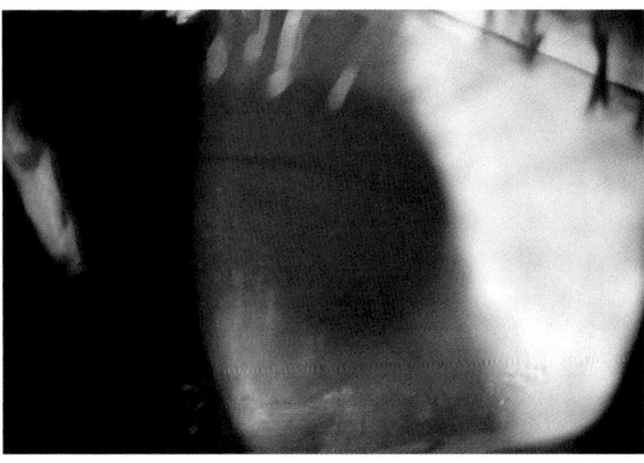

Figure 20.3 Fleischer's ring is the faint brown ring, probably of ferrous deposits, sometimes found around the base of the cone in keratoconus. Note also the corneal scarring. (Courtesy of A. J. Phillips)

In 1906, Fleischer described the iron pigment ring, which bears his name. This ring (Fig. 20.3), often only partial, is characterized by accumulations of ferritin (iron-containing protein) particles in the widened intercellular spaces and/or in the cytoplasmic vacuoles of the basal or wing cell layers of the corneal epithelium (Iwamoto and de Moto, 1976). In its early stages it may be more easily detected with blue light. The majority of keratoconus patients eventually show some corneal scarring, quite unrelated to, but possibly exacerbated by, contact lens wear. These scars may be small focal opacities, sub-Bowman's or pre-Descemet's membrane or Bowman's reticular scarring (Figs 20.3 and 20.4).

A small percentage of patients will develop corneal hydrops, sometimes incorrectly called 'acute keratoconus'. Here (Figs 20.5, 20.6) a sudden gross corneal oedema follows a rupture of Descemet's membrane, usually in a vertical or vertically oblique direction. Most of these cases resolve spontaneously by Descemet's membrane resurfacing over the split. Hydrops is painful and causes reduced vision due to increased scarring but the corneal curvature may flatten, rendering corneal lens fitting

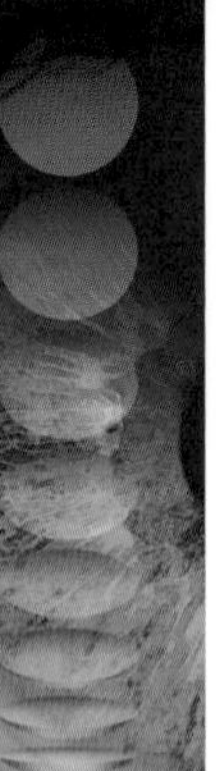

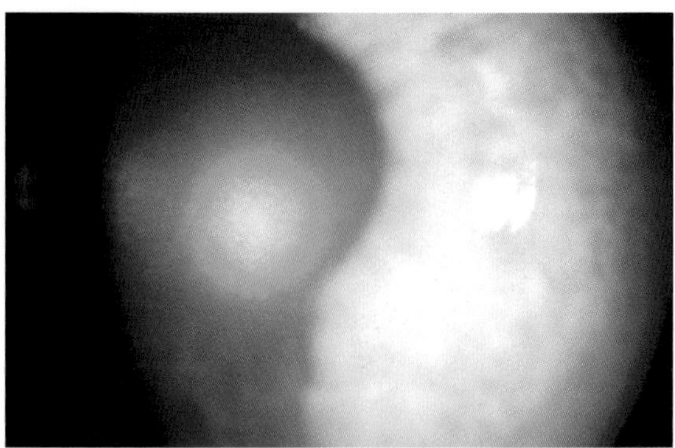

Figure 20.4 Central scarring – here showing staining with sodium fluorescein. The dense, but diffuse, nature of the staining indicates that Bowman's layer has been eroded and that the fluorescein is diffusing into the surrounding stroma. (Courtesy of A. J. Phillips)

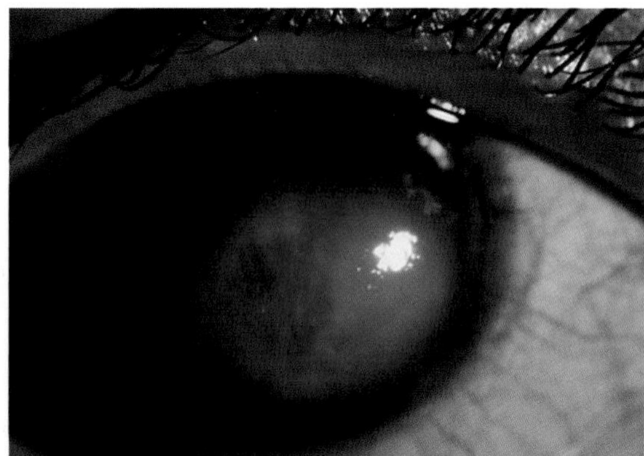

Figure 20.5 Corneal hydrops

simpler (see p. 462). Lens wear does not induce hydrops although vigorous eye-rubbing can cause it (Ionnidis et al. 2005).

MANAGEMENT

Many patients are apprehensive about their long-term prognosis so it is important to be as reassuring as possible. In a long-term study of keratoconus patients, Cox (1984) showed that over 70% retained a visual acuity of 6/9 or better over a 5-year period with contact lens wear, and 89% were able to see well enough to drive. In addition, many patients retain adequate spectacle-corrected vision in at least one eye.

The management of the condition varies considerably with location, depending on the availability of a contact lens service capable of dealing with the more advanced cases and alternative strategies such as keratoplasty and epikeratoplasty.

Tuft et al. (1994a) carried out a 7-year retrospective study of 2723 keratoconus patients at Moorfields Eye Hospital. At the end of the study period, 757 eyes (21%) had received at least one keratoplasty. In the United Kingdom the percentage of eyes requiring corneal transplants is probably between 10 and 20%, varying with centre. Criteria for a transplant or explant vary (see Grafting/Transplantation p. 465).

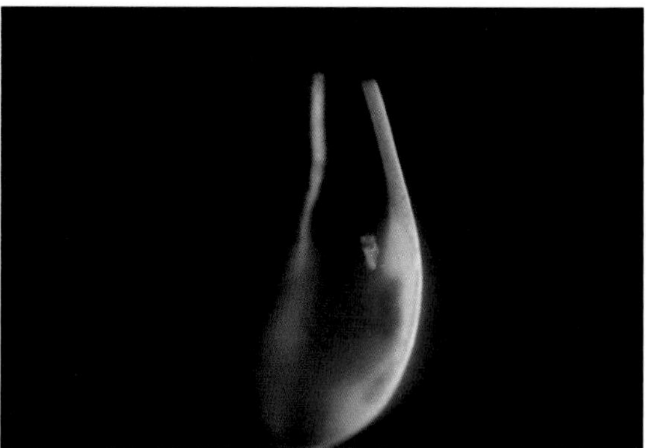

Figure 20.6 Corneal hydrops (optic section)

Keratoconus was the most common indication for penetrating keratoplasty in Australia in 2004 – 31% of all transplants (Australian Corneal Graft Registry 2004).

In one long-term study, Smiddy et al. (1988) reported that 60% of patients having penetrating keratoplasty required corneal lenses afterwards. These figures have reduced greatly since laser and other refractive procedures (e.g. relaxing incisions and compression sutures) have been used to correct post-graft refractive errors.

In terms of a clear graft, success rates are very high (Marechal-Courtois & Prijat 1972, Pouliquen et al. 1972, Davies et al. 1977). In the Moorfields series of patients with grafts, 70% achieved a best acuity of 6/6 or better and 95% achieved 6/12 or better (Cox 1984). Up to 2003, 89% of transplants carried out for keratoconus in Australia achieved better vision postoperatively (Australian Corneal Graft Registry 2004). However, Tuft et al. (1994b) found that corneas transplanted after an episode of hydrops stand a significantly greater risk of rejection.

Several alternatives to keratoplasty have been reported. Woolensak et al. (2003) described the application of riboflavin to corneas where the epithelium had been removed. The result was an improvement in visual acuity and keratometry values. Boxer-Wachler et al. (2003) implanted intrastromal corneal segments to improve visual acuity, and Nepomuceno et al. (2003) assessed the feasibility of fitting rigid gas-permeable (RGP) or hydrogel lenses to these eyes.

Contact lens wear is not found to affect the progression of keratoconus (Ruben & Trodd 1976, Woodward 1980a) but claims for retardation, remission or reversal being produced by contact lens wear have all been based on keratometry. This is inevitably misleading because contact lens wear can produce a temporary flattening of the cornea. As keratoconus is essentially a disease of corneal thinning it can only properly be monitored by serial topographical pachometry. Where this has been done, contact lens wear has been shown to have no effect on the progression of the condition. In some cases corneal thinning progresses very little, but in the majority of cases corneal thickness stabilizes at approximately 60% of normal (Woodward 1980b).

Patients may think that contact lens fitting will control the disease and that this is an indication for fitting as early as possible. It should be explained that the only purpose of fitting contact lenses in keratoconus is visual rehabilitation.

It has also been suggested that contact lens wear may precipitate keratoconus. Gasset et al. (1978) compared the number of patients in their clinics who developed keratoconus after having worn either hard or soft contact lenses and went on to claim an association between hard contact lens wear and the risk of developing keratoconus. However, the soft lens wearers were analysed prospectively and were compared with a group of patients who had been wearing rigid corneal lenses for some time. Although the refractive errors of the two groups were said to be similar in terms of spherical equivalents, it seems unlikely that the proportion of cases with irregular or high astigmatism were equal, since these conditions would suggest the use of rigid lenses. In the early stages of keratoconus, many cases show high regular astigmatism. A population of rigid lens wearers is thus much more likely to contain undiagnosed keratoconic patients than a population of soft lens wearers.

In another study, Macsai et al. (1990) considered that, in some cases, long-term rigid lens wear may be a risk factor for keratoconus. However, their patients had not been evaluated by computerized photokeratoscopy, nor was corneal thickness measured prior to fitting. It is known that contact lens wear over a period of years can produce stromal thinning and that atopic patients with normal vision have an abnormal distribution of corneal thickness skewed to the thinner end of the range (Kerr-Muir et al. 1987); hence, it is possible that prolonged contact lens wear in atopic patients could precipitate latent keratoconus.

The mechanical trauma of eye rubbing is, in some cases, a trigger for the changes noted in keratoconus (McMonnies & Boneham 2003, Jafri et al. 2004, Ionniddis et al. 2005). Excessive eye rubbing can be attributed to increased ocular itchiness, as occurs with atopic disease. In other allergic eye disease, such as vernal conjunctivitis or atopic dermatitis, the tissue most profoundly affected by eye rubbing is the superior tarsal conjunctiva, not the cornea or bulbar conjunctiva. McMonnies and Boneham (2003) found that where keratoconus patients admitted to eye rubbing, it was 'severe and prolonged'.

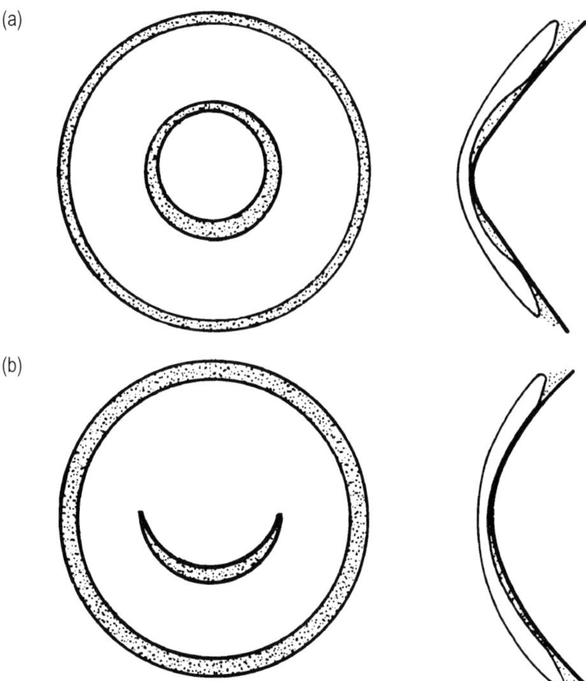

Figure 20.7 Fitting with the weight of the lens distributed (a) in developed keratoconus; (b) in early keratoconus. The left-hand diagrams show a representation of the fit where the dotted areas indicate corneal clearance. The right-hand diagrams show the same fit (exaggerated) in cross-section

CONTACT LENS OPTIONS

Corneal lenses

The majority of keratoconic patients are fitted with corneal lenses and the most appropriate fitting philosophy has been debated for many years.

OLDER DESIGNS

In the early days of corneal lens fitting, large relatively flat-fitting lenses were advocated and in a modified form this approach still has its proponents, mainly in the Scandinavian- and German-speaking countries. The recent development of limbal and paralimbal lenses reverts somewhat to this fitting philosophy (see p. 458), although with the older designs there was a specific intention to reshape the cornea using a flat lens and depending entirely on the plasticity of the cornea (Clifford-Hall 1963).

Flatter-fitting lenses often give a superior visual performance, which may remain enhanced for some time after lens removal due to the cornea remaining relatively flattened. The CIBA Persecon E Keratoconus lens is an example of this approach (Achatz et al. 1985, Astin 1987). There are reservations concerning this fitting philosophy as it can affect the natural history of the disease.

The majority of patients with keratoconus exhibit corneal scarring whether or not they have worn contact lenses (Bron et al. 1978, Barr et al. 2000), but wearing flat-fitting lenses only hastens the rate of scarring in sub-Bowman's stroma (see Fig. 20.4) (Ruben 1975, Korb et al. 1982). Although it would not be ethically viable to test whether flat-fitting corneal lenses exacerbate corneal scarring in keratoconus, the debate has been comprehensively reviewed by Edrington et al. (1999) and Leung (1999).

While the large flat-fitting philosophy was being propagated in Europe, an alternative approach was favoured in the USA and South America. This was to fit small, thin, tricurve lenses from 6.00 to 8.00 mm in total diameter, with back optic zone radii from 5.00 to 7.50 mm (Arias 1963). The disadvantages with this philosophy are mainly visual, and monocular diplopia was a common complaint. Furthermore, in all but the earliest cases, such lenses need to be of high negative power with attendant edge thickness problems.

The most widely accepted corneal lens fitting philosophy is one where the weight of the lens is distributed between the cone and the more peripheral cornea (Fig. 20.7a) with an apical contact area of 2–3 mm, an intermediate clearance zone, a

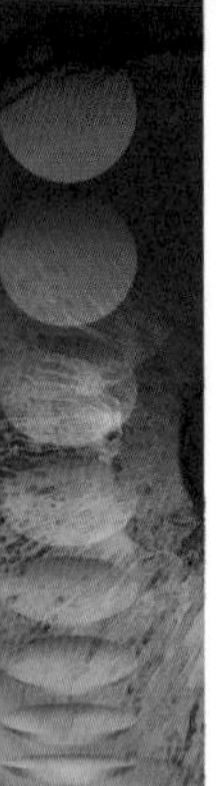

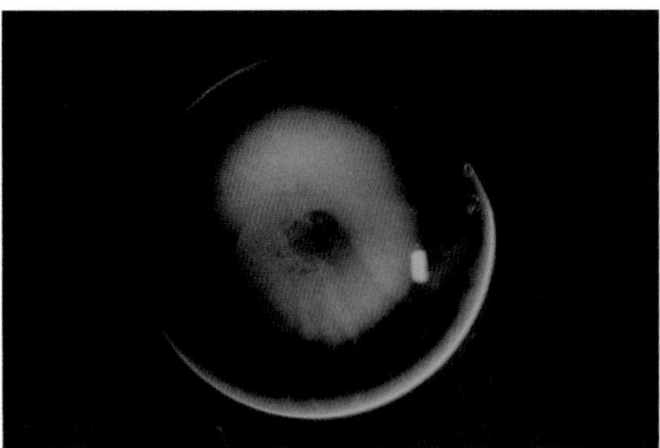

Figure 20.8 A classic 'three-point touch' alignment fit in keratoconus, i.e. alignment of the majority of the peripheral curve and capillary contact with the cone apex by the central back optic zone. (Courtesy of A. J. Phillips)

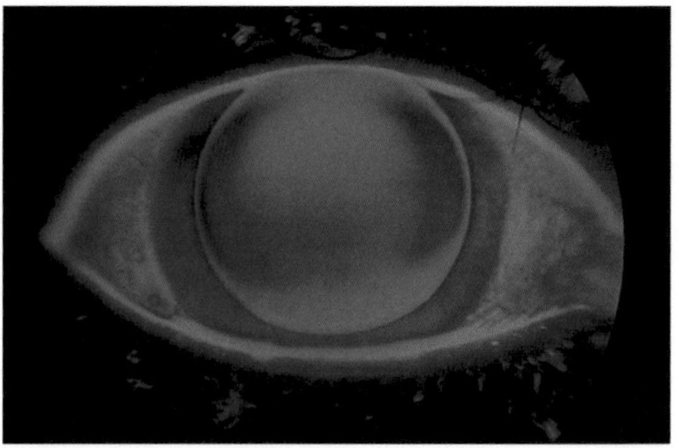

Figure 20.9 Keratoconic corneas frequently show marked with-the-rule toricity. This fluorescein fit shows minimal cone contact just below the lens centre, with peripheral curves aligning (to borderline tight) in the horizontal meridian but with marked edge standoff vertically. The use of a toroidal periphery increases the area of alignment and may avoid the optical complications of a fully toric lens. (Courtesy of A. J. Phillips)

mid-peripheral contact or bearing annulus, and conventional edge clearance at the periphery (Fig. 20.8). The peripheral cornea does thin in keratoconus but only at half the rate of the centre (Woodward 1980b). In the earlier stages of the condition, owing to the vertical asymmetry of the cone, the intermediate zone may form a crescent rather than an annulus, as shown in Figure 20.7b. With the exception of very early cases, it is necessary to use specifically designed lenses to achieve this type of fit. If lenses of a conventional design are used, the lens with the desired central fit usually has insufficient edge clearance.

TORIC LENSES

Conventional fully toroidal back surface corneal lenses are rarely used in fitting keratoconus, although newer designs can work well in toric designs (see Dyna Intra-Limbal p. 459). The cornea is highly astigmatic but the astigmatism is irregular and asymmetrical in any one meridian. Toroidal back peripheral curves can be used to enhance lens centration.

Lenses frequently show reasonable edge clearance except in the inferior quadrant where it is excessive (Fig. 20.9), sometimes allowing air under the lens edge (Fig. 20.10a). Such lenses are unstable and are often blinked out by the patient or fall out when the patient looks from side to side. Here a lens with a toric periphery may improve the situation, although the inferior clearance always exceeds the superior because of the meridional asymmetry. As this is less peripherally than centrally, a compromise fit can often be achieved, as seen in Figure 20.10b (see also Varying edge clearance, p. 458).

The degree of peripheral toricity can be estimated from a spherical set such as that designed by Woodward (Table 20.1). Phillips suggested modifying this design in order to increase the zone of mid-peripheral alignment (Tables 20.2a and b). A toric periphery fitting set designed by Phillips is shown in Table 20.3.

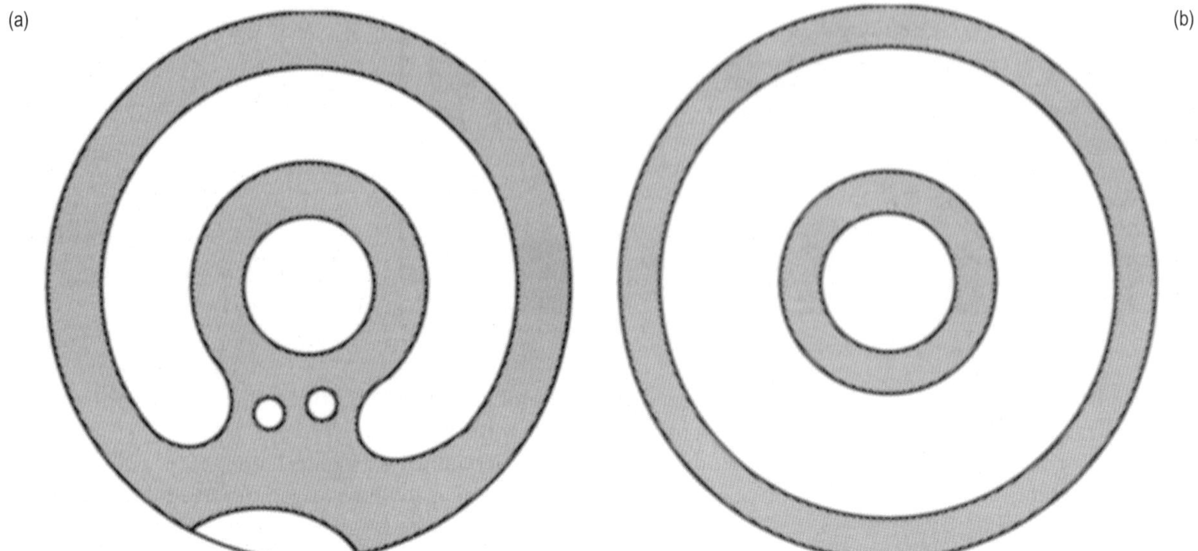

Figure 20.10 Keratoconic cornea fitted with (a) a spherical corneal lens, showing bubbles under the lower edge, the shaded areas indicating corneal clearance; (b) a corneal lens with a toroidal periphery showing much more uniform clearance at the edge

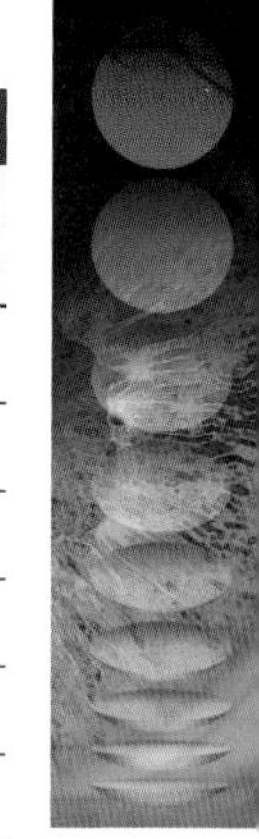

Table 20.1: Tricurve keratoconus fitting set (Woodward)

BOZR (mm)	BOZD (mm)	BPR_1 (mm)	BPD_1 (mm)	BPR_2 (mm)	TD (mm)	BVP (D)
5.50	5.60	6.50	7.60	8.50	8.60	–11.00
5.60	5.60	6.60	7.60	8.60	8.60	–10.00
5.70	5.70	6.70	7.80	8.70	8.80	–9.50
5.80	5.70	6.80	7.80	8.80	8.80	–9.00
5.90	5.80	6.90	7.80	8.90	8.80	–8.50
6.00	5.80	7.00	8.00	9.00	9.00	–8.00
6.10	5.90	7.10	8.00	9.10	9.00	–7.50
6.20	5.90	7.20	8.00	9.20	9.00	–7.00
6.30	6.00	7.30	8.00	9.30	9.00	–6.50
6.40	6.00	7.40	8.00	9.40	9.00	–6.00
6.50	6.00	7.50	8.00	9.50	9.00	–5.50
6.60	6.00	7.60	8.00	9.60	9.00	–5.00
6.70	6.00	7.70	8.00	9.70	9.00	–4.50
6.80	6.00	7.80	8.20	9.80	9.20	–4.00
6.90	6.00	7.90	8.20	9.90	9.20	–3.50
7.00	6.00	8.00	8.20	10.00	9.20	–3.00

MORE RECENT DESIGNS

A number of new products have entered the market in recent years, for example the Rose K (Betts et al. 2002) and the CLEK lens (Edrington et al. 1996), both based on sagittal height (sag); the Shepherd K lens (Acuity Contact Lenses, UK), a design available in both rigid and soft lenses; the Profile lens (Pullum 2003), and many others. All these designs have claimed advantages, both in terms of ease of fitting and patient comfort, and are particularly useful for those doing only small amounts of keratoconic fitting. The main disadvantages are typically:

- Lack of information about the full lens parameters.
- Lack of the ability to alter the lens parameters by known amounts.
- Lack of the ability to check the lenses other than the basic (supplied) parameters.
- Supply is restricted to the laboratory fabricating the fitting sets.

Other examples of newer designs include the following.

Profile lenses (Jack Allen Contact Lenses, UK)

The Profile lens (Pullum 2003) is fitted differently from other corneal lenses in that the lens parameters are specified according to the axial profile of the individual cornea rather than specific measurements of curvature, much like the preformed scleral lens designed by Pullum (see Chapter 15).

- Each trial lens increases 0.1 mm apical sag from the previous lens, and lenses are numbered from 1 to 13 with 1 having the smallest sag.

Table 20.2a: Keratoconus tetracurve fitting set I (Phillips)

BOZR (mm)	BOZD (mm)	BPR_1 (mm)	BPD_1 (mm)	BPR_2 (mm)	BPD_2 (mm)	BPR_3 (mm)	TD (mm)	BVP (D)
5.00	6.00	7.20	8.00	10.50	8.60	12.25	9.00	–17.00
5.10	6.00	7.30	8.00	10.50	8.60	12.25	9.00	–16.50
5.20	6.00	7.40	8.50	10.50	8.60	12.25	9.00	–16.00
5.30	6.00	7.50	8.00	10.50	8.60	12.25	9.00	–15.50
5.40	6.00	7.60	8.00	10.50	8.60	12.25	9.00	–15.00
5.50	6.00	7.70	8.00	10.50	8.60	12.25	9.00	–14.50
5.60	6.00	7.70	8.00	10.50	8.60	12.25	9.00	–14.00
5.70	6.00	7.70	8.00	10.50	8.60	12.25	9.00	–13.50
5.80	6.00	7.80	8.00	10.50	8.60	12.25	9.00	–13.00
5.90	6.00	7.90	8.00	10.50	8.60	12.25	9.00	–12.50
6.00	6.50	8.00	8.50	10.50	9.10	12.25	9.50	–12.00
6.10	6.50	8.10	8.50	10.50	9.10	12.25	9.50	–11.50
6.20	6.50	8.20	8.50	10.50	9.10	12.25	9.50	–11.00
6.30	6.50	8.30	8.50	10.50	9.10	12.25	9.50	–10.50
6.40	6.50	8.40	8.50	10.50	9.10	12.25	9.50	–10.00
6.50	6.50	8.00	8.50	10.50	9.10	12.25	9.50	–9.50
6.60	6.50	8.10	8.50	10.50	9.10	12.25	9.50	–9.00
6.70	6.50	8.20	8.50	10.50	9.10	12.25	9.50	–8.50
6.80	6.50	8.30	8.50	10.50	9.10	12.25	9.50	–8.00
6.90	6.50	8.40	8.50	10.50	9.10	12.25	9.50	–7.50
7.00	6.50	8.50	8.50	10.50	9.10	12.25	9.50	–7.00

Table 20.2b: Keratoconus tetracurve fitting set II (Phillips)

BOZR (mm)	BOZD (mm)	BPR_1 (mm)	BPD_1 (mm)	BPR_1 (mm)	BPD_2 (mm)	BPR_3 (mm)	TD (mm)	BVP (D)
6.00	6.80	7.50	8.80	10.50	9.40	12.25	9.80	–12.00
6.10	6.80	7.60	8.80	10.50	9.40	12.25	9.80	–11.50
6.20	6.80	7.70	8.80	10.50	9.40	12.25	9.80	–11.00
6.30	6.80	7.80	8.80	10.50	9.40	12.25	9.80	–10.50
6.40	6.80	7.90	8.80	10.50	9.40	12.25	9.80	–10.00
6.50	6.80	8.00	8.80	10.50	9.40	12.25	9.80	–9.50
6.60	6.80	8.10	8.80	10.50	9.40	12.25	9.80	–9.00
6.70	6.80	8.20	8.80	10.50	9.40	12.25	9.80	–8.50
6.80	6.80	8.30	8.80	10.50	9.40	12.25	9.80	–8.00
6.90	6.80	8.40	8.80	10.50	9.40	12.25	9.80	–7.50
7.00	6.80	8.30	8.80	10.50	9.40	12.25	9.80	–7.00
7.10	6.80	8.40	8.80	10.50	9.40	12.25	9.80	–6.50
7.20	6.80	8.50	8.80	10.50	9.40	12.25	9.80	–6.00
7.30	6.80	8.60	8.80	10.50	9.40	12.25	9.80	–5.50
7.40	6.80	8.70	8.80	10.50	9.40	12.25	9.80	–5.00

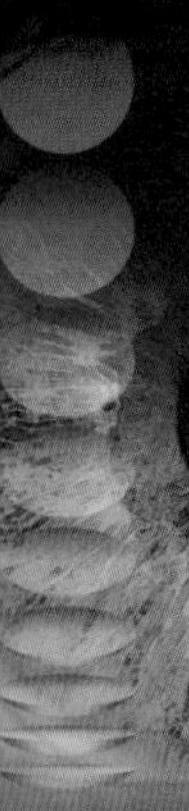

Table 20.3: Toric periphery keratoconus fitting set (Phillips)

BOZR (mm)	BOZD (mm)	BPR_1 (mm)	BPD_1 (mm)	BPR_2 (mm)	BPD_2 (mm)	BPR_3 (mm)	TD (mm)	BVP (D)
5.80	6.50	7.80 × 7.40	8.50	10.50 × 10.10	9.10	12.25 × 11.85	9.50	−13.00
5.90	6.50	7.90 × 7.50	8.50	10.50 × 10.10	9.10	12.25 × 11.85	9.50	−12.50
6.00	6.50	8.00 × 7.60	8.50	10.50 × 10.10	9.10	12.25 × 11.85	9.50	−12.00
6.10	6.50	8.10 × 7.70	8.50	10.50 × 10.10	9.10	12.25 × 11.85	9.50	−11.50
6.20	6.50	8.20 × 7.80	8.50	10.50 × 10.10	9.10	12.25 × 11.85	9.50	−11.00
6.30	6.50	8.30 × 7.90	8.50	10.50 × 10.10	9.10	12.25 × 11.85	9.50	−10.50
6.40	6.80	7.90 × 7.50	8.80	10.50 × 10.10	9.40	12.25 × 11.85	9.80	−10.00
6.50	6.80	8.00 × 7.60	8.80	10.50 × 10.10	9.40	12.25 × 11.85	9.80	−9.50
6.60	6.80	8.10 × 7.70	8.80	10.50 × 10.10	9.40	12.25 × 11.85	9.80	−9.00
6.70	6.80	8.20 × 7.80	8.80	10.50 × 10.10	9.40	12.25 × 11.85	9.80	−8.50
6.80	6.80	8.30 × 7.90	8.80	10.50 × 10.10	9.40	12.25 × 11.85	9.80	−8.00
6.90	6.80	8.40 × 8.00	8.80	10.50 × 10.10	9.40	12.25 × 11.85	9.80	−7.50
7.00	6.80	8.50 × 8.10	8.80	10.50 × 10.10	9.40	12.25 × 11.85	9.80	−7.00
7.10	6.80	8.10 × 7.70	8.80	10.50 × 10.10	9.40	12.25 × 11.85	9.80	−6.50
7.20	6.80	8.20 × 7.80	8.80	10.50 × 10.10	9.40	12.25 × 11.85	9.80	−6.00
7.30	6.80	8.30 × 7.90	8.80	10.50 × 10.10	9.40	12.25 × 11.85	9.80	−5.50
7.40	6.80	8.40 × 8.00	8.80	10.50 × 10.10	9.40	12.25 × 11.85	9.80	−5.00

- The two peripheral edge lifts are standard, and reduced (R) which is 0.1 mm less than standard.
- There are three total diameters: normal (N) = 9.30 mm; small (S) = 8.70 mm; large (L) = 9.80 mm.

The first lens chosen is in the middle of the range, lens number N5, which is equivalent to 6.64 mm (50.83 D) back optic zone radius (BOZR). Lenses are then altered according to:

- How steep/flat the lens is.
- The edge clearance.
- The total diameter (TD).

Observing the fit of the N5 lens, the following alterations can be made:

- Lens is too flat – refit with lens N7.
- TD is too small – select lens LN5.
- Too much edge clearance – change to LR5, and so on.

The fit of the lens must be observed not only with straight-ahead gaze but also with left and right versions as a lens that appears to fit well in straight-ahead gaze may lift off when the eye moves to the side.

Aspheric designs

An example of this is the KBA (Keratoconic Bi-Aspheric) design by Mountford and Noak (Capricornia Contact Lenses, Australia). The back surface is highly aspheric (e = 0.98) with a front surface curve that corrects for induced radial astigmatism and a typical TD of 10.20 mm. The back surface asphericity can be varied to match the individual cornea (up to e = 1.30). The lens centre and periphery are fitted separately, with the final, combined design being derived from a practitioner computer program. The initial lens design can also be derived from the Medmont E-300 Topographer data. Lenses with different eccentricities in the two principal meridians can be ordered for cones with a pseudo-astigmatic shape, this information again being derived from the Medmont Topographer.

Varying edge clearance

The latest lathing technology also allows practitioners to specify the edge lift to be different in one quadrant from the others. A useful rule of thumb is to order the (typically) inferior quadrant (on a spherical or toroidal lens) 0.3 mm steeper if there is simple inferior underhang and 0.4–0.5 mm steeper if there is bubble entry. Care is necessary in the manufacture of these 'quadrant' lenses as the steeper inferior zone will be slightly thicker and this may increase patient awareness. Prism ballast is not usually necessary, although it is incorporated in the Dyna Intralimbal lens. It is also important to ascertain whether the lens design enables steepening of just the peripheral curve(s) (which may be very narrow in some designs), or all lens curves.

Large-diameter lenses

As a general 'problem-solving' device, large-diameter corneal RGP lenses have become more popular for cases where smaller-diameter corneal lenses do not fit well or are uncomfortable, and scleral lenses are either not available or unsuccessful. In particular:

- Steep corneal topography.
- Highly eccentric/displaced cones; in pellucid marginal degeneration (degeneration and thinning of the inferior cornea); and

Terrien's marginal degeneration (progressive degeneration and thinning in the superior cornea).

- Those with very sensitive eyes.

Examples include:

- *S-Limlens (Jack Allen Contact Lenses, UK):* The lens is available in TDs of 13.50–14.75 mm and material Dks of 70 and 120. The EpiCon LC lens (Capricornia Contact Lenses, Australia) is similar, with a 13.5 mm TD.
- *Dyna Intra-Limbal (DIL) by Lens Dynamics, Inc. (USA):* The standard diameter is 11.2 mm, but is available from 10.8 to 12.0 mm and is fitted within the limbus. These lenses can be ordered in toric or bitoric parameters if necessary.
- *The EyCon (Australia) Mini-Scleral lens:* This is 16.5 mm in diameter and resembles the fenestrated lenses for optic measurement (FLOM) design described in Chapter 15.

The increase in contact surface area and reduced lid interference can produce a marked improvement in both lens fit and stability, and also in patient comfort. With modern gas-permeable materials and the use of fenestrations, the disadvantages of large occlusive lenses are greatly reduced. This approach has many of the advantages of scleral lenses but supply of lenses is quicker, and insertion and removal easier.

FITTING PROCEDURES

It has been suggested over the years that keratoconic corneas may be classified by shape and cone apex position into distinct groups and that such a classification is of value in deciding which design of corneal lens to fit. However, computerized photokeratoscopy (Rabinowitz & McDonnell 1989, Wilson et al. 1991, Young et al. 1991) shows that keratoconus produces a spectrum of change with no clearly defined taxonomy. In addition, consideration of the shape changes produced by eccentric thinning of the cornea does not support the concept of classifiable changes (Edmund 1987).

Keratometry

Keratometers are calibrated on the assumption that the areas from which the mire images reflect lie on a spherical surface. In keratoconus, as the curvature differs in each area and the areas do not have a common centre of curvature, the measurements will be incorrect.

Keratometry is a useful indicator of corneal topographic change in keratoconus but results must be considered as qualitative rather than quantitative. Except in the early stages of the condition, keratometry gives only minimal help in deciding on the first trial lens.

As the condition progresses and the irregularity of the cornea increases, keratometry readings become increasingly meaningless. Where readings can still be taken, the optimum fitting lens is often found to be only slightly steeper than the flattest *K* reading. More information is gained from corneal topography maps or fluorescein pictures with trial lenses.

Whatever type of lens is used, the classic three-point touch, keratoconic fit as shown in Figure 20.8 may not always be achievable. Bubble formation and retention below the apex of the cone is not uncommon (Fig. 20.11) and it may be necessary to use fenestrations if static bubbles produce dimple veiling. However, with some of the newer designs this is not so much of a problem (see above).

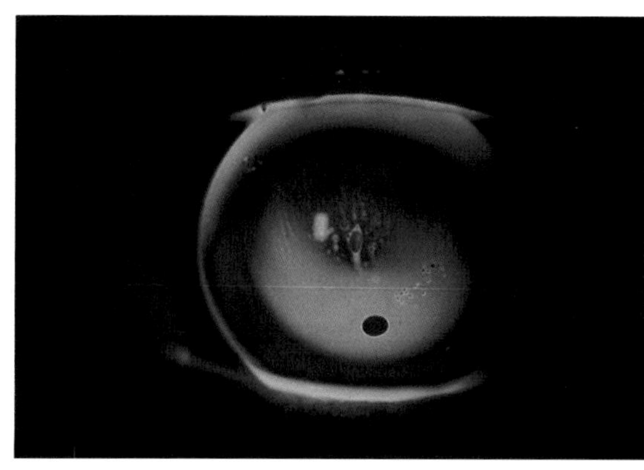

Figure 20.11 As keratoconus advances, the cornea becomes so steep centrally that the sharp change in curvature between the back optic zone and aligning periphery produces bubbles under the optic zone area that cannot escape. These break up to form froth centrally. Dimple 'staining' is shown under the lens here and dimple veiling usually results. Fenestrating the lens may help but often worsens the situation. Utilizing a flatter BOZR may reduce the frothing but at the risk of causing increased cone pressure and possible subsequent central scarring. Just above the cone apex can be seen vertical epithelial wrinkling due to pressure on the cone apex. Fluorescein collects in the channels with the lens in situ but runs out on lens removal. The wrinkles can then only be seen by indirect illumination. Epithelial wrinkling can also occur after wearing thin hydrogel lenses. (Courtesy of A. J. Phillips)

Lens material

A low wetting angle and dimensional stability are of greater importance than the maximum permeability to oxygen, especially in the severely atopic patient where tears may be significantly affected. In such cases, it may even be necessary to consider the use of polymethylmethacrylate (PMMA) as a material because of its excellent wetting properties. PMMA also finds occasional use in the case of keratoconic wearers with recalcitrant giant papillary conjunctivitis due to its good resistance to surface deposition. The steep high minus lens, usually necessary in keratoconus, is prone to distortion if made from materials with a high siloxane content.

Corneal topographers (see also Chapter 7)

The concept of ordering contact lenses by computer analysis of photokeratograms or videokeratographs is an attractive one. This was first suggested using the Wesley–Jessen PEK System 2000 which made use of an ellipsoidal configuration of the illuminated rings. Computer-assisted videokeratoscopes such as the EyeSys or TMS Corneal Topography systems use many more rings and have a highly sophisticated system of analysis, but the illuminated targets are in a fixed configuration. Because of this, as astigmatism increases, the precision of the output values is beyond the capability of the instrument (McCarey et al. 1992). The accurate analysis of corneal topography in keratoconus

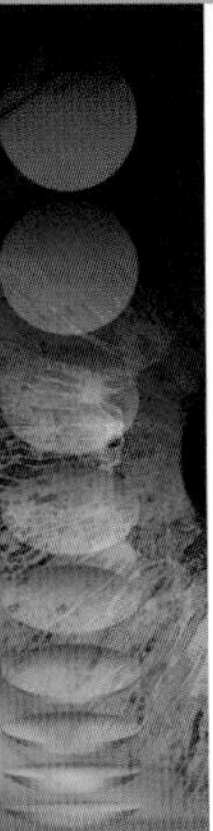

is only possible using projection rather than reflecting techniques, such as rasterstereography (de Cunha & Woodward 1993). Because of these constraints, the prescribing of contact lenses for keratoconus using such systems is generally only of use in very early cases. Soni et al. (1991) suggested that they could be used for evaluating the front surface of the soft lens when fitting piggyback systems.

Nevertheless, topographic devices have become a vital tool for those doing significant amounts of keratoconic fitting for the following reasons.

- Confirmation of diagnosis.
- Location of the cone apex.
- Locating the width of the cone area.
- Obtaining simulated *K* readings and other curvature values.
- Measurements of corneal eccentricity (the value of this will depend upon the topographer in use).
- For some lenses the topographer will design the first lens – for example the KBA design described above.
- Monitoring progression of the disease.
- Differential diagnosis of displaced cones, Terriens or pellucid degeneration (see above).
- Demonstration to the patient of their problem.

Lens fitting

With conventional fitting sets the fitting routine can be summarized as follows.

- Attempt *K* readings. Asking the patient to shift fixation until the mire pattern is at its most regular will often give a more accurate idea of curvature.
- Carry out topography if available. Again, move fixation until the mires are at their most regular. This will give simulated *K* readings, the position of the cone apex, and the width of the cone. (Some lens manufacturers advise that the measurement 4–5 mm temporal to the centre of the cornea gives the approximate BOZR of the first trial lens.)
- Select a dedicated trial fitting set. Lenses with conventional TDs (e.g. 9–10.0 mm) will provide the greatest comfort and optimal vision because of their larger back optic zone diameter (BOZD). Where possible use only fitting sets where *all* parameters are known and specified.
- Select a BOZR nearly as flat as the flattest *K*, or the topographical measurement 4–5 mm temporal to the central cornea. Place the lens on the anaesthetized cornea and assess the fit. Ensure that the peripheral fit of this lens either aligns or is slightly flat in order not to affect the central fit. Modify the BOZR until light central contact is achieved.
- If this lens is comfortable, an over-refraction may be performed.
- Knowing the back peripheral radius (BPR_1) of the trial lens used to assess the BOZR, estimate the trial lens required to give good peripheral alignment. Assess the periphery with a lens having the BOZR sufficiently steep not to affect the peripheral fit. Aim for alignment over a bandwidth of 0.75–1.00 mm depending upon the design.
- Modify this secondary curve until good alignment is achieved. If necessary, consider the need for a toric periphery or full toric.
- Ensure that the very edge of the lens shows good clearance, usually by the addition of two flat, narrow outer curves (normally part of the fitting design).

Soft hydrogel lenses

Soft lenses are not the lens type of first choice as the optical results are usually inferior to rigid lenses. Occasionally they are the only lenses tolerated and certain lens types (e.g. Keratosoft, see below) can give reasonable vision. Alternatively, a conventional soft lens used in conjunction with a spectacle overcorrection may provide better vision than spectacles alone.

Corneal sensitivity is reduced in keratoconus (Bleshoy 1986), but the sensitivity of the upper lid margins is not affected. In patients with abnormal lids and palpebral conjunctivae associated with atopic eczema and vernal conjunctivitis, the thickened lids may render rigid lens wear difficult. For these patients, large limbal or paralimbal lenses (see p. 458) or scleral lenses (see Chapter 15) may prove easier to wear.

In the early stages of the disease, a medium-water-content lens of positive power (with a significant centre thickness of at least 0.35 mm) can be fitted, together with a negative astigmatic spectacle overcorrection. However, this cannot be regarded as anything more than a short-term expedient in view of the possible long-term deleterious effects of wearing thick hydrogel lenses for long periods.

Some may think that there is a role for toric soft lenses in the fitting of keratoconus. Except occasionally in forme fruste (where corneal thinning and irregular astigmatism do not proceed to complete keratoconus), this is not the case, because:

- The asymmetry along a single meridian makes it difficult to obtain a satisfactory fit.
- In order to obtain a satisfactory visual result with materials of a low refractive index, large meridional differences in curvature are required with large differences in lens thickness. These can lead to localized corneal oedema and corneal neovascularization, which can affect any future keratoplasty. Blood vessels in the cornea provide easy access between donor antigen and host lymphocytes, thus removing most of the immunological privilege normally enjoyed by the cornea.

A number of soft lenses are designed for use in keratoconus. These are mid-water-content lenses with a geometry designed to reduce the normal 'draping' effect in order to produce better visual consistency. Examples of this type of lens are Kerasoft (Ultravision CLPL, UK) and Acuity Soft K (Acuity Contact Lenses, UK).

The parameters of the Keratosoft lens are shown in Table 20.4. The lens is designed to produce stability from the scleral topography so that the corneal correction is more reliable. The manufacturers claim that the acuity is comparable with a rigid lens but that is often not the case. Initially Series A and B are supplied, with Series B being the flatter of the two. The first lens chosen depends on the *K* readings. For steeper cones, Series A is first choice and the total diameter can be altered if it needs to be tighter. Series C is used if Series B is too tight.

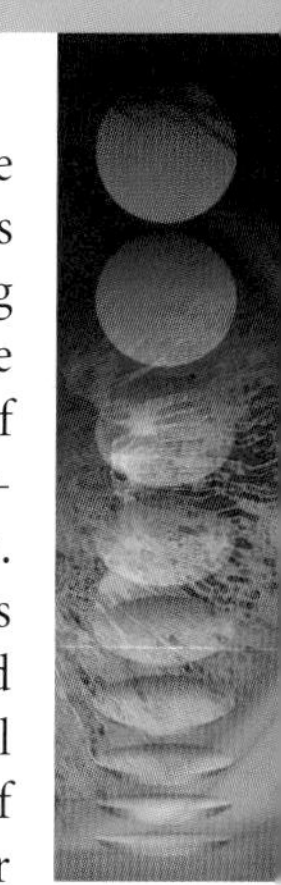

Table 20.4: Parameters of the Keratosoft lens	
Diameter	**14.50 ± 0.5 mm**
BOZR	Series A, B or C (see text)
Powers	Unlimited spherical power Cylinder up to −11.00 D
Axes	Any in 0.5° steps
Near add	Up to +2.50 D
Prism	Up to 2.00 D at any axis
Design	Back surface toric
UV and handling tint	Possible
Material	Hioxifilcon B11
Water content	49%
Dk (35°C Fatt units)	15

Lim and Vogt (2002) and Kapur et al. (2003) carried out clinical audits and found that only around 1% of patients use hydrogel lenses. Furthermore, patients initially fitted with soft lenses often find it difficult to convert to rigid lens wear if the condition progresses.

Scleral lenses (see Chapter 15)

The use of scleral lenses in keratoconus is not high, but is of significance because for many patients they are the only alternative to keratoplasty. The main candidates for scleral lens fitting are those whose corneas have steepened too much for a corneal lens to be retained on the eye, yet with minimal corneal scarring and hence the possibility of a reasonable level of acuity.

Where the apex of the cone is decentred down more than usual, a corneal lens may not centre sufficiently near the visual axis for good acuity, and similarly penetrating keratoplasty would require a larger graft with the consequential increased risk of graft rejection. Down's syndrome patients usually find scleral lenses easier to cope with.

Until recently, scleral lenses for keratoconus were invariably fitted by the impression technique. This was because with lenses fabricated from PMMA the clearance of the optic portion of the lens was crucial in determining success, and hours of painstaking modification were usually required to achieve this. If a preformed fitting technique was used, the eccentricity of the cone in relation to the corneal axis and its asymmetry made the modifications required even more numerous. The advent of RGP scleral lenses has changed this situation. These lenses are much more forgiving in terms of corneal clearance and it is possible to fit preformed scleral lenses in either a sealed or fenestrated form. Sealed preformed RGP lenses in particular may offer a relatively straightforward option. Pullum and Buckley (1997) reported that 53% of eyes, which could not be fitted with other contact lens types, were successfully fitted with RGP scleral lenses for the management of primary corneal ectasias, the majority being keratoconus.

There are still a significant number of patients who have been wearing PMMA scleral lenses for many years, sometimes fitted prior to the availability of dedicated corneal lens fitting sets for keratoconus. These patients can present considerable management problems. Usually they wear their lenses most of their waking hours and the inevitable consequence is a low-grade but chronic hypoxia and ensuing neovascularization. Furthermore, these patients may have good contact lens tolerance and be asymptomatic, only complaining of a reduced level of vision when vessels and infiltrates reach the central corneal area. Generally scleral lenses give a higher quality of vision than the equivalent corneal lens because of their flatter back optic zone radii and larger back optic zone diameters. It can therefore be difficult to wean such scleral lens wearers from their lenses when they are beginning to exhibit undesirable contact lens-induced changes but relatively minor symptoms. A clear explanation must be given that they are putting in jeopardy any future keratoplasty by increasing the possibility of rejection.

Combination lenses and systems

A lens combining the visual acuity of a rigid lens with the comfort of a soft lens is very attractive. This may be achieved with two separate lenses, usually known as a 'piggyback lens', or a single lens fabricated from two different materials (Westerhout 1973, 1985, Baldone 1985).

PIGGYBACK LENSES (see also Chapters 22 and 23)

The piggyback lens system consists of a soft lens fitted underneath a well-fitted rigid lens. Nowadays, a plano or low-power daily-wear silicone hydrogel lens is commonly used (such as PureVision (Bausch & Lomb) or Acuvue Oasys (Johnson & Johnson). In steeper cones, if these lenses do not drape the cornea adequately, a soft lens of medium or high water content is used – for example, a Proclear (CooperVision) monthly lens or an Acuvue (Johnson & Johnson) daily lens. The TD of the rigid lens is between 9.0 and 10.0 mm and the fit is the optimum keratoconic fit (O'Donnell & Maldonado-Codina 2004). The fit of the system is assessed using high-molecular-weight fluorescein (see Chapter 5) although with low-water content silicone hydrogel materials, conventional fluorescein penetrates only slowly.

Unfortunately, the rigid lens may ride low on the soft lens with little or no movement. In order to overcome this problem, the corneal lens can be fitted onto a low positive soft lens or into a recessed portion cut into the front surface of a soft lens (Fig. 20.12). An alternative method is to fit a minus-powered soft or silicone hydrogel lens in order to artificially flatten the cornea and take *K* readings over this lens in order to fit the RGP lens (Caroline & Andre 2004).

Corneal hypoxia and neovascularization are greatly reduced with modern materials and strategies (Glasson et al. 2001), but, if such signs become evident, this lens system should be abandoned. A common reason for the discontinuation of wear is the patient's inability to handle and maintain two different types of lens.

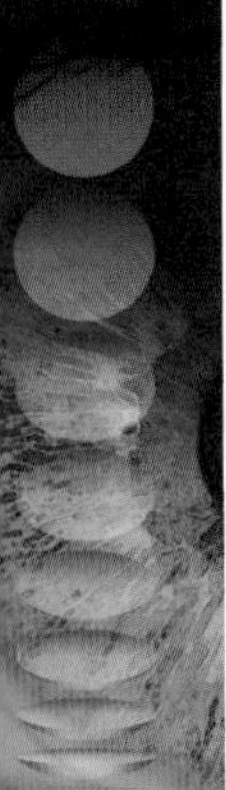

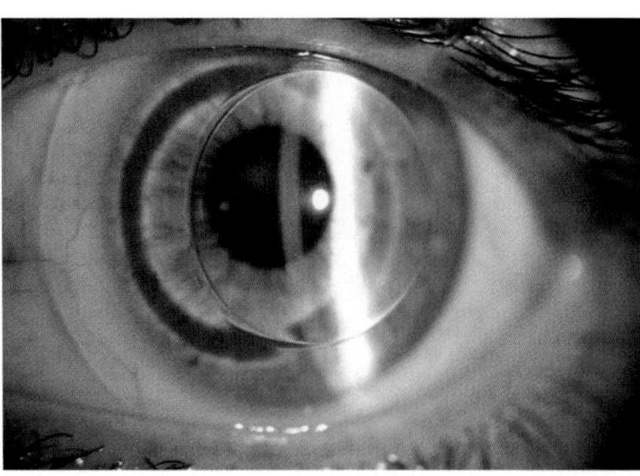

Figure 20.12 Sunken piggyback lens. In cases of gross corneal irregularity and high sensitivity, such as advanced keratoconus, an RGP lens may have to be fitted over a soft carrier lens. In order to prevent lens decentration the RGP lens has been inset into a recess cut into the soft lens (lenses by Hydron (Australia) Ltd). (Courtesy of A. J. Phillips)

HYBRID LENSES

The first commercially available hybrid lens manufactured from two different materials was the Saturn lens initially designed by Precision Cosmet Inc. in 1977. This lens was composed of a rigid central segment made of PMMA and a silicone skirt.

Currently available is the SoftPerm lens (CIBA Vision). The lens comprises:

- Pentasilcon-P RGP centre of 8 mm with a Dk of 17.
- 25% water content modified HEMA skirt (Dk 7) giving a TD of 14.3 mm.
- BOZR available are 6.5 to 8.1 mm, in 0.1 mm steps.
- The chord width of the rigid portion of the lens is fixed, as is the relationship between the radii of curvature of the rigid and flexible portions.

Success in fitting mild to moderate cases has been reported with this lens (Hewett & Hewett 1991) and it can be useful for fitting 'difficult' keratoconic eyes (Rubinstein & Sud 1999). However, it is common for the lens to tighten with wear, leading to hypoxia and corneal neovascularization (Owens et al. 2002). Because the design of the lens cannot be varied, if the corneal portion fits well, the peripheral flange is usually too tight and patients exhibit corneal oedema after a few hours wear. This tendency is exacerbated by the low Dk (Morgan 1992).

The SynergEyes (Quarter Lambda Technologies, USA) is a hybrid lens with higher Dk. For details, see Chapter 23.

PATIENT MANAGEMENT

Contact lens fitting should be initiated at an appropriate time, when there is significant visual gain, otherwise patients may not persevere with lens wear. During an active phase of keratoconus, refitting as frequently as every 3 months may be necessary, as the lens becomes unstable, leading to fluctuating vision, and lens decentration and loss from the eye. The fluorescein fit will demonstrate heavy pressure on the cone with no peripheral bearing surface.

CORNEAL HYDROPS (see Figs 20.5 and 20.6)

This condition occurs in approximately 3% of keratoconic eyes (Tuft et al. 1994b). Descemet's membrane splits and allows aqueous ingress into the corneal stroma resulting in marked oedema, pain and loss of lens tolerance. Lens wear must be discontinued until all the stromal oedema has resolved, which may take several months. Refitting is not always necessary following an episode of hydrops but the visual acuity is often reduced due to scarring of Descemet's membrane. If refitting is necessary, the resultant lens may be flatter than the pre-hydrops lens, harking back to the treatment suggested by Nottingham of inducing scarring to strengthen the cornea (see p. 464).

After-care problems in keratoconus

Several problems specific to keratoconus are seen during fitting or at after-care visits. Some have already been mentioned but for reference are summarized here, together with the necessary clinical action.

TOROIDAL PERIPHERIES (see p. 456 and Table 20.3)

Keratoconus commonly produces a form of pseudo-with-the-rule astigmatism. A spherical lens will often rock along the horizontal meridian or lag low. In milder cases, and where a spherical trial lens gives good acuity, the use of a toric periphery should be considered. Typically, the toricity should be between 0.4 and 0.6 mm.

- Determine the secondary curve that gives good alignment in the flatter meridian by using either a toric periphery trial set or a standard spherical trial lens.
- If a spherical set only is available, order the first lens 0.10 mm flatter than the BPR_1 (since a toric periphery steepens immediately from the flattest point, effectively tightening the fit) and, empirically, 0.40 mm toric. Thus, if the trial lens used was:

  C4/6.50:6.80/**7.50**:8.80/10.50:9.40/12.25:9.80

  then the first lens ordered would be:

  C4/6.50:6.80/**7.60** × **7.20**:8.80/10.50 × 10.10:9.40/12.25 × 11.85:9.80

Toroidal peripheries have the advantage that, since the cornea is invariably with-the-rule, the oval optic so produced is orientated vertically on the eye, thereby reducing blur from the edge of the BOZD on vertical lens movement. Peripheral curves more than 0.6 mm toric will leave an insufficient bearing surface in the vertical meridian and a full toric design should be used.

CHANGES IN BVP WHEN THE BOZR IS CHANGED

As discussed in Chapter 9, a useful clinical rule-of-thumb is that changing the BOZR by 0.05 mm produces a change in liquid lens power of 0.25 D. This, of course, only applies over the normal range of corneal radii.

If the BOZR of a trial or subsequent lens needs changing, the compensating change in BVP can be deduced from the CD-ROM accompanying this book. However, a useful approximation is as follows:

		BOZR change	*BVP change*
If the BOZR is:	>7.20 mm	0.10 mm	0.50 D
	6.20–7.20 mm	0.10 mm	0.75 D
	5.50–6.20 mm	0.10 mm	1.00 D
	5.00–5.50 mm	0.10 mm	1.25 D

INFERIOR UNDERHANG

Cones are commonly inferocentral. The effect is to produce a flatter superior and steeper inferior cornea. This produces a horseshoe-shaped pattern of alignment and shows inferior clearance. This may produce:

- Bubbles entering into the inferior back optic zone.
- Awareness of the lower edge.
- Lens instability.
- Low lens lag.
- Lens ejection.

Action

Refit with a:

- Compromise toric periphery or full toric lens.
- Smaller lens TD.
- Piggyback design.
- Combination lens (e.g. SoftPerm) or semi-scleral.
- Lens design that allows a steeper curve in the inferior lens quadrant.

APICAL STAINING/CONE PRESSURE

Apical staining may be present even before lens fitting commences and is probably due to cell separation over the stretched corneal apex, i.e. the stain is present *between* the cells. However, this stain worsens, especially with pressure on the cone, producing a classic vortex or fleck stain (Fig. 20.13). If considered to be due to the lens fit, then it typically indicates excessive cone pressure. If left untreated, and particularly if severe, it may produce localized epithelial loss and possible scarring or ulceration.

Excessive cone pressure is likely to produce apical staining and may eventually lead to:

- Central erosion.
- Lens instability.
- Loss of tolerance.
- Photophobia.
- Central scarring if excessive and prolonged.

Action

- Steepen the BOZR in 0.10 or 0.20 mm steps.
- Warn the patient that, as the pressure is taken off the cone, further steepening may occur, requiring further changes until stability is reached.

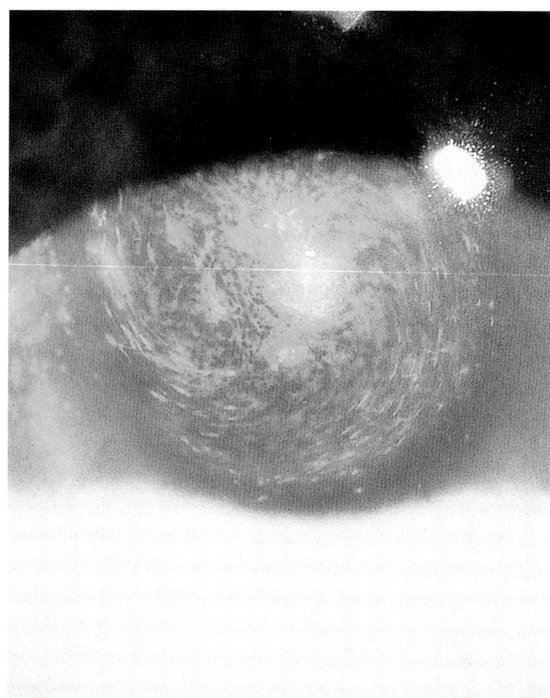

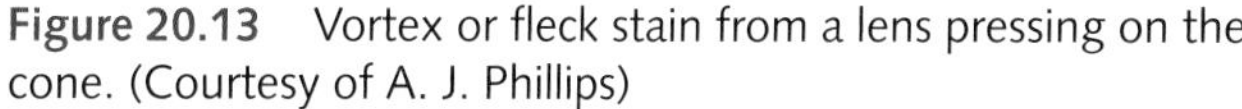

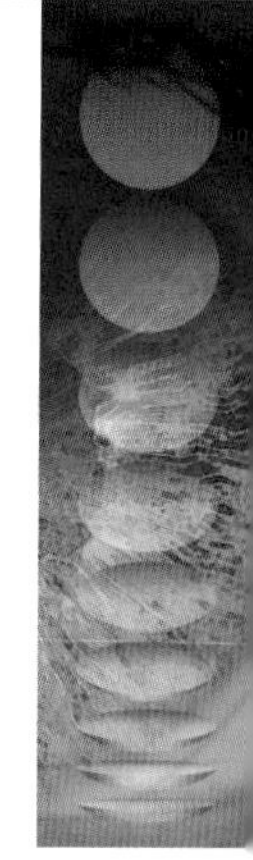

Figure 20.13 Vortex or fleck stain from a lens pressing on the cone. (Courtesy of A. J. Phillips)

- Warn the patient that the acuity may reduce as flat-fitting lenses can sometimes mould the cornea to the shape of the lens back surface, producing a more regular shape. Nevertheless, the risk of excessive cone pressure must be explained.
- Resist the temptation to make large changes to the BOZR in one step, otherwise excessive cone clearance will result, with the risk of bubbles and froth occurring under the back optic portion.

FROTHING

The patient will typically complain of their acuity deteriorating as the day goes on. Removing the lens and cleaning it will give short-term improvement only. Fluorescein will pool in the dimples produced by the bubbles (dimple veiling).

The causes may be:

- Inferior underhang.
- Sharp transitions.
- Too steep a BOZR.
- Spherical lens on an astigmatic cornea.
- Too flat a periphery.

Action

Depending on the cause:

- Flatten the BOZR.
- Steepen the periphery.
- Reduce the TD.
- Fit a toroidal design.
- Utilize a lens allowing a steeper curve in the inferior quadrant.

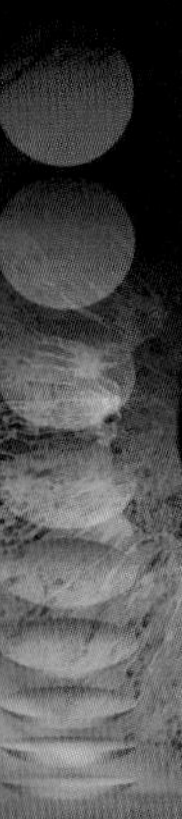

RESIDUAL ASTIGMATISM

Sometimes a well-fitting spherical lens will leave an uncorrected cylinder. To incorporate this into the lens would be impractical due to lens rotation. A toroidal lens design can sometimes be utilized but, due to the narrower area of alignment in keratoconic lens designs, these may still be unstable.

Action

- Consider a *compensated* bitoric lens.
- Prescribe supplementary spectacles to correct the astigmatism. These may be necessary for concentrated visual tasks such as driving and may be usefully made as photochromic lenses so that they double-up as sunglasses.

DISPLACED CONES

In the early stages, displaced cones are often missed, particularly if the vision is good. Pupil dilatation may show the classic retinoscopy reflex distortion at the pupil margin. Corneal topography will usually show that the cone is displaced low and often slightly nasally.

Displaced cones are notoriously difficult to fit. All RGP lenses centre over the corneal apex and in these cases the 'apex' is displaced downwards. Exposure of the lens superior edge makes them uncomfortable. Equally, displaced cones require larger grafts and if adjacent to the limbal vessels, they are more likely to reject. Other peripheral thinning conditions such as Terriens marginal degeneration and pellucid marginal degeneration also fall into this category.

Action

Fit with a:

- Large TD lens (10.00–11.00 mm).
- Large TD lens and prism ballast and truncate to prevent the lens lagging low (and possibly binding).
- Decentred BOZD.
- Piggyback design.
- Combination lens (e.g. SoftPerm) or scleral lens.
- Semi-scleral design.
- Scleral lens.

LOSS OF TOLERANCE

The atopy commonly associated with keratoconus often means that these patients are very sensitive to lens wear from the start. Subsequent loss of tolerance may be due to:

- Prolonged 3 and 9 o'clock staining.
- Prolonged or excessive apical staining or pressure.
- Persistent drying.
- Giant papillary conjunctivitis (GPC)/contact lens-induced papillary conjunctivitis (CLPC).
- Chronic low-grade oedema.

Action

- Refit to avoid staining or GPC/CLPC.
- Treat the underlying cause.
- Consider grafting.

CONTACT LENS-INDUCED DISEASE

If CLPC develops, it may be impossible to persuade patients to cease lens wear because they find it difficult to manage without their lenses. All that can be done is to initiate the appropriate management and try to persuade the patient to reduce their lens wear as much as possible.

Seasonal allergic conjunctivitis and, less commonly, vernal conjunctivitis are often found in conjunction with keratoconus.

Action

- For GPC/CLPC – see Chapters 17 and 18.
- For seasonal allergic conjunctivitis – mast cell stabilizers and mild topical steroids during the summer months.

MONOCULAR KERATOCONUS

True monocular keratoconus has been shown by corneal topographical devices to be rare (see p. 452). However, some 15% of keratoconus cases are *effectively* monocular, i.e. they require a correction in one eye only.

Action

- Fit only if well motivated.
- Fit a single RGP lens if tolerance is good and/or a high level of acuity is required.
- Consider a soft lens.
- Consider a combination or semi-scleral lens.

ADVANCED KERATOCONUS

Keratoconus becomes increasingly more difficult to manage as the cone advances, particularly below 5.50 mm (61.36 D).

Action

- Smaller, very steep BOZR lenses, up to approximately 4.80 mm (70.30 D), depending upon the BOZD.
- Scleral lenses.
- Consider grafting.

CORNEAL HYDROPS (see p. 462)

After an episode of hydrops (see Figs 20.5, 20.6) the contact lens may no longer fit.

- No contact lens wear (or graft) should be attempted until the cornea has resolved, which may take more than 3 months.
- Vision may be reduced due to scarring.
- The cornea often flattens, making refitting easier.

CORNEAL 'PIPS' OR 'CORNS'

These are tiny (0.50–1.00 mm) raised lumps of scar tissue on or close to the cone apices. They are probably keratinized epithelial or scar tissue. They stain easily or collect stain and can be very uncomfortable, presumably due to pressure or rubbing from the lens.

Action

- Refer for 'pipectomy' (superficial keratectomy or phototherapeutic keratectomy) (Moodaley et al. 1994).

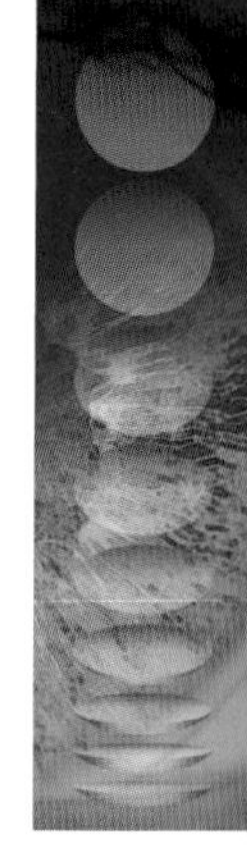

- A temporary hydrogel therapeutic lens may then be necessary (Moodaley et al. 1991).
- Refit post-surgery if necessary.

PRESCRIBING SPECTACLES

As already mentioned, supplementary spectacles are often used to correct residual astigmatism. However, keratoconic lens wearers will often request spectacles for when they are not wearing their lenses or when ill, etc.

Action

- Warn the patient that their acuity will be only around 50% of what it is with contact lenses. Keep expectations down!
- Do not proceed with spectacles unless a useful improvement can be made.
- Warn the patient that their spectacles may by high powered and therefore not cosmetically attractive. Also advise that there may be a difficult adaptive period.
- Use a ±0.75 D cross-cylinder rather than the normal ±0.25 D for determining astigmatism.
- After completing the refraction, it may be possible to reduce the cylindrical component without a loss of acuity.
- Put the final trial lenses in a trial frame and have the patient rotate the cylinder to determine the best subjective axis. This does not always correspond with the refraction result!

GRAFTING/TRANSPLANTATION

Counsel the patient that a corneal transplant is not a straightforward option. It takes many months to settle, is always at risk of rejection and may need a contact lens to improve acuity afterwards.

Refer for keratoplasty when there is:

- Poor visual acuity (typically 6/12–6/18 or poorer).
- Contact lens intolerance.
- Contact lens management problems (e.g. Down's syndrome).
- Unresolved corneal hydrops.
- Chronic hypersensitivity – check that a 'pipectomy' (see above) is not possible.
- Difficulty in achieving a good contact lens fit (e.g. cornea extremely steep, decentred cone, etc.).

Fees and charges

Keratoconus fitting requires great skill and time. Changes to the lens fit are frequent and often changes between lens types are necessary. All this must be explained to the patient before the commencement of fitting. The practitioner's fees and charges must be structured to cover this.

CONCLUSION

Contact lens care for the keratoconic patient is challenging and the chair-time required, as well as the number of diagnostic lenses used, may be extensive (Zhou et al. 2003). However, success rates are good and both patient and practitioner satisfaction is high. Keratoconic patients have gained the reputation with many eye care professionals of being difficult. This has been shown not to be due to any psychoneurotic traits (Mannis et al. 1987, Cooke et al. 2003) but that compared with the typical ophthalmic patient, they are more likely to have received higher education and to be more articulate, younger and more willing to voice their doubts and fears concerning the management of their condition. It should also be remembered that keratoconus patients have to cope continually with reduced contrast sensitivity and some lens discomfort, as well as flare and glare problems, even with well-fitting lenses and good Snellen acuity. Even though their problems may not be resolvable, a certain amount of sympathy and explanation will help.

Acknowledgement

The authors would like to thank Tony Phillips and Lynne Speedwell for their help in the preparation of this chapter.

References

Achatz, M., Escmann, R., Rockert, H., Wilkens, B. and Grant, R. (1985) Keratoconus: a new approach using bi-elliptical contact lenses. Contactologia, 7, 17–21

Amsler, M. (1961) Quelques données du problème du keratocone. Bull. Soc. Belg. Ophthalmol., 129, 331–334

Arias, V. C. (1963) El queratocono su correccion por medio de lente de contacto. Arch. Soc. Oftal. Optom., 4, 41–44

Astin, C. (1987) Bi-elliptical contact lenses for keratoconus. J. Br. Contact Lens Assoc., 10(1), 24–28

Australian Corneal Graft Registry (2004) Report 2004. eds. K. A. Williams, N. B. Hornsby, C. M. Bartlett, H. K. Holland, A. Esterman and D. J. Coster. Adelaide: Australian Corneal Graft Registry

Baldone, J. A. (1985) Piggy-back fitting of contact lenses for keratoconus. Contact Lens Assoc. Ophthalmol. J., 11(2), 130–134

Barr, J. T., Zadnik, K., Edrington, T. B. et al. (2000) Factors associated with corneal scarring in the Collaborative Longitudinal Evaluation of Keratoconus (CLEK) Study. Cornea, 19(4), 501–507

Barth, J. (1948) Statisk uben 300 keratoconusfalle mit 557 befallen augen. MD Thesis. University of Zurich

Beardsley, T. and Foulks, G. (1982) An association of keratoconus and mitral valve prolapse. Ophthalmology, 89, 35–37

Betts, A. M., Mitchell, L. and Zadnik, K. (2002) Visual performance and comfort with the Rose K lens for keratoconus. Optom. Vis. Sci., 79(8), 493–501

Bleshoy, H. (1986) Corneal sensitivity in keratoconus. Trans. BCLA Conference, 9–13

Blix, M. (1880) Oftalmometriska studier. Uppsala Lakareforenigs Farhandiglingar, 15, 349–420

Boxer-Wachler, B. S., Chandra, N. S., Chou, B., Korn, T. S., Nepomuceno, R. and Christie, J. P. (2003) Intacs for keratoconus. Ophthalmology, 110(5), 1031–1040

Bron, A. J., Tripathi, R. C., Harding, J. J. and Crabbe, M. J. C. (1978) Stromal loss in keratoconus. Trans. Ophthalmol. Soc. UK, 98(3), 393–396

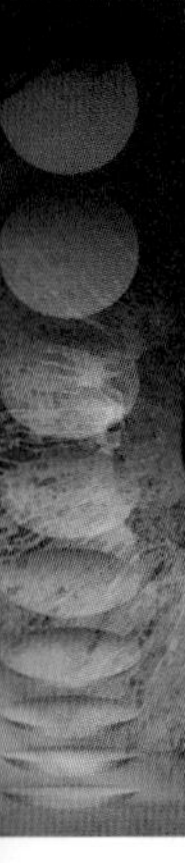

Caroline, P. J. and Andre, M. P. (2004) Masking irregular astigmatism with soft contact lenses. Contact Lens Spectrum, 19, 56

Clifford-Hall, K. G. (1963) A comprehensive study of keratoconus. Br. J. Physiol. Opt., 20(4), 215–256

Cooke, C. A., Cooper, C., Dowds, E., Frazer, D. G. and Jackson, A. J. (2003) Keratoconus, myopia and personality. Cornea, 22(3), 239–242

Cox, S. N. (1984) Management of keratoconus. J. Br. Contact Lens Assoc., 7(2), 86–92

Cullen, J. F. and Butler, H. J. (1963) Mongolism (Down's syndrome) and keratoconus. Br. J. Ophthalmol., 47(6), 321–330

Davies, P. D., Ruben, M. and Woodward, E. G. (1977) Keratoconus: an analysis of the factors which affect the optical results of keratoplasty. Trans. Eur. Contact Lens Soc. Ophthalmol. (Ghent), 97–99

de Cunha, D. and Woodward, E. G. (1993) Measurement of corneal topography in keratoconus. Ophthalmic Physiol. Opt., 13(4), 377–382

Edmund, C. (1987) Assessment of an elastic model in the pathogenesis of keratoconus. Acta Ophthalmol. (Kbh), 65, 376–380

Edrington, T. B., Barr, J. T., Zadnik, K. et al. (1996) Standardised rigid contact lens fitting protocol for keratoconus. Optom. Vis. Sci., 73, 369–375

Edrington, T. B., Szczotka, L. B., Barr, J. T. et al. (1999) Rigid contact lens fitting relationships in keratoconus. Optom. Vis. Sci., 76(10), 692–699

Edwards, M., McGhee, C. N. and Dean, S. (2001) The genetics of keratoconus. Clin. Exp. Ophthalmol., 29(6), 345–351

Elschnig, A. (1894) Uber den keratoconus. Klin. Monatsbl. Augenheilk., 32, 25–26

Fick, A. E. (1888) Eine contactbrille. Arch. Augenheilk., 18, 279–288

Fleischer, H. (1906) Uber keratoconus unt eigenartige pigmentbildung in der kornea. Münch. Med. Wochenschr., 53, 625–627

Forrest, J. (1929) The Recognition of Ocular Disease, p. 77. London: J. H. Taylor

Gasset, A. R., Haude, W. L. and Garcia-Bengochia, M. (1978) Hard contact lens wear: an environmental risk in keratoconus. Am. J. Ophthalmol., 85(3), 39–41

Georgiou, T., Funnell, C. L., Cassels-Brown, A. and O'Conor, R. (2004) Influence of ethnic origin on the incidence of keratoconus and associated atopic disease in Asians and white patients. Eye, 18(4) 379–383

Glasson, C. J., Perrault, N. and Brazeau, D. (2001) Oxygen tension beneath piggyback contact lenses and clinical outcomes of users. CLAO J., 27(3), 144–150

Gonzalez, V. and McDonnell, P. J. (1992) Computer-assisted corneal topography in parents of patients with keratoconus. Arch. Ophthalmol., 110(10), 1413–1414

Hewett, L. and Hewett, P. (1991) Clinical impressions of the Softperm contact lens. Clin. Exp. Optom., 74(4), 130–132

Ihalainen, A. (1986) Clinical and epidemiological features of keratoconus: genetic and external factors in the pathogenesis of the disease. Acta Ophthalmol. (Kbh), Suppl. 178, 1–64

Ionnidis, A. S., Speedwell, L. and Nischal, K. K. (2005) Unilateral keratoconus in a child with chronic and persistent eye rubbing. Am. J. Ophthalmol., 139(2), 356–357

Iwamoto, T. and de Moto, D. G. (1976) Electron microscopical study of the Fleischer ring. Arch. Ophthalmol., 94(9), 1579–1584

Jaensch, P. A. (1929) Keratoconus die engebrisse de forschung de cetzen 20 jahre. Zbl. Ophthalmol., 21, 305–327

Jafri, B., Lichter, H. and Stulting, R. D. (2004) Asymmetric keratoconus attributed to eye rubbing. Cornea, 23(6), 560–564

Kapur, S., Rubinstein, M. and Wolffsohn, J. (2003) Managing keratoconus – a hospital clinic audit. Optician, 226, 26–27

Kennedy, R. H., Bourne, W. M. and Dyer, J. A. (1986) A 48-year clinical and epidemiological study of keratoconus. Am. J. Ophthalmol., 101, 267–273

Kerr-Muir, M. K. M., Woodward, E. G. and Leonard, T. (1987) Corneal thickness, astigmatism and atopy. Br. J. Ophthalmol., 71(3), 207–211

Korb, D. R., Finnemore, D. M. and Herman, J. P. (1982) Apical changes and scarring in keratoconus as related to contact lens fitting techniques. J. Am. Optom. Assoc., 53(3), 199–205

Kornerup, T. and Lodin, L. (1959) Ocular changes in 100 cases of Bodriens prurigo atopic dermatitis. Acta Ophthalmol. (Kbh), 37, 508–512

Leung, K. K. Y. (1999) RGP fitting philosophies for keratoconus. Clin. Exp. Optom., 82(6), 230–235

Lim, N. and Vogt, U. (2002) Characteristics and functional outcomes of 130 patients with keratoconus attending a specialist contact lens clinic. Eye, 16, 54–59

Macsai, M. S., Varley, G. A. and Krachmer, J. H. (1990) Development of keratoconus after contact lens wear: patient characteristics. Arch. Ophthalmol., 108, 534–538

Mannis, M. J., Morrison, T. L., Zadnik, K., Holland, E. S. and Kracher J. H. (1987) Personality traits in keratoconus. Arch. Ophthalmol., 105, 798–800

Marechal-Courtois, C. and Prijat, E. (1972) Relative values of contact lenses and keratoplasty in the treatment of keratoconus. Contact Lens J., 3(6), 36–37

Maumenee, I. (1975) Hereditary connective tissue diseases involving the eye. Trans. Ophthalmol. Soc. UK, 94, 753–763

McCarey, B., Zurawski, C. and O'Shea, D. S. (1992) Practical aspects of a corneal topographical system. CLAO J., 18, 248–254

McDonnell, P. (1991) Current applications of the corneal modelling system. Refrac. Corneal Surg., 7, 87–91

McMonnies, C. W. and Boneham, G. C. (2003) Keratoconus, allergy, itch, eye-rubbing and hand-dominance. Clin. Exp. Optom., 86(6), 376–384

Moodaley, L. C., Buckley, R. J. and Woodward, E. G. (1991) Surgery to improve contact lens wear in keratoconus. CLAO J., 17(2), 129–131

Moodaley, L. C., Woodward, E. G., Liu, C. S. C. and Buckley, R. J. (1992) Life expectancy in keratoconus. Br. J. Ophthalmol., 76(10), 590–592

Moodaley, L., Liu, C., Woodward, E. G. et al. (1994) Excimer laser superficial keratectomy for proud nebulae in keratoconus. Br. J. Ophthalmol., 78(6), 454–457

Morgan, P. (1992) A new soft/RGP combination lens. Optician, October, 16–22

Negris, R. (1992) Floppy eyelid syndrome associated with keratoconus. J. Am. Optom. Assoc., 63(5), 316–319

Nepomuceno, R. L., Boxer-Wachler, B. S. and Weissman, B. A. (2003) Feasibility of contact lens fitting on patients with INTACS inserts. Cont. Lens Anterior Eye, 26(4), 175–180

Nottingham, J. (1854) Practical Observations on Conical Cornea. London: Churchill

Nuel, J. P. (1900) Systems of Diseases of the Eye, vol. IV, pp. 249–253, eds. E. Norris and J. Oliver. London: Lewin

O'Donnell, C. and Maldonado-Codina, C. (2004) A hyper-Dk piggyback contact lens system for keratoconus. Eye Contact Lens, 30(1), 44–48

Obrig, T. E. and Salvatori, P. (1958) Contact Lenses, pp. 145–146. New York: Chilton

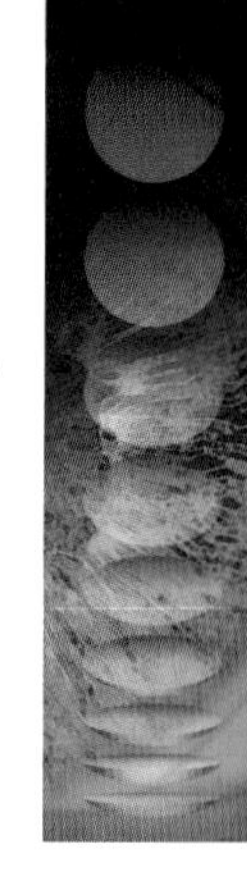

Owens, H., Watters, G. and Gamble, G. (2002) Effects of SoftPerm lens wear on corneal thickness and topography : a comparison between keratoconic and normal corneae. CLAO J., 28(2), 83–87

Pearson, A. R., Soneji, B., Sarvananthan, N. and Sandford-Smith, J. H. (2000) Does ethnic origin influence the incidence or severity of keratoconus? Eye, 14(4), 625–628

Phillips, A. J. (2003) Can true monocular keratoconus occur? Clin. Exp. Optom., 86(6), 309–402

Pouliquen, Y., Bellivet, J., Lecoq, J. and Clay, C. (1972) Keratoplastic transfixante dans le traitment du keratocone. A propos de 60 cas. Arch. Opthalmol. Paris, 32, 735–744

Pullum, K. (2003) A keratoconus fitting system using the axial profile to establish optimum lens parameters. Cont. Lens Anterior Eye, 26, 77–84

Pullum, K. W. and Buckley, R. J. (1997) A study of 530 patients referred for rigid gas permeable scleral contact lens assessment. Cornea, 16(6), 612–622

Rabinowitz, Y. S. and McDonnell, P. (1989) Computer-assisted corneal topography in keratoconus. Refract. Corneal Surg., 5(6), 400–408

Ruben, M. (1975) Contact Lens Practice, pp. 283–284; 339–341. London: Baillière-Tindall

Ruben, M. (1978) Treatment of keratoconus. Ophthalmol. Opt., 3(18), 64–72

Rubinstein, M. P. and Sud, S. (1999) The use of hybrid lenses in management of the irregular cornea. Cont. Lens Anterior Eye, 22(3), 87–90

Ruben, M. and Trodd, C. (1976) Scleral lenses in keratoconus. Contact Interoc. Med. J., 2(1), 18–20

Sharif, K. and Casey, T. (1992) Prevalence of mitral valve prolapse in keratoconus patients. J. R. Soc. Med., 85(8), 446–448

Smiddy, W. E., Hamburg, T. R., Kracher, G. P. and Stark, W. J. (1988) Keratoconus: contact lenses or keratoplasty. Ophthalmology, 95(4), 487–492

Soni, P. S., Gerstman, D. R., Horner, G. and Heath, G. G. (1991) The management of keratoconus using the corneal modelling system and a piggyback system of contact lenses. J. Am. Optom Assoc., 62(8), 593–597

Tuft, S. J., Moodaley, L. C., Gregory, W. M., Davison, C. R. and Buckley, R. J. (1994a) Prognostic factors for the progression of keratoconus. Ophthalmology, 101(3), 439–477

Tuft, S. J., Gregory, W. M. and Buckley, R. J. (1994b) Acute corneal hydrops in keratoconus. Ophthalmology, 101(10), 1738–1743

Walsh, S. Z. (1981) Keratoconus and blindness in 469 institutionalised subjects with Down's syndrome and other causes of mental retardation. J. Ment. Defic. Res., 25, 243–251

Westerhout, D. (1973) The combination lens and therapeutic uses of soft lenses. Contact Lens J., 4(5), 3–10

Westerhout, D. (1985) Combination and piggy-back lenses. Trans. BCLA Conference, 49–51

Wilson, S. E., Lin, D. T. C. and Klyce, S. D. (1991) Corneal topography of keratoconus. Cornea, 10(1), 2–8

Woodward, E. G. (1980a) Keratoconus: the disease and its progression. Doctoral Thesis. The City University, London

Woodward, E. G. (1980b) The cornea in health and disease. Trans. 16th Congr. Eur. Soc. Ophthalmol., 40(1), 531–536

Woodward, E. G. (1981) Keratoconus: maternal age and social class. Br. J. Ophthalmol., 65(2), 104–107

Woodward, E. G. and Morris, M. (1990) Joint hypermobility in keratoconus. Ophthalmic Physiol. Opt., 10(4), 360–363

Woolensak, G., Spoeri, E. and Seiler, T. (2003) Treatment of keratoconus by collagen cross linking [Behandlung von Keratokonus durch Kollagenvernetzung]. Ophthalmologe, 100(1), 44–49

Young, S., Lundegan, M. and Olson, D. J. (1991) The spectrum of topography found in keratoconus. CLAO J., 17(3), 198–204

Zhou, A. J., Kitamura, K. and Weissman, B. A. (2003) Contact lens care in keratoconus. Cont. Lens Anterior Eye, 26, 171–174

Chapter 21

High prescriptions

Lynne Speedwell

CHAPTER CONTENTS

INTRODUCTION

Most patients with high prescriptions benefit both optically and cosmetically from contact lenses, more so than patients with low prescriptions. Fitting the lenses is not always straightforward and lens wear has unique problems relating in part to the different lens parameters but also to the medical aspects of the condition causing the high prescription. Extra vigilance is required at after-care to ensure that both the health of the eyes and the state of the contact lenses are adequately assessed.

GENERAL POINTS

Patients requiring high prescriptions are at a disadvantage when dealing with their lenses, as their unaided acuity is especially poor.

Lens handling

- Insertion: Everything needs to be set up to insert the lenses and the spectacles removed at the last moment. If the patient cannot manage at all without their glasses, an empty frame can be glazed in one eye only and the first contact lens inserted through the empty side of the frame.
- Removal: Spectacles need to be at hand when lenses are to be removed.
- A mislaid lens is harder to find so it is safer to work over a clean towel on a designated surface.
- Thick (positive) lenses are easily scratched. Thin (negative) lenses, both soft and rigid gas-permeable (RGP), can distort with handling. The back vertex power (BVP), especially in thin high-minus lenses, may alter with energetic lens cleaning.
- Ordering different tints helps differentiate left and right lenses.
- Provide a lens case with different colour tops or mark one top with indelible ink or nail varnish.

Vision

- Spectacle aberrations are more obvious when alternating between spectacles and contact lenses and the pincushion effect of aphakic spectacles is especially difficult to cope with.
- Objects appear larger with hypermetropic spectacles and smaller with myopic spectacles (see Chapter 6).

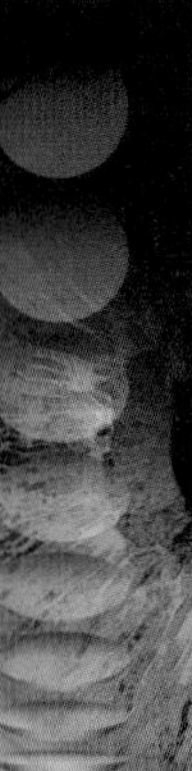

- Distance judgement is likewise affected when alternating between the two forms of correction and patients who drive need to be warned about this.
- Where acuity is good, normal parameter tolerances are not always adequate and replacement lenses may be unacceptable to the patient, even when a new lens is ordered with exactly the same parameters as the previous lens.
- Patients with good vision in only one eye may find it helpful if both eyes are fitted with a similar prescription so the lens in the eye with poorer vision acts as a spare lens for the better eye.

Lens ordering

- Lenses are likely to be tailor-made to each prescription, as 'off the peg' lenses are not available. Errors are more likely to occur in the manufacture of such lenses.
- Disposable lenses are available in limited powers only (although the range of parameters is improving all the time).
- Thick lenses develop deposits more than thin ones. Disposable lenses are not usually available in the prescriptions required but, although more expensive, it is advisable that lenses are replaced at regular 6- or 12-monthly intervals as all high-powered lenses are prone to scratching and excessive build-up of deposits.
- Before reordering lenses that have been worn for some time, recheck parameters as they are liable to have altered.

Ordering high-power lenses (see Chapter 6 and the accompanying CD-ROM)

Lens power

- Careful refraction is needed and the back vertex distance (BVD) must be measured.
- The lens power at the cornea equals the BVP of the contact lens to be ordered. This is either calculated or read off a chart (see Appendix A and CD-ROM).
- For astigmatic corrections, the power of the lens at the cornea must be calculated in the two principal meridians.

Lens material

The ideal material used for high-power lenses should have the following properties:

- High oxygen permeability.
- Good wettability.
- Good deposit resistance.
- Good scratch resistance.

In addition, extra properties of RGP lenses are:

- High refractive index (for thinner lenses).
- Low specific gravity (positive lenses less likely to drop).

Extra properties of soft lenses are:

- Bound water.
- Silicone hydrogel if available.

Unfortunately, the properties required are frequently not available in a single material.

MANUFACTURE OF HIGH PRESCRIPTIONS

The manufacture of lenses is covered in Chapters 6 and 27 but there are some differences to be noted when manufacturing high prescriptions.

- The lenses are all made in lenticular form (see Fig. 21.3).
- Junction thickness needs to be calculated to ensure that it is not too thin in hypermetropic or aphakic prescriptions and not too thick in myopic prescriptions (see below).
- If the lenticular or front optic zone diameter (FOZD) is made smaller, the lens may fit better; however, if it is too small, flare will be a problem. With multicurve RGP lenses, the FOZD is made the same or up to 0.5 mm larger than the BOZD to avoid the problem of flare.
- Soft lenses are made in the dry state (xerogel) and high powers are difficult to check accurately. The lenses need to be left longer to hydrate after manufacture before checking and inaccuracies are commonly found once the material is fully hydrated.

APHAKIA

General points

- The natural crystalline lens is absent, so more ultraviolet light is able to reach the retina.
- The risk of retinal detachment and glaucoma is increased.
- Contact lenses can have a dual purpose – for example, to correct the refractive error and as a therapeutic lens for an aphakic patient with mild bullous keratopathy (see Chapter 26).

Nowadays, the usual surgical procedure is to have an intraocular lens (IOL) inserted, so that neither thick spectacles nor contact lenses are required. For those patients who cannot have an IOL, a corneal section is performed to remove the lens. This often results in varying degrees of with-the-rule astigmatism (Reading 1984).

Most aphakic patients fall into the following categories:

- Elderly patients who had cataracts removed before IOLs were the norm.
- Those where a problem occurred at the time of the initial operation such that it was not possible to insert an IOL.
- Traumatic aphakes where an IOL is not viable. Traumatic aphakia often occurs in manual labourers who are not very dextrous or diligent when it comes to lens handling and care. It is frequently associated with other ocular trauma, which can affect the appearance of the eye (Fig. 21.1), and also makes the eye photophobic. An aphakic lens with a tint or a prosthetic lens may then be required (see 'Unilateral ametropia', below and Chapter 25).
- Infants and children born with cataracts who are unable to have IOLs at the time of surgery (see Chapter 24).

These patients have particular problems with contact lenses:

- Handling difficulties.
- Poor tears.
- Low endothelial cell count.

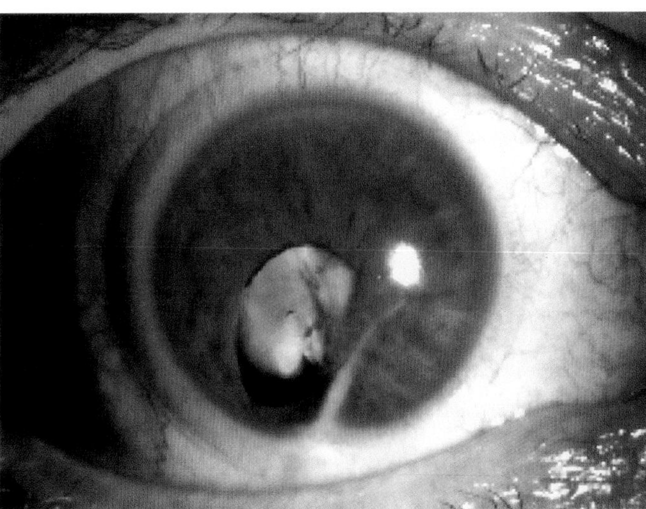

Figure 21.1 Traumatic aphakia. A contact lens improves the vision but the cosmesis is poor. A prosthetic lens would improve the appearance but would be difficult to fit as the useable pupil is displaced downwards. This patient later had further surgery to remove more of the lens matter

- Lid problems
  - epiphora.
  - entropion/ectropion.
  - loose lids
    a. poor lower lid support.
    b. low upper lid (ptosis).
    c. poor lid closure/blink.
- Other ocular pathology
  - glaucoma.
  - retinal detachment.
  - corneal problems
    a. dystrophy.
    b. keratitis.

Trauma and surgery

Eyes where trauma or surgery has rendered the eye difficult to fit:

- Failed IOLs.
- Glaucoma surgery.
- Pupil off-centre or enlarged.
- Multiple pupils (polycoria).
- Apex of cornea not central.
- Induced astigmatism.

Advantages of contact lenses over spectacles

- Better field of vision.
- Fewer peripheral aberrations.
- Cosmetically more acceptable (see Fig. 24.3).

Disadvantages of contact lenses over spectacles

- Acuity is not as sharp, due to the reduction in image size – this can be a problem in cases of impaired vision.
- Spectacles are still required over the lenses for reading.

Lens fitting

- Choose a material that incorporates an ultraviolet inhibitor as the natural protection from the crystalline lens has been removed.
- Consider extended wear (whether soft or RGP), especially in an elderly patient where handling is a problem and if there is no carer available to remove the lenses regularly. However, the risks of infection are high and the elderly are not always keen to ask for help if they have problems with their lenses (Carpel & Parker 1985).
- More neovascularization is acceptable in elderly patients, as life expectancy is less.
- In infants and young children, short periods of extended wear may be necessary but it is always advisable to encourage daily lens removal from the outset as problems such as infections and scarring developed in childhood can lead to amblyopia. These, and any neovascularization that develops, will affect the patient for life (see Chapter 24).
- Bifocal lenses, although good in theory, are not always effective in practice as the thick lenses move too much with blinking and there may be a compromise in the vision. However, some patients do well with bifocals so they should not be dismissed altogether (see Chapter 14).

As with conventional lenses for low prescriptions, aphakic lenses must fit well and cause no adverse reactions. Lenses can be made of any material but they are all thick in the centre. This results in several factors including the following.

- Lenses are liable to drop (Fig. 21.2).
- The lenses move more with blinking. This is especially a problem when only one eye is aphakic, as the image from the aphakic eye may appear to move at each blink.
- The oxygen permeability of the lens is poor compared to a low-power lens of the same material.
- Unwanted long-term effects are more likely. Optimum fitting is even more important than for low prescriptions because patients are more dependent on their contact lenses as alternating with spectacles is not usually practical or convenient (see 'General points', above).
- Deposits are common and protein may build up, particularly at the junction between the lenticular portion of the lens and the carrier (Fig. 21.3).
- Lenses are more likely to become scratched with handling.

RGP LENSES

- The centre thickness is typically 0.30–0.40 mm.
- As previously mentioned, lenses are manufactured in lenticular form in order to reduce the weight. This helps to shift the centre of gravity back towards the eye, which helps improve centration, thus causing the lens to drop less (see Fig. 9.3).
- Fitting the lenses minimally steep will also help centration but not so steep as to cause bubbles to become lodged under the back optic zone.
- The junction thickness needs to be adequate to prevent the lens from flexing or breaking at the junction.
- Larger total diameters can improve comfort and stabilize acuity.

APEX LENSES

So named as they were originally designed for aphakic experimental purposes (Bagshaw et al. 1966).

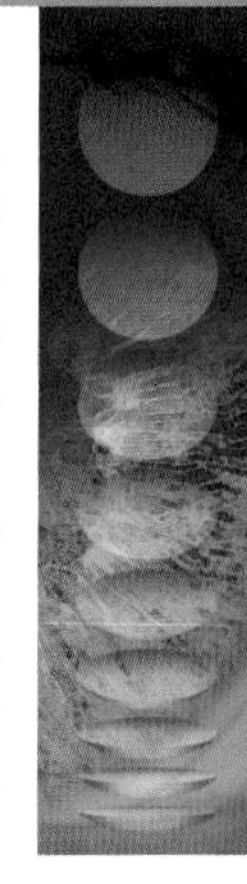

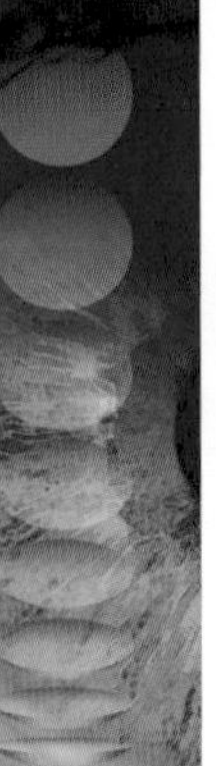

(a)

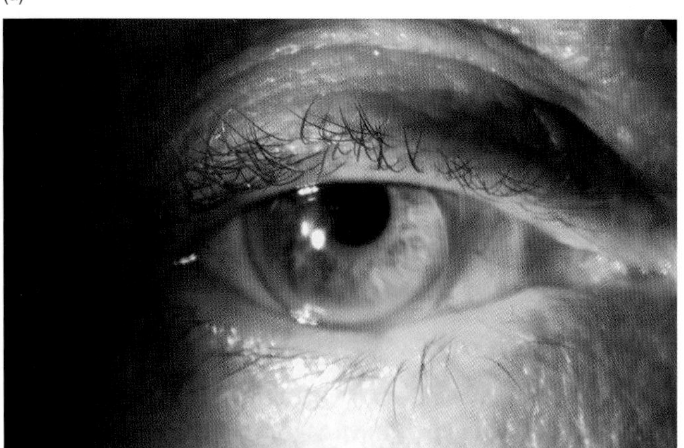

(b)

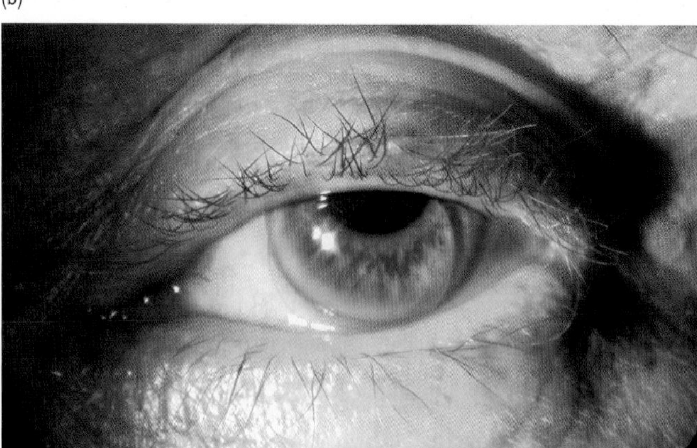

(c)

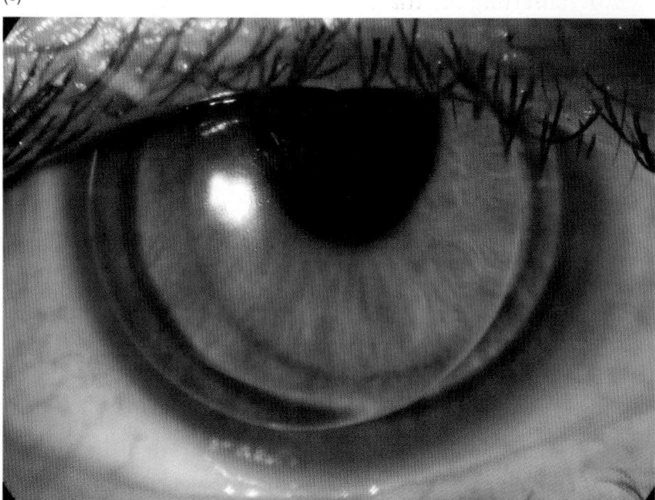

Figure 21.2 (a) The right and (b) the left eye of a bilateral aphake with ptosis. Both lenses sit low on the cornea, but the left eye also has an updrawn pupil with a superior iridectomy resulting in poor vision. The patient underwent surgery for the ptosis and the lenses were refitted to encourage better centration. (c) Aphakic eye with updrawn pupil. Lens is fitted with negative carrier to provide lid hitch. There is good pupil cover which reduces flare

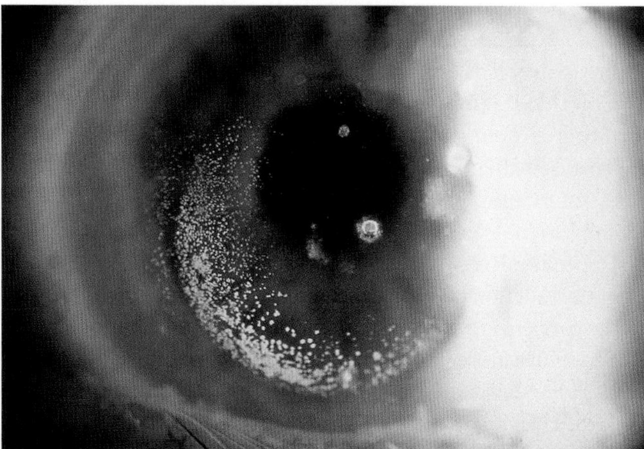

Figure 21.3 Aphakic lens showing deposits around the lenticular portion. (Courtesy of A. J. Phillips)

- These lenses have a large total diameter (TD), typically between 10.50 and 13.5 mm, which aids centration and reduces movement on blinking (Fig. 21.4).
- The BOZD is typically 8.5–10.0 mm and the lens is usually made as a bicurve with the second curve at least 0.7 mm flatter than the BOZR. If tear exchange is found to be inadequate, a third peripheral curve can be added later.
- Lenses may need to be fenestrated in order to facilitate tear exchange and lens removal.
- Lenses can be manufactured in very high-Dk materials to reduce hypoxia.

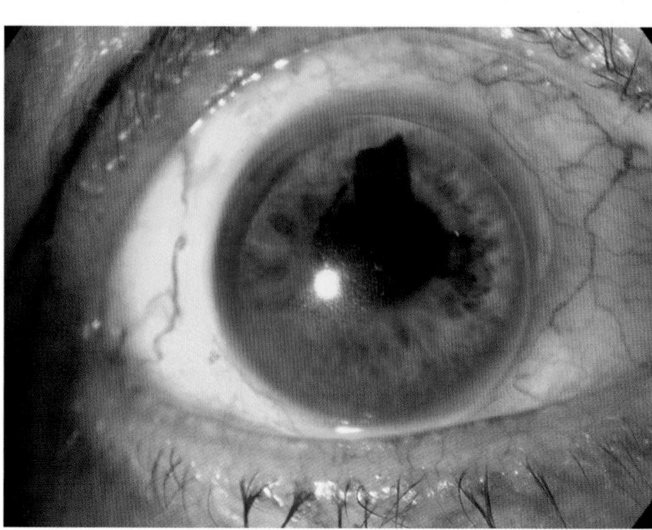

Figure 21.4 Apex lens fitted to an aphakic eye to improve centration of a low-riding lens. This lens has a total diameter of 11.50 mm and is still sitting low on the cornea but provides adequate pupil cover

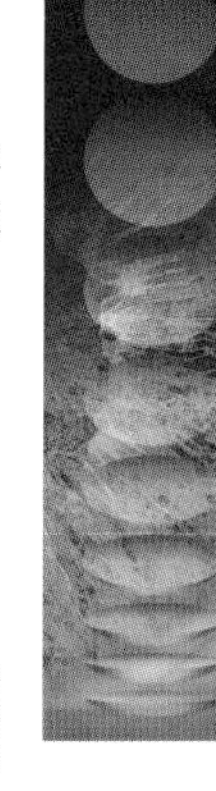

- Apex lenses are particularly useful in cases of traumatic aphakia where the cornea is irregular and the pupil abnormal.

SOFT LENSES (see Chapter 11)

- The junction must not be too thin or the carrier is liable to evert on lens insertion or to break with lens handling.
- Likewise, the carrier should not be too thin.
- As with rigid lenses, large TDs are used to aid centration.
- High-power soft lenses exhibit bending effects when the lens is on the eye which can cause fluctuations in the vision (Chaston & Fatt 1980).

Thicker lenses do not drape the cornea in the same way as thin lenses. A greater range of lens parameters is therefore needed in order to achieve a satisfactory fit. Trial lenses are usually necessary.

After inserting the trial lens, it should be allowed to settle for at least 30 minutes. Thick lenses take longer than thin lenses to equilibrate. When carrying out an over-refraction, the BVD should be measured and the correct power calculated.

If single-vision lenses are fitted, reading spectacles should be prescribed. Alternatively, bifocal or progressive lenses or monovision contact lenses can be prescribed (see Chapter 15).

Troubleshooting

Poor centration – lenses drop

Soft lenses

- Fit larger TD.
- Make lenses thinner.
- Reduce FOZD.
- Fit aspheric lenses.

RGP lenses (see Fig. 21.2)

- Reduce FOZD.
- Fit a multicurve lens with increased edge lift.
- Order a lens with a negative or parallel carrier (see Figs 9.16, 9.28).
- Fit a larger TD or Apex.
- Change material
  - higher refractive index.
  - lower specific gravity.

Lenses move excessively on blinking

- Make lenses thinner.
- Fit larger TD or Apex.

Signs of hypoxia

- Higher Dk material.
- Thinner lens.
- Fit silicone hydrogel if available.
- Fit the nearest silicone hydrogel and overcorrect with spectacles.

Lenses scratch centrally with handling

RGP lenses

- Use harder material (e.g. Boston ES).
- Change storage case design.

Soft and RGP

- Replace lenses more frequently.

Protein deposits

- Use protein remover tablets regularly.
- Try aspheric lenses – these lenses have a more uniform thickness profile (Bleshoy & Guillon 1984) and the junction is not so well circumscribed, so deposits may build up less.
- Replace lenses more frequently.

Handling difficulties or poor stability of image

- Consider scleral lenses (see Chapter 15).

HIGH HYPERMETROPIA

Unless the hypermetropia is extremely high (e.g. in nanophthalmos – see Chapter 24), the problems found when fitting high hypermetropes are similar, but to a lesser degree, to those found in aphakia. Many disposable lenses are available in these prescriptions and can be used to overcome some of the problems associated with aphakia. There are some differences, however.

General points

- Eyes may be smaller and steeper than normal.
- Often associated with strabismus and amblyopia. Extra care is needed where one eye is amblyopic. Rigorous hygiene is required to help prevent contact lens-induced infection as effects on the better eye will affect overall vision.
- If the high refractive error is not corrected from a young age, varying degrees of bilateral amblyopia can occur and, even when fully corrected, normal acuity may not develop.
- High hypermetropia is associated with closed-angle glaucoma. There is a theoretical possibility that tight soft lenses might increase the IOP by compression of the limbal drainage vessels.

Advantages of contact lenses over spectacles

- A better field of view (see Fig. 6.2).
- Less accommodation and convergence required for close work (see Chapter 6).

Disadvantages of contact lenses over spectacles

- The visual acuity is not as good for both distance and near: this is a particular problem where the spectacle acuity is less than 6/6 Snellen.

HIGH MYOPIA

General points

- Prevalence figures for myopia of more than 6.00 D range from 5 to 15% in the general population (Saw 2005).
- Pathological myopia, where there is elongation of the eyeball and degenerative changes of the retina and choroid, has a prevalence of 1–3% (Saw 2005).
- It may be dominantly transmitted (Coscas & Soubrane 1993).
- There is a higher incidence in premature infants (Larsson et al. 2003).
- Figures for incidence of unilateral myopia vary.

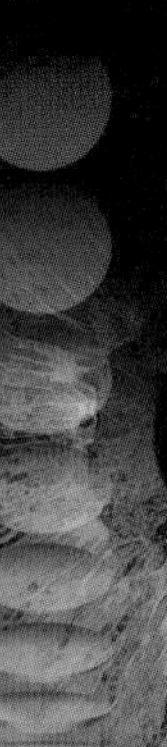

- It can be associated with other syndromes such as Stickler's or Marfan's syndrome.
- Most high myopia is axial (Grosvenor & Scott 1991).

Ophthalmic problems of high myopia

- Enlarged globe.
- Exophthalmia.
- Fundus changes
  - myopic crescents.
  - straightening of the retinal vessels.
  - tessellated background.
  - peripapillary atrophy.
  - chorioretinal degeneration, often leading to loss of vision.
  - risk of retinal detachment.

Problems with enlarged exophthalmic eyes include:

- Poor blink.
- Dry eyes.
- Flat, large corneas.

Advantages of contact lenses over spectacles

- Better acuity.
- Better field. Although the field is theoretically greater with spectacles than with contact lenses, the peripheral field is distorted so contact lenses provide a better usable field. In addition, the spectacle frame limits the field (see Chapter 6 and Fig. 6.1).

Disadvantages of contact lenses over spectacles

- More accommodation and convergence are exerted for close work (see Chapter 6).
- Cosmetic effect may be poor if eyes are exophthalmic (Fig. 21.5). It may be worthwhile to fit the greater part of the prescription with contact lenses and the remainder in spectacles. For example, a –20.00 DS myope can be fitted with, say, –15.00 DS contact lenses and –5.00 DS spectacles over the top.
- High myopia combined with astigmatism requires lenses that are especially thick in one meridian. This frequently leads to neovascularization, particularly with soft lenses. Correcting the astigmatism in spectacles may be preferable.
- Where hypoxia is a problem and silicone hydrogel lenses are not available in high enough prescriptions, a compromise lens can be fitted in silicone hydrogel material and the remainder prescribed in spectacles.
- High myopes with poor acuity may prefer to read unaided rather than using a low visual aid. This is not always convenient.

Presbyopes

For presbyopic patients, supplementary reading spectacles still need to be prescribed. As with aphakia, bifocal contact lenses do not always work in high prescriptions. Early presbyopes may benefit from having a reduced prescription in contact lenses and the remainder in spectacles as they are then able to remove the glasses whenever they wish to read or do any close work.

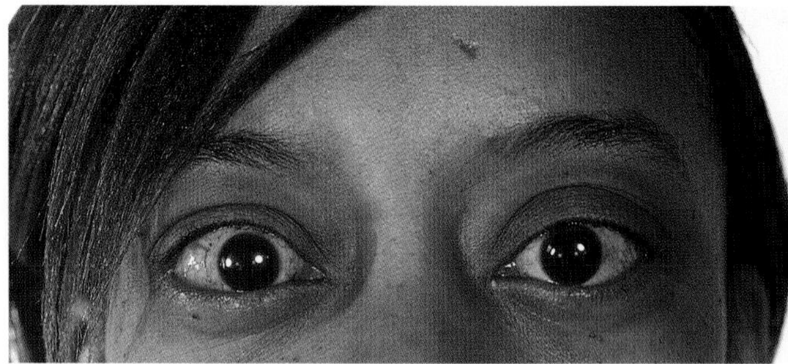

Figure 21.5 Exophthalmos in high myopia. This patient would benefit from wearing supplementary spectacles with a low-minus prescription to reduce the exophthalmic appearance

Lens fitting

- All types of lenses can be fitted – RGP, soft, scleral.
- Lenses are thin centrally and thick peripherally.
- Oxygen is reduced at the limbus and hypoxia can lead to neovascularization.
- Thin lenses break easily when handling, and the power can alter or become distorted with lens cleaning.

High-minus contact lenses are occasionally used as the eyepiece together with a high-plus lens in spectacles as a Galilean telescope (see Chapter 29) although they are rarely successful.

RGP LENSES

Thick edges cause displacement

- Upwards – the lid is hitched up with each blink (Fig. 21.6). This can cause desiccation of the cornea below the lens. If the lens is hitched up too high, it can result in flare as the peripheral zone or even the lower edge of the lens fails to cover the lower part of the pupil adequately.
- Downwards – an interpalpebral fitting lens can be pushed downwards with each blink as the upper lid pushes on the thick junction between the lenticular and the carrier zone.

Requirements

- A thinned junction is preferable (see CD-ROM) to prevent too much movement on blink, too much lid hitch or the lens being pushed down with tight lids (Mandell 1974). This can also be achieved by careful polishing although nowadays it is more common to input the required thickness into a computer program attached to a lathe (Moore & Mandell 1989) (see also Chapter 27).
- Aspheric lenses may be preferable as the junction is not as pronounced.
- Use a material with good dimensional stability to prevent lens changes due to wear on the thin optic zone and the thick peripheral zones.

Fitting lenses to large myopic eyes

- Corneas are often flat so lenses tend to drop; however, in moderate myopia of less than 10.00 D, the corneas may actually be steeper (Carney et al. 1997).

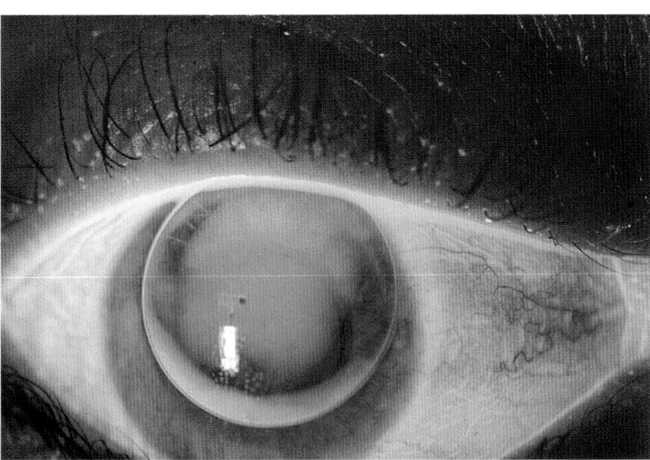

Figure 21.6 High-riding lens. The high-minus lens has thick edges which cause it to be hitched up by the upper lid, resulting in desiccation of the inferior cornea and poor pupil cover, giving rise to flare. (Courtesy of A. J. Phillips)

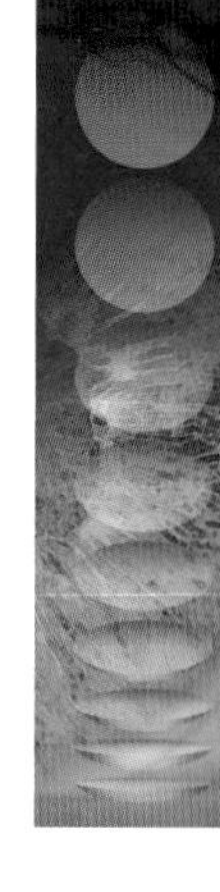

- Large corneas require large TDs.
- Small lenses can sometimes be successful as the mid-periphery can be made thinner; however, if the lens fits interpalpebrally, it will tend to sit low. Many high myopes have large pupils and small RGP lenses may result in flare, which is problematic, especially with night driving.

SOFT LENSES

- Ultrathin soft lenses, unless otherwise contraindicated, are ideal, although problems associated with RGP lenses also affect soft lenses.
- The transition between the lenticular portion of the lens and the carrier portion is thick, resulting in excess movement as the lid pushes the lens downwards or hitches it up, and reduced oxygen to the peripheral cornea can result in neovascularization:
  - small TDs exacerbate this problem and large TDs of 15.00 mm or more may be necessary.
  - large aspheric lenses may centre better.
- A tight lens may still move excessively with each blink due to edge thickness.

TROUBLESHOOTING

Poor centration – lid hitch (RGP lenses)

- Fit an aspheric lens.
- Use material with higher specific gravity.
- Fit a reduced FOZD and a thin lens carrier.

Poor centration – lenses pushed down by action of tight lids on thick junction

Soft and RGP lenses

- Increase TD.
- Reduce FOZD.
- Fit aspheric lenses.

RGP lenses

- Fit a multicurve lens with increased edge lift.
- Order a lens with a negative or parallel carrier (see Fig. 9.16).
- Change material
  - higher refractive index.
  - lower specific gravity.

Lenses move excessively on blinking

- Make junction thinner.
- Smaller lenticular diameter.
- Refit with an aspheric lens.
- Larger TD.

Poor oxygen permeability

- Higher-Dk material.
- Fit silicone hydrogel to maximum power available and overcorrect with spectacles.

Protein deposits

- Use protein remover tablets regularly.
- Try aspheric lenses – the junction is not so well circumscribed in aspheric lenses so deposits may build up less.
- Replace lenses more frequently.

Handling difficulties or poor stability of image

- Consider scleral lenses (see Chapter 15).

HIGH ASTIGMATISM

General points

Astigmatism can be any or all of the following:

- Corneal.
- Lenticular.
- Retinal.

Astigmatism can be either regular or irregular, although most cases of the latter are related to keratoconus or trauma and are covered in Chapters 20 and 26.

Where there is a high degree of regular astigmatism, it is common to find that the major component is corneal astigmatism and that the axes of the astigmatism, as measured with a keratometer, correspond to the axes of ocular astigmatism.

Where the astigmatism is congenital, if not corrected from a young age, meridional amblyopia is likely.

Advantages of contact lenses over spectacles

- Field less distorted.

Disadvantages of contact lenses over spectacles

- Small dislocation of lens axes causes large visual effect.

Lens fitting

For comprehensive information about fitting toric lenses, see Chapter 13.

Lens requirements

- Stable lenses.
- Good oxygen permeability.
- High refractive index (RGP).

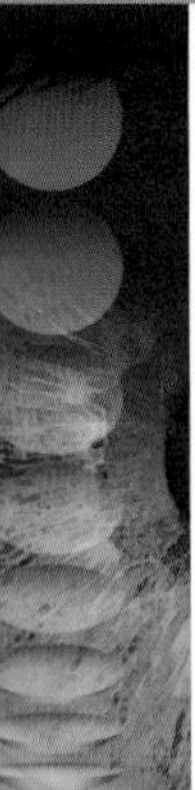

Contact lenses can provide good acuity but it may be difficult to achieve a fit that is stable and at the same time cause no corneal compromise. Fitting with a rigid lens usually requires a bitoric design in a material that has good oxygen permeability and wets well.

Lens stability is critical when fitting toric soft lenses and this may lead to long-term corneal compromise. The thick areas of the contact lens lead to meridional hypoxia and neovascularization, and these lenses are prone to deposit formation in the thicker parts of the lens. Encourage weekly enzymatic cleaners from the outset to reduce this build-up.

UNILATERAL AMETROPIA (see also Chapter 8)

Myopia

In cases of unilateral ametropia or aphakia, there is a better chance of stereopsis with a contact lens than with a spectacle lens. Aniseikonia is reduced for both axial and refractive myopia (Winn et al. 1988). These authors suggested that each retina has the same number of photoreceptors, and in the longer eye these are more widely spaced than in the shorter eye, as might be expected during the growth process. Thus the larger retinal image in the longer eye is thought to cover the same number of receptors as the smaller retinal image in the shorter eye, giving rise to better binocular fusion.

Patients who have achieved some stereoacuity with spectacles may not appreciate any improvement when a contact lens is fitted and their stereoacuity may be disrupted.

Where the unilaterally myopic eye is larger than the fellow eye, it may look better cosmetically to continue to wear all or part of the myopic correction in the form of a spectacle lens as the size of the eye will appear reduced.

Aphakia

Many unilateral aphakes are not able to achieve stereopsis, especially if the cataract had been long-standing. Even with a contact lens, because the lens is in front of the nodal point of the eye, binocular vision is, at best, poor. Guillon and Warland (1986) found that most unilateral aphakes achieved only 140 seconds of arc and 80% had intermittent suppression. However, patients may prefer to wear the lens as it may increase the field of vision and help to keep the eye straight where it might otherwise converge or, more commonly, diverge.

If the cataract resulted from trauma, other components of the eye and orbit may have been damaged, including extraocular muscles. Binocular single vision may be impossible and intractable diplopia may result (see Chapter 26).

SPORT

The better field and stereopsis afforded by contact lenses to high ametropes is particularly beneficial in sport. However, in certain sports (e.g. squash and badminton) safety spectacles should always be worn over the lenses. Patients who change from spectacles to contact lenses lose the protection provided by the spectacle frame and indeed by the lenses if they are made of a toughened material.

Swimming is particularly inadvisable in contact lenses. As well as a general risk of infection and irritation, there is an increased risk of *Acanthamoeba* keratitis (see Chapter 18). For contact lens-wearing swimmers, therefore, either goggles over the lenses or preferably swimming goggles with the spectacle prescription should be worn.

AFTER-CARE

After-care is covered in Chapter 17 and the detail is the same whatever the power of the lenses. However, eyes with high refractive errors are at risk of concomitant pathology, and signs and symptoms of ocular pathology must not be mistaken for an adverse response to contact lenses. For example, corneal oedema can result from contact lens-induced hypoxia but may equally be caused by a closed angle glaucoma attack; likewise poor vision may be a contact lens problem but could also result from a retinal detachment.

An adverse response is more likely with high-power lenses and careful observation is necessary. Lens parameters and/or lens type should be altered accordingly. However, where optimum fitting has been achieved and some small degree of ocular change still pertains, the practitioner must feel competent enough to decide whether it is acceptable for the patient to continue thus, to reduce lens wear or even to stop it altogether.

CONCLUSION

Fitting high degrees of ametropia can be especially rewarding. Many patients have been totally dependent on spectacles for as long as they can remember, and have no idea of what life will be like without them. Because of some of the difficulties encountered with high prescription contact lenses, instruction on lens care and potential eye problems are even more important than with low prescriptions. The lens of choice is often not available in the required power and some compromise may be necessary in order to enable the patient to wear lenses.

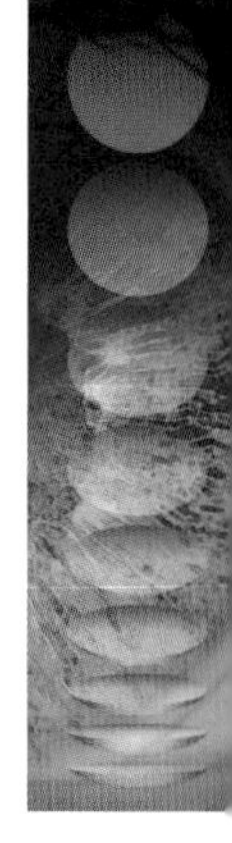

References

Bagshaw, J., Fordon, S. P. and Stanworth, A. (1966) A modified corneal contact lens: binocular single vision in unilateral aphakia. Br. Orthopt. J., 23, 19–30

Bleshoy, H. and Guillon, M. (1984) Soft lens design – clinical results. J. Br. Contact Lens Assoc., 7(1), 41–47

Carney, L., Mainstone, J., Henderson, B. (1997) Corneal topography and myopia. A cross-sectional study. Invest. Ophthalmol. Vis Sci., 38(2), 311–320

Carpel, E. and Parker, P. (1985) Extended wear aphakic contact lens fitting in high risk patients. Contact Lens Assoc. Ophthalmol. J., 11, 231–233

Chaston, J. and Fatt, I. (1980) The change in power of soft lenses. Optician, 180, 12–21

Coscas, G. and Soubrane, G. (1993) Myopie fort ou myopie maladie. Rev. Practicien, 43(14), 1768–1772

Grosvenor, T., and Scott, R. (1991) Comparison of refractive components in youth-onset and early adult-onset myopia. Optom. Vis. Sci., 68(3), 204–209

Guillon, M. and Warland, J. (1986) Aniseikonia and binocular function in unilateral aphakes wearing contact lenses. J. Br. Contact Lens Assoc., 3(1), 36–38

Larsson, E. K., Rydberg, A. C. and Holmstom, G. E. (2003) A population-based study of the refractive outcome in 10-year-old preterm and full-term children. Arch. Ophthalmol., 121(10), 1430–1436

Mandell, R. B. (1974) What is the gravity lens? Int. Contact Lens Clin., 18, 267–273

Moore, C. and Mandell, R. B. (1989) The design of high minus lenses. Contact Lens Spectrum, 11, 43–47

Reading, V. (1984) Astigmatism following cataract surgery. Br. J. Ophthalmol., 68, 97–104

Saw, S.-M. (2005) Refraction and refractive errors. In: Pediatric Ophthalmology and Strabismus, eds D. Taylor and C. S. Hoyt. Philadelphia, Elsevier

Winn, B., Ackerley, R. G., Brown, C. A., Murray, F. K., Prais, J. and St John, M. F. (1988) Reduced aniseikonia in axial anisometropia with contact lens correction. Ophthalmic Physiol. Opt., 8(3), 341–344

Chapter 22

Post-keratoplasty contact lens fitting

Christopher F. Steele

CHAPTER CONTENTS

INTRODUCTION

Fitting contact lenses after keratoplasty can be one of the greatest challenges to the contact lens practitioner. Keratoplasty involves the replacement of abnormal host tissue by healthy donor corneal tissue. A corneal graft may be partial thickness (lamellar or deep lamellar) or full thickness.

Lamellar keratoplasty (LK) is a surgical technique in which donor corneal stroma with overlying epithelial cells is transplanted. It was first successfully performed in 1886 by von Hippel. Although recent advancements in surgical techniques have resolved many of the earlier problems encountered in LK, including interlamellar opacification and irregular astigmatism, it is not as popular as penetrating keratoplasty (PK), which still accounts for the majority of corneal transplants today (Fig. 22.1). This is mainly due to:

- Technical difficulty of LK.
- Relatively poor postoperative visual outcome.
- Thin corneas (such as those found in keratoconus), where there is a risk of corneal perforation.
- LK not being possible in recurrent corneal disease.

Deep lamellar keratoplasty (DLK) was introduced in 1984 to improve postoperative visual performance while maintaining the other advantages of LK. The principle of DLK is to remove all recipient stromal tissue to Descemet's membrane and place a donor cornea over the bed. DLK can be applied in most causative diseases treated by PK. DLK is, however, technically difficult and very time consuming. A comparison of the various transplantation procedures is shown in Table 22.1.

Despite advances in surgical techniques for PK (Sugar & Sugar 2000), postoperative ametropia and high irregular astigmatism remain common. Earlier studies (Ruben & Colebrook 1979) give figures of around 65% of post-graft patients requiring contact lenses for optimal vision although better operative techniques and postsurgery refractive modification (see below) have reduced this figure to around 9% (Australian Corneal Graft Registry 2004).

INDICATIONS FOR KERATOPLASTY

Indications for LK include marginal corneal thinning or infiltration, for example recurrent pterygium, Terrien's marginal degeneration or limbal dermoids (see Fig. 22.3), and where the superficial third of the corneal stroma is opacified, as long as it is not caused by potentially recurrent disease.

Indications for DLK include cases involving diseased cornea up to 95% of total corneal thickness, with intact endothelium and Descemet's membrane being free of breaks or scars.

The indications for PK may be divided into the following categories:

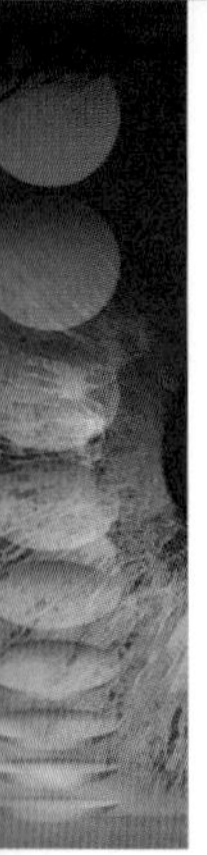

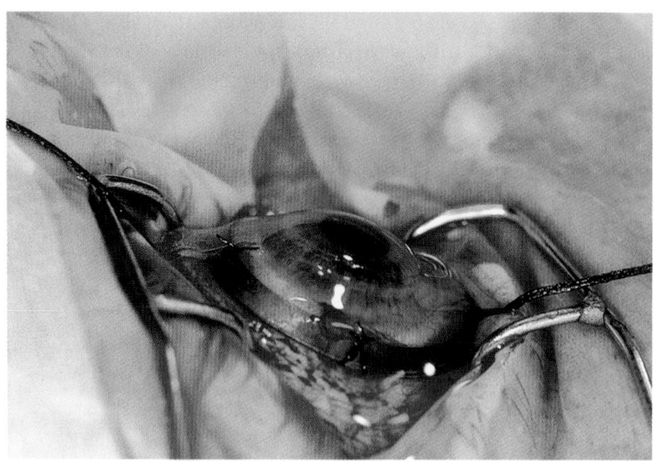

Figure 22.1 Side profile of penetrating keratoplasty at the end of the procedure. Note the interrupted sutures. (Courtesy of S. J. Morgan)

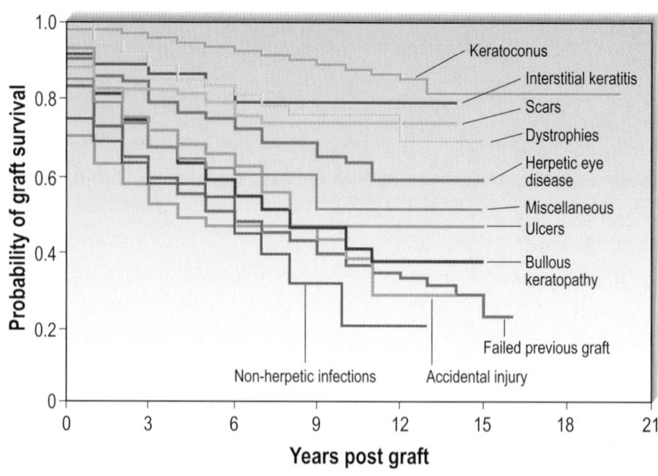

Figure 22.2 The probability of graft survival for the various conditions for which grafting was performed. (From Australian Corneal Graft Registry 2004)

Table 22.1: A comparison of the various corneal transplantation procedures

Condition	LK	DLK	PK
Good-quality donor cornea required	No	No	Yes
Ease of technique	Yes	No	Yes
Visual prognosis	Acceptable	Good	Good
Complications during surgery	Rare	Occasionally	Occasionally
Endothelial rejection	No	No	Occasionally
Irregular astigmatism	Occasionally	Occasionally	Occasionally
Endothelial decompensation	No	No	Occasionally
Other complications	Interface opacification	Double anterior chamber	Cataract, glaucoma, infection

DLK, deep lamellar keratoplasty; LK, lamellar keratoplasty; PK, penetrating keratoplasty.

- *Optical* – where keratoplasty is most commonly performed to improve vision; for example, keratoconus, pseudophakic bullous keratopathy, corneal dystrophies, degenerations and localized scarring. These grafts seldom reject.
- *Tectonic* – this is carried out to restore or preserve corneal integrity in situations involving severe structural changes; for example, stromal thinning in pellucid marginal degeneration or descemetoceles.
- *Therapeutic* – sometimes performed to remove infected corneal tissue which is unresponsive to antibiotic therapy. Grafts performed for post-inflammatory disease reject more often (Fig. 22.2).

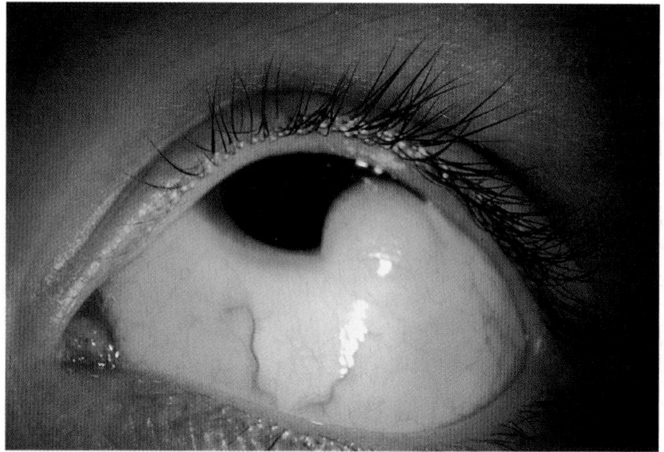

Figure 22.3 Limbal dermoid cyst in a young child. This was excised and a PK performed. The eye was densely amblyopic and the procedure was carried out simply to improve the cosmesis. (Courtesy of Department of Medical Illustration, Great Ormond Street Hospital, London)

- *Cosmetic* – rarely a PK may be performed to improve cosmesis (Fig. 22.3).

More recently, there has been a change in the leading indications for corneal transplant surgery in different regions of the world (Dandona et al. 1997, Frucht-Pery et al. 1997, Cursiefien et al. 1998). The number of PKs performed in the United States each year has slowly decreased since 1990 (Cosar et al. 2002), and the most common indication for PK is pseudophakic bullous keratopathy. Of those, 65% result from posterior intraocular lenses (IOLs), 34% anterior chamber IOLs and 1% iris-fixated IOLs. Regraft is the second most common indication, followed by keratoconus and Fuchs' endothelial dystrophy. Similar findings have been reported in South East Asia (Wong et al. 1997). In Australia and New Zealand, however, keratoconus is the most common indication for PK (Edwards et al. 2002). In many countries, religious beliefs prevent tissue donation for transplants.

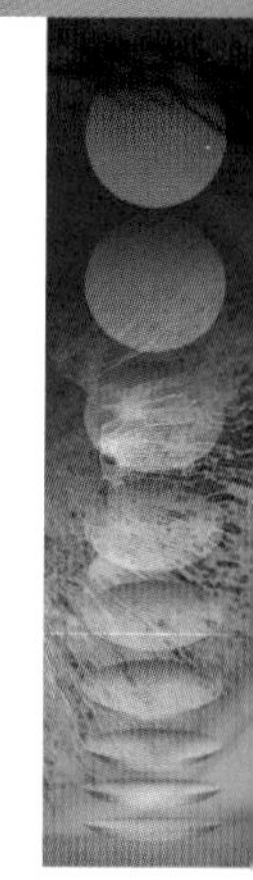

THE POST-KERATOPLASTY CORNEA

Post-keratoplasty corneal thickness

Immediately after transplantation, the donor button may be extremely oedematous, with thickness gradually returning to normal levels over a few days or weeks. In the year after surgery, while steroids are still being used and sutures are in situ, the grafted cornea may be thinner than normal (Bourne 1983). Once all treatment has ceased and the sutures have been removed, the vast majority of transplants show increased thickness.

Post-keratoplasty endothelial morphology

Some endothelial cell damage occurs at the time of PK surgery with more cells being lost from the peripheral graft and recipient cornea nearer the junction compared with the centre of the graft. The central graft cell population then gradually reduces as cells migrate to the peripheral region. Corneal thickness measurements may remain within normal limits, even with endothelial cell counts down to one-third of normal, although the eye will be more vulnerable to oedema developing. For this reason, appropriate contact lens materials with sufficient Dk/t values should always be used. Speaker et al. (1991) demonstrated that well-fitting rigid gas-permeable (RGP) lenses with a high Dk/t have little or no effect on graft endothelial cell survival in the first few years after keratoplasty.

Post-transplant sensitivity

Central corneal sensitivity in the normal cornea is significantly greater than in the periphery but the reverse is true for the post-graft cornea. Generally, resensitization of transplanted corneas slowly progresses over 3–5 years, although there is considerable individual variation where recovery may be full, partial or non-existent (Macalister et al. 1993). However, although the majority of patients have reduced corneal sensitivity, lid sensation remains normal and post-keratoplasty patients are generally more sensitive than normal, with psychological factors often exacerbating symptoms of sensitivity.

Post-transplant corneal topography

Designing a rigid contact lens for a patient who has undergone keratoplasty requires careful consideration of all the relevant features of the corneal graft (Lindsay 1995) including:

- Corneal topography of both graft and host.
- Graft size.
- Graft centration.
- Suturing technique.

The post-PK patient requires careful evaluation of the central and peripheral cornea, which is best undertaken using computer-assisted corneal topography (see Chapter 7). The most appropriate contact lens options will depend on the classification of corneal topography present (Tripoli et al. 1990).

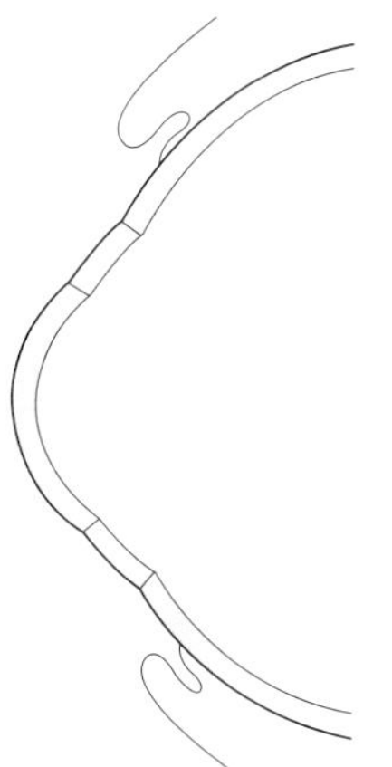

Figure 22.4 Corneal transplant in section: seen to be steeper than the host cornea, giving the effect of a nipple-like protrusion

The topography of a post-graft cornea invariably differs from the normal corneal shape (Bogan et al. 1990). Corneal astigmatism may be as high as 15.00 D. The corneal topography may be prolate where the central 'nipple-like' cornea is steeper (depicted by a central red bow tie pattern) than the increasingly flatter periphery (Fig. 22.4). Approximately 30% of cases (Karabatsas et al. 1999) are referred to as 'proud' (Fig. 22.5), i.e. where the thicker graft stands slightly forward or proud of the thinner host (Figs 22.6, 22.7). A further 30% have a plateau or oblate-shaped cornea, i.e. the graft is flat or appears sunken, and a central blue bow tie pattern is seen (Lagnado et al. 2004). Mixed prolate and oblate corneal topographies present in 18% of patients with a flat side and a steep side, and possibly symmetrical astigmatism, although in many cases the astigmatism is far from symmetrical. Some grafts exhibit only a small amount of astigmatism but contact lenses will not centre and excessive edge stand-off may be apparent in one particular area. This is usually caused by the graft being tilted in relation to the host cornea.

Suturing technique and the sizing of the corneal graft have a significant effect on the corneal topographical profile. Interrupted sutures, which are relatively long on the host side, are used more commonly nowadays, the result of which can be a flattening or drumhead effect (Assil et al. 1992) owing to the radial direction of pull. In contrast, continuous or double continuous sutures cause a tangential direction of pull, which may give rise to a 'purse-string' effect and a steep corneal profile (Fig. 22.8).

The diameter of the graft zone is usually between 7.5 and 8.5 mm for the best prognosis; survival rates of corneal grafts less than 7.5 mm or greater than 8.5 mm are poorer (Australian Corneal Graft Registry 2004). The sizing of the host trephine depends on a number of factors including corneal size, pathology involved and risk of rejection. The diameter of donor tissue cut with a trephine from the endothelial surface measures 0.25 mm smaller than that of the recipient corneal tissue cut with the same instrument from the front surface. Consequently, the donor tissue trephine is routinely sized 0.25 mm larger than the host (Olson 1979). In cases with severe peripheral corneal thinning, caused by, for example, keratoconus, active infection or pellucid marginal degeneration, the graft may need to be decentred and possibly oversized to encompass this pathology. In such cases, aligning the

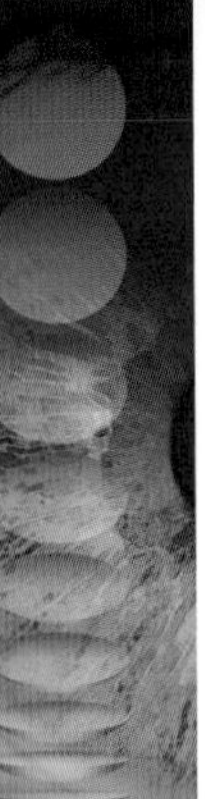

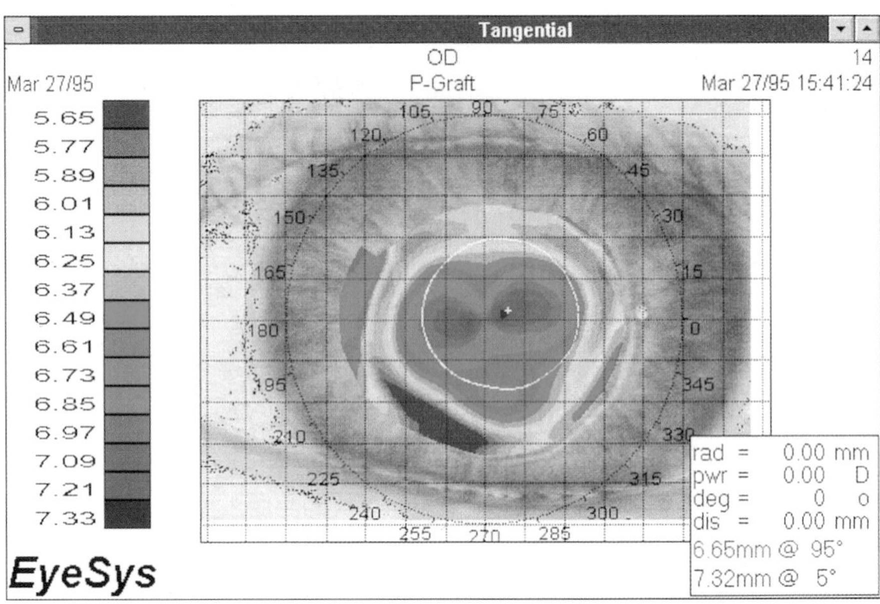

Figure 22.5 A tangential corneal topographical plot of a transplant showing with-the-rule astigmatism in the pupil area and a proud ridge at the transplant margin. The flat edge of the host cornea can just be seen beyond the graft. (Courtesy of A. J. Phillips)

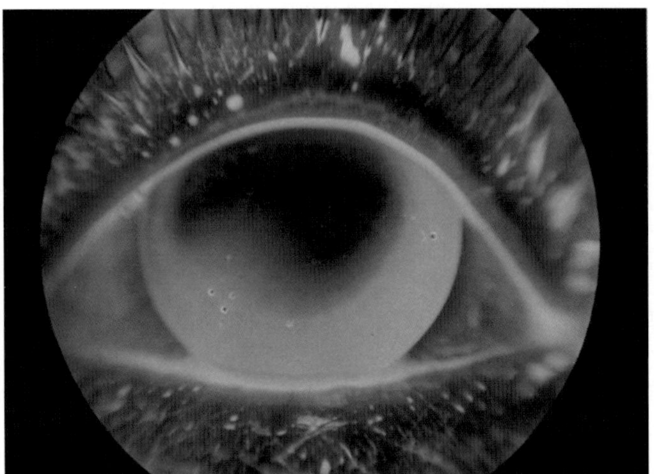

Figure 22.6 Corneal transplants commonly stand slightly proud of the host tissue. This is illustrated here by using a conventional tricurve lens to align the graft. The clearance around the transplant area is easily visible. (Courtesy of A. J. Phillips)

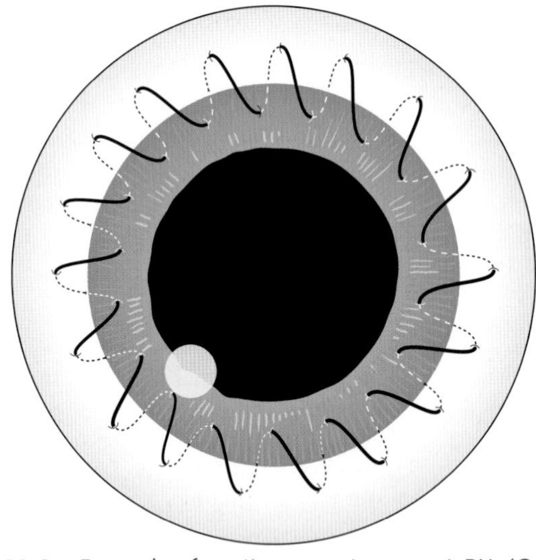

Figure 22.8 Example of continuous sutures post-PK. (Courtesy of S. J. Morgan)

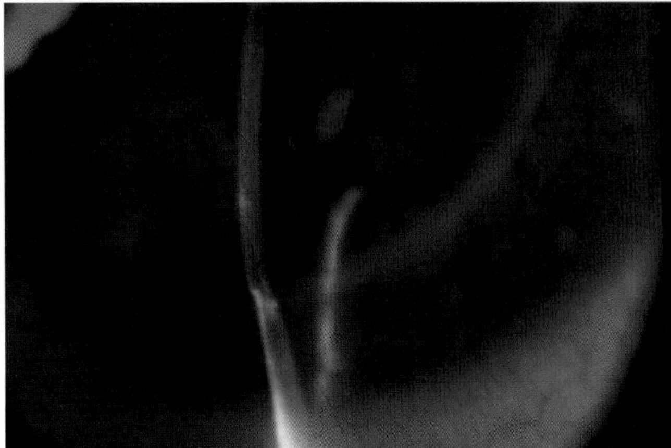

Figure 22.7 Optic section viewing by slit-lamp microscopy of the graft–host junction in keratoplasty. The raised nature of the graft in this instance can be seen. (Courtesy of A. J. Phillips)

graft over the centre of the pupil (which approximates to the line of sight) is physically impossible (Fig. 22.9). Small amounts of decentration do not cause significant problems although more decentration can result in high astigmatism (Van Rij et al. 1985).

In a small percentage of cases, the natural progression of the disease means that, some years after grafting, keratoconus will appear in the host. For those patients wearing spectacles there may be a sudden increase in their astigmatism and, for those wearing contact lenses, a change in lens fitting. Careful slit-lamp examination may show thinning in one portion of the host adjacent to the graft and newer instruments, such as the Oculus Pentacam, will show thinning by both pachometry and optical cross-section (Fig. 22.10). Compression sutures, wedge resection (removing an arc of the affected tissue) or regrafting may then be necessary.

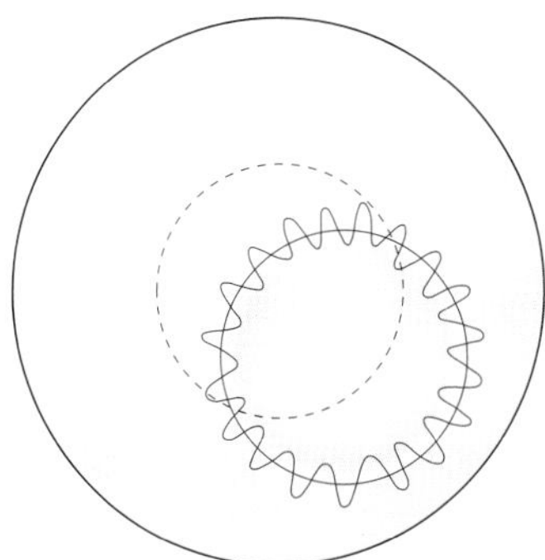

Figure 22.9 An eccentric transplant shown relative to pupil position, making contact lens centring relative to the visual axis extremely difficult to achieve

OPTICAL CONTACT LENS FITTING AFTER KERATOPLASTY

Despite advances in surgical techniques, postoperative ametropia and large degrees of irregular astigmatism remain problems, and contact lens correction is often better than spectacles (Woodward et al. 1990a). If postoperative astigmatism is regular then spectacles may suffice or else refractive surgical procedures may be considered. These include relaxing incisions, wedge resections or, more commonly, laser keratectomy to decrease or even correct the astigmatism.

Where contact lens fitting becomes essential, no one particular type of lens fitting philosophy works in all cases. RGP lenses are the most commonly used and provide the best visual performance and patient tolerance for cases of irregular astigmatism. However, several different lens fitting designs are needed as each will fit only a small proportion of post-graft cases. Many lens designs may have to be trialled before an acceptable one can be found. Practitioners will therefore need a wide range of lenses available, many of which will be eclectic lenses from previous failures!

Commencement of contact lens fitting

Post-PK, the corneal epithelium is intact after about 4 days although the whole cornea will not be fully healed for at least 18–24 months. Contact lens fitting is usually started 6–12 months after surgery. Occasionally, to provide some functional vision, it is possible to fit contact lenses as early as 3 months postoperatively, but this may require several lens changes as corneal sutures are removed and may increase the risk of graft rejection.

Contact lens wear after PK has a potential risk of complications including:

- Epithelial defects.
- Corneal ulcers.
- Neovascularization.
- Graft rejection or failure.

Close monitoring is required, particularly in the early stages when steroids are being reduced and sutures are still in place. Patients must be educated to seek urgent attention should they develop any pain, redness or decreased vision, and regular follow-up is essential (Dart 1993).

Post-PK rigid contact lens fitting

Contact lenses are usually fitted after PK to improve visual acuity. According to Wietharn and Drieb (2004), reasons for fitting contact lenses after PK are multifactorial, although irregular astigmatism (62.9%), spherical anisometropia (57.1%) and astigmatic anisometropia (54.3%) are the main indicators.

Prior to contact lens fitting, the following should be undertaken:

- A full refraction with best-corrected visual acuity.
- Full slit-lamp examination recording all clinically relevant details
  - the presence or absence of any sutures, and whether fully or partially buried.
  - any neovascularization.
- Keratometry.
- Computer-assisted corneal topography where possible.

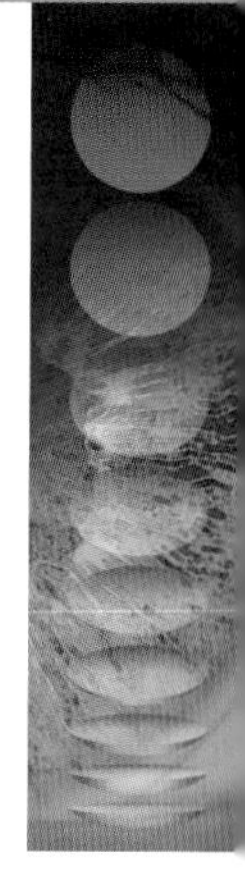

In earlier years it was considered best to fit rigid lenses within the borders of the graft as lenses were only available in polymethylmethacrylate (PMMA), which often resulted in significant graft oedema. A common method of dealing with this was to fenestrate the lens.

Although it is feasible to fit a rigid lens within the donor graft area, particularly where the donor button is greater than 8.0 mm in diameter, this is not usually successful. The graft–host junction is often irregular (Fig. 22.11) and the lenses may cause mechanical irritation at this junction, inducing neovascularization into donor tissue (Shovelin 1995). To avoid this, a larger-diameter lens, more than 10 mm total diameter, is fitted so that it vaults the graft (Winkler 1999) and rests on host peripheral cornea or sclera (see below).

CONVENTIONAL RGP LENSES

In regular and near regular grafts, and where the corneal curvature begins to approach normal, a conventional fitting technique may be employed. A toric back surface is often necessary. This simple approach should always be made first because it often works. In addition, a regular curved lens will usually give a fluorescein picture of the entire corneal surface and so will demonstrate proud or tilted areas (see Fig. 22.6). From this, a more logical decision as to the next step can be made.

LARGE-DIAMETER RGP LENSES

Many grafts are proud of the host tissue, or show raised areas around the graft–host junction such that lenses with conventional total diameters (TD) frequently decentre. It is necessary, therefore, to use lenses with large TDs, especially when fitting proud, tilted or displaced grafts (Figs 22.12 and 22.13). To provide good-quality vision, they should have a back optic zone diameter (BOZD) which is at least the same size as or larger than the corneal transplant. There are a number of specialist lenses available that are designed to be fitted in this way (see below). The goal of fitting RGP lenses is to maintain the best possible alignment and to maximize lens bearing (Collins et al. 2002, Wietharn & Drieb 2004). One of the problems with large TD lenses is inadequate lens

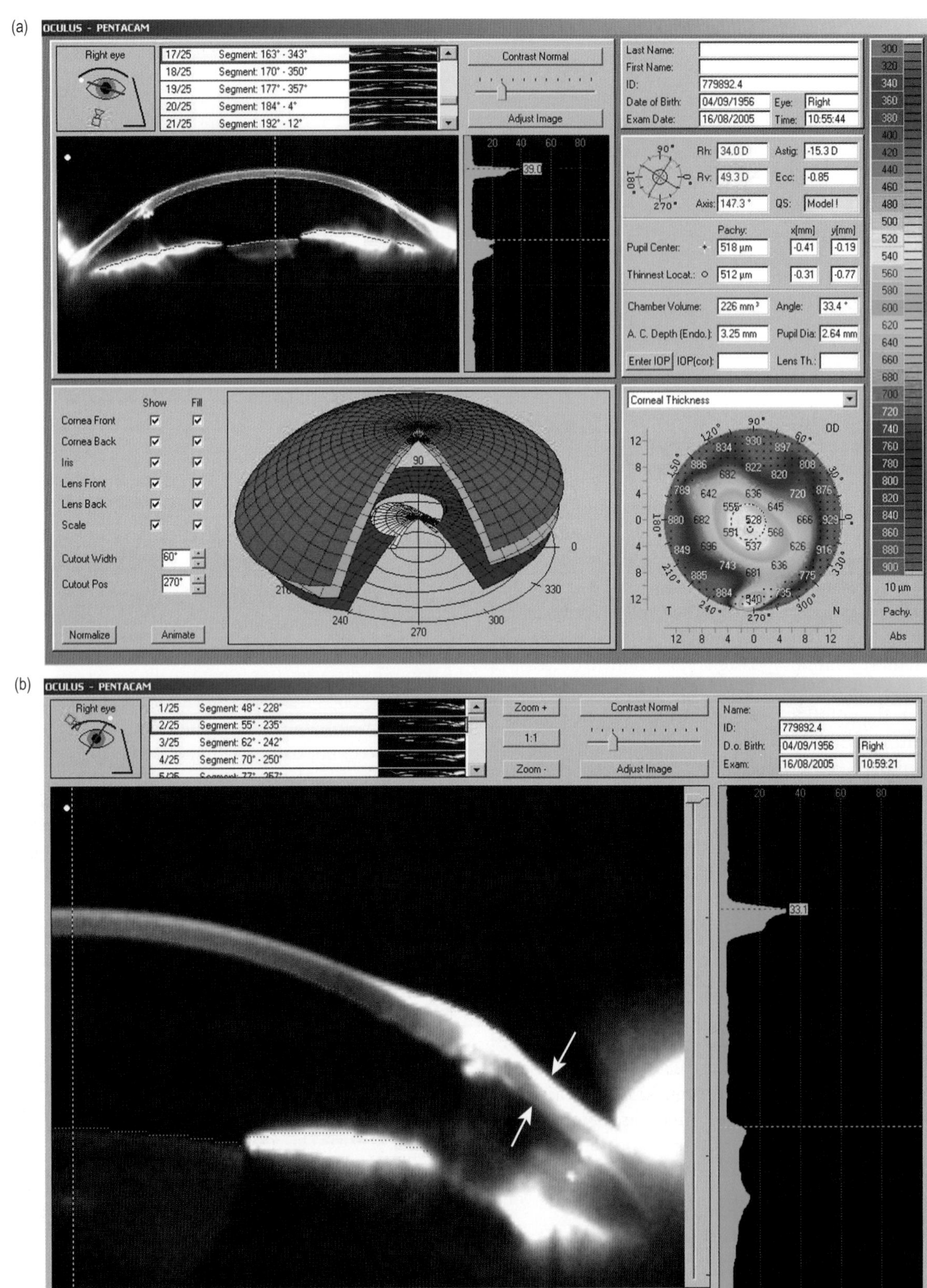

Figure 22.10 (a) Corneal pachymetry taken with an Oculus Pentacam showing thinning of the host at 250–270°. (b) An optical cross-section taken along this meridian shows thickening at the graft–host junction but thinning in the adjacent host tissue due to the appearance of keratoconus (arrowed). (Courtesy of K. Pesudovs)

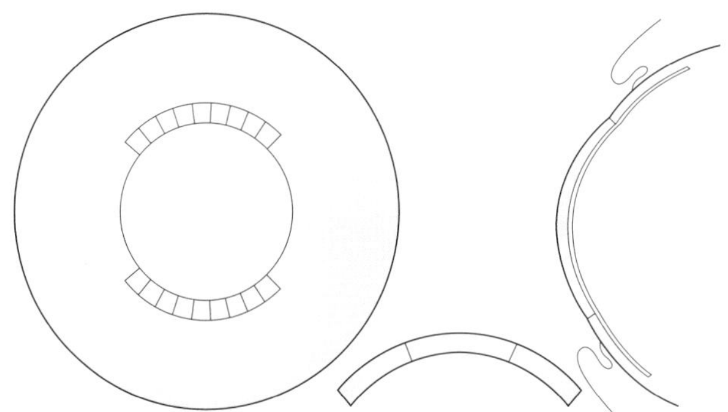

Figure 22.11 Guttering (shown hatched in the left-hand diagram) at the upper and lower graft–host junctions due to the host cornea being spherical whereas the graft is toroidal. The cross-sectional diagrams show the guttering in the vertical meridian (right) and the smooth graft–host junction in the horizontal meridian (centre)

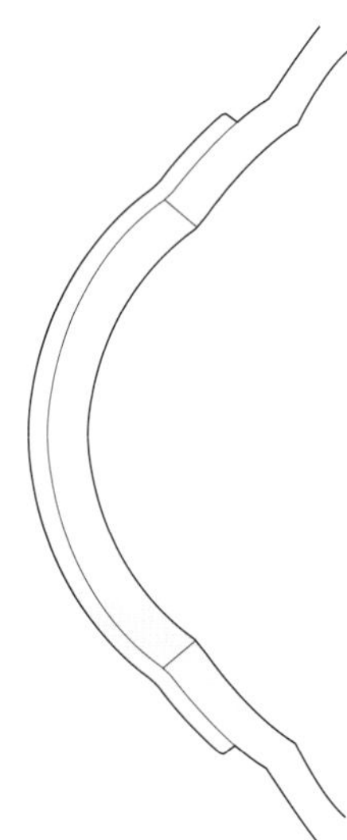

Figure 22.13 Irregular graft–host junction being spanned by the back optic zone of a corneal lens

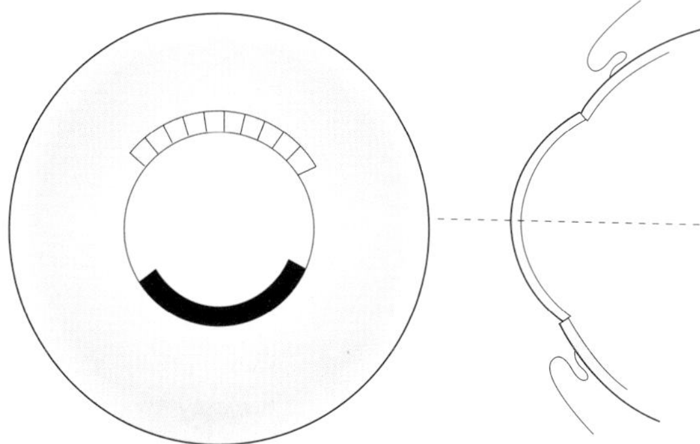

Figure 22.12 Tilted transplant. The hatched area (left) shows where the transplant tissue is proud while the black area shows where it is recessed. This can be seen more clearly in the right-hand diagram

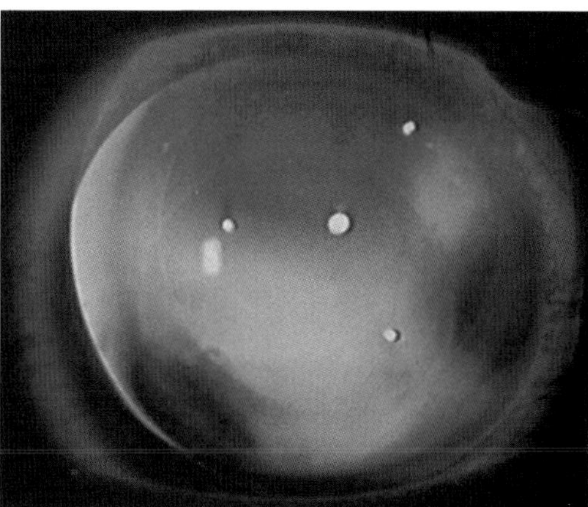

Figure 22.14 In some cases of corneal transplant a grossly irregular surface is produced, such that, although a contact lens is the only means of producing reasonable vision, it is equally impossible to provide a normally fitting lens. The fluorescein fit shown is an example of a bizarre fitting sometimes necessary. Four fenestrations have been provided to prevent tear liquid stagnation in the gutter zones

movement which may result in poor retro-lens tear flow and corneal staining, requiring fenestrations and/or ocular lubricants (Fig. 22.14) may solve these problems.

The diameter of these lenses is typically 10.50–12.00 mm. High-Dk/t lens materials, such as Boston XO (DK/t 100), are recommended. Many laboratories produce post-graft designs but typical examples of prescription are:

8.20:9.50/10.00:11.00/12.25:11.50 *or*
8.20:10.00/11.00:11.50/13.50:12.00.

Examples of post-graft design lenses are shown in Figures 22.15–22.18.

Fitting large-diameter lenses

The use of trial lenses is essential, assessing the fluorescein fit both centrally and peripherally.

- The BOZD should show good or close alignment of the graft.
- Postsurgically, the graft is nearly always flatter than the graft–host interface, which often has raised areas of scar tissue significantly steeper than the central cornea. This can cause the lens to decentre towards the steepest part of the cornea (see Fig. 22.18). To overcome this, steeper or larger lenses can improve the fit, an increase of 0.5 mm producing a significant effect.
- In the periphery, an optimum fit over the host tissue will give a fluorescein band 0.5–0.7 mm wide with no excessive stand-off and a uniform peripheral band.
- A reduction in lens diameter should be considered if the lens is riding too high and encroaching onto the upper sclera (see Fig. 22.16).

Postoperative astigmatism should be ignored, initially, and spherical trial lenses should be used. If a toric lens is necessary, it must be determined whether the toricity is required over the entire lens or just over the graft. In the latter case, a toric back optic zone radius (BOZR) with spherical peripheral curves will provide the optimum fit (see Fig. 22.18).

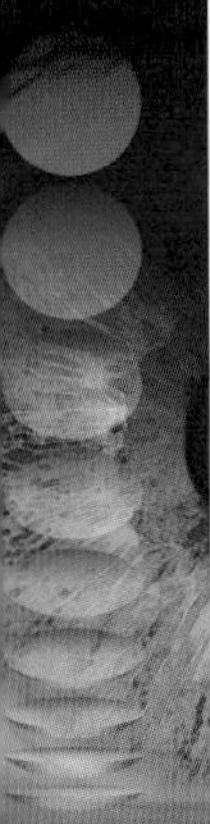

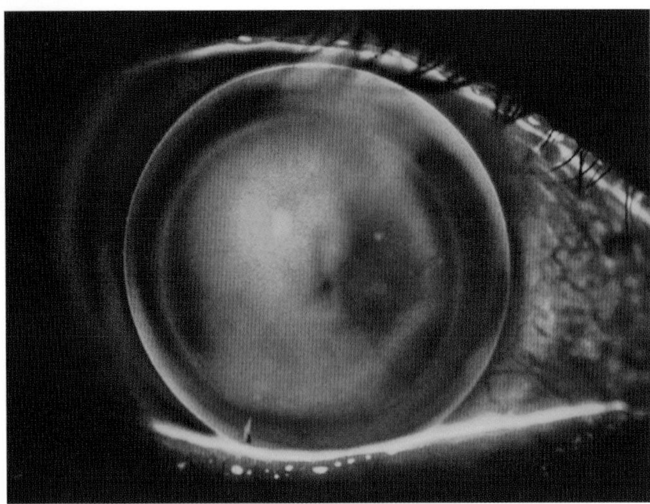

Figure 22.15 Rose K 2 lens centring well with central clearance. Note the area of touch due to a slightly tilted/proud graft on the right side causing nasal displacement of the lens. (Courtesy of Nova Contact Lenses)

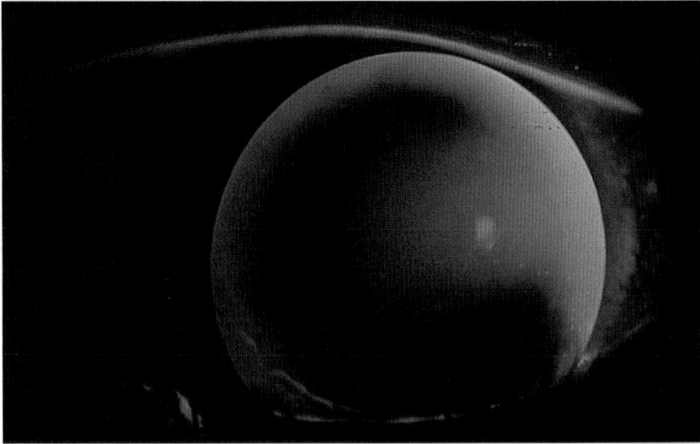

Figure 22.17 An example of a sunken graft along the 50° axis. An acceptable area of alignment has been maintained over the rest of the graft but with some edge stand-off on the right-hand side. (Courtesy of Nova Contact Lenses)

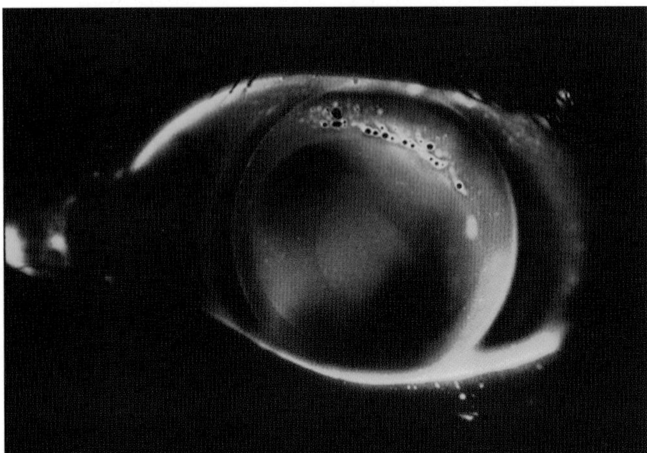

Figure 22.16 A large TD RGP lens fitting in alignment centrally but with air bubbles present superiorly due to graft–host junction guttering. (Courtesy of Nova Contact Lenses)

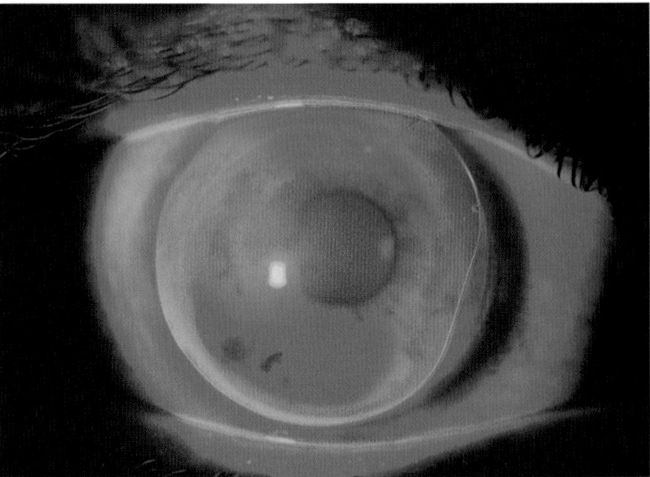

Figure 22.18 Dyna Z Intra-Limbal lens vaulting a corneal graft. Because of the graft topography, the lens is decentred. A toric lens may fit better. (Courtesy of No. 7 Contact Lenses)

REVERSE GEOMETRY LENSES

A reverse geometry lens (RGL) is one in which the first peripheral curve is *steeper* than the BOZR. As mentioned earlier, grafts are commonly proud or have a proud area at the graft–host interface. In these cases, a conventional multicurve RGP (i.e. one that flattens progressively from centre to periphery) may be unsuccessful, showing good graft alignment but excessive edge clearance. Similarly, when the central graft is relatively flat and the peripheral cornea is more than 4.0 D steeper, the peripheral fit may be satisfactory but central clearance excessive and bubbles may result (Figs 22.17 and 22.20).

A RGL may solve this problem as it can be made to align the graft centrally, while the second peripheral curve(s) align(s) with the host tissue.

RGLs were originally developed for use in orthokeratology (Jessen 1962) and later for post-refractive surgery (see Chapters 19 and 23). Some of the best-known types include the OK series (Contex) and the Plateau lens (Menicon) (Szczotka & Aronsky 1998, Mathur et al. 1999, Lim et al. 2000).

- Typically, the secondary reverse curve is 0.60 mm (3.00 D) to 1.60 mm (8.00 D) steeper than the BOZR.
- BOZDs range from 6.0 to 8.5 mm.
- TDs range from 10.5 to 11.5 mm to aid stability of the lens fit.

The aim is to achieve:

- Good centration with central alignment or slight clearance.
- A narrow band of clearance at the graft margin.
- Mid-peripheral alignment.
- Adequate edge clearance (Fig. 22.20) (see Chapter 9) (Szczorka 1998).

In most designs the degree of steepening of the first peripheral curve can be varied to achieve alignment of the host by the outer curves. The use of fitting sets is essential.

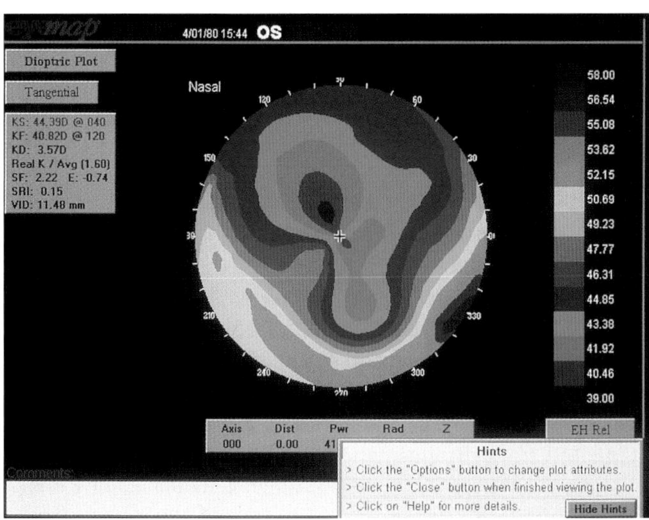

Figure 22.19 EyeMap corneal topography demonstrating a flat post-PK cornea. (Courtesy of Nova Contact Lenses)

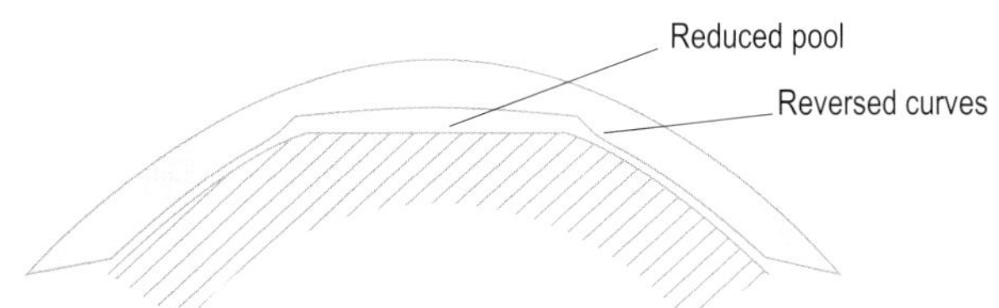

Figure 22.20 Reverse curve lens in relation to the flattened corneal profile often seen following PK

As previously mentioned, the BOZD should be close to or slightly larger than the graft diameter, typically around 8 mm. Examples include the OK85A (Contex) and the PCS (UltraVision Capricornia, Australia).

The main disadvantages of RGLs are:

- The mid-peripheral thickness which can exacerbate lens awareness.
- The risk of neovascularization with the larger, thicker lens, especially if there is inadequate movement.
- The lack of toric designs in most cases.

COMBINATION OR PIGGYBACK LENSES

Soft lenses are often required where there is hypersensitivity to RGPs or where lid sensation is a problem. However, good visual acuity may not be achievable with hydrogels alone. The increasing use of the piggyback concept, an RGP lens fitted on top of a soft lens, has resulted from the growing popularity of silicone hydrogels (Edwards 2002) (Fig. 22.21). The increased rigidity and enhanced oxygen transmission of these lenses compared with conventional soft lenses make silicone hydrogels a good choice for piggyback combinations. Second-generation silicone hydrogels are used more commonly as they drape the cornea better.

Fitting procedure

- Fit a best-fit silicone hydrogel or conventional soft lens with a Plano or low-plus back vertex power.
- Take keratometry measurements with the soft lens in situ and fit the BOZR of the RGP slightly flatter than K.
- The BOZD should be approximately 7.8–8.0 mm.
- TD is determined by practitioner preference and lid aperture.
- The RGP lens should centre well over the soft lens. The fit can be assessed with fluorescein and if the soft lens is discolored it can be discarded after use. Alternatively, high-molecular-weight fluorescein (e.g. Fluorosoft – see Chapter 5) can be used.
- Hydrogen peroxide solutions may be used for disinfection of both sets of lenses (Loveridge 2004).

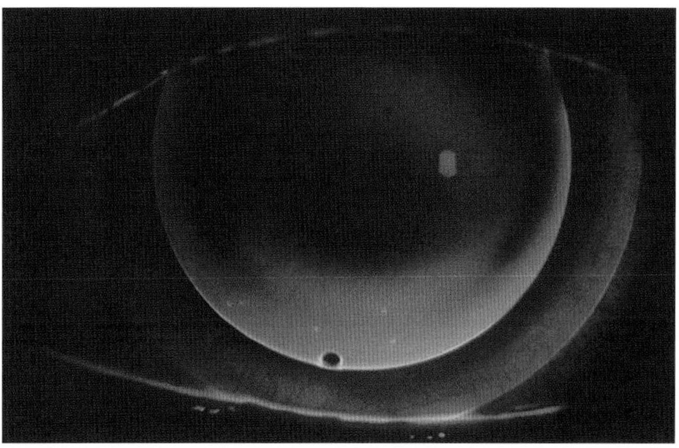

Figure 22.21 Silicone hydrogel and large TD post-graft lens used in piggyback combination centring well over the graft. (Courtesy of Nova Contact Lenses)

HYBRID COMBINATIONS

The SoftPerm lens (CIBA Vision) consists of an 8.0 mm RGP centre made of a silicone acrylate tertiary butylstyrene copolymer, surrounded by a soft 25% water content HEMA hydrophilic skirt with a TD of 14.3 mm. The SoftPerm lens is useful in some cases of decentred grafts, highly irregular corneal topographical profiles, tilted grafts or highly sensitive eyes. The main problem with this lens type is its limited oxygen transmissibility (Dk/t) with the inevitable consequence that, with time, neovascularization into the graft occurs. Unacceptable lens tightening, leading to inadequate lens movement, is also common. Shortened wearing periods are therefore advisable.

For details of an alternative hybrid lens, the SynergEyes lens (Quarter Lambda Technologies, California, USA), see Chapter 23.

SOFT LENSES

Conventional toric soft lenses may well be satisfactory where the graft astigmatism is reasonably regular. These should be tried initially to determine whether more complex lens options are required. Care is needed to ensure that there is adequate oxygen supply and no neovascularization develops. High-water-content or, where available, silicone hydrogel materials are essential in the thinnest design commensurate with adequate vision. Restricted wearing times may be advisable.

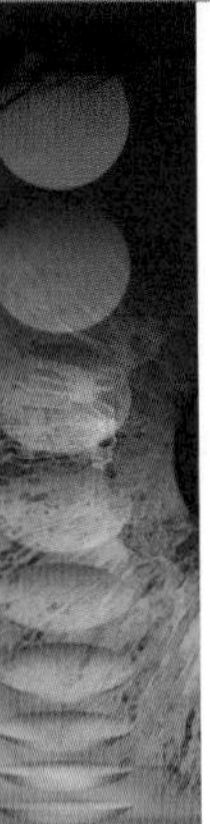

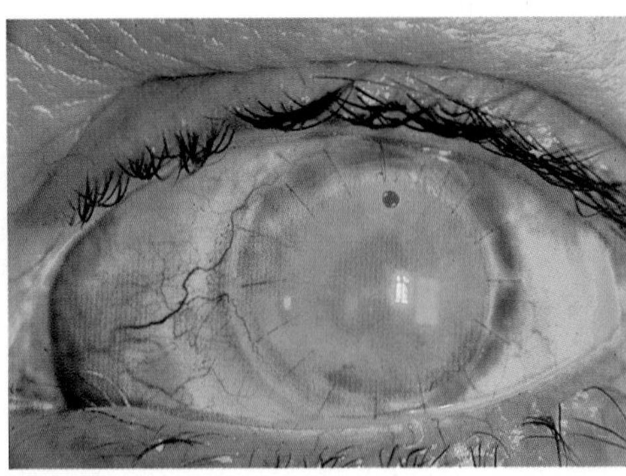

Figure 22.22 Scleral lens used to vault a PK where the weight of the lens is supported entirely on the sclera. Note interrupted sutures still in situ. (Courtesy of K. Pullum)

EXTRALIMBAL LENSES

Where grafts are grossly decentred, or comfort or handling is a major problem, rigid lenses that extend beyond the limbus may prove helpful. By resting or aligning the perilimbal area, good centration and comfort are normally possible.

Examples include:

- S-Lim lens (Jack Allen Contact Lenses, UK) – TD 13.5–14.75 mm.
- Epicon LC (UltraVision Capricornia, Australia) – TD 13.5 mm.
- Mini-Scleral (Eycon, Australia) – TD 16 mm.

Here again, it is necessary to use a fitting set.

The disadvantages of these lenses are similar to those of scleral lenses (see below) but they may also cause an increase in intraocular pressure.

SCLERAL LENSES (see Chapter 15)

With the continued development and improved availability of scleral lenses with good oxygen permeability, these are another option for post-keratoplasty patients (Pullum 1997). They are supported almost entirely by the sclera (Fig. 22.22) and generally centre well. They are simple to maintain, relatively easy to handle and almost impossible to lose.

In some cases, sealed scleral lenses are unsatisfactory and impression moulding is needed to produce a shell that fits the irregular cornea (see Chapter 15).

The disadvantages of scleral lenses are:

- Greater risk of neovascularization compared to corneal RGP lenses.
- Poor retro-lens tear flow.
- Longer time involved in fitting.
- Higher cost.
- Occasionally, poorer cosmesis of the thicker lens.

THERAPEUTIC LENSES (see also Chapter 25)

Therapeutic contact lenses (TCLs) are used occasionally after keratoplasty, especially in the early postoperative phase, but caution must be exercised in their application as the cornea is immunosuppressed and completely denervated (Saini et al. 1988).

TCLs are fitted after corneal transplant for a variety of reasons:

- When the size of an epithelial defect fails to decrease or is persistent beyond 6–7 days (Brightbill & Lazorik 1999). Rapid epithelialization of a corneal keratoplasty is important to re-establish a barrier to infection and to prevent subepithelial scarring. Medical management of epithelial defects seen on the first postoperative visit usually results in complete healing.
- Protruding sutures causing discomfort and attracting mucus. If these cannot or must not be removed, they may act as a nidus for infection and stimulate vessel growth.
- Protecting the corneal surface against the abrasive effects of an abnormal eyelid or against exposure in patients with incomplete eyelid closure (Treumer 1986).
- There may be a leak because of faulty suturing, demonstrated by a positive Seidel's test (fluorescein instilled into the eye appears in the anterior chamber after a few minutes).

In a series of 522 PKs at the Rotterdam Eye Hospital (Beekuis et al. 1991), 77 (14.8%) were fitted with contact lenses after surgery. In 28 cases (36%), TCLs were utilized for the following reasons: delayed epithelial healing (more than 1 week), epithelial filaments, steps in the graft–host junction or a loose running suture requiring tightening at a later stage.

Where an existing graft has perforated, a disposable hydrogel or silicone hydrogel TCL may be used to reform the anterior chamber. Silicone rubber lenses were formerly used (Woodward 1984) but these are not currently available in plano prescriptions.

Good corneal coverage is essential, requiring relatively large flat-fitting lenses having a TD of more than 15.0 mm and a BOZR greater than 9.0 mm. Again, this is because, in the early stages post-keratoplasty, some grafts are flatter than the host cornea (see above). Woodward et al. (1990b) suggested that after keratoplasty, TCLs may provide mechanical support and actually mould the corneal surface, thus helping to reduce corneal irregularity.

Several publications advocate the use of disposable soft contact lenses (Gruber 1991, Suleweski et al. 1991, Rubinstein 1995, Bouchard & Trimble 1996, Spraul & Lang 1997, Srur & Dattas 1997) because of the much lower costs compared to conventional hydrogel TCLs; however, the parameters are limited and therefore not suitable in all cases after keratoplasty (Bourne 1983). The maximum TD of most disposable lenses is 14.5 mm with a BOZR range of 8.3–9.1 mm: larger TDs and flatter BOZR are often necessary. Soflens 66 (Bausch & Lomb) has been recommended as a good choice of disposable lens after keratoplasty owing to its incorporation of a reverse geometry style design. This makes the lens particularly useful when fitting a centrally flat graft (Szczotka & Lindsay 2003).

First-generation silicone hydrogel lenses are relatively thick and have a lower water content than standard hydrogels but they have very high oxygen transmissibility. Second-generation silicone hydrogels drape better over proud graft margins and produce less edge stand-off, with a high Dk material being preferable. In a prospective open-ended randomized clinical trial involving 54 eyes with various conditions including PK, Lim et al. (2001) reported good safety and efficacy with continuous wear (average 1.1 months) of PureVision lenses used therapeutically.

AFTER-CARE

Although highest in the first year or two after surgery, the risk of graft rejection is always present. The major factors triggering rejection are:

- Inflammation.
- Endothelial cell failure.
- Increased intraocular pressure.
- Infection.

The risk of inflammation from an ill-fitting lens, inadequate oxygen supply, poor retro-lens tear flow, or host and graft neovascularization are all present after corneal transplantation. The importance of regular after-care cannot be overemphasized. This should include a general check of the ocular health and IOP. Close liaison with the surgeon is also essential.

Figure 22.23 shows the significantly reduced life of second and subsequent grafts. For a younger person to lose a graft may mean total loss of sight in old age if subsequent grafts fail. For this reason every effort should be made to ensure the safety and life of the first graft.

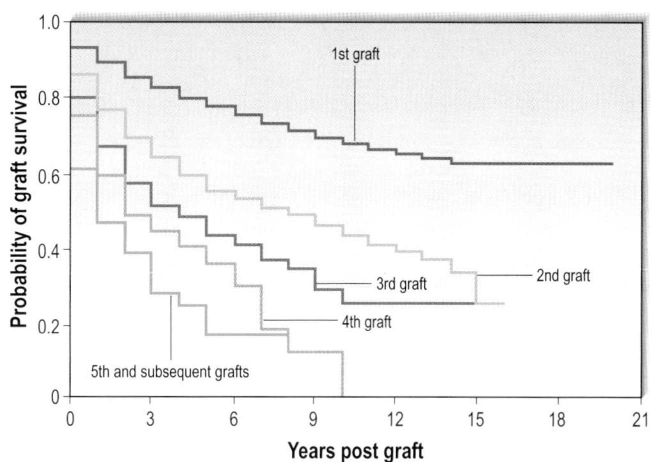

Figure 22.23 The probability of graft survival showing the marked reduction for subsequent grafts. (From Australian Corneal Graft Registry 2004)

CONCLUSION

Improvements in surgical techniques have reduced the number of patients requiring contact lenses after keratoplasty. However, fitting these patients demands great flexibility in the use of appropriate lens designs and materials, including some that have been especially developed for this purpose.

Post-keratoplasty fitting represents one of the greatest challenges to the contact lens practitioner. Every facet of skill, lens design, visual optics, knowledge of corneal physiology and the results and complications of corneal surgery is called upon. The risks of infection, neovascularization, graft rejection or failure should never be forgotten.

References

Assil, K. K., Zarnegar, M. D. and Schanzlin, M. D. (1992) Visual outcome after penetrating keratoplasty with double or combined interrupted and continuous suture wound closure. Am. J. Ophthalmol., 114, 63–71

Australian Corneal Graft Registry (2004) Report 2004. eds. K. A. Williams, N. B. Hornsby, C. M. Bartlett, H. K. Holland, A. Esterman and D. J. Coster. Adelaide: Australian Corneal Graft Registry

Beekhuis, W. H., Van Rij, G., Eggink, F. A. G. J. et al. (1991) Contact lenses following keratoplasty. CLAO J., 17, 27–29

Bogan, S. J., Waring, G. O. and Ibrahim, O. S. (1990) Classification of normal corneal topography based on computer assisted videokeratography. Arch. Ophthalmol., 108, 945–949

Bouchard, C. S. and Trimble, S. N. (1996) Indications and complications of therapeutic disposable Acuvue contact lenses. CLAO J., 22, 106–108

Bourne, W. M. (1983) Morphological and functional evaluation of the transplanted cornea. Trans. Am. Ophthalmol. Soc., 81, 403–450

Brightbill, F. S. and Lazorik, R. J. (1999) Contact lens fitting. In Corneal Surgery: Theory, Technique and Tissue, 3rd edition, Chapter 55, ed. F. S. Brightbill. London: Mosby

Collins, R. S., Jarecke, A. J. and Traver, R. (2002) Contact lens stability after penetrating keratoplasty. Contact Lens Spectrum, 17(12), 26–30

Cosar, C. B., Sridhar, M. S. and Cohen, E. J. (2002) Indications for penetrating keratoplasty and associated procedures. Cornea, 21, 148–151

Cursiefien, C., Kunchle, M. and Naumann, G. O. (1998) Changing indications for penetrating keratoplasty: histopathology of 1250 buttons. Cornea, 17, 468–470

Dandona, L., Ragu, K., Janarthanan, M. et al. (1997) Indications for penetrating keratoplasty in India. Ind. J. Ophthalmol., 45, 163–168

Dart, J. K. G. (1993) Disease and risk associated with contact lenses. Br. J. Ophthalmol., 77, 49–53

Edwards, K. (2002) Silicone hydrogel contact lenses. Part 2: Therapeutic applications. Optom. Today, 42(2), 26–29

Edwards, M., Clover, G., Brookes, N. et al. (2002) Indications for corneal transplantation in New Zealand: 1991–1999. Cornea, 21, 152–155

Frucht-Pery, J., Shtibel, H., Solomon, A. et al. (1997) Thirty years of penetrating keratoplasty in Israel. Cornea, 16, 16–20

Gruber, E. (1991) The Acuvue disposable lens as a therapeutic bandage lens. Ann. Ophthalmol., 23, 446–447

Jessen, G. N. (1962) Orthofocus techniques. Contacto, 6, 200–204

Karabatsas, K. H., Cook, S. D. and Sparrow, J. M. (1999) Proposed classification for topographic patterns seen after penetrating keratoplasty. Br. J. Ophthalmol., 83, 403–409

Lagnado, R., Rubinstein, M. P., Maharajan, S. et al. (2004) Management options for the flat corneal graft. Cont. Lens Anterior Eye, 27, 27–31

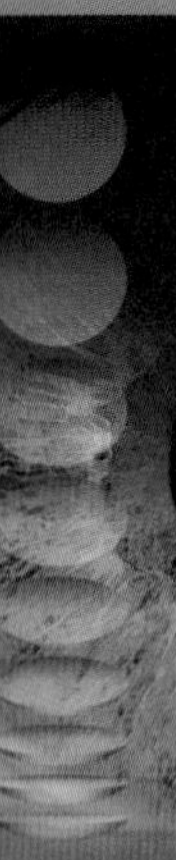

Lim, L., Siow, K. L., Sakamoto, R. et al. (2000) Reverse geometry contact lens wear after photorefractive keratectomy, radial keratectomy or penetrating keratoplasty. Cornea, 19, 320–324

Lim, L., Tan, D. T. and Chan, W. K. (2001) Therapeutic use of Bausch & Lomb Pure Vision contact lenses. CLAO J., 27, 179–185

Lindsay, R. G. (1995) Post keratoplasty contact lens management. Clin. Exp. Optom., 78, 223–226

Loveridge, R. (2004) What's new in the world of RGPs? Current status and new opportunities. Optom. Today, May 21, 34–39

Macalister, G. O., Woodward, E. G. and Buckley, R. J. (1993) The return of corneal sensitivity following transplantation. J. Br. Contact Lens Assoc., 16, 99–104

Mathur, A., Jones, L., Sorbara, L. et al. (1999) Use of reverse geometry rigid gas permeable contact lenses in the management of the post radial keratotomy patient: review and case report. Int. Contact Lens Clin., 26, 121–127

Olson, R. J. (1979) Variation in corneal graft size related to trephine technique. Arch. Ophthalmol., 97, 1323–1325

Pullum, K. (1997) A study of 530 patients referred for rigid gas permeable scleral contact lens assessment. Cornea, 16, 612–622

Ruben, M. and Colebrook, E. (1979) Keratoconus, keratoplasty curvatures and lens wear. Br. J. Ophthalmol., 63, 268–273

Rubinstein, M. P. (1995) Disposable contact lenses as therapeutic devices. J. Br. Contact Lens Assoc., 18, 95–97

Saini, J. S., Rao, G. N. and Aquavella, J. V. (1988) Post keratoplasty corneal ulcers and bandage lenses. Acta Ophthalmol., 66, 99–103

Shovelin, J. P. (1995) Vaulting success on post-PKP fits. Online. Available: www.lensdynamics.com

Speaker, M. G., Cohen, E. J., Edelhauser, H. F. et al. (1991) Effects of gas permeable contact lenses on the endothelium of corneal transplants. Arch. Ophthalmol., 109, 1703–1706

Spraul, C. W. and Lang, G. K. (1997) Contact lenses and corneal shields. Curr. Opin. Ophthalmol., 8, 67–75

Srur, M. and Dattas, D. (1997) The use of disposable contact lenses as therapeutic lenses. CLAO J., 23, 40–42

Sugar, A. and Sugar, J. (2000) Techniques in penetrating keratoplasty. A quarter century of development. Cornea, 19, 603–610

Suleweski, M. E., Kracher, G. P., Gottsch, J. D. et al. (1991) Use of disposable contact lens as a bandage contact lens. Arch. Ophthalmol., 109, 1341–1346

Szczotka, L. (1998) Contact lenses for the irregular cornea. Spectrum, 13, 21–27

Szczotka, L. B. and Aronsky, M. (1998) Contact lenses after LASIK. J. Am. Optom. Assoc., 69, 775–784

Szczotka, L. B. and Lindsay, R. G. (2003) Contact lens fitting following corneal graft surgery. Clin. Exp. Optom., 86(4), 244–249

Treumer, H. (1986) Therapeutic and optical contact lenses following keratoplasty. Contactologia, 8, 71–76

Tripoli, N. K., Ibrahim, O. S., Coggins, J. M. et al. (1990) Quantitative and qualitative topography classifications of clear penetrating keratoplasties. Invest. Ophthalmol. Vis. Sci., 30(Suppl), 480–485

Van Rij, G., Cornell, F. M., Waring, G. O. et al. (1985) Postoperative astigmatism after central versus eccentric penetrating keratoplasty. Am. J. Ophthalmol., 99, 317–320

Wietharn, B. E. and Drieb, W. T. (2004) Fitting contact lenses for visual rehabilitation after penetrating keratoplasty. Eye Contact Lens, 30, 31–33

Winkler, T. D. (1999) Case report of a corneo-scleral RGP lens. Contact Lens Spectrum, 14(9), 41–43

Wong, T. Y., Chan, C., Lim, L. et al. (1997) Changing indications for penetrating keratoplasty; a newly developed country's experience. Aust. N. Z. J. Ophthalmol., 25, 145–150

Woodward, E. G. (1984) Therapeutic silicone rubber lenses. J. Br. Contact Lens Assoc., 7, 42–49

Woodward, E. G., Moodaley, L. C. M., Lyons, C. et al. (1990a) Post keratoplasty dimensional and refractive change in the contact lens and spectacle corrected cases. Eye, 4, 689–692

Woodward, E. G., Moodaley, L. C. and O'Hagan, A. (1990b) Predictors for likelihood of cornea transplantation in keratoconus. Eye 4, 493–496

Chapter 23

Postrefractive surgery

Patrick J. Caroline and Jennifer D. Choo

CHAPTER CONTENTS

INTRODUCTION

For the past 30 years, visual scientists from around the world have struggled with the challenge of surgically correcting human refractive error. While great strides have been made in recent years, the nature of ocular surgery and its inherent complications has left in its wake a growing number of patients with suboptimal visual results. For a number of these patients, contact lenses may provide the best means for visual correction and restoration of binocular vision (McDonnell et al. 1989a, Szczotka 2001).

Throughout the evolution of refractive surgery, many experimental and poorly understood procedures have been attempted on millions of patient eyes. These included such procedures as keratophakia, keratomileusis, epikeratophakia, thermal keratoplasty, automated lamellar keratoplasty and radial keratotomy (RK).

Some patients have successful outcomes but others are left with permanently scarred and/or irregular corneas. More recent surgical procedures such as photorefractive keratectomy (PRK) and laser-assisted in situ keratomileusis (LASIK) have provided improved outcomes. However, a study by Stulting et al. (1999) involving 14 surgeons found that 4.8% of 1062 eyes lost two or more lines of best spectacle corrected visual acuity.

Since 1999, in the United States alone, approximately one million people per year have undergone refractive surgery. If 3% of these patients are experiencing significant postoperative visual problems, this represents 30,000 patients a year. When this number is added to the previous 25 years of refractive surgery failures, the pool of potential patients requiring postsurgical contact lens correction is significant.

Currently, the various refractive surgery procedures can be classified into one of six categories (Table 23.1).

Most modern refractive procedures modify corneal shape to achieve the desired refractive outcome because the cornea is the most powerful refracting surface of the eye (approximately 7.85 mm radius or 43.00 D). A small change in corneal curvature can result in a large change in refractive error, so measuring postoperative corneal shape is often how optical success or failure of a given procedure is assessed.

Postoperative corneal shape is influenced by:

- Type of refractive error being corrected (myopia, hyperopia, astigmatism or presbyopia).
- Surgical technique employed.
- Individual wound healing response.
- A wide range of potential intraoperative and postsurgical complications.

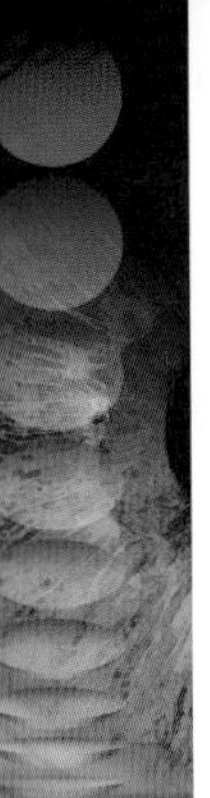

Table 23.1: Types of refractive surgery procedure

Tissue addition	Tissue subtraction	Tissue coagulation
Incisional keratotomy	LASIK/LASEK PRK	Thermal keratoplasty
Keratophakia	Wedge resection	Conductive keratoplasty
Epikeratophakia	Clear lens extraction	Laser thermal keratoplasty
Intracorneal implants	Keratomileusis	
Tissue modification	**Intraocular implant**	**Extraocular implant**
Crystalline lens modification	Phakic intraocular lens	Scleral expansion
Corneaplasty	Aphakic intraocular lens	Intrastromal implants

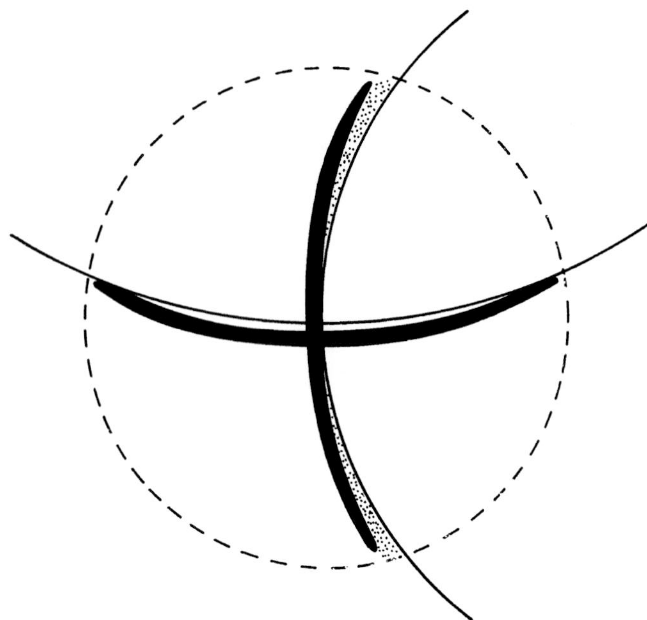

Figure 23.1 Optimum lens-to-cornea fitting relationship on a normal, unoperated eye with with-the-rule astigmatism. Note the central apical clearance, the mid-peripheral lens bearing at 3 and 9 o'clock and the clearance along the steeper vertical meridian

GENERAL PRINCIPLES OF POSTSURGICAL CORNEAL TOPOGRAPHY

It is not within the scope of this chapter to describe each refractive surgical procedure in detail. Instead, the focus is on postsurgical corneal topographies and the contact lens designs required for each.

The ultimate success of any rigid contact lens, regardless of its design, is predicated on the establishment of three fitting criteria:

- The back optic zone radius (BOZR) must be just steep enough to clear the apex of the cornea (see Chapter 9).
- An area of lens bearing (contact point) should be present in the mid-periphery along the horizontal meridian, approximately 3.0–4.0 mm from the centre of the cornea.
- The lens should maintain unobstructed movement along the vertical meridian (Fig. 23.1) (Caroline & Andre 2000a).

Apical clearance is a necessary design feature to prevent the contact lens from rocking on the corneal apex. Any amount of apical touch can result in lens decentration.

The bearing areas, or 'touch', at 3 and 9 o'clock lock the lens into position along the horizontal meridian to restrict lateral decentration; this is the primary design feature responsible for centration of the lens on the eye.

Finally, a BOZR is required that will allow unobstructed movement of the lens along the vertical meridian with each blink.

When approaching a postrefractive surgery cornea:

- A topographical map should be obtained and viewed in axial display mode.
- The measuring cursor of the topographer should be moved 4.0 mm from centre and curvature readings recorded in the areas of the nasal, temporal, superior and inferior mid-peripheral cornea.
- An appropriate BOZR can then be selected from the average of these four readings to accomplish the three fitting criteria described above.

CORNEAL TOPOGRAPHY CHANGES AFTER RADIAL KERATOTOMY

Radial keratotomy (RK) involves cutting deep (90% corneal thickness), equally spaced, radial incisions into the cornea. The incisions begin in the paracentral area of the cornea 1.5–2.5 mm from the centre and extend out just short of the limbus. Over the years, RK evolved from 16 to eight or four incisions.

The radial incisions result in a central corneal flattening while transverse or arcuate incisions have been used to correct astigmatism. In the past, hexagonal incisions were used to correct hyperopia by steepening the central cornea (Ward 2003).

Throughout the years there have been a number of explanations presented for the central flattening effect noted in RK. Fyodorov and Durnev (1979) proposed that the mechanism for the corneal flattening was related to a severing of a (yet undiscovered) circular ligament located near the limbus. Ivashina (1987) proposed that the central cornea was stretched, secondary to a bulging of the mid-peripheral cornea.

Holladay and Waring (1992) used mathematical modelling and modern corneal mapping techniques to indicate that a wound gape model presents the best explanation as to how RK works. The radial incisions create wounds that gape open under the force of the intraocular pressure and stresses within the

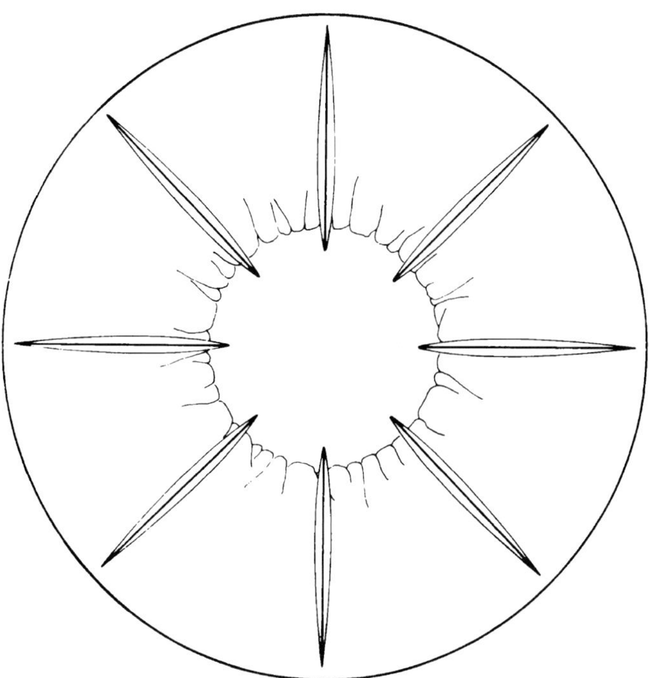

Figure 23.2 Corneal wound gape created by eight symmetrically placed radial incisions

corneal tissue (Fig. 23.2). These gaping incisions are first filled with an epithelial plug and finally with scar tissue (Fig. 23.3).

Salz (1986) found this process resulted in an overall increase in corneal surface area. Figure 23.4 shows a cornea with preoperative *K* readings of 7.70 along 180/7.65 along 90 and the outer ring chord of the photokeratoscope image measuring 37.5 mm with an equivalent mid-peripheral radius of curvature of 7.80 mm. Six months after eight-incision RK the central *K* readings were 8.70 along 180/8.50 along 90 and the outer ring chord now measured 38.0 mm with an equivalent mid-peripheral radius of curvature of 7.90 mm, i.e. 0.10 mm (0.50 D) flatter than the preoperative cornea.

It is therefore possible to state that RK is a diffuse (limbus-to-limbus) flattening procedure. The postoperative corneal topography will demonstrate considerable flattening in the centre, a lesser degree of flattening mid-peripherally and very little flattening peripherally. In addition, the postoperative mid-peripheral cornea will be steeper than the adjacent central cornea, although it will be flatter (in the same area) than the preoperative cornea.

The amount of wound gape and the subsequent corneal flattening will be influenced by a number of biological and surgical factors that include:

- Patient age at the time of surgery.
- Number, length and depth of the incisions.
- Preoperative shape factor (*e* or *p*) (see Chapter 9).
- Intraocular pressure, stresses and biochemical properties within the corneal tissue.
- Individual wound healing response (Rowsey 1986).

RIGID LENS FITTING

The post-RK cornea presents a number of challenges when fitting contact lenses including:

- Central versus mid-peripheral corneal topography.
- Anisometropia and aniseikonia.
- Irregular astigmatism.
- Elevation of incisional scars.
- Corneal neovascularization.
- Fluctuating refractive error.
- Postoperative glare and photophobia.

(a)

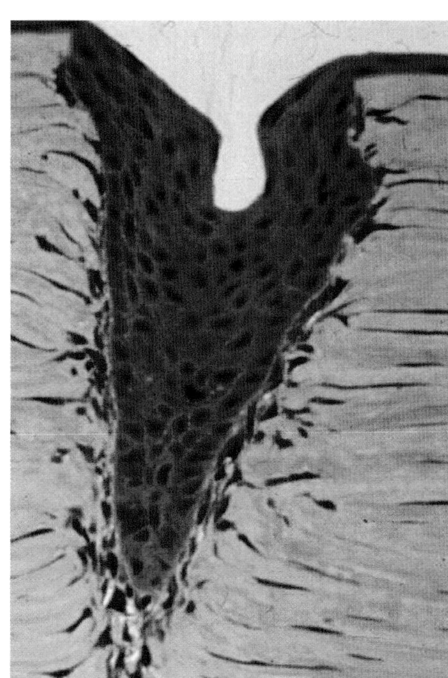

(b)

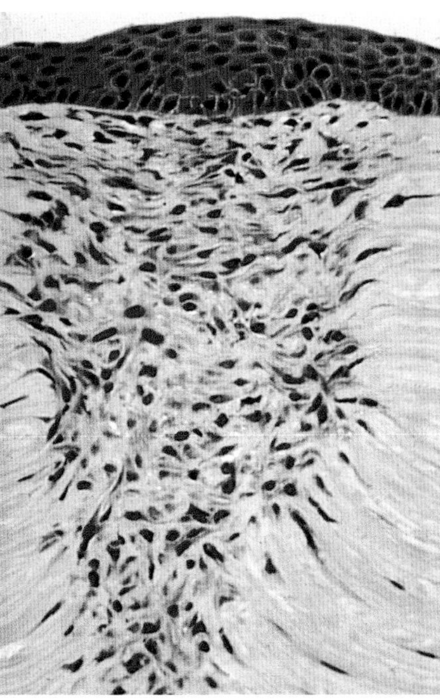

Figure 23.3 (a) With incisional wound gape, an epithelial plug is formed. (b) With time, the epithelium is pushed out and replaced with stromal scar tissue

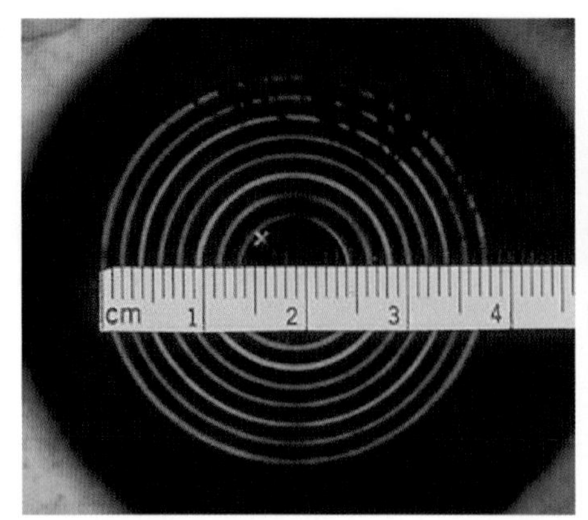

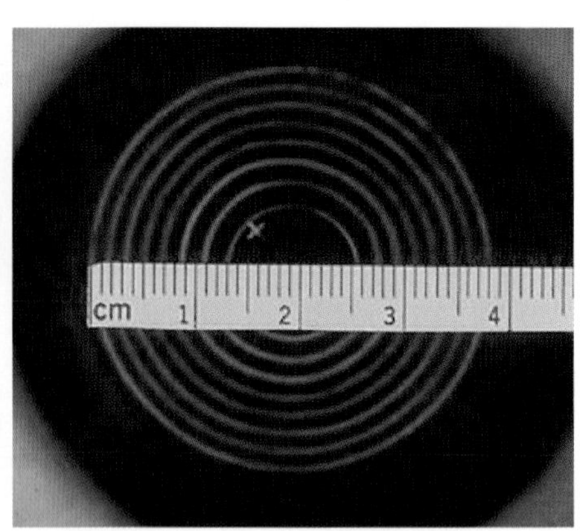

Figure 23.4 (a) Presurgical, ninth ring, chord diameter = 37.5 mm, with an equivalent mid-peripheral radius of curvature of 7.80 mm. (b) Six months post-eight-incision RK; the ninth ring chord now measures 38.0 mm with an equivalent mid-peripheral radius of curvature of 7.90 mm, i.e. 0.10 mm (0.50 D) flatter than the preoperative cornea

Waring et al. (1994), reporting on 10-year data from the Prospective Evaluation of Radial Keratotomy (PERK) study, identified a refractive condition unique to RK called 'hyperopic shift'. This occurred in approximately 43% of individuals where hyperopia increased by 1.00 D or more over a period of between 6 months and 10 years. It was unrelated to any ageing phenomenon, i.e. latent hyperopia, but was an unexplained ongoing effect of the flattening procedure. The aetiology and mechanisms responsible for this hyperopic shift are unknown.

When to fit lenses

Following RK, contact lens fitting should be delayed until the incisions have completely epithelialized and corneal topography and refraction have stabilized. Some fluorescein pooling may be present around the incision sites but the epithelium should be intact.

Clinical experience has shown that contact lens fitting can usually begin 6 weeks postoperatively. Additional time may be required for corneal sensitivity to return to its preoperative level and for all incisions to heal. They must withstand the minor trauma of lens movement and daily lens insertion and removal.

BOZR selection following RK

As discussed earlier, following RK, the cornea will exhibit significant central flattening with only minimal topographical changes in the mid-periphery. Therefore, it is important to select a BOZR steep enough to land or 'touch' the mid-periphery of the cornea approximately 4.0 mm from centre. This will invariably result in apical clearance across the flatter central cornea (Fig. 23.5).

Following refractive surgery, any of three techniques can be used to determine the radius of curvature of the mid-peripheral cornea:

- Computerized corneal mapping.
- Peripheral keratometry.
- Preoperative keratometric readings.

COMPUTERIZED CORNEAL MAPPING

This is the most accurate technique (McDonnell & Garbus 1989, McDonnell et al. 1992). The BOZR of the diagnostic lens is chosen to equal the corneal curvature 4.0 mm temporal to the centre of the cornea. For example:

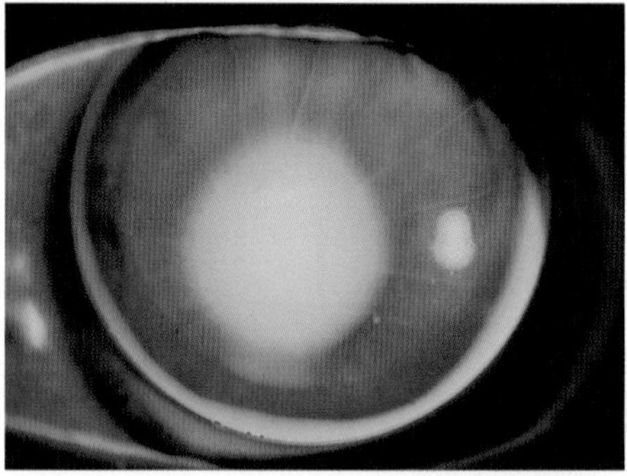

Figure 23.5 Following RK a BOZR is selected that is steep enough to align the mid-peripheral cornea. This will result in apical clearance and fluorescein pooling beneath the centre of the lens

Central *K* readings along 8.90 along 180/8.60 along 90 and radius of curvature 4.0 mm temporal to the centre of the cornea is 7.85 mm. Therefore, the BOZR of the diagnostic lens is 7.85 mm (Fig. 23.6) (Campbell & Caroline 1997).

PERIPHERAL KERATOMETRY

Following traditional central keratometry, the patient is instructed to direct fixation eccentrically in order to measure the mid-peripheral cornea directly. Caroline and Norman (1997) found that, with the Bausch & Lomb keratometer, a strong correlation existed between the mid-peripheral readings obtained by corneal mapping and those obtained by peripheral keratometry.

The keratometer can be modified by placing 1.0 mm fixation dots onto the faceplate 4.0 mm from the outside rim of the centre viewing port. With the patient viewing the fixation dots, central and peripheral *K* readings are taken and a numeric profile of the mid-peripheral cornea established.

As with corneal mapping, a diagnostic lens is selected with a BOZR equal to the temporal radius of curvature (Campbell & Caroline 1994).

PREOPERATIVE KERATOMETRY TECHNIQUE

The radius of the mid-peripheral cornea after RK is estimated from the *preoperative* central *K* readings.

(a)

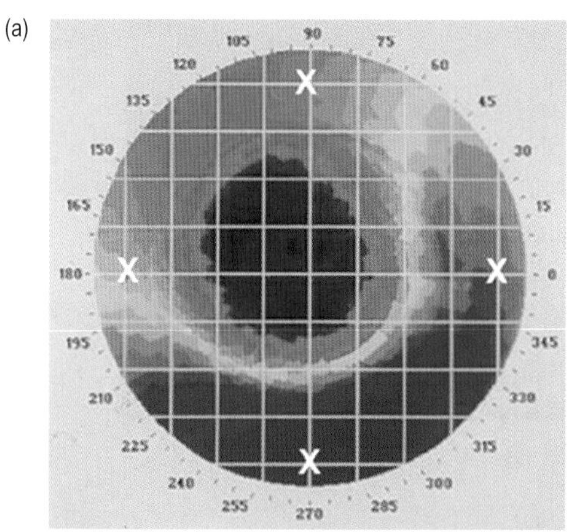

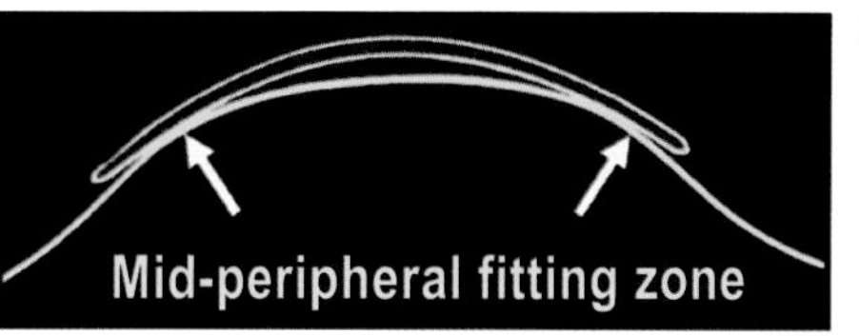

(b) **Figure 23.6** The initial BOZR of an RGP lens is selected by determining the radii of the mid-peripheral cornea 4.0 mm from centre (shown by the white crosses)

(a)

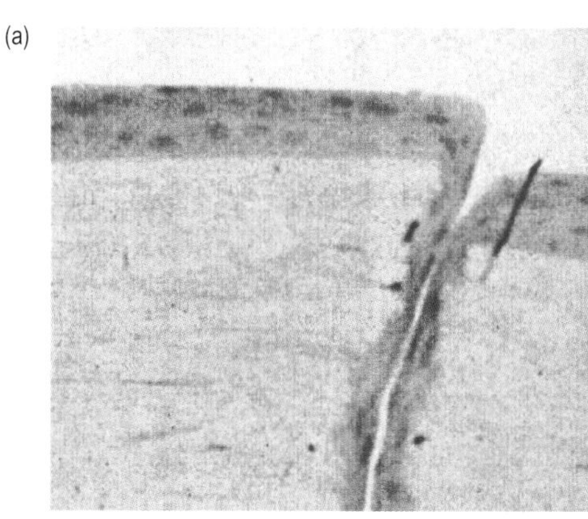

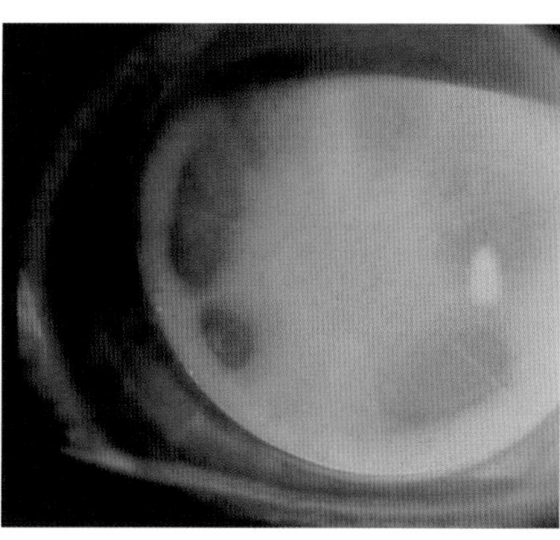

(b) **Figure 23.7** (a) Histological section of a primate cornea illustrating uneven incisional wound healing. (b) RGP lens decentration secondary to the resulting pivot points

The normal cornea flattens approximately 0.10 mm from centre to mid-periphery. If, for example, preoperative *K* readings were 7.70 along 180/7.50 along 90, then mid-peripheral *K* readings will be typically 7.80 mm along 180.

Topographical studies indicate that, after RK, the cornea flattens a further 0.10 mm (approximately) in the mid-periphery (Caroline 2002a). Therefore, a lens can be selected with a BOZR that is 0.20 mm flatter than the preoperative 'flattest *K*'.

In the above example, the flat *K* is 7.70 mm, so an initial diagnostic lens with a BOZR of 7.90 mm would be selected. Alternatively, if only one eye has undergone surgical treatment, a diagnostic lens with a BOZR 0.20 mm flatter than the flat *K* of the unoperated eye should be selected.

Total diameter

Lens decentration is common following RK, resulting most often from uneven healing of the incisions. As discussed earlier, when radial incisions are made in the cornea, the wound gapes and the walls become separated, initially by an epithelial plug and eventually by stromal collagen. If the walls of the incision do not heal in apposition, geographic surface elevations occur (Fig. 23.7) (Jester et al. 1992). As a rigid lens will pivot on these elevations, forcing the lens to decentre, any post-RK lens design must have a large total diameter (TD).

Diagnostic lenses used after RK (Table 23.2) have a TD of 10.0–11.0 mm. This, together with a large back optic zone diameter (BOZD) of 9.0 mm, helps to stabilize the lenses (Pederson & Coral-Ghanem 2003).

FITTING PROCEDURE

- The appropriate diagnostic lens (equal to the radius of curvature in the mid-peripheral cornea) is placed on the eye and the fit evaluated with fluorescein.
- The BOZR should clear the central cornea and align the mid-peripheral cornea 4–5 mm from centre, providing good centration.
- If decentration occurs, sequentially steeper BOZR should be placed on the eye until good centration is established.
- If the lens rides high, the lower edge will project forward, resulting in blink-induced irritation to the lower lid margin (Astin 1997). This leads to frothing, dimpling and increased mucus production.
- A spherocylinder over-refraction is performed to determine final lens power and *K* readings are taken over the front surface of the rigid gas-permeable (RGP) lens. If either measurement is unstable or fluctuates with blinking, it may indicate lens flexure, which can be minimized by increasing the centre thickness by approximately 0.05 mm.

Large-diameter semi-scleral rigid lenses

Traditional rigid lens designs may not always provide the required centration, optics or comfort. The patient may then

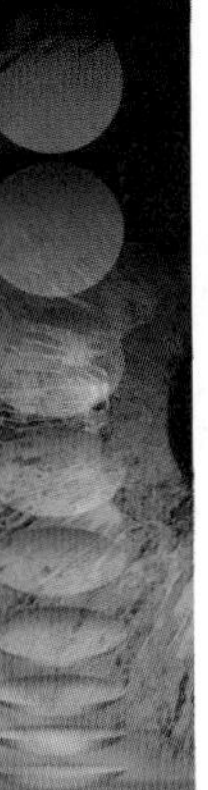

Table 23.2: Postrefractive surgery diagnostic set

BOZR	Power	Diameter (mm)	BOZD (mm)	Thickness (mm)
8.50	Plano	10.4	9.0	0.14
8.40	Plano	10.4	9.0	0.14
8.30	Plano	10.4	9.0	0.14
8.20	Plano	10.4	9.0	0.14
8.10	Plano	10.4	9.0	0.14
8.00	Plano	10.4	9.0	0.14
7.90	Plano	10.4	9.0	0.14
7.80	Plano	10.4	9.0	0.14
7.70	Plano	10.4	9.0	0.14
7.60	Plano	10.4	9.0	0.14
7.50	Plano	10.4	9.0	0.14
7.40	Plano	10.4	9.0	0.14
7.30	Plano	10.4	9.0	0.14
7.20	Plano	10.4	9.0	0.14

benefit from a large diameter (13.5–15.5 mm) semi-scleral lens design, manufactured in a wide range of parameters from high-Dk (100+) materials (see also Chapters 21 and 22).

Semi-scleral lenses are fitted using a diagnostic set of 12 lenses, incorporating a large limbal fenestration to reduce lens adhesion and facilitate lens removal (Caroline & Andre 1999a, 2000a).

FITTING PROCEDURE

- Select a diagnostic lens with a BOZR equal to the radius of the mid-peripheral cornea 4.0 mm from centre.
- The ideal fluorescein pattern should exhibit apical clearance across the central cornea, a 1.0 mm band of pooling adjacent to the limbus and alignment in the area of the scleral curve (Fig. 23.8).

Semi-scleral lenses are beneficial for postrefractive surgery patients with highly irregular and/or asymmetric corneas, as they reduce many of the comfort and centration complications

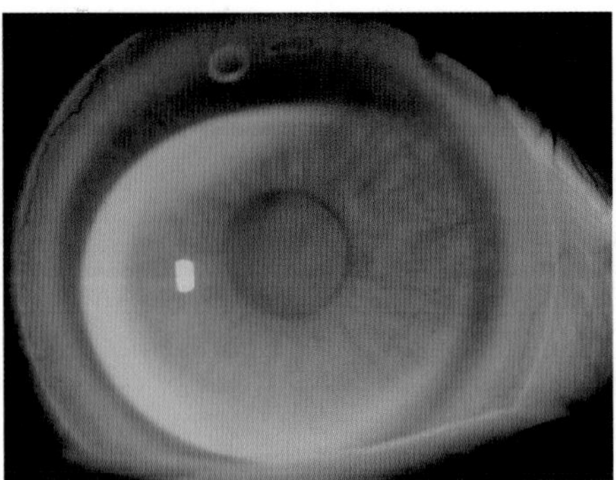

Figure 23.8 Semi-scleral RGP, Jupiter Lens design

associated with more traditional rigid lens designs. The main disadvantages are:

- An appropriate fitting set is required.
- Adequate post-lens tear flow may be restricted.

Reverse geometry lenses (see also Chapter 22)

Due to the oblate shape of the post-RK cornea (see 'Anterior aspheric soft lens designs', below), once mid-peripheral alignment has been established with a diagnostic lens, excessive apical clearance and fixed bubbles may be present beneath the centre of the lens. It may then be necessary to use a reverse geometry lens design in which the central radius of the lens is *flatter* than the mid-periphery. The lens creates a 'plateau' configuration, thereby decreasing the volume of tears beneath the centre of the lens (El Hage & Baker 1986, Shin et al. 1993, Kame 1996).

FITTING PROCEDURE

- Corneal topography is carried out; for example, central *K* readings of 8.90 along 6/8.50 along 96 and a 4.0 mm temporal mid-peripheral radius of 7.75 mm (Fig. 23.9).
- The 7.70 mm BOZR diagnostic lens (see Table 23.2) is placed on the eye and evaluated with fluorescein.
- If the fluorescein pattern exhibits mid-peripheral lens alignment and no central bubble, an over-refraction can be performed and the appropriate lens ordered.

(a)

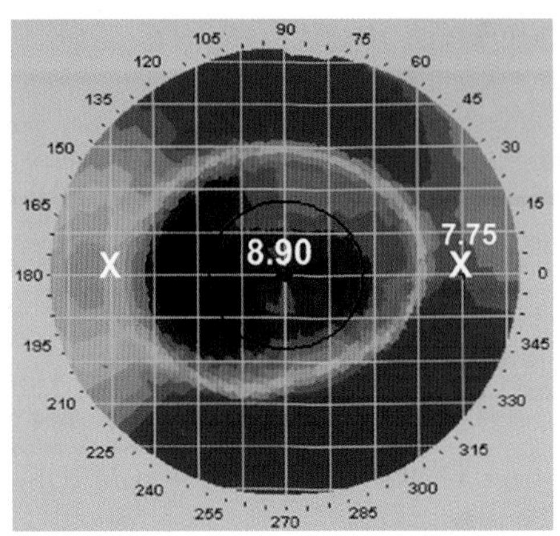

(b)

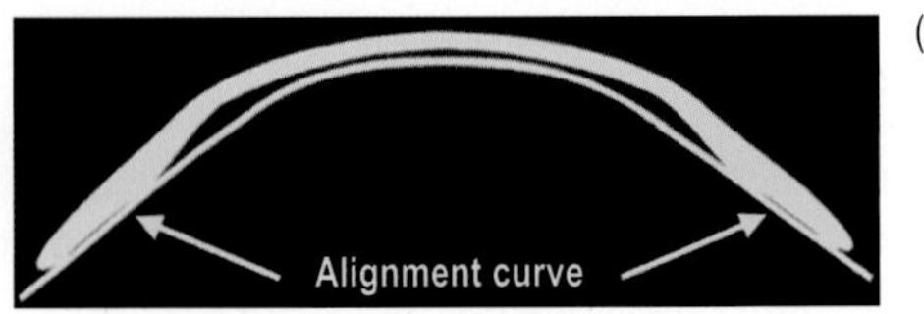

Figure 23.9 Corneal mapping is used to determine the BOZR and mid-peripheral alignment curve of the reverse geometry lens. Central keratometric readings in this example are 8.90 along 6/8.50 along 96 and a 4.0 mm temporal mid-peripheral radius of 7.75 mm (indicated by the white crosses)

(a)

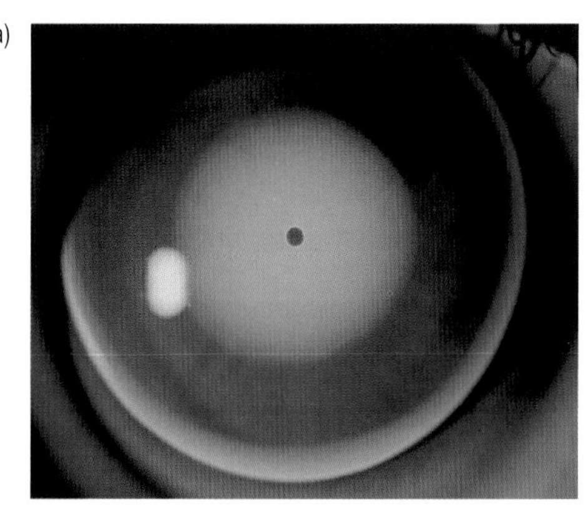

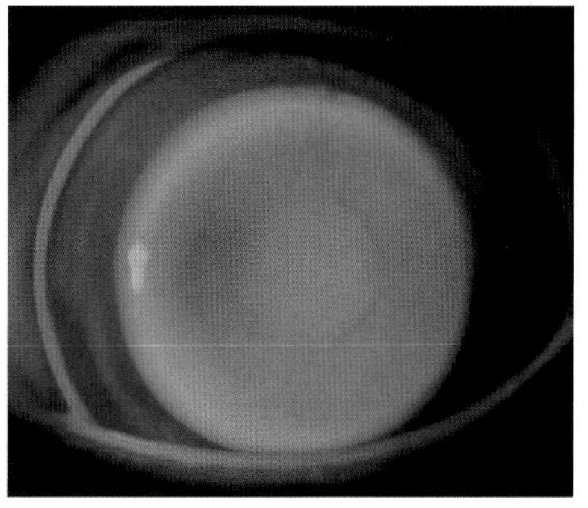

(b) **Figure 23.10** (a) Standard RGP lens design postrefractive surgery; note the apical clearance and fixed bubble. (b) Reverse geometry lens design on the same eye

- If a central bubble is present, a reverse geometry lens design will be required (Fig. 23.10a).
- The desired BOZR (equal to flattest *K*) and the radius of the mid-peripheral alignment curve (equal to the corneal curvature 4.0 mm from centre) are entered into a commercial computer program, and the computer selects a reverse curve that joins the BOZR with the mid-peripheral alignment curve (Caroline & Andre 2001a,b).
- The ideal lens provides a small degree of apical clearance and mid-peripheral lens alignment (Fig. 23.10b).

SOFT CONTACT LENSES AFTER RADIAL KERATOTOMY

A wide range of inventory soft lens designs can be used following RK. The lens material preferred by the authors is silicone hydrogel. The high Dk of these lenses (50–170) may reduce some of the visual symptoms such as fluctuating vision, which could be related to mechanical bending of the lens or to corneal hypoxia. Shivitz et al. (1986, 1987) reported that high-Dk lenses might help prevent incisional neovascularization, a common complication associated with the wearing of lower-Dk soft lenses after RK.

FITTING PROCEDURE

Postsurgical fitting techniques are similar to those used in normal, unoperated eyes.

- A TD is selected 2.0 mm larger than the cornea. For example, a 14.00 mm TD would be selected for a 12.00 mm horizontal visible iris diameter in order that the lens extends approximately 1 mm beyond the limbus.
- The BOZR is selected 0.70 mm flatter than the *preoperative* flat *K*. For example, a patient with a preoperative flat *K* of 7.90 mm and a corneal diameter of 12.0 mm would require a post-RK diagnostic lens with a BOZR of approximately 8.60 mm and a TD of 14.0 mm.
- The diagnostic lens should centre well and move approximately 0.25 mm on blink.
- After settling, the parameters can be altered as necessary
  - loose: increase TD or decrease BOZR.
  - tight: reduce TD or increase BOZR.
  - poor acuity: spherocylinder over-refraction.

Vision may fluctuate with soft lenses after RK, due to various physical and physiological factors including:

- Uncorrected refractive error.
- Dehydration.
- Blink-induced lens flexure across the flatter central cornea.
- Corneal hypoxia.

Normal diurnal fluctuations in vision and corneal shape are frequently experienced following RK (Schanzlin et al. 1986, Wyzininski 1987, McDonnell et al. 1989b).

Anterior aspheric soft lens designs

Following refractive surgery, a complex relationship exists between:

- Visual acuity.
- Defocus.
- Diffraction.
- Optical aberration.

The normal preoperative cornea exhibits a positive, aspheric (prolate) shape factor (*e* value) of +0.10 to +0.30, while the postrefractive surgery cornea has a negative (oblate) shape factor of –0.50 to –3.50, with '0' being spherical.

The lack of postoperative asphericity can create aberrations in a number of patients, especially those with large pupils. Clinical experience has shown that lenses that incorporate anterior aspheric optics can reduce patient symptoms from spherical aberration. Patients wearing these lenses often report less flare and glare, especially at night (Caroline & Andre 1999b, 2004c).

Customized reverse geometry soft lens designs

The primary concerns in fitting soft contact lenses after RK are:

- Hypoxia.
- Incisional neovascularization.
- Excessive apical vaulting over the flattened central cornea.

Recent advances in latheable, high-Dk, silicone hydrogel lenses (e.g. from Lagado Corporation, Colorado and Innovations in Sight Inc., Virginia, USA) have dramatically lessened the physiological concerns related to hypoxia and neovascularization. Excessive apical clearance can be managed with a customized soft

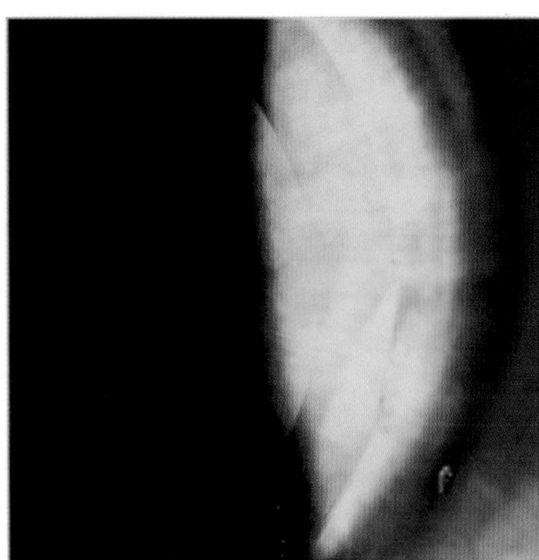

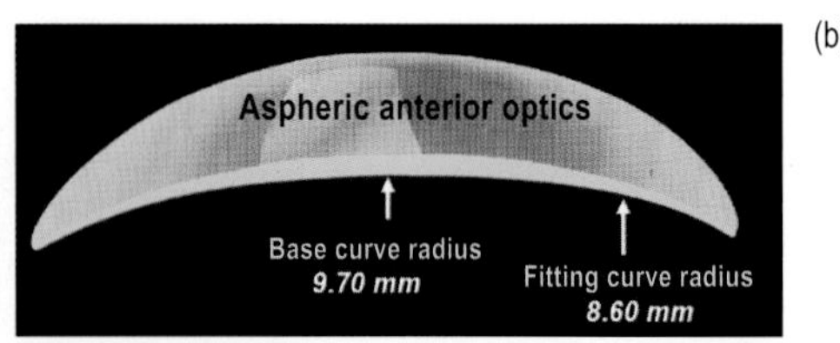

Figure 23.11 Customized reverse geometry soft contact lens design. The reverse curve can be seen in (a)

Table 23.3: Soft lens reverse geometry diagnostic set

BOZR/fitting curve	Power	Diameter (mm)	Centre thickness (mm)
9.1/8.6	Plano	14.5	0.25
9.4/8.6	+2.00	14.5	0.25
9.7/8.6	+4.00	14.5	0.25
10.0/8.6	+6.00	14.5	0.25

lens design that incorporates a reverse geometry configuration, i.e. flatter central radius of curvature and a steeper periphery (Caroline & Andre 2002). This is further enhanced by incorporating anterior aspheric optics to address the surgically induced spherical aberration (Caroline & Andre 2003), and can be improved by increasing the centre thickness by an additional 0.05 to 0.10 mm (Fig. 23.11) (Caroline & Andre 2004b).

FITTING PROCEDURE

- The lens is fitted from a four-lens diagnostic set (Table 23.3).
- The BOZR is selected by adding 0.40 mm to the postoperative flat *K*. For example, if the flat *K* is 9.20 mm, add +0.40 mm for a suggested BOZR of approximately 9.60 mm.
- Insert the 9.7/8.6 diagnostic lens and evaluate movement and centration.
- The two posterior lens radii and TD can be adjusted independently to optimize the lens fit.
- Over-refract with spherocylinders to determine the final lens power. If any residual cylinder is present, three options are available:
  - lens centre thickness can be adjusted by up to 0.35 mm to further optimize visual acuity.
  - additional power can be provided in spectacle lenses.
  - cylindrical power can be incorporated into the lens as a toric, reverse geometry soft lens.

Piggyback soft lenses

The technique of placing a rigid contact lens onto a soft lens (piggyback) was first reported in the mid 1970s (Baldone 1973). Early piggyback systems consisted of thick, low-Dk soft lenses and low-Dk rigid lenses. Not surprisingly, this combination frequently resulted in corneal oedema and neovascularization, limiting the usefulness of the modality. With the introduction of high-Dk silicone hydrogel lenses and stable high-Dk RGP materials, the dual lens system is enjoying a rebirth, particularly for patients experiencing discomfort or poor lens centration following refractive surgery (Caroline 2002b) (see also Chpaters 20 and 22).

Traditional piggyback lens system

This consists of a high-Dk silicone hydrogel soft lens over which a high-Dk RGP lens is fitted.

FITTING PROCEDURE

- A silicone hydrogel soft lens is selected of low to moderate plus power. The anterior surface of the soft lens now better emulates the prolate shape of the normal cornea (see below) (Caroline & Andre 2004d).
- Keratometry or videokeratography is performed over the anterior surface of the soft lens to determine the radii of the 'new' corneal surface.
- Select an RGP lens with a BOZR equal to the flattest *K* and a diameter of approximately 9.0–9.5 mm and adjust until an appropriate lens-to-lens fitting relationship is established. This can be assessed using high-molecular-weight fluorescein (see Chapter 5).
- Carry out an over-refraction to determine the final power of the RGP lens.

The RGP lens can be manufactured in a high-Dk material and the periphery and edge configurations customized (Fig. 23.12).

In a number of situations it may be helpful to create a new anterior fitting surface to the cornea by manipulating the power of the soft lens. Thus, if a flatter anterior surface is desired, a minus-powered soft lens can be used; if a steeper anterior surface is desired (which is often the case following myopic refractive surgery), a plus-powered soft lens can be used (Fig. 23.13). Figures 23.14 and 23.15 show the effect of using silicone hydrogel soft lenses of differing powers to provide a new base onto which an RGP lens can be fitted.

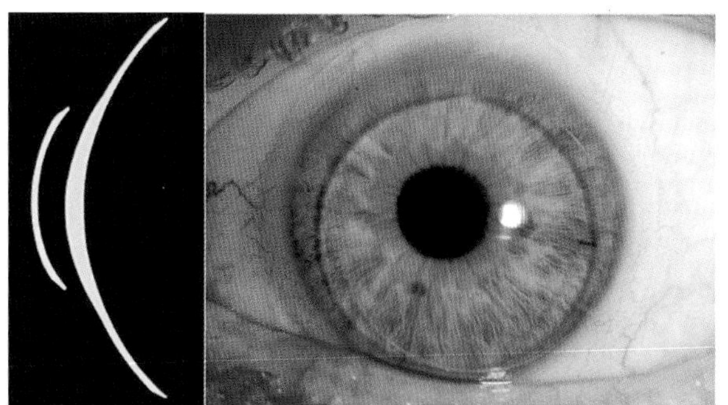

Figure 23.12 Traditional 'piggyback' lens system post-RK, with a +6.00 D silicone hydrogel soft contact lens

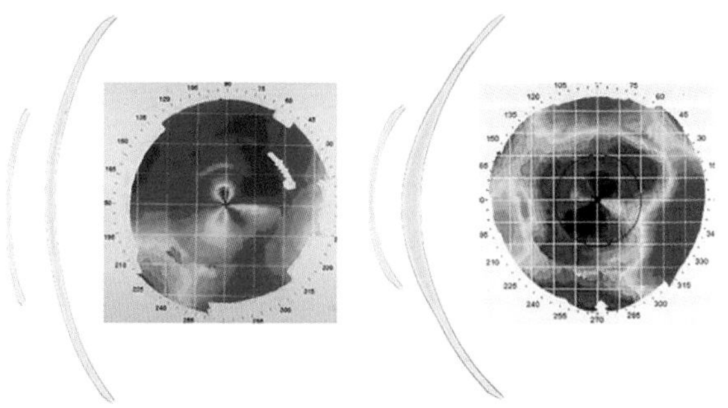

Figure 23.13 The anterior fitting surface of the cornea can be altered by the anterior surface power of the soft lens (flattened with minus-powered lenses and steepened with plus-powered lenses)

Customized piggyback lens system

A circular depression is recessed into the centre of the anterior surface of the soft lens (see Chapter 20) and a high-Dk RGP lens is fitted within the boundaries of the recess. The system provides optimal performance as the RGP is better centred,

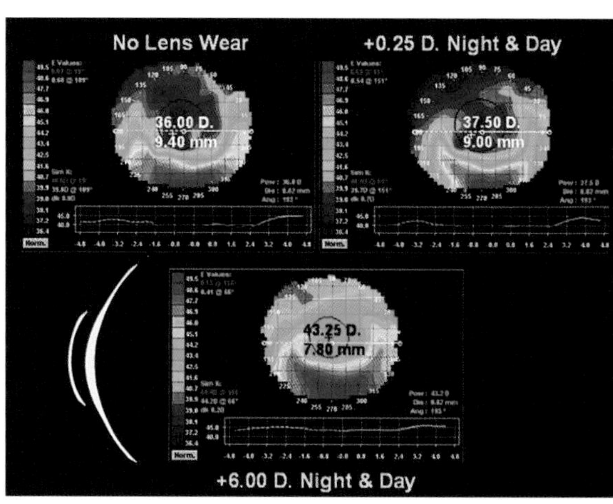

Figure 23.15 Post-RK: central apical radius of curvature of 9.40 mm (top left). A silicone hydrogel lens of +0.25 D steepens the central corneal radius to 9.00 mm (top right) and to 7.80 mm with the +6.00 D soft lens (lower centre). The patient was ultimately fitted with a +6.00 D silicone hydrogel soft lens with a 7.80 mm RGP lens on top

providing better optics and enhanced comfort through the bandage effect of the soft lens.

X-Cel Laboratories (Georgia, USA) produce a customized piggyback soft lens. It is available in a wide range of parameters, including BOZR from 6.00 to 11.00 mm and TDs from 12.5 to 16.5 mm. The recessed cut-out can be manufactured in diameters of 7.5–11.5 mm. Further designs are available from other laboratories.

FITTING PROCEDURE

The soft lens fitting is identical to that of any soft lens, with good movement and centration.

(a) (b)

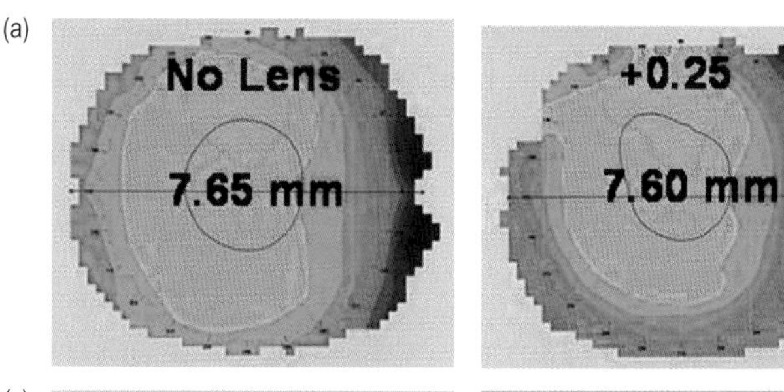

(c) (d)

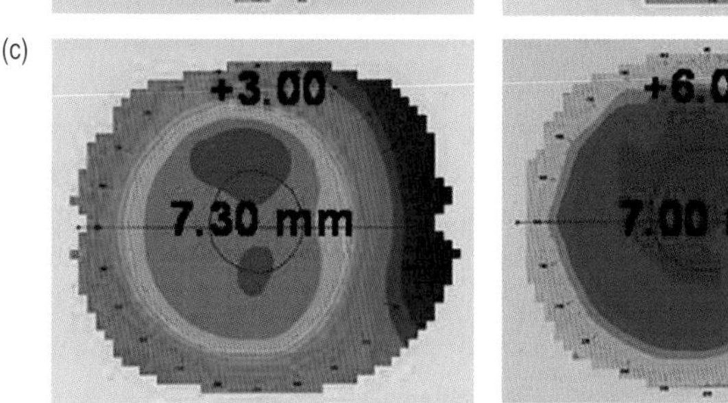

Figure 23.14 The anterior surface of a normal cornea can be effectively steepened with the fitting of hyperopic silicone hydrogel soft lenses. With no lens in place, the apical radius of curvature of the patient's cornea is 7.65 mm. The central radius steepens with the increased plus power, +0.25 D (7.60 mm), +3.00 D (7.30 mm) and +6.00 D (7.00 mm)

Diagnostic fitting is enhanced by inserting any rigid lens into the recessed cut-out of the soft lens to better mimic final lens weight and lid/lens interaction.

Once the appropriate soft lens fit has been established, the rigid lens can be removed and *K* readings performed over the central portion of the soft lens.

A diagnostic RGP lens with a BOZR equal to the flattest *K* is inserted into the cut-out and its fitting relationship evaluated and adjusted. The TD of the RGP should be 1.0 mm smaller than the cut-out diameter to allow for some lens movement and tear exchange. For example, if the cut-out diameter is 9.5 mm, the RGP lens diameter should be 8.5 mm (Fig. 23.16) (Caroline & Andre 1998).

(a)

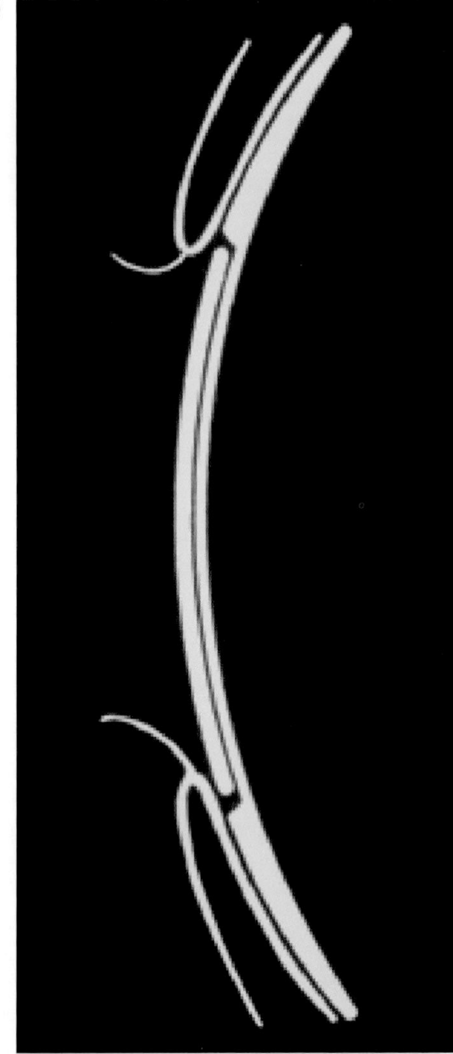

(b)

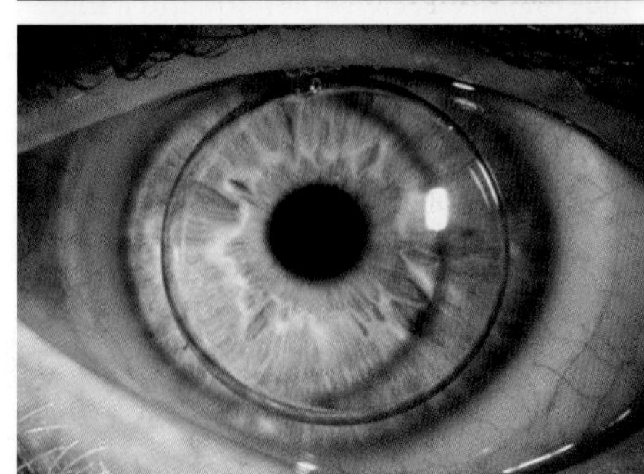

Figure 23.16 The Flexlens customized piggyback lens design

Hybrid lenses

SynergEyes (Quarter Lambda Technologies, California, USA) is a high-Dk hybrid lens that has been used successfully by the authors. It incorporates an 8.2 mm Paragon HDS 100 (Dk 100) rigid centre and a non-ionic 31% water content, soft lens skirt. The TD is 14.5 mm.

The lens is available in three designs for the postrefractive surgery cornea, in particular for patients with irregular astigmatism or comfort and centration issues with traditional RGP lens designs.

- *SynergEyes A* is the standard aspherical design, ideal for postsurgical corneas in which there is minimal topographical difference between the central and mid-peripheral cornea.
- *SynergEyes PS* incorporates a flatter radius of curvature in the centre of the RGP lens and a steeper curve in the mid-peripheral radius, ideal for patients with highly oblate corneas following refractive surgery.
- *SynergEyes KC* has been designed specifically for keratoconus, although it has proven extremely valuable in managing patients with LASIK-induced keratectasia, where the thinned post-LASIK cornea begins to bulge anteriorly, similar to that seen in keratoconus.

FITTING PROCEDURE

- Each SynergEyes design has a 12-lens diagnostic set.
- Select a diagnostic lens with a BOZR equal to the radius of the mid-peripheral cornea approximately 4.0 mm from the centre.
- Insert the lens into the eye with high-molecular-weight fluorescein in the bowl of the lens and allowed to equilibrate.
- The RGP portion of the lens should exhibit central apical clearance and mid-peripheral lens bearing (Fig. 23.17).
- The soft lens skirt should move 0.25 mm on blinking.

LASER PHOTOREFRACTIVE PROCEDURES

Laser procedures such as PRK and LASIK are tissue subtraction or ablation techniques in which an argon-fluorine excimer laser is used to remove tissue to alter the shape of the cornea. The high-energy ultraviolet light (193 nanometres) is delivered to the cornea through a pulsating spot or slit.

A single pulse of focused light enters the corneal tissue and within 1 picosecond the intermolecular bonds (holding the tissue together) are broken. The intense build-up of energy and pressure ejects the fragmented tissue off the surface of the cornea and the pulse then terminates. Repeated laser pulses ablate the corneal tissue to allow a remodelling of the corneal shape to correct myopia, hyperopia, astigmatism or presbyopia (Seiler et al. 1992).

Worldwide, LASIK is now the most commonly performed refractive procedure. The principal indication for postsurgical contact lenses is residual refractive error including:

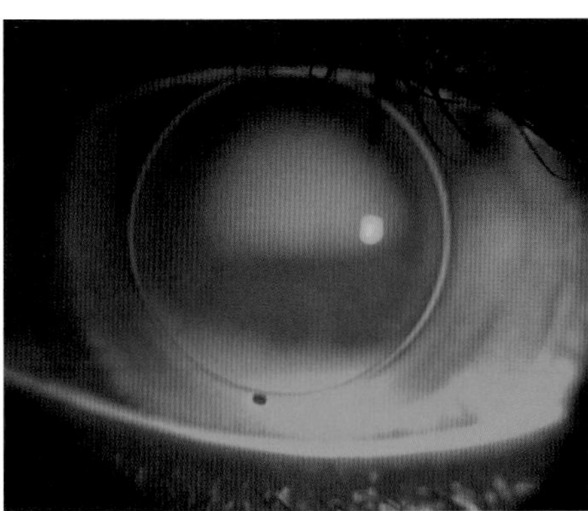

Figure 23.17 SynergEyes hybrid lenses with an 8.2 mm high-Dk, RGP centre and a 31% soft lens skirt, viewed using high-molecular-weight fluorescein

- Undercorrection.
- Overcorrection.
- Residual or induced astigmatism.

Other less common indications include:

- Decentred ablations.
- Central islands.
- Keratectasia.

Corneal topography after PRK and LASIK

The hallmark of corneal topography after PRK and LASIK is a flattened central cornea over a chord of 5–7 mm. This ablated area is surrounded by a 0.5–1.5 mm zone that extends across the treated portion of the cornea into the normal untreated mid-peripheral cornea. As with all surgical procedures, complications can compromise the depth, position and contour of the ablation zone.

PRK and LASIK complications can be divided into three categories: intraoperative, postoperative and refractive.

- *Intraoperative* complications are seen more commonly in LASIK due to the added complexity associated with the microkeratome, and include microkeratome or suction ring malfunction resulting in incomplete or irregular cuts, laser malfunction and human data entry errors.
- *Postoperative* complications include flap perforation, dehiscence or detachment, epithelial ingrowth, foreign bodies within the flap interface and infection.

  While intra- and postoperative complications are rare, they can significantly jeopardize the surgical outcome.
- *Refractive* complications form the majority and include undercorrections, overcorrections, regression of effect, irregular astigmatism or surface irregularities, stromal haze, central islands, decentration of the ablation and corneal ectasia (Ward 2001).

When to fit

As with all refractive procedures, contact lens fitting should be delayed until the cornea has completely epithelialized and the refractive error is stable. PRK and LASIK epithelialization is usually completed within 1 week but the refractive error and corneal topography may not stabilize for 6 weeks. By then, the integrity of the cornea and, in the case of LASIK, the stability of the flap interface is usually sufficient to withstand the minor trauma associated with contact lens wear.

Several authors (Ang et al. 2001, Benitez-del-Castillo et al. 2001, Toda et al. 2001) have found that post-LASIK patients sometimes experience severe dry eye symptoms. While the exact mechanism(s) responsible for this complication remains unclear, ocular dryness has obvious implications if contact lenses are to be worn after LASIK. The symptoms of dryness appear to lessen with time but some patients experience chronic dry eye symptoms for many years and others never return to their baseline level.

Contact lens fitting after PRK and LASIK

FITTING PROCEDURE

- The rigid lens fitting procedure is similar to that described earlier after RK.
- Corneal topography is performed and a diagnostic lens is selected with a BOZR equal to the temporal corneal curvature 4.0 mm from centre.
- The lens is placed on the cornea and evaluated with fluorescein.
- The optimum BOZR is the radius that aligns the mid-peripheral cornea at 3 and 9 o'clock, locks the lens along the horizontal meridian and prevents nasal or temporal decentration.
- Significant pooling of fluorescein may be present beneath the centre of the lens, which is directly related to the amount of central tissue ablated at the time of surgery, for example:
  - a patient with a –3.00 D refractive error will require an ablation depth of 36 microns, an amount less than the thickness of the human epithelium. The minimal difference between the central and mid-peripheral cornea creates few fitting problems in the area of the central cornea and conventional RGP lenses can often be used.
  - a patient with –9.00 D of preoperative refractive error will require the removal of approximately 110 microns of corneal tissue. In this case the difference between the central and mid-peripheral cornea is such that a diagnostic lens designed to align the mid-peripheral cornea may exhibit excessive apical clearance and bubble formation. A reverse geometry lens may be indicated (see Reverse geometry lenses, p. 496).

The wide range of soft lens designs used after RK (see p. 496) can also be used for PRK and LASIK patients. Postoperative complications include:

- Undercorrection.
- Overcorrection.
- Irregular astigmatism.
- Anisometropia.
- Keratectasias.

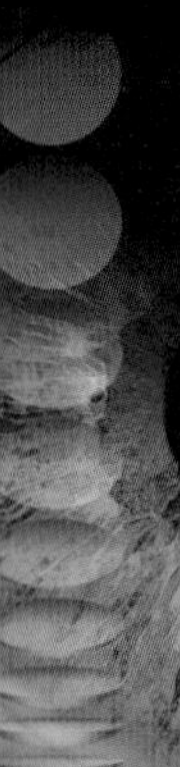

Corneal reshaping after LASIK
(see also Chapter 19)

The most common complication associated with modern refractive surgery is unplanned under- or overcorrection of the targeted refractive error. Where the error is significant, additional surgery in the form of laser re-treatment or conductive keratoplasty can be performed. However, where the residual refractive error is low (1.00 D or less), patients are frequently advised that additional surgery may not be in their best interest.

Advances in RGP corneal reshaping show that tissue in the central portion of the cornea can be safely and effectively remodelled overnight to correct myopia (corneal flattening) and hyperopia (corneal steepening). For a number of patients, overnight corneal reshaping (ortho-k) has been the ideal method for managing their postsurgical refractive error (Caroline & Andre 2004a).

FITTING PROCEDURE

- The parameters of the initial corneal reshaping lens are selected by first identifying the spherical equivalent of the postsurgical refractive error to be corrected. For example, if the residual refractive error was –1.00/–0.50 × 180, the spherical equivalent power to be corrected would be –1.25 D.
- Carry out corneal topography and identify the apical radius (r_0). For example, if the postsurgical apical radius is 8.55 mm (39.50 D) and an additional –1.25 D of corneal flattening is required, select a BOZR 1.25 D flatter than r_0, i.e. 8.80 mm (38.25 D).
- Select a mid-peripheral fitting curve equal to the radius of curvature 4.0 mm from centre on the temporal side of the cornea – for example, 7.90 mm (42.75 D).
- Laboratory software will calculate the appropriate reverse curve to join the BOZR with the mid-peripheral fitting curve radius.

The combination of curves should result in a lens that centres and moves well. Within 5–7 days of overnight lens wear, fluid forces beneath the reverse geometry lens should flatten the cornea the additional 1.25 D, resulting in a more acceptable uncorrected visual acuity throughout the patient's waking hours.

SUMMARY

Refractive surgery procedures will continue to be a cornerstone in the delivery of modern eye care throughout the world. With ongoing technological advances, the number of patients undergoing current and future refractive procedures staggers the imagination. However, as with any cosmetic surgery, suboptimal results will continue to be an ever-present reality. Despite the industry's most valiant efforts, complications secondary to surgical errors, equipment malfunction and individual patient healing response will continue with an incidence of approximately 3%.

Fortunately, today's contemporary contact lens practice is equipped with a wide range of lens designs and materials to cope successfully with the complex challenges presented by these patients.

References

Ang, R. T., Dartt, D. A., Tsubota, K. (2001) Dry eye after refractive surgery. Curr. Opin. Ophthalmol., 12, 318–322

Astin, C. L. (1997) Radial keratotomy and photorefractive keratectomy. In Contact Lens, 4th edn, Chapter 20.4, eds. A. J. Phillips and L. Speedwell. Oxford: Butterworth-Heinemann

Baldone, J. A. (1973) The fitting of hard contact lenses onto soft contact lenses in certain diseased conditions. Contact Lens Med. Bull., 6, 15–17

Benitez-del-Castillo, J. M., del Rio, T., Iradier, T. et al. (2001) Decrease in tear secretion and corneal sensitivity after laser in-situ keratomileusis. Cornea, 20, 30–32

Campbell, R. and Caroline, P. (1994) A unique technique for fitting post-RK patients. Contact Lens Spectrum, December, 56

Campbell, R. and Caroline, P. (1997) Correcting irregular astigmatism after RK/PRK. Contact Lens Spectrum, August, 64

Caroline, P. J. (2002a) Post refract surgery. In Contact Lens Practice, Chapter 31, ed. N. Efron. Oxford: Butterworth-Heinemann

Caroline, P. J. (2002b) Piggyback lenses. Global CONTACT, 34, 34–35.

Caroline, P. J. and Andre, M. P. (1998) Custom soft contact lenses. Contact Lens Spectrum, April, 38–43

Caroline, P. J. and Andre, M. P. (1999a) Fitting after refractive surgery. Contact Lens Spectrum, June, 56

Caroline, P. J. and Andre, M. P. (1999b) Visual rehabilitation for post-refractive surgery patients. Contact Lens Spectrum, December, 56

Caroline, P. J. and Andre, M. P. (2000a) Empirical RGP fitting. Contact Lens Spectrum Supplement, August, 8–12

Caroline, P. J. and Andre, M. P. (2000b) An RGP solution for LASIK gone wrong. Contact Lens Spectrum, October, 56

Caroline, P. J. and Andre, M. P. (2001a) Software aids in lens design for post LASIK patients. Contact Lens Spectrum, March, 56

Caroline, P. J. and Andre, M. P. (2001b) Fitting reverse geometry lenses post ALK. Contact Lens Spectrum, September, 56

Caroline, P. J. and Andre, M. P. (2002) A reverse geometry soft lens for post-RK patients. Contact Lens Spectrum, January, 56

Caroline, P. J. and Andre, M. P. (2003) Fitting contact lenses after RK surgery. Contact Lens Spectrum, May, 56

Caroline, P. J. and Andre, M. P. (2004a) Fitting corneal reshaping post-LASIK. Contact Lens Spectrum, April, 56

Caroline, P. J. and Andre, M. P. (2004b) Masking irregular astigmatism with soft contact lenses. Contact Lens Spectrum, February, 56

Caroline, P. J. and Andre, M. P. (2004c) Correcting human error. Contact Lens Spectrum, May, 56

Caroline, P. J. and Andre, M. P. (2004d) Sometimes two lenses are better than one. Contact Lens Spectrum, March, 56

Caroline, P. J. and Norman, C. W. (1997) The case for adding corneal topography. Rev. Optom., April, 24–26

El Hage, S. and Baker, R. N. (1986) Controlled keratoreformation for post-operative radial keratotomy patients Int. Eyecare, 2, 49–53

Fyodorov, S. N. and Durnev, V. V. (1979) Operation of dosaged dissection of corneal circular in cases of myopia of mild degree. Ann. Ophthalmol., 11, 1885–1890

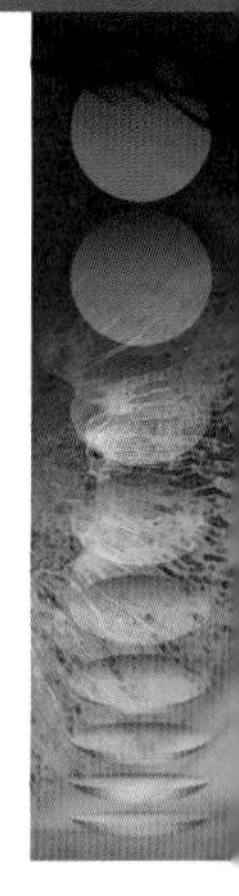

Holladay, J. T. and Waring, G. O. (1992) Optics and topography of radial keratotomy. In Refractive Keratotomy for Myopia and Astigmatism, ed. G. O. Waring. St Louis: Mosby

Ivashina A. I. (1987) Radial keratotomy as a method of surgical correction of myopia. In Microsurgery of the Eye, pp. 46–80, ed. S. Fyodorov. Moscow: Mir Publishers

Jester, J. V., Villasensor, R. A., Schanzlin D. J. and Cavanagh, H. D. (1992) Variations in corneal wound healing after radial keratotomy in non human primate eyes. Am. J. Ophthalmol., 92, 153–171

Kame, R. (1996) Reverse geometry lenses, improved rigid gas permeable lens technology. Prim. Care Optom. News, 1(11), 12

McDonnell, P. J. and Garbus, J. (1989) Corneal topographic changes after radial keratotomy. Ophthalmology, 96, 45–49

McDonnell, P. J., Caroline, P. J. and Salz, J. J. (1989a) Irregular astigmatism after radial keratotomy. Am. J. Ophthalmol., 107, 42–46

McDonnell, P. J., Fish, L. A. and Garbus, J. (1989b) Persistence of diurnal fluctuation after radial keratotomy. Refract. Corneal Surg., 5, 89–93

McDonnell, P. J., Garbus, J. J., Caroline, P. J. and Yoshinaga, P. D. (1992) Computer analysis of corneal topography as an aid in fitting contact lenses after radial keratotomy. Ophthalmol. Surg., 23, 55–59

Pederson, K. and Coral-Ghanem, C. (2003) Fitting contact lenses after refractive surgery. In Contact Lenses in Ophthalmic Practice, Chapter 15, eds. M. Mannis, K. Zadnik, C. Coral-Ghanem and N. Kara-Jose. New York: Springer-Verlag

Rowsey, J. J. (1986) Corneal topography and astigmatism. In Refractive Corneal Surgery, Chapter 12, eds. D. Sanders, R. Hofmann and J. Salz. New Jersey: Slack

Salz, J. J. (1986) Pathophysiology of radial and astigmatic keratotomy incisions. In Refractive Corneal Surgery, Chapter 8, eds. D. Sanders, R. Hofmann and J. Salz. New Jersey: Slack

Schanzlin, D. J., Santos, V. R., Waring, G. O. et al. (1986) Diurnal change in refraction, corneal curvature, visual acuity and intraocular pressure after radial keratotomy on the PERK study. Ophthalmology, 93, 167–175

Seiler, T., Fantes, F. E., Waring, G. O. et al. (1992) Laser corneal surgery. In Refractive Keratotomy for Myopia and Astigmatism, ed. G. O. Waring. St Louis: Mosby

Shin, J., Ackley, K. and Caroline, P. (1993) Use of 'plateau' designed lenses to improve corneal health in a post-operative radial keratotomy patient. Optom. Vis. Sci., 72, 82–83

Shivitz, I. A., Russell, B. M., Arrowsmith, P. N. et al. (1986) Optical correction of post-operative radial keratotomy patients with contact lenses. CLAO J., 12, 59–62

Shivitz, I. A., Arrowsmith, P. N. and Russell, B. M. (1987) Contact lenses in the treatment of patients with overcorrected radial keratotomy. Ophthalmology, 94, 899–903

Stulting, R. D., Carr J. D., Thompson K. P. et al. (1999) Complications of laser in situ keratomileusis for the correction of myopia. Ophthalmology, 106, 13–20

Szczotka, L. B. (2001) Corneal topography and contact lenses after LASIK. In LASIK, Clinical Co-management, Chapter 10, ed. M. M. Hom. Woburn, MA: Butterworth-Heinemann

Toda, I., Asano-Kato, N. and Komai-Hori, T. K. (2001) Dry eye after laser in situ keratomileusis. Am. J. Ophthalmol., 132, 1–7

Ward, M. A. (2001) Visual rehabilitation with contact lenses after laser in situ keratomileusis. J. Refract. Surg., 17, 433– 440

Ward, M. A. (2003) Contact lens management following corneal refractive surgery. Ophthalmol. Clin. North Am., 16, 395–403

Waring, G. O., Lynn, M. J. and McDonnell, P. J. (1994) Results of the PERK study 10 years after surgery. Arch. Ophthalmol., 112, 1298–1308

Wyzininski, P. (1987) Diurnal cycle of refraction after radial keratotomy. Ophthalmology, 94, 120

Chapter 24

Paediatric contact lenses

Lynne Speedwell

CHAPTER CONTENTS

INTRODUCTION

Children requiring contact lenses fall into two main categories with some overlap between them.

- Refractive
  - myopia.
  - hypermetropia.
  - astigmatism.
  - coloured contact lenses.
- Pathological
  - congenital refractive conditions.
  - cosmetic conditions.
  - traumatic effects.
  - therapeutic.

FITTING CHILDREN IN PRACTICE

Refractive contact lens fitting requires procedures and lens parameters similar to those for adults although there are certain differences in technique and patient management.

The practitioner is likely to be the one to introduce the idea of contact lenses. Remember that the child is the patient: treat each on their own merits and avoid generalizations. In most instances, if the child is keen to wear lenses, they should be able to insert or at least remove the lenses for themselves.

Many children initially appear keen to try lenses; however, on closer questioning, some do not actually know what contact lenses are or that they have to be inserted into the eye! The practitioner therefore must discuss with the child what they want out of their lenses, why they want to wear them, and to try to stop the parent from answering for them.

Peer pressure or bullying, even in young children, can be the reason, although changing to a cosmetically more acceptable frame may be preferable to being fitted with contact lenses. Conversely, the practitioner may feel it is worth fitting lenses to a child who might not otherwise be an ideal candidate. The psychological effects of having to wear thick spectacles should be considered (Barnard 1991) and where there are no obvious contraindications, contact lens fitting can be initiated.

If a child is keen to wear lenses but the parent is against the idea, as long as the practitioner thinks the child is suitable, the

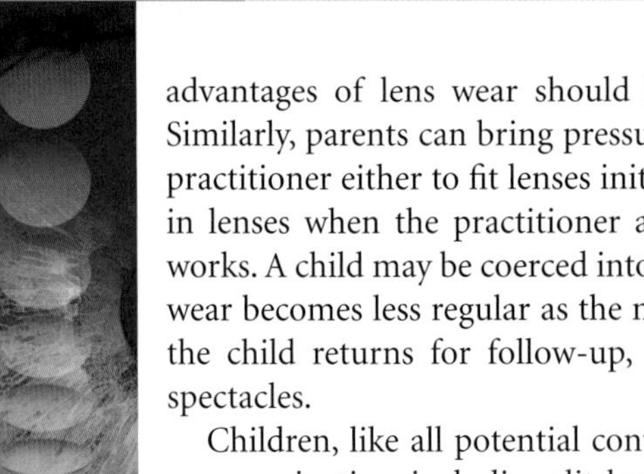

advantages of lens wear should be explained to the parent. Similarly, parents can bring pressure to bear on both child and practitioner either to fit lenses initially or to maintain the child in lenses when the practitioner advises otherwise: this rarely works. A child may be coerced into trying lenses but day-to-day wear becomes less regular as the novelty wears off. By the time the child returns for follow-up, they have often reverted to spectacles.

Children, like all potential contact lens patients, need a full eye examination, including slit-lamp, prior to commencing lens wear. This can show how cooperative a child is likely to be. For example, if fluorescein instillation proves difficult, it is unlikely that the child will allow contact lens insertion. Conversely, most children who allow eversion of the upper eyelids will not be difficult when a contact lens is being inserted. Bear in mind that if lenses are fitted to a child who cannot be examined adequately, it may prove impossible to carry out a thorough after-care examination.

As with all dealings with children, several short appointments are usually better than one lengthy one. Be patient and positive. If the patient finds lens insertion difficult, the following may help:

- Ask the parents to instil artificial tears for a few weeks.
- Encourage the child to touch their conjunctiva with a clean finger.
- Use an eye bath filled with normal saline while keeping the eye open.

By the subsequent appointment the child is usually more relaxed and keen to show off their achievements.

Age to fit lenses

There is no a particular age at which lenses should be first attempted. Some 5 year olds are excellent candidates for lens wear and some 15 year olds are definitely not. The decisions about whether to fit lenses are similar to those in adults, i.e. on an individual basis. Only if the best contact lens type or modality is out of reach financially for the parent need fitting be postponed for a child who is otherwise suitable.

Lens type and material

No one type of lens suits all children. They can do remarkably well with rigid gas-permeable (RGP) lenses if these are deemed to be the best lens of choice. Before commencing lens wear, explain both to the parent and to the child about the different types of lens available and the advantages and disadvantages of each. Always give reasons for your decisions. Provide as much information as possible, preferably in written form so that they can go home and discuss what they have been told. If the reason not to fit is reluctance on the part of the child, leave the way open to trying again at a later date.

Stressing lens hygiene cannot be overemphasized. Children over the age of 5 years are often enthusiastic and are prepared to clean their own lenses. Parental supervision is advisable initially, but after a time children should be capable of caring for their own lenses. Allow both child and parent time to ask questions. Remember that, when dealing with children, although they may be young, they can still understand. Some of them are very astute and their level of comprehension astounding.

It can help with cooperation, especially if RGP lenses are to be fitted, to instil local anaesthetic drops first. Ask the patient whether they prefer to have drops or not. If anaesthetic drops are instilled and the lenses left to settle for more than 15 minutes, the drops will have worn off by the time the patient returns. If at that stage the lenses are comfortable, the practitioner can explain that that is how they will feel when they are worn regularly.

Sometimes it is advisable to start with a lens that does not necessarily give the optimum vision. A child with myopic astigmatism may do better initially with spherical soft lenses, even though the vision may not be as good, rather than toric soft or RGP lenses. This can build confidence and keep expenses down. Once they have mastered the handling and shown that they are keen to wear lenses, the lens type can be changed to give better acuity.

Refractive error (see also p. 507)

The visual benefits that children with refractive errors derive from contact lenses are the same as those for adults.

Contact lenses fitted for anisometropia or unilateral ametropia will reduce aniseikonia and provide better stereopsis than spectacles (Winn et al. 1986). They also produce better vision in cases of amblyopia (Abdulla et al. 1998) and should, where possible, be attempted.

Fitting young myopes with rigid lenses may retard any increase in refractive error (Stone 1976, Perrigin et al. 1990), although this is open to conjecture (Walline et al. 2004; see also Chapter 30). However, as long as lenses are fitted without corneal compromise and hygiene is maintained, it is up to the individual practitioner to decide whether or not to try.

Orthokeratology can be carried out on young myopes and can be successful (see Chapter 19) but only if the children are themselves compliant. Parents must have the risks explained to them and should sign an informed consent form (see also Chapter 32). In China, orthokeratology is frequently carried out on very young children and microbial keratitis has been reported in several cases (Ruston & van der Worp 2004). In the United States, where regulations are much stricter, Lang and Rah (2004) and Macsai (2005) have reported on adverse responses to orthokeratology including microbial keratitis.

Coloured lenses

Children and parents will at times request tinted contact lenses because they find sunlight too bright, but unless they are severely photophobic or have some pathological condition in one or both eyes, it is inadvisable to prescribe them (see Photophobic conditions, p. 514). A pair of sunglasses worn over the lenses on bright days is more beneficial.

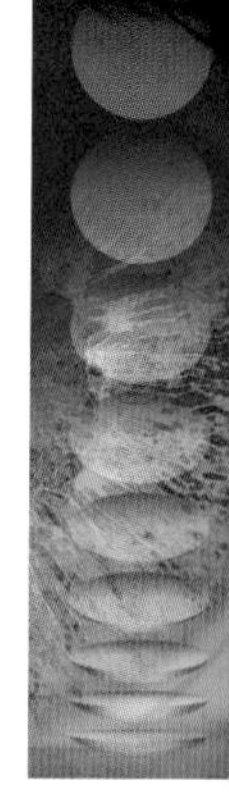

CORNEAL TOPOGRAPHY AND PHYSIOLOGY

- The infant has a large eye:head ratio.
- The length of the eyeball is approximately 17 mm compared to 24 mm in the adult (Larsen 1971, Blomdahl 1979).
- The average corneal diameter at birth is 10 mm: by the age of 2 years it has grown to 11.7 mm, which is almost adult size (Sorsby & Sheridan 1960).
- Many figures have been quoted for the refractive error in babies, ranging from slightly myopic in the premature infant to moderately hypermetropic and astigmatic in many normal neonates (Molnar 1970, Marshall & Grindle 1978, Weale 1982, Table by Grounds in Speedwell 2003).
- The corneal radius is approximately 7.1 mm, which gradually flattens to an adult average of 7.86 mm (Asbell et al. 1990), although other authors (Wood et al. 1996) have suggested that the infant corneal radius may be somewhat flatter.
- The corneal physiology differs little from that of the adult except that there are a greater number of endothelial cells per unit area (Speedwell et al. 1988). This may account for the apparent ability of the infant cornea to recover rapidly from a hypoxic reaction. Anecdotally, infants appear less sensitive to lens wear than older children and adults, and RGP lenses can easily be fitted to young babies.
- Blink rate is lower in infants than in adults; the mean rate of spontaneous blinking is less than two per minute in early infancy, increasing steadily during childhood up to 14–20 per minute by the mid teens (Zametkin et al. 1979).

CONGENITAL AND PATHOLOGICAL CONDITIONS

Most infants and young children who require lenses for congenital and pathological conditions are seen in hospital clinics but the ability to cope with both the patient and their parents remains the lynchpin around which successful fitting is based.

Whatever the condition or type of lens to be fitted, it is advisable that the lenses are removed daily to reduce the risk of infection or hypoxia.

INDICATIONS FOR CONTACT LENSES

Refractive conditions

These include:

- High myopia and hypermetropia (see also Chapter 21).
- Unilateral ametropia.
- Strabismus with a high refractive error.
- Anisometropia.
- Corneal irregularity as a result of trauma (without aphakia).

HIGH MYOPIA

There are two types of high myopia: intermediate myopia and pathological myopia (Saw 2004).

Intermediate myopia

- Excessive enlargement of the posterior segment of the globe.
- Clinical changes of the fundus (myopic crescents, straightening of the retinal vessels and tessellated background).
- Visual function is usually normal for a child although it may be reduced due to an amblyogenic effect of defocus.

Pathological myopia

- The globe continues to grow and posterior staphyloma can develop.
- Peripapillary atrophy, straightening of the retinal vessels and chorioretinal degeneration, often leading to loss of vision.
- Complications such as retinal detachments are common.
- Can be associated with some syndromes (e.g. Stickler syndrome).

Choice of lens type

Although visual acuity is better with contact lenses due to the enlarged retinal image size (see Chapter 6), visual development is likely to be just as good with either form of correction. It is, therefore, not always advisable to fit lenses with all their inherent problems to the very young myope.

High-water-content soft or silicone hydrogel, where available, are the first lenses of choice as they are more comfortable initially, but RGP lenses should also be considered.

The axially myopic eye is larger than normal and the cornea flatter. Infants may start with lenses of 8.00 mm radius in a high-water-content material and as large as 13.50 or even 14.00 mm diameter.

As mentioned previously, and as discussed in Chapter 30, the retarding effect of rigid lenses is open to debate, so lenses should not be fitted on this basis alone. However, there may be other justifications for fitting lenses – for example, if a young child will not wear glasses or cannot tolerate the full spectacle prescription.

HIGH HYPERMETROPIA, STRABISMUS AND ANISOMETROPIA

Children with these types of refractive error can do well with contact lenses although hypermetropes do not see as well as with spectacles due to the magnifying effect of the spectacle lenses (see Chapter 6).

Unilateral ametropes

Unilateral ametropes, be they myopes or hypermetropes, are reluctant to wear spectacles: they rarely derive any visual benefit from them, as the ametropic eye is usually amblyopic and vision from that eye is suppressed. Contact lenses, together with extensive patching to the good eye, are a better option. Where there is resistance to lens wear, spectacles and patching can work just as well in reducing amblyopia, especially if there is no binocular vision and no risk of aniseikonia preventing comfortable fusion.

Unilateral myopes are more successful than unilateral hypermetropes (Morris 1979). Myopia in children is thought to be only axial (Grosvenor & Scott 1993) and since aniseikonia has

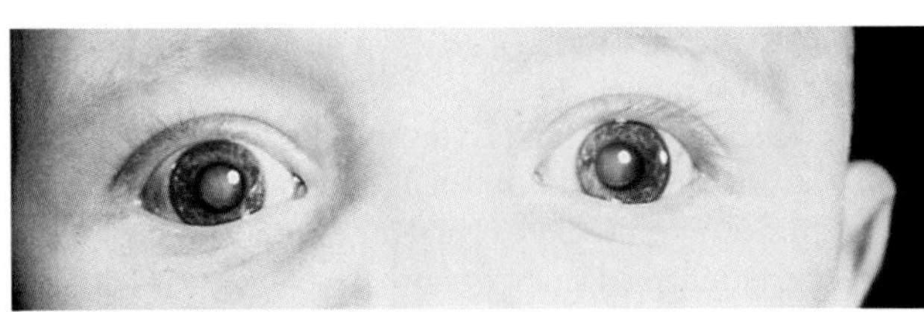

Figure 24.1 Congenital cataracts in an infant

been shown to be less for both axial and refractive anisometropia when contact lenses are employed (Winn et al. 1986), better stereopsis should develop if lenses can be prescribed early. However, Roberts and Adams (2002) found that unilateral high myopia, more than –9.00 D, does not respond well to patching.

Strabismus

Patients with accommodative esotropias benefit from contact lenses simply as a replacement to spectacles and older children with a high AC/A ratio who would normally be fitted with bifocal spectacles can be fitted with bifocal contact lenses as an alternative (Rich & Glusman 1992).

Choice of lens type

The most comfortable lens may prove to be the best, so the initial choice of material is again high-water-content soft or silicone hydrogel where parameters are available; however, RGPs should also be considered.

PATHOLOGICAL REASONS FOR CONTACT LENSES

Cataracts and aphakia

- The largest group of infants and children fitted with contact lenses.
- The number of aphakes is reducing as more intraocular lenses are used.
- Cataracts can be congenital or traumatic, unilateral or bilateral.
- The most common surgical procedures are lensectomy and aspiration producing small scars near the limbus which induce a minimal degree of astigmatism. Topography is only slightly altered by surgery.

Infants born with congenital cataracts (Figs 24.1, 24.2), posterior hyperplastic primary vitreous (PHPV) and posterior lenticonus should have surgery as early as possible, preferably before 3 months of age to reduce the amblyogenic effect (Taylor et al. 1979). Infants who develop cataracts in the first few months of life need to be carefully monitored in order that surgery can be performed as soon as the cataracts start to interfere with vision.

As soon as the inflammation has settled after surgery, not usually less than one week postoperatively, contact lenses are fitted where possible as they provide a more normal visual environment for the aphake as well as overcoming the mechanical difficulties of wearing spectacles (Fig. 24.3). To ensure continuous visual stimulation, back-up glasses should also be prescribed for periods when the contact lenses cannot be worn. Where parents have difficulty handling the lenses, possibly because they themselves are visually impaired, spectacles are the only option and it should be stressed that visual acuity develops just as well with either form of correction.

Lenses do not need to be fitted under anaesthetic, although if the child is having an anaesthetic for another reason, measurements can be taken at the same time.

Lens power

- Carry out retinoscopy, taking care to refract on axis.
- As there is no active accommodation, cycloplegia is not needed and a mydriatic only necessary if the pupil is very small.
- No trial frame is used, as it is impractical on a baby's small features.
- The first spectacle trial lens should be +20.00 D. If a much lower power is used, the pupil area can be filled with light,

(a)

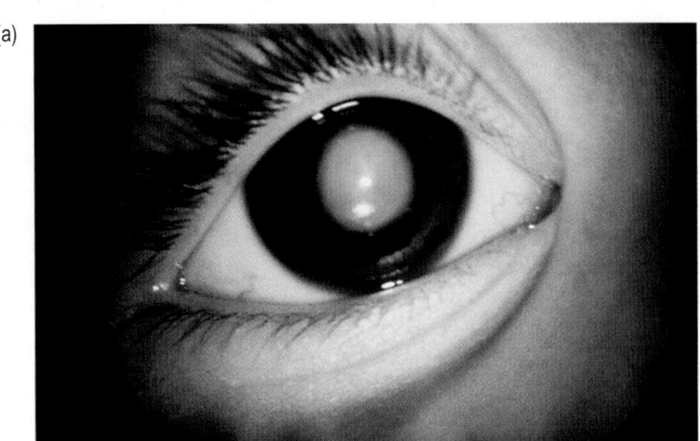

(b)

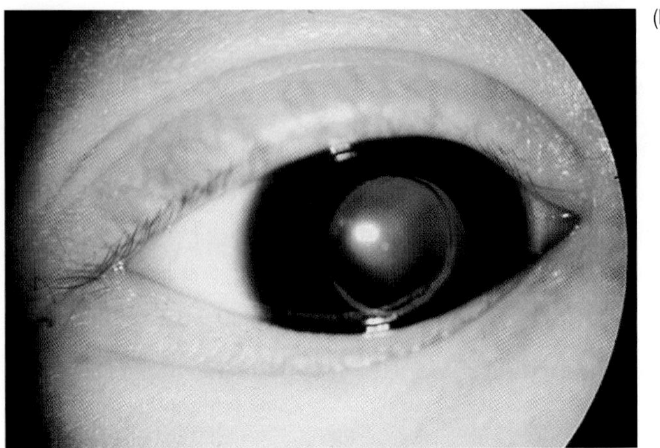

Figure 24.2 Congenital cataracts do not always show as white pupils, as in (a). As with adults, it may be easier to recognize them with a retinoscope or ophthalmoscope held away from the eye as in (b)

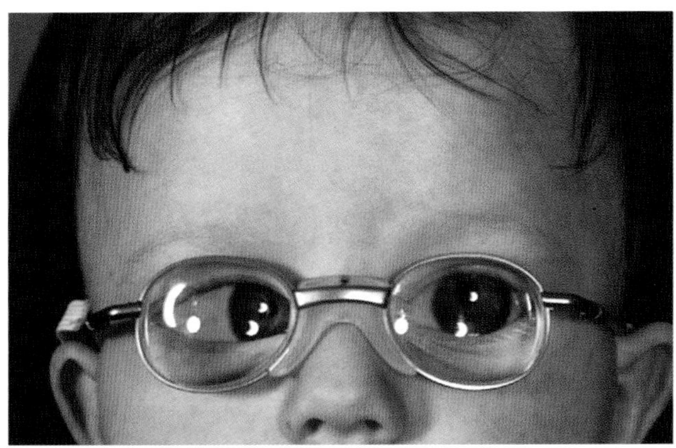
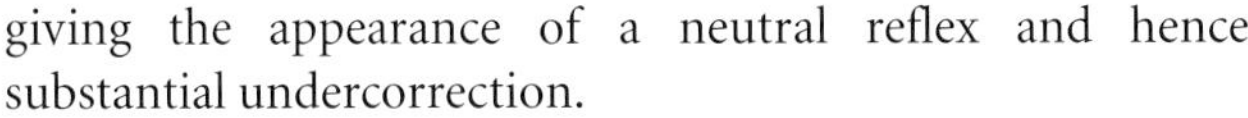

Figure 24.3 Infant in aphakic spectacles. Note the right esotropia, which results in poor centration of a spectacle lens in front of that eye – a contact lens provides much better centration

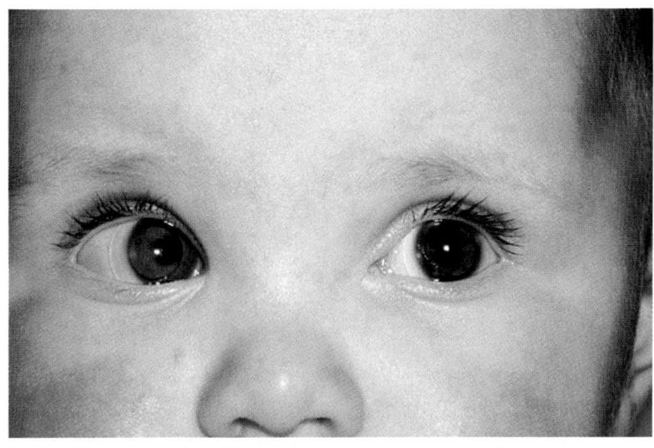

Figure 24.4 Bilateral aphake wearing contact lenses. The right lens did not centre perfectly but the pupil was covered by the lenticular part of the lens all the time. Note the scars from surgery

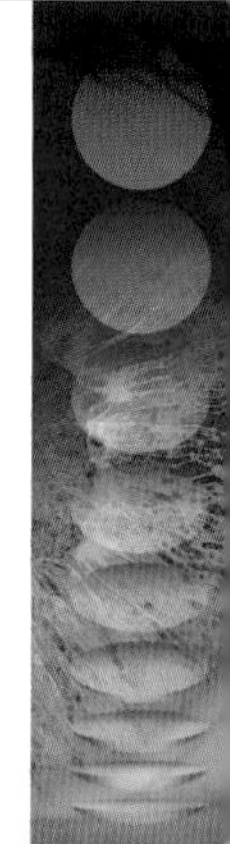

giving the appearance of a neutral reflex and hence substantial undercorrection.

- Hold the lens close to the eye as a small increase in back vertex distance (BVD) induces a large increase in effective power; +20.00 D at 16 mm BVD requires a +29.41 D contact lens on the eye (see Chapter 6 and Appendix A, or the CD-ROM accompanying this book).
- The back vertex power (BVP) at the cornea is typically around +30.00 D.
- Infants are motivated and attracted by objects that are close to them (e.g. faces, feeding bottle, toys, etc.) and as they are unable to accommodate, the lenses should be focused at approximately a third of a metre, i.e. an overcorrection of +3.00 D, reducing to distance prescription by school age (or earlier), when reading spectacles are prescribed.
- The first lens is therefore of the order of +33.00 D (although some eyes require lower powers and microphthalmic, aphakic eyes can require lens powers of +50.00 D or more).
- Lenses are thick: 1 mm centre thickness is not uncommon in soft lenses, and hence overnight wear can result in corneal hypoxia. This is less likely if RGP lenses are fitted.

Because of the potential danger to the retina caused by ultraviolet light in an aphakic eye, where possible, lenses with an ultraviolet inhibitor should be prescribed.

SOFT AND SILICONE HYDROGEL LENSES

Manufacture of small, high-powered lenses is difficult:

- The refractive index of the xerogel soft lenses is 1.524, giving very high powers in the dry state. As these are difficult to measure, the BVP may be less accurate and more difficult to check on the focimeter.
- Lens parameters are likely to steepen more than lower powers as the lenses hydrate.
- The carrier lens and junction need to be thick enough to allow for reasonable handling.

Advantages

- Available in a wide range of parameters so can fit any size of eye.
- Available in different water contents.
- Can be biocompatible.
- Relatively cheap.

Disadvantages

- Break and get lost easily.
- Dry out and fall out.
- Can lead to corneal desiccation.

Wearing the lenses

- High-water-content lenses are fitted for comfort and convenience (they are impractical to remove every time the baby sleeps).
- Explain the risks of overnight wear to the parents and encourage daily removal and disinfection from the outset.
- If daily removal is not possible, lenses should be removed at least once a week initially and increase frequency to every day.
- Stress the importance of removing the lens if there is any sign of infection or redness.
- For older children who do not sleep during the day, lower-water-content lenses may be used in order to reduce lens turnover, but these have a lower Dk.

Astigmatism is not corrected until the child is older, except where RGP lenses are fitted, but it is usually only of a small degree induced by lensectomy or aspiration (note scars in Fig. 24.4). It is not practical to fit these infants with anything other than spherical lenses, and many emmetropic adults start life with varying degrees of astigmatism (Atkinson et al. 1980).

Back optic zone radius (BOZR)

- Keratometry measurements are not always done, although if a hand-held keratometer is available, it is a useful starting point especially when fitting silicone hydrogel lenses (Fig. 24.5).

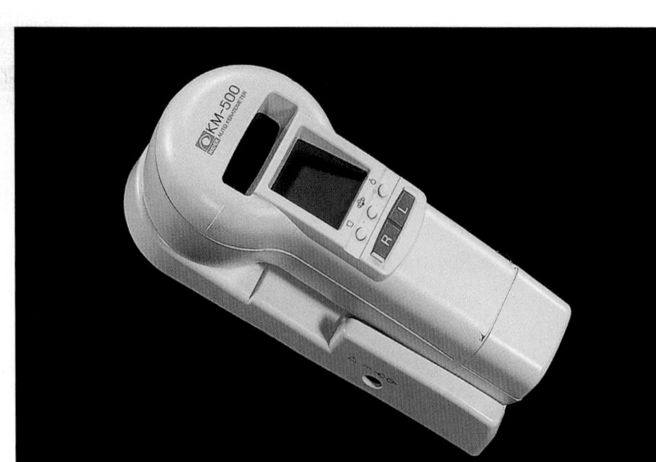

Figure 24.5 A Nidek hand-held keratometer

- The BOZR of the first lens is fitted according to age, on known average *K*, i.e. 7.10 mm (47.54 D) for a neonate.

Total diameter (TD)

- This depends on corneal diameter, which is approximately 10 mm at birth, growing to 11.7 mm by the age of 2 years (Sorsby & Sheridan 1960).
- Fit 2 mm larger than the horizontal visible iris diameter (HVID), i.e. 12.00–12.50 mm TD depending on age and corneal appearance.
- If the lens does not centre well, try a larger or smaller TD.
- Tight lids on the thick lens may result in lens displacement into the upper fornix when the child sleeps or cries.
- Thinner aspheric lenses or lenses with a reduced front optic zone diameter (FOZD) minimize displacement.
- Standard FOZD is 8.00 mm on a 12.00 mm TD; this can be reduced to 6.00 mm FOZD where appropriate.

Microphthalmic eyes

- Congenital cataract and PHPV frequently occur in microphthalmic eyes, having an HVID of 8 mm or less.
- A smaller TD may be necessary in order to achieve adequate centration: 10.50 mm or less, depending on the peripheral corneal and scleral topography.
- Larger TDs may centre better where there is poor differentiation between corneal and scleral topography.

Lens insertion and removal

- Insert lens by holding between finger and thumb and posting it up underneath the top eyelid.
- Remove as for rigid lenses by scooping it out (see Handling of lenses, p. 515, and Figs 24.12 and 24.13).

Assessing the lens fit

- Insert lenses and, if the eyes look comfortable, allow to settle for 20 minutes.
- First lenses do not always fit well.
- Slit-lamp assessment of lens fit may not be possible; instead watch eye/lens movement while showing toys, lights, etc.

Table 24.1: Back vertex powers (D) and appropriate BOZR and TD values for an infant aphakic soft lens fitting set

	TD (mm)				
BOZR (mm)	12.00	12.50	13.00	13.50	14.00
7.00	**+34.00** +30.00	**+32.00** +28.00	**+30.00**		
7.20	**+32.00**	**+30.00** +26.00	**+28.00** +24.00	+22.00	
7.40		**+28.00**	+26.00 +22.00	**+24.00** +20.00	+22.00
7.60			+24.00	**+22.00**	+18.00
7.80				+20.00	+16.00

- Some compromise on centration may be necessary as long as:
  - the lenticular portion covers the pupil.
  - the edge does not knock the limbus.

Lens cleaning

There are numerous contact lens solutions available to clean and disinfect lenses. For children, it may be safer to advise surfactant cleaning as well as lens soaking when using multipurpose solutions and to prescribe only large-molecular-weight preservatives. Allergies can occur, albeit infrequently, and parents should be warned accordingly. Hydrogen peroxide systems may be best avoided until the parents are comfortable with lens handling and hygiene.

Alternatively, if parents have a steam sterilizer for babies' bottles, the lenses can be cleaned with a surfactant cleaner, such as Miraflow (CIBA), rinsed and placed in a watertight case with unpreserved saline, and disinfected during a cycle in the sterilizer.

Inventory

It is useful to keep a stock of lenses available. The ideal set contains 44 lenses (Table 24.1), but if infant aphakes are only rarely seen, the number can be reduced to 18 (figures in bold type). Two of each set of parameters will ensure that lenses can be issued at the first visit. Where possible, the parents should have a spare pair to keep at home against loss or breakage.

SILICONE RUBBER LENSES

Silicone rubber is a hydrophobic material that is coated to make it hydrophilic and comfortable to wear (see Chapter 3). Lenses made of this material can be used as an alternative to hydrogel. The only silicone rubber lenses currently available are Silsoft lenses from Bausch & Lomb (Table 24.2).

Advantages

- Hydrophobic material that does not require good tears or blinking, so it does not dry out and fall from the eye.
- Lens not easily rubbed out.
- Excellent oxygen permeability (Koch et al. 1991; see also Chapter 3).

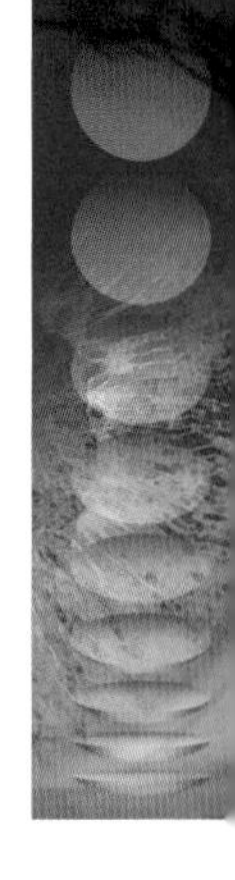

Table 24.2: Available parameters of Silsoft lenses from Bausch & Lomb

Total diameter (mm)	11.3 mm	12.5 mm
BOZR (mm)	7.50, 7.70, 7.90	7.50, 7.70, 7.90, 8.10, 8.30
Power (D)	+23.00, +26.00, +29.00, +32.00	+7.50 to +20.00 (0.50 steps)

Disadvantages

- May be difficult to remove if the eye is sore.
- Hydrophilic lens coating can become scratched or deposited with lipid (Huth & Wagner 1981) (Fig. 24.6). This may occur rapidly in some patients.
- Expensive.
- Limited parameters, with steepest available being too flat for many infant aphakes.
- Time consuming to fit. If not fitted carefully, lenses can bind to the cornea (Refojo & Leong 1981).
- Not available with ultraviolet inhibitor.

Fitting the lenses

- Take *K* readings. If the child is anaesthetized and lying on their side, and only a conventional keratometer is available, the horizontal and vertical measurements should be interchanged.
- Fit on flattest *K* for toric corneas and flattest *K* +0.1 mm (0.50 D) for spherical corneas.
- If a keratometer is not available, fit steepest available, i.e. 7.50 mm (45.00 D) as a first trial lens.
- Total diameter is 11.30 mm for powers over +20.00 D. If this does not fit, a different lens modality is needed.
- Insert lens and assess immediately using fluorescein and an ultraviolet lamp; remove the lens at once if it shows central pooling.
- Fit should be minimally flat initially as the lens may tighten and a steep lens is difficult to remove. It is safer to err on the flat side than have difficulty removing a tight lens.
- Check again 10 minutes later before allowing the lens to settle for at least 45 minutes when final assessment and over-refraction can be carried out.
- The ideal fitting lens shows minimal central touch with slight edge clearance (Fig. 24.7).
- Lenses that are too flat cause no apparent corneal damage (Cutler et al. 1985) but do dislodge and fall out.

Lens insertion and removal (see also p. 515)

- Insert as for soft lenses. Hold the lens and 'post' it under the upper eyelid; alternatively, loosely attach the lens to the index finger using rigid lens wetting solution. Hold the lids apart and place the lens directly onto the cornea.
- Remove by scooping the lens out as with rigid lenses.
- Occasionally, a rubber suction holder may be necessary.

Lens cleaning

- Rub lens with surfactant cleaner for soft lenses.
- Rinse with unpreserved saline.
- Soak overnight in RGP soaking solution.

Inventory

Very few trial lenses are needed: a pair of 7.50/11.30 and 7.70/11.30 in high powers and a pair of 7.70/12.50 in a lower power is adequate (see Table 24.2). Because of the high cost of these lenses it may not be possible to have parameters available to issue; the lenses can be ordered at the fitting appointment.

RIGID GAS-PERMEABLE LENSES

Most infants can do well with RGP lenses (Amos et al. 1992). Young children anecdotally appear to have reduced corneal sensitivity compared to older children and adults, so fitting them does not evoke the same response as with adults. Older children vary in their response to rigid lenses.

Advantages

- Easier for parents to handle.
- Good range of materials.
- Available in high Dk.
- Less likely to induce GPC (CLPC).
- Provide best acuity in cases of corneal trauma or opacity.
- Useful where soft lenses dry out.

Disadvantages

- Can cause corneal abrasions if the child squeezes their eyes on lens insertion.

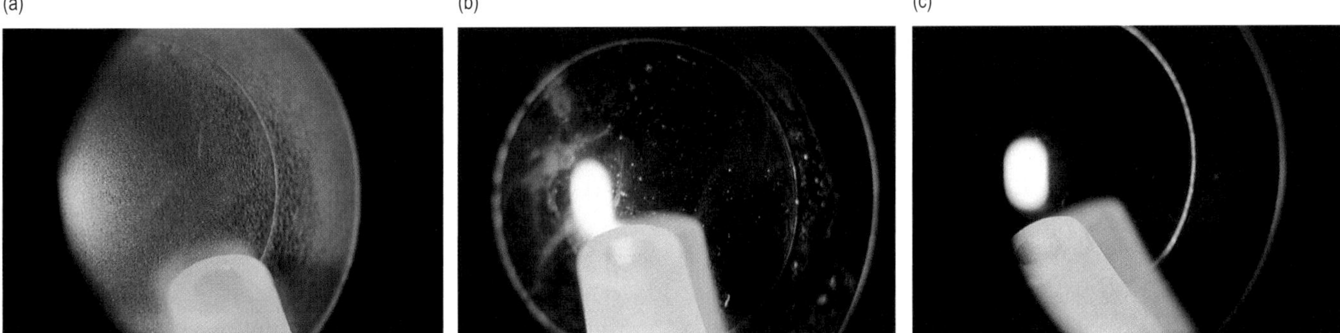

Figure 24.6 (a) A silicone rubber lens with the surface degraded after 3 months of use. (b) The lens after cleaning in 5% sodium hypochlorite and (c) after further rinsing in distilled water. Although much of the surface degradation of silicone rubber lenses is due to the coating being damaged, some lenses are salvageable. (Courtesy of D. Westerhout)

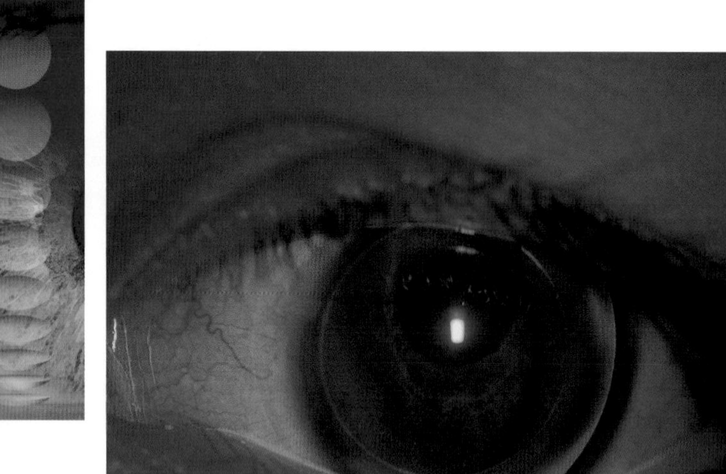

Figure 24.7 Well-fitting silicone rubber lens

- Not always possible to fit to microphthalmic corneas.
- Can be lost from the eye.

Fitting the lenses

- Take *K* readings if possible.
- If *K* readings are not available, the first lens can be fitted empirically on known average *K*, i.e. 7.1 mm for a neonate.
- Instil a local anaesthetic before inserting the first trial lens.
- Using aspheric or partially aspheric aphakic trial lenses (preferably with variable edge lift), fit on the flattest *K*, or 0.1–0.2 mm (0.50–1.00 D) steeper if corneal astigmatism is more than 0.3–0.5 mm (1.50–2.50 D).
- The diameter of the lens should be approximately 1–1.5 mm smaller than HVID. This relatively large diameter, coupled with the aspheric design, aids comfort and reduces the risk of the lens being rubbed out.
- Edge clearance should be only just adequate in order to reduce lens loss further. When the child is older the amount of edge lift may need to be increased.
- Check fit using fluorescein and an ultraviolet lamp or the blue filter on a slit-lamp, then allow to settle for 20 minutes.
- Assess the fit and carry out an over-refraction.

Lens insertion and removal

- For lens insertion, the child can be sitting or lying down.
- Loosely attach the lens to the index finger using lens wetting solution, hold the lids apart and place the lens directly onto the cornea.
- Remove the lens by scooping it out (see Fig. 24.13).

Lens cleaning

Practitioner's system of choice.

RGP SCLERAL LENSES

These can be fitted using Pullum's controlled clearance RGP scleral lenses of +30.00 D power (see Chapter 15) or impression lenses. They are useful in cases where there is an irregular corneal surface due to injury or surgery and they can be modified as the prescription changes (Ezekiel 1995). Fitting may be better managed with a sedated infant.

Unilateral aphakia

Unilateral aphakes are treated in much the same way as bilateral cases, except that they usually need a lens in one eye only and patching is necessary for up to half the waking hours for the first 7 years of life (Lloyd et al. 1995).

Where patching is difficult, an occlusive black-tinted contact lens or a high-powered lens may be used in the good eye, although the risk to the health of that eye needs to be carefully considered. These lenses are not usually successful as the child soon learns to move or remove them.

With mild amblyopia a cycloplegic can be instilled into the good eye. This is of no use with dense amblyopia, as the better eye is still the preferred eye.

Traumatic aphakia

It can be impossible to regain the confidence of a child of 18 months to 3 years who has suffered corneal trauma and general anaesthesia may be necessary even to measure the eye. If a lens is fitted while the child is anaesthetized, it may subsequently be possible to remove the lens while the child is asleep. However, spectacles may be a better option initially, together with patching, in an effort to rehabilitate the vision. With time, the child may be more prepared to try contact lenses. A soft lens is then a good starting point. Where the injury occurs at less than 3 years of age, the resultant amblyopia is usually too dense to respond much to treatment but it should still be attempted in most instances.

Intraocular lenses (IOLs)

Where IOLs are inserted in infancy, the prescription is often not accurate, especially as an allowance has to be made for eye growth. Contact lenses and/or spectacles may be fitted to correct the remaining ametropia, particularly in cases of anisometropia. The lenses may need to be specially ordered although disposable lenses may fit older children if the eyes are of normal size.

Aphakia after-care (see also After-care, pp. 516–517)

There are certain differences in after-care between children and adults. If problems occur, lens wear should be discontinued for a period and the child should wear spectacles full-time.

A particular problem in infant aphakia is the risk of glaucoma. This can manifest itself as:

- Hazy cornea.
- Enlarged cornea.
- Reduction in plus power.

In a bilateral aphake, where the refraction in one eye has suddenly become more myopic than that in the other eye, glaucoma should be suspected. Once the pressure is controlled, a lens with a larger TD, flatter BOZR and lower back vertex power may be required.

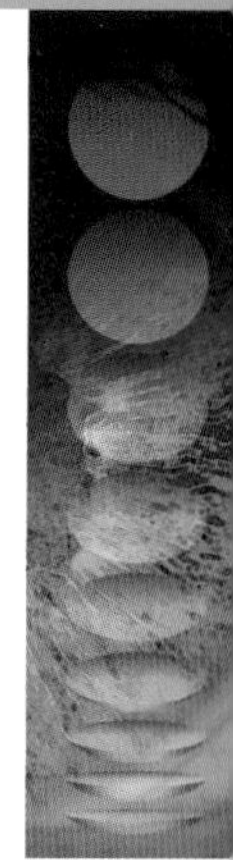

Alterations with age

Eye changes

- Axial length grows so BVP reduces.
- Corneal diameter increases.
- Corneal radius flattens.

Lens changes

- A lens for a 2-year-old aphake may be similar in size to that of an adult but with greater back vertex power.
- Before school age the prescription is changed to a distance correction; bifocals, incorporating any astigmatic correction, are prescribed in conjunction.
- Soft lens wearers may be refitted with RGP lenses to improve vision and corneal health.

Other points to note

- Aphakes have better acuity with spectacles but a worse field of vision due to the effect of the back vertex distance (see Chapter 6). They may therefore prefer to wear spectacles for school or work and lenses for outdoors and social activities.
- Too great a reduction in plus power, especially in young children, may indicate high intraocular pressure.
- It is not practical to fit young children with bifocal contact lenses, as the fitting relies too much on subjective responses and the lenses do not always provide optimum focus for distance and/or reading.
- Any adverse effect of lens wear on visual acuity in a young child will affect them for life.
- In bilateral aphakes up to 18 months old, where one contact lens needs to be removed because of infection or lens loss, it is a good idea to remove both lenses, as the uncorrected eye can quickly become amblyopic, even within a few days. In cases of infection, back-up spectacles should be worn.

Microphthalmic eyes

- These eyes grow very little.
- A microphthalmic adult patient may need lenses similar to those worn as a child except that the power is likely to have reduced.
- Prosthetic lenses may be useful for the older child and/or low-plus spectacles to magnify the eye (see Chapter 25).

Ectopia lentis (dislocated lenses)

Characteristics of eyes with dislocated lenses include:

- High myopia which is either
  - axial, or
  - lenticular
    - caused by a weak zonule.
    - resulting in a micropehricized lens (i.e. steeper and smaller).
- High degree of irregular astigmatism.
- Risk of retinal detachment.

Dislocated lenses occur in 60–80% of people with Marfan's syndrome (Evain et al. 1986); these eyes usually have flat corneas, possibly as flat as 9.50 mm. Large soft lenses are the first lens of choice (Speedwell & Russell-Eggitt 1994), although if *K*s are less flat, RGP lenses can be fitted. These should have a large TD with a parallel or negative carrier to try to improve centration (see Chapter 9). Similar lenses are used to fit adults with dislocated lenses.

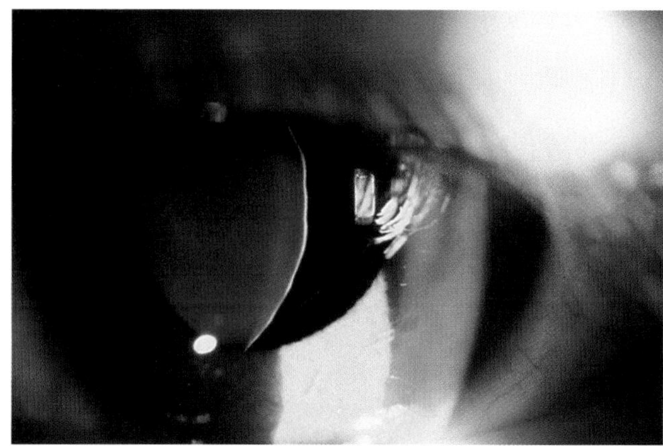

Figure 24.8 Dislocated lens cutting across the visual axis

The natural lens is often tilted and dislocated off axis, resulting in irregular astigmatism. This is not fully corrected by toric contact lenses, and spectacles (or spectacles over contact lenses) are necessary to correct the total astigmatism.

When one eye is rendered aphakic or the lens has dislocated sufficiently to use the aphakic portion of the pupil (Fig. 24.8), there is gross anisometropia. Contact lenses will provide binocularity, although where the child is completely averse to lens wear, spectacles can be supplied as an interim measure. Amblyopia can slowly improve with either form of correction (Speedwell & Russell-Eggitt 1995).

If the lens is mobile or if the edge of the lens cuts across the visual axis (see Fig. 24.8), it should be removed surgically as good acuity is not otherwise possible.

Staphylococcus blepharitis and keratoconjunctivitis

Staphylococcus aureus and *Staphylococcus epidermidis* can cause severe infection at a critical time in visual development. The result can be corneal scarring and neovascularization, leading to amblyopia (Fig. 24.9). Once the infection is under control, high-Dk RGP lenses are fitted. These patients are not good candidates for corneal grafts.

Nystagmus

Contact lenses do not provide better acuity but have been found to reduce the amplitude of the nystagmus (Abadi 1979), especially rigid lenses (Golubovic et al. 1989). They are normally well tolerated and allow the child to move their eyes to find the nystagmoid null-point, which may be beyond the edge of any spectacle correction.

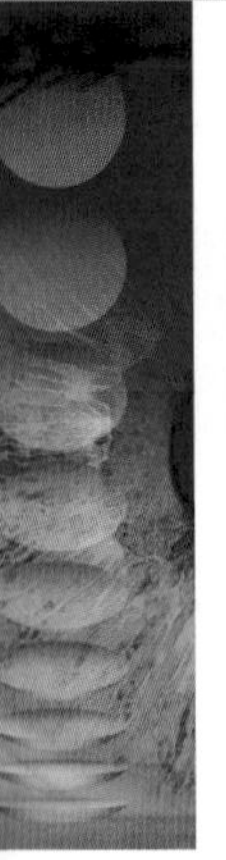

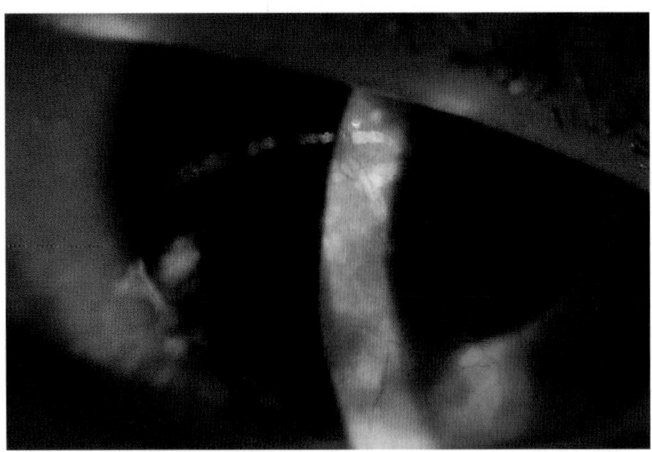

Figure 24.9 Corneal scarring and neovascularization resulting from a staphylococcal infection. (Courtesy of K. K. Nischal)

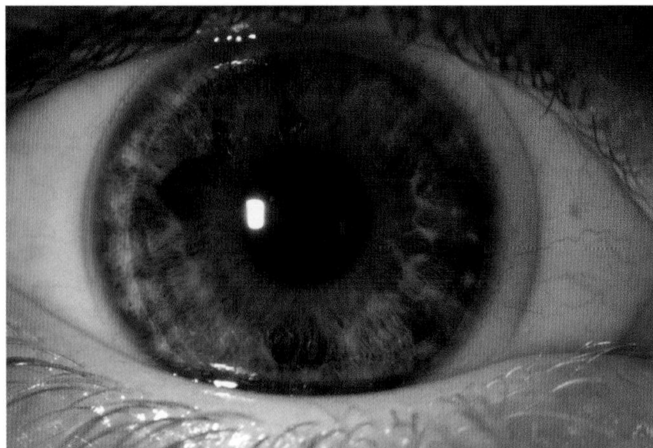

Figure 24.10 A standard lens with a light all-over tint worn by an ocular albino

COSMETIC CONDITIONS

Pathological conditions requiring cosmetic lenses are similar in both adults and children although the distribution of pathology is different (see Chapter 25). Soft lenses are most commonly fitted, although other types are used.

Tinted soft lenses must be thoroughly cleaned with a product that is not likely to affect the tint (e.g. Quattro [Abatron Ltd, UK]), although a surfactant cleaner and/or protein remover tablets may also be necessary (check with the manufacturing laboratory).

Conditions requiring cosmetic lenses fall largely into two categories:

- Photophobic
  - aniridia.
  - iris coloboma.
  - albinism.
  - cone dystrophy.
- Unsightly
  - microphthalmos.
  - scars and opacities.

Photophobic conditions

ANIRIDIA

Tinted lenses do not improve acuity in congenital aniridia. However, older children do appear more comfortable with tinted soft lenses, especially where lens opacities develop. Care is needed as aniridics have a corneal stem cell deficiency and pannus is common (Nishida et al. 1995). In adulthood, the cornea may become opacified and RGP lenses are better physiologically, give better acuity and may delay the need for a corneal or stem cell graft.

In cases of traumatic aniridia, a prosthetic iris lens can be helpful (see Chapter 25 and Fig. 25.19).

IRIS COLOBOMA

Iris coloboma rarely produces a cosmetic appearance bad enough to warrant fitting tinted lenses. In the older child, if either the appearance or the photophobia requires cosmetic lens fitting, the lens is fitted as for an adult (see Fig. 25.20).

ALBINISM

Infants with oculocutaneous albinism appear more sensitive and resistant to having contact lenses inserted. Lenses, even scleral lenses with an opaque sclera (Ruben 1967), do not improve visual acuity and the dark tints required are cosmetically unacceptable (unless hand-painted lenses are used). The lack of pigment in the retina and foveal hypoplasia, together with the abnormal percentage of fibres partially decussating at the optic chiasm, preclude any recordable visual improvement. Wearing dark glasses and a hat or shading the pram is usually more beneficial.

Tinted lenses, RGP or soft, do benefit some older children. For those who are only mildly photophobic, a lightly tinted iris and pupil is adequate (Fig. 24.10).

When fitting lenses, correcting the with-the-rule astigmatism that is common in albinos does not usually produce much improvement in acuity, so soft spherical lenses are adequate. Where an astigmatic correction proves beneficial, RGP or toric soft lenses can be fitted.

ACHROMATOPSIA

People with achromatopsia are particularly photophobic and a tint is needed constantly. Although tinted pupil lenses (which leave the iris colour unaffected) can be used, light can enter the pupil obliquely. If that causes difficulties, an iris tint lens can be substituted. Dark glasses should be worn over the lenses outdoors.

As with spectacle tints, the optimum colour of the tint varies between individuals. Some older children (and adults) may have a pair of sunglasses with their 'perfect' colour (usually dark red, brown or grey): a sample spectacle lens can be sent to the contact lens laboratory to match.

Unsightly conditions

MICROPHTHALMOS

This can occur with or without cataracts (see 'Aphakia', above). Where only one eye is microphthalmic, fitting a cosmetic soft

(a)

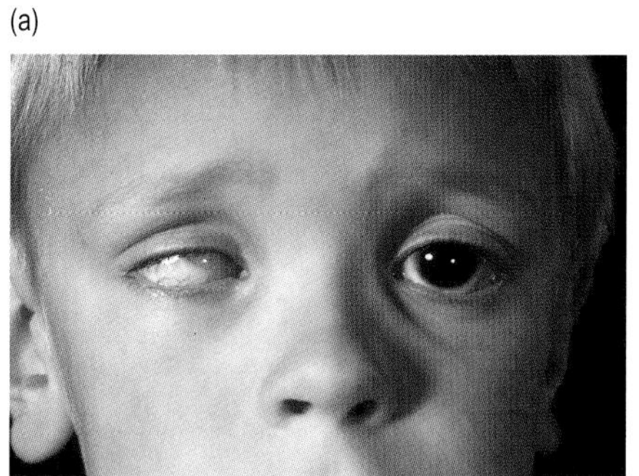

(b)

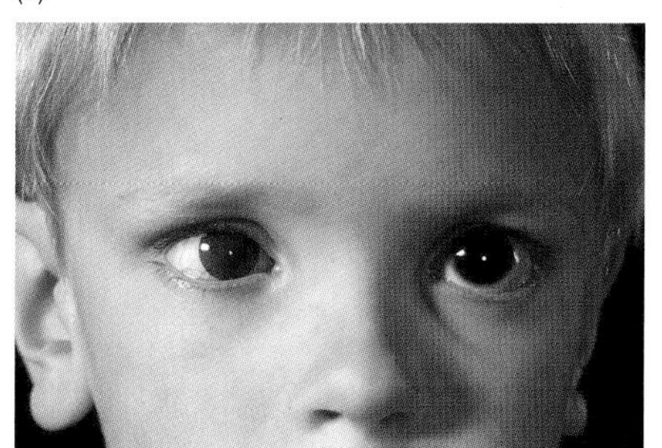

(c)

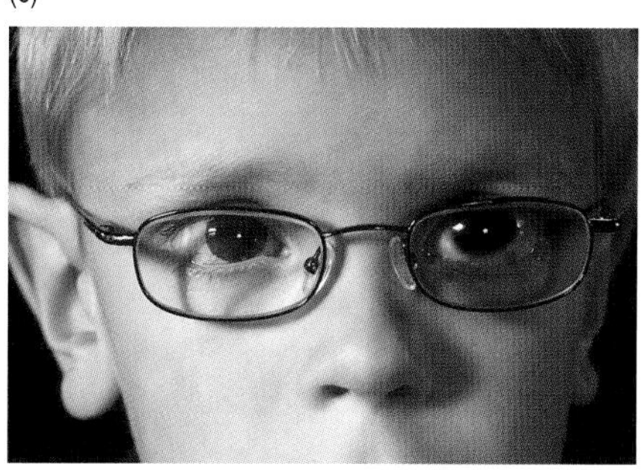

Figure 24.11 (a) Opaque buphthalmic eye; (b) fitted with a tinted lens 9.00/22.00/–4.00. (c) Same child wearing overcorrection in spectacles which provides a better cosmetic appearance. This lens was later changed for one that was slightly darker.

lens with the iris size matching the fellow eye will improve cosmesis. A prescription can be incorporated into the lens for a sighted eye; for a severely amblyopic eye, a plano cosmetic lens is prescribed. Where the axial length is much smaller than the fellow eye, a cosmetic shell may be preferable. Congenital microphthalmic and nanophthalmic (see below) eyes do not grow much from the size they are in infancy. It is worth remembering when fitting adults with these conditions that they usually require lenses of similar parameters to those used for young children.

NANOPHTHALMOS

Nanophthalmic eyes have a steep radius of curvature and are highly hypermetropic, possibly as high as +25.00 D. Lens fitting and follow-up are similar to young aphakes, except that the distance correction is prescribed as the eyes can accommodate.

UNSIGHTLY SCARS AND OPACITIES

These are caused by a variety of conditions, including penetrating injuries, developmental anomalies and dermoid cysts.

In the first months and years of life, children with unsightly eyes may be fitted more for the parents' sake than any other reason (Fig. 24.11). However, an older child may develop worries about the disfigurement and a cosmetic lens will help to overcome this. Many children refuse to go to school when they are unable to wear their cosmetic lens.

Initially an iris tint lens is prescribed, even if it does not exactly match the good eye. This can be made of a high-water-content material that can be worn during sleep. There is an extensive range of colours available and with these the cosmesis is usually acceptable. When the child is older, a full prosthetic lens will produce a better appearance. In cases where some vision has been retained, the cosmetic lens must not compromise the cornea. A clear soft lens can be fitted initially to teach lens handling and check for adverse reactions, and a cosmetic lens ordered later.

In a blind eye, the lens can be ordered with a prescription, say +14.00 D, in order to make the lens easier to handle. This also has the effect of making the eye look larger or the lids wider open.

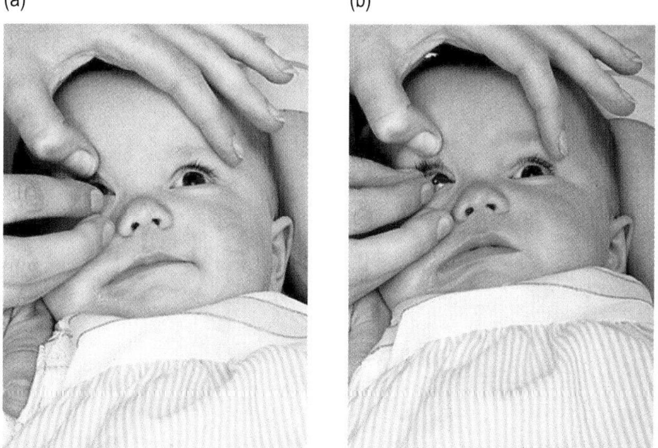

(a) (b)

Figure 24.12 Inserting lenses in a baby's eyes

THERAPEUTIC LENSES

Therapeutic lenses (see Chapter 26) are used for conditions similar to those in adults – corneal dystrophies, leaking blebs, grafts and perforations. They are worn temporarily while the eye heals or until alternative treatment is available.

HANDLING OF LENSES FOR INFANTS

At the first visit, the practitioner inserts the lenses while the parent cradles the child or holds them supine on a couch. The upper lid is raised, close to the lashes and the lens slotted underneath (Fig. 24.12). Removal of a soft lens is as for a corneal lens (Fig. 24.13) because an adult's fingers are too large to remove the lens by the conventional method of pinching it.

Occasionally, lenses (of any material) may need to be removed using a hollow rubber suction holder, especially in cases where the eyes are deep-set or microphthalmic. Lens centration must be confirmed before attempting lens removal. The suction holder must be regularly disinfected. A rubber suction holder is not easy to manipulate on a fractious child.

Most parents, once they have been told of the potential dangers of extended wear, are keen to remove their child's lenses

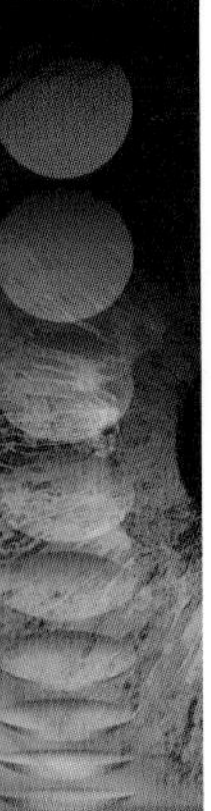

(a)

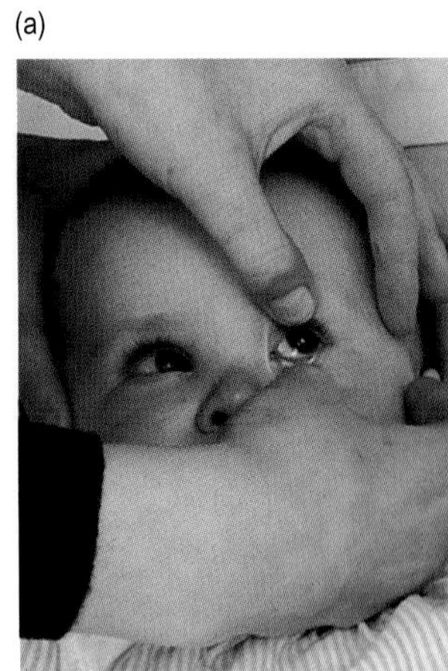

(b)

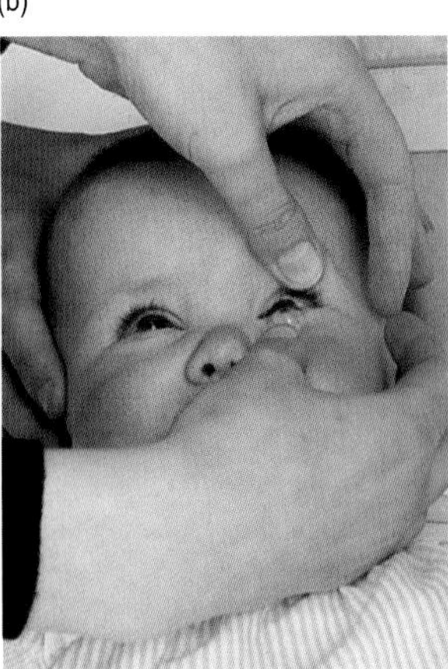

Figure 24.13 Removing lenses from a baby's eyes

regularly. Time spent in explaining and demonstrating lens insertion and removal at the beginning can save many emergency visits later. Emphasize that the lenses do not cause pain to the child and parents should try to be relaxed when the lenses are to be handled: if the parent is tense, the child senses it and also tenses up, making lens insertion or removal more difficult.

Lens handling is easier if:

- One parent holds the baby and the other handles the lenses.
- The lenses are inserted/removed when the child is asleep.
- The child has just started to feed or certain music is playing.
- The child is wrapped in a blanket.
- In an older child, they are asked to help (e.g. by holding their lower lid).

Other points to note

- If daily handling is not possible or difficult, start removing and cleaning weekly (as long as the eyes remain clear) and build up to daily removal.
- If lens insertion is too traumatic for parent or child, spectacles should be substituted. It is better for a child to wear anisometropic spectacles together with a patch than the family being continuously distressed. Contact lenses can always be tried when the child is older.
- Some toddlers become uncooperative at around 18 months and should be refitted with spectacles. Parents are often reluctant to give up contact lenses, but soon appreciate the wisdom of the decision. Indeed, many aphakic children prefer to wear spectacles if their visual acuity is poor, as they see better due to the magnifying effect induced by the back vertex distance of the glasses.
- Children aged 2–5 years who have not worn lenses previously are not usually cooperative and, where spectacle wear is adequate at this stage, it may be advisable to remain thus corrected.
- Many children who have had lenses since infancy are able to remove soft lenses by the age of 5 years, although they need to be older to insert them.

AFTER-CARE

After-care in children is similar to that in adults (see Chapters 17 and 18) with a few extra precautions.

- Children are just as likely as adults to develop giant papillary conjunctivitis or contact lens-induced papillary conjunctivitis, and disposable lenses are not available for most of the conditions discussed. Protein remover tablets should be used and, if necessary, the lenses changed to RGP or the child prescribed full-time spectacles.
- Poor hygiene can lead to infections in all lens wearers and the risks should be stressed to both parent and child. Corneal scars in infancy, however caused, can result in amblyopia and will affect the vision for life, especially if the scar is central. Corneal scars lead to neovascularization, which can leak lipid and reduce vision.
- Children's tears are usually adequate, but blink rate may be low, especially in infants: soft lenses then dry and fall out. In these cases, and also in many Down's syndrome patients where the tears are poor, it may be advisable to instil normal saline drops or contact lens rewetting drops (without preservative) every few hours. Alternatively, refit with silicone rubber or RGP lenses.
- Older children can develop blepharitis or meibomitis, which requires lid hygiene.
- Where lenses are not replaced frequently, deposit formation can occur.
- Most medical and nursing personnel have no training in contact lens removal in adults let alone children; therefore the parents are advised to remove the lenses themselves before taking the child to the local eye specialist for treatment.
- Anoxia can lead to vessel growth, especially with soft lenses. In cases where parents cannot remove lenses daily, or where the child is too uncooperative to be refitted with rigid lenses, it may be necessary to change to spectacle wear for a time.

LENS LOSS AND BREAKAGE

The number of soft lenses lost or broken, especially in the first few months of wear, can be very high. Spare lenses should be available against such events to ensure continuity of lens wear. Contact lens loss from the eye is a common reason for refitting with silicone rubber lenses (if parameters are available) or RGP lenses as they are lost less often. Alternatively, spectacles can be worn.

In the early months of life, soft lenses usually need to be changed or replaced before any build-up of deposits or protein occurs but, once the lens parameters have stabilized, it is worth initiating a planned replacement system so that new lenses are issued every 3–6 months, thereby avoiding the problems of deposited lenses.

EXAMINING THE CHILD

Infants and young children need to be reviewed frequently. Their lenses need changing and necessary objective observations made, as subjective information is less available. A hand-held slit-lamp provides one method of examination (Fig. 24.14), but a good view with a conventional slit-lamp can be obtained by holding the infant in the 'flying baby' position (Fig. 24.15).

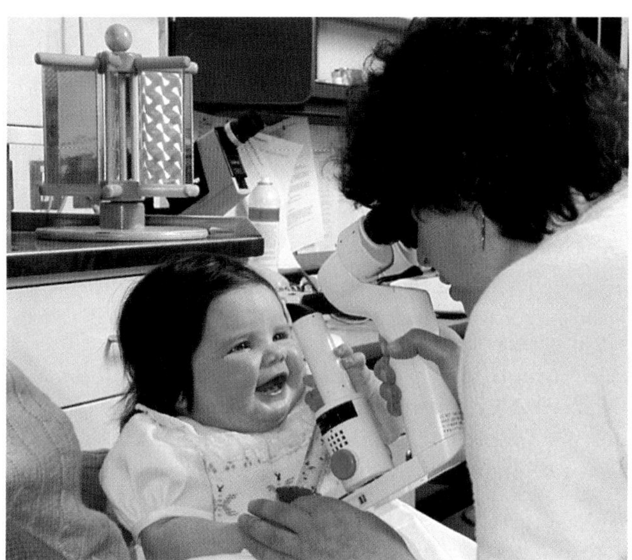

Figure 24.14 Examination using a hand-held slit-lamp

Concurrent eye disease

At follow-up, care must be taken to exclude any developing eye disease. For example, a red or watery eye may not be contact lens-induced but due to an increase in intraocular pressure or irritation from a loose suture. The eye condition itself requires regular follow-up in conjunction with the contact lens assessment, in particular:

- Aphakia (see Aphakia after-care, p. 512)
  - fundus.
  - intraocular pressure as infant aphakes have a 25% risk of developing glaucoma (Simon et al. 1991, Johnson & Keech 1996).
- Ectopia lentis
  - fundus checks, especially in Marfan's syndrome, as retinal detachment occurs in between 10 and 25% of patients (Nelson & Maumenee 1982).
- Aniridia
  - intraocular pressure.
  - peripheral corneal assessment as stem cell deficiency results in pannus (Nishida et al. 1995).
- Nanophthalmos
  - intraocular pressure. These patients have a high risk of glaucoma (Calhoun 1976).

Swimming and holidays

The same advice should be given for children as for adults. It is safer to remove lenses altogether for swimming or to wear closely fitting goggles (though not for diving). Prescription goggles can be provided or an ordinary pair of spectacles with a sportsband to hold them in place. On holiday it is prudent to remove lenses for the duration of any flight and on the beach.

One particular problem for toddlers is wearing lenses in dusty environments such as sandpits or on the beach. Lenses are then best avoided.

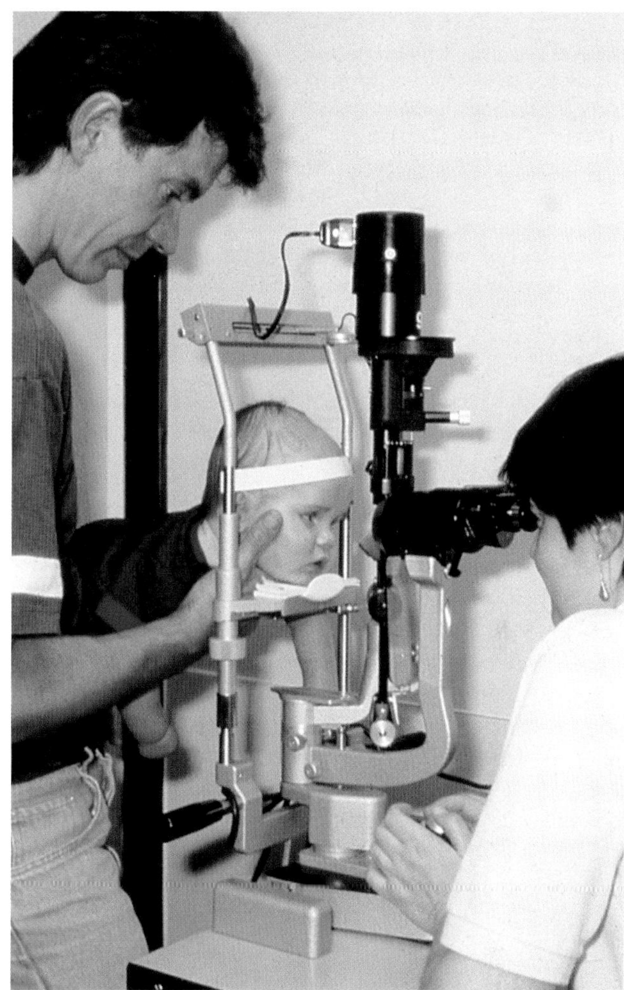

Figure 24.15 The 'flying baby' position used to examine young infants at a conventional slit-lamp

SUMMARY

Although most of the problems of contact lens fitting and wear can be overcome and parents' questions answered, the long-term visual outcome remains elusive. Results differ in every case. Many children with congenital visual problems improve beyond expectation, whereas others, unfortunately, do not. Even with the sophisticated equipment now available – visual evoked potentials, electroretinograms and preferential looking techniques – it is still not possible to answer with anything other than a calculated guess.

The age at which implants are used for young children has dropped dramatically in recent years. Modern surgical techniques obviate the need for contact lens fitting in many cases but for the foreseeable future, the contact lens practitioner will still be an essential part of the vision-care team.

Acknowledgement

Thanks are due to the Department of Medical Illustration, Great Ormond Street Hospital for Children, London, for the photographs included in this section.

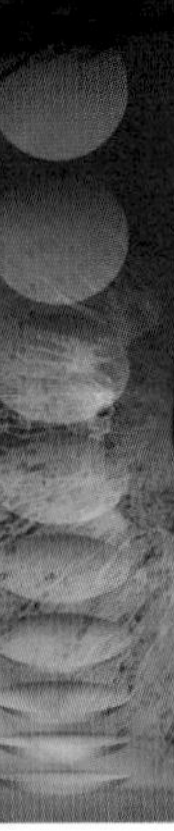

References

Abadi, R. V. (1979) Visual performance with contact lenses and congenital idiopathic nystagmus. Br. J. Physiol. Opt., 33(3), 32–37

Abdulla, N., O'Malley, D., Bowell, R. and O'Keefe, M. (1998) Childhood anisometropia and contact lenses. Optician, 5654(215), 36–37

Amos, C. F., Lambert, S. R. and Ward, M. A. (1992) Rigid gas permeable contact lens correction of aphakia following congenital cataract removal during infancy. J. Pediatr. Ophthalmol. Strab., 29(4), 243–245

Asbell, P., Chiang, B., Somers, M. and Morgan, K. (1990) Keratometry in children. CLAO J., 16(2), 99–102

Atkinson, J., Braddick, D. and French, J. (1980) Infant astigmatism: its disappearance with age. Vision Res., 20, 891–893

Barnard, N. A. S. (1991) The psychological effect of contact lenses on a seven year old. Contact Lens J., 18(10), 282

Blomdahl, S. (1979) Ultrasonic measurements of the eye in the newborn infant. Acta Ophthalmol. (Copenhagen), 57, 1048–1056

Calhoun, F. P. Jr. (1976) The management of glaucoma in nanophthalmos. Trans. Am. Ophthalmol. Soc., 73, 97–122

Cutler, S. I., Nelson, L. B. and Calhoun, J. H. (1985) Extended wear contact lenses in pediatric aphakia. J. Pediatr. Ophthalmol. Strab., 22, 85–91

Evain, B., Langlois, M. and François, P. (1986) Decollement de retine et syndrome de Marfan. Bull. Soc. Ophtalmol. Fr., 86(6–7), 875–882

Ezekiel, D. (1995) A gas-permeable paediatric aphakic scleral contact lens. Optician, 35(5), 25–27

Golubovic, S., Marjanovic, S., Cvetkovic, D. and Manic, S. (1989) The application of hard contact lenses in patients with congenital nystagmus. Fortschr. Ophthalmol., 86(5), 535–539

Grosvenor, T. and Scott, R. (1993) Three-year changes in refraction and its components in youth-onset and early adult-onset myopia. Optom. Vis. Sci., 70(8), 677–683

Huth, S. and Wagner, H. (1981) Identification and removal of deposits on polydimethylsiloxane silicone elastomer lenses. Int. Contact Lens Clin., 7/8, 19–26

Johnson, C. P. and Keech, R. V. (1996) Prevalence of glaucoma after surgery for PHPV and infantile cataracts. J. Pediatr. Ophthalmol. Strab., 33, 14–17

Koch, J. M., Refojo, M. F. and Leong, F. L. (1991) Corneal edema after overnight lid closure of rabbits wearing silicone rubber contact lenses. Cornea, 10(2), 123–126

Lang, J. and Rah, M. J. (2004) Adverse corneal events associated with corneal reshaping: a case series. Eye Contact Lens, 30(4), 231–233; discussion 242–243

Larsen, J. S. (1971) The sagittal growth of the eye. Parts I–IV. Acta Ophthalmol. (Copenhagen), 49, 873–886

Lloyd, I. C., Dowler, J. G., Kriss, A. et al. (1995) Modulation of amblyopia therapy following early surgery for unilateral congenital cataracts. Br. J. Ophthalmol., 79(9), 802–806

Macsai, M. S. (2005) Corneal ulcers in two children wearing paragon corneal refractive therapy lenses. Eye Contact Lens, 31(1), 9–11

Marshall, J. and Grindle, C. F. J. (1978) Fine structure of the cornea and its development. Trans. Ophthalmol. Soc. UK, 98, 320–328

Molnar, L. (1970) Refraktionsanderung des Auges im Laufe des Lebens. Klin. Monatsbl. Augenheilkd., 156, 326–339

Morris, J. (1979) Contact lenses in infancy and childhood. Contact Lens J., 8, 15–18

Nelson, L. B. and Maumenee, I. H. (1982) Ectopia lentis. Surv. Ophthalmol., 27, 143–160

Nishida, K., Kinoshita, S., Ohashi, Y., Kuwayama, Y. and Yamamoto, S. (1995) Ocular surface abnormalities in aniridia. Am. J. Ophthalmol., 120(3), 368–375

Perrigin, J., Perrigin, D., Quintero, S. and Grosvenor, T. (1990) Silicone-acrylate contact lenses for myopia control: 3-year results. Optom. Vis. Sci., 67(10), 764–769

Refojo, M. F. and Leong, F. L. (1981) Water pervaporation through silicone rubber contact lenses: a possible cause of complications. Contact Intraoc. Lens Med. J., 7(3), 226–233

Rich, L. S. and Glusman, M. (1992) Tangent streak RGP bifocal contact lenses in the treatment of accommodative esotropia with high AC/A ratio. CLAO J., 18(1), 56–58

Roberts, C. J. and Adams, G. G. (2002) Contact lenses in the management of high anisometropic amblyopia. Eye, 16(5), 577–579

Ruben, M. (1967) Albinism and contact lenses. Contact Lens J., 1(2)

Ruston, D. and van der Worp, E. (2004) Is Otho-K OK? Fitting techniques and safety issues. Optom. Today, 44(24), 25–31

Saw, S-M. (2005) Refraction and refractive errors. In Pediatric Ophthalmology and Strabismus, eds. D. Taylor and C. Hoyt. London: Elsevier

Simon, J. W., Mehta, N., Simmons, S. T. et al. (1991) Glaucoma after pediatric lensectomy/vitrectomy. Ophthalmology, 98(5), 670–674

Sorsby, A. and Sheridan, M. (1960) The eye at birth: measurement of the principal diameters in forty-eight cadavers. J. Anat., 94, 192–195

Speedwell, L. (2003) Optometric management of children. Optom. Today, 43(14), 32–34

Speedwell, L. and Russell-Eggitt, I. (1994) The long and the short and the tall. J. Br. Contact Lens Assoc., 17, 135–139

Speedwell, L. and Russell-Eggitt, I. (1995) Improvement in visual acuity in children with ectopia lentis. J. Pediatr. Ophthalmol. Strab., 32(2), 94–97

Speedwell, L., Novakovic, P. and Sherrard, E. (1988) The infant corneal endothelium. Arch. Ophthalmol., 106(6), 771–775

Stone, J. (1976) The possible influence of contact lenses on myopia. Br. J. Physiol. Opt., 31, 89–114

Taylor, D., Morris, J., Rogers, J. E. and Warland, J. (1979) Amblyopia in bilateral infantile and juvenile cataract. Trans. Ophthalmol. Soc. UK, 99, 170–176

Walline, J. J., Jones, L. A., Mutti, D. O. and Zadnik K. (2004) A randomized trial of the effects of rigid contact lenses on myopia progression. Arch. Ophthalmol., 122, 1760–1766

Weale, R. A. (1982) A Biography of the Eye. Development, Growth, Age. London: H. K. Lewis

Winn, B., Ackerley, R. G., Brown, C. A. et al. (1986) The superiority of contact lenses in correction of all anisometropia. Trans. BCLA Conference, 95–100

Wood, I. C. J., Mutti, D. O. and Zadnik, K. (1996) Crystalline lens parameters in infancy. Ophthalmic Physiol. Opt., 16(4), 310–317

Zametkin, A. J., Stevens, J. R. and Pittman, R. (1979) Ontogeny of spontaneous blinking and of habituation of the blink reflex. Ann. Neurol., 5(5), 453–457

Chapter 25

Cosmetic and prosthetic contact lenses

Mark Lazarus

CHAPTER CONTENTS

In this chapter, coloured contact lenses are differentiated into *cosmetic* lenses, i.e. tinted contact lenses that simply change the colour of the eyes, and *prosthetic* lenses, i.e. lenses that change the appearance of an unsightly eye, although cosmetic lenses are often used for the latter purpose.

The fact that contact lenses can provide benefits other than visual is often overlooked and their ability to change a patient's appearance should not be trivialized. People with unsightly eyes are often self-conscious and uncomfortable about appearing in public or meeting strangers. Prosthetic lenses offer an increased sense of confidence about their appearance.

A practitioner who wishes to provide prosthetic lenses for patients with disfigured eyes should have experience in fitting normal tinted cosmetic lenses. The basic principles in both cases are the same: the lenses should be tailored to each person and should make them feel comfortable about their image.

Coloured lenses can also provide more physical benefits. Patients with conditions such as photophobia, diplopia, coloboma and aniridia can be helped with opaque lenses and some conditions requiring therapeutic lenses can benefit from having a tint incorporated to improve the appearance (see Chapter 26).

A HISTORY OF COSMETIC LENSES

Glass and polymethylmethacrylate (PMMA) lenses were originally clear. Later, corneal PMMA lenses were tinted for a variety of reasons:

- As an aid to handling, making lens insertion and removal easier.
- To differentiate lenses from each other.
- To enhance or alter eye colour.
- To reduce photophobia.

PMMA buttons or rods are tinted in a wide range of colours, prior to lathing. Each tint has a specific density and number, two of which are of clinical quality (CQ). These are very light grey/brown and light grey/brown and were annotated as 911CQ and 912CQ (now 9042 and 9043) respectively. They use inert carbon particles within the monomer (Gasson & Morris 2003) to ensure that there are no toxic effects on the eye.

It was only in the 1980s that soft tinted lenses became available. These were initially pale blue to act as a 'visibility tint' but they did not change the natural colour of the eye. A slight

Figure 25.1 *Left*: CIBA Color. *Right*: Bausch & Lomb Optima

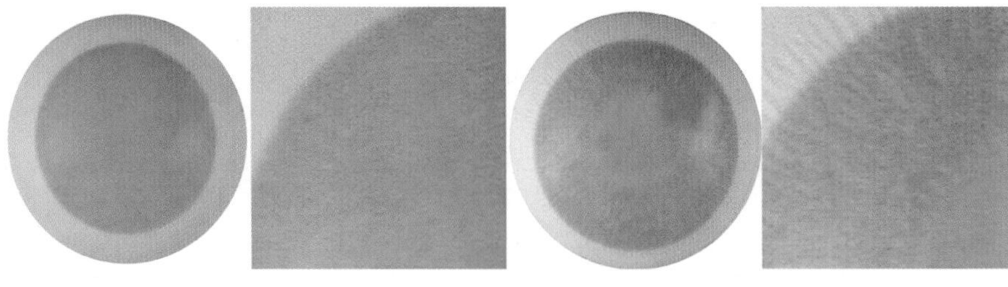

Figure 25.2 Dot matrix pattern on early opaque lenses

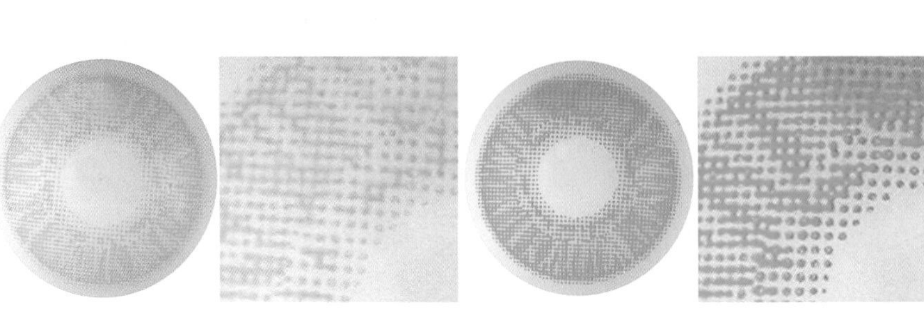

cosmetic change could be achieved by deepening the dye, which would enhance the colour in blue or green eyes, but have no effect on brown eyes (CLACO 1984) (Fig. 25.1).

A lens with a printed single colour dot matrix pattern (see p. 521) was produced in the 1990s using a photographic technique, but was only available in limited colours (CLACO 1984). In this process, the tinted portion of the lens was opaque and stopped the transmission of light. Unlike the blue-tinted variety, these opaque lenses were able to change the colour of eyes from brown to blue (Fig. 25.2).

The pioneering companies in the development of prosthetic soft contact lenses were the Toyo Lens Company (now Menicon Ltd), Titmus Eurocon Contact Lens and Wesley–Jessen (both now CIBA Vision).

MANUFACTURE OF COLOURED LENSES

Cosmetic contact lenses are now produced by all the major lens manufacturers and are available in a wide spectrum of colours and prescriptions (Tables 25.1, 25.2). Due to improved manufacturing techniques, more recent opaque cosmetic lenses have a much more natural appearance as three or more colours are used to produce each lens.

Coloured lenses are made using a variety of methods:

- *Dye dispersion* – usually for rigid lenses. The dye is added to the monomer matrix and mixed to disperse the colour.
- *Vat dye tinting* – the finished soft contact lens is soaked in a water-soluble dye to produce a uniform surface tint.
- *Chemical bond tinting* – the lens is soaked in a dye solution together with a catalyst, which produces a chemical bond between the dye and the polymer (Efron 2002).
- *Printing* – the iris pattern is printed onto the lens much like printing on paper except the pigment is now enclosed within the lens matrix.

In order to make the cosmetic lens appear more natural, the pigment is printed to match the fibrous elements within the human iris. A black limbal band can be incorporated, along

Table 25.1: Enhancer contact lenses

	CIBA Vision Focus 2 Weekly Softcolors	CIBA Vision FreshLook Dimensions	CIBA Vision Focus Monthly Softcolors
Base curve	8.4, 8.8	Median	8.6, 8.9
Power range	Plano to –6.00 D	+6.00 to –8.00 D	+6.00 to –8.00 D
Diameter	14.0 mm	14.5 mm	14.0 mm
Material	Vifilcon	Phemfilcon A	Vifilcon
Water content	55%	55%	55%
Thickness (–3.00)	0.06 mm	0.06 mm	0.10 mm
Colour diameter	11.0 mm	12.5 mm	11.0 mm
	Johnson & Johnson Acuvue 2 Colours Enhancer	**CooperVision Expressions Accents**	**Bausch & Lomb Optima Colors**
Base curve	8.3, 8.7	8.7	8.4, 8.7
Power range	–0.50 to –6.00 D	+4.00 to –6.00 D	Plano to –6.00 D
Diameter	14 mm	14.4 mm	14 mm
Material	Etafilcon A	Methafilcon A	Polymacon
Water content	58%	55%	38%
Thickness (–3.00)	0.84 mm	0.08 mm	0.06 mm
Colour diameter	11.4 mm	11.0 mm	12.5 mm

Table 25.2: Cosmetic and prosthetic contact lenses

	Johnson & Johnson Acuvue 2 Colours Opaque	CIBA Vision Freshlook ColorBlends	CIBA Vision Freshlook Color	CIBA Vision Dura Soft 3 Colors and Dura Soft Color Blend
Base curve	8.3	8.6	8.6	8.3, 8.6, 9.0
Diameter	14 mm	14.5 mm	14.5 mm	14.5 mm
Iris print diameter	12.4 mm	12.5 mm	12.5 mm	12.5 mm
Pupil aperture	5.4 mm	5.0 mm	5.0 mm	5.0 mm
Central thickness (–3)	0.84 mm	0.8 mm	0.08 mm	0.06 mm
Material	Etaficon A	Phemfilcon A	Phemfilcon A	Phemfilcon A
Water content	58%	55%	55%	55%
Power range	+6.00 to –9.00 D	+6.00 to –8.00 D	+6.00 to –8.00 D	+6.00 to –8.00 D Made to order +20.00 to –20.00 D
	CIBA Vision Elegance	**CIBA Vision Wild Eye**	**EyCon EyColours**	**EyCon Prosthetic Lens, any parameters**
Base curve	8.4, 8.7	8.6	Any BC	8.6
Diameter	13.8 mm	14.5 mm	14.3 mm	14.3 mm
Iris print diameter	12.0 mm	12.5 mm	11.5 mm	12.0 mm
Pupil aperture	5.0 mm	5.0 mm	5.0 mm	4, 5 or 6 mm clear Black pupil 4 mm
Central thickness (–3)	0.08 mm	0.06 mm	0.11, 0.06 mm	0.11, 0.06 mm
Material	Polymacon	Phemfilcon A	Polymacon	Polymacon
Water content	38%	55%	38%	38%
Power range	+1.00 to –6.00 D	Plano to –6.00 D	+25.00 to –25.00 D	+25.00 to –25.00 D
	CooperVision Expressions	**CooperVision Crazy Lens**	**CooperVision Prosthetic Lens**	**Innova Vision Calaview**
Base curve	8.7	8.6	8.3, 8.7, 9.0	8.6
Diameter	14.4 mm	14.2 mm	14.5 mm	14 mm
Iris print diameter	12.6 mm	13.0 mm	12.00 mm	12.5 mm
Pupil aperture	5.2 mm	5.2 mm	3, 4, 5 or 6 mm Black pupil 4 mm	N/A
Central thickness (–3)	0.08 mm	0.07 mm	0.07 mm	N/A
Material	Methafilcon A	Methafilcon A	Polymacon	HEMA and MAA
Water content	55%	55%	38%	60%
Power range	+4.00 to –6.00 D	Plano to –4.00 D	+25.00 to –25.00 D	N/A

HEMA, hydroxyethyl methacrylate; MAA, methacrylic acid.

with colour variation from the pupil edge to the limbus (Figs 25.3, 25.4).

The above methods are used for translucent tints. There are also different methods of producing opaque tints including:

- *Dot matrix tinting* (Fig. 25.4) – an opaque coloured dot matrix is applied to the front surface of a soft lens and chemically fixed to make it permanent.
- *Opaque backing* – an opaque white backing of barium sulphate is precipitated into the matrix of the back surface of the lens. The iris colour is then painted onto the front surface and bonded (see Fig. 25.17c).
- *Laminating* – this method is not often used now. The colour or front surface of a soft lens button is lathed and polished, either tinted or hand-painted (see below) and sandwiched with a further layer of polymer.

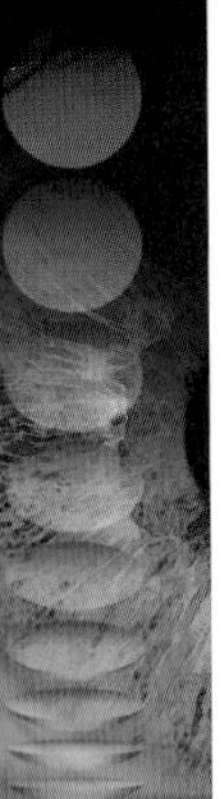

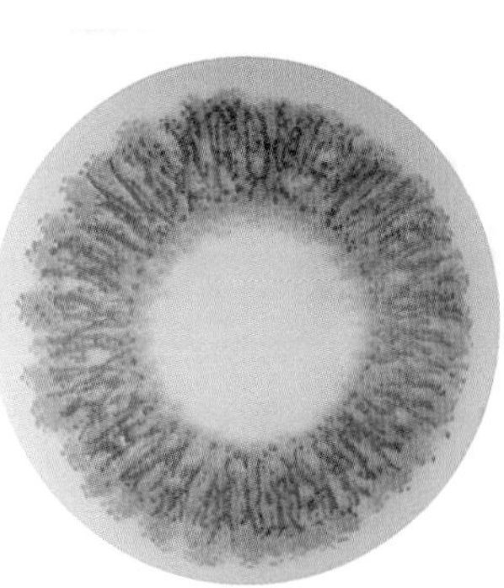

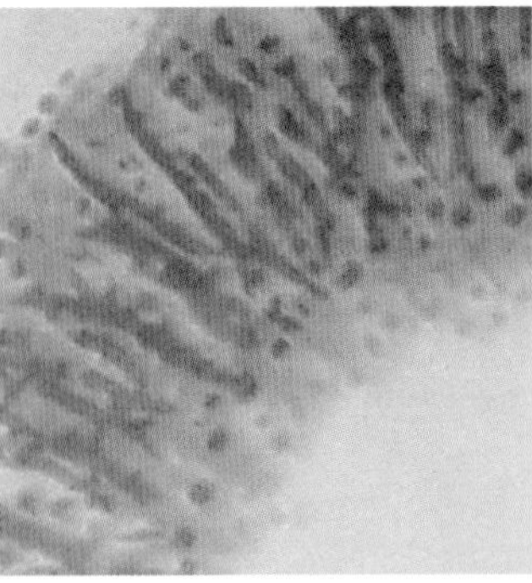

Figure 25.3 Enclosed pigment within the lens matrix

COMMON USES OF COSMETIC LENSES

Cosmetic coloured lenses have an advantage over other forms of vision correction, such as refractive surgery, as they can correct vision and alter appearance. Various types of these lenses are available, from simple tints that enhance the original eye colour, to opaque lenses made with multicoloured patterns that provide a natural-looking new eye colour. Generally, the opaque lenses are used to change the colour of dark irides or for use as prosthetic lenses (see p. 523), while transparent tints are useful for deepening the colour of light blue or blue–green irides.

Lenses are also available that make the eyes look deliberately unnatural (see Fig. 29.18). These have been standard wear for actors in Hollywood vampire movies and musicians in rock videos for many years (Greenspoon 1969). Yet unnatural lenses are not just limited to the entertainment industry. The production and popularity of cosmetic lenses has become so widespread that there are now lenses with team emblems for football fanatics, cats' eyes for attention-seekers and various other dramatic patterns. These lenses are often available without prescription over the internet and even at markets.

Risks and problems associated with cosmetic lenses

Given that cosmetic lenses have become so readily available, it is important to promote good lens hygiene. People who irregularly use these lenses tend to be less careful about lens hygiene. For example, distinctive unnatural lenses are sometimes exchanged among young people, leading to eye infections (Gagnon & Walter 2006). Significantly, these lenses can be distributed directly to consumers without instructions about correct care (Steinemann et al. 2003). To help prevent damage to the eye, the US Food and Drug Administration (FDA) has cautioned consumers against using decorative contact lenses that have not been prescribed and fitted by a qualified eye-care professional (FDA 2002).

After-care

It is essential that anyone using plano cosmetic lenses is taught how to look after their lenses and have regular follow-up consultations with their practitioner, just as patients wearing contact lenses for refractive correction. If there is any doubt about a patient's reliability or understanding regarding infection, they should not be supplied with lenses (see also Chapter 32).

There are also visual issues for patients wearing cosmetic lenses.

- Colour-tinted contact lenses are associated with a reduction of contrast sensitivity (Ozkagnici et al. 2003).
- The visual field is slightly reduced (Josephson & Caffery 1987, Albarran Diego et al. 2001). This can be overcome by making the iris pattern less dense near the pupil.
- It has been shown that the corneal topography can be altered after just 1 hour of cosmetic lens wear (Voetz et al. 2004).

Patients who wear coloured contact lenses should be informed about the possible reduction in visual function, both during lens wear and for several hours after removing the lenses. It is especially important that patients are aware that they may be affected, especially in dim illumination, such as driving at night. For safety reasons, pilots should not use cosmetic contact lenses when flying (Nakagawara et al. 2002).

FITTING THE LENS

For patients already wearing corrective contact lenses and who simply wish to change or highlight their eye colour, fitting a lens from the same company as their current lenses can work well. For example, those wearing Focus (CIBA Vision) or Acuvue (Johnson & Johnson) lenses should be fitted with the same brand of cosmetic lenses so that they do not have to adjust to a new lens type. This can eliminate fitting and adaptational problems.

To prevent the risk of cross-contamination, trial lenses should be discarded after one use and should not be sterilized and reused.

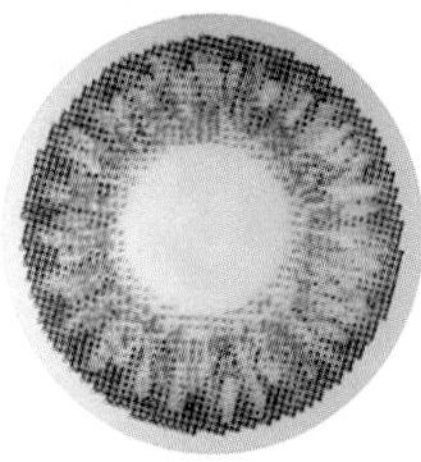

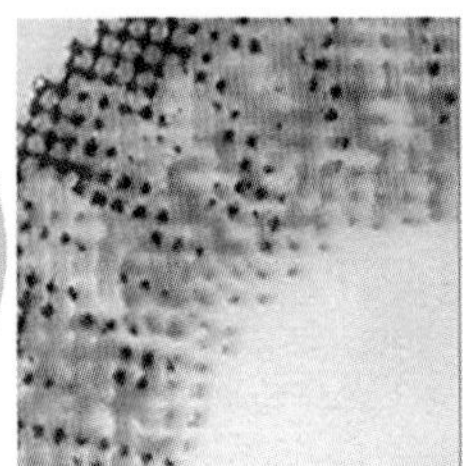

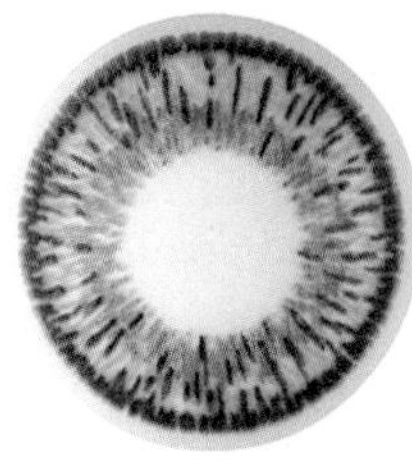

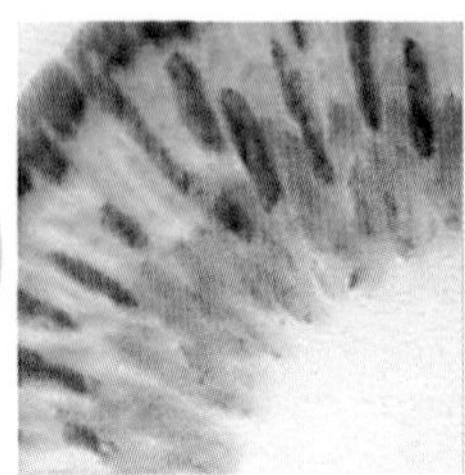

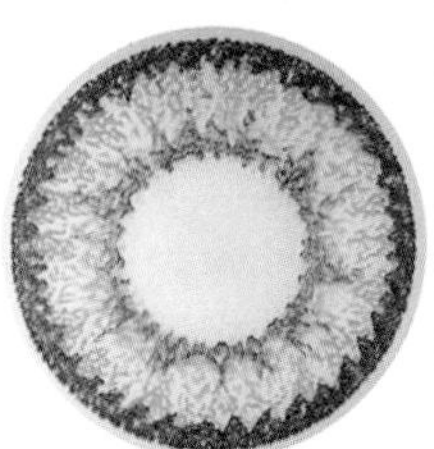

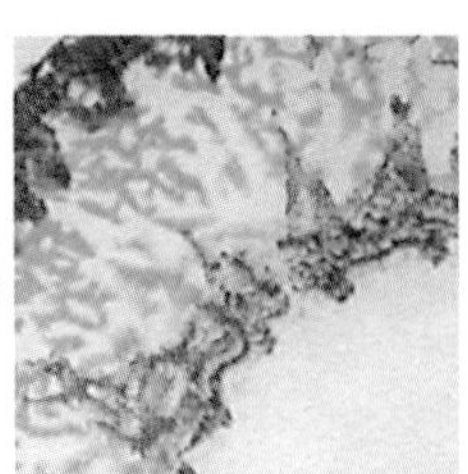

Figure 25.4 Dot matrix and printed lenses showing limbal bands

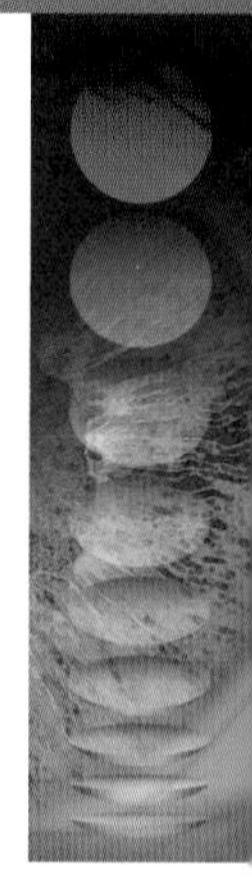

Choice of colour

- Spend time choosing the colour that the patient feels suits them.
- It can be difficult to gauge whether a pigment will suit a patient until they are actually wearing the cosmetic lens, so encourage them to try various colours.
- The majority of patients only want a subtle change in eye colour but it can take some time for them to make their decision.
- Let the patient sit and discuss the different lenses with their friends or your receptionist before deciding. This may seem trivial, but it can be a light-hearted way to interact with patients and although the initial fitting will be prolonged and involve multiple lenses, most patients continue to use the same type of cosmetic lens once they are satisfied.

Occasionally practitioners may encounter patients with body dysmorphic disorder (BDD). These usually young patients are anxious or depressed about their bodily appearance and continually request unnecessary procedures. The most common complaints involve facial blemishes, which sufferers may think would be improved with cosmetic contact lenses. These patients should be referred to a psychiatrist for help.

Finally, care is needed when fitting any patients who have had successful refractive surgery as the cornea is no longer normal and fitting lenses can be more difficult (see Chapter 23).

As mentioned earlier, the more experience in fitting patients with cosmetic lenses, the better the practitioner will be able to handle prosthetic lenses.

PROSTHETIC CONTACT LENSES

Ocular prostheses have been fitted for thousands of years. Recent developments in both ophthalmic surgery and prosthetic contact lenses merge the role of the prosthetic eye maker and the contact lens practitioner. For those practitioners who fit prosthetic contact lenses, it is worthwhile knowing about the historic development of artificial eyes.

The history of prostheses and damaged eyes

In ancient Egypt 2000 BCE, the dead were provided with artificial eyes fixed in their coffin cases in order to see in the after-life. The Ancient Greeks and Romans decorated statues of their heroes and gods with artificial eyes made of glass paste or enamel (Lawrence 1972). In the Roman period, the manufacturer of these artificial eyes was known as a *faber ocularis*. In contrast, the eye doctor, or *medicus ocularius*, fitted artificial eyes for patients. At this stage, there were two types of artificial eye: one worn in front of the lids, known as an *ekblephara*, and the other worn under the eyelids and called *hypoblephara*. The unknown medicus ocularis who first fitted a *hypoblephara* is the originator of the modern craft of fitting prosthetic contact lenses to blind and disfigured eyes (Tonkellaar et al. 1991).

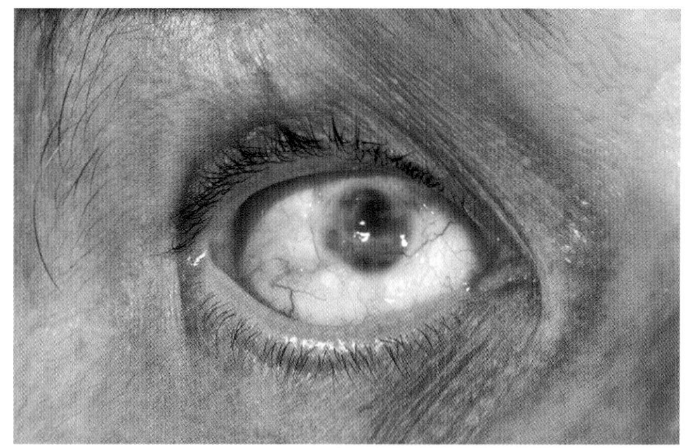

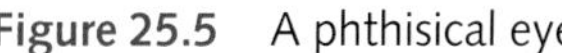

Figure 25.5 A phthisical eye

Typically, the normal result of an untreated penetrating injury to an eye is phthisis bulbi. The name is derived from the Greek *phthisis* – 'decay' or wasting, and the Latin *bulbus* – a bulb or sphere. When phthisis bulbi occurs after a penetrating injury, the eye is blind and shrinks, losing its normal architecture (Fig. 25.5).

Until recent times, penetrating eye injuries were not repaired surgically, so phthisis bulbi usually followed this sort of damage to the eye. Prosthetic eye manufacturers make use of this eye shrinkage to fit the artificial eye within the orbit. Prosthetic eyes or shells are fitted under the lids, so that they completely fill the orbit and extend the lids over the shell, giving the patient a normal appearance.

Ocular prostheses and cosmetic shells

An ocular prosthesis is an artificial eye, fitted after an eye has been lost, surgically removed, or the contents eviscerated. In the 1850s, the enamel prosthesis was introduced, but these were expensive and did not last more than a few months, and in 1892, Snellen introduced a hollow glass prosthesis called the 'Reform-Auge'. The modern ocular prosthesis is similar, in principle, to Snellen's but made of PMMA, although glass is still sometimes used (e.g. in cases of giant papillary conjunctivitis) (Fig. 25.6).

A small ball of plastic or coral is inserted to replace the eye and maintain the volume of the orbit (Fig. 25.7). This mimics phthisis bulbi and, generally, the volume needs to be 2 ml less to allow room for the prosthesis. It is important to note that in purely cosmetic cases, the only reason that the eye is enucleated is to make enough room to fit the prosthesis. Standard ophthalmic surgical textbooks still give cosmesis as an indication for the enucleation of a blind eye. Fortunately, the recent development of soft and rigid prosthetic contact lenses has removed this long-standing need.

Cosmetic shells are more likely to be fitted to a blind shrunken eye. A mould is taken of the eye and a PMMA cast made from the mould in a similar way to scleral impressions (Pullum 1997). The cast is then painted with an iris pattern and sclera to match the fellow eye (if present).

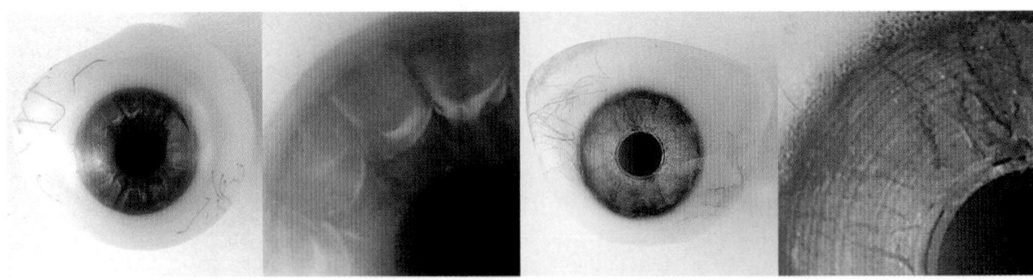

Figure 25.6 *Left*: Glass prosthesis. *Right*: PMMA prosthesis

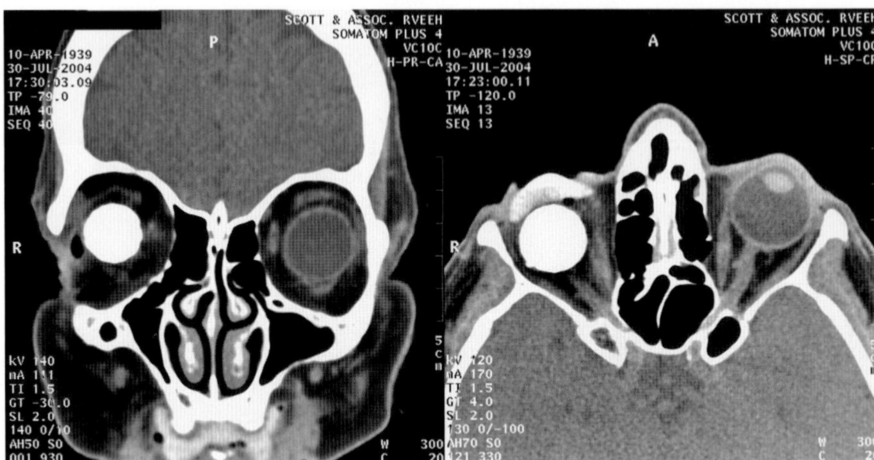

Figure 25.7 CT scan showing a coral insert and prosthesis

An artificial eye manufacturer (oculist or ocular prosthetist) is usually a member of an ophthalmology department involved in the treatment of disfigured eyes. They are artists who have both the skill and training to help match the injured eye with a prosthetic contact lens and the experience with patients who have recently lost an eye. They should work closely with the contact lens practitioner.

Modern surgical developments

Before current techniques of vitreoretinal surgery, a significant percentage of eyes that had complicated penetrating ocular injuries were enucleated within a week of injury (Thordarson et al. 1979) because of poor visual prognosis and to prevent the loss of the other eye from sympathetic ophthalmia, a bilateral granulomatous panuveitis (Lubin et al. 1980). Today, complex penetrating injuries that involve the cornea, lens, vitreous and retina are treated by specialist surgeons who can safely remove vitreous and preretinal membranes. Many of these eyes end up with useful vision and, even when the visual prognosis is poor, patients avoid the psychological trauma of having their eye removed.

Unfortunately, some eyes that have suffered a penetrating injury end up with no vision and are significantly disfigured. As long as there is no ocular pain or risk to health, the eye should not need to be removed. Where eyes must be enucleated, it can result in significant cosmetic sequelae of a deep superior sulcus and ptosis of the upper lid.

In cases where a blind eye is also painful, such as bullous keratopathy or sterile ulcer, if a therapeutic lens is of no benefit, a thin flap of conjunctiva is surgically drawn over the damaged cornea to make the eye comfortable. This is called a Gundersen's flap (Fig. 25.8).

Patients who require prosthetic lenses

There is ongoing research on new eyes and artificial retinas that depend on an intact optic nerve and normal anterior segment. As medical technology advances, some patients believe that their blind eye may once again become sighted and are therefore very reluctant to give consent to have an eye removed. The total number of enucleations and enviscerations has decreased in Australia, from 576 in 1994 to 522 in 2003, in spite of an increase in the Australian population (www.medicareaustralia.gov.au and www.abs.gov.au), hence the increased need for prosthetic contact lenses.

Realistically, blind eyes requiring prosthetic contact lenses are almost certainly unsuitable for any of these developments although it is inadvisable to disillusion patients. Their mental well-being tends to be significantly better if they can preserve some hope of returning to normal health and it is the responsibility of cosmetic lens practitioners to help ensure that eyes are not unnecessarily enucleated for cosmetic reasons (Zimmerman & McLean 1975, Dortzbach & Woog 1985).

Patients need to be warned from the outset that the lens will not look perfect. Those with long-standing disfigurements have a certain view of themselves as do those around them. They may be upset when the lens is fitted, as it is not as good as they want and refuse to wear it even though cosmetically it may be excellent.

The process of fitting a prosthetic contact lens is more involved than simply matching the lens to the patient's good eye. Where the loss of the eye is recent, the practitioner should

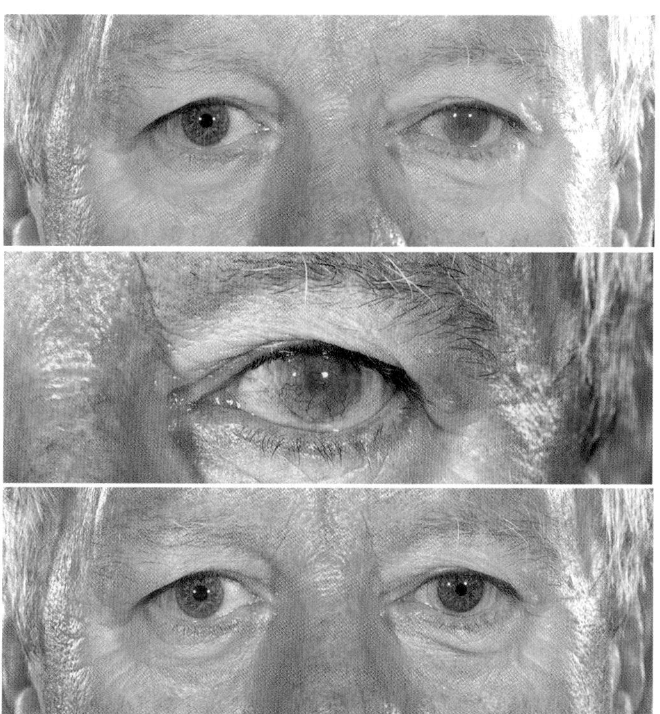

Figure 25.8 (Top and middle) Left eye with a failed corneal graft with a Gundersen's flap and (Bottom) wearing a prosthetic lens

advise on the problems that arise from it and provide information on everyday matters, such as local laws regarding driving with one eye (e.g. see www.austroads.com.au). Counselling can sometimes be necessary and patients may need to discuss their injury with a psychologist as well as their ophthalmologist (see www.visionaustralia.org.au).

IMPROVING OCULAR COSMESIS

There are various different lens tint designs that can be used to improve cosmesis and the optimum lens depends on the appearance of the eye and whether the pupil is normal or not (see Fig. 25.13).

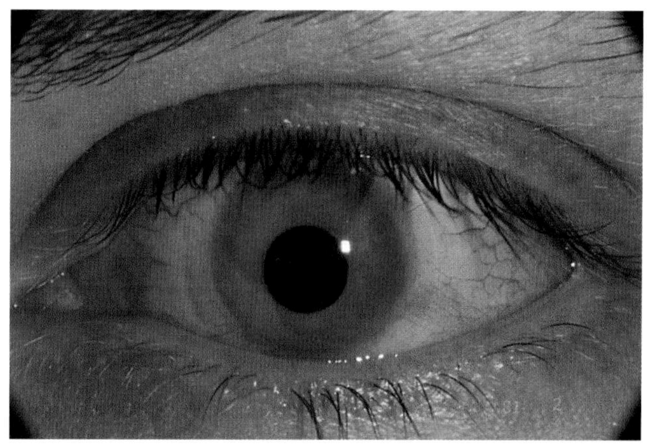

Figure 25.10 Fuchs' dystrophy. The loss of a normal black pupil draws attention to the condition. A black pupil soft lens is a simple and effective remedy

For iris colours, manufacturers usually provide a set of lenses with homogeneous tints and their own codes for the practitioner to use when ordering (e.g. Brown 4 or Grey–blue 1042).

It is best to keep a prosthetic lens as simple as possible. In some cases, a lens with a 4 mm black pupil may be all that is needed for an excellent cosmetic effect (Figs 25.9, 25.10).

Cosmetic lenses should always be tried on the eye, as the colour appears different from that on, say, a white opacified cornea from that on a large iridectomy. In addition, an eye that has suffered trauma may be redder than the fellow eye. This can affect the appearance of a coloured lens when matching it to the fellow eye.

In-office tinting of lenses and making cosmetic pupils

It is useful to be able to tint lenses in the practice. Patients may request a small pupil for the daytime and another lens with a larger pupil for the evening in order to match the normal eye better. A black pupil can also be useful as an occlusive lens for patients with intractable diplopia (see Diplopia, p. 528). Where necessary, the pupil of the lens can be tinted grey, instead of

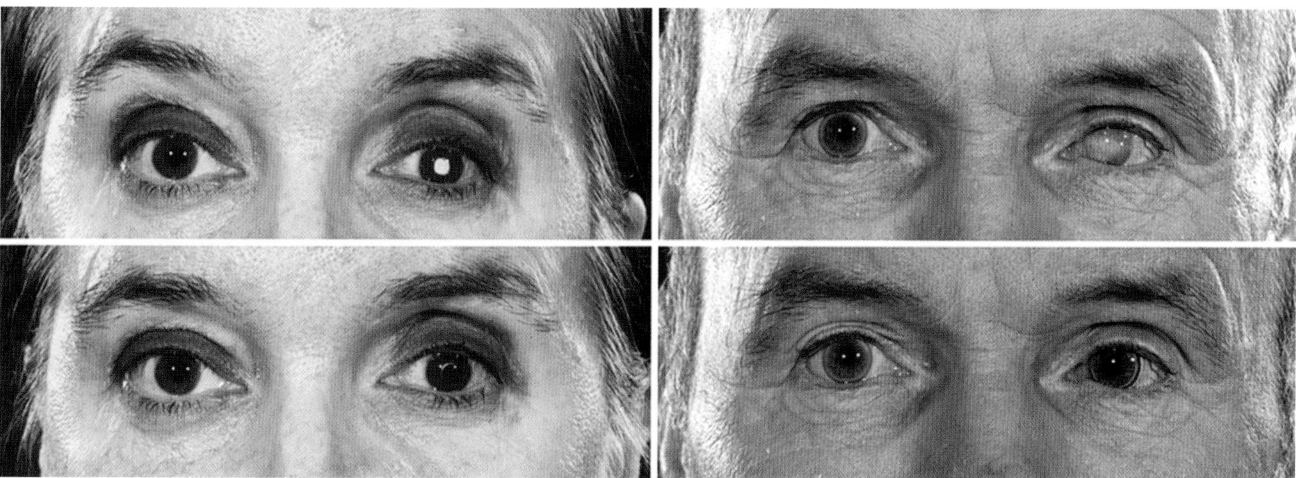

Figure 25.9 *Left*: Prosthetic contact lens with a simple 4 mm black pupil. *Right*: Full prosthetic lens with black pupil

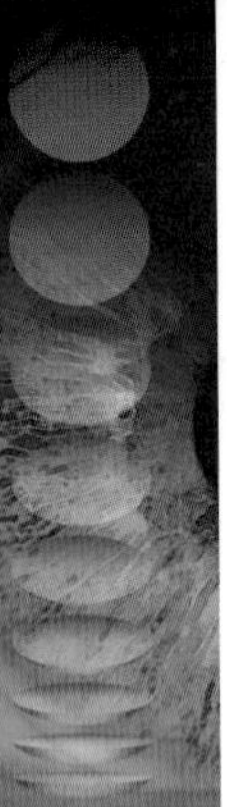

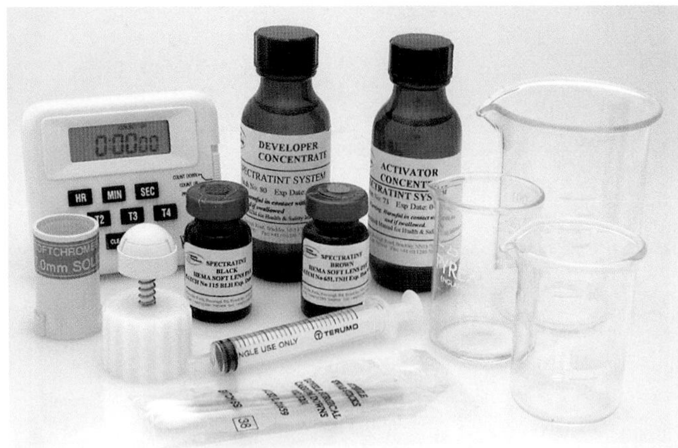

Figure 25.11 Practitioner tinting kit

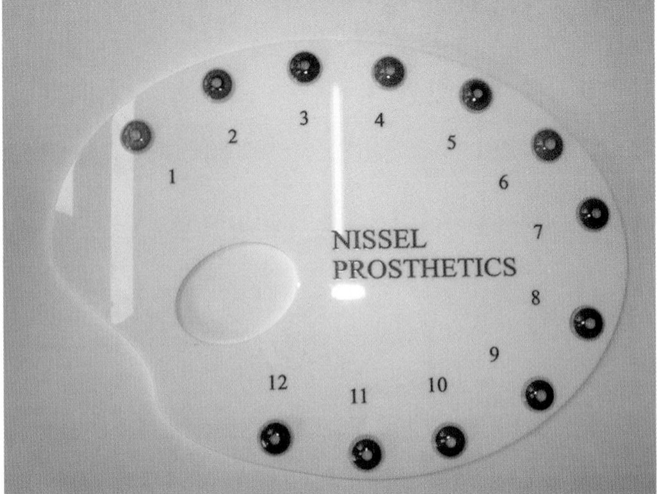

Figure 25.13 Nissel prosthetic palette for matching. (Courtesy of Steve Lennox, Cantor & Nissel, UK)

black, simply to cut down the amount of light entering a photophobic eye.

Tinting lenses is not difficult and only requires the appropriate equipment and dyes (Fig. 25.11).

Nevertheless, experience is needed when dyeing lenses in order to produce a realistic-looking pupil. The depth of colour depends on time, which itself depends on the ambient temperature and the age of the vial of dye (if over a year old, this should be replaced). Depth of colour also depends on water content. Higher-water-content materials are required for darker tints because the large pigment molecules are unable to penetrate the matrix of the lower-water-content materials. Altering the water content will therefore affect the colour of the lens as will changing the material.

For a black pupil on a clear or cosmetic lens:

- Place the lens on a silicone domed tinting jig.
- Mask the required pupil size and inject the black dye into the reservoir.
- Wait 7–8 minutes.
- Remove the mask and rinse the lens under tap water.
- Using separate syringes, measure 2.5 ml of developer and fixer with 5 ml of distilled water.
- Place the tinted lens in a beaker with the pre-mixed developer and fixer solution.
- The developing and fixing process can be speeded up if the beaker is placed in an ultrasound bath. If the room temperature is low, a hotplate should be used.

Dyes can be purchased that are suitable for either 38% hydroxyethyl methacrylate (HEMA) or 58% HEMA polymer lenses. In practice, it is simpler to choose only to use either low- or high-water-content lenses. A low-plus lens is ideal to use for tinting to take advantage of the increase in central thickness (Fig. 25.12). Although it is not yet possible to tint high-Dk silicone hydrogel lenses, such as Bausch & Lomb's PureVision or CIBA's Night & Day, Johnson & Johnson's Acuvue Advance lenses can be tinted.

Hand-painted corneal and soft lenses

Many patients can be fitted with commercial prosthetic or cosmetic lenses or in-office tinted lenses. If neither of these types of lens provides a good match for the normal eye, lenses can be hand-painted to order by the manufacturer. This can be done in one of two ways.

- A photograph or digital image can be sent or emailed to the laboratory. Care is needed to take the photograph in daylight, otherwise the colour rendering can be poor.
- Some laboratories have a palette of iris 'buttons' (Fig. 25.13), which can be matched to the patient's eye and the relevant number of the button sent with the lens order. Descriptive modifications can be made on the order form; for example, 'enhance the green tone' or 'darker ring around pupil'.

These lenses can be made as PMMA semi-scleral lenses (sometimes called a mini-prosthesis – Fig. 25.14) or more commonly in a soft lens.

Because the lenses become thicker with the hand-painted, high-water-content materials are usually used to improve oxygen permeability. Lenses can be made in diameters up to

Figure 25.12 *From left to right*: Contact lens with 4 mm black pupil; brown periphery, clear pupil; black pupil in brown cosmetic lens; clear space filled in with brown dye

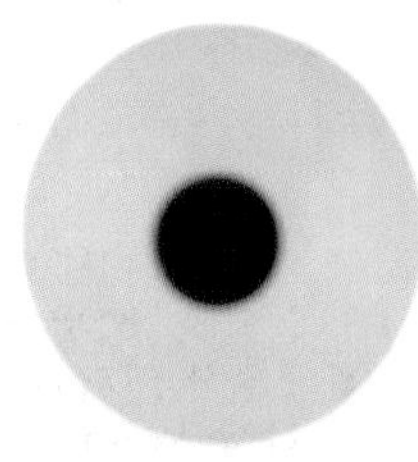

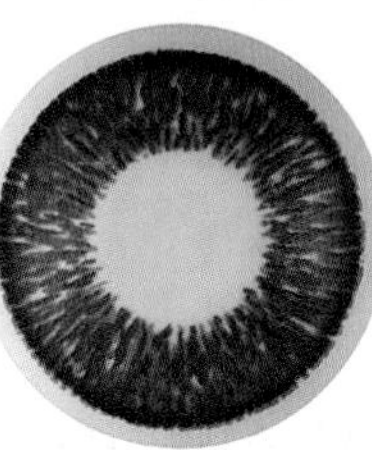

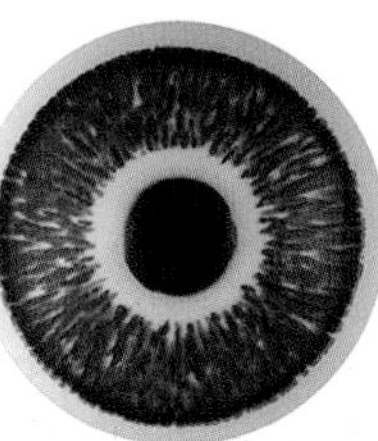

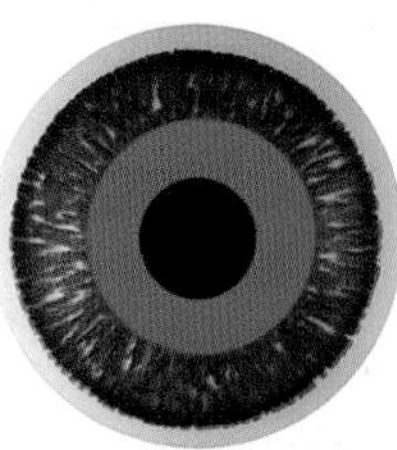

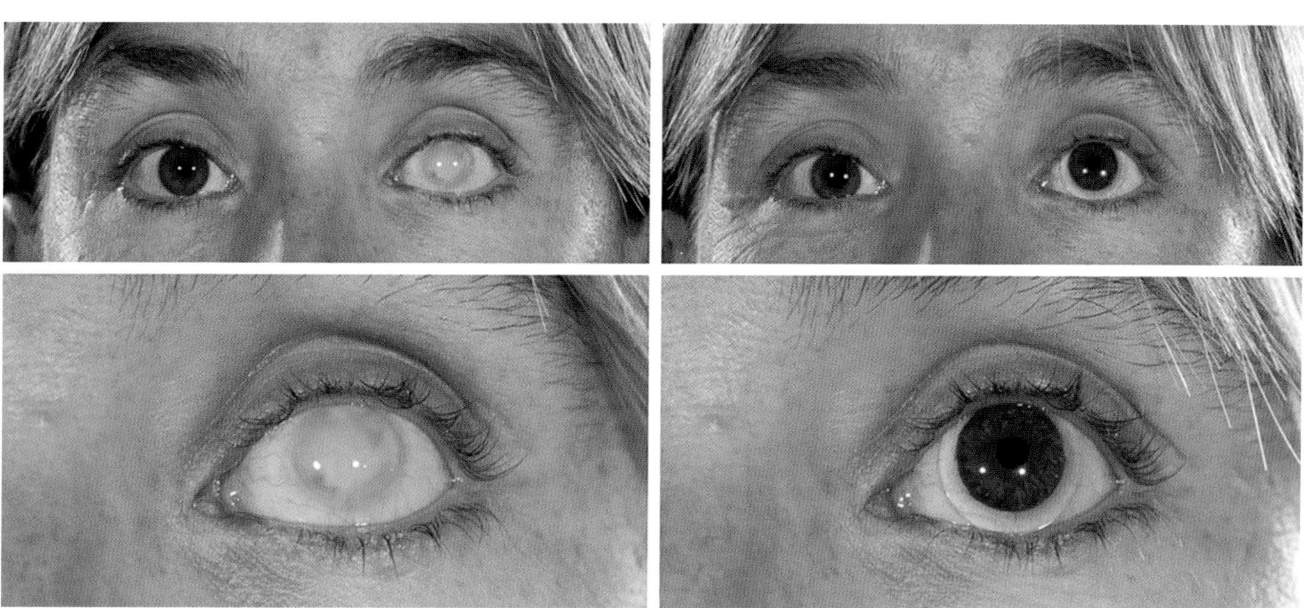

Figure 25.14 Patient fitted with a mini-prosthesis

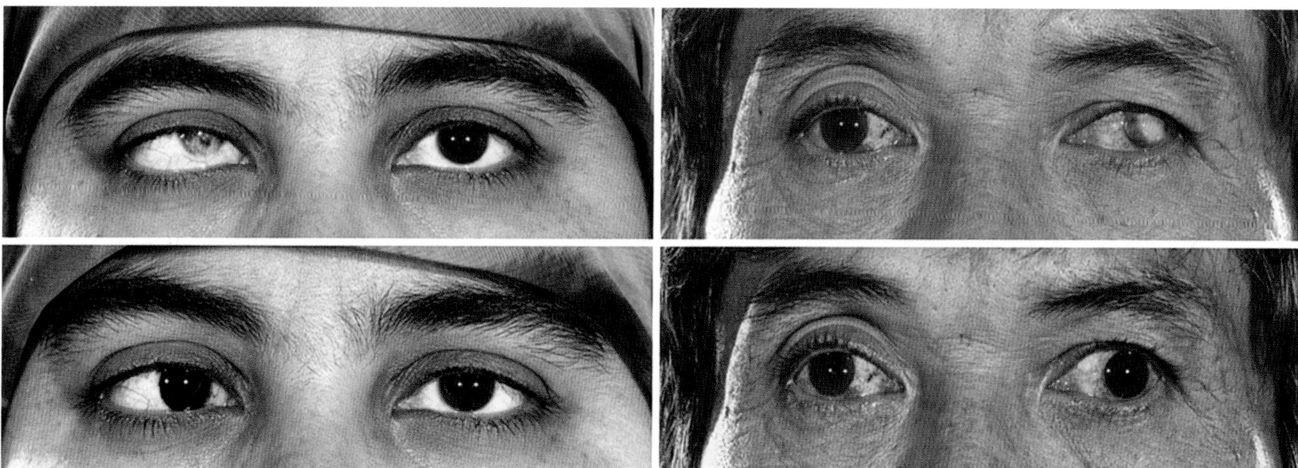

Figure 25.15 Prosthetic lenses in patients with strabismus

24 mm although these large lenses do not always move sufficiently on the eye.

The colour is applied on the front surface of the lens and a chemical reaction used to produce an opaque white pigment in the lens matrix to make the colour look effective. The white area can be extended beyond the iris, if necessary, to mask a discolored sclera.

A number of companies manufacture individual soft prosthetic lenses. These include the Narcissus Foundations and Adventures in Color in the USA, EyCon and UltraVision Capricornia in Australia, and Cantor & Nissel and UltraVision CLPL in the UK.

STRABISMUS

Eyes with poor vision following injury often become divergent. If the eye looks unsightly, a prosthetic lens can make it look more natural, but will not correct the strabismus (Fig. 25.15).

Likewise, amblyopic eyes can be either convergent or divergent and although the eye may appear normal itself, with both eyes open, the patient is very conscious of the appearance. Botulinum toxin injections are commonly used to improve the appearance of a strabismic eye but where surgery is not possible the only option may be a displaced prosthetic lens (Fig. 25.16).

It is possible to mask a squint with a cosmetic scleral shell or a large total diameter (TD) soft lens (16–22 mm) and a displaced 'cornea' (Phillips 1989). Cantor & Nissel (UK) issue an opaque white trial lens (or a clear lens if no scleral tinting is required) which employs dynamic stabilization (i.e. thinned top and bottom) to achieve orientation and stability. It is marked with a dot at the lens top and centre (Fig. 25.17a). This lens is the basis of the prosthetic fitting.

- Insert the lens and allow it to settle fully.
- Check the general fit.
- Lift the lid and note the degree of rotation of the upper dot (Fig. 25.17b).

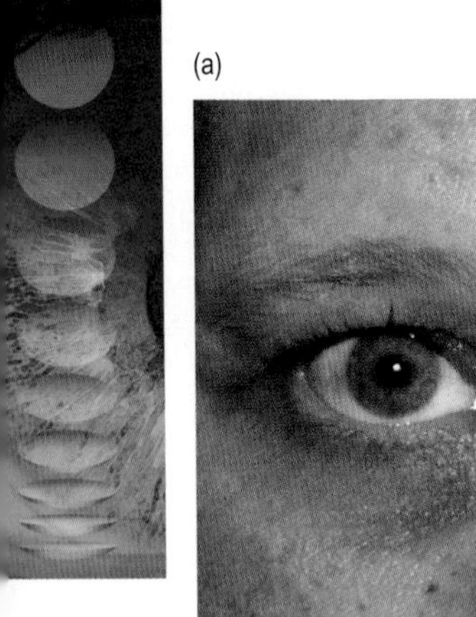

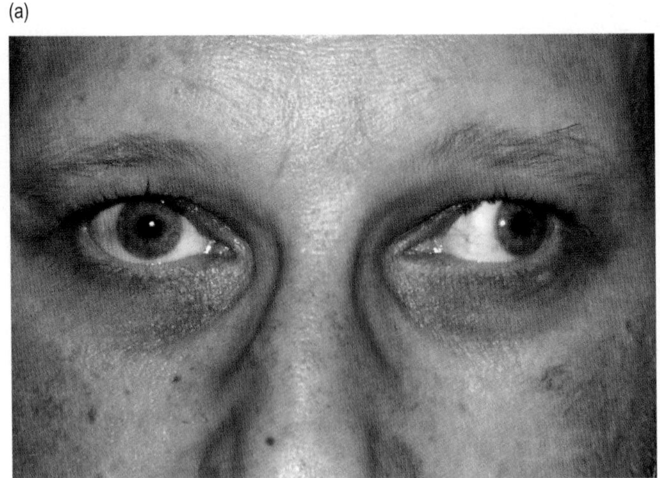

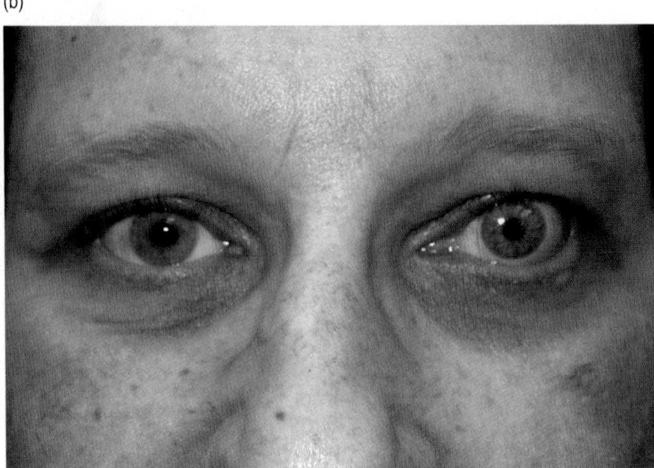

Figure 25.16 (a) Patient with a divergent strabismus; (b) same patient wearing a large cosmetic 74% hydrophilic lens manufactured using the method described in the text and demonstrated in Figure 25.17. (Courtesy of Steve Lennox, Cantor & Nissel, UK)

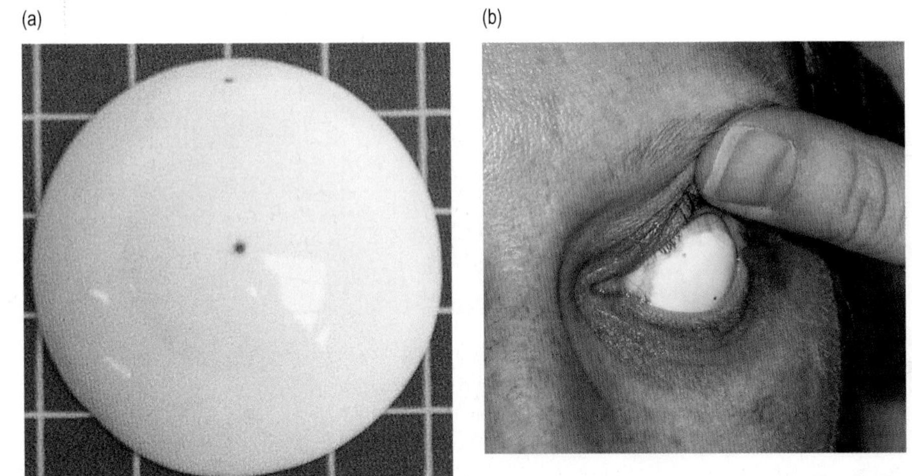

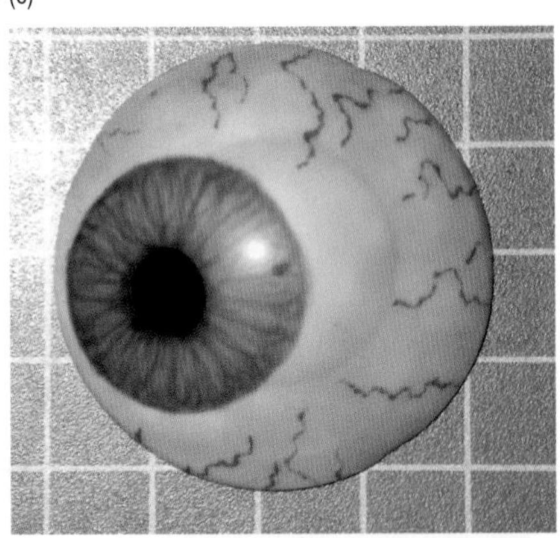

Figure 25.17 (a) Large opaque trial lens marked with dots at the top and in the centre; (b) same lens in situ. (c) Lens manufactured from the measurements taken (see Fig. 25.16b for the final lens in situ). (Courtesy of Steve Lennox, Cantor & Nissel, UK)

- Note the position of the central dot relative to the required position.
- Transmit this information with a good-quality photograph, slide or digital image of the eye to be matched, to the manufacturing laboratory.

The final lens is shown in Figure 25.17c.

DIPLOPIA

Patients with intractable double vision within the central 20° can benefit from a cosmetic lens with a black pupil. However, a large pupil (greater than 7 mm) may be necessary, as light can still enter the eye obliquely behind the prosthetic pupil, causing some diplopic patients great annoyance. An unusually large pupil may be unacceptable cosmetically and an opaque iris may be required.

MICROPHTHALMOS

The microphthalmic eye is invariably amblyopic. A prosthetic lens, matching the fellow eye, can give excellent results, especially if fitted in conjunction with a pair of safety glasses with a plano lens in the normal eye and approximately +3.00 D in front of the microphthalmic eye to enlarge the small eye further (Fig. 25.18) (see also Chapter 24).

ANIRIDIA

Patients with congenital aniridia are very difficult to fit with prosthetic contact lenses. The corneal epithelium is poor due to stem cell deficiency and this, coupled with the negligible oxygen permeability of prosthetic lenses and the desire for long-wearing schedules, can lead to hypoxic corneal stress (see also Chapter 24).

Traumatic or surgical aniridics can benefit from prosthetic lenses. The aniridia may be partial or total, possibly together with aphakia and/or a central scar causing corneal distortion. Visually, these patients benefit most from a rigid lens. Unfortunately, prosthetic PMMA corneal lenses are not always comfortable and often result in hypoxia. A soft iris tint lens can be fitted (Fig. 25.19), together with spectacle over-correction. Alternatively, by using a piggyback prosthetic lens and a

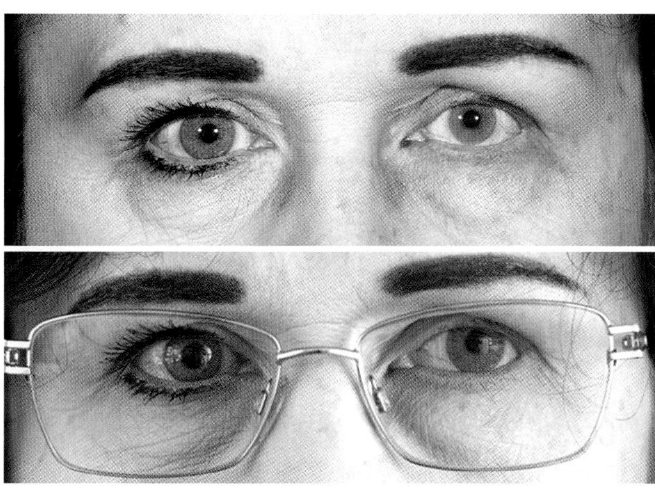

Figure 25.18 (Top) Patient with left microphthalmos and (Bottom) wearing a cosmetic lens and over-spectacles with plano in the right and +3.00 D sphere in the left

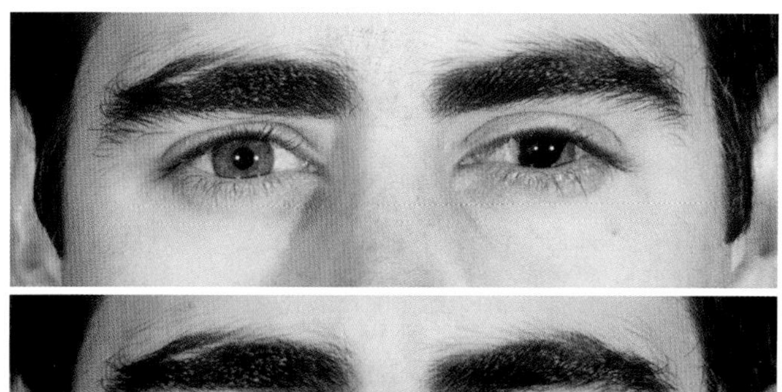

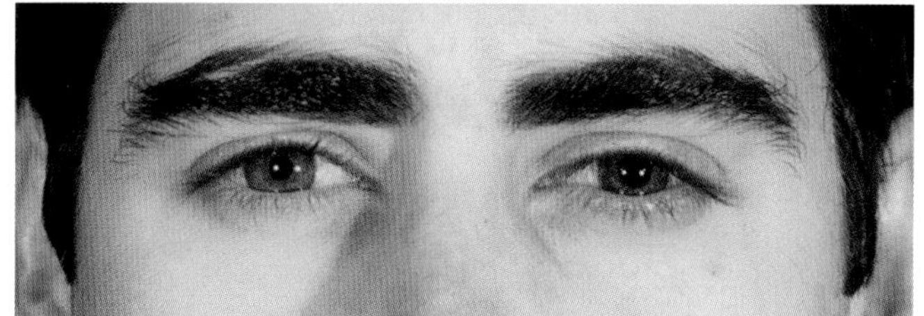

Figure 25.19 (Top) Patient with traumatic iridectomy and (Bottom) with a prosthetic lens

gas-permeable lens, the vision can usually be optimally corrected, while considerably reducing problems of glare and improving the eye's cosmesis. The patient should be encouraged to keep the wearing time down, as the level of hypoxia is likely to induce neovascularization into the scar tissue.

COLOBOMA

Using a stabilized lens, an iris coloboma or iridectomy can be masked using a segment of iris painted onto the lens (Phillips 1990) (Fig. 25.20).

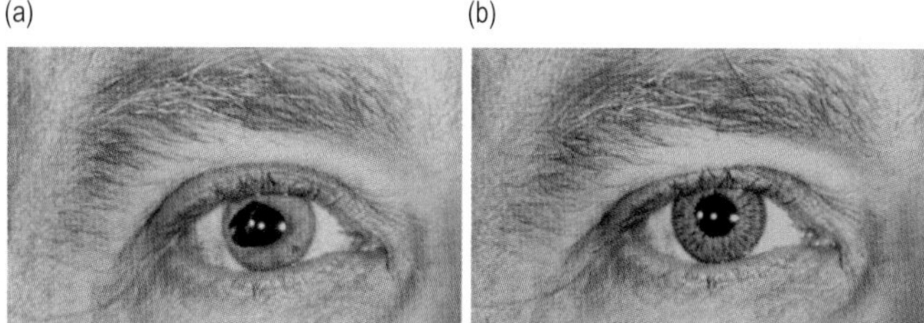

Figure 25.20 (a) A patient with an iridectomy (b) fitted with an iris segment in a prosthetic lens

Scleral prosthetic lenses

In an eye that retains useful vision, where a soft lens is inadvisable and a corneal prosthetic lens will not stabilize on the eye, a transparent scleral lens can be made. This can later have an iris hand-painted onto it to match the normal eye, leaving the pupil area clear for vision.

FITTING AND ORDERING PROSTHETIC LENSES

When fitting prosthetic lenses, care is needed to ensure that there are no adverse reactions. Fit a clear lens first to assess the lens fit and alter it accordingly. This is particularly useful in PMMA lenses where the patient can wear the lenses for a few weeks to make sure that they are comfortable and their vision stable.

The TD in PMMA prosthetic lenses should be made larger than standard (approximately 10.50–11.00 mm) to ensure stability. One or more fenestrations can be incorporated to provide some oxygen transmission.

The fitting requirements of prosthetic lenses are the same as for clear lenses but some extra information should be included on the order.

- Measure the iris diameter of the fellow eye and order it the same.
- Note the iris colour and what type of tint is required (e.g. homogeneous tint or blue dot matrix).
- Measure the diameter of the pupil of the fellow eye in bright and dim illumination and order it halfway between the two. For light-coloured irides a difference in the size of the pupils will be noticeable. Explain this to the patient. Two different lenses can be ordered with different pupil sizes; however, this is very expensive, especially for hand-painted lenses.
- Specify whether a black, clear or tinted pupil is required. As well as reducing glare, a tinted pupil is more natural looking as it softens the demarcation between coloured iris and pupil.
- When re-ordering tinted lenses, keep the lens material the same, otherwise the tint will be different (see p. 526).

LENS CARE

Most currently available soft lens solutions can be used safely with disposable cosmetic contact lenses. However, for prosthetic lenses and tinted lenses that are not thrown away at least monthly, some solutions (although safe) may affect the lens colour – in particular, hydrogen peroxide with long soaking

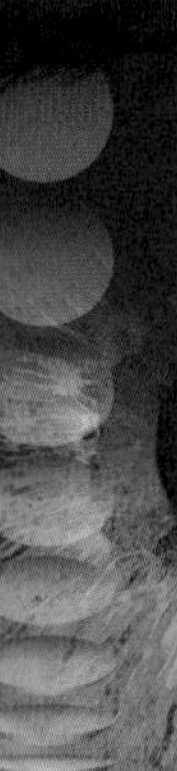

times, and alcohol-based cleaners. Conversely, some opaque tints are *best* stabilized in hydrogen peroxide and advice should always be sought from individual manufacturers.

AFTER-CARE

As with cosmetic lenses, patients must be taught how to look after their lenses. They may find it tempting to overwear their lenses and to wear them even if damaged. At after-care, this advice can be reaffirmed.

The practitioner needs to monitor for signs of hypoxia, especially in a sighted eye, and take action to avoid it. This is not always easy as the best cosmesis may be from lenses with the lowest oxygen transmissibility.

CONCLUSION

The availability of reasonably priced cosmetic lenses and the ease of tinting lenses in practice make the fitting of cosmetic lenses readily available. Prosthetic lens fitting requires time and patience but patients' lives can be substantially enhanced by improving the cosmesis of disfigured eyes.

Acknowledgements

I would like to thank the Photographic Department at the Royal Victorian Eye and Ear Hospital in Melbourne for their help with the illustrations in this chapter. Thanks also to Steve Lennox and Josie Barlow of Cantor & Nissel, UK and, in particular, to Lynne Speedwell.

References

Albarran Diego, C., Montes-Mico, R., Pons, A. M. and Artigas, J. M. (2001) Influence of the luminance level on visual performance with a disposable soft cosmetic tinted contact lens. Ophthalmic Physiol. Opt., 21(5), 411–419

CLACO (1984) Guide to Basic Science and Clinical Practice, 2nd edn, 37.5. Orlando: Grune and Stratton

Dortzbach, R. K. and Woog, J. J. (1985) Choice of procedure. Enucleation, evisceration, or prosthetic fitting over globes. Ophthalmology, 92(9), 1249–1255

Efron, N. (2002) Contact Lens Practice. London: Butterworth-Heinemann

FDA. (2002) Public Health Web Notification: Non-Corrective Decorative Contact Lenses Dispensed without a Prescription. October, 23

Gasson, A. and Morris, J. (2003) Lenses for presbyopia. In The Contact Lens Manual: A Practical Fitting Guide, 3rd edn, eds. A. Gasson and J. Morris. London: Butterworth-Heinemann

Greenspoon, M. K. (1969) History of the cinematic uses of cosmetic contact lenses. Am. J. Optom. Arch. Am. Acad. Optom., 46(1), 63–67

Gagnon, M. R. and Walter, K. A. (2006) A case of Acanthamoeba as a result of a cosmetic contact lens. Eye Contact Lens, 32(1), 37–38

Josephson, J. E. and Caffery, B. E. (1987) Visual field loss with colored hydrogel lenses. Am. J. Optom. Physiol. Opt., 64(1), 38–40

Lawrence, A. W. (1972) Greek and Roman Culture, p. 38. London: Jonathan Cape

Lubin, J. R., Albert, D. M. and Weinstein, M. (1980) Sixty-five years of sympathetic ophthalmia. A clinicopathologic review of 105 cases (1913–1978). Ophthalmology, 87(2), 109–121

Nakagawara, V. B., Montgomery, R. W. and Wood K. J. (2002) Aviation accidents and incidents associated with the use of ophthalmic devices by civilian airmen. Aviat. Space Environ. Med., 73(11), 1109–1113

Ozkagnici, A., Zengin, N., Kamis, O. and Gunduz, K. (2003) Do daily wear opaquely tinted hydrogel soft contact lenses affect contrast sensitivity function at one meter? Eye Contact Lens, 29(1), 48–49

Phillips, A. J. (1989) The use of a displaced, tinted zone, prosthetic hydrogel lens in the cosmetic improvement of a strabismic, scarred cornea. Clin. Exp. Optom., 72(1), 1–2

Phillips, A. J. (1990) Iris coloboma managed with a prosthetic contact lens: a case report and review. Clin. Exp. Optom., 73(2), 55–57

Pullum, K. (1997) The role of scleral lenses in modern contact lens practice. In Contact Lenses, 4th edn, pp. 566–608, eds. A. J. Phillips and L. Speedwell. Oxford: Butterworth-Heinemann

Steinemann, T. L., Pinninti, U., Szczotka, L. B., Eiferman, R. A. and Price, F. W. Jr (2003) Ocular complications associated with the use of cosmetic contact lenses from unlicensed vendors. Eye Contact Lens, 29(4), 196–200

Thordarson, U., Ragnarsson, A. T. and Gudbrandsson, B. (1979) Ocular trauma. Observation in 105 patients. Acta Ophthalmol. (Copenhagen), 57(5), 922–928

Tonkellaar, D., Henkes, H. E. and Van Leersum, G. K. (1991) Herman Snellen (1834–1908) and Muller's 'Reform-Auge'. Doc. Ophthalmol., 77, 349–354

Voetz, S. C., Collins, M. J. and Lingelbach, B. (2004) Recovery of corneal topography and vision following opaque-tinted contact lens wear. Eye Contact Lens, 30(2), 111–117

www.abs.gov.au – Australian Bureau of Statistics

www.austroads.com.au – Association of Australian and New Zealand road transport and traffic authorities

www.medicareaustralia.gov.au – Medicare Australia (formerly Health Insurance Commission)

www.visionaustralia.org.au – Vision Australia Foundation

Zimmerman, L. E. and McLean, I. W. (1975) Changing concepts of the prognosis and management of small malignant melanomas of the choroid (Montgomery Lecture). Trans. Ophthalmol. Soc. UK, 95(4), 487–494

Chapter 26

Contact lenses in other abnormal ocular conditions

Sheila B. Hickson-Curran

CHAPTER CONTENTS

INTRODUCTION

Contact lenses are now well established in the field of ophthalmology as useful devices to assist in the treatment of many ocular conditions. When lenses are fitted primarily to protect or promote healing of the cornea, rather than to provide refractive correction, they are known as therapeutic or bandage lenses. Soft lenses (conventional and silicone hydrogel) provide the majority of therapeutic lens applications, but other lens modalities also have a role. Although the application of a contact lens to a diseased cornea seems to be a contraindication, the idea of introducing a foreign body to an eye in order to act as an ocular bandage is not new. In the first century AD, Celsus was purported to have applied honey-soaked linen to the conjunctival fornices to prevent symblepharon formation following pterygium removal.

In modern times, scleral lenses were the first lens type to be used as a protective device in diseased or injured tissues (Ridley 1962) and these lenses are still widely used for therapeutic purposes, particularly in patients for whom other lens types have failed (see Chapter 15). Gas-permeable scleral lenses are a more recent development (Ezekiel 1983) and their introduction has at least partially eliminated some of the hypoxic problems encountered with conventional scleral lenses, giving them new therapeutic applications (Schein et al. 1989).

In 1970, Gassett and Kaufman published the first report of hydrogel lens use for therapeutic purposes, and the introduction in the late 1990s of silicone hydrogel lenses added a further option (see Chapter 10). The high oxygen transmissibility of these lenses offers theoretical advantages over conventional hydrogels and have been successfully used for therapeutic applications in a variety of ocular surface disorders and postsurgical cases (Lim et al 2001).

THERAPEUTIC MECHANISMS OF CONTACT LENSES

Contact lenses can act as a therapeutic device by a variety of different mechanisms.

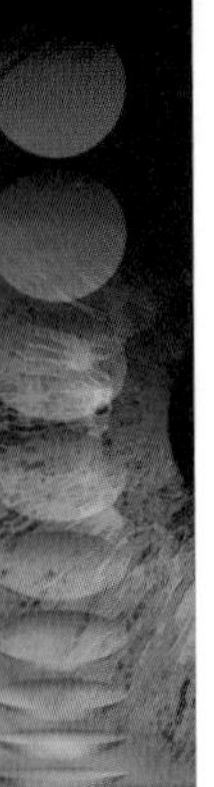

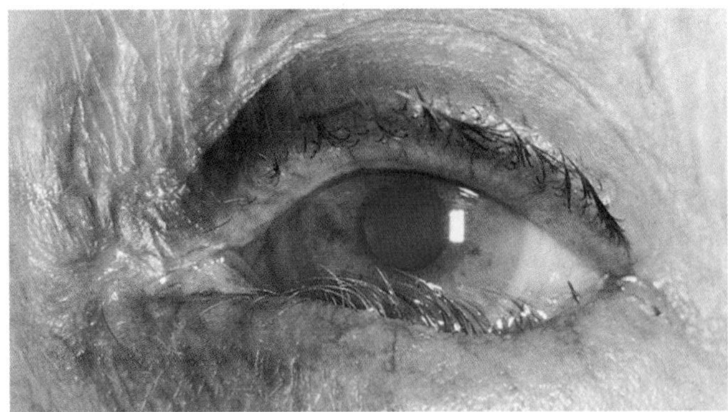

Figure 26.1 Severe entropion and trichiasis associated with blepharitis. A bandage soft lens allowed regeneration of damaged corneal epithelium and prevented further disturbance prior to surgery. (Courtesy of D. Westerhout)

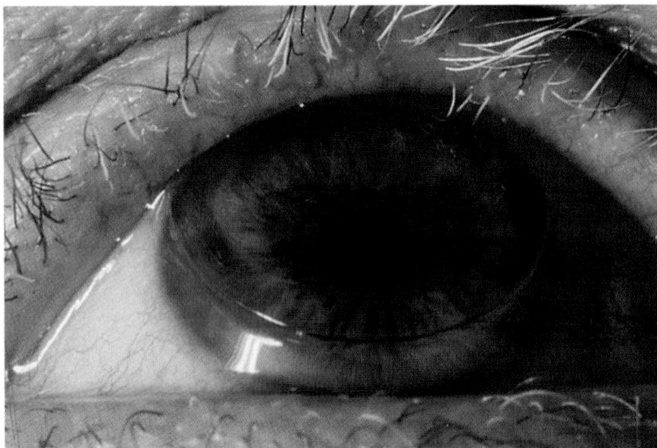

Figure 26.2 Trichiasis with RGP prescription lens. The lens sat superiorly on the cornea, thus protecting it from the misaligned lashes. (Courtesy of L. Speedwell)

Mechanical effects

- As a mechanical barrier
  - where eyelid loss or dysfunction leads to exposure keratitis.
  - in trichiasis where the presence of a contact lens protects the cornea from trauma caused by the lashes (Figs 26.1, 26.2).
  - in conditions where re-epithelialization is taking place a lens can protect the new tissue from the 'windshield wiper' effect of the eyelids.
- As a splint
  - in corneal perforation or where a descemetocele has formed, a contact lens can act as a splint providing structural support to these weak areas.

Symptom relief

- To alleviate symptoms in conditions such as bullous keratopathy (Fig. 26.3), the presence of a lens alleviates pain.

Adjunct to healing

- To assist healing in conditions such as recurrent epithelial erosions and persistent epithelial defects. The lens permits re-epithelialization to occur beneath it and protects vulnerable new epithelial cells from lid action.

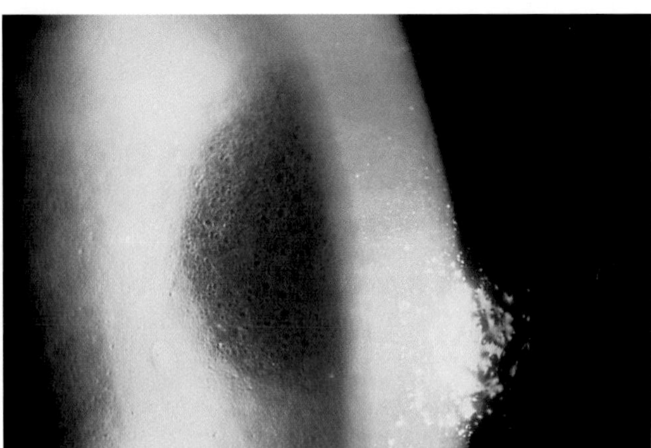

Figure 26.3 Bullous keratopathy. (Courtesy of A. J. Phillips)

Drug delivery

Hydrogel lenses may be used to deliver ophthalmic drugs to the eye. They allow a variety of different drugs to remain in contact with the ocular tissues for longer periods than with topical application.

Maintaining corneal hydration

Therapeutic soft lenses can be used to maintain corneal hydration in severe dry eye conditions, together with regular instillation of ocular lubricants.

Scleral lenses can maintain a fluid reservoir underneath the lens which is useful in dry eye conditions when the tear film is supplemented by ocular lubricants.

SELECTION OF THERAPEUTIC LENSES

Selection of an appropriate therapeutic lens requires an understanding of the primary ocular disorder as well as the available therapeutic lens types and their effects on the cornea.

Lenses can affect corneal physiology in three ways:

- By inducing variable degrees of hypoxia.
- By altering the tear film distribution over the corneal surface.
- By inducing low-grade mechanical trauma to the corneal epithelium.

The ideal lens fit minimizes these effects while aiding the recovery of the condition under treatment.

- It should allow the maximum possible oxygen to reach the cornea except in the case of a blind eye where comfort becomes the primary concern (see 'Lens fitting', below). High oxygen permeability is particularly important for therapeutic applications where the primary aim is corneal healing.
- Adequate lens movement is important but, if excessive, it will exacerbate any pain.

- Physiological considerations are of particular importance because, in most cases, therapeutic lenses are worn continuously.

Also to be considered is the desired mechanism of the therapeutic lens and the primary ocular condition under treatment. For example, if the therapeutic goal is protection and healing of the corneal epithelium, hypoxic complications should be avoided and an optimum fit achieved. Foulks et al. (2003) suggested that a silicone hydrogel lens may be the best option.

In summary, general fitting principles should always apply when choosing an appropriate lens for therapeutic purposes and each case should be considered individually. Appropriate caution should be applied so that the lens fits well and acts in the intended manner.

LENS MATERIALS AND FITTING (see also Chapters 10 and 13)

The oxygen permeability of hydrogel lenses depends on water content and thickness.

The first generation of silicone hydrogel lenses had much lower water contents than most conventional hydrogel lenses and, therefore, a higher modulus or 'stiffness'. However, the incorporation of silicone resulted in extremely high levels of oxygen transmissibility, 5–10 times greater than low-Dk disposable hydrogels (Compan et al. 2002). The newer silicone hydrogels, used for daily wear, have a much higher water content (comparable to conventional water content hydrogels) and are much less stiff. The materials maintain flexibility, hydration and oxygen transmissibility nearly three times that of a conventional hydrogel (Steffen & Schnider 2004). The centre thicknesses of silicone hydrogel lenses range from 0.07 to 0.09 mm.

Lens design and manufacturing technique affect how a lens centres and moves on the eye. Small changes in back optic zone radius (BOZR) have less influence on lens movement and centration in moulded lenses than in lathe-cut and some silicone hydrogel lenses. With these, steeper BOZR fit more tightly than lenses with flatter back optic radii made to the same total diameter (TD) and design.

Excessive lens movement of a therapeutic lens may retard healing of the epithelial surface or cause pain (e.g. in bullous keratopathy) and such a lens may displace or fall out of the eye. Conversely, tight lenses can induce oedema and discomfort and trap cellular debris behind the lens, which can break down to release toxic substances that, in turn, could lead to an inflammatory response (Zantos & Holden 1978, Mertz & Holden 1981).

As with all soft lens fitting, the TD should be large enough to cover the limbus completely and provide optimum movement during versions. Some conditions, however, need particularly large lenses (e.g. a leaking filtration bleb) or are required to aid the healing process of a peripheral corneal lesion.

Disposable hydrogel contact lenses

Disposable lenses have been used extensively as therapeutic devices to treat a wide variety of conditions such as recurrent corneal erosions, filamentary keratitis, bullous keratopathy and neuroparalytic keratitis (Weinstock 1990, Gruber 1991, Sulewski et al. 1991, Tanner & DePaolis 1992). They offer many advantages over conventional hydrogel lenses when used for therapeutic purposes. In particular, their low cost allows regular replacement so excessive lens spoilation is prevented. However, these lenses still carry the risks of conventional lenses such as hypoxia and infectious keratitis, and some are not labelled for use in diseased eyes.

Silicone hydrogel lenses

Conventional hydrogel contact lenses have been the most common type of lens used for therapeutic purposes (Rubinstein 2003) but their oxygen transmissibility does not meet the minimum level required to avoid corneal swelling in overnight wear (Holden & Mertz 1984, Harvitt & Bonnano 1999). Since most therapeutic lenses are worn overnight, this is a significant limitation.

The high oxygen transmissibility of silicone hydrogel lenses has made them an increasingly popular choice for therapeutic applications. Even before these lenses received CE Mark and US Food and Drug Administration approval for therapeutic use, they were already widely prescribed on an 'off-label' basis (Foulks et al. 2003) and are now among the most popular choices for bandage lenses (Karlgard et al. 2004).

Advantages

- High oxygen transmissibility.
- Low water content of silicone hydrogels reduces dependence on tear quality and quantity (Ehrlich 2001) and makes them less prone to dehydration (Lim et al. 2001).
- Surface treatment or internal wetting agents render the lens surface hydrophilic and helps to resist deposition.
- Fluid transport helps prevent binding and facilitates lens movement (Edwards & Atkins 2002, Fonn et al. 2002).
- Less binding of *Pseudomonas aeruginosa* results in lower levels of corneal epithelial thinning and less effect on tear lactate dehydrogenase (Ren et al. 2002), factors that may contribute to reduce corneal infections.

Several studies have investigated the therapeutic use of silicone hydrogel lenses. Lim et al. (2001) evaluated balafilcon A lenses (PureVision, Bausch & Lomb) in subjects with a variety of corneal and ocular surface diseases and concluded that the lenses showed good performance and therapeutic efficacy.

Kanpolat and Ucakhan (2003) found that lotrafilcon A lenses were safe and effective in patients requiring bandage contact lens use for ocular surface disorders and observed that infrequent replacement of these lenses was especially advantageous in patients for whom lens insertion and removal may be associated with epithelial trauma, pain and a potential increase in infection risk. Ambroziak et al. (2004) reported that lotrafilcon A lenses were effective and well tolerated in selected therapeutic cases and Szaflik et al. (2004) found that these lenses offered advantages over conventional hydrogels when used as a bandage after laser-assisted subepithelial keratomileusis (LASEK) surgery.

Randleman et al. (2003) and O'Donnell and Maldonado-Codina (2004) described cases where a high-Dk rigid gas-permeable (RGP) lens was fitted over a silicone hydrogel lens in a piggyback system for therapeutic purposes (see Chapter 20).

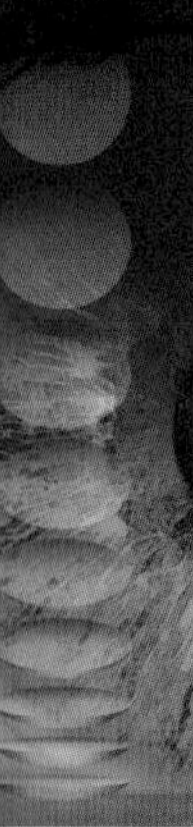

Silicone rubber lenses

Silicone rubber lenses have played an important role in therapeutic lens work in the past as the material is highly oxygen permeable and does not require the hydration of a soft lens. Indications for silicone rubber lenses include keratinized mucous membranes, trichiasis and incomplete lid closure (Woodward 1979). Plano lenses are not currently available, which has greatly reduced the use of this material but some of those patients may now be able to wear silicone hydrogel lenses. Where silicone rubber is the only option in a seeing eye, a prescription lens can be fitted with the addition of a spectacle over-correction.

Scleral lenses

Scleral lenses have been used for therapeutic purposes for over 100 years and in cases of dry eyes with cicatricial tissue, no other lens is as useful. Their main drawback is that of convenience. Impression sclerals are time consuming to fit and require special equipment and expertise although preformed RGP scleral lenses are more straightforward (see Chapter 15 on fitting techniques).

Corneal lenses

Occasionally, a rigid lens may be used for such conditions as trichiasis (see Fig. 26.2), lid keratinization or multiple palpebral concretions. The lenses may become scratched with use and should be polished or replaced at regular intervals.

Collagen bandage lenses

Collagen degrades in a foreign biological environment and eventually disappears, leaving no permanent residue. This property lends itself to many medical applications such as dissolving sutures, in dressings for burns, and injections for facial augmentation. In ophthalmology, uses of collagen include scleral buckling devices, lacrimal drainage plugs and external eye patches.

At present, collagen shields are not available but in the past were used successfully to treat many corneal disorders and to promote wound healing after anterior segment surgery (DePaolis et al. 1987, Aquavella et al. 1988, Ruffini et al. 1989).

PATIENT FOLLOW-UP

After-care is particularly important because the risks of contact lens complications are greater in a compromised eye than a healthy eye. After-care provides an opportunity to review the condition under treatment and to exchange any bandage lens. Many gross corneal conditions can be examined through the lens but extra care should be employed when inserting or removing lenses.

The frequency of appointments depends on the condition and the patient. Astin (1989) suggested initial after-care after 1 day, 3–7 days, 1 month and 2–3 months depending on the progress of the condition. Needless to say, each patient and condition should be assessed individually to ensure adequate monitoring.

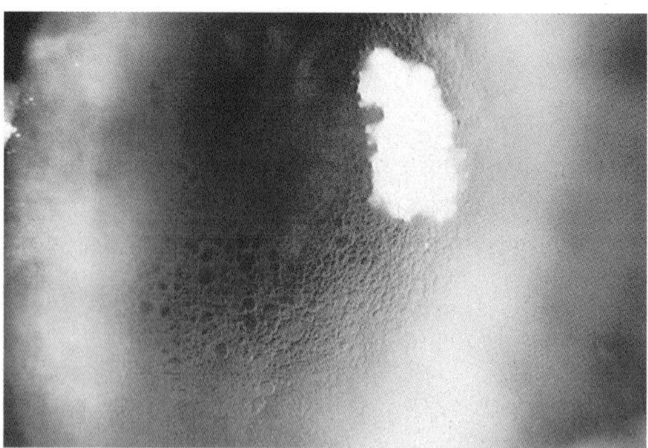

Figure 26.4 Bullous keratopathy. (Courtesy of C. McMonnies)

CONDITIONS THAT CAN BENEFIT FROM THE USE OF THERAPEUTIC CONTACT LENSES

Bullous keratopathy

Condition

A condition of chronic corneal oedema, caused by endothelial dysfunction, characterized by symptoms of pain, epiphora, blepharospasm and photophobia. The cornea is totally or partially involved and appears hazy or opaque due to the severe oedema, which also reduces vision. Small fluid-filled vesicles, known as bullae, form in the epithelium and rupture on the corneal surface (Figs 26.3, 26.4). The severe pain experienced by patients with this condition is thought to be due to exposure of nerve endings once bullae rupture, or stretching of nerve endings due to acute swelling of the epithelium (Liebowitz & Rosenthal 1971a).

Lens type

Hydrophilic lenses may provide almost immediate relief as well as significant visual improvement, particularly in less severe and recent-onset cases which mainly affect the epithelium (Gasset & Kaufman 1970, 1971a, Liebowitz & Rosenthal 1971a, Takahashi & Liebowitz 1971, Høvding 1984, Rehim & Samy 1989). Prescription lenses can be fitted to correct the refractive error as well as improve the comfort, for example to aphakic patients (Fig. 26.5) (Speedwell 1991); however, where gross stromal oedema and Descemet's folds are present, the visual improvement may be minimal (Liebowitz & Rosenthal 1971a).

Lenses are worn on a continuous-wear schedule because pain recurs immediately the lenses are removed. The duration of lens wear varies, depending on the severity of the condition, but may be permanent, as surgery may be contraindicated due to underlying ocular pathology or patient age.

Lens fitting

The guiding parameter is patient comfort, although any neovascularization in an eye with visual potential may affect the

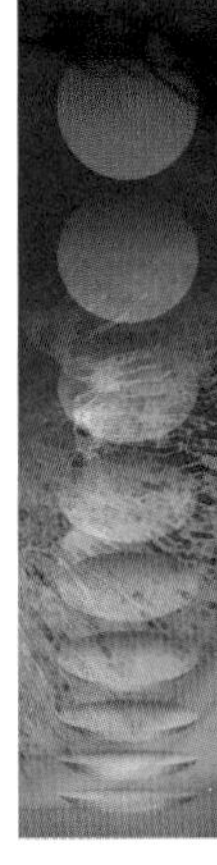

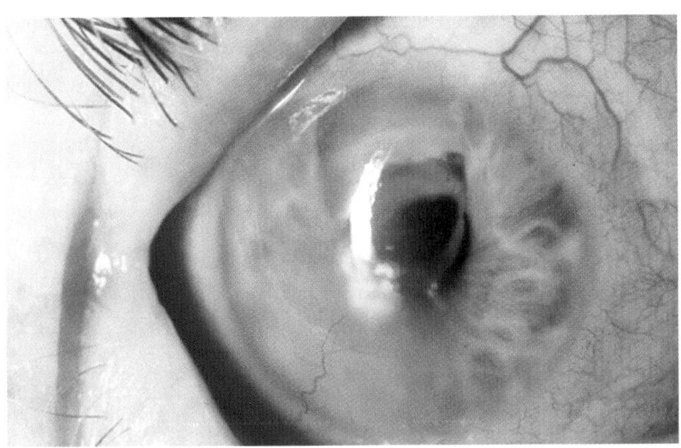

Figure 26.5 Aphakia with bullous keratopathy. This eye was fitted with an extended-wear high-water-content aphakic soft contact lens which acted as a bandage and gave the patient a visual acuity of 6/12. (Courtesy of L. Speedwell)

success of a future penetrating keratoplasty. Hence, when choosing a lens, the oxygen transmissibility should be considered and a silicone hydrogel lens may be the best choice. Two studies described the use of silicone hydrogel lenses for therapeutic purposes in bullous keratopathy (Montero et al. 2003, Ambroziak et al. 2004). Some patients find the stiffness of silicone hydrogel materials makes them less comfortable than conventional hydrogels, but second-generation lenses are much more comfortable.

Alternative treatment

Hypertonic saline on its own or in conjunction with therapeutic lenses.

Fuchs' endothelial dystrophy

Condition

A slowly progressive disorder characterized by bilateral dysfunction of the corneal endothelium, which leads eventually to corneal oedema and bullous keratopathy.

Lens type

Hydrophilic bandage lenses may be used to relieve pain, often until penetrating keratoplasty can be carried out. Kanpolat and Ucakhan (2003) included two cases of Fuchs' endothelial dystrophy among patients fitted with lotrafilcon A lenses for therapeutic use (see also Fig. 25.10).

Lens fitting

As bullous keratopathy (see above).

Alternative treatment

Treatments include the use of hypertonic drops and ointment and the use of a hairdryer directed at the eyes for a few minutes each morning in an attempt to increase tear evaporation and draw fluid from the eye.

Recurrent corneal erosions

Condition

These occur in many different conditions including certain stromal dystrophies, and some viral or bacterial infections. The most common cause is mild trauma to the cornea (such as a child's finger in a parent's eye), which can result in a chronic recurrence of the erosion (recurrent erosion syndrome). This can lead to chronic, intermittent attacks of painful epithelial cell loss lasting for several months due to incomplete reformation of the underlying basement membrane.

Lens type

Soft bandage lenses allow healing and re-epithelialization by protecting the delicate regenerating epithelium from the windshield wiper effect of the lids. Once epithelialization is complete, the hydrogel lens allows the epithelial layer to stabilize and provides optimum conditions for hemidesmosomal formation, which can take many months to regenerate completely (Gipson et al. 1989). The lenses therefore need to be worn for long periods to ensure healing is complete, and as epithelial detachment generally occurs during the night or immediately on waking, lenses should be worn on a continuous basis.

Disposable contact lenses are a good option to treat recurrent erosions and offer a convenient and cost-effective alternative to conventional hydrogel lenses (Weinstock 1990, Gruber 1991, Tanner & DePaolis 1992, Levy & Nguyen 1993). Ambroziak et al. (2004) found that 15 of their 19 cases of 'non-healing' corneal erosions or postoperative keratoepitheliopathy showed full corneal healing when fitted with silicone hydrogel lenses. Both of these studies used the lotrafilcon A lens.

Again, second-generation silicone hydrogels are more comfortable.

Alternative treatment

Ocular lubricants, hypertonic agents, topical antibiotics, mydriatics. Phototherapeutic keratectomy (PTK). Occasionally mechanical debridement and pressure patching may also be helpful but the healing period may last for several days and is associated with continuing pain and further disability from the dressing.

Anterior membrane dystrophies

Condition

Recurrent erosions from intermittent epithelial breakdown are common in epithelial dystrophies such as map-dot-fingerprint and Reis-Buckler, or stromal dystrophies such as lattice dystrophy.

Lens type

As recurrent erosions (see above).

Thygeson's superficial punctate keratitis

Condition

A rare corneal condition characterized by distinctive central corneal lesions in the absence of conjunctival inflammation

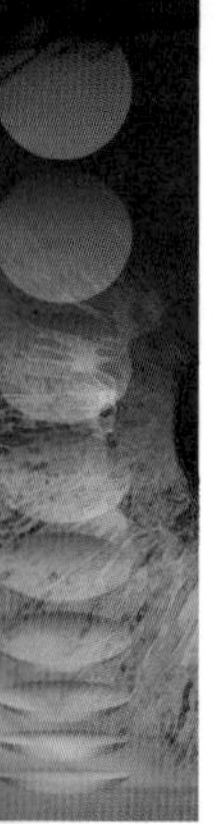

(a)

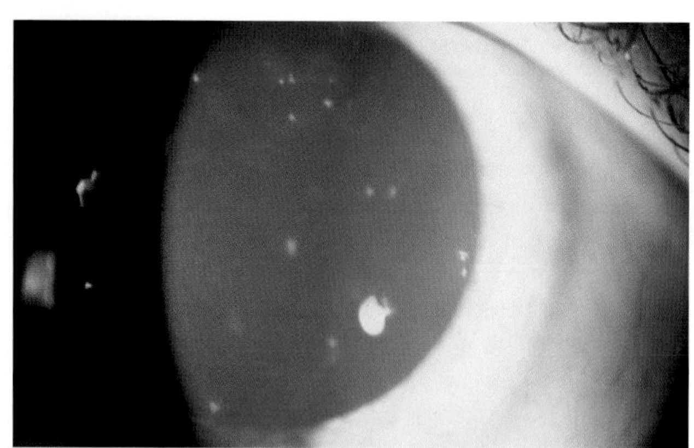

(b)

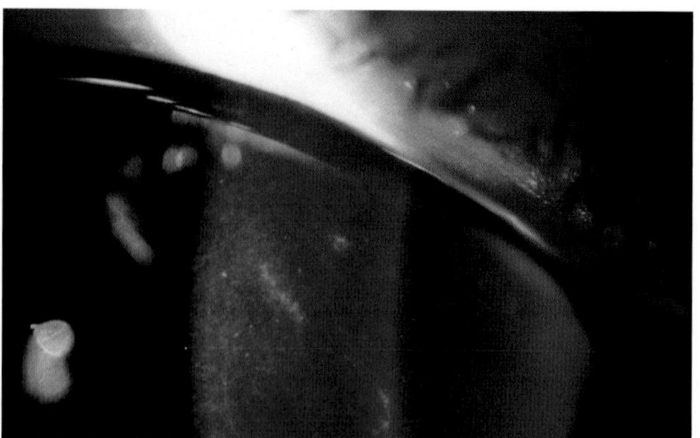

Figure 26.6 (a) Thygeson's superficial punctate keratitis showing corneal infiltrates. The patient in (b) was fitted bilaterally with extended-wear ultrathin therapeutic lenses as the eyes were too painful to remove the lenses while the infiltrates were present. The patient had previously used steroid drops to no avail. The eyes immediately became more comfortable and the lenses were removed a few weeks later. (Courtesy of (a) A. J. Phillips and (b) L. Speedwell)

(Fig. 26.6). It is generally chronic and typified by periods of exacerbation and remission lasting for weeks or months at a time (Thygeson 1950, Marshall and Holdeman 1992).

It is bilateral and asymmetric, with each eye presenting a different clinical picture at any time (Thygeson 1961). During the active phase of the condition, patients complain of photophobia, foreign body sensation, tearing, and possibly decreased vision, depending on the site of the lesions. Symptoms may be disproportionately severe in relation to the clinical picture. Biomicroscopic examination reveals distinctive stellate or snowflake-like infiltrates in the corneal epithelium. The epithelial surface is raised over the lesions, creating an irregular corneal area that stains incompletely with fluorescein dye. It is this irregularity that results in reduced visual acuity. During remission, patients are asymptomatic and the corneal lesions appear as flat, faint grey opacities or may be completely absent.

Lens type

Soft bandage lenses relieve symptoms and can also improve the optical characteristics of the irregular corneal surface and hence improve visual acuity (Forstot & Binder 1979, Goldberg et al. 1980). In particular, ultrathin, low-water-content hydrogels alleviate symptoms (Speedwell 1991) and silicone hydrogels can also prove beneficial (Caroline & Andre 2001).

Filamentary keratitis

Condition

A condition in which fine threads of mucin and corneal epithelium, which are attached at their base to the surrounding epithelium, form (Fig. 26.7). Symptoms usually consist of foreign body sensation and pain. It is associated with keratoconjunctivitis sicca, superior limbic keratoconjunctivitis and systemic disorders such as rheumatoid disease (Kowalik & Rakes 1991).

The exact cause is unknown but the filament formation occurs when there is damage to the basal epithelial cells, epithelial basement membrane or Bowman's layer with subsequent focal epithelial basement membrane detachment. This results in a slightly elevated area that acts as a receptor site for mucus produced by the eye, which in turn attracts loose epithelial cells and debris, thus forming a filament (Zaidman et al. 1985).

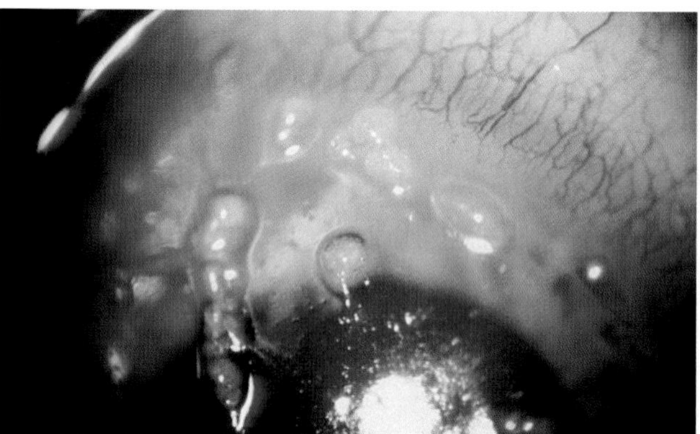

Figure 26.7 Severe filamentary keratitis. (Courtesy of A. J. Phillips)

Lens type

A soft bandage lens protects the epithelial surface from the shearing effect of the eyelids and offers protection from further trauma to any damaged areas of epithelial basement membrane. However, they are not ideal in dry eyes. Low-water-content silicone hydrogels are more useful as treatment. The basal epithelial cells can then reattach to the epithelial basement membrane, preventing the formation of elevated receptor sites for further filament formation. Ocular lubricants are used in conjunction with the lenses and the lower water content of silicone hydrogels can prove useful as treatment.

Alternative treatment

Mechanical removal of filaments, the application of 0.5% silver nitrate solution, hypertonic agents.

Persistent epithelial defects and stromal ulceration

Condition

Persistent epithelial defects (PED) can have numerous different aetiologies including:

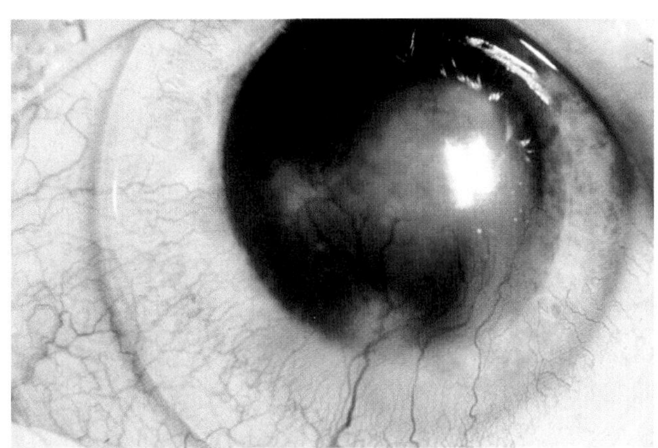

Figure 26.8 Healed herpes ulcer after treatment with a hydrogel bandage lens. (Courtesy of L. V. Prasad Eye Institute)

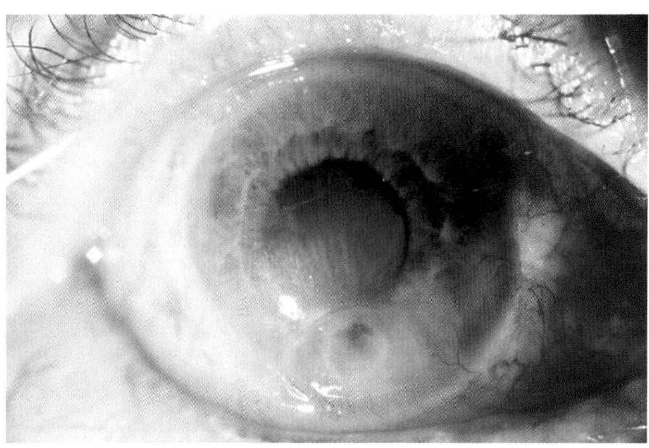

Figure 26.9 Neurotrophic keratopathy. (Courtesy of A. J. Phillips)

- Bacterial, viral or fungal corneal infections.
- Following chemical or thermal burns.
- As a result of poor healing after surgery.
- In association with neuroparalytic keratitis.

PED frequently follows herpes simplex virus (HSV) where an epithelial defect results either from a geographic ulcer during the active viral disease or from epithelial breakdown over an area previously damaged by HSV.

An epithelial defect can result from toxicity of topical antiviral agents (McDermott & Chandler 1989).

Lens type

Soft bandage lenses are occasionally used to protect the epithelium, allowing it to regenerate. However, wearing a soft bandage lens in cases of HSV can exacerbate the condition and it can then be difficult to differentiate between lesions from the disease and a PED.

Indolent corneal ulcers

Condition

A long-standing corneal ulcer that does not heal.

Lens type

A hydrophilic lens protects the corneal surface from lid trauma and splints the healing epithelium (Fig. 26.8). They reduce pain and allow rapid epithelialization (Liebowitz & Rosenthal 1971b, Høvding 1984). After several months of well-monitored soft lens bandage treatment, the cornea has usually healed well and in some cases useful vision can be restored.

Once fully healed, an RGP lens can be fitted to improve the vision in a scarred irregular cornea.

Alternative treatment

Tarsorrhaphy or (in the past) enucleation.

Neuroparalytic and neurotrophic conditions

Condition

Fifth or seventh cranial nerve damage can lead to neurotrophic keratopathy or neuroparalytic keratitis. When damage to the sensory branch of the fifth cranial nerve (e.g. by a virus) results in an anaesthetic cornea, it can lead to neurotrophic keratopathy (Fig. 26.9). The loss of neural influences affects epithelial mitosis that in turn leads to exfoliation and oedema of the corneal epithelium. This can occur even if the blink reflex and lacrimal secretions are normal.

In seventh nerve paralysis, incomplete eyelid closure can lead to exposure keratitis that manifests initially as punctate epithelial erosions but can eventually lead to corneal ulceration.

Lens type

Espy (1971) reported that patients with fifth nerve lesions and neurotrophic keratitis could be treated successfully with hydrophilic bandage lenses, resulting in complete clearing of epithelial irregularities and associated visual improvement. Great care is needed when fitting any type of lens to an anaesthetic cornea as the patient is unaware of problems.

In seventh nerve palsies, a silicone rubber or silicone hydrogel lens protects the cornea from drying and is used in conjunction with ocular lubricants. Lenses may be worn on an extended-wear schedule if incomplete lid closure occurs during sleep, or alternatively, complete eye closure can be achieved by taping the lids together at night. Alternatively, an RGP scleral or semi-scleral lens can be fitted.

Alternative treatment

In order to prevent keratopathy occurring prior to neurosurgery being performed, tarsorrhaphy may be carried out.

Corneal thinning and perforation

Condition

Corneal perforation can occur due to accidental injury or surgical trauma of the cornea or following a persistent epithelial defect after a corneal ulcer. A common cause of corneal thinning is rheumatoid arthritis resulting in keratolysis which destroys the corneal stroma. Where perforation is imminent, a descemetocele often forms (Fig. 26.10) and a therapeutic lens can prevent perforation by reinforcing the cornea and preventing distension of the descemetocele by intraocular pressure.

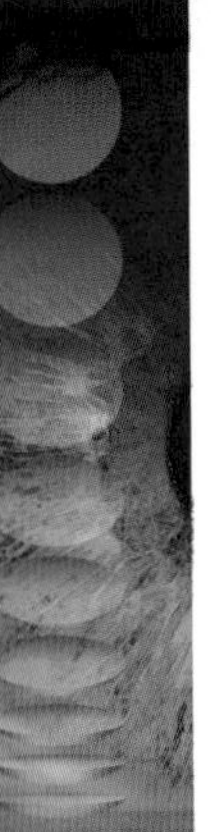

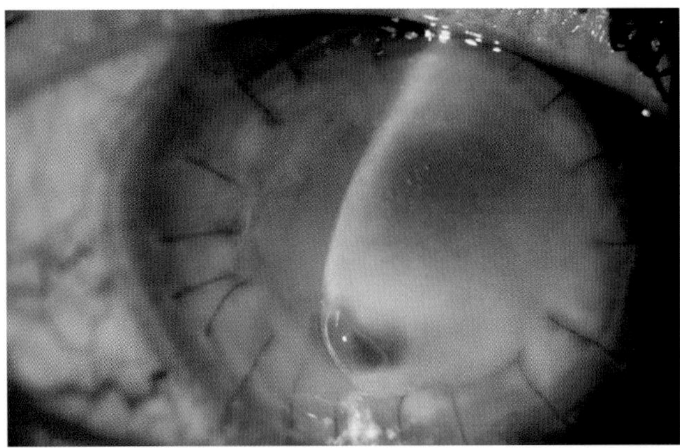

Figure 26.10 Descemetocele in a failed graft. (Courtesy of A. J. Phillips)

Lens type

When the cornea thins or perforates, the main aim of therapy is to maintain or restore the corneal integrity, so that the anterior chamber either reforms or remains formed. Therapeutic lenses allow small perforations to heal themselves, provided the wound edges are in good apposition and there is no incarceration or prolapse of the uvea or the crystalline lens.

Rehim et al. (1990) reported a high success rate when non-infected perforations, less than 3 mm in size, were treated with thin, high-water-content lenses worn for 1–2 weeks. Larger perforations were not as successful and generally required surgical repair.

Silicone hydrogel may now be a safer option or silicone rubber lenses if available.

Lens fitting

When fitting a perforated cornea, the anterior chamber may be shallow or flat. The initial lens should be fitted slightly tight and, as the anterior chamber reforms, the lens becomes less tight. Over a period of a few hours the lens may need to be changed to a steeper lens, which should be comfortable and move well. Strict hygiene is required as such an eye is particularly susceptible to infection.

Alternative treatment

Lenses are used to act as a splint until surgery or tissue adhesive can be applied. After gluing, a bandage contact lens may be used over the adhesive, both to protect the 'seal' from being displaced by the lids and to decrease eyelid irritation from the rough surface of the dried adhesive.

Weiss et al. (1983) studied 80 cases treated with tissue adhesive. Almost half healed with tissue adhesive alone or tissue adhesive and a bandage contact lens. Eiferman and Snyder (1983) used cyanoacrylate glue and later inserted a bandage lens to treat infected corneal ulcers that had perforated. Intensive antibiotic therapy was also employed, and the incidental bacteriostatic effect of cyanoacrylate adhesive against Gram-positive organisms was thought to expedite healing in these patients.

Therapeutic contact lens uses following ocular surgery

Hydrophilic lenses can be used to assist epithelial healing, to protect the eyelids from suture ends (Fig. 26.11) and to reduce pain.

Following penetrating keratoplasty, punctate epithelial keratitis may develop. Lenses protect the ocular surface and promote healing (Zadnik 1990, Beekhuis et al. 1991). Where rapid visual rehabilitation is required, powered lenses can provide refractive correction as well as acting as a bandage, although corneal astigmatism often means that vision will be poor unless an RGP lens is used. However, it should be borne in mind that fitting lenses in the early postoperative stages may increase the risk of graft rejection due to physiological stress on the vulnerable graft tissue.

Wound dehiscence after penetrating keratoplasty can be successfully managed with medium-water-content, stiff, steep-fitting soft lenses. However, due to the length of time these have to be left in place, and the consequential risk of oedema and neovascularization, nowadays low-water-content silicone hydrogel lenses are more commonly used.

Various postsurgical complications can be managed with bandage lenses including:

- Wound dehiscence.
- Leaking blebs require soft bandage lenses with large TDs of 18.00–22.00 mm.
- Stem cell grafts also require large soft therapeutic lenses to protect the lid from thick sutures.
- Pain relief and promotion of epithelial healing after
  - excimer laser photorefractive keratectomy (PRK) (Eiferman et al. 1991, Sher et al. 1992, Talley et al. 1994).
  - epikeratoplasty (Zadnik 1990).
  - superficial keratectomy (Moodaley et al. 1991).

Silicone hydrogel lenses are used as continuous-wear bandage lenses after corneal refractive surgery. Lim et al. (2001) fitted 36 patients with balafilcon A lenses following penetrating or lamellar keratoplasty, LASIK or PRK. Szaflik et al. (2004) evaluated the therapeutic use of the lotrafilcon A lens in post-LASEK cases and found that the lenses were effective and well tolerated.

Cicatrizing conjunctival diseases

In cicatrizing conjunctival diseases, therapeutic lenses can relieve pain and provide corneal protection from exposure, entropion and trichiasis. They can help maintain the conjunctival fornices in such conditions as ocular pemphigoid (Fig. 26.12), chemical and thermal burns (Fig. 26.13), trachoma and Stevens–Johnson syndrome by preventing symblepharon (adhesions between bulbar and palpebral conjunctiva) and ankyloblepharon (fusion of lid margins).

Lens type

All types of lens can be useful in these disorders:

(a)

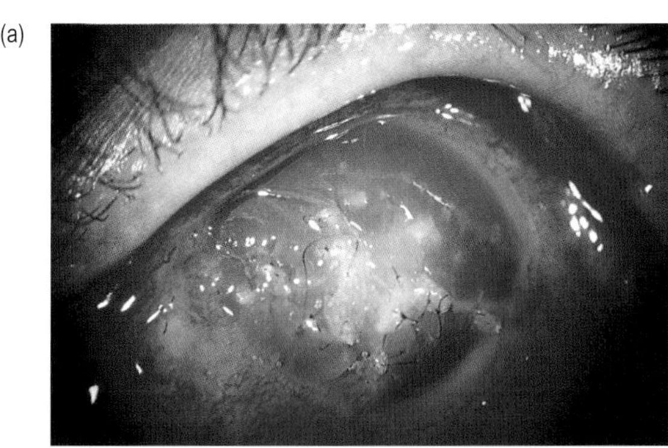

(b)

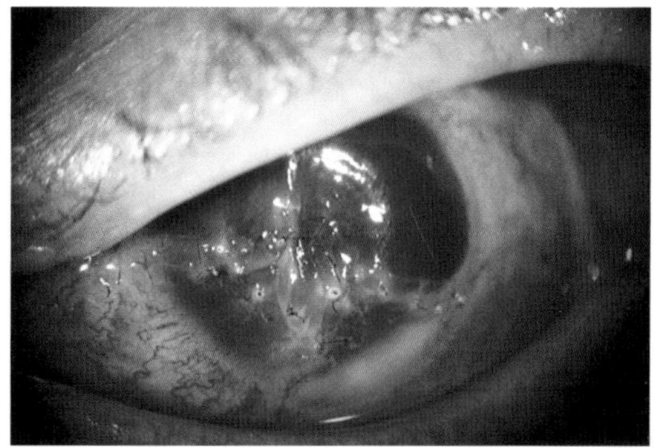

(c)

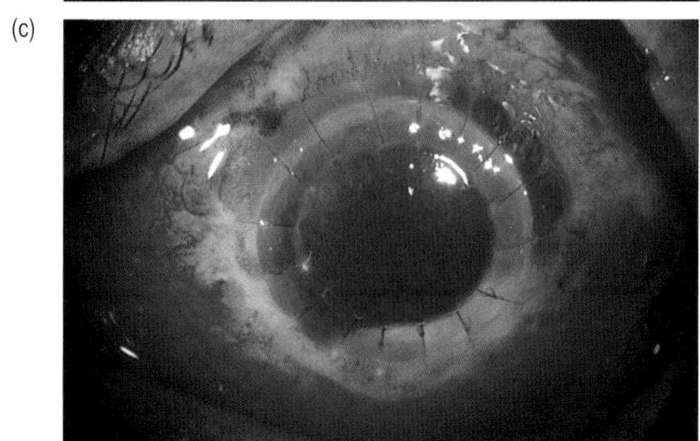

Figure 26.11 (a) Primary care of this corneal wound was carried out at a remote hospital. The corneal surface was grossly irregular and the suture ends exposed. (b) A bandage lens was used for comfort. When the cornea had healed and the inflammation settled, (c) keratoplasty was performed with good results. (Courtesy of D. J. Coster)

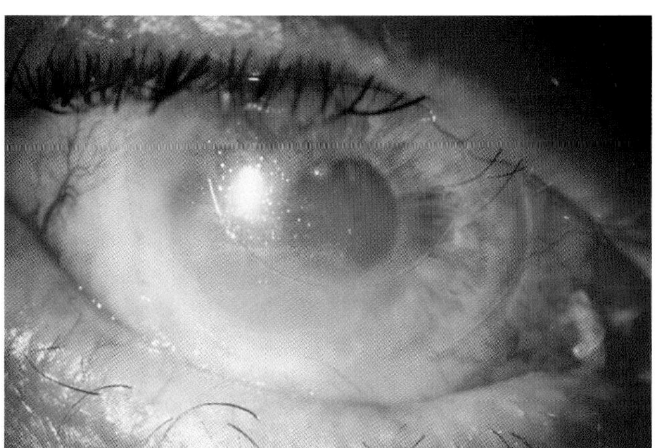

Figure 26.12 A silicone rubber therapeutic contact lens on ocular pemphigoid. (Courtesy of L. Speedwell)

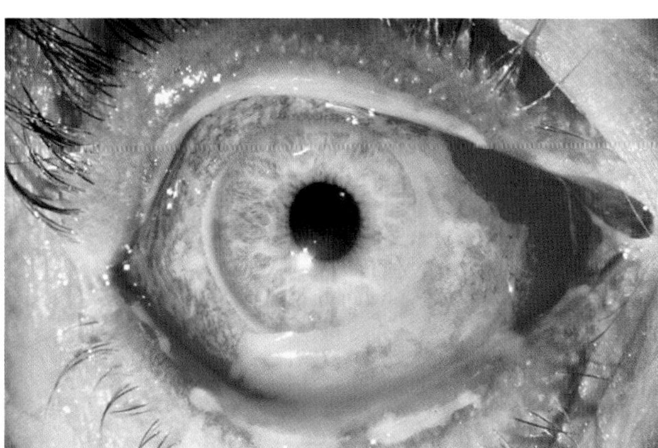

Figure 26.13 Chemical burn caused by paraquat. (Courtesy of A. J. Phillips)

- Hydrogel lenses used in association with ocular lubricants offer protection to the cornea from drying, and entropion and trichiasis.
- Low-water-content silicone hydrogel or silicone rubber lenses are preferable as they do not need such frequent lubricant drop instillation.
- Scleral lenses maintain a good fluid reservoir between the lens and cornea when supplemented with ocular lubricants. They can be used for refractive correction of scarred and irregular eyes and, because they cover most of the ocular surface, they protect both the cornea and conjunctiva while maintaining the fornices.
- Scleral rings (the outer ring of a scleral lens cut off and polished) (Fig. 26.14) can be similarly used.
- In advanced cases of ocular pemphigoid, symblepharon may prevent the insertion of scleral lenses and in such cases,

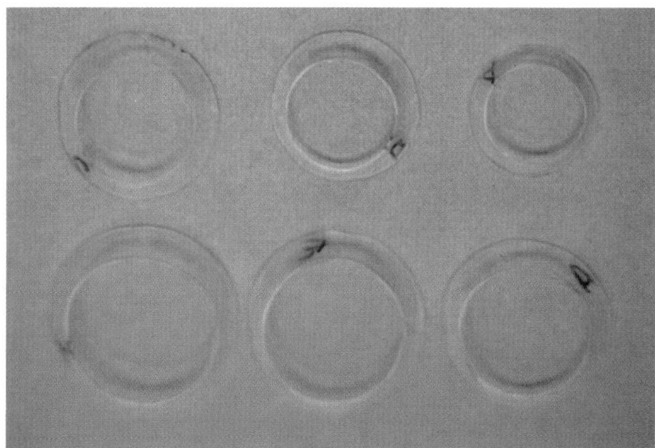

Figure 26.14 Scleral rings: these are cut from different-sized scleral lenses and are used in cases of symblepharon. (Courtesy of N. Sapp)

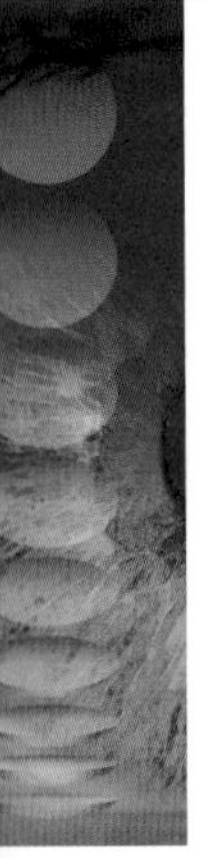

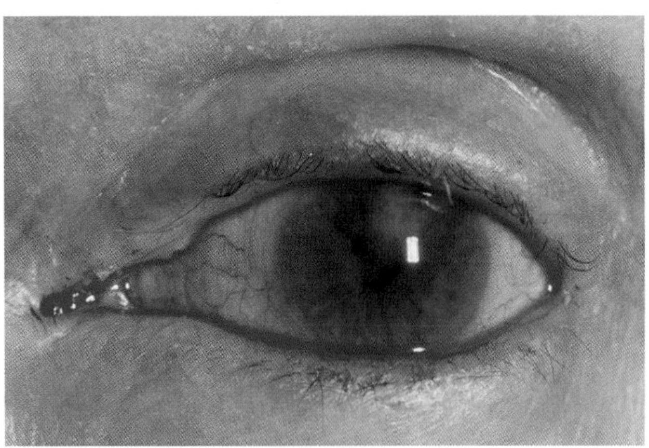

Figure 26.15 Keratoconjunctivitis sicca associated with chronic blepharitis. (Courtesy of D. Westerhout)

silicone rubber or rigid gas-permeable lenses can be successful in visual rehabilitation of patients with ocular surface irregularities (Pesudovs & Phillips 1992).

The dry eye

The use of therapeutic lenses in the management of keratoconjunctivitis sicca (Fig. 26.15) and other dry eye conditions is controversial. Dart (1987) and Mackie (1985) suggest they should be used rarely in keratoconjunctivitis sicca whereas other practitioners advocate their controlled use (Gassett & Kaufman 1971b, Gassett 1978, Høvding 1984).

A therapeutic contact lens is generally only considered in the treatment of dry eye patients when other modes of therapy have failed. In most mild cases, artificial tear solutions or ointment, or punctal occlusion are prescribed.

Lens fitting

Contact lens options include silicone hydrogel (Ambroziak et al. 2004) scleral and RGP lenses with good wettability where there is associated surface disease and irregularity (O'Callaghan & Phillips 1994).

As the risk of ocular infection secondary to contact lens wear in dry eye patients is high (Mackie 1985), regular follow-up is essential. Lenses alone do not usually alleviate dry eye symptoms and the frequent instillation of ocular lubricants is still required.

Alternative treatment

Frequent application of ocular lubricants (drops, gels, ointments), eye closure and, if necessary, taping the lids at night.

DRUG DELIVERY

When a drug is instilled into the eye in drop or ointment form, there is an initial high concentration, followed by a rapid decrease and the efficacy is limited by the short contact time. If higher concentrations are used to try to overcome this problem, adverse effects may occur.

Hydrophilic contact lenses have the potential to provide slow and prolonged delivery of low drug dosages to the eye, thereby increasing drug efficacy while reducing the risk of toxicity.

Drugs can be incorporated into hydrogel lenses in a number of ways.

- Soaking the lens in a water-soluble form of the drug, saturating the aqueous component of the lens (most common method).
- Employing a water-soluble pro-drug, which biodegrades into its active form upon diffusion from the hydrogel and exposure to the ocular environment.
- Attaching the drug to the lens polymer molecules. Upon contact with the tears and ocular tissues the bonds between the drug molecules and the lens polymer break down, thereby releasing the drug.

Waltman and Kaufman (1970) investigated the use of hydrophilic lenses for drug delivery using sodium fluorescein dye, and concluded that hydrophilic lenses were a useful method of maintaining a high drug concentration in the anterior segment of the eye. Since this report, many investigators have used hydrogel lenses to deliver a variety of different drugs to the eye including the glaucoma drug pilocarpine (Ramer & Gasset 1974, Ruben & Watkins 1975), the antibiotic gentamicin (Busin & Spitznas 1988) and the antiviral agent, 5-iodo-2-desoxyuridine (IDU) (Praus et al. 1976).

Karlgard et al. (2003) reported that the exceptional oxygen transmission characteristics of silicone hydrogel materials warranted further studies to determine their applicability as sustained drug-delivery devices.

The molecular size of a drug affects its ability to be taken up by a hydrophilic lens because large molecules penetrate the material less well than smaller molecules. High-water-content materials hold more drug than those with low water content and may deliver drugs more rapidly.

MISCELLANEOUS APPLICATIONS OF THERAPEUTIC CONTACT LENSES

Hydrogel contact lenses can be used to provide corneal protection during ocular procedures, such as specular microscopy and tonometry, which require direct contact of an instrument with the cornea.

Patients may need to have their intraocular pressure (IOP) monitored regularly, and although lenses can be removed for such a procedure, removal may have a detrimental effect on the condition under treatment, such as in patients who are being treated for recurrent erosions. In these cases, applanation tonometry carried out through the bandage lens using white light or high-molecular-weight fluorescein (see Chapter 4) or, alternatively, non-applanation tonometry, can be used. Measurements taken through ultrathin lenses were very close to those taken without a lens (Meyer et al. 1978, Rubenstein & Deutsch 1985, Mark et al. 1992), although other authors have not reported such a good correlation, particularly when powered lenses are worn (Insler & Robbins 1987). Allen et al.

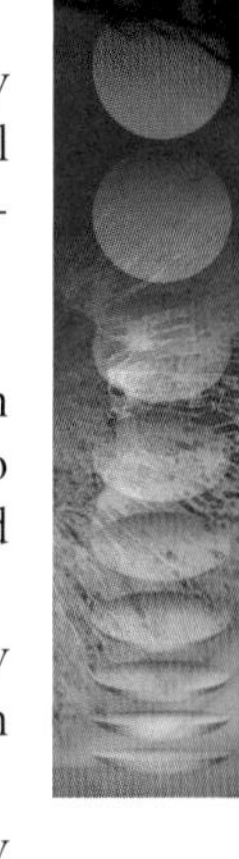

(2004) found that Goldman tonometry measurement of IOP through silicone hydrogel lenses was closely correlated to that of measurements taken without contact lenses.

Other uses of bandage lenses include:

- Protection of the epithelium in diabetic patients during photocoagulation (Arentsen & Tasman 1981).
- Protection of the cornea for scleral impression (Westerhout 1975).
- Increasing patient comfort in the 'piggyback' fitting of keratoconics and other unusually shaped corneas (see Chapter 20).
- Prevention of lens loss in a keratoconic patient when a hydrogel lens is worn over a rigid lens for contact sports (McKinnon 1989).

COMPLICATIONS OF THERAPEUTIC LENS USE

As mentioned above, complications are more likely in a compromised eye.

Complications range from minor to severe. These include:

- Ocular redness and irritation, possibly associated with a minor anterior chamber reaction and early vascularization (Dohlman et al. 1973).
- Superficial neovascularization which usually regresses once lenses are removed. Thermal burns or stromal ulceration can benefit from new vessels, which have a positive effect on surface healing (Conn et al. 1980). These eyes have a poor visual prognosis so vascularization is not detrimental.
- Lens-induced corneal oedema can be overlooked, especially if it is a prominent feature of the condition (Thoft & Mobilia 1981). Although silicone hydrogel lenses have virtually eliminated the hypoxic problems associated with conventional hydrogels, inflammation, infection and mechanical complications remain (Dumbleton 2002) (see Chapters 10 and 13).
- Lens deposition (Høvding & Seland 1984).
- Lens discoloration, possibly from certain drugs used in conjunction with soft contact lenses (Sugar 1974) (see also Chapter 4). Lenses should be replaced regularly to avoid further complications such as papillary conjunctivitis.
- Sterile corneal infiltrates (see Chapters 13, 17 and 18) usually resolve after lens removal without sequelae, but may be an early sign of microbial keratitis.
- Microbial keratitis. Kent et al. (1990), in a retrospective study of corneal ulcers secondary to bandage lens use, found the majority of ulcers occurred in patients treated for bullous keratopathy, with neurotrophic and exposure keratitis the second most common indication. More than two-thirds of the ulcers in this study were culture positive. Saini et al. (1988) reported a 9% incidence of corneal ulcers with low-Dk bandage lenses following keratoplasty (see also Chapter 18).

These complications emphasize the need for regular after-care and suggest that therapeutic lenses should only be prescribed when patients can attend such visits. Prior to fitting, the risks of therapeutic lens wear should be weighed against the likely benefits and explained to the patient.

ACKOWLEDGEMENTS

I wish to thank Alison Ewbank for her assistance, and Stephen and Henry Curran for their general support in the writing and updating of this section.

References

Allen, R. J., De Witt, D. and Saleh, G. (2004) Applanation tonometry in silicone hydrogel contact lens wear. ARVO Poster, April 2004

Ambroziak, A. A., Szaflik, J. P. and Szaflik, J. (2004) Therapeutic use of a silicone hydrogel contact lens in selected clinical cases. Eye Contact Lens, 30(1), 63–67

Aquavella, J. V., Musco, P. S., Ueda, S. and Locascio, J. A. (1988) Therapeutic applications of a collagen bandage lens: a preliminary report. Contact Lens Assoc. Ophthalmol. J., 14, 47–50

Arentsen, J. J. and Tasman, W. (1981) Using a bandage contact lens to prevent recurrent erosion during photocoagulation in patients with diabetes. Am. J. Ophthalmol., 92, 714–716

Astin, C. (1989) Clinical appraisal of therapeutic contact lenses. Contact Lens J., 17, 186–189

Beekhuis, W. H., van Rij, G., Egginnk, F. A. G. J., Vreugdenhil, W. and Schoevaart, C. E. (1991) Contact lenses following keratoplasty. Contact Lens Assoc. Ophthalmol. J., 17, 27–29

Busin, M. and Spitznas, M. (1988) Sustained gentamicin release by presoaked medicated bandage contact lenses. Ophthalmology, 95, 796–798

Caroline, P. J. and Andre, M. P. (2001) When the eye needs a bandage. Contact Lens Spectrum, 16(12), 56

Compan, V., Andrio, A., Lopez Alemany, A., Riande, E. and Refojo, M. F. (2002) Oxygen permeability of hydrogel contact lenses with organosilicon moieties. Biomaterials, 23, 2767–2772

Conn, H., Berman, M., Kenyon, K., Langer, R. and Gage, J. (1980) Stromal vascularization prevents corneal ulceration. Invest. Ophthalmol. Vis. Sci., 19, 362–370

Dart, J. (1987) Therapeutic contact lenses. Contax, March, 11–17

DePaolis, M. D., Musco, P. M., Aquavella, J. V. and Shovlin, J. P. (1987) The collagen bandage lens. Contact Lens Spectrum, 2(6), 39–40

Dohlman, C. H., Boruchoff, S. A. and Mobilia, E. F. (1973) Complications in the use of soft contact lenses in corneal disease. Arch. Ophthalmol., 90, 367–370

Dumbleton, K. (2002) Adverse events with silicone hydrogel continuous wear. Cont. Lens Anterior Eye, 25, 137–146

Edwards, K. and Atkins, N. (2002) Silicone hydrogel contact lenses. Part 2: Therapeutic applications. Optom. Today, 42(20), 26–29

Ehrlich, D. (2001) Therapeutic contact lenses. Optician, 224(5808), 28–32

Eiferman, R. A. and Snyder, J. W. (1983) Antibacterial effect of cyanoacrylate glue. Arch. Ophthalmol., 101, 956–960

Eiferman, R. A., O'Neill, K. P., Forgey, D. R. and Cook, Y. D. (1991) Excimer laser photorefractive keratectomy for myopia: six month results. Refract. Corneal Surg., 7, 344–347

Espy, J. W. (1971) Management of corneal problems with hydrophilic contact lenses. Am. J. Ophthalmol., 72, 521–526

Ezekiel, D. (1983) Gas permeable haptic lenses. J. Br. Contact Lens Assoc., 6, 158–161

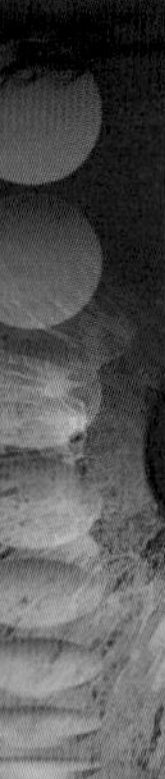

Fonn, D., Dumbleton, K., Jones, L., Du Toit, R. and Sweeney, D. (2002) Silicone hydrogel material and surface properties. Contact Lens Spectrum, 17, 24–28

Forstot, S. L. and Binder, P. B. (1979) Treatment of Thygeson's superficial punctate keratopathy with soft contact lenses. Am. J. Ophthalmol., 88, 186–189

Foulks, G. N., Harvey, T. and Raj, C. V. (2003) Therapeutic contact lenses: the role of high-Dk lenses. Ophthalmol. Clin. North Am., 16, 455–461

Gassett, A. R. (1978) Corneal diseases and soft contact lenses. In Soft Contact Lenses: Clinical and Applied Technology, pp. 245–254, ed. M. Ruben. London: Baillière Tindall

Gassett, A. R. and Kaufmann, H. E. (1970) Therapeutic uses of hydrophilic contact lenses. Am. J. Ophthalmol., 69, 252–259

Gassett, A. R. and Kaufmann, H. E. (1971a) Bandage lenses in the treatment of bullous keratopathy. Am. J. Ophthalmol., 72, 376–380

Gassett, A. R. and Kaufmann, H. E. (1971b) Hydrophilic lens therapy of severe keratoconjunctivitis sicca and conjunctival scarring. Am. J. Ophthalmol., 71, 1185–1189

Gipson, I. K., Spurr-Michaud, S., Tisdale, A. and Keough, M. (1989) Reassembly of the anchoring structures of the corneal epithelium during wound repair in the rabbit. Invest. Ophthalmol. Vis. Sci., 30, 425–434

Goldberg, D. B., Schanzlin, D. J. and Brown, S. I. (1980) Management of Thygeson's superficial punctate keratitis. Am. J. Ophthalmol., 89, 22–24

Gruber, E. (1991) The Acuvue disposable contact lens as a therapeutic bandage lens. Ann. Ophthalmol., 23, 446–447

Harvitt, D. and Bonnano J. (1999) Re-evaluation of the oxygen diffusion model for predicting minimum contact lens Dk/t values needed to avoid corneal anoxia. Optom. Vis. Sci., 76, 712–719

Holden, B. and Mertz, G. (1984) Critical oxygen levels to avoid corneal oedema for daily and extended wear. Invest. Ophthalmol. Vis. Sci., 25, 1161–1167

Høvding, G. (1984) Hydrophilic contact lenses in corneal disorders. Acta Ophthalmol., 62, 566–576

Høvding, G. and Seland, J. H. (1984) Deposits on hydrophilic 'bandage' lenses. Acta Ophthalmol., 62, 849–858

Insler, M. S. and Robbins, R. G. (1987) Intraocular pressure by noncontact tonometry with and without soft contact lenses. Arch. Ophthalmol., 105, 1358–1359

Kanpolat, A. and Ucakhan, O. O. (2003) Therapeutic use of Focus Night & Day contact lenses. Cornea, 22, 726–734

Karlgard, C. C., Jones, L. W. and Moresoli, C. (2003) Ciprofloxacin interation with silicone-based and conventional hydrogel lenses. Eye Contact Lens, 29, 83–89

Karlgard, C. S., Jones, L. W. and Moresoli, C. (2004) Survey of bandage lens use in North America. Eye Contact Lens, 30, 25–30

Kent, H. D., Cohen, E. J., Laibson, P. R. and Arentsen, J. J. (1990) Microbial keratitis and corneal ulceration associated with therapeutic soft contact lenses. Contact Lens Assoc. Ophthalmol. J., 16, 49–52

Kowalik, B. M. and Rakes, J. A. (1991) Filamentary keratitis – the clinical challenges. J. Am. Optom. Assoc., 62, 200–204

Levy, B. and Nguyen, N. (1993) Therapeutic utilization of disposable lenses. Int. Contact Lens Clin., 20, 181–183

Liebowitz, H. M. and Rosenthal, P. (1971a) Hydrophilic contact lenses in corneal disease. II. Bullous keratopathy. Arch. Ophthalmol., 85, 283–285

Liebowitz, H. M. and Rosenthal, P. (1971b) Hydrophilic contact lenses in corneal disease. I. Superficial, sterile, indolent ulcers. Arch. Ophthalmol., 85, 163–166

Lim, L., Tan, D. T. and Chan, W. K. (2001) Therapeutic use of Bausch & Lomb PureVision contact lenses. Contact Lens Assoc. Ophthalmol. J., 27, 179–185

Mackie, I. A. (1985) Contact lenses in dry eyes. Trans. Ophthalmol. Soc. UK, 104, 477–483

Mark, L. K., Asbell, P. A., Torres, M. A. and Failla, S. J. (1992) Accuracy of intraocular pressure measurements with two different tonometers through bandage contact lenses. Cornea, 11, 277–281

Marshall, W. L. and Holdeman, N. R. (1992) Thygeson's superficial punctate keratopathy: a case report. Clin. Eye Vis. Care, 4, 151–154

McDermott, M. L. and Chandler, J. W. (1989) Therapeutic use of contact lenses. Surv. Ophthalmol., 33, 381–394

McKinnon, T. J. (1989) Case report: contact lens correction of keratoconus for contact sports. Clin. Exp. Optom., 72, 179–180

Mertz, G. W. and Holden, B. A. (1981) Clinical implications of extended wear research. Can. J. Optom., 43, 203–205

Meyer, R. F., Stanifer, R. M. and Bobb, K. C. (1978) Mackay–Marg tonometry over therapeutic soft contact lenses. Am. J. Ophthalmol., 86, 19–23

Montero, J., Sparholt, J., Mély, R. and Long, B. (2003) Retrospective case series of therapeutic applications of Lotrafilcon A silicone hydrogel soft contact lenses. Eye Contact Lens, 29(2), 72–75

Moodaley, L., Buckley, R. J. and Woodward, E. G. (1991) Surgery to improve contact lens wear in keratoconus. Contact Lens Assoc. Ophthalmol. J., 17, 129–131

O'Callaghan, G. J. and Phillips, A. J. (1994) Rheumatoid arthritis and the contact lens wearer. Clin. Exp. Optom., 77, 137–143

O'Donnell, C. and Maldonado-Codina, C. (2004) A hyper-Dk piggyback contact lens system for keratoconus. Eye Contact Lens, 30, 44–48

Pesudovs, K. and Phillips, A. J. (1992) The use of a rigid gas permeable lens in ocular cicatricial pemphigoid. Clin. Exp. Optom., 75, 188–191

Praus, R., Krejci, L., Brettschneider, I. and Mikova, M. (1976) Use of hydrophilic contact lens for application of IDU. Study on rabbits with artificial cornea lesions and herpetic keratitis. Ophthalmol. Res., 8, 362–366

Ramer, R. M. and Gasset, A. R. (1974) Ocular penetration of pilocarpine: the effect of hydrophilic soft contact lenses on the ocular penetration of pilocarpine. Ann. Ophthalmol., 12, 1325–1327

Randleman, J. B., Ward, M. A, and Stulting, R. D. (2003) Visual rehabilitation after severe alkali injury with piggyback hyper O_2 contact lenses. Cornea, 22(2), 181–183

Rehim, M. H. A. and Samy, M. (1989) The role of therapeutic soft contact lenses in treatment of bullous keratopathy. Contact Lens J., 17, 119–125

Rehim, M. H. A., Shafik, M. A. A. and Samy, M. (1990) Management of corneal perforation by therapeutic contact lenses. Contact Lens J., 18, 107–111

Ren, D. H., Yamamoto, K., Ladage, P. M. et al. (2002) Adaptive effects of 30-night wear of hyper-O2 transmissible contact lenses on bacterial binding and corneal epithelium. Ophthalmology, 109, 127–140

Ridley, F. (1962) Therapeutic uses of scleral contact lenses. Int. Ophthalmol. Clin., 2, 687–716

Ruben, M. and Watkins, R. (1975) Pilocarpine dispensation for the soft hydrophilic contact lens. Br. J. Ophthalmol., 59, 455–458

Rubinstein, M. (2003) Applications of contact lens devices in the management of corneal disease. Eye, 17, 872–876

Rubenstein, J. B. and Deutsch, T. A. (1985) Pneumatonometry through bandage contact lenses. Arch. Ophthalmol., 103, 1660–1661

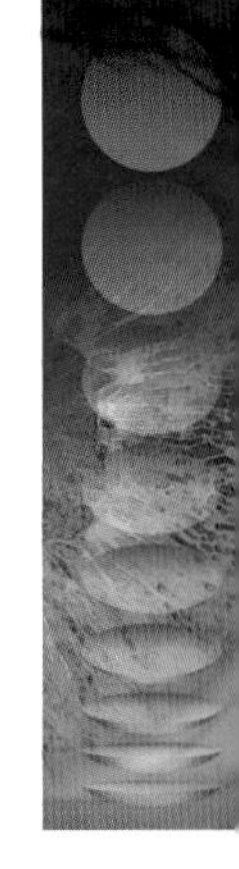

Ruffini, J. J., Aquavella, J. V. and Locascio, J. A. (1989) Effect of collagen shields on corneal wound healing following penetrating keratoplasty. Ophthalmol. Surg., 20, 21–25

Saini, J. S., Rao, G. N. and Aquavella, J. V. (1988) Post-keratoplasty corneal ulcers and bandage contact lenses. Acta Ophthalmol., 66, 99–103

Schein, O. D., Rosenthal, P. and Ducharme, C. (1989) A gas permeable scleral contact lens for visual rehabilitation. Am. J. Ophthalmol., 109, 318–322

Sher, N. A., Barak, M., Daya, S. et al. (1992) Excimer laser photorefractive keratectomy in high myopia. Arch. Ophthalmol., 110, 935–943

Speedwell, L. (1991) A review of therapeutic lenses. Optician, 202(5341), 25–30

Steffen, R. and Schnider, C. (2004) A next-generation silicone hydrogel lens for daily wear. Part 1: Material properties. Optician, 224(5958), 23–25

Sugar, J. (1974) Adrenochrome pigmentation of hydrophilic lenses. Arch. Ophthalmol., 91, 11–12

Sulewski, M. E., Krachner, G. P., Gottisch, J. D. and Stark, W. J. (1991) Use of the disposable contact lens as a bandage contact lens. Arch. Ophthalmol., 109, 318

Szaflik, J. P., Ambroziak, A. M. and Szaflik, J. (2004) Therapeutic use of a silicone hydrogel contact lens as a bandage after LASEK surgery. Ophthalmology, 30, 59–62

Takahashi, G. H. and Liebowitz, H. M. (1971) Hydrophilic contact lenses in corneal disease. III. Topical hypertonic saline in bullous keratopathy. Arch. Ophthalmol., 86, 133–137

Talley, A. R., Sher, N. A., Kim, M. S. et al. (1994) Use of the 193nm excimer laser for photorefractive keratectomy in low to moderate myopia. J. Cataract Refract. Surg., 20(Suppl), 239–242

Tanner, J. B. and DePaolis, M. D. (1992) Disposable contact lenses as alternative bandage lenses. Clin. Eye Vis. Care, 4, 159–161

Thoft, R. A. and Mobilia, E. F. (1981) Complications with therapeutic extended wear soft contact lenses. Int. Ophthalmol. Clin., 21, 197–208

Thygeson, P. (1950) Superficial punctate keratitis. J. Am. Med. Assoc., 18, 1544–1549

Thygeson, P. (1961) Further observations of superficial punctate keratitis. Arch. Ophthalmol., 66, 34–38

Waltman, S. R. and Kaufman, H. E. (1970) Use of hydrophilic contact lenses to increase ocular penetration of topical drugs. Invest. Ophthalmol., 9, 250–255

Weinstock, F. J. (1990) Management of corneal erosions with the Acuvue disposable lens. Contact Lens Forum, 15(6), 47–55

Weiss, J. L., Williams, P., Lindstrom, R. L. and Doughman, D. J. (1983) The use of a tissue adhesive in corneal perforations. Ophthalmology, 90, 610–615

Westerhout, D. I. (1975) The use of soft lenses in the fitting of haptic lenses. Optician, 169(4363), 13–16

Woodward, E. G. (1979) Therapeutic contact lenses: forms and materials. Contacto, 23(5), 14–17

Zadnik, K. (1990) Postoperative use of bandage soft contact lenses. Contact Lens Update, 9(3), 1–4

Zaidman, G. W., Geeraets, R., Paylor, R. R. and Ferry, A. P. (1985) The histopathology of filamentary keratitis. Arch. Ophthalmol., 103, 1178–1181

Zantos, S. G. and Holden, B. A. (1978) Ocular changes associated with continuous wear of contact lenses. Aust. J. Optom., 61, 418–426

Chapter 27

Contact lens manufacturing

John H. Clamp

CHAPTER CONTENTS

This chapter will discuss the various manufacturing options for producing both soft and rigid gas-permeable (RGP) contact lenses dispensed either as disposable or durable lenses. In this instance, disposable refers to lenses that are designed to be used for up to 1 month; durable refers to lenses that are designed to last more than 1 month, typically designed for annual replacement.

Contact lens manufacturing has changed tremendously and many processes are covered by patents or simply kept private. Therefore, the chapter does not aim to be comprehensive but will attempt to describe the basic concepts.

Moulding and lathe cutting

There are three main manufacturing methods:

- Moulding – mainly the mass production of lenses of limited parameters at low cost.
- Lathe cutting – the production of individually specified lenses.
- Hybrid lens manufacture – a combination of the two, which not only has the benefit of low cost mass production, but also goes some way to producing lenses that are more specific.

In general, lenses sold under the disposable modality tend to be moulded and lenses sold under the durable modality tend to be lathe cut. Of course, there are exceptions, such as specialist moulded RGP lenses, and there is a potential to sell disposable fully lathe-cut lenses using the latest state-of-the-art lathing systems (see Automation, p. 560).

As moulding is becoming more of a mainstream process, the parameters available are increasing; for example, moulded soft toric and multifocal lenses are now common. However, inventories of moulded lenses are limited, not by the ability to manufacture but by that of logistical control and storage.

Table 27.1 shows that a full inventory of Frequency aspheric lenses (CooperVision) will have 104 stock allocations and for the Frequency XCEL XR toric, 6156 stock allocations would be necessary. This has the knock-on cost effect of large stock inventories and increased logistical control.

MOULDING

The moulding of lenses can be performed using a number of different methods. These are described in general without reference to each manufacturer. Others are more particular to individual companies, in which case the company will be referenced.

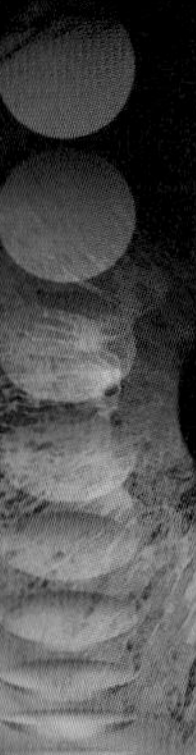

Table 27.1: Comparison of stock profiles for CooperVision lenses

	Number of variations						
	Manufacturing process	BOZR	Diameter	Spherical power	Cylindrical power	Cylindrical axis	Total number of variations
Frequency 55 aspheric	Cast moulding	2	1	68 (8.7 Base curve) 36 (8.4 Base curve)	n/a	n/a	104
Frequency XCEL toric	Hybrid	1	1	57	4	18	4104
Frequency XCEL XR toric	Hybrid	1	1	57	3	36	6156

Cast moulding

This is a general method used for manufacturing spherical, toric and multifocal disposable contact lenses. Plastic injection moulding machines are used to create female and male casts in which the contact lens is moulded. It has 12 stages (Fig. 27.1):

- *Stage 1* – Within a typical injection-moulding machine are two operating faces known as bolsters. These effectively close together to form the cavity into which the moulding material, in this case polypropylene, is injected. The majority of contact lens applications require two injection-moulding machines configured to create either female or male casts. The former is used to form the front surface of the contact lens and the latter the back surface. The insert tools create the cast surface, which then forms the contact lens. The insert tool is generally manufactured from a nickel-based alloy and the working surface is lathe cut. As these tools produce thousands of contact lenses, their preparation is critical. Typically, these are cut using state-of-the-art lathes such as a Precitech Inc., Optoform 50 or Optoform 80. The surface reflects the final contact lens design but is adapted to take into account the expansive material properties of the lens and account for changes in the casts following the injection moulding process.

  During Stage 1 the bolsters are brought together at high pressure to form the cavity. Typically, this would be in the order of 50–80 tonnes depending on the number of cavities within each bolster. This force is required to counteract the forces of the plastic injected into the mould. The injection-moulding machine is designed to ensure that the bolsters meet in exactly the same orientation every time the process is performed.
- *Stage 2* – Once the cavity is formed, hot polypropylene is injected into the mould at very high pressure to ensure that the complete cavity is filled. In many applications, the number of cavities within the bolster totals six or eight. These are linked together in a 'petal' arrangement, forming the cavity in which the contact lens cast is formed, the runners (stalks) connecting the petals being the channels through which the polypropylene is transferred (see Fig. 27.1b).

  Once the polypropylene has been injected, the plastic cools and solidifies to make the cast mould. The critical factors that ensure consistent results are:
  - the temperature of the bolster, which controls the cooling profile of the plastic.
  - the pressure with which the plastic is injected.
  - the time the plastic is allowed to cool.
- *Stage 3* – Once cooled, the bolsters are moved apart to allow access to the cast.
- *Stage 4* – The cast is removed from the bolster, generally using a robotic system and vacuum-assisted suction pads. The robotic system then transfers the cast onto a conveyor belt system where it is stocked for the next stage.
- *Stages 5 and 6* – A precise quantity of contact lens material monomer is placed on the female cast mould. Immediately after dosing the mould, the male cast mould is placed on the female to form an individual contact lens cavity containing the monomer. The casts are squeezed together at a predetermined pressure to ensure that the monomer flows throughout the cavity and any excess is extruded. If the lens being manufactured is a stabilized toric lens, the front and back casts may be rotated relative to each other to determine the axis of the lens.
- *Stages 7 and 8* – The combined female and male mould containing the contact lens monomer is transferred from the conveyor system into a polymerization process. Each contact lens material uses a different polymerization process to cure the monomer (examples include ultraviolet light and temperature exposure) and an annealing process may be employed to reduce any stresses in the material matrix.
- *Stages 9 and 10* – Once fully cured and annealed, the casts are mechanically bent and separated to reveal the contact lens. The lens is then removed by mechanically 'pinching' the lens from the mould, or by immersing the lens and cast into a hydrating fluid such as saline and hydrating the lens from the mould.
- *Stage 11* – The lens is hydrated and washed in a hydrating fluid, such as saline, and a cleaning solution, in a suitable bath. This process also removes any excess monomers that have not been polymerized.
- *Stage 12* – Quality inspection and final packaging. Lenses produced by this method are visually inspected in the wet state for:
  - surface blemishes.
  - edge defects, profile and consistency.
  - tears.
  - any deformation that would compromise the quality of the lens.

  This is carried out using a wet cell projection device such as the Optimec JCF Contact Lens Analyser (Fig. 27.2), although

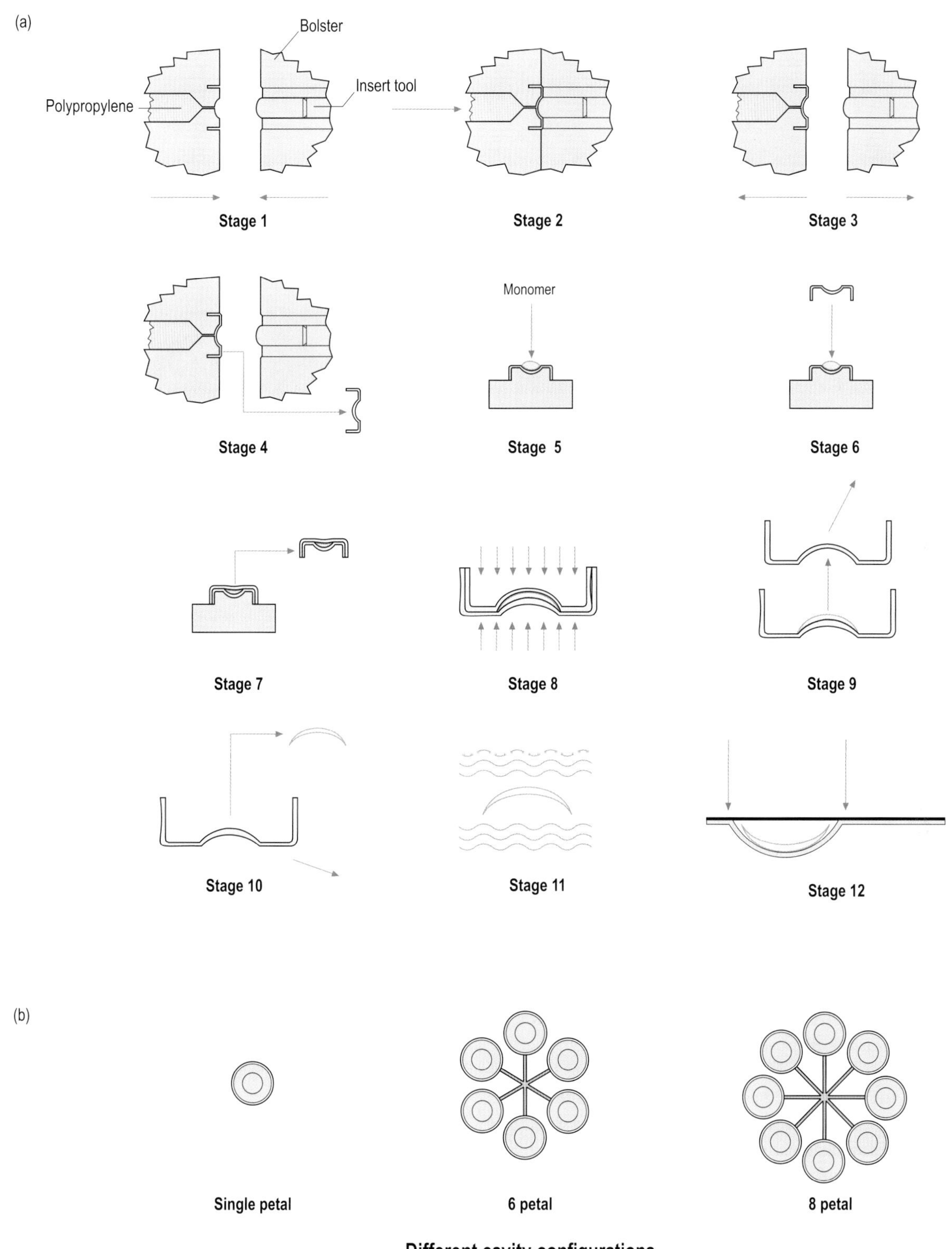

Figure 27.1 (a) Illustration of the cast moulding process. Stages 1–4, preparation of the mould. Stages 5–10, manufacture of the lens. Stages 11–12, hydration and inspection. (b) Cavities formed in bolster (see Stage 2 in text)

automated visual inspection systems that detect blemishes using video camera and computer imaging systems are becoming more common. Additional quality checks, generally performed on a sampling basis are also carried out, including:

- power.
- back optic zone radius (BOZR).
- total diameter (TD).
- lens edge profile assessment.
- material properties verification.

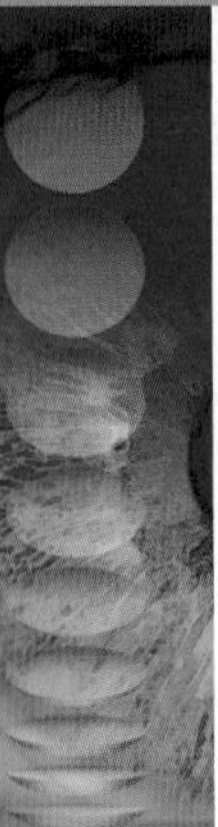

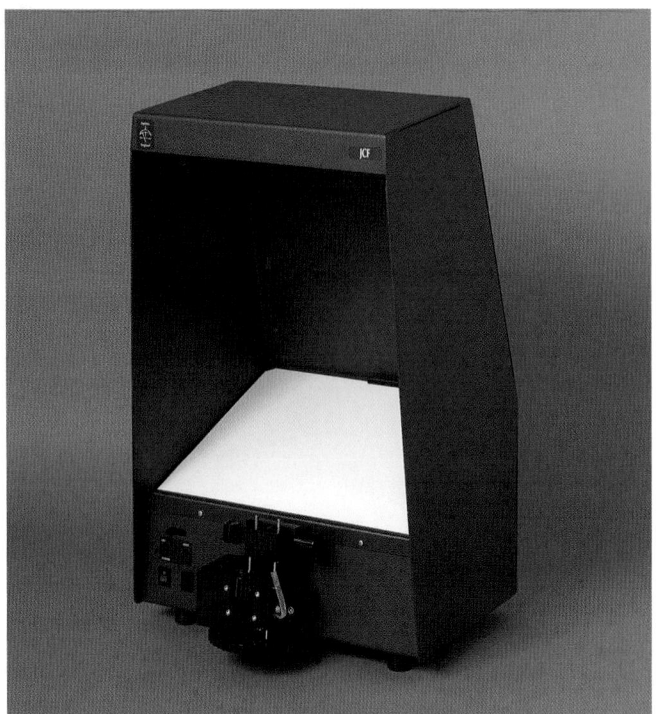

Figure 27.2 The Optimec JCF Contact Lens Analyser

The contact lens is then placed into a preformed blister pack with a predetermined amount of saline solution and sealed using a foil glued around the periphery of the contact lens compartment.

Finally, the label is attached and the lens stocked ready for despatch.

Spin casting

Bausch & Lomb refined the original method of moulding developed in 1963 and 1964 by Dr Otto Wichterle, a polymer chemist at the Czechoslovak Academy of Sciences (see Chapters 3 and 10). The contact lens monomer is injected into a precast mould and spun at a predetermined speed. The centripetal force causes the monomer to spread out against the front surface towards the edge of the mould. The front surface shape is fixed by the mould geometry and the back surface shape by the rate of spin and the viscous nature of the monomer, both of which determine the power of the lens.

Limited spin-casting moulds are required to achieve a complete power range, as the speed of rotation controls the power. However, there is a trade-off between the number of moulds used and the back surface variation across the complete power range. In order to add more plus to the power of the lens, the mould has to rotate faster to produce a flatter back surface radius in relation to the front. Likewise, a slower rotation will result in a more negative lens, which can affect the fitting characteristics. Having a larger number of moulds would reduce this effect, but increase manufacturing costs.

The back surface of these lenses is aspheric rather than spherical, which also affects the fitting characteristics, although this can be beneficial.

The formed dehydrated lens may need to be edged before the lens is hydrated in a process similar to Stages 11 to 12 described above, although this can be done within the spin-casting moulds.

By using a spin-casting mould that is configured to present a toric surface and the necessary stabilization zones on the front of the lens, moulded front surface toric lenses may be manufactured. However, this process is limited with respect to the cast-moulding method described previously, as the spin-casting mould determines the axis. The numbers of spin-casting moulds necessary are increased to cover the complete range of toric lenses, although the one spin-casting mould can be used for several spherical powers. Hydron UK, currently owned by CooperVision, manufacture the ActiFresh 400 toric using this method.

Further advances in this process are in the automation and the use of the spin-casting mould as part of the packaging (e.g. ClearLab, Plymouth, UK, formerly VisionTec CL Ltd).

Specialized moulding techniques

Moulding of contact lenses has clearly changed the contact lens marketplace by introducing the concept of disposable lenses. Indeed, mainly due to these processes, the four largest contact lens companies (Vistakon, CIBA Vision, CooperVision Inc. and Bausch & Lomb) have increased their sales to around US$3.6 billion (estimated 2004) of which less than 10% was manufactured using lathe-cutting processes.

CIBA Vision's LightStream Technology moves away from conventional moulding techniques in a number of areas. The technology meets the requirements to manufacture daily disposable lenses at a competitive cost and ensures good repeatability.

Unlike spin casting and cast moulding, the process does not use an intermediary cast to form the lens. Each lens is formed directly from tooling to the correct dimensions before being inserted in the final packaging. This removes a number of stages and the need to use large injection moulding machines that require close controls to ensure repeatability. The company utilizes this process to manufacture its Focus daily disposable soft lenses.

The LightStream Technology uses a number of innovations:

- As contact lens material is polymerized prior to casting, only a process of cross-linking is required to stabilize the material in its cast form. This avoids any necessary hydration and monomer extraction prior to final packaging.
- Moulds are made from high-quality quartz and glass and are cycled constantly throughout the process.
- Edges – the lenses are cross-linked in the moulds by controlled exposure to ultraviolet light. An opaque mask is used to prevent cross-linking at the periphery, thus forming the lens edge.

THE PROCESS

- The polymer is metered into the female glass mould and the male mould is brought into close proximity until the correct lens thickness is obtained.

(a)

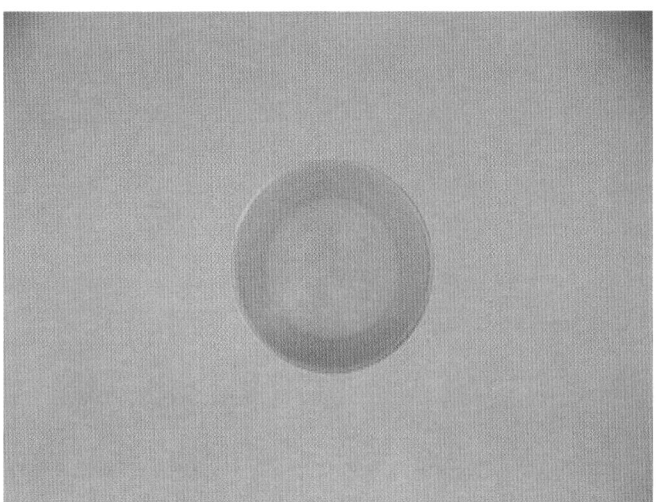

(b)

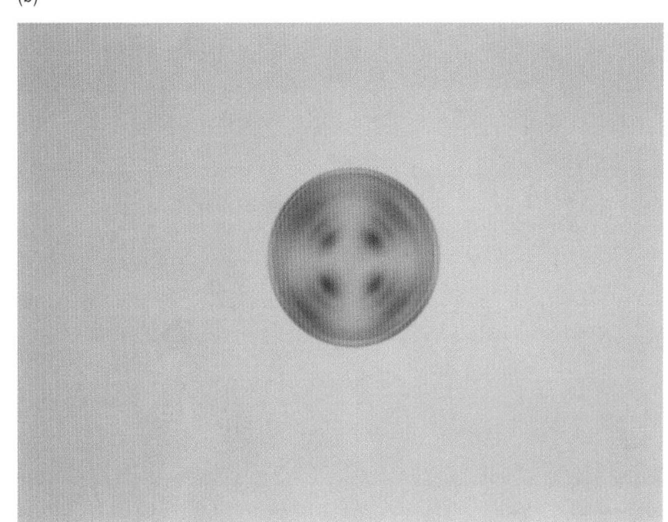

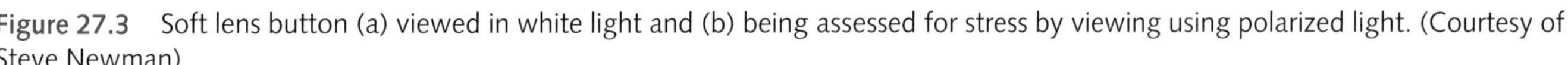

Figure 27.3 Soft lens button (a) viewed in white light and (b) being assessed for stress by viewing using polarized light. (Courtesy of Steve Newman)

- Once the cavity is formed, ultraviolet light is passed through the quartz tool to cross-link the polymer, but masked at the periphery to form the edge.
- Any unlinked polymer is washed away using purified water.
- As the moulds separate, a static electrical force ensures that the lens remains on the glass mould.
- Vacuum grippers remove the lens from the mould and pass it into an inspection cell for an automated inspection process, designed to detect any imperfection. Batches are sampled in the normal way for volume production.
- To complete the manufacturing process, the lenses are placed into strips of five blister packs ready for autoclaving.
- While the lens is being inspected, the moulds are cleaned using purified water and then returned to the beginning of the process ready for the next batch of polymer.

LATHE CUTTING

Lathe cutting is a technique favoured throughout the world as a method for the manufacture of both specialist and durable RGP and soft lenses. The advantage of this method over a moulding process is the ability to manufacture lenses on an individual basis to specific requirements. Since soft lenses are manufactured in the dehydrated state, the method of manufacture for soft and RGP contact lenses is virtually the same. Differences occur for soft lenses where swell factors have to be taken into account – for example, polishing the lenses, where moisture-free polishes are used, and in the final processes such as hydration and sterilization.

The process described below features manual loading of computer numerical controlled (CNC) lathes with polishing and finishing processes. Potential process variations, including submicron and automation machining, are discussed on p. 560.

LENS DESIGN

From the initial lens order, machining parameters are determined taking into account the specified parameters of the lens, the design of the lens and the material properties including refractive index and swell factors (for soft lens materials). Mostly these are computed using software written specifically for the contact lens company. The machining parameters include all the necessary geometric data to specify the front and back surfaces, the thicknesses and any other data that are relevant to the production of the particular contact lens. Depending on the level of automation, the machining parameters are transferred into the contact lens laboratory via fabrication sheets and/or lathe data files for automatic lathe-cutting cycles. Each fabrication sheet or lathe data file would have a unique identifier to ensure traceability throughout the process. Typically, this would be in the form of a barcode.

ANNEALING

RGP blanks are either individually cast or cast in rods, whereas PMMA blanks are made from cast sheet, cast block or rod turned from cast block. All casting introduces strain, which needs to be released from the material to ensure consistent results in rigid lens fabrication. This is done by annealing which involves heating the material to a temperature between 140 and 150°C for a short period and slowly returning it to room temperature. This does not cause any difficulty when done with sheet material but with thick material the temperature has to be low enough to prevent depolymerization of the surface but heated long enough to ensure the centre of the block reaches at least 130°C. Annealing is usually carried out by the supplier of the blank.

STRESS TESTING

Stress may already be a component in the blank prior to lathing, but good material manufacture has helped to minimize this problem. Even so, the lens laboratory still has to ensure that the blank reaches the quality claimed by the material manufacturer and so material stress analysis is an essential part of the initial manufacturing process – any stress present in the blank will later cause distortion to the finished lens. Blanks are assessed for stress by viewing with a polarized light strain tester (Fig. 27.3).

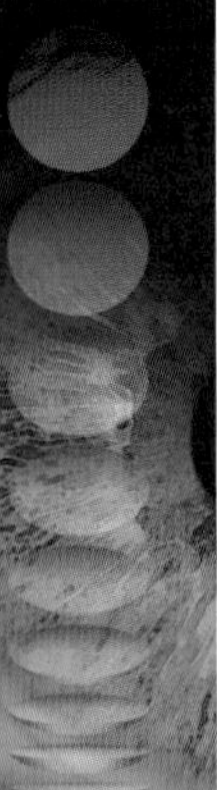

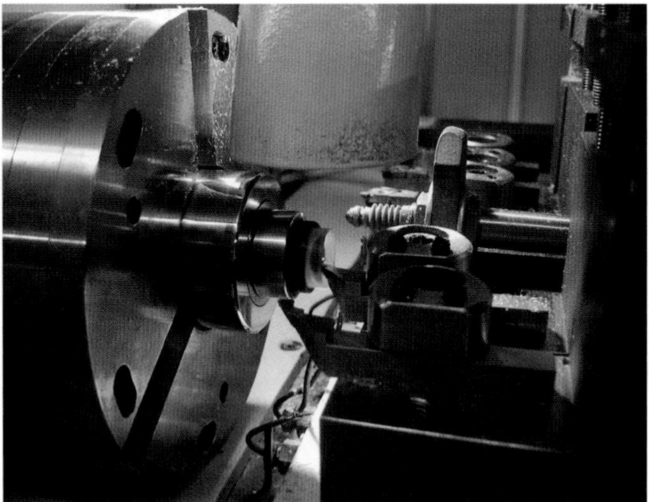

Figure 27.4 Back surface cutting on an Optoform 30 2-axis lathe

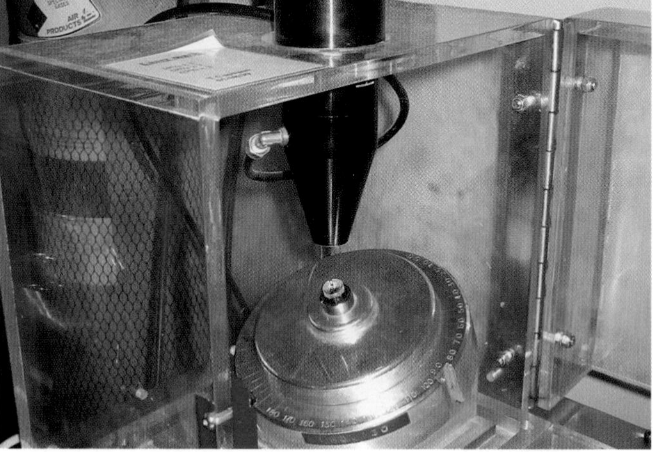

Figure 27.5 Back surface marking using a laser system

Back surface lathing

The material blank is held in the spindle of the lathe using either a dolly (Fig. 27.4) or directly by the spindle collet. The consistency of the overall size of the blanks and the tightness of the collet will determine whether any stress is introduced as the collet tightens on to the blank. Too tight a collet, which causes the blank to be crimped during cutting, will result in a toric surface once the cut blank is released from the collet. Too loose a collet, which allows the blank to slip during machining, will produce a poor-quality surface.

Once the blank is held by either a dolly or collet the technician will start the cutting process, ensuring that the correct data have been uploaded into the lathe. The lathe computer will then calculate the various cutting paths necessary to create the back surface geometry specified from the fabrication sheets or lathe data files. These cutting paths will include:

- Rough cuts.
- Intermediate cuts.
- Final cuts.
- Diameter cuts.

The final cut creates the final back surface geometry and removes only 0.005–0.02 mm of material. The speed at which the diamond traverses the surface is much slower than previous cuts in order to produce the best surface finish. It is at this stage that some lathes form an edge shape by generating a curve continuous with the back periphery and terminating a short way on to the front surface.

The feed rate, depth of cuts and spindle speeds are pre-programmed according to the particular characteristics of the material being machined. Machining can also introduce stress if too great an amount of material is removed with each cut. If the speed of cutting is too fast, the surface may overheat, causing changes to the surface polymer with a higher risk of back surface parameter changes on hydration and poorer back surface wetting. The cycle time of the lathe will depend on these parameters and the amount of material removed. This can be reduced by using blanks that are preformed, with some of the material already removed, and by using materials that can be cut at higher feed rates and depths of cut without being adversely affected.

The movement and speed of the spindle and the diamond cutting tools are controlled from the computer via the drive system. The tools and lens blank are cooled by a constant stream of cool air blown across the cutting surface via narrow metal pipes and the swarf is extracted by a vacuum system positioned directly above the tip of the diamond tool.

When the generation of the back surface is complete, the blank is removed from the collet and replaced with the next blank.

MARKING

Some contact lens designs include the requirement for markings (e.g. orientation marks on toric lenses). These marks can be applied in a number of ways to either the front or back surface. In the example in Figure 27.5 the marks are produced by laser light focused to create a series of axis alignment marks. Other methods include engraving using a diamond tool held against the surface with a specific force and moved to create the required mark. The depths of mark are carefully controlled to ensure that the lens is not weakened, but the mark is clearly visible.

SUBSTANCE MEASUREMENT

The back of the lens blank is classed as the reference surface and the distance from the back to the apex of the cut surface determines the substance thickness. This can be measured using a simple digital dial gauge mounted for ease of use (Fig. 27.6). During the front lathing process, the lathe probes the reference surface and then calculates the amount of material to remove by subtracting the desired centre thickness from the substance thickness.

Other production systems rely on a dead stop, which makes measuring the substance thickness unnecessary. Effectively, if the back lathe always removes the same amount from the blank to create the back surface, and the front surface blocking system employs a dead stop to ensure that the thickness of the chuck and blank together remain constant, the substance thickness

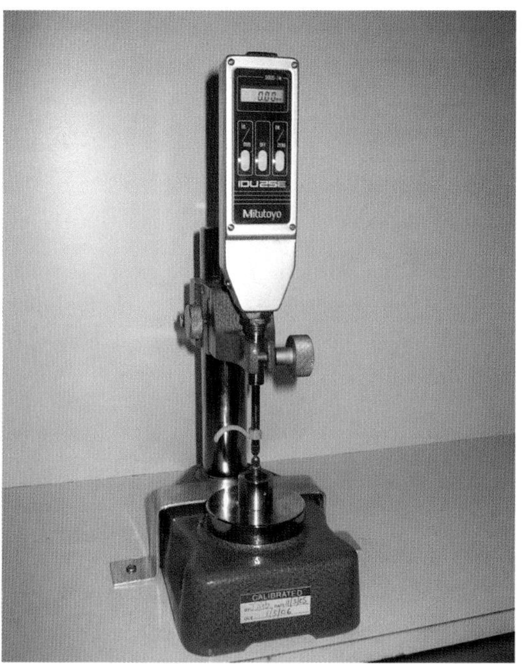

Figure 27.6 Substance measurement gauge

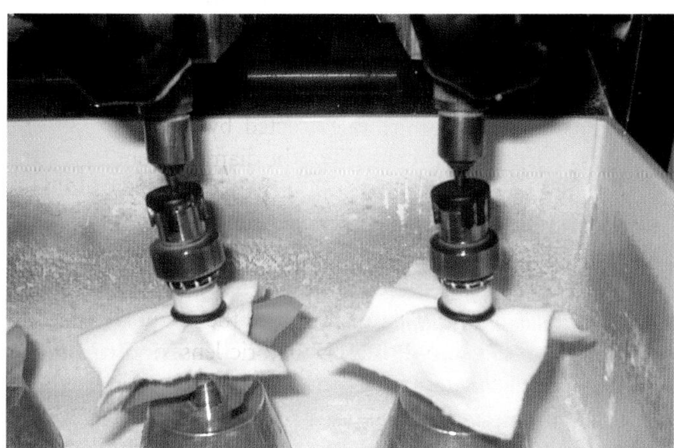

Figure 27.7 Back surface polishing

will always be the same. This system is more difficult to set up but removes the risk of operator error.

BACK SURFACE POLISHING

The back surface of the blank will usually need to be polished and this is carried out in the conventional manner by mounting the blank or dolly in a plastic 'clippy' (Fig. 27.7). The polishing tool may be formed from a spherical convex tool covered with foam, and a polishing cloth held on to the tool by an O-ring.

During polishing care is needed to prevent the material from overheating. This is done by ensuring that the blank is not polished for too long and that there is sufficient polish between the blank and the polishing tool – the better the surface finish after lathe cutting, the shorter the polishing cycle.

FRONT SURFACE BLOCKING

To allow the front lathe to cut the front surface accurately, the blank must be presented on a chuck designed to fit within the spindle collet and remain optically concentric (unless a prism is required) and parallel to the spindle axis. There are three ways to achieve this:

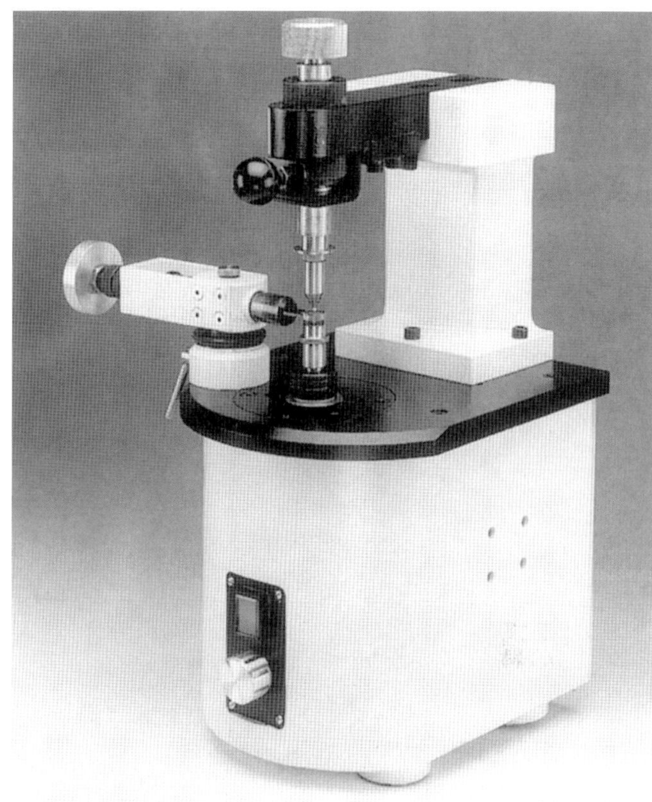

Figure 27.8 Nissel blocker

- Static.
- Dynamic.
- Optical.

All methods use wax to secure the back surface of the lens blank onto a brass chuck that is designed to fit into the front lathe collet. The chuck will have a convex surface that is matched closely to the cut back surface of the lens blank.

DYNAMIC BLOCKING

This process relies on a rotating spindle and the ability to correct the wobble of the lens blank while the wax is still soft. The simplest method requires a rotating spindle. A small amount of wax is melted on a hot chuck and the lens blank placed onto the chuck so that the cut back surface aligns the convex surface of the chuck. This is then placed into the collet of a spindle. Once in position, the spindle is started and a pointed object is held against the cut diameter of the back surface to reduce the wobble to zero. The accuracy of this method depends solely on the skill of the technician.

The process has been automated by a number of contact lens companies. Nissel (now Cantor & Nissel) developed the blocker shown in Figure 27.8. In this instance, a controlled device is used to reduce the wobble of the lens.

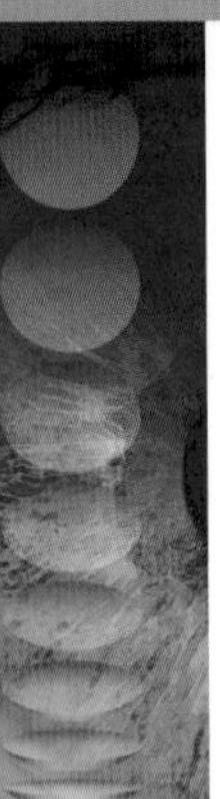

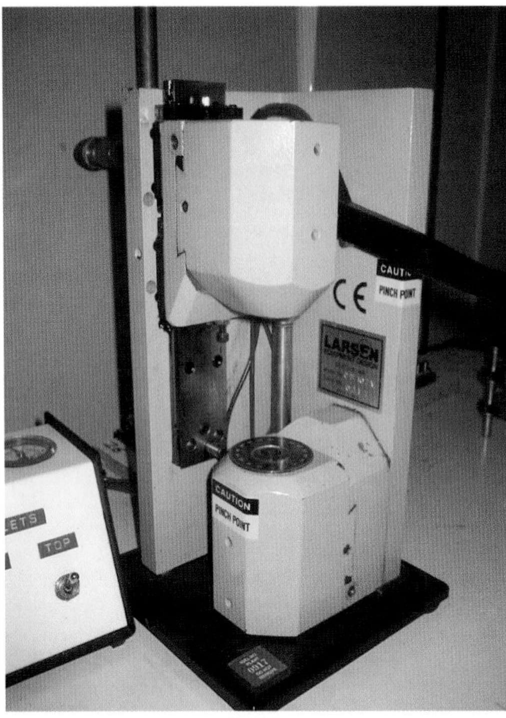

Figure 27.9 Larson static blocker

STATIC BLOCKING

By using high-precision parts and machinery, the location of the back surface is aligned accurately with the front surface. Figure 27.9 shows such a configuration, which uses collets similar to those used in the actual lathe spindle. The vertical slide is engineered so that the top and bottom collets remain concentric at all times. This system can be configured to use a dead stop as discussed previously.

One static blocking system originally developed by Polytech (UK) is based on disposable, low-cost injection-moulded inserts. These are machined for either back or front surface blank blocking and are designed to take the skill out of blocking while retaining the accuracy.

- The insert has an internal taper that matches the lathe spindle taper.
- The uncut blank, machined to 12.70 mm, is fitted into the back surface insert and sits firmly on an internal stop.
- This assembly is fixed into a carousel to hold it in position, inverted and loaded into the wax dispenser.
- Heated wax, at a controlled temperature, is then injected into the back of the insert/blank assembly.
- After cooling, the insert is removed from the carousel and placed on the taper of a back surface lathe.
- The back surface is then machined (Fig. 27.10) and an 'insert fit' diameter cut on the blank to enable correct location in the front surface insert.
- The blank, still in the back insert, is then polished and transferred to a front surface insert (Fig. 27.11) with a bore diameter into which the lathed 'insert fit' diameter is mounted. There must be no more than 10–20 μm diameter difference between the bore diameter and the lathed blank 'insert fit' diameter, to produce a maximum of 5–10 μm decentration.

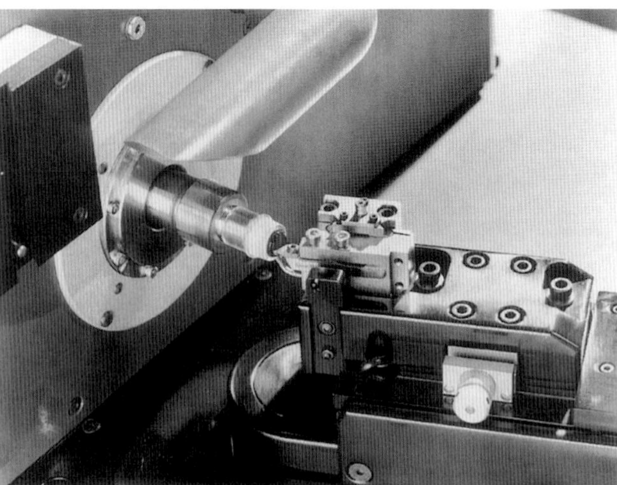

Figure 27.10 Polytech back surface insert blocker being machined on a Polytech air-bearing spindle lathe

- The assembly is then loaded into the carousel, inverted and blocked with wax as before. The machined diameter and the shoulder on the blank ensure that the semi-finished blank is located squarely into the insert, thus virtually eliminating unwanted prism and decentration.
- Once cool, the assembly is placed on a front surface lathe taper and cut to the required radius and thickness (see Fig. 27.11). The front surface can then be polished with the lens still fixed in the insert.

OPTICAL BLOCKING

This method uses an optical system to determine the optical centre of the cut back surface of the lens blank and then allows for the positioning of the chuck relative to the optical centre. The advantage of this system is that external references are not required. One example is the Optical Precision Blocker, developed by Benz Research and Development, which can be used in conjunction with state-of-the-art lathes for a fully automated manufacturing cell.

FRONT SURFACE LATHING

The chuck carrying the lens blank is placed into the collet of the front surface lathe. Once it is correctly located and the appropriate information loaded into the lathe, including the substance thickness measured previously, cutting is started.

The cutting process is similar to that of the back surface except that an initial probing routine is used to determine the back reference surface of the lens blank as previously described (see Substance measurement, p. 550).

Feed rates and depths of cut will again affect the overall surface quality and material performance.

In general, CNC lathes can cut both front and back surfaces. In practice, however, certain lathes are dedicated to certain processes. In this case, the diamond position is configured to optimize the front cutting process.

FRONT SURFACE POLISHING

Once the front surface has been machined to the required radius and thickness, it is polished (Fig. 27.12). This process, as

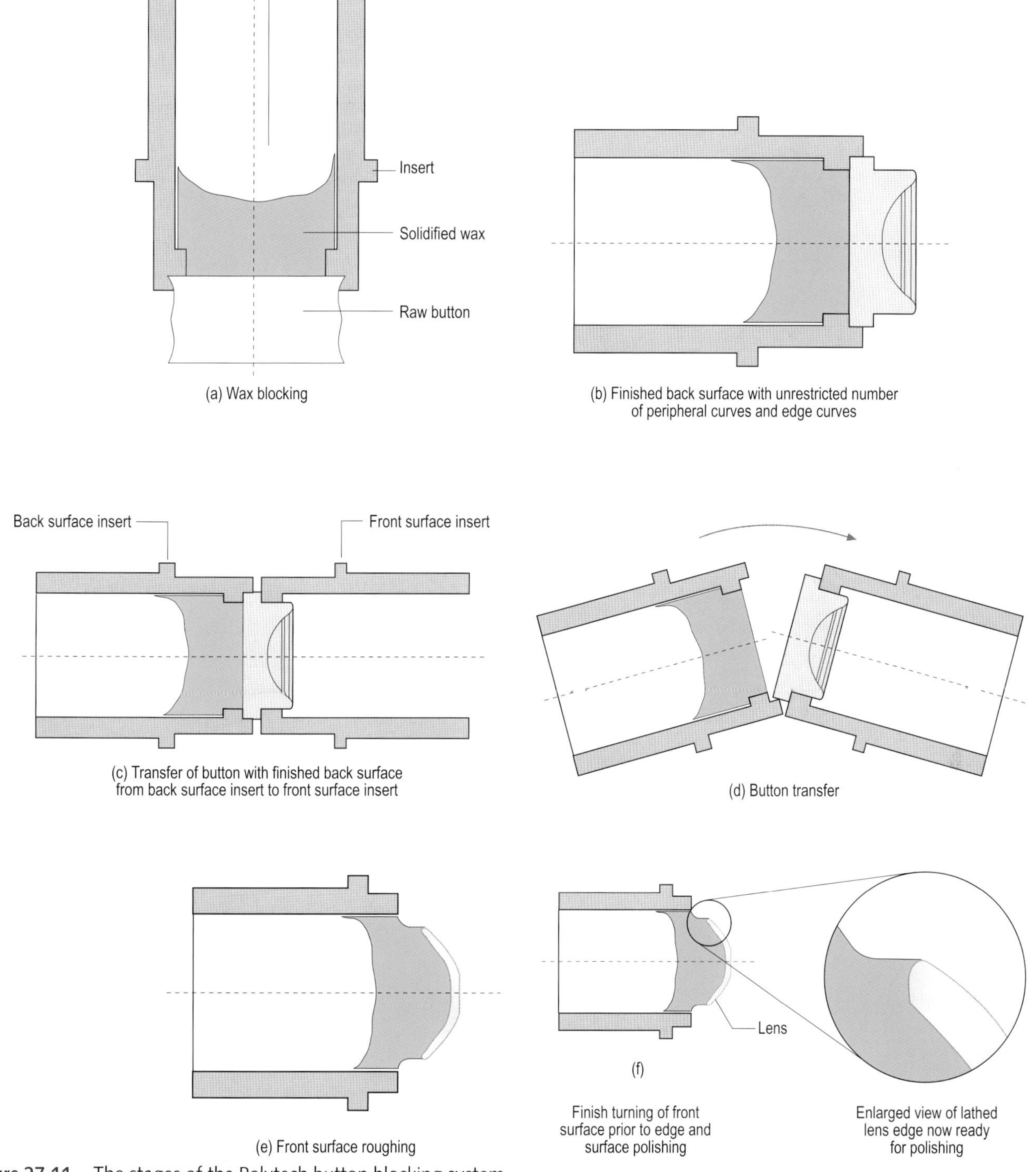

Figure 27.11 The stages of the Polytech button blocking system

with the back surface, should be for the shortest time possible as excessive polishing and/or insufficient polish will damage the surface and lead to poor lens wetting. The front surface polisher may be formed from a small drum tool filled with foam and covered with a polishing cloth held on to the tool by an O-ring.

To remove the lens, the chuck is either gently heated until the wax just melts or the wax is dissolved using an ultrasonic bath containing a suitable solvent (for soft lenses) or water (for RGP lenses). All residual wax adhering to the lens is then dissolved. During this process care is needed to ensure that a minimum amount of heat is transferred from the chuck to the lens and also to ensure compatibility of the solvent with the soft lens material.

BACK SURFACE BLENDING

This is carried out on multicurve RGP lenses (see Chapters 9 and 28). The number of curves can vary between two and six. In

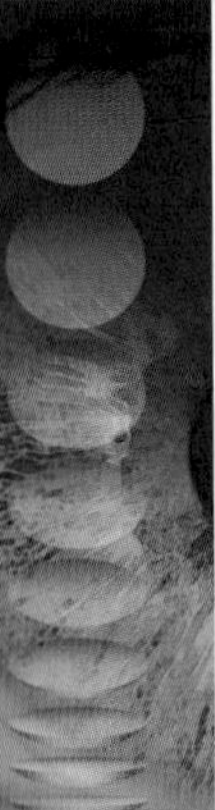

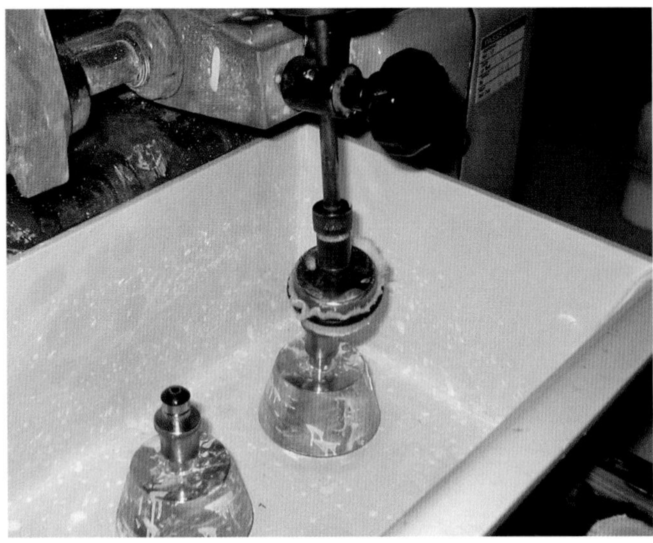

Figure 27.12 Front surface polishing

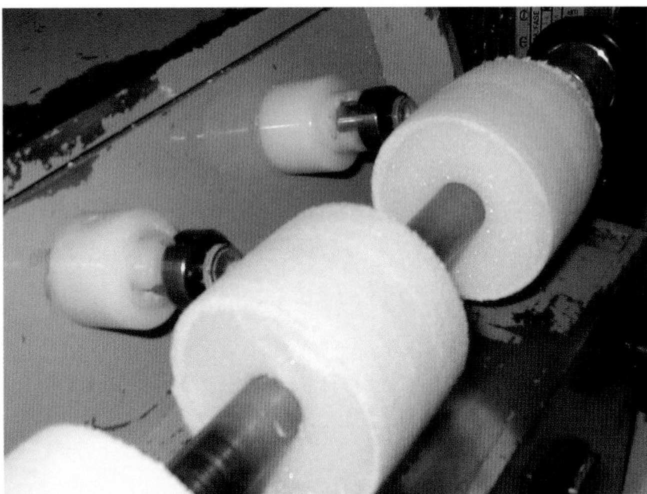

Figure 27.13 Back edge polishing

order to smooth the transitions, it is necessary to blend between each successive curve using a convex polishing tool with a radius determined as the average radius of the successive curves. The contact lens is held on a suction holder against the vertical spindle carrying the convex tool. Using plenty of polishing compound, the lens is moved from side to side and removed for frequent inspection. The amount of blending can be increased if requested by the practitioner.

EDGE POLISHING

Edge polishing differs between soft and RGP lenses mainly due to the material strength and design edge thicknesses.

Soft lens edges tend to be polished as additional processes prior to back and front surface polishing. Figure 27.13 shows the back edge being presented almost directly against the polishing sponge and polish compound to round the inside edge and allow for easier lens handling. Figure 27.14 shows the front edge being polished, bringing the surface down to meet the back polished edge.

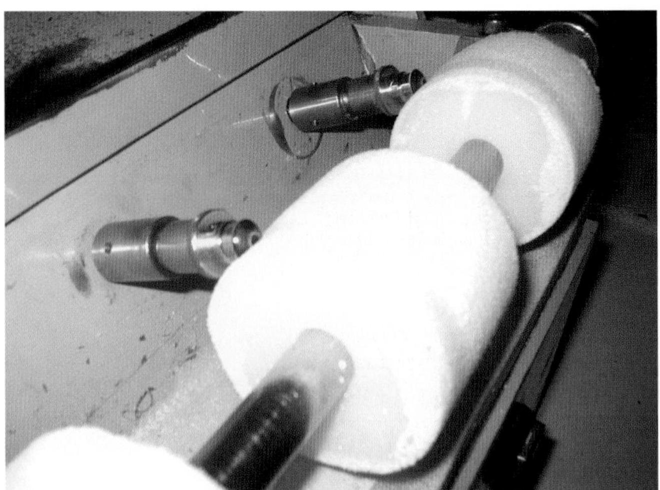

Figure 27.14 Front edge polishing

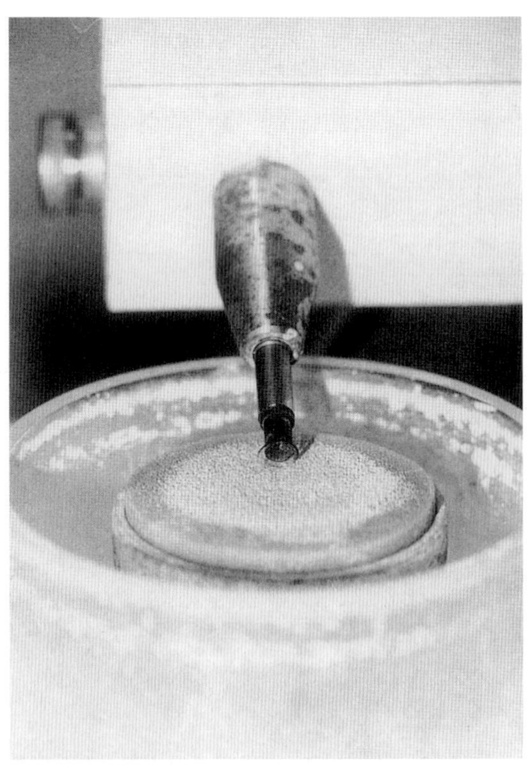

Figure 27.15 Edge polishing

Most laboratories use an automatic edge polisher (Fig. 27.15) to polish RGP lenses. The lens is held in a suction cup and rotated on a revolving sponge, which contains polish. This produces good results, provided the edge has already been shaped, and the process is suitable for mass stock lens production. However, it may result in the edge being polished but poorly shaped if the edge was poorly shaped prior to polishing (e.g. the lens may have a polished square edge).

The edge may also be polished by hand on a rotating velveteen-covered drum, the lens being held in a suction holder and rotated by hand with first the concave and then the convex surface facing the direction of rotation of the drum. This is followed by apical polishing of the edge with the lens rotated

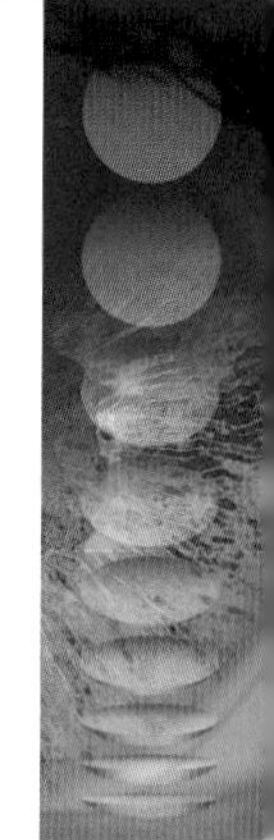

parallel to the edge of the drum. Although labour intensive, shaping and polishing of the edge by a skilled technician can give good results. The lens is checked regularly so that allowances can be made for the different thicknesses of individual prescriptions.

FINAL CHECKING

The checking of the final lens includes:

- Thickness.
- Diameter.
- Radius.
- Back vertex power measurements.
- Surface and edge quality.

At this stage, minor modification can be made to:

- Total diameter.
- Edge shape and polish.
- Blending of peripheral curves (RGP).
- Power.

LENS CLEANING AND PACKAGING

Once an RGP lens completes final inspection, it is cleaned using a laboratory contact lens cleaning solution, which removes all traces of polish and detritus likely to affect the surface wettability of the lens. The lens is then rinsed in purified water, to ensure that it is perfectly clean, and placed into its final container either as a dry lens or with a disinfecting wetting solution. The cleaning process should be performed in either a laminar flow cabinet or a clean room environment.

Soft lenses should be cleaned using an ultrasonic bath (see Front surface polishing, pp. 552–553).

Additional processes for soft lenses

HYDRATION

To hydrate a soft contact lens, the lens is placed in a 0.9% wv saline solution. This may be in single vials or in suitable baths depending on the numbers of lenses processed at one time. Different contact lens materials require different hydration times, varying from 5 minutes for a thin biomimetic lens, such as Proclear (CooperVision) to 1 day for an aphakic 38% HEMA lens. Once hydrated, the saline is replaced to remove any monomer extractables.

SOFT LENS FINAL CHECKING

Lathe-cut soft lenses are inspected manually or by an automated imaging system to detect any defects or blemishes. Manually, this is achieved using a wet cell projection device such as the Optimec JCF (see Fig. 27.2). This equipment can also measure the TD of the lens and the BOZR. However, the BOZR measurement derives from the sagittal depth of the back surface assuming a spherical surface. Measurement of toric or aspheric back curves would require allowances to be made.

Power is read using a standard projection focimeter such as a Nikon PL2 (Fig. 27.16). The soft lens is blotted dry before being placed on the stage of the focimeter, otherwise inconsistent power readings will be obtained. It is important not to allow the lens to dry out while taking the reading as this will result in inconsistencies.

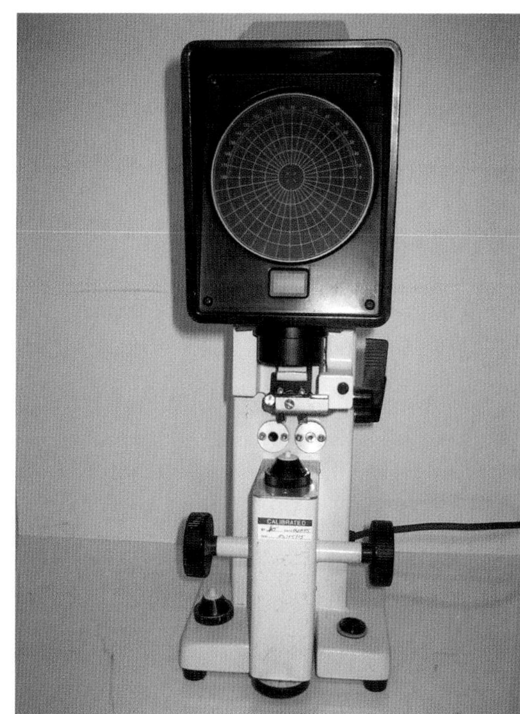

Figure 27.16 Nikon PL2 projection focimeter

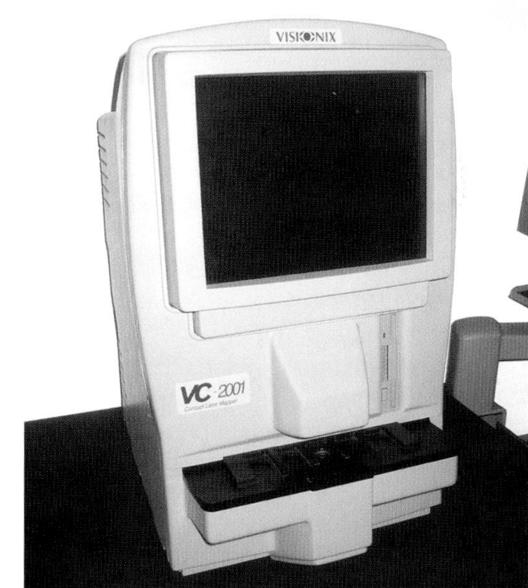

Figure 27.17 Visionix VC2001 contact lens mapper

Electronic methods of assessing power are available – for example, the Visionix Power Mapper VC2001 (Fig. 27.17), which uses a Shack–Hartmann grid to determine lens aberrations and hence powers, or the Rotlex ConTest (see Chapter 16) which uses interference fringes.

Electronic instruments reduce potential operator error, but must be set up correctly. The lens is immersed in a wet cell during the measurement process and the instrument measures

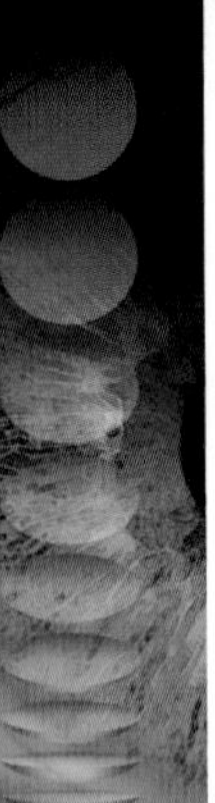

the wavefront deviation between the lens and the solution. The refractive index of the lens is typically around 1.43, and the solution around 1.33, which is a relatively small difference; therefore any set-up error is increased.

CLEANING AND PACKAGING

Once hydrated, the soft lens is cleaned either manually or using a series of cleaning baths. Again, a thorough rinsing process is employed to remove all traces of cleaning fluid. The lens is then inserted into a pre-washed vial with purified saline and sealed with a bung and crimp top.

STERILIZATION

Generally, pressurized steam is used to sterilize the contact lenses in their vials. This process is carefully controlled to ensure that all contact lenses undergo a time/temperature sequence approved by the Medical Devices Agency (MDA) – for example, 121°C for 15 minutes (see Chapter 4). Controls to verify this include autoclave performance qualification trials, using specific load patterns and recording temperature and pressure during the cycle.

Toric lens production

Concave and convex toric surfaces can be produced in one of two ways:

- Manual methods such as crimping, polishing or grinding – these are of historical interest only. For details, see Proctor (1997).
- Lathe cutting, which can be subdivided into:
  - direct lathing using oscillating tool technologies.
  - toric generation using fly-cutting techniques.
  - automatic crimping techniques.

TORIC LATHE CUTTING

Oscillating tool technology

First developed by Beauford Council and patented in 1987, under US patent 4680998, Council described a method for oscillating the diamond-cutting tool on a contact lens lathe. The oscillations are sinusoidal and the period is synchronized to the rotation of the lathe spindle, such that the lathe cuts a toric surface directly onto the contact lens blank.

Euro Precision Technology (EPT) commercialized the first lathing system using the rapid oscillating technology. Moving away from oscillating the diamond-cutting tool, EPT oscillated the spindle to create non-rotationally symmetrical forms that are not restricted to purely toric surfaces. These lathes are capable of machining complex surfaces designed for stabilizing the lens on the eye as well as correcting for astigmatism.

Other notable lathe manufacturers that incorporate the oscillating tool technologies are:

- Precitech Inc. (USA) manufacture and sell the Optoform range of contact lens lathes and the Variform, Varimax and FTS1000 oscillating tool technologies. The Variform and Varimax units rely on mechanically amplified dual piezoelectric actuators that allow for very high response rates and tool stiffness, but reduced tool movement range. The latest FTS1000 drives the tool using opposing linear motors, which allows for a greatly increased range of movement while maintaining high response rate and tool stiffness.
- DAC International Inc. (USA). DAC's oscillating tool technologies are based again on rapid movement of the diamond, but are controlled using voice coils. This system allows for large tool movements, again with high response rates and stiffness.
- Contamac B.V. (Netherlands) manufacture the Opteq 2-axis submicron lathe, on which the voice coil operated oscillating tool system permits three diamond tools to be controlled. This allows for greater flexibility in lens design as edge shapes can also be based on non-rotationally symmetrical geometries.
- Lamda Polytech Ltd. (UK) Multiform 40 2-axis lathe incorporates an oscillating tool system.

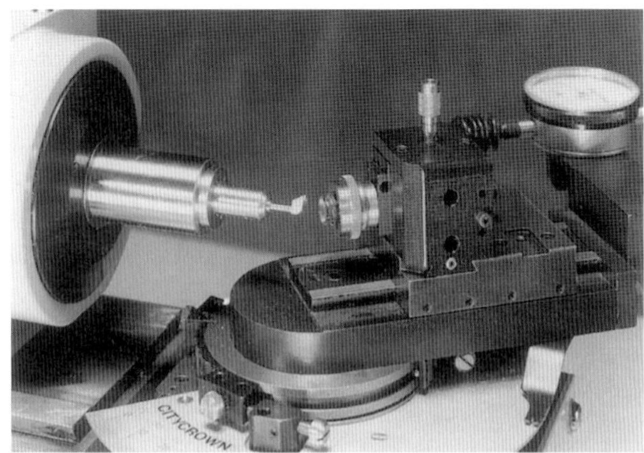

Figure 27.18 City Crown back surface toric lathe showing fly-cutter diamond tool and lens blank

The closed loop control systems to drive the oscillating tools are all software controlled and synchronized with the spindle using spindle encoders. Typically, lens design software is provided with these lathes as non-rotationally symmetrical contact lens designs contain many more complexities than standard spherical lens designs, although this can be commercially restrictive and in-house control over the designs may be preferable.

Toric generation using fly-cutting techniques

Back surface toric generator lathes use a diamond fly cutter – a diamond tool with its cutting tip at right angles to the axis of its shank. The shank of the fly cutter is held in the spindle collet while the lens blank is held in a collet in the radius cartridge (where the diamond would normally be in a conventional spherical lathe). The positions of the blank and cutting tool are therefore reversed (Fig. 27.18). When the spindle rotates the fly-cutter tip describes, in the vertical plane and at right angles to the spindle axis, a circle whose radius is the distance from the centre of the spindle to the tip of the diamond. The radius of the vertical circle, which is the flatter radius (axis horizontal) of the toric surface, can be altered by:

- Changing the size of the cutting tool.
- Offsetting the axis of the fly-cutting tool centre line in relation to the centre line of the radius cartridge.

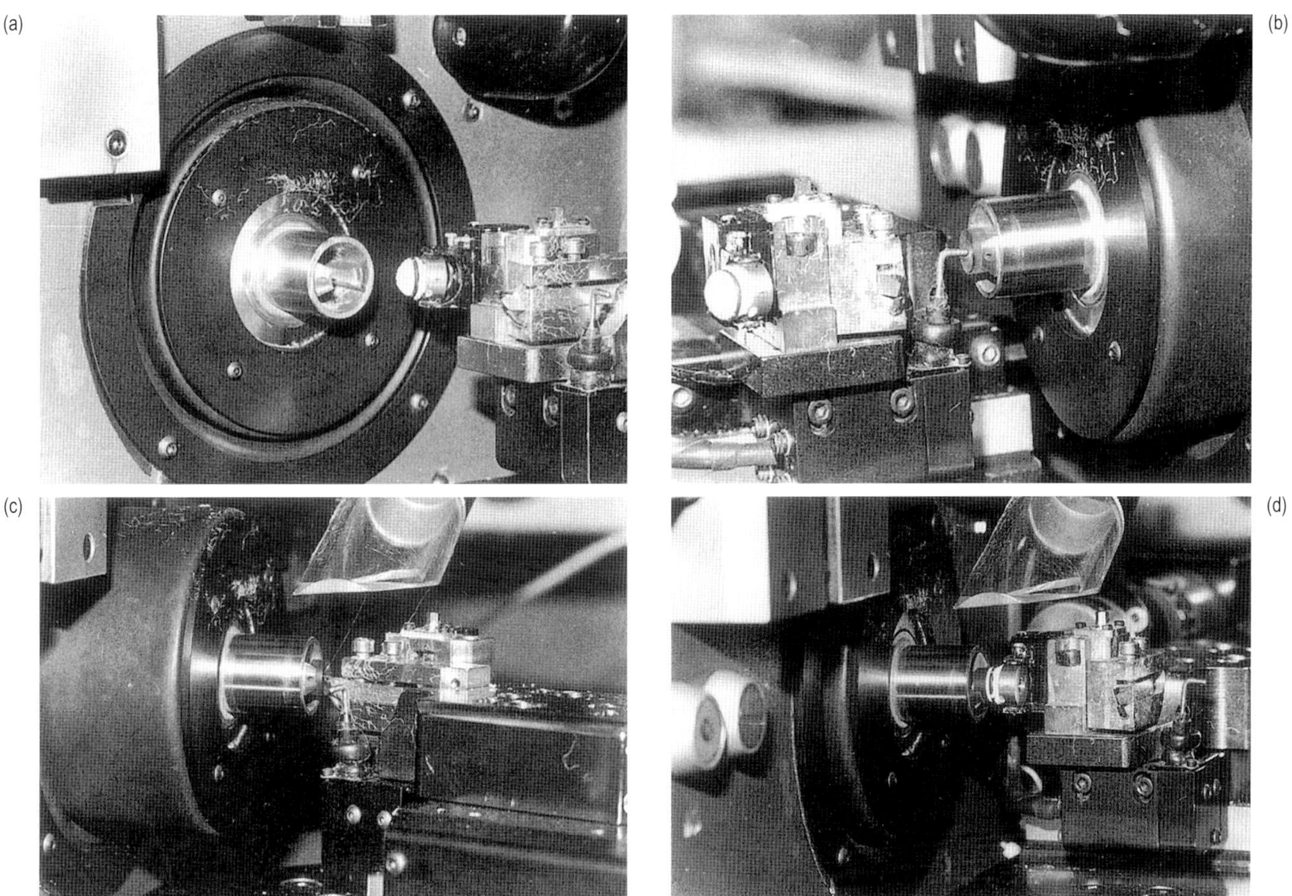

Figure 27.19 Polytech toric lathe: (a) showing the two jaw collet and polishing tool; (b) the sensor probe making contact to find the reference datum; (c) cutting the crimped base curve; (d) polishing the cut surface while still crimped

In all back surface toric lathes, the cutting tool remains constant for the flatter radii between 6.0 and 10.0 mm (Gfeller, Switzerland) and 6.0 and 12.0 mm (City Crown, UK). For flatter radii outside this range, the fly-cutting tool has to be changed.

In the Gfeller back surface toric lathe, the offset of the centre line is achieved by the special offset collet fixed to the spindle. The fly-cutting tool is held in this offset collet which effectively helps to extend the size (radius) of the cutting tool. The City Crown lathe achieves the offset of the centre line by a facility on the radius cartridge. This offset facility enables the whole radius cartridge assembly to be displaced at right angles to the spindle centre line, thus effectively offsetting the spindle to the radius cartridge centre line.

The toric surface is produced by presenting the non-rotating blank to the tip of the rotating fly-cutter tool. The non-rotating blank held in the collet of the radius cartridge describes an arc, along the horizontal plane, whose radius, when it passes through the tip of the fly-cutter diamond, is at right angles to the spindle axis. This horizontal arc represents the steeper curve (axis vertical) of the toric surface. This radius can be varied by altering the distance by which the centre of radius of the cutting tool extends beyond the pivot point of the radius cartridge.

Front surface toric lathes, such as that produced by Gfeller, work on a similar principle to the back surface toric lathes. They also use offsets of spindle axis in relation to the cutting tool centre line. However, the diamond-cutting tool is held in its conventional position and the work piece is mounted on the spindle but with its central axis at right angles to the spindle axis – similar to the fly-cutter tool of the back surface lathe. This has a special small front surface chuck onto which the lens blank is blocked. The blank rotates with the apex of its front surface describing a vertical circle at right angles to the spindle axis. The process is similar to the cutting of toric grinding and polishing wheels originally used by Nissel.

Automatic crimping techniques

Lamda Polytech Ltd. toric lathe

The Polytech back and front surface toric lathe (Fig. 27.19) induces toricity by a double-toothed jawed collet, crimping the blank in situ. The degree of crimp and hence toricity is controlled by computer which automatically adjusts the hydraulic pressure to the jaws of the collet by previously determined amounts. Once the requisite amount of crimp is achieved, the lens blank is machined using conventional spherical lathing. The machine has air bearings; it produces a high-quality surface finish, which is then lightly polished using the integral polishing tool. Front surface toric lenses can be generated in a similar fashion to the back surface with finishing carried out using the Polytech blocking system.

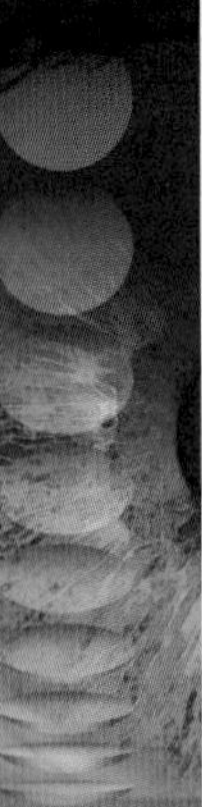

Miscellaneous techniques

FENESTRATION

Fenestration involves forming a hole, typically 0.20–0.30 mm diameter, with a vertical drill (or laser) while the lens is mounted convex surface uppermost on a chuck containing a small depression (or hole) which receives the penetrating drill. Both sides of the fenestration must be countersunk and polished. This is best done with a sharpened boxwood stick which is rotated in a circular fashion in the opposite direction to the vertical spindle on which the chuck and lens are rotating. To polish and countersink the back surface of the fenestration, the lens is placed on a concave chuck with the fenestration hole at its centre. The lens may be held in place by wax or double-sided adhesive tape, avoiding the central depression in the chuck. The central part of the fenestration is polished by running the lens up and down a length of polish-soaked cotton sewing thread passed through the fenestration hole (see also Chapter 28).

PRISMS

A prism may be incorporated into the lens either to correct a vertical extraocular muscle imbalance or more frequently to stabilize the lens, i.e. to prevent a front surface toric lens from rotating on the eye.

The optical axis of the front of the lens is offset in relation to the back of the lens. Methods vary but include the following:

- Offset collets – Spindle collets are machined with a defined offset, typically 0.156 mm to equate to 1 dioptre of optical prism, depending on BOZR and back vertex power (BVP). Usually, the back surface of the lens would be prepared and blocked onto a standard chuck, and then held in an offset collet for front lathe cutting.
- Variable offset adapters – Mechanically more complex, these tools have the same effect as an offset collet but with the ability to vary the offset distance.
- Offset blocking – Blocking systems may be adapted to induce a level of offset between the chuck and the lens back surface. The chuck is prepared so that the spherical surface will match the offset back surface of the cut lens blank, or a suitable amount of wax is used to fill the gap and support the lens.
- Oscillating tool technology – The prismatic surface can be manufactured with an oscillating tool system without the need to offset the front surface relative to the back; however, two factors need to be considered:
  - the tool movement is considerably greater than that required to machine a toric surface and may be out of range for particular systems.
  - a discontinuity may occur in the centre of the lens depending on the diamond tool radius used.

TRUNCATING

Lens truncation is usually carried out to help stabilize a toric or bifocal lens and is nearly always combined with prism ballast. Most frequently it involves only the lower edge. The edge is removed using an emery board or a diamond-impregnated tool. It is then polished with a felt wheel rotating in a flexible drive or on a rotating velveteen drum chuck, while the lens is mounted on an edging chuck. The corners of the truncation are rounded to minimize discomfort to the lower lid. With a bifocal lens, the edge is left fairly square to assist the lower lid in raising the lens when the gaze is depressed.

HYBRID PROCESSES

Hybrid processes bring together the volume and cost-saving aspects of moulding and the flexibility of lathe cutting. They are used for production of durable soft stock lenses as well as disposable toric lenses.

To simplify the process, lenses are manufactured using the cast-moulding technique with a defined back surface geometry and a generic front surface, to a thickness that will allow the front surface to be lathe-cut into all the required designs. Once the mould is split, the cast lens is then lathe-cut while remaining attached to the back surface mould (Fig. 27.20).

- *Stages 1–8* of the previously described cast-moulding process (see Fig. 27.1) apply to the hybrid process with the exception that the female cast mould is not designed for a specific contact lens power.
- *Stages 9 and 10* – The cast contact lens has a prepared moulded back and a thickness that will allow the front surface to be lathe cut to produce the correct lens geometry. The generic female cast mould is removed, exposing the front of the cast lens.
- *Stage 11* – Using a breach-loading system, the male cast mould and moulded lens are held concentrically on the lathe spindle. Once in place, the lathe will cut the correct front surface geometry onto the moulded lens in a similar fashion to the lathe-cutting process described previously. As the amount of material to be removed is small, the cutting cycle is short compared to standard lathe-cutting processes. The lathe is automatically loaded and unloaded to maximize production efficiency.
- *Stages 12–14* – These stages are similar to Stages 10–12 of the cast moulding process described on page 546.

Lathe technology

Lathe technology is the most common way of defining the surfaces of contact lenses, whether it be by machining the contact lens directly or machining the insert tools for cast moulding manufacture. The exceptions include the forming of the back surface using spin-casting techniques (although the front cast is manufactured using tools cut on lathes) and CIBA Vision's LightStream Technology, which employs a grinding technique to manufacture the quartz and glass tools.

3-AXIS AND 2-AXIS LATHES

Generally, lathes are available in 3-axis or 2-axis configurations, the former being able to produce spherical surfaces mechanically

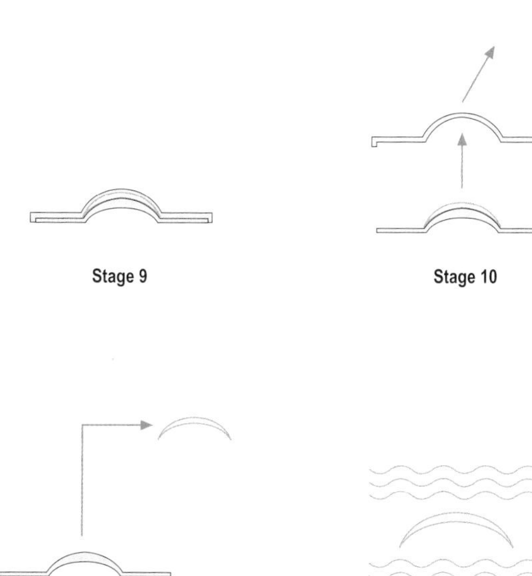

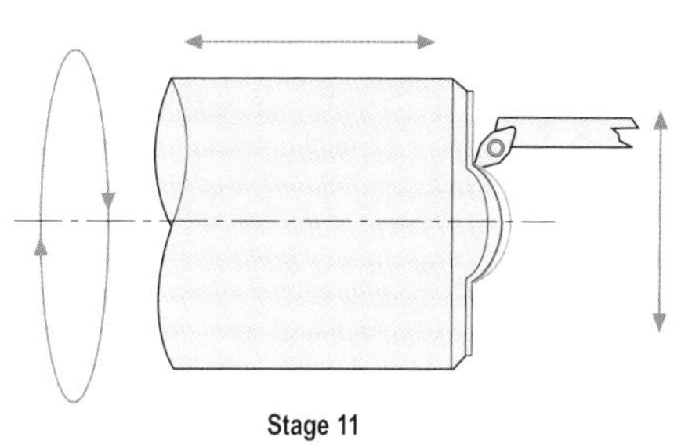

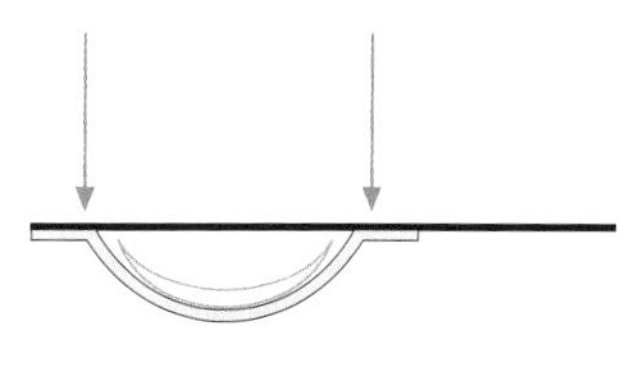

Figure 27.20 Illustration of hybrid process. This follows on from Stage 8 in Figure 27.1. (See text for explanation)

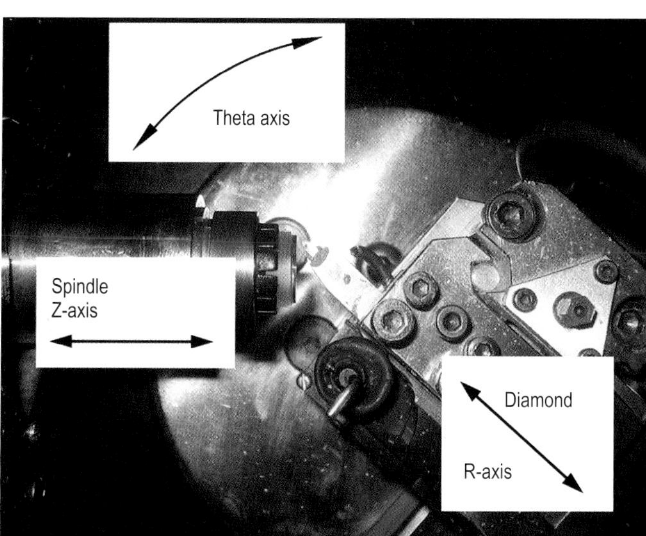

Figure 27.21 Polytech P1800 aspheric lathe showing axis details

without the need for computer control. Additionally, 4-axis lathes are available for specialist manufacturing such as the production of intraocular lenses.

3-axis lathes

The first 3-axis lathes consisted simply of a ball-bearing spindle, mounted on a dovetail slide (Z-axis) and a radius slide (R-axis) mounted on a theta bearing (theta axis) (Fig. 27.21). The radius slide is set to cut the correct radius curve into the contact lens material to position the spindle axis and ensure that the correct depth of cut is achieved, and to control the speed of cut by moving the radius slide around the theta axis by manipulating the radius slide lever.

Advances to this lathe configuration have been many and inventive and include the following:

- *Motor-driven radius slide* – The addition of a motor drive to the theta bearing to allow for greater control over the cutting movement.
- *Lenticular slides* – An additional slide mounted onto the radius slide, configured to cut a lenticular and an optic radius.
- *Aspheric surfaces* – Gfeller developed a system of cams to change the radius slide in relation to the theta position, allowing various aspheric surfaces to be cut.
- *Semi-automatic* – Using a series of motor drives on the Z-axis and theta axis. Once the optic radius, lenticular radius and angle are manually set, the technician can programme the lathe to take a series of cuts at specified speeds, rates and depths to complete the process.
- *Full CNC control* – Manufacturers such as Lamda Polytech, Chase and City Crown developed a number of fully automatic CNC lathes that offer aspheric surface capabilities by mapping the R- or Z-axis slides to the theta axis. Combined with air-bearing spindles, these lathes are used in large numbers worldwide. To achieve high levels of reproducibility, closed loop servo controls are used on all axes. Figure 27.21 indicates the axis positions on a full CNC lathe.

2-axis lathes

With the advent of computer numerical control systems, 2-axis lathes became possible. The axes in the lathe configuration are set at 90° to each other, typically with the spindle axis along the Z-axis and the diamond mounted on a tool plate which moves along the X-axis (Fig. 27.22).

To machine any surface other than flat requires a high degree of coordination between both axes of the lathe. This is achieved by incorporating:

- High-precision motion controllers.
- Amplifiers.
- Optical grating linear transducers.
- Linear drive systems.

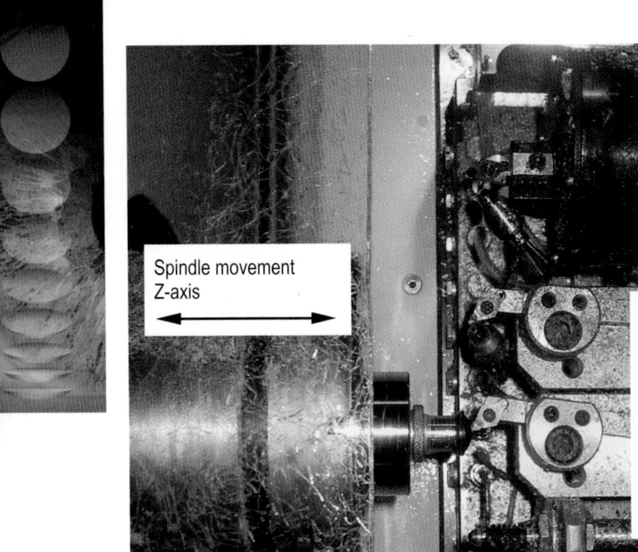

Figure 27.22 Optoform 80 lathe showing axis details

These are all tuned to a particular lathe. Additionally, complex mathematical algorithms are used to determine the diamond tool path, compensating for the radius of the diamond tool tip, as the majority of cutting will be done using the side of the tool. In this respect the diamond tool has to have a closely controlled radius, nominally deviating less than 0.5 μm from a perfect spherical curve.

Two-axis lathes are now considered superior for a number of reasons:

- *Simplicity* – Mechanically, 2-axis lathes offer a simpler configuration than 3-axis lathes, which allows more robust design methodology, thereby reducing set-up times.
- *Multiple tools* – It is common to position a number of tools on the tool plate, each configured for a different purpose (e.g. roughing tools, finishing tools and edging tools).
- *Oscillating tool capability* – Oscillating tool units can be placed on the tool plate, enabling non-rotationally symmetrical surfaces to be cut.
- *Suited to insert tool manufacture* – Many insert tools require additional geometric features in order to produce, for example, the edge profile and meeting surfaces of the cast. The 2-axis machines allow for this.
- *More accurate form definition and higher surface quality* – 2-axis lathes tend to be stiffer.

SUBMICRON MANUFACTURE

A number of companies worldwide are currently achieving the manufacture of polish-free contact lenses, and others will follow. It does, however, rely on a complete revision of the total manufacturing process from raw materials and contact lens design through to final inspection and packaging. Along with the obvious cost saving of a labour-intensive polishing process, there are a number of additional benefits:

- Complete definition of the contact lens includes polishing, blending and edging, processes that can introduce a reduction in process repeatability. Polish-free lenses are defined in their entirety, including any junction blending geometries and edge profiles.
- Reduction in lens contamination – in particular for RGP lens manufacture, over-polishing may modify the contact lens surface and reduce the wettability of the lens.
- Elimination of toric and aspheric polishing – polishing toric and aspheric surfaces tends to reduce the process flexibility and introduce greater variations.
- Allows for great automation (see below).

AUTOMATION

Cost of manufacture tends to dictate the modality and parameter range of the contact lens. The lower the cost, the more likely the lens is to be sold as frequent replacement but in a limited parameter range: the higher the cost, the more likely the lens is to be sold as a durable lens but to the patient's own prescription. Hybrid processes may go someway to cover the middle ground but fail to fulfil the goal of full prescription lenses based on a disposable modality.

Recent advances in submicron manufacture and robotic automation can potentially reduce the cost of manufacture to a level where it may be commercially viable to sell fully bespoke lenses as a disposable modality.

Benz Research and Development (USA) have developed a system based on cellular manufacturing units, consisting of two or three state-of-the-art submicron lathes and a robotic feed system. Using such a system, it is possible to manufacture lathe-cut lenses 24 hours a day, 7 days a week with minimal supervision and intervention.

Although the capital cost of such manufacturing systems is high, it is likely that forward-thinking contact lens laboratories will move towards automated manufacture in order to remain competitive.

References

Council, B. (1987) Toric lenses, method and apparatus for making same. US Patent 4680998

Proctor, E. (1997) Contact lens manufacturing. In Contact Lenses, 4th edn, pp. 791–792, eds. A. J. Phillips and L. Speedwell. Oxford: Butterworth-Heinemann

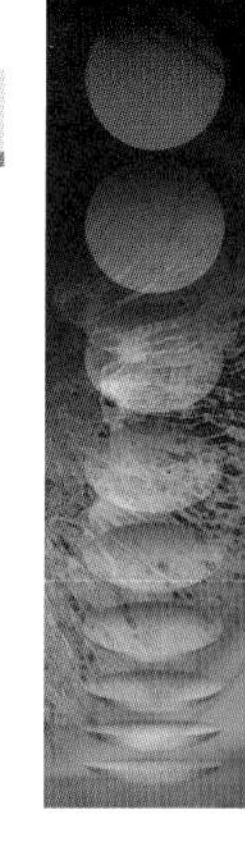

Further reading

Cordrey, P. (1973) Technical and economic effects of contact lens production methods. Ophthal. Opt., 13, 230–236

Crundall, E. J. (1977) Spun to curve. Optician, 173(4483), 15–16, 19–20, 23, 28

Haynes, P. R. (1965) Modification procedures. In Contact Lens Practice: Basic and Advanced, pp. 252–280, ed. R. B. Mandell. Springfield: C. C. Thomas

Hicks, M. (1975) More than a million. Optician, 170(4407), 18–26

Hodd, F. A. B. (1974) Bifocal contact lens practice. Ophthal. Opt., 13, 315–320, 325–326, 378–380, 385–388

Hough, A. (1994) Technology leaps light years ahead. Optician, 214(5626), 16–18

Inman, D. R. (1974) Peripheral design of toric corneal lenses. Optician, 167(4318), 13–17

Nissel, G. (1975) Manufacturing techniques. In Contact Lens Practice: Visual, Therapeutic and Prosthetic, pp. 314–342, ed. M. Ruben. London: Baillière Tindall

Chapter 28

Modification procedures

A. J. Phillips

CHAPTER CONTENTS

THE IMPORTANCE OF THE PRACTITIONER BEING ABLE TO CARRY OUT MODIFICATIONS

Nowadays, when modifications can be carried out relatively quickly and cheaply by laboratories, it is often difficult to impress on students, and even qualified practitioners, the following reasons why contact lens practitioners should be able to carry out their own modifications.

- There is no interruption to the patient's wearing schedule or necessity for extra visits.
- Often only the practitioner knows exactly what is required and it may be difficult to describe this to the laboratory (particularly so with scleral lenses).
- Modifications can be done in increasing stages, with the effect on the fit of the lens noted at each stage.
- Subsequent modifications may become apparent and can be done immediately.
- Practitioners who carry out modifications are better able to evaluate lenses that have been made or modified by a laboratory.
- Patients are more satisfied because they do not have to be without their lenses.

Against these advantages must be set the cost of the equipment involved. However, much of this cost can be redeemed, not only from tax relief but also on the savings of doing the modification oneself. Further, most of the equipment, especially the more expensive items, will last a lifetime (see Points to note when modifying RGP lenses, p. 571).

MODIFICATION EQUIPMENT FOR CORNEAL LENSES

Corneal lens holders

GLASS TUBE AND DOUBLE-SIDED ADHESIVE TAPE

A glass tube of approximately 6 mm in diameter, with rounded ends, has a small strip of double-sided adhesive tape stretched over one end, on to which the lens is lightly pressed. An inverted glass tube from a dropper bottle is ideal.

MODIFIED SCLERAL LENS HOLDER

An ordinary scleral lens suction holder is cut down and thinned on a rotating rough grinding stone to an internal diameter of approximately 7.5 mm and an edge thickness of approximately 0.5 mm (Figs 28.1, 28.2). A corneal lens holder may also be used

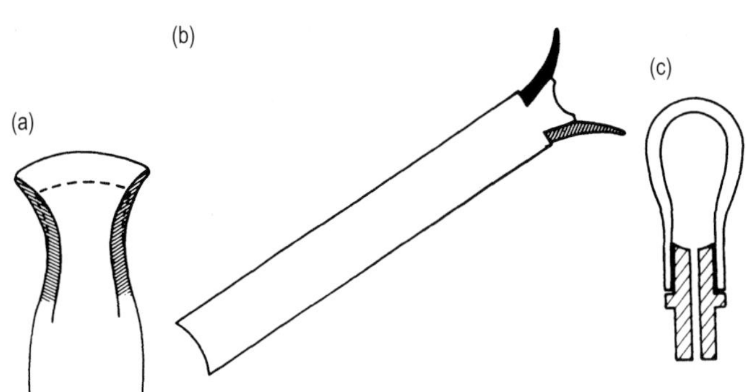

Figure 28.1 Cross-sections of corneal lens holders. (a) Scleral lens suction holder with the dotted line indicating the reduced size suitable for holding corneal lenses. (b) The end of a corneal lens suction holder mounted on a Perspex or nylon rod. (c) A double-ended suction holder. The lower shaded portion is removable and reversible, having a flat end and a concave end for holding back and front surfaces of corneal lenses, respectively

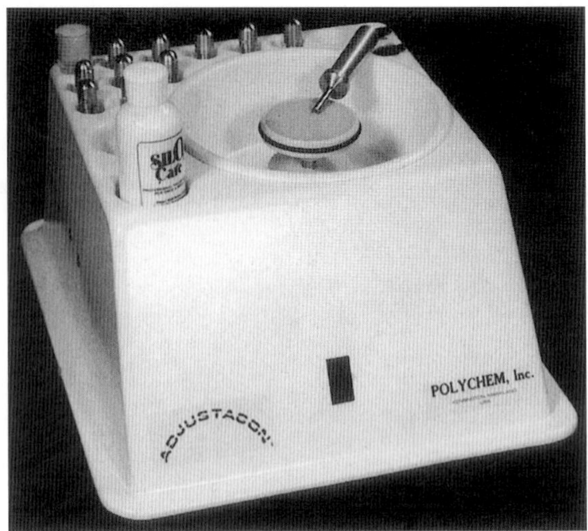

Figure 28.3 Vertical spindle or Office Modification Unit by PolyChem Inc. (Coburn Optical Industries Inc.)

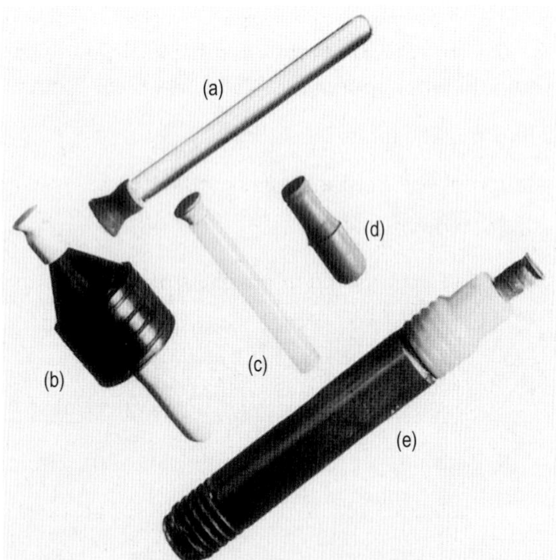

Figure 28.2 Corneal lens holders. (a) Corneal lens suction holder cup mounted on a Perspex handle; (b) spinner (Madden & Layman Ltd); (c) corneal lens suction holder cup mounted on a nylon handle; (d) modified scleral lens suction holder; (e) spinner

with a hollow plastic tube in the stem to give support (Haynes 1965). These holders are best used filled with water and rotated manually to prevent oval optics.

MODIFIED CORNEAL SUCTION HOLDER

The end of a corneal lens suction holder is placed over a short nylon or Perspex rod cut (see Figs 28.1b and 28.2c). Again, best used with the open end full of water, this type gives good control and spins easily with one finger resting lightly on the upper end.

SPINNER

A more efficient version of the previous holder, this consists of a rotatable spindle with a corneal lens suction holder at the end, mounted in a handle (see Fig. 28.2b,e). The lens can rotate freely on the end of the spindle while the handle is held still.

DOUBLE-ENDED SUCTION HOLDER

This has one end for attachment to convex surfaces and one for concave surfaces (see Fig. 28.1c). As this is the only type of lens holder, apart from those using adhesive tape, which will attach to the back surface of a corneal lens, it finds particular application in the alteration of lens power and removal of front surface abrasions (see below). Suction holders have the disadvantage that the lens may flex, particularly with thinner lenses, and the curves may be produced slightly steeper than desired, or slightly distorted. In addition, care must be taken when removing the lens from the holder.

Vertical spindle or Office Modification Unit (Fig. 28.3)

A speed of between 500 and 1500 rev/min is required – ideally, variable over this range, especially in the slower region.

The unit should be mounted in a bench or unit with the part shown situated above the level of the bench (Fig. 28.3). This enables the operator to rest with the elbows on the tabletop and steady the hands, and to roll the cutting blade and smoothing tools around the edge of the lens when shaping the edge or reducing the total diameter.

Spindle lens chuck or edging chuck (Fig. 28.4)

This is used for edge and total diameter modifications and should be carefully chosen so that the taper fits the practitioner's own vertical spindle (e.g. standard or 0-morse tapers). It is preferable to have a chuck, approximately 6 mm wide and 2 cm long, held by a stem that is not too short or thick.

The same chuck may also be used for holding lenses for peripheral curve modification of the back surface. The lens is stuck on to the chuck with wax or double-sided adhesive tape

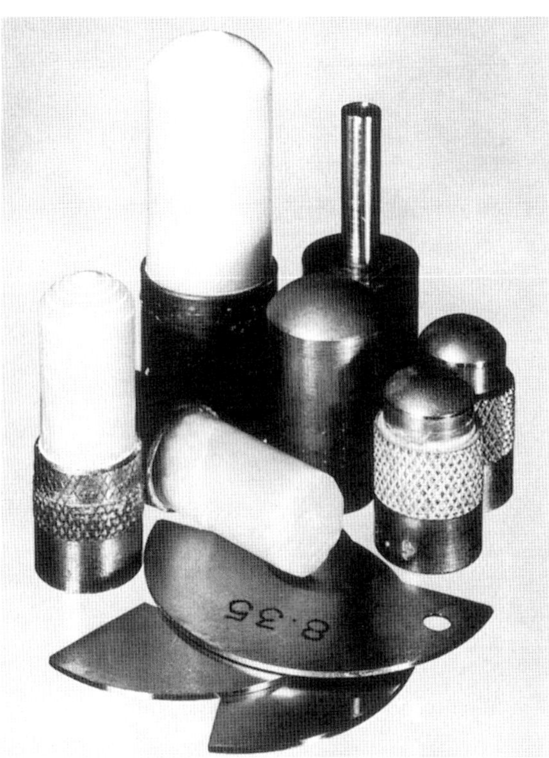

Figure 28.4 *Left to right*: (*rear*) large wax tool and spindle lens holder (or edging chuck); (*centre*) small wax tools, cut and uncut, and large and small diamond-impregnated brass tools; (*front*) female gauges

and held rigid on the tool so that no flexing occurs during polishing; however, if the stem is very narrow the periphery of a large corneal lens may still flex.

Adhesive wax and Bunsen burner

Adhesive wax, obtainable in stick form, is one way of attaching the lens to the spindle lens chuck. A Bunsen or compressed butane burner is used to melt the wax. More sophisticated electric heaters are also available to heat the metal chucks. Low-melting-point wax should be used for rigid gas-permeable (RGP) materials.

Centring devices

These are necessary when double-sided adhesive tape is used on the spindle lens chuck instead of beeswax, and where the lens must be accurately centred on the chuck.

The lens is placed in the well of the device. The centring part is carefully lowered on to the lens and slowly rotated to centre the lens within the well. It is then withdrawn.

These devices are not usually as accurate as centring by hand (see below).

Wax polishing tools

The practitioner makes these tools by pouring molten wax into moulds and allowing this to set. They are used for accurate polishing to a specific radius (see Fig. 28.4). Instructions for their manufacture are given by the laboratory supplying them; alternatively, they may be made up by the laboratory. Normally, only convex curves are cut on these tools.

Female gauges

These cut wax tools to their required radius (see Fig. 28.4). Stainless steel gauges are the most accurate and long lasting. A razor blade should be used to cut the wax cylinder to approximately the correct radius, and the female gauge used only for final 'truing-up' in order to prevent excessive wear.

Metal or plastic tools and adhesive tape

As an alternative to the wax polishing tools, adhesive cloth zinc oxide 'sticking plaster' is stretched over a suitable tool, and used for polishing lens peripheries, an allowance of approximately 0.2 mm (depending on the tape used) being made for the thickness of the tape. When using this type of tool, check with the manufacturing laboratory whether an allowance has been made for an average tape thickness when constructing the tool.

This method has the advantage that it is not normally necessary to put on a separate transitional curve as with the wax tools. However, the accuracy of curves polished by 'cloth polishing' cannot be guaranteed.

Tools may also be covered in muslin, stretched taut and held in place with a rubber band.

Polishing liquids

The polishing liquid used most frequently for polymethylmethacrylate (PMMA) lenses is the metal polish Silvo. Allow the container to stand for 2 or 3 days, then pour off most of the excess clear fluid and use the slightly thicker polishing fluid.

The ammonia in Silvo acts as a solvent for most RGP materials and should not therefore be used on these types of lens, nor should solvents or polishing compounds containing alcohol, esters, chlorinated hydrocarbons, ammonia, etc. Suitable polishes are X-Pal, Linde A, SPI, Hyprez, Boston, Silo2 Care polish, etc., but ideally consult the individual material manufacturers.

For soft lenses, a good standard polish that will give an excellent surface finish is CCPI polishing compound mixed with silicone oil.

Paraffin oil

Ordinary paraffin oil (kerosene) is used to remove any wax that remains attached to a lens after removal from a chuck. It may also be used as a lubricant with diamond-impregnated tools when putting on the peripheral curve of a corneal lens prior to final polishing, or grinding out the back optic surface of a scleral lens. Being more viscous than water, it prevents such deep scratches (although grinding is slower), enabling the final polishing to be done more quickly.

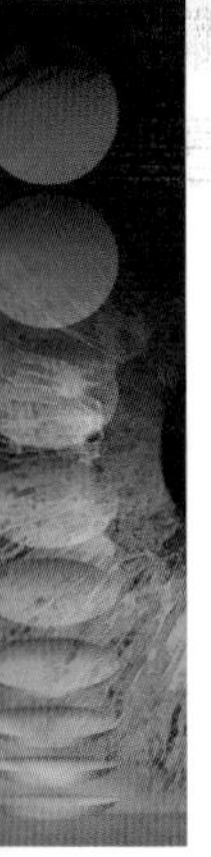

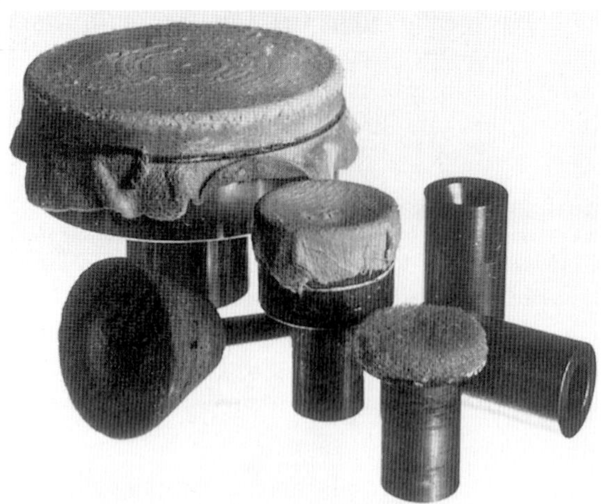

Figure 28.5 *Left to right*: (*rear*) large polishing drum; (*centre*) carborundum tool for reduction of total diameter, small polishing drum, and conlish tools; (*front*) flat plate sponge chuck

Razor and scalpel blades

Single-edge ('safety') razor blades and scalpel blades (straight and curved) are useful for certain modifications (see below). Alternatively, a thicker square-edged cutter may be used.

Carborundum tool for total diameter reduction

This is an internally tapering cone, held in a Jacob's chuck (Fig. 28.5). The tool is soaked in water and the lens must be placed centrally to remove peripheral material. If it is not central, material will be removed unequally (Haynes 1959). With lenses incorporating a prism, more material may be removed from the thinner lens edge.

Assorted carborundum or diamond-impregnated burrs

These (Fig. 28.6) are used for final edge shaping. Very fine emery paper may also be used.

Polishing cloth

This very soft cloth (e.g. 'Selvyt' cloth) is used for adding small amounts of power to lenses. Suitable cloth may be obtained from any contact lens laboratory at little cost; alternatively, ordinary velveteen material may be purchased.

Flat plate and sponge or drum chucks

These chucks (see Fig. 28.5) are used on a vertical spindle for adding positive and negative power to lenses, removing surface scratches and edge polishing. The drum chuck is a hollow chuck over which a piece of chamois leather or similar material is stretched and held in place with a rubber band or wire. The flat plate chuck has an upper flat portion with a thin piece of sponge rubber or moleskin attached.

Chamois leather

A large piece of chamois leather (e.g. 15 × 15 cm) is a useful backing to the polishing cloth mentioned above, and is sometimes used as an alternative.

A smaller piece of thinner chamois leather or sponge rubber may be used for edge polishing while the lens remains mounted on the spindle lens chuck.

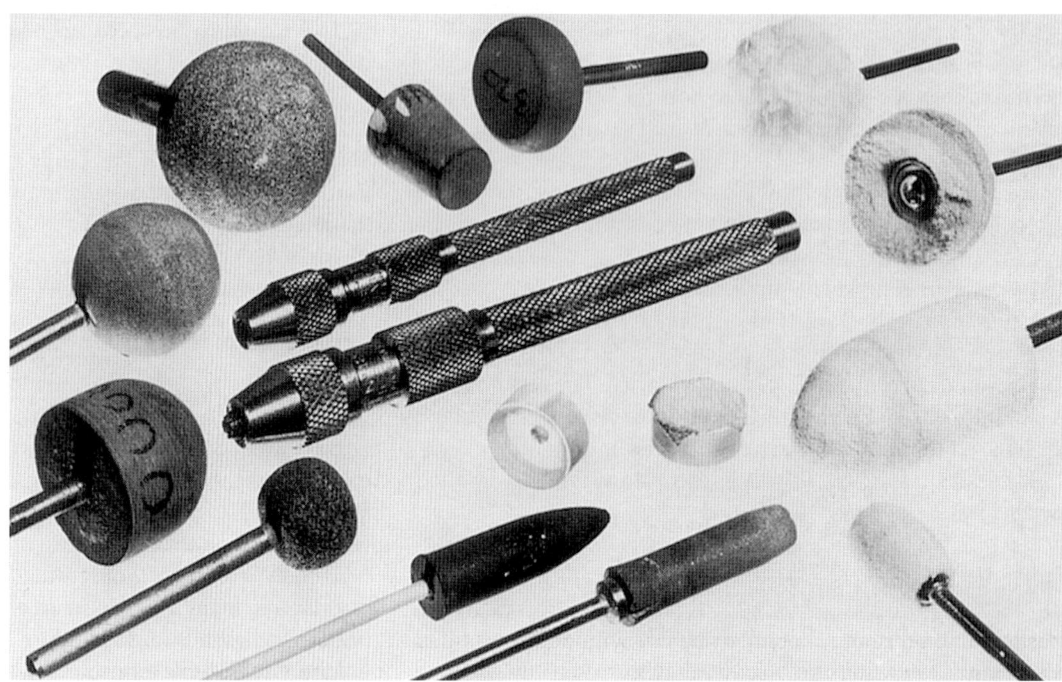

Figure 28.6 Assorted grinding tools and polishing buffs. *Top centre*: large and small pin-vice holders for drills. *Lower centre*: corneal lens buttons with one surface cut for use as scleral lens runners. The left button shows a guide hole on the rear surface; the right button has double-sided adhesive tape on the concave surface

Conlish tools (from conical and polish)

These are a series of hollow cone tools of varying angles (see Fig. 28.5) lined with adhesive cloth tape and used on a vertical spindle.

The lens can be mounted on a glass tube and the edge polished for a specific number of seconds on each tool.

Drills

Drills bits of 0.10–0.30 mm diameter mounted in hand drill or pin-vice holders (see Fig. 28.6) are used to fenestrate corneal lenses.

Countersinking fenestrations are carried out using the finest dental countersink rose (size 0 or 1) then several finely sharpened boxwood sticks for hand polishing the countersink.

For scleral lenses the following additional tools are required.

Scleral lens runners

Scleral lens runners are attached to the front optic scleral lens surface with broad (12 mm) double-sided adhesive tape on the concave runner surface. They are used with a pencil or ballpoint pen tip in the guide hole on the upper flat surface (see Fig. 28.6) to control the lens on wax or diamond tools.

Rough grinding stone and buff (Fig. 28.7)

These are used for reducing lens total diameters and edge polishing, respectively. The grinding stone is not essential since file and emery papers serve the same function, though more slowly; alternatively, a 25 mm carborundum ball may be used (see Fig. 28.6, top left).

Horizontal spindle with Jacob's chuck fitting or flexible drive (Fig. 28.7)

This is necessary for holding many of the tools used for back scleral zone surface modifications and in fenestrating. A Jacob's chuck attachment may also be obtained for the vertical spindle. Alternatively, some practitioners prefer to use a small motor with flexible drive attachment, which should have a foot-operated speed control to allow both hands freedom for lens and tool manipulation.

Grinding balls and polishing buffs

A selection of grinding balls and polishing buffs of various sizes and shapes are necessary (see Fig. 28.6).

Tripoli or Buffite polishing compound

The initial polishing after grinding is carried out more quickly with these compounds, but with some danger of burning the plastic. Final polishing is best carried out with Silvo or similar compounds suitable for RGP lenses as discussed above.

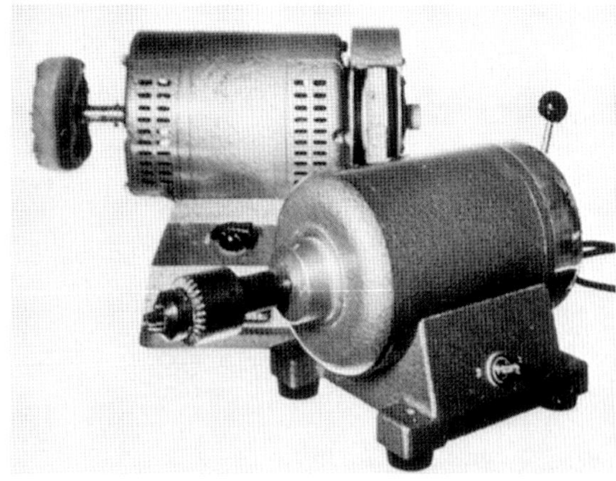

Figure 28.7 Grinding stone and buff (*rear*), and variable speed horizontal spindle with Jacob's chuck fitting (*front*). A flexible drive may be attached to the right-hand end of the grinding stone and buff motor

Diamond-impregnated brass tools

Used with or without a runner, back optic zone and spherical transition grind-outs are performed with these tools (see Fig. 28.4). Radii commonly used for transitional curves include 7.80, 8.00, 8.20, 8.40, 8.60, 8.90, 10.00 and 11.00 mm but a comprehensive range includes tools of radii from 5.00 to 15.00 mm.

Large wax tools

These (see Fig. 28.4) are used for polishing spherical transitions.

Drills and dental burrs

Drills of 0.50, 0.75 and 1.00 mm diameter may be required for making fenestration holes in scleral lenses. Slightly larger round or flame-shaped dental burrs or a larger drill may be used for countersinking.

CORNEAL LENS MODIFICATIONS

Reducing the total diameter of a lens

Reduction of the lens total diameter (TD) is carried out for the following reasons.

- To reduce excessive edge clearance.
- To reduce edge thickness of a high negative lens.
- To reduce lens weight.
- To eliminate a small edge chip.

Procedure

- Check the total diameter on a magnifying or V-gauge and note the amount to be removed.
- Heat a spindle lens holder at its upper end with a Bunsen burner for a few seconds, and remove any old wax polishing compound with a tissue.

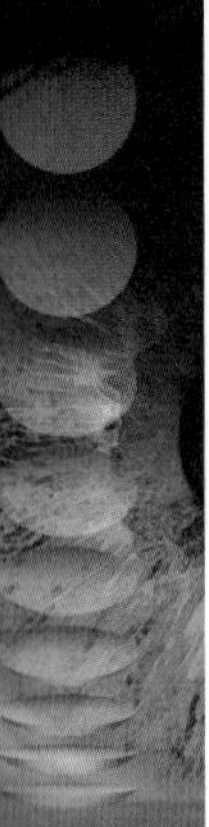

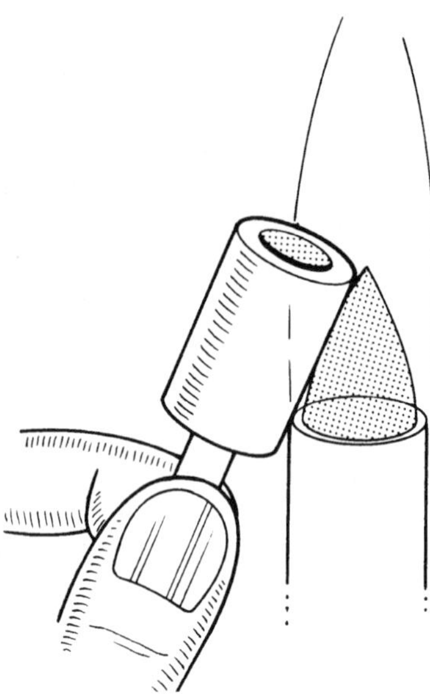

Figure 28.8 Heating the spindle lens chuck. The chuck is held by the stem and the base placed in the lower part of the Bunsen burner flame

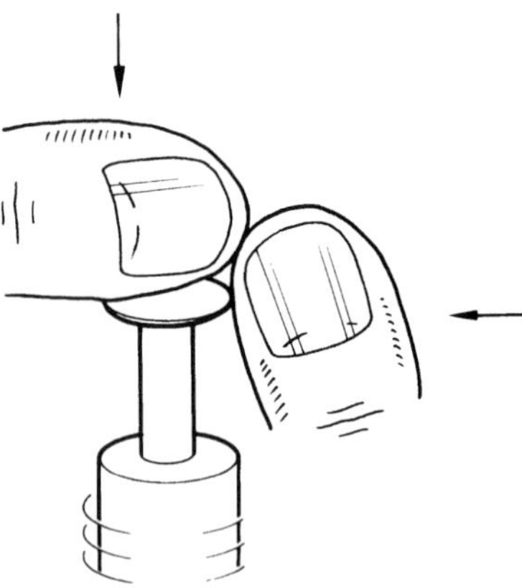

Figure 28.9 Centring the lens. While the adhesive wax is still soft, the lens is centred on the edging chuck by gently touching the top edge with one thumb and the side edge with the other

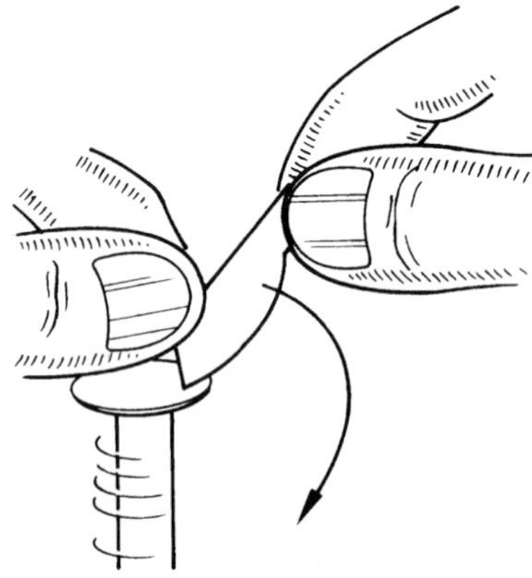

Figure 28.10 Shaping the edge. The blade or cutter is arching around the lens working from the back surface to just over the mid-edge, and then again from the front surface to slightly over the mid-edge position

- Direct the Bunsen flame on to the top of the chuck and touch the end of the adhesive wax stick on to the upper end of the chuck stem so that one small drop of the wax is left in the concavity. Too much wax causes it to spread over the underside of the lens when placed on the stem, making the edge difficult to modify or check and clean.
- While the wax is still soft (reheat for a second, if necessary), place the lens convex side down on the chuck as near centrally as possible. Setting the spindle in motion will show that the lens is not yet centred about the axis of rotation. Cutting it now would give a non-circular lens. The lens must, therefore, be centred.
- The wax on the chuck, if not still soft, must be softened without burning the lens (Fig. 28.8). Hold the inverted chuck by the stem, with the base in the lower part of the flame until the stem is too hot to hold. Place it firmly on the spindle, and set the spindle in motion. Using two smooth rods or one finger of each hand, touch one on the side, and the other on the opposite top edge (Fig. 28.9) until an object (such as a strip light) mirrored by the concave lens surface appears stationary while the lens rotates. (Centring is difficult in prismatic lenses.)
- Hold the chuck as near vertical as possible and run cold water over the base. Do not allow water to enter the spindle recess or knock the lens off the chuck.
- Replace the lens on the spindle and set it in motion. To reduce the TD, a single-edge razor blade or hard, carborundum-impregnated rubber tool is carefully brought into contact with the lens edge in line with the centre, with its cutting edge vertical and slightly trailing to the direction of rotation of the lens edge (Fig. 28.10).
- Check the TD every few seconds and stop cutting when it is about 0.20–0.30 mm more than required to allow for the edging.

Edging, re-edging and edge polishing

Edging and re-edging is the most useful modification to be able to carry out oneself. Re-edging is necessary in the following circumstances.

- When the TD is reduced.
- If there is a small chip in the edge of the lens, re-rounding that portion of the edge, although making the lens slightly 'truncated', may save having to order a new lens.
- If a replacement lens has a different edge shape from the original or from the lens in the other eye, reshaping can restore comfort.
- If the edges indent the cornea or conjunctiva and cause epithelial damage.

Procedure

Mount the lens on a spindle lens chuck, as described above, and examine the edge by the plasticine impression and binocular microscope (or slit-lamp) method. Note the points to be altered.

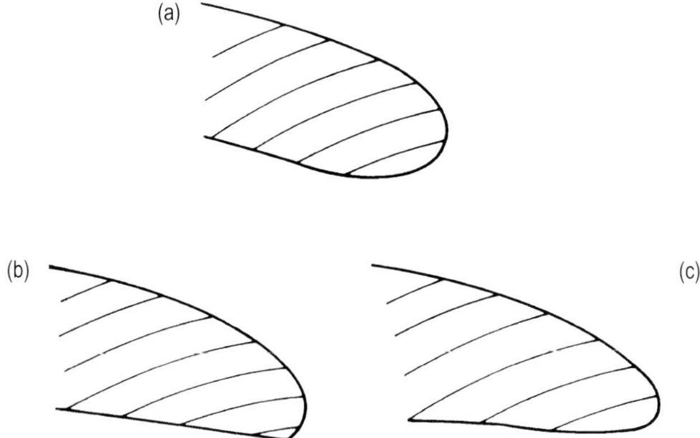

Figure 28.11 Corneal lens edge profiles. (a) Profile of initial monocurve lens prior to the addition of peripheral curves. (b) The same lens after the addition of a small peripheral curve (no edge treatment). (c) The final edge profile

A thick square-edged cutter or large curved scalpel blade with the tip removed (see Fig. 28.10) or a single straight-edged razor blade is held gently against the rotating lens with the first finger and thumb of both hands, as shown, noting the following points.

- Start cutting on either the back or the front surface of the lens, working round the outside of the edge and slightly over to the opposite surface.
- When cutting on the front surface, take care not to cut more than 0.5–1.0 mm in from the lens edge as scratches caused by the blade can be difficult to remove. Similarly, when cutting on the back surface edge, take care not to scratch any peripheral curve.
- If the lens has yet to have a peripheral curve put on, the edge must be shaped as in Figure 28.11a, with a very rounded rear edge to allow for the material that will be removed when polishing the peripheral curve (Fig. 28.11b).
- Left and right lens edge thicknesses should be matched for optimum patient comfort (Farnum 1959).

Any scratches on the edge and any sharp points remaining (e.g. those at the junction between the peripheral curve and edge curve) must be removed using a hard rubber burr. This should be cylindrical or conical and impregnated with carborundum or diamond. The burr is carefully rolled around the edge a few times in the same manner as the cutting blade.

Inspection should show the lens edge is ready for polishing, with a profile as in Figure 28.11c.

Wrap a double-folded piece of thin chamois leather around a forefinger. Dip it in polish and rub the edge of the lens for several minutes on a spindle.

To remove the lens from the chuck, lightly flick it with the finger on the front surface. Wet the front lens surface with paraffin to remove any adhesive wax and rub it gently.

A sewn rag wheel buff can be used for polishing truncated edges. It should be only lightly applied with buffing compound. Mount the lens on a spinner-type holder and hold lightly against the edge of the rotating buff (Haynes 1959), barely penetrating the fibres. If not mounted on a spinner, slowly and evenly rotate the holder and lens round the full edge curve then polish, using a piece of chamois leather and the appropriate polishing compound.

The edge can also be polished (or the TD reduced) on a drum tool or flat sponge pad. Mount the lens by its front surface and press lightly into the drum surface, perpendicular to the direction of rotation, then arch around the edge profile, parallel to the direction of drum travel, while continually rotating the lens. This is then repeated with the lens mounted on its back surface.

Reduction of the back optic zone diameter (BOZD), alteration of peripheral radii, addition of new curves and transition blending

These are necessary:

- To improve tear flow under the lens.
- To remove sharp transitions.
- To flatten peripheral curves.

Procedure

- Cut a wax tool, free from cracks and air bubbles, to the required radius using a razor blade for rough shaping and then a female gauge of the correct radius. This is held vertically and stationary on the centre of the wax tool rotating on a spindle. With stainless steel tools, in order to avoid damaging the wax tool, incline them very slightly towards the operator initially, and gradually approach the vertical as the wax tool is cut to the correct radius.
- Cut two or three small circular grooves in the surface of the wax with a pin point while the tool is rotating (see Fig. 28.4). These maintain the polish on the tool surface, prevent the lens adhering to the tool by suction and prevent surface waves forming, due to build-up of polish on the tool, during polishing. Cut a small indentation in the centre of the tool to position the female gauge during final cutting. The female gauge is then retouched on the wax tool to smooth off the surface of the grooves. Alternatively, tape- or cloth-covered tools may be used.
- Place the lens on one of the corneal holders or an edging chuck as described earlier. Apply a few drops of polishing liquid every few seconds to the rotating wax tool and slowly oscillate the lens either backwards and forwards from near the edge to near the centre of the tool, or across one side of the slowly rotating tool.

The BOZD should be measured with a scale and magnifier. A narrow peripheral curve may be impossible to measure and is best judged by means of a slit-lamp or other high-powered magnifier, or by optical projection. The degree of blending can be judged by inspecting the reflection of a strip light from the back of the lens surface using a loupe (see Figs 17.44 and 17.45).

An approximate measurement of curves can be made by coating the lens back surface with a waterproof 'instant drying' ink, which is removed where the lens is being polished, making the curve easily seen. This method is useful when blending

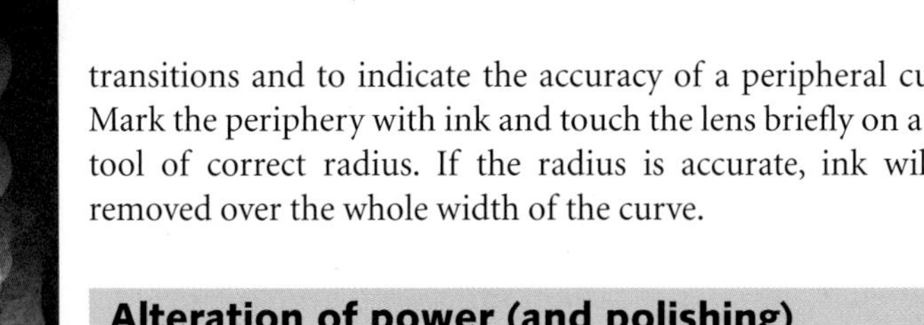

transitions and to indicate the accuracy of a peripheral curve. Mark the periphery with ink and touch the lens briefly on a wax tool of correct radius. If the radius is accurate, ink will be removed over the whole width of the curve.

Alteration of power (and polishing)

ADDING NEGATIVE POWER

Addition of negative power becomes necessary as the refractive error changes and alterations of up to 1.00 D are possible.

Negative power modifications are easier than positive ones. For this reason, most practitioners err on the positive side when ordering lenses.

Procedure

- Spread a 15 cm square of soft, clean, moistened polishing cloth over a similar-sized piece of chamois leather or moleskin laid on a smooth flat surface.
- Spread a small amount of polish in a circle on the cloth, using a finger.
- Position the dry back surface of the lens on a suitable lens holder preferably, or on the tip of a finger.
- Hold the front surface of the lens on the polishing cloth in the polish and describe circular movements of about 5–8 cm in diameter, exerting light pressure on the lens and taking care not to tilt the lens holder or finger.
- After every six complete circular movements, reverse the direction of rotation to counteract the effect of any tilting, which can produce distortion or cylindrical power.

Approximately 12 rotations are needed for every –0.25 D increase, and when nearing the end of a power alteration, the pressure should be gradually lessened to almost zero. Even when adding more than –0.25 D, the power must be checked frequently.

A more accurate method is to mount the lens, at about 20° from the horizontal (Fig. 28.12a), on a holder by its back surface and place it near the edge of the rotating 10 cm chuck (Isen 1959). The drum 'skin' should be kept continually moist with polishing fluid with one hand while the lens is kept slowly rotating. Pressure on the lens should be just sufficient to contour the drum material to the lens shape. Excessive pressure will cause vibration of the lens and holder. RGP materials polish faster than PMMA and should be held nearer the drum centre with the drum rotating at less than 1000 rev/min to prevent surface degradation (Morgan et al. 1992).

ADDITION OF POSITIVE POWER

To add positive power, the lens is placed at or near the centre of the drum just described. Since the drum's speed of rotation is zero at its centre, more lens material is removed from the lens edge and, consequently, positive power is added. Provided the chamois leather surface is kept moist with suitable polish, the addition of positive power is straightforward; as long as the lens is gently rotated, no cylindrical effect should be introduced.

With conditions as for the addition of negative power, the lens is slowly moved in a small circle of approximately 3 or 4 mm or

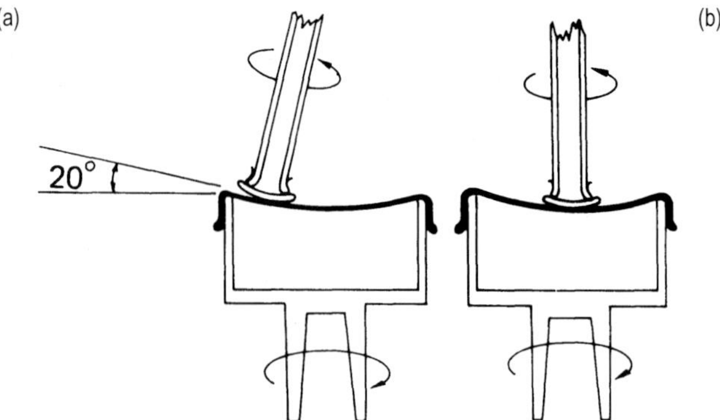

Figure 28.12 The use of a drum chuck for power alterations (cross-sections). (a) Addition of negative power. The lens is held near the drum edge at approximately 20° from the horizontal. The lens is slowly rotated in either the same or the opposite direction to drum movement. (b) Addition of positive power. The lens is held vertically close to the drum centre and again slowly rotated

less around the drum centre, in either the same or the opposite direction to that of drum rotation (Fig. 28.12b). This avoids the small 'pip' sometimes obtained in the centre of the lens if it is held stationary at the drum centre, where there is no polishing action.

In adding positive power, occasionally a 'haze' may appear round the target image of the focimeter when checking the lens power. If this occurs, the diameter of the circle that the lens is being moved in should be increased to approximately 8 or 9 mm to give more even polishing over the entire front surface. This should add neither positive nor negative power. If this does not remove the 'haze', add about +0.12 D too much positive power and then remove this by adding –0.12 D.

REPOLISHING THE LENS FRONT SURFACE

Either of the two methods described in the preceding paragraph will also remove superficial front surface scratches.

Fenestration

If corneal oedema occurs with RGP lenses, especially large-diameter limbal lenses (see Chapter 21), central fenestration holes – up to five in number – may encourage tear flow, but only where the lens is fitted apically clear of the cornea, otherwise each hole can provide an additional meniscus of tears between lens and cornea, thus discouraging tear flow but aiding lens centration and reducing movement.

A typical fenestration is 0.20–0.30 mm in diameter.

- Place the lens on the tip of the forefinger and mark the position of the hole(s) with a waterproof fibre pen.
- Hold the fine drill in a pin-vice and drill from the front by hand. This keeps the drill at the correct angle, perpendicular to the convex surface.
- Rotate the pin-vice slowly. Do not use excessive pressure as this may break the drill or crack the lens. To minimize the risk of the drill slipping and scratching the front surface of the lens, it should protrude as little as possible from the pin-vice.
- The hole can be drilled through sticky tape stuck to the front surface of the lens.

The edge of the hole is then countersunk on both sides by gently rotating a dental burr, size 0 or 1, anticlockwise in the fenestration. Only a touch is needed and the countersunk effect is then examined using a suitable magnifier.

Carefully polish the hole by hand using a finely sharpened boxwood stick and a trace of suitable polishing fluid, with as rapid rotation as possible. Several changes of sticks may be needed in order to maintain a sharpened point. For larger fenestrations, a fine-pointed felt buff in a spindle may be used for a few seconds. Finally, inspect the fenestration carefully.

An alternative method is to:

- Mount the lens, using double-sided adhesive tape, onto first a convex then a concave chuck so that the fenestration hole is positioned over a small central depression in each chuck.
- As the chuck rotates on the vertical spindle, apply a drop of polish in the hole, and gently hold a boxwood stick, sharpened to a suitably angled point, in the fenestration hole.
- Rotate the boxwood stick slowly in a small circle in the opposite direction to the spindle rotation. This both countersinks and gives a fine polish (Mackie 1968).
- If necessary, polish the inner part of the fenestration by running a length of polish-covered cotton sewing thread though the fenestration hole.

A fenestrating machine formerly available to the practitioner is shown in Figure 28.13. It is still used by some laboratories although lasers are the most common method.

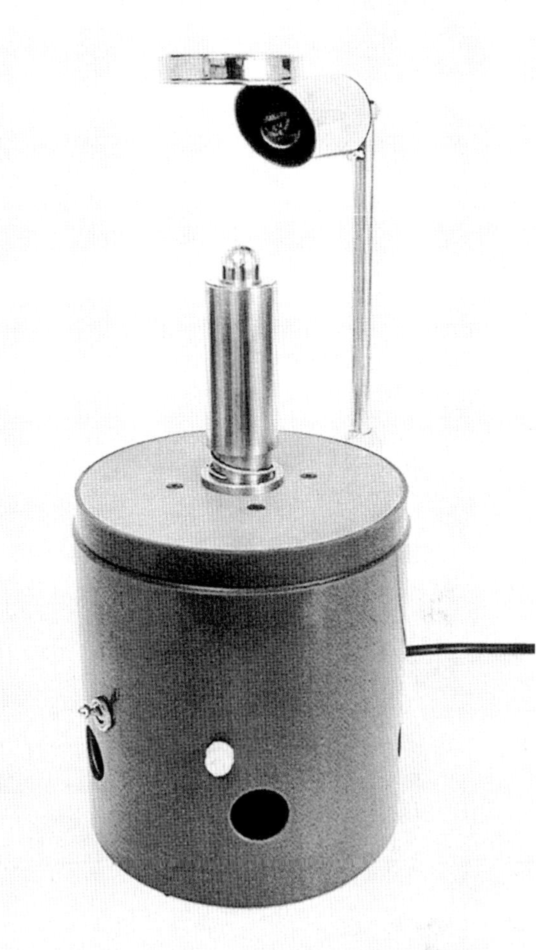

Figure 28.13 Fenestrating machine developed for the practitioner and suitable for both corneal and scleral lenses. (Courtesy of Focus Contact Lens Laboratory Ltd)

Truncation

Truncation may be necessary:

- If existing truncation does not line up correctly with the eyelid margin.
- If the lens edge is damaged in one place.
- To improve axis location of a round, front surface toric lens.
- If a truncated bifocal lens needs more truncation to lower the segment height when the latter interferes with distance vision (see Chapter 14).

Before truncating a lens, the final edge thickness of the truncation must be considered (Haynes 1959, 1965). For instance, truncating a high-powered negative lens with minimal centre thickness will produce an edge that is too thin to modify and can be damaged.

- Mark the relevant portion with a suitable marking agent, such as 'instant drying' ink.
- Hold the lens between the fingers and remove the marked material with either a pin-file, a hand-manipulated abrasive stone or a rotating fine abrasive wheel.
- Contour using a pin-file or fine emery paper.
- Polish with a rag-wheel buff, a drum chuck or a foam rubber pad. Protect the part of the lens not being modified with adhesive tape.

The lens may also be truncated by the edge being held firmly against the material of a rotating drum chuck and the edge shape rounded as previously described. In some instances truncation should be kept relatively square in cross-section to prevent the lens moving under the lid margin.

POINTS TO NOTE WHEN MODIFYING RGP LENSES

With many different RGP materials available, the following are important.

- Surface-treated lenses should not be modified.
- The higher-Dk materials (e.g. fluorosilicone acrylates) warp and burn easily and are best done by a skilled laboratory technician.
- Various polishes (e.g. Silvo) should not be used (see Polishing liquids, p. 565).
- Overheating RGP lenses induces material stress, which causes subsequent lens flattening (Schwartz 1986). Cutting and polishing should therefore be done slowly and gently and at a relatively slow spindle speed.
- RGP lenses should not be allowed to dry out during polishing. Surface 'burning' caused by drying out may show as poor wetting areas when the lens is dispensed and may add to stress-induced flattening.

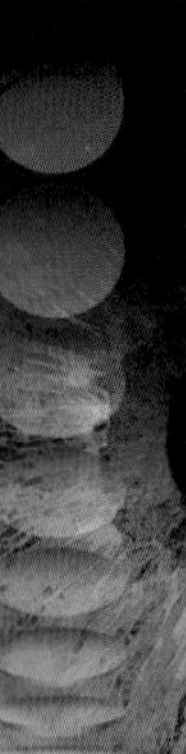

- Preheated blocks or high melting point waxes should be avoided. Suction holder attachments should be used where possible.
- Newman (S., personal communication, 1987) recommends the use of more than one type of polishing medium for modification to the optic zone in order to obtain a good surface finish (e.g. CCPI polishing compound in water followed by Boston finishing solution). Another method of maintaining good polishing medium viscosity is to add some dishwashing liquid to the medium. A mixture of dishwashing liquid and water also makes an excellent finishing solution.
- In order to prevent burning or 'orange peeling' of the lens surface, abrasive-cloth-type coverings of tools such as velveteen or pellan pads should be treated with respect. Velvet, cotton, chamois leather and vinyl can all be used.
- Grind and polish lenses with the absolute minimum of pressure.
- Never wipe polish off a lens with a dry tissue. Keep a bowl of water and detergent mix available for washing the lens. Rubbing the lens between fingers while submerged in this solution will clean the lens adequately. The lens can then be gently blotted dry for inspection.
- Store polishing cloths and polishing powders in clean, airtight containers to keep them dust-free, thereby avoiding lens scratching.

SCLERAL LENS MODIFICATIONS

Indications for carrying out modifications to scleral lenses made from eye impressions are given in Chapter 15.

A general reduction in TD is indicated:

- When a lens remains stationary as the eye moves behind it, i.e. the lens appears a 'steep fit'.
- Localized reductions of diameter may be made if, for example, the lower scleral zone is too big for the lower fornix.
- If a horizontal oval fluorescein pool shows against-the-rule astigmatism with edge stand-off nasally and temporally and edge blanching at upper and lower edges, making the vertical meridian smaller effectively flattens it in that meridian, allowing it to settle back. Scleral zone grinding out may also be necessary.
- Conversely, a vertical oval lens for with-the-rule astigmatism is not normally satisfactory cosmetically unless the palpebral aperture is particularly small.

Reducing an equal amount from all round the lens edge, in the case of a regular preformed lens, is carried out by simply rubbing the lens against a piece of medium-grade sandpaper placed on a flat surface. Care must be taken to maintain an even pressure around the whole lens edge.

Localized or overall reductions in lens TD may be carried out by means of either a rotating grinding stone or an ordinary hand file.

As mentioned earlier, since scleral lenses may be made from either PMMA or RGP materials, care should be taken in selecting the appropriate polish.

Edging

Edging is necessary:

- When total diameter reductions have been carried out.
- If the edge has been damaged.
- If scleral zone modifications have altered the edge shape.

Use a stone grinding ball of 2.54 cm diameter, soaked in water and held in a horizontal spindle, for rounding both front and back edge surfaces. Alternatively, an ordinary small hand file, followed by fine emery paper, may be used for the front surface and a large rounded rubber tool impregnated with diamond or carborundum for the back surface.

Polish with a rag-wheel buff and the lens edge held vertically and in line with the rotating buff to polish the back edge surface. The lens should be held lightly and continually rotated during polishing to avoid burning the plastic. This also prevents a ridge of plastic building up on the back edge. The final edge should be of a blunt, rounded form.

Alternatively, the lens may be edged and polished by tools held in a flexible drive.

Back optic zone grind-out

This is done to increase the clearance of the back optic zone from the cornea. A steeper radius may be required if heavy central touch exists with a large annular bubble at the limbus. A flatter back optic zone radius is indicated if central corneal touch and mid-peripheral corneal or limbal touch occur together. Changing the BOZR alters the power of the contact lens and liquid lens (see Chapters 6 and 15). Where possible, therefore, the BOZR should be kept the same.

Procedure

- Measure the central optic zone thickness and mark the front surface with a waterproof mark at this point.
- Attach a 'runner' to the centre of the front surface of the optic zone with double-sided adhesive tape. Set a diamond-impregnated brass tool of the desired radius in motion on a vertical spindle.
- Grind the back optic zone using paraffin or water as the lubricating agent and a pencil point or similar in the runner guide hole.
- Allow the lens to rotate freely and move it slowly backwards and forwards across one side of the head of the diamond tool, keeping it lubricated with polishing fluid. Check the rate of reduction in central thickness regularly.
- Final grinding is best performed with paraffin as the lubricating agent. It is slightly more viscous than water and there is less risk of abrading the surface but the increased viscosity slows the grinding rate.

Paraffin is inconvenient with fenestrated lenses as it leaks through the fenestration, dissolving the adhesive, and causing the runner to become detached from the lens. Approximately 0.02 mm thickness should be allowed for final polishing of the back optic zone. This is carried out in exactly the same way as for corneal lenses – retaining the lens on the runner and using a

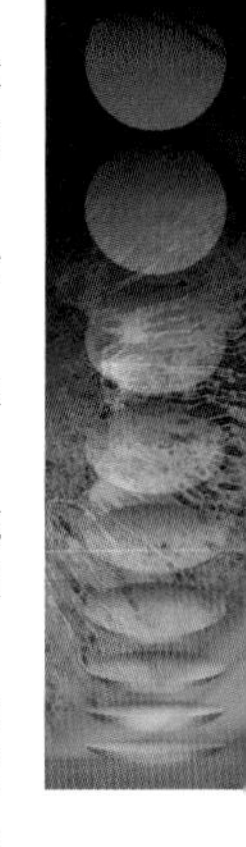

wax-, tape- or cloth-covered tool of the correct radius with suitable polish (see above).

Transitional grind-out or extension

This is done:

- If the transitions are sharp and cause frothing of the bubble.
- If limbal touch occurs.
- Where there is insufficient clearance beyond the limbus, as indicated by the extent of the fluorescein pool.
- After a back optic zone grind-out owing to the reduction in width of the transitional curve(s).

It is carried out as for 'Reduction of the BOZD' (p. 569) using the large-size diamond-impregnated tool. The widths of transition are measured rather than thickness removed, and final polishing is carried out using a large wax tool or felt ball; any fenestration will then need re-countersinking and polishing.

A transitional grind-out is best performed after the back optic zone has been polished to facilitate measurement of the transition width. Alternatively, mark the area with ink to show the border between the transition and optic zones during grinding. (Paraffin cannot be used as a lubricant if it dissolves the inks used.)

Polishing the rough ground transition extends its width slightly. This becomes important when extending a transition well into the back optic zone, and especially when making a double curve back optic zone.

Localized scleral zone and transition grind-outs

Localized grind-outs are performed in regions where the scleral zone or transition touches the eye heavily, as evidenced by blanching of the conjunctival blood vessels. If the optic zone gives too much clearance from the cornea, the whole back scleral zone surface is ground out to settle the lens. More substance should be removed from near the transition region to maintain the same curvature and give the most effective settling.

A temporal scleral zone grind-out near the transition is often required to permit the lens to settle and move slightly nasally. This is indicated when a large temporal static bubble occurs at the limbus accompanied by nasal corneal touch from the optic. A slight reduction in nasal scleral zone size may also be needed to permit the nasal shift of the lens.

Procedure

- Mark the area to be ground on the back surface (or front, according to preference) with a suitable quick-drying ink or grease pencil. For the beginner, it is useful to measure the average thickness of the area to be ground out – at several noted points if the area is large. This can be checked during the grind-out to determine the amount of material removed and, in a large area, to check that the material is being removed evenly. If necessary, the back optic zone may be protected with a small piece of plasticine (Bier 1957) or adhesive tape pressed firmly into it.
- Place a spherical, cigar-shaped or wheel-shaped stone into a Jacob's chuck on a horizontal spindle. The size of the stone depends on the area to be ground out and it should be kept moist throughout the operation to prevent deep scratches in the scleral zone.
- Move the lens back and forth continually, until the ink over the area (if on the back surface) is removed.
- Remove surplus lens material and polish regularly with a tissue; check the scleral zone thickness before continuing.
- If necessary, the rough area is now smoothed with a rotating hard rubber burr and polishing carried out with a felt buff and polishing compound or, more slowly, with a soft mop buff.
- Finally, polish with a soft mop and polishing compound to give a better finish. To save time, this may be omitted until the lens has been checked on the eye and has been found to fit satisfactorily.
- Examine the lens under magnification to show areas which have not been polished completely. For equal scleral zone settling, relatively more plastic must be removed from near the transition than from the periphery (Forknall 1953).

Fenestration

Most PMMA scleral lenses are fenestrated to permit tear flow and oxygen exchange behind the lens. If a fenestration hole becomes covered by the upper lid regularly, or otherwise blocked as by loose conjunctival tissue or mucus, then a further hole (or holes) may be required within the palpebral aperture.

Procedure

- Determine the position as explained in Chapter 15.
- With a 0.50 or 0.75 mm drill (typically), held in a pin-vice with a minimum length of drill protruding, drill a hole normal to the surface (to minimize its length and give greater control over positioning), taking care not to slip and scratch the optic zone surface. Alternatively, the drill is held in a Jacob's chuck on a horizontal spindle, which lessens the risk of the drill or lens slipping and scratching the optic zone surface, and the lens is 'fed' on to the drill.
- Turn a flame-shaped dental burr anticlockwise (to give a finer cut) in the hole to countersink (Fig. 28.14); a few turns initially using a 1.50 or 2.00 mm drill will speed up the process. Countersinking should be continued equally on both sides of the lens until examination under magnification (e.g. a slit-lamp) shows the two countersinks almost meeting. Funnel shaping is essential to create an even tear flow and prevent turbulence likely to remove epithelium from the corneal surface.
- Use a slightly larger spherical dental burr, as before, to taper the outer edges of the countersinking.
- Polish the countersinks at low speed to avoid burning, using a pointed soft felt burr soaked in polishing compound, until a high polish is obtained.
- Inspection under magnification should show a fenestration polished all the way through and with tapered edges as shown in Figure 28.14d. Any remaining polishing residue may be removed with a tapered stick (e.g. a toothpick), tissue or bristle.

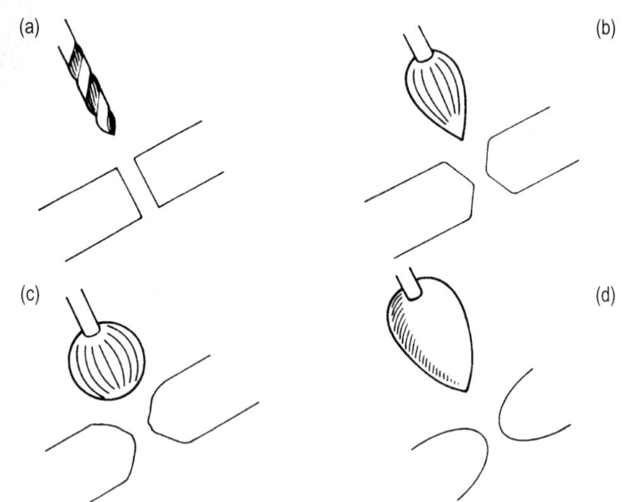

Figure 28.14 The four stages of fenestrating a scleral lens

Channelling

Channelling is an alternative to fenestration, and may be indicated:

- If the limbal region is irregular and the introduction of a bubble would lead to frothing.
- If the limbal conjunctiva is loose and blocks the fenestrations.

Although not always as successful as fenestration, it may be necessary under certain conditions. Various uses and designs of channel were discussed by McKay Taylor (1969).

The channel is cut in the same way as a local back surface scleral zone grind-out, along a specific line or curve, and, where possible, using a sharp-edged wheel-shaped grinding tool. This is usually from the upper temporal lens edge into the mid-transition, although an inferior channel and/or other channels may become necessary. The channel should occupy about half the lens thickness and have well-blended edges to prevent conjunctival abuse.

Fluorescein examination should show a clear channel from the lens edge into the back optic zone.

Alternatively, glue a suitable piece of nylon film along the desired line of the channel on the cast of an eye impression or a preformed lens and then press the shell over the cast. This method enables the shell to be pressed from a thinner sheet initially.

Power alterations

Power alterations must be made if the refraction changes or if a change in BOZR is carried out for fitting purposes (see Adding negative power, p. 570). These are normally carried out by the laboratory as the front surface must be recut each time. Minor front surface alterations may be made on a drum, as for corneal lenses.

By reducing the thickness of the optic zone, a back optic zone grind-out will effectively add a small amount of negative power to the lens. In order to prevent unnecessary modification, +0.25 to +0.50 D should be added to the power required if back optic zone grind-outs are likely to become necessary (see Chapters 6 and 15).

MODIFICATION OF SOFT CONTACT LENSES

Soft lenses can be modified in a number of ways. These range from simple dotting of lenses to aid identification to complicated cut-outs to circumnavigate pingueculae or fluid drainage blebs.

Most modifications are best done by skilled technicians at the manufacturing laboratory. This ensures that the modifications are performed by those with an intimate knowledge of both the lens material and design.

A simple modification is to dot lenses either to identify left and right, or to enable orientation of a toric lens on the eye by the patient.

Blot the lens with lint-free tissue and mount on the convex dome of a suitable soft lens container. Apply a single dot (right lens) or two dots (left lens) to the lens edge with a fine waterproof marking pen – for example, Sanford's Sharpie No. 3000 or Nikko Permanent Ink Marker No. 150. Allow the lens to dry for a further 1–2 minutes before thorough surfactant cleaning and rinsing. Dots applied by this method will gradually fade but are easily reapplied at after-care visits (Hallock 1980).

Laboratory modification procedures

While it is possible to carry out many modifications to soft lenses, the increase in the prescribing of planned replacement and disposable lenses (both spherical and toric) makes the need to modify existing lenses uncommon. In addition, the cost of laboratory modifications may be more expensive than simply replacing the lens. One technique still frequently carried out by the laboratory is tinting or retinting lenses.

The major factor controlling soft lens modifications is the dehydration techniques used. The laboratory must be able to dehydrate the lens completely and still maintain the original surface geometry.

CONCLUSION

Practitioners are advised to obtain a selection of reject lenses on which to practise modifications. The majority of modifications may be accurately carried out with only a little practice, but practitioners are urged to maintain their own standards to at least those that they would expect from their laboratory.

Acknowledgement

I am indebted to Stephen Newman for his technical advice.

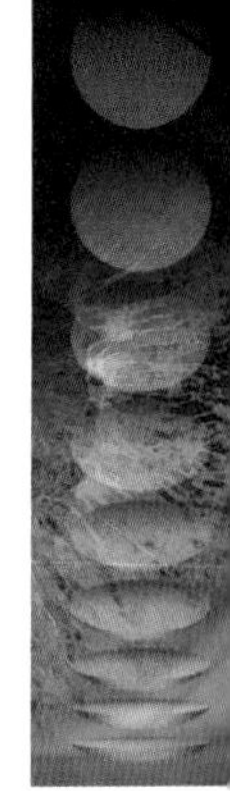

References

Bier, N. (1957) Contact Lens Routine and Practice, 2nd edn. London: Butterworths

Farnum, F. E. (1959) Refinements in contact lens adjustments to increase wearing time. Am. J. Optom., 36, 382–384

Forknall, A. J. (1953) Conversion of sealed to ventilated contact lenses. Optician, 125, 327–330, 356–358

Hallock, S. J. (1980) Dotting soft contact lenses. J. Am. Optom. Assoc., 51(3), 237

Haynes, P. R. (1959) Modification of contact lenses. In Encyclopaedia of Contact Lens Practice vol. 22, pp. 1–97, ed. P. R. Haynes. South Bend, IND: International Optics Publishing

Haynes, P. R. (1965) Modification procedures. In Contact Lens Practice, Basic and Advanced, ed. R. B. Mandell. Springfield: C. C. Thomas

Isen, A. (1959) Spherical power changes in contact lenses. In Encyclopaedia of Contact Lens Practice, vol. 22, pp. 72–74, ed. P. R. Haynes. South Bend, IND: International Optics Publishing

McKay Taylor, C. (1969) The S-bend and other channelled haptic lenses. Ophthal. Opt., 9, 1256–1258

Mackie, I. A. (1968) Lecture to The Contact Lens Society

Morgan, G. W., Henry, V. A., Bennett, E. S. and Casoline, P. S. (1992) The effect of modification procedures on rigid gas permeable contact lenses: the UM-St Louis study. J. Am. Optom. Assoc., 63, 201–214

Schwartz, C. A. (1986) Radical flattening and RGP lenses. Contact Lens Forum, 11(8), 49–52

Chapter 29

Special types of contact lens and their uses

Janet Stone and Judith Morris

CHAPTER CONTENTS

Special types of contact lens not covered elsewhere in this book are described in this chapter.

LENSES TO AID DIAGNOSIS AND SURGERY

Various special contact lenses have been developed to assist observation of the eye in diagnosing eye disease.

Contact lenses for corneal observation

The bright reflection observed with a slit-lamp biomicroscope when examining corneal endothelium using specular reflection is intrusive. Haag–Streit's Eisner Contact Glass is a thick aplanatic plano-convex lens used for this purpose (Eisner et al. 1985). The plane face contacts the cornea using a solution such as Celluvisc (Allergan) and transfers the annoying reflex to the front of the lens, out of the field of view of the microscope (Fig. 29.1).

Tsubota (1988) used a two-part specular microscope-contact lens consisting of a tube with an annular curved base held by surface tension to the front surface of a rigid contact lens. This is placed on the eye following local anaesthesia and a wide-field specular microscope applied to the base contact lens via the tube.

Fundal examination with corneal abnormalities

Although slit-lamp examination of the fundus can be carried out using a Volk lens, even if the cornea is irregular, a contact lens facilitates ophthalmoscopic examination of the media and fundus, by removing the irregularities.

The fundus of a high myope is also more easily observed through a high-minus contact lens which reduces the high magnification obtained in direct ophthalmoscopy.

Assessment of corneal thickness (see Chapter 7)

If a soft lens of known thickness is placed on the eye, the corneal thickness can be gauged by comparing lens thickness to corneal thickness. Instillation of fluorescein makes this more obvious.

Friedman (1967) developed a corneal lens with a stepped thickness: central portion 0.8 mm, intermediate portion 0.6 mm and an outer portion 0.4 mm. Using a narrow slit

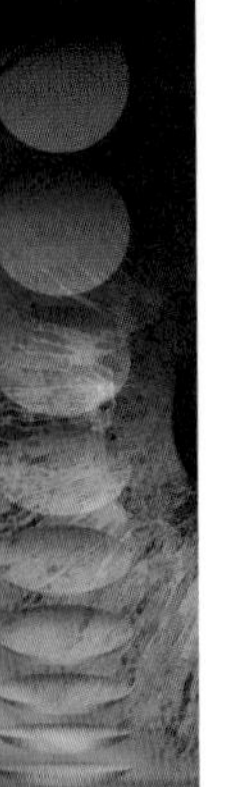

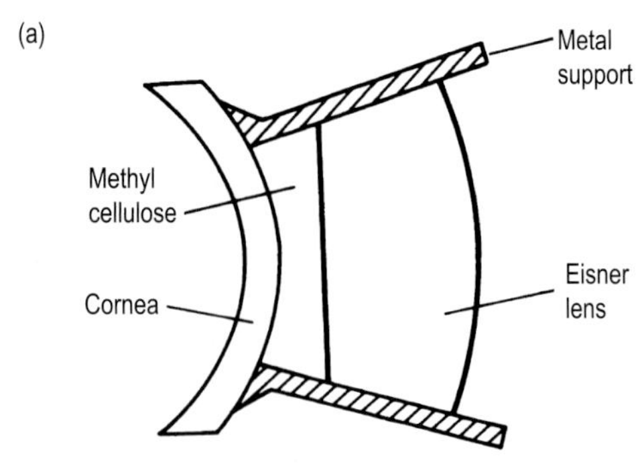

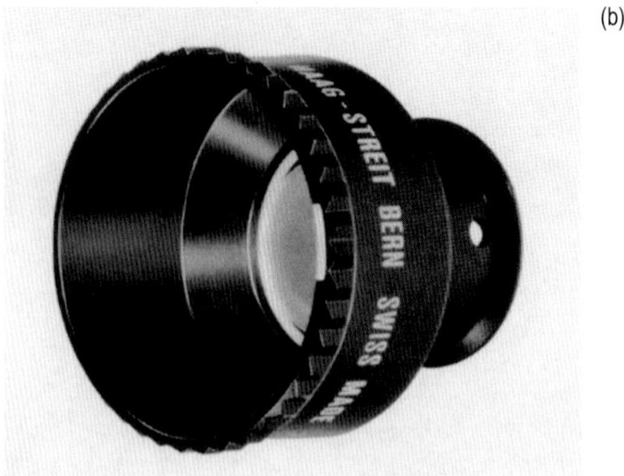

Figure 29.1 The Eisner Contact Glass: (a) cross-section on the cornea showing its plano-convex form which gives a 32.2 magnification of the corneal endothelium. The bright anterior corneal reflex is removed by its presence and transferred to the front surface of the Eisner lens, out of the field of view of the slit-lamp microscope. (After Eisner et al. 1985.) (b) The supporting structure which holds the eyelids apart and permits easy handling of the lens so that it can be tilted in situ to get rid of any reflections from its plane back surface separated from the cornea by a solution such as methyl cellulose. (Reproduced by kind permission of Haag–Streit AG., Switzerland)

beam, corneal thickness was compared to the different lens portions.

Gonioscopy contact lenses

Observation of the anterior chamber angle is made possible by the use of a lens incorporating mirrors that either partially or completely neutralizes the power of the cornea. Most modern gonioscopy lenses are based on the designs introduced by Koeppe (1919), Uribe Troncoso (1921) and Goldmann (1938). The Goldmann lens incorporates a mirror and is used in conjunction with a slit-lamp biomicroscope (Fig. 29.2). The angle of the anterior chamber is seen by reflection.

To see the entire angle, the lens must be rotated on the eye and the slit beam rotated with it but perpendicular to it, a horizontal slit being used when the mirror is vertical and vice versa. Magnification is given by the biomicroscope. The need for all but small amounts of rotation of the lens has been overcome by the use of multiple mirrors, as in the Zeiss pyramid or four-mirror gonioscope (Fig. 29.3); the fundus can also be viewed through one of these lenses (see below).

The Lovac Direct Goniolens is shown in Figure 29.4. The angle is viewed directly without reflection through the flat surface of the goniolens, which is angled at 45° to the patient's visual axis, allowing about half the anterior chamber angle to be viewed at one time.

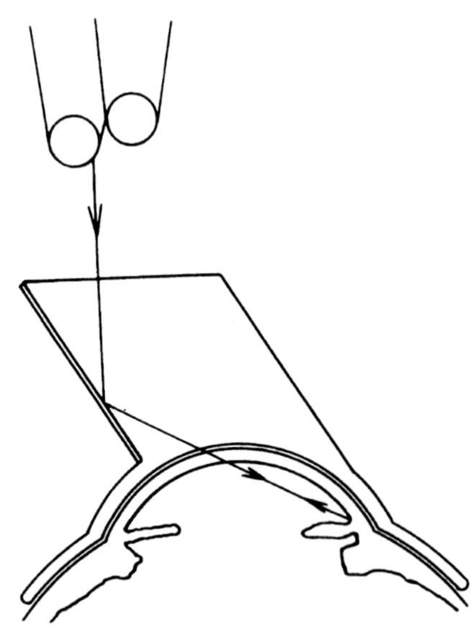

Figure 29.2 Cross-section of a Goldmann gonioscopy lens. Light from a slit-lamp is reflected, as shown, into the anterior chamber angle, and returns along the same path to be viewed through the microscope

Contact lenses for examination of the fundus

Viewing the fundus binocularly with a slit-lamp allows a three-dimensional magnified view of the fundus. A contact lens with a flat front surface is used with a Volk lens to eliminate corneal refraction (Fig. 29.5). The macula region of the fundus is observed directly with such a high negative lens, and mirrors used to observe the mid-periphery and extreme periphery of the fundus.

Richards et al. (1993) described a lens with a flat front surface incorporating a fixation light-emitting diode angled at approximately 17° to the observation axis. It is used in slit-lamp observation of the optic nerve head in functionally monocular patients and those glaucomatous patients with fixed miotic pupils.

Haag–Streit makes a lens with a plane face and three mirrors inclined to it. A 59° mirror is used for gonioscopy, a 66° mirror for the region around the equator, a 73° mirror from there to within 30° of the posterior pole, and the posterior pole itself is viewed through the plane face of the lens. An ora serrata attachment depresses the sclera to aid observation just behind the ciliary body (Fig. 29.6).

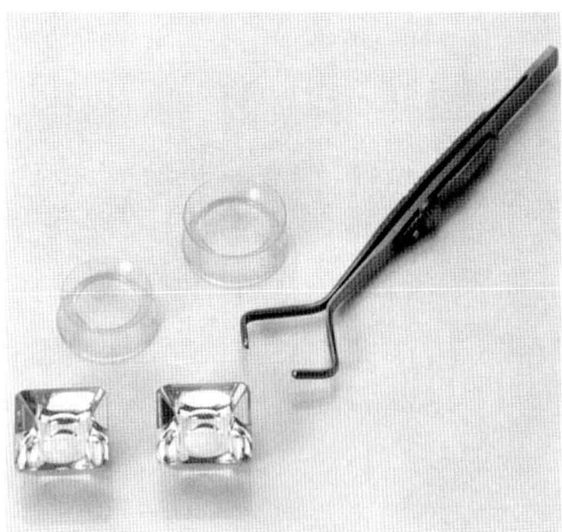

Figure 29.3 The Zeiss four-mirror gonioscope with special forceps, and scleral holders that keep the lids apart. (Reproduced by kind permission of Carl Zeiss, Oberkochen)

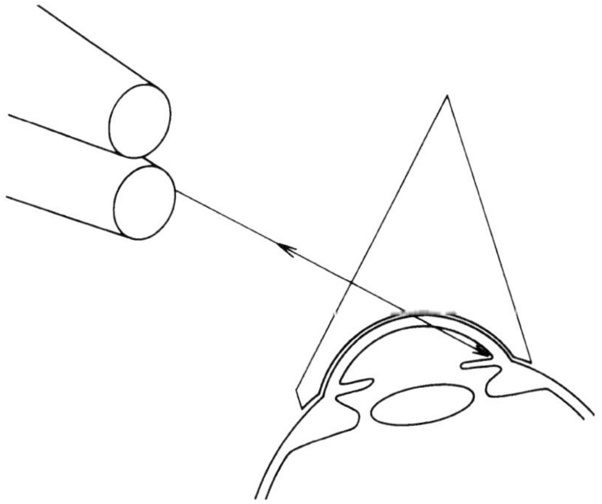

Figure 29.4 Cross-section of the Lovac Direct Goniolens being used with the biomicroscope. The direction of illumination and observation are the same

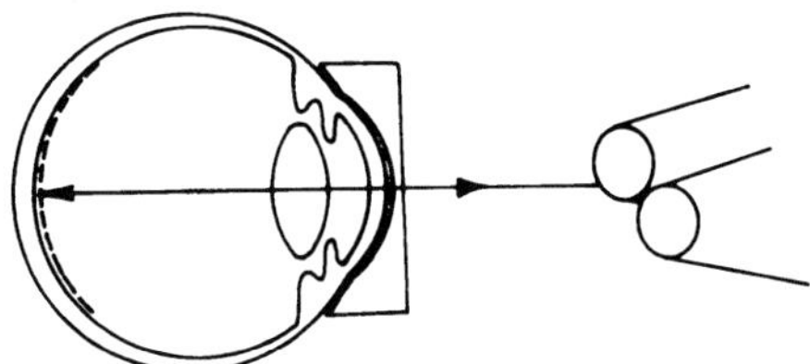

Figure 29.5 Fundus observation with the biomicroscope, by means of a contact lens with a flat front surface

Haag–Streit's paediatric three-mirror lens is available in two sizes: newborn and under 4 years old.

The Rodenstock Panfunduscope (Fig. 29.7) has a two-element optical system comprising a spherical lens and a high-positive lens. This allows the entire central fundus to be viewed simultaneously using the slit-lamp. A solution such as methylcellulose is used between the high-positive lens and the cornea and forms a real inverted image of the fundus, reduced in size by about 30%.

Contact lenses for laser surgery

Argon laser photocoagulation used for iridectomy and trabeculotomy, and neodymium:yttrium–aluminium–garnet (Nd:YAG) lasers used in capsulotomy and vitrectomy, must avoid laser damage to areas of the eye not being treated. Special contact lenses, which are antireflective coated to give maximum transmission of the low-energy beam, are used. These:

- Magnify the image seen through the slit-lamp biomicroscope, enabling accurate location of the laser beam focus.
- Increase the cone angle of the beam (Fig. 29.8), dissipating its energy, thereby avoiding tissue damage.
- Form a pinpoint focus rather than a comatic blur.

PROTECTIVE LENSES

Radiation treatment

For malignant tumours of the orbital region, a plastic-covered lead scleral shell can be used to protect the eye. Where the tumour is ocular, a partial lead shell can be specially constructed to cover the entire anterior eye except the part to be irradiated.

Visible light

Ball (1964) postulated that some of the photophobia experienced by new contact lens wearers, transferring from spectacles to contact lenses, may be due to increased ultraviolet (UV) radiation reaching the cornea, which is most sensitive to radiation of 288 nm. Most plastics, tinted or otherwise, have a cut-off at 290 nm.

Soft and rigid gas-permeable (RGP) lenses are available with varying amounts of ultraviolet absorption. Corneal lenses do not cover the whole cornea and leave the limbus unprotected, whereas soft lenses cover the entire cornea and circumlimbal conjunctiva, providing UV protection for the cornea, crystalline lens, retina and epithelial stem cells – the source of new corneal epithelial cells, located in the limbus and adjacent conjunctiva (Meyler & Schnider 2002).

Acuvue (Johnson & Johnson) and Precision UV (CIBA Vision) lenses block most wavelengths below 400 nm. Lunelle aphakic and standard ES70 UV lenses (CooperVision) have a light transmission cut-off at 350 nm. Other UV-absorbing disposable soft lenses are available, or individual lenses can be made up to prescription.

Many UV-absorbing RGP lenses are also available (see also Chapter 9). These materials typically block the peak wavelength (365 nm) emitted by UV Burton lamps, so that the fluorescein pattern cannot be satisfactorily seen. The fitting must be assessed using a blue filter on the slit-lamp biomicroscope (see Chapter 9).

A study by Chou et al. (1988) of soft and rigid UV-inhibiting materials concluded that none was as effective in

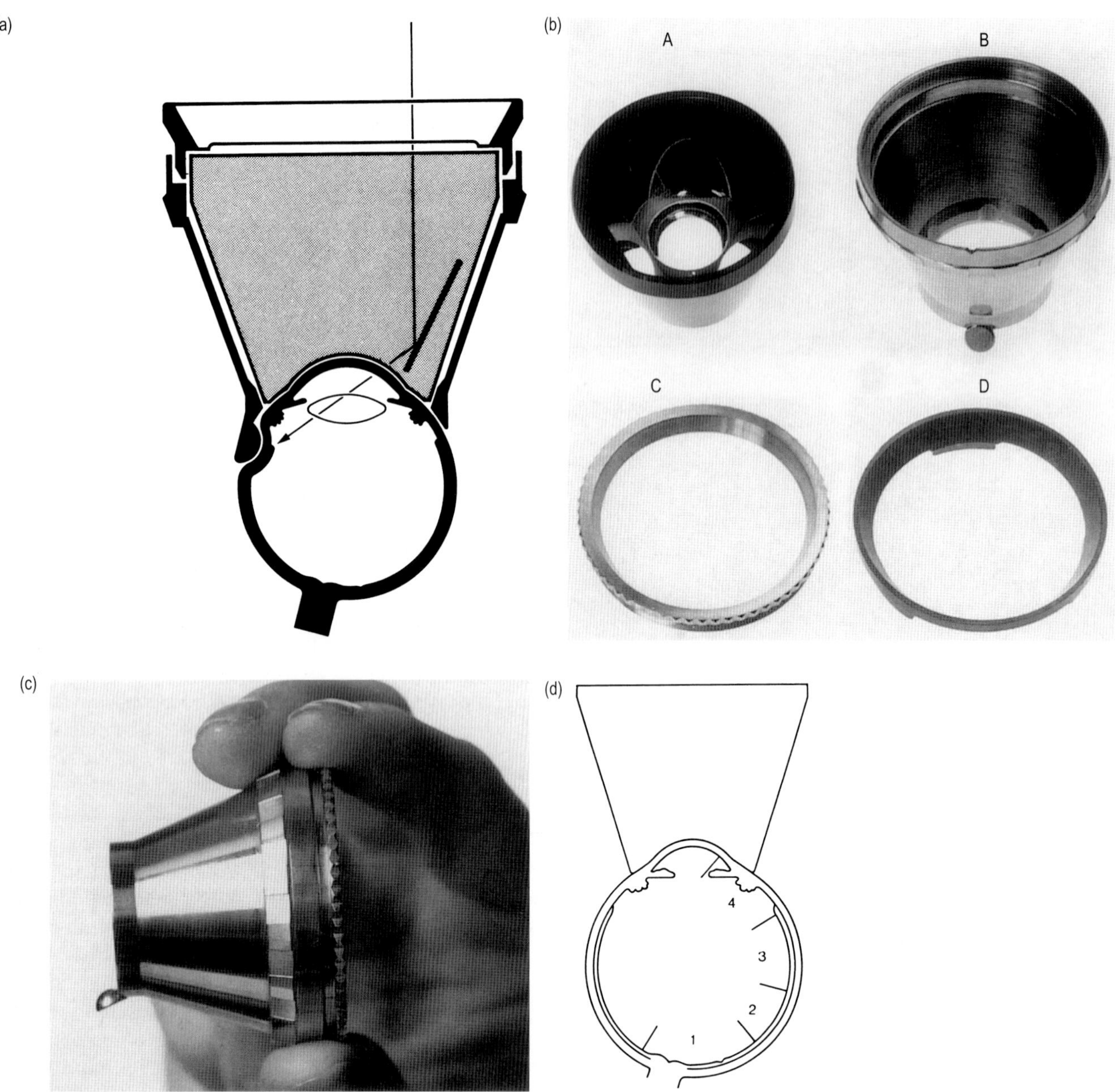

Figure 29.6 The Haag–Streit three-mirror diagnostic lens. (a) Observation of the ora serrata using a 6 mm ball scleral depressor attached to the mount opposite the 59° mirror. (b) The three mirrors can be seen in A, the mount with scleral depressor in B, a locking ring C to hold the two together, and a plastic protection ring D, to prevent scratching of the front surface of the lens. (c) Side view showing scleral depressor which is rotated by the middle finger on the milled ring, the lens being held by thumb and forefinger on the notched locking ring or plastic protective ring if in place. (d) Areas of the eye seen with the lens. Area 1 is seen through the plane face, 2 via the 73° mirror, 3 via the 66° mirror, and 4 via the 59° mirror. (Reproduced by kind permission of Haag–Streit AG., Switzerland)

blocking UV light as proper sports and industrial eyewear but that the contact lenses probably afforded ocular protection against normal lifelong exposure to environmental UV radiation.

THERAPEUTIC LENSES

Contact lenses are used in treating certain eye conditions, and fall into several categories.

Bandage and special soft lenses
(see also Chapter 26)

Hydrophilic and silicone hydrogel contact lenses are used as bandage lenses for many conditions. Although rare now because of the success of intraocular implants, aphakic continuous-wear hydrophilic lenses were successfully applied at the time of operation for cataract extraction, acting as a splint and bandage and permitting immediate good vision postoperatively (Kersley 1975).

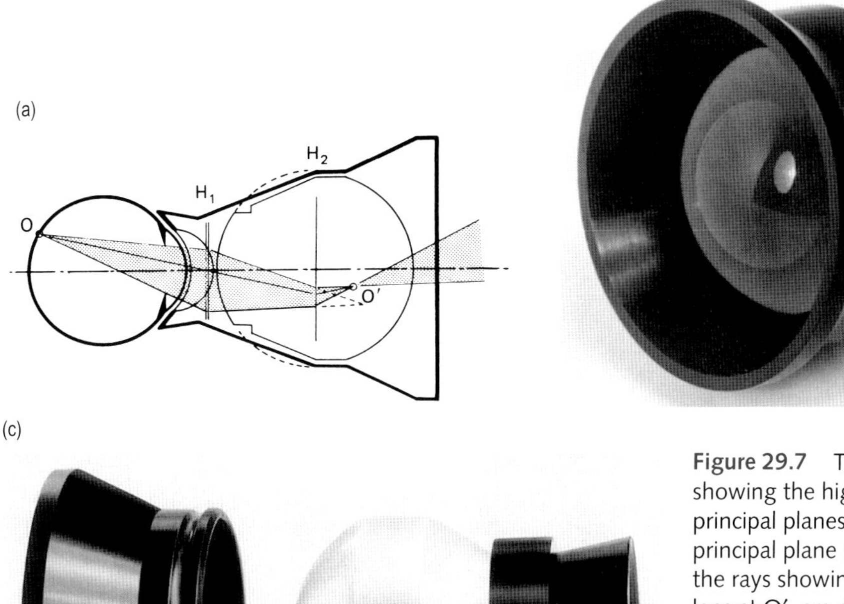

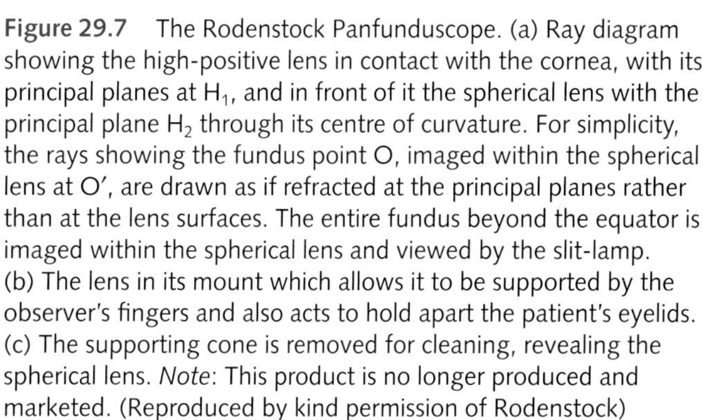

Figure 29.7 The Rodenstock Panfunduscope. (a) Ray diagram showing the high-positive lens in contact with the cornea, with its principal planes at H_1, and in front of it the spherical lens with the principal plane H_2 through its centre of curvature. For simplicity, the rays showing the fundus point O, imaged within the spherical lens at O′, are drawn as if refracted at the principal planes rather than at the lens surfaces. The entire fundus beyond the equator is imaged within the spherical lens and viewed by the slit-lamp. (b) The lens in its mount which allows it to be supported by the observer's fingers and also acts to hold apart the patient's eyelids. (c) The supporting cone is removed for cleaning, revealing the spherical lens. *Note*: This product is no longer produced and marketed. (Reproduced by kind permission of Rodenstock)

Astin (1987) described fitting specially shaped soft lenses, cut with an upper crescent or truncation to avoid impinging on surgically induced drainage blebs above the upper limbus.

Medical applicators (see also Chapter 26)

Hydrophilic lenses have been used as medical applicators in the application of several drugs (Hillman 1976). The lens, usually a high-water-content material, is saturated in the drug for about 2 hours. When placed on the eye there is a slow release into the conjunctival sac over the following 2 hours.

The Klein applicator (Klein 1949) (Fig. 29.9) was an example of a medical applicator that maintained a reservoir of a drug in contact with the eye. It was a modified scleral lens with two tubes extending from the optic.

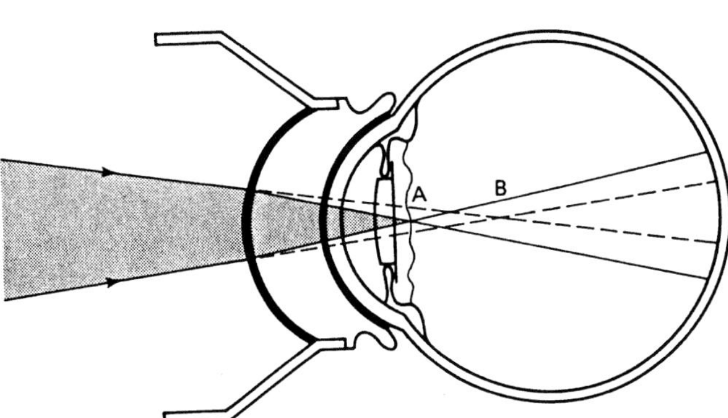

Figure 29.8 Lens used for laser capsulotomy. The spherical front surface refracts the beam to a larger angle at A, thereby diffusing the energy in the surrounding tissues. This gives less risk of damage than with a plane front surface which would give a smaller angle of beam, B, with less spread and more concentration of energy in the surrounding tissues

Splints (see also Chapters 16 and 18)

Scleral shells or scleral rings (the outer annulus only of a scleral lens) (see Fig. 26.14) can be applied to the eye following facial burns or episodes of Stevens–Johnson syndrome to prevent the

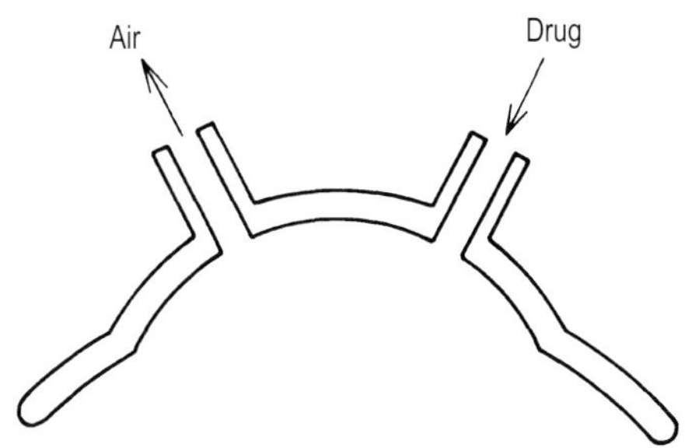

Figure 29.9 The Klein applicator in cross-section

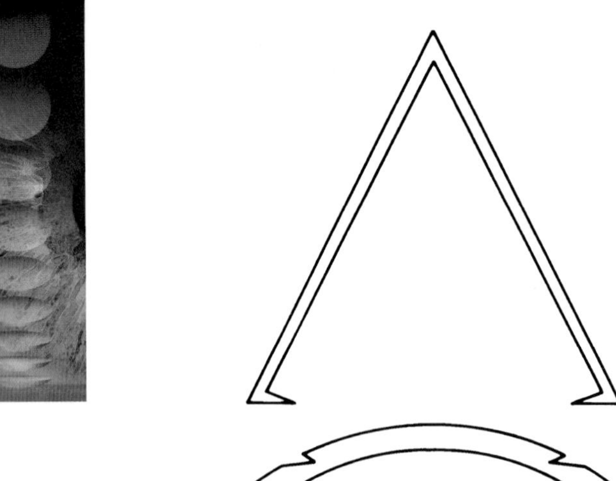

Figure 29.10 A contact lens splint and toothed forceps in cross-section

lids sticking to the globe (symblepharon) or to each other (ankyloblepharon). They are left in place during healing to maintain the fornices. Alternatively, large soft or silicone hydrogel lenses can be used. Silicone rubber lenses can be fitted but these are currently available only in high-plus prescriptions.

A large corneal lens can act as a splint to hold a corneal graft in place following keratoplasty. The front surface of the cornea is not held by stitches, but by the smooth spherical back surface of the contact lens. The splint itself is held by stitches to the bulbar conjunctiva. When these are cut, the splint is removed by special toothed forceps that fit into small slots on the front surface of the splint (Fig. 29.10).

Orthoptic uses (see Chapters 24 and 25)

A contact lens may act as an occluder in cases of intractable diplopia. Complete occlusion can only be achieved by having an opaque iris and pupil but an opaque pupil in an otherwise clear lens may be sufficient.

In squint treatment, contact lens occluders are used on the better eye instead of a sticky patch to treat amblyopia. Alternatively, adequate occlusion may be achieved with a high-negative or positive lens (Catford & Mackie 1968). However, the risk of infection in the better eye, although small, makes this form of treatment controversial. It is mainly of value where young children will not cooperate in the wearing of a patch.

The fitting of anisometropic amblyopes with contact lenses can improve the visual acuity and assist in the orthoptic treatment of squints in such cases.

Control of refractive errors

The effect of contact lenses on controlling myopia progression is covered in Chapter 30.

As an aid to defective colour vision and specific learning difficulties (dyslexia)

THE X-CHROM LENS

The X-Chrom lens is a red contact lens, with peak transmission of 595 nm and worn in one eye only (La Bissoniere 1974). It attempts to overcome certain red–green colour deficiencies by allowing a comparison of the different contrasts perceived by the two eyes. The eyes have a different perception of hues, altering their saturation or brightness, or imparting a lustre that the wearer learns to relate to a particular colour name.

Ciuffreda (1980) reported on the Pulfrich effect, elicited when subjects first wore the lens, being equivalent to the effect of a 0.57 neutral density filter or of 27% light transmission. Until adaptation has taken place, patients should be advised of some misjudgement of depth.

Clear soft lenses with a red-tinted pupil area are cosmetically more acceptable and comfortable than smaller rigid lenses and almost as effective in improving colour perception (Wood & Wood 1991).

CHROMAGEN LENSES

ChromaGen contact lenses are a range of soft lenses with precision-tinted pupils of varying hue and saturation which, when used singly or sometimes in combination, enhance colour perception in colour defectives. The ChromaGen system is also recommended in cases of specific learning difficulties.

- The fitting set contains 25 lenses and so-called diagnostic Haploscopic filters, in conjunction with an optional computerized test (Burnett Hodd 1998).
- Tints used are violet, purple, orange, yellow, green, amber and magenta.
- Three intensities of tint and three diameters are available ranging from 5 to 7 mm.
- A spectacle lens filter is held in front of the non-dominant eye and the patient decides which colour enhances a rainbow test screen the most. There may be two or three colours that enhance the colour range seen and make certain colours fluoresce.
- The appropriate soft contact lens with this optimum tint is inserted into the non-dominant eye.

The authors' experience is that only one in four patients finds the lens suitable for use and many do not order lenses because of the visual effects. Swarbrick et al. (2001) found that ChromaGen lenses significantly reduced errors on both the D15 and the Ishihara tests. However, particularly for deutan subjects, lens wear had no significant effect on Farnsworth Lantern test performance and vision was reported to be poor in dim light. To suggest that the wearer could pass Health and Safety tests for occupations where good colour differentiation is needed would be ethically unsound.

The use of colour to ease reading problems for those with specific learning difficulties is well documented (Wilkins et al. 1994) and, not surprisingly, the ChromaGen system is promoted for these cases. However, a wide range of precisely

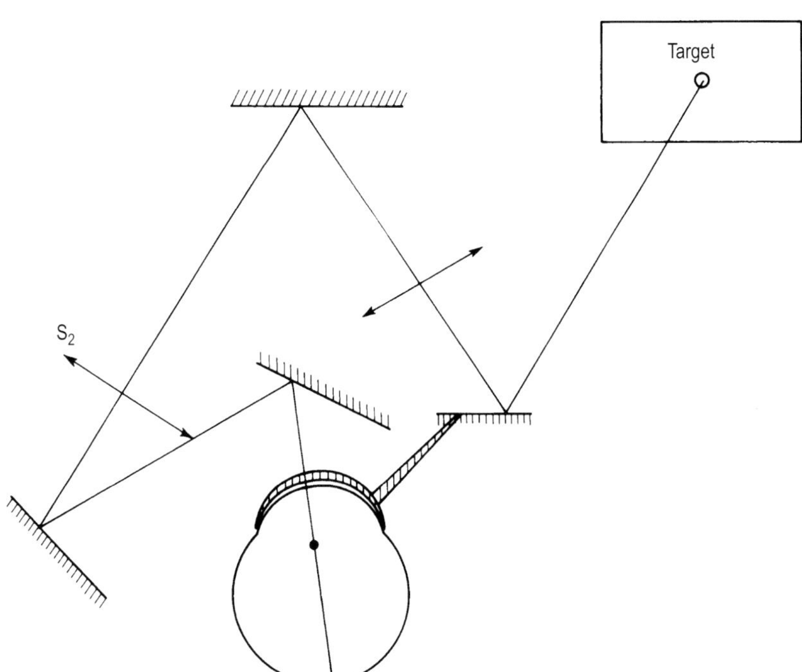

Figure 29.11 A contact lens with projecting stalk and mirror attached, used to produce a stabilized retinal image by means of a mirror and lens system. (After Millodot 1965)

chosen colours must be available as evaluated by the Wilkins rate of reading test (Harris & MacRow-Hill 1999).

CONTACT LENSES USED FOR RESEARCH INTO VISUAL FUNCTION

Contact lenses can maintain devices in contact with the eye for research purposes. These include electrodes, thermistors, oxygen probes, mirrors and telescopes.

Electrodes

Electroretinography (ERG) is the most common use of electrodes in contact lenses. Most electrical activity in the eye takes place in the retina, and the potential difference in the retina is measured as different light stimuli are applied. Electrodes used are of silver or platinum inserted into a small scleral lens.

An electrode incorporated into a contact lens may be used in iontophoresis for therapeutic purposes.

Stabilized retinal images

A better understanding of the physiological and psychological aspects of seeing has been achieved by studying what happens when the retinal image of an object remains stationary on the retina, i.e. when small movements of the retinal image, due to saccadic movements of the eye, are prevented. Two basic contact lens systems have been employed for this purpose. One utilizes a tightly fitting contact lens with a protruding stalk, on the end of which is a plane mirror. The mirror is used to reflect light from a target through a compensating optical system into the eye. Such a system was originally devised by Ditchburn and Ginsborg (1952); another system (Millodot 1965) is depicted in Figure 29.11.

Any movement of the eye causes a corresponding movement of the mirror, and the reflected image of the target is moved through twice this angle. To compensate for this, lenses S1 and S2 reduce magnification by half; thus, light is always imaged on the same portion of retina, regardless of eye movements.

The alternative system (Evans & Piggins 1963, Evans 1965) incorporates a small telescopic device into the contact lens (Fig. 29.12). A suitably illuminated target is placed approximately in the anterior focal plane of a high-positive lens,

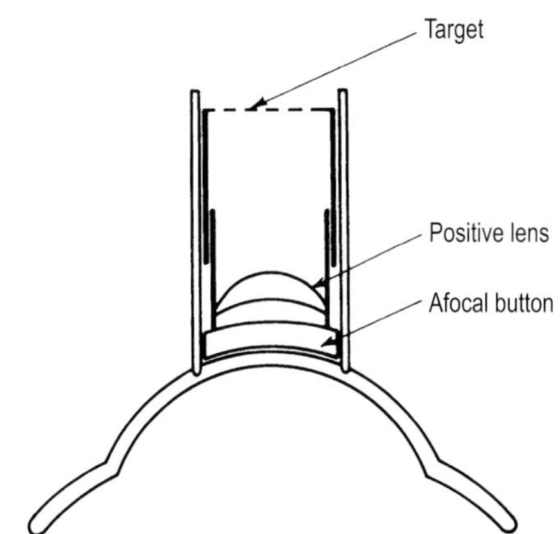

Figure 29.12 A contact lens incorporating a small telescopic device, used in the study of stabilized retinal images. The target is in the focal plane of a positive lens. Sliding supports allow some latitude in focusing. The positive lens is separated from the eye by an afocal button

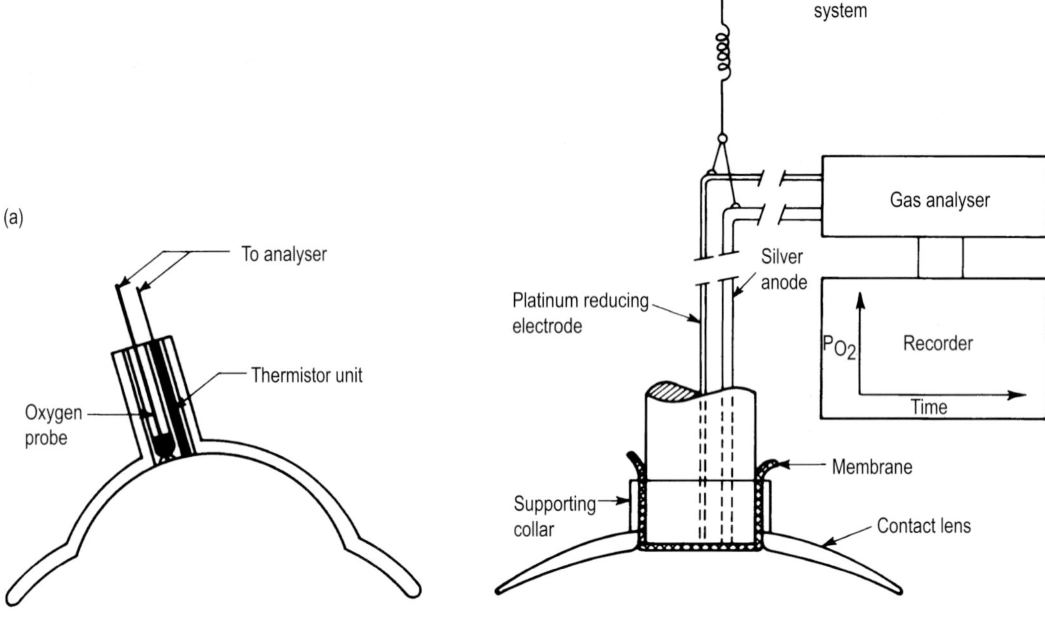

Figure 29.13 (a) A scleral contact lens incorporating a probe for recording oxygen tension. (After Hill & Fatt 1966). (b) A corneal lens used for measurement of oxygen uptake. (After Fatt & Hill 1970)

separated from the contact lens by an afocal button. The entire optical system is contained in aluminium tubing and the target and positive lenses move relative to each other to facilitate accurate focusing on the retina.

Temperature measurement

Temperature changes due to palpebral aperture, lid closure, eye position and the presence of the contact lens itself can be monitored using a thermistor – a tiny electrical device sensitive to temperature changes. Thermistors can be incorporated in scleral and corneal lenses. Hill and Leighton (1965) described the temperature changes of the eye wearing a scleral contact lens containing a thermistor, and showed how the rise in temperature behind a lens affects corneal metabolism.

Gas exchange of the cornea during contact lens wear

Scleral lenses were used to hold an oxygen probe against the cornea (Hill & Fatt 1966) (Fig. 29.13a). The probe is a polarographic oxygen electrode covered by an oxygen-containing membrane. As the oxygen from the membrane is lost to the cornea or surrounding liquid, the current in the electrode drops. Figure 29.13b shows a similar system in a corneal lens (Fatt & Hill 1970). The output of carbon dioxide by the corneal epithelium can also be recorded.

LENSES FOR SPORTS

Contact lenses worn for sports must satisfy the following criteria.

- They must not move when accidental foreign pressure is applied.
- The optic must remain centred.
- The tear lens must remain completely free of bubbles in front of the pupil area.
- Corneal metabolism must be adequately maintained during the period required for the sport.

With current materials and lens designs, a fairly tight-fitting RGP corneal lens or a well-fitted soft lens satisfies the above criteria most of the time, although a slight risk of lens displacement remains. To minimize this risk a slightly tight soft lens with a minimal total diameter (TD) of 14.50 mm is desirable.

Large soft lenses are manufactured specifically for sports purposes such as the Cantor & Nissel Sportlens, TD 14.90 mm. This has an aspheric front surface and large optical zone with aberration-controlled optics designed to reduce flare under adverse lighting conditions. Custom-made soft lenses are available in larger diameters and can incorporate a tint if required.

The S-Lim design (Jack Allen, UK), an aspheric semi-limbal RGP lens of 14.0 mm TD with a back optic zone radius (BOZR) range of 5.80–9.10 mm, is fitted according to sagittal depth. This and other large rigid lenses can be used for sports.

Tint manipulation is also available:

- Varichrome photochromic lens (Visiontech) changes from light blue/green to deep blue/violet, having a light transmission of 200–430 nm.
- SportSight GP (Paragon Vision Sciences) is very dark in appearance and provides better contrast sensitivity than normal rigid lens materials.
- Soft lenses are also available: the Solaire (Cantor and Nissel, UK) with a UV inhibitor is available in two densities of brown tint, 35% and 70%. It is used for sports such as sailing and skiing.

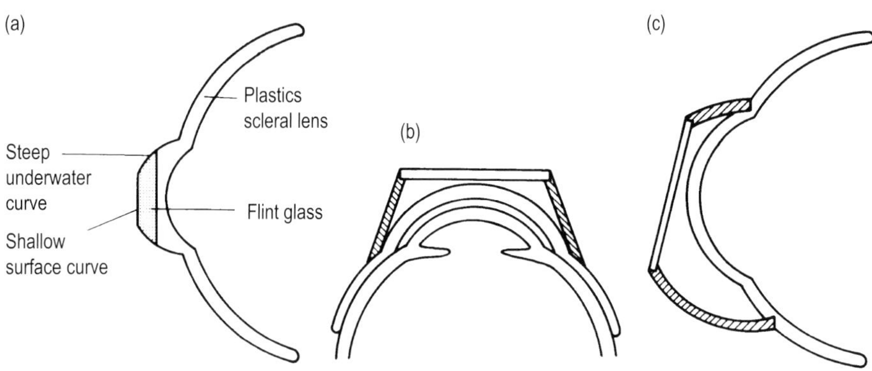

Figure 29.14 Underwater contact lenses. (a) Douthwaite's bifocal flint glass button lens (reproduced by kind permission of W. A. Douthwaite). (b) Lens containing an air space. The flat front surface has dark tinted supports to prevent distortion and glare. (c) An air space with tilted front surface, which gives added comfort and is supported by the lower lid during wear

CIBA Vision's Softperm lenses (see Chapter 10) with a central RGP zone and a 14.3 mm soft periphery may prove useful for sports, particularly if corneal astigmatism requires correction, toric soft lenses are unsuccessful and the comfort of a soft lens is needed (Minarik 1987).

Where corneal lenses are necessary, soft or silicone hydrogel lenses can be worn on top of the rigid lenses during sporting activities to reduce the risk of lens loss. This can be particularly useful in keratoconus.

Scleral lenses are ideal as they are unlikely to dislodge but are now rarely an economic option. For all professional sports, the contact lenses fitted must satisfy the standards laid down by the authorizing body of that particular sport in the country concerned.

Climbing and cold weather sports and activities

Socks (1983) found no significant problems when lenses were worn for cold weather activities and contact lenses had the advantage over spectacles: they did not mist up, become brittle or break as spectacles may do when cold. Contact lenses protect the eye from wind-driven ice and snow and have been worn successfully up to 26,000 feet on Mount Everest (Clarke 1975).

Most difficulties occur with the cleaning fluids and procedures, as the liquids may freeze and contact lenses become difficult to handle with cold fingers. Extended-wear silicone hydrogel lenses would be better.

Swimming

Contact lenses should not be worn while swimming as there is a risk of both infection and lens loss (Choo et al. 2005). In fresh water, the saline content of soft lenses becomes more hypotonic with time, resulting in possible corneal oedema and difficulty removing the lenses. However, sealed scleral lenses provide almost complete protection of the eye while swimming, and no risk of loss.

Lenses for scuba diving

Under water, the power of the eye is reduced by approximately 42.00 D. This is due to water replacing air in front of the cornea. If the front surface of the cornea is assumed to have a radius of curvature of 8.0 mm, then the reduction in power is as follows.

$$\begin{pmatrix}\text{Power of front corneal}\\\text{surface in air}\end{pmatrix} - \begin{pmatrix}\text{Power of front corneal}\\\text{surface in water}\end{pmatrix}$$

$$\frac{(1.376 - 1)\ 1000\ \text{D}}{8.0} - \frac{(1.376 - 1.333)\ 1000\ \text{D}}{8.0}$$

$$= 41.50\ \text{D}$$

The emmetropic eye therefore becomes hypermetropic to this extent. Douthwaite (1971) described a concentric lens designed to replace this power loss. A flint glass button was fused by the 'Uniseal' method to a plastic scleral lens with a flat interface (Fig. 29.14a). The steep outer curve on the front of the flint button permits vision under water where the illumination is low and the pupil dilated, while the flatter central surface curve provides vision in air when the pupil is likely to be more constricted in daylight. The lens gives a full, unrestricted field of view. Its disadvantages are slight displacement on the eye that can cause a loss of vision above water, and the out-of-focus image formed by the peripheral zone in air giving rise to haze and reducing contrast and acuity.

The air-cell type of lens has a plane front surface enclosing an air space in front of a conventional scleral lens sighted to correct the wearer's normal refractive error. It is like a tiny 'face mask' worn in front of the eye only (Fig. 29.14b). The optical effect is the same as looking through any plane surface into water.

Refraction of light from water to air causes objects to appear at three-quarters of their real distance, giving a magnification of 31.333. Due to total internal reflection at the plane face, the visual field is restricted to 97.2° in air and approximately 55–60° in water (Cockell 1967). If the side supports are left transparent, there is considerable distortion of the peripheral visual field.

Mossé (1964) described a lens in which the front plane face is tilted (Fig. 29.14c) and the supports opaque, eliminating the distortion of the peripheral field. The tilt of the plane face makes upper lid movement more comfortable and prevents the lens from sagging as it is better supported by the lower lid.

The mode of attachment of the plane face to the lens is important so that the air chamber does not collapse at pressures experienced under water. Figure 29.15 shows Cockell's construction in which all but the plane face is made from one solid piece of plastic.

Attempts have been made to fill the space with air under pressure. The incorporation of a little silica gel in the air space

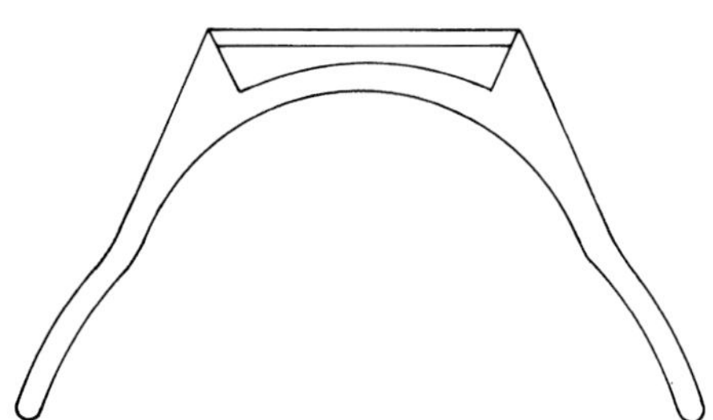

Figure 29.15 Cockell's underwater contact lens (developed at The City University, London)

prevents condensation. The plane face should be as close as possible to the front optic surface of the scleral lens, but not sufficiently close to cause interference fringes. The advantage of such a lens is that it gives adequate vision both above and below water without allowing the diver to be seen from afar from the reflections from a plane facemask. This type of lens can be worn satisfactorily for periods of approximately 4 hours.

According to Bennett (1985), soft lenses, with their greater adhesion, are preferable to rigid lenses while wearing a facemask during normal diving procedures. Should the facemask be lost, the diver would be able to surface and see his support vessel.

Where deep diving is undertaken, rigid lenses are contraindicated (Molinari & Socks 1986) as bubbles and oedema form underneath. When diving in a chamber or bell, contact lenses should not be worn at all (Bennett 1985) because divers live for long periods under high pressure and *Pseudomonas aeruginosa* (see Chapters 4 and 18) is known to thrive in diving chambers.

LENSES FOR THE PARTIALLY SIGHTED

Partially sighted people need extra magnification to see detail. This can be provided in the form of a Galilean telescope device, in which a high-minus contact lens forms the eyepiece and a conventional spectacle lens the objective (Fig. 29.16).

Since the eyepiece contacts the cornea, the magnification (for an emmetropic eye) is given directly by

$$\frac{w_2}{w_1} = \frac{f_1'}{f_2'} = \frac{f_1'}{f_1' - d} = \frac{1}{1 - dF_1'} \text{ (d in metres)}$$

With a typical power for F_1' of +25.00 D and a vertex distance, d, of 12 mm

$$\text{Magnification} = \frac{1}{1 - 3/10} = \frac{1}{0.7} = \times 1.4$$

The powers of the two lenses and their separation must correct the patient's refractive error, K, where

$$K = \frac{F_1'}{1 - dF_1'} + F_2' \text{ (d in metres)}$$

This system has been used with soft, scleral and corneal lenses forming the eyepiece, soft and scleral lenses being more satisfactory as they are more stable. The weight of the high-positive spectacle lens can be further relieved by the use of a Fresnel press-on lens (Gerstman & Levene 1974).

The advantages over the telescopic type of spectacle aid are:

- Reduction in weight.
- Psychological benefit of improved cosmesis.

However, the contact lens system cannot be removed as quickly and conveniently as spectacles although this is less of a disadvantage when the system is worn on one eye only. The patient then has a normal visual field with one eye, while the other eye receives the magnified image for detailed vision (Moore 1964). However, the patient must be able to suppress each eye alternately.

Magnification reduces the visual field and can cause disorientation. This may be minimized by magnifying only a small central portion of the visual field using a carefully fitted contact lens which corrects refractive error and has a flat central portion producing a high negative power centrally. The diameter of this portion must be approximately two-thirds of the pupil diameter in normal illumination, typically between 3.5 and 4.0 mm, and approximately –50.00 D power (Filderman 1964). This is the high-negative eyepiece of power F_2' used in conjunction with a positive segment of approximately 10 mm diameter and +25.00 D power, cemented on to the back surface of an afocal spectacle lens of 12.00 D base. Below this, a near addition may be cemented on to the carrier lens (Fig. 29.17). Fresnel press-on segments may be used as an alternative to cemented segments.

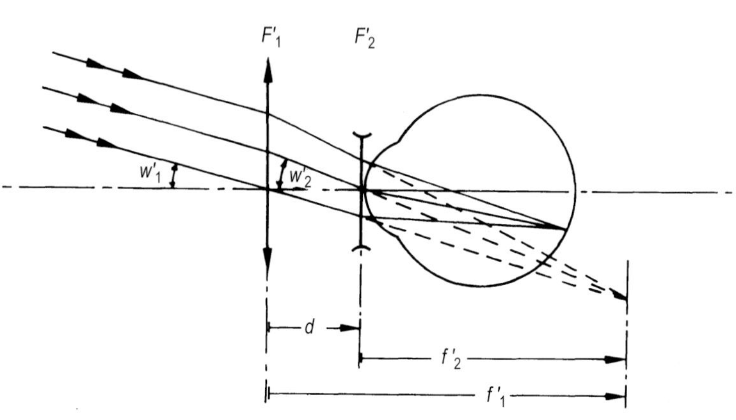

Figure 29.16 A Galilean telescope system incorporating a contact lens of power F_2' as eyepiece, and a spectacle lens of power F_1' as objective

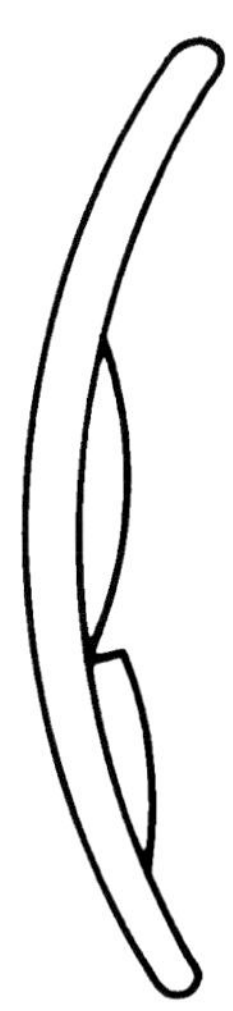

Figure 29.17 A spectacle lens used as the objective for a Galilean telescope system, having separate portions for distance and near vision, cemented on to an afocal carrier lens

F_2' depends on the thickness and BOZR of the contact lens. Since

$$K = \frac{F_1'}{1 - dF_1'} + F_2'$$

and d can be measured, F_1' may be determined. The magnification may then be computed from

$$\frac{1}{-dF_1'}$$

Filderman (1964) described a small corneal lens, prism ballasted to rest on the lower lid, with the optic zone displaced to sit in front of the pupil and the upper edge just above the upper pupil margin. Best results were obtained with scleral lenses but soft lenses can also be used (Stone & Breakspear 1977). A large lenticulated RGP lens fitted to give minimal movement provides superior optical quality.

Feinbloom (1961) attempted to incorporate both positive objective and negative eyepiece in one scleral lens with an air space between the two but the lenses were thick, heavy and uncomfortable.

Drasdo (1970) developed a similar lens to be used in conjunction with a spectacle lens, which he described as a 'feedback corrected' lens system. It produced magnification without increasing the eye movements usually needed to fixate peripheral objects. It therefore overcame the major disadvantage of disorientation.

Bier (1960) described a reversed telescope system, useful for restricted peripheral vision or hemianopia in which a high-positive contact lens and a high-negative spectacle lens produced a reduction in magnification. This allowed more to be seen in the existing visual field but reduced the visual acuity.

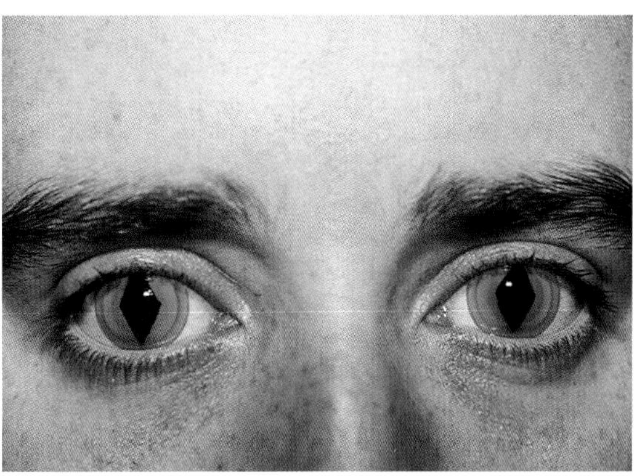

Figure 29.18 An example of soft lenses used for effect in dramatic productions

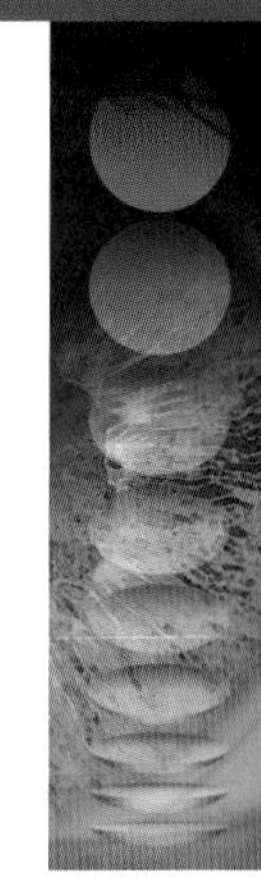

ANIMALS' LENSES

Animal treatment with contact lenses falls into three categories.

- *Experimental lenses* – Animal experimentation assesses aspects of visual function in several species and special contact lenses are used for this purpose.
- *Utilitarian lenses* – Chickens and turkeys fitted with opaque and coloured contact lenses to reduce acuity and prevent feather pecking (Anon 1967).
- *Therapeutic lenses* – Tammeus et al. (1983) reported the use of a 72% water-content soft lens of 34 mm TD and 18 mm BOZR for a horse with an injured cornea. It was worn therapeutically for 6 days following corneal perforation. Schmidt et al. (1977) reported the use of soft lenses to treat corneal conditions in dogs and cats.

MISCELLANEOUS LENSES

Certain lenses or types of lens do not fall into any of the above categories, and yet some mention of them should be made.

Tinted lenses

RGP and soft lenses are available with handling tints. While RGP tints are limited in density, soft lenses can be made to any colour, density or light absorption (see Chapters 9 and 10). Care is needed for patients with colour vision difficulties and these lenses should not be worn when driving.

Lenses for stage and screen

Various effects, for use by actors, can be made in scleral, corneal or soft lenses (Fig. 29.18). All designs of 'fun' lenses are available, while hand-painted options extend the choice for film roles.

This concludes the details of special contact lenses but no doubt many more types of lens will be developed as the need arises.

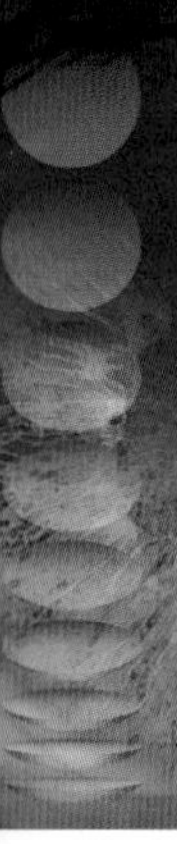

References

Anon (1967) Contact lenses for turkeys – report. Optician, 154, 575

Astin, C. (1987) Case report: three cases of fitting a superiorly truncated hydrophilic lens. J. Br. Contact Lens Assoc., 10(2), 27–28

Ball, G. V. (1964) Characteristics of tinted contact lenses. Br. J. Physiol. Opt., 21, 219–223

Bennett, Q. M. (1985) Contact lenses for diving. Aust. J. Optom., 68(1), 25–26

Bier, N. (1960) Correction of Subnormal Vision, p. 87. London: Butterworths

Burnett Hodd, N. (1998) Putting ChromaGen to the test. Optom. Today, 38(14), 39–42

Catford, G. V. and Mackie, I. A. (1968) Occlusion with high plus corneal lenses. Br. J. Ophthalmol., 52, 342–345

Choo, J., Vuu, K., Bergenske, P., Burnham, K., Smythe, J. and Caroline, P. (2005) Bacterial populations on silicone hydrogel and hydrogel contact lenses after swimming in a chlorinated pool. Optom. Vis. Sci., 82(2), 134–137

Chou, B. R., Cullen, A. P. and Dumbleton, K. A. (1988) Protection factors of ultraviolet-blocking contact lenses. Int. Contact Lens Clin., 15, 244–251

Ciuffreda, K. J. (1980) Binocular space perception and the X-Chrom lens. Int. Contact Lens Clin., 7, 71–74

Clarke, C. (1975) Contact lenses at high altitude: experience on Everest south-west face 1975. Br. J. Ophthalmol., 60, 479–480

Cockell, R. R. (1967) A survey of underwater visual problems. Paper read to The Contact Lens Society, January 1967

Ditchburn, R. W. and Ginsborg, B. L. (1952) Vision with a stabilized retinal image. Nature, 170, 36–37

Douthwaite, W. A. (1971) Bifocal underwater contact lenses. Ophthal. Opt., 11, 10–14

Drasdo, N. (1970) The effect of high powered contact lenses on the visual fixation reflex. Br. J. Physiol. Opt., 25, 14–22

Eisner, G., Lotmar, W. and Papritz, F. (1985) A new contact glass for slit-lamp examination of the cornea, especially in specular reflection. Ophthalmology (Instrument and Book Supplement), 92, 72–83

Evans, C. R. (1965) A universally fitting contact lens for the study of stabilized retinal images. Br. J. Physiol. Opt., 22, 39–45

Evans, C. R. and Piggins, D. J. (1963) A comparison of the behaviour of geometrical shapes when viewed under conditions of steady fixation, and with apparatus for producing a stabilized retinal image. Br. J. Physiol. Opt., 20, 261–273

Fatt, I. and Hill, R. M. (1970) Oxygen tension under a contact lens during blinking – a comparison of theory and experimental observation. Am. J. Optom., 47, 50–55

Feinbloom, W. (1961) Feinbloom miniscope contact lens. Described by Allan Isen, Encyclopaedia of Contact Lens Practice III, Supplement 13, Appendix B, 53–55. South Bend, IND: International Optics Publishing

Filderman, I. P. (1964) The spectacle lens – contact lens system. Br. J. Physiol. Opt., 21, 195–196

Friedman, B. (1967) A contact lens for estimating corneal thickness. Eye Ear Nose Throat Mon., 46, 344–345

Gerstman, D. R. and Levene, J. R. (1974) Galilean telescope for the partially sighted. Br. J. Ophthalmol., 58, 761–765

Goldmann, H. (1938) Zur Technik der Spaltlampenmikroskopie. Ophthalmologica, 96, 90

Harris, D. A. and MacRow-Hill, S. J. (1999) Application of ChromaGen haploscopic lenses to patients with dyslexia: a double-masked, placebo-controlled trial. J. Am. Optom. Assoc., 70(10), 629–639

Hill, R. M. and Fatt, I. (1966) Oxygen measurements under a contact lens. Am. J. Optom., 43, 233–237

Hill, R. M. and Leighton, A. J. (1965) Temperature changes of human cornea and tears under a contact lens, I, II & III. Am. J. Optom., 42, 9–16, 71–77, 584–588

Hillman, J. S. (1976) The use of hydrophilic contact lenses. Optician, 172(4458), 9–11

Kersley, H. J. (1975) Continuous wear lenses after aphakic operation. Optician, 170(4393), 12–18

Klein, M. (1949) Contact shell applicator for use as a corneal bath. Br. J. Ophthalmol, 33, 716–717

Koeppe, L. (1919) Die Theorie und Anwendung der Stereomikroskopie des lebenden menschlichen Kammer-winkels in fokalen Lichte der Gullstrandschen Nernst-spaltlampe. Münch Med. Wochenschr., 66, 708

La Bissoniere, P. E. (1974) The X-chrom lens. Int. Contact Lens Clin., 1(4), 48–55

Meyler, J. and Schnider, C. (2002) The role of UV-blocking soft CLs in ocular protection. Optician, 223(5854), 28–32

Millodot, M. (1965) Stabilized retinal images and disappearance time. Br. J. Physiol. Opt., 22, 148–152

Minarik, K. R. (1987) Using Saturn II lenses to manage toric soft lens 'failures'. Contact Lens Forum, 12(9), 80–81

Molinari, J. F. and Socks, J. F. (1986) Effects of hyperbaric conditions on corneal physiology with hydrogel contact lenses. J. Br. Contact Lens Assoc. Scientific Meetings, pp. 17–19

Moore, L. (1964) The contact lens for subnormal visual acuity. Br. J. Physiol. Opt., 21, 203–204

Mossé, P. (1964) Underwater contact lenses. Br. J. Physiol. Opt., 21, 250–255

Richards, D. W., Murphy, K. A. and Cartwright, M. J. (1993) Ophthalmic contact lens with internal fixation light for examination of the optic nerve head. Ophthalmol. Physiol. Opt., 13, 320–321

Schmidt, G. M., Blanchard, G. L. and Keller, W. F. (1977) The use of hydrophilic contact lenses in corneal diseases of the dog and cat: a preliminary report. J. Small Anim. Pract., 18, 773–777

Socks, J. F. (1983) Use of contact lenses for cold weather activities: results of a survey. Int. Contact Lens Clin., 10, 82–91

Stone, J. and Breakspear, H. R. (1977) Two interesting cases of low visual acuity seen at The London Refraction Hospital. Contact Lens J., 6(3), 3–4, 6

Swarbrick, H. A., Nguyen, P., Nguyen, T. and Pham, P. (2001) The ChromaGen contact lens system: colour vision test results and subjective responses. Ophthalmol. Physiol. Opt., 21(3), 182–196

Tammeus, J., Krall, C. J. and Rengstorff, R. H. (1983) Therapeutic extended wear contact lens for corneal injury in a horse. J. Am. Vet. Med. Assoc., 182, 286

Tsubota, K. (1988) A contact lens for specular microscopic observation. Am. J. Ophthalmol., 106(5), 627–628

Uribe Troncoso, M. (1921) Gonioscopy with the electric ophthalmoscope. New York Academy of Medicine. Referred to in Gonioscopy, by Troncoso. Philadelphia, PA: Davis (1947)

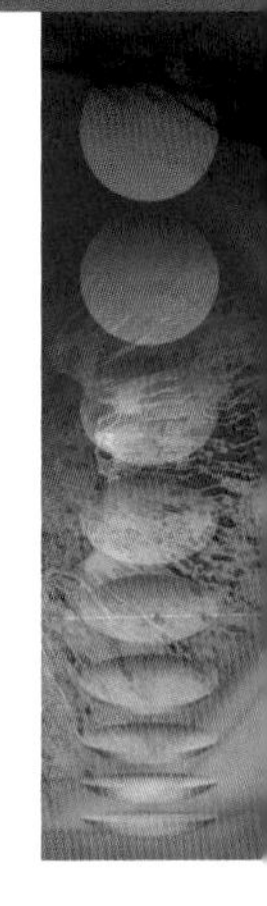

Wilkins, A. J., Evans, B. J. W., Brown, J. et al (1994) Double-masked placebo controlled trial of precision tinted spectral filters in children who used overlays. Ophthalmol. Physiol. Opt., 14, 365–370

Wood, S. and Wood, J. M. (1991) Red pupil soft lens aids colour perception, provides comfort. Rev. Optom., 128(2), 96–98

Chapter 30

Contact lens correction and myopia progression

Nicola Logan and Bernard Gilmartin

CHAPTER CONTENTS

INTRODUCTION

Whereas genetic modelling and studies of family history confirm that heredity predominates in the genesis of myopia (Pacella et al. 1999, Hammond et al. 2001), the quality of the retinal image and its role in myopia onset and progression has featured in many research reports over the last decade. The consensus, based principally on animal models of myopia (Smith 1998), is that myopia in humans can be induced by:

- Hyperopic and myopic blur due to inaccurate accommodation.
- Lag of accommodation at near.
- Transient myopia following near vision.
- Deficits in integrative/adaptive oculomotor responses that incorporate accommodation as a response component (Gilmartin 2004).

Each of these sources of retinal blur can be differentially affected by contact lens wear when compared to spectacles and, coupled with differences in peripheral image formation, engender the hypothesis that the superior imaging properties offered by contact lens correction may in some way retard myopia progression.

It is not known how retinal blur generates excessive elongation of the posterior vitreous chamber, but this is generally accepted to be the principal structural correlate of myopia (Wildsoet 1998). Nevertheless, contact lenses are likely to be important as a technique that optimizes optical and visual performance, and is a well-established, reasonably safe, accessible and relatively inexpensive mode of correction.

The epidemiological pressure to further understand the aetiology of myopia and putative methods of amelioration is immense. The prevalence of myopia in adolescent eyes has increased substantially over recent decades and is now approaching 10–25% and 60–80% in industrialized societies of the West and East, respectively (Saw 2003). Worldwide, the condition is the leading cause of visual impairment (World Health Organization 2000). It is widely acknowledged that a myopic eye, over 6.00 D, is a vulnerable eye and is especially susceptible to a range of ocular pathologies (Curtin 1985, Tano 2002).

Of special interest is the relative efficacy of contact lenses in retarding myopia progression in the young developing eye and the adult eye; congenital myopia is not included in this group. Early-onset (or school/juvenile) myopia represents around 60% of myopia. Onset is between 9 and 11 years, progressing throughout the early teenage years and reducing in the late teens or early twenties to stabilize at approximately 3.00–4.00 D. Late-onset (or early adult-onset) myopia, representing between 8 and 15% of myopes (Edwards 1998), occurs when coordinated biological growth of the eye ceases, typically between 15 and 18 years (Zadnik et al. 2003) and occasionally in the early twenties. It progresses slowly to levels rarely in excess of 2.00 D. Corneal curvature changes do not appear to be correlated with myopia onset and progression in either early- or late-onset myopia

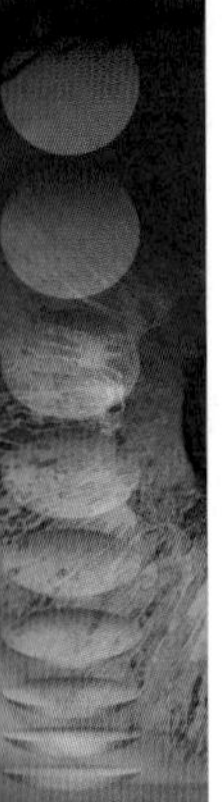

Table 30.1: Selection of recent studies on the prevalence of myopia and hyperopia in children and young adolescents

Country	No. subjects	Age (years)	Prevalence of myopia		Prevalence of hyperopia	
			Criteria	Percentage	Criteria	Percentage
UK[1]	7600	7	<–1.00 D	1.1	>+2.00 D	5.9
Sweden[2]	1045	12–13	≤–0.50 D	45	≥+1.00 D	8.4
USA[3]	2583	6–14	≤–0.75 D	10.1	≥+1.25 D	8.6
USA[4]	2523	5–17	≤–0.75 D	9.2	≥+1.25 D	12.8
African–American	534			6.6		6.4
Asian	491			18.5		6.3
Hispanic	463			13.2		12.7
White	1035			4.4		19.3
Australia[5]	2571	5	<–0.50 D	2.8	>+0.50 D	46.1
		12	<–0.50 D	8.7	>+0.50 D	24.1
Hong Kong[6]	7560	5–16	≤–0.50 D	36.7	≥+2.00 D	4.0
Singapore[7]	1453	7	≤–0.50 D	29.0	Data not reported	
		8	≤–0.50 D	34.7		
		9	≤–0.50 D	53.1		
Hong Kong[8]		13–15	≤–0.50 D		Data not reported	
Local school	335			85–88		
International school	789			43 in non-Chinese		
				65 in mixed Chinese		
				80 in Chinese		

[1] Barnes et al. (2001); [2] Villarreal et al. (2000); [3] Zadnik et al. (2003); [4] Kleinstein et al. (2003); [5] Junghans & Crewther (2003); [6] Fan et al. (2004); [7] Saw et al. (2002a); [8] Lam et al. (2002).
After Gilmartin (2004), with permission of Blackwell Publishing.

(Bullimore et al. 1992, McBrien & Adams 1997, Zadnik et al. 2003).

This chapter outlines current estimates of myopia prevalence, the characteristics of its progression and attempts to retard its progression with contact lenses.

PREVALENCE OF MYOPIA

Figures on the prevalence of myopia vary because of differences in population samples, discrepancies in methodology (Weale 2003), variations across nations and differences with age (Saw 2003). To some extent these discrepancies are offset by international initiatives to standardize sampling and measurement protocols (Negrel et al. 2000, Ellwein 2002). A group of researchers have proposed a protocol for refractive error study in children that comprises obtaining population-based cross-sectional samples of children aged 5–15 years through cluster sampling (Negrel et al. 2000). The main outcome measures include uncorrected and best-corrected visual acuity and cycloplegic autorefraction.

Prevalence of myopia in children

Refractive error has a wide distribution in newborn infants, with myopia present in approximately 19% of Caucasian infants (Cook & Glassock 1951). However, in the first few years of life an active emmetropization process reduces this distribution. Consequently, in pre-school children there is a low prevalence of myopia (2–3% for Caucasian children), but by the age of 6 years the prevalence rises to approximately 6% (Robinson 1999, Junghans & Crewther 2003, Kleinstein et al. 2003).

The prevalence of myopia differs by geographical location but the data are confounded by other factors including ethnicity, age, education and socioeconomic status. Examples of recent studies on myopia prevalence in children are given in Table 30.1, showing a 60–80% prevalence in urban areas of Asia such as Hong Kong, Singapore and Taiwan, and approximately 10% in Australia and USA; however, values for Sweden approach those seen in the East.

To date, seven centres have adopted the Refractive Error Study in Children protocol and the findings are summarized in Table 30.2. These surveys were conducted in populations with different ethnic origins and environments and it is evident that there is a substantial difference in myopia prevalence between these populations.

Prevalence of myopia in adolescents

The prevalence of myopia varies with age, with much higher values reported for adolescents than for children. For example, myopia has been found in 30% of 6–7-year-old Chinese children and up to 70% in 16–17-year-old males (Lam & Goh 1991). Similarly, 15–20% of Japanese 7-year-olds and 66% of 17-year-olds are myopic (Matsumura & Hirai 1999). In Taiwanese

Table 30.2: Studies on the prevalence of myopia in children (>–0.50 D spherical equivalent cycloplegic autorefraction in either eye) using the Refractive Error Study in Children sampling and measurement protocols*

			Myopia prevalence (% [95% CI])	
Country	Region	Sample size	5 years	15 years
China[1]	Shunyi District (rural)	5884	M + F: 0.0	M: 36.7 [29.9–43.4]; F: 55.0 [49.4–60.6]
Nepal[2]	Mechi Zone (rural)	5067	M + F: ~0.5	M: ~2.9; F: ~1.0[†]
Chile[3]	La Florida (suburban)	5303	M + F: 3.4 [1.72–5.05]	M: 19.4 [13.6–25.2]; F: 14.7 [10.1–19.2]
India[4]	Andra Pradesh (rural)	4074	M + F: 2.80 [1.28–4.33]	M + F: 6.72 [4.31–9.12]
India[5]	New Delhi (urban)	6447	M + F: 4.86 [2.54–6.83]	M + F: 10.80 [6.71–14.80]
South Africa[6]	Durban (metropolitan)	4890	M + F: 3.2 [0.6–5.7]	M + F: 9.60 [6.4–12.7]
China[7]	Guangzhou (urban)	4363	M + F: 3.3 [0.4–6.3]	M + F: 73.1 [68.0–78.2]

[1] Zhao et al. (2000); [2] Pokharel et al. (2000); [3] Maul et al. (2000); [4] Dandona et al. (2002); [5] Murthy et al. (2002); [6] Naidoo et al. (2003); [7] He et al. (2004). M, male; F, female; [†] Extrapolated data.
* See Negrel et al. (2000). After Gilmartin (2004), with permission of Blackwell Publishing.

children a prevalence of 61% at the age of 12 years increased to 84% for 16–18-year-olds (Lin et al. 2001).

Prevalence of myopia in adults

Approximately 25% of Caucasian young adults develop myopia (Sperduto et al. 1983) and, based on population surveys, approximately 26% of West Europeans over 40 years old are myopic (Kempen et al. 2004). In a study in Norway, myopia was found in 35% of adults aged 20–25 years and in 30.3% of adults aged 40–45 years (Midelfart et al. 2002). The discrepancy between different races is not as great in adult populations although slightly higher prevalence data have been reported: myopia prevalence for Chinese adults aged 40–81 years is 34.4% (Wong et al. 2003) and for Japanese adults aged 40–79 years is 45.7% (Shimizu et al. 2003).

MYOPIA PROGRESSION

Progression of myopia is influenced by a variety of factors: age of onset, ethnicity, gender and visual environment (Zadnik et al. 2004). One important question is whether myopia prevalence in Europe, Australia and the USA will increase to the levels currently seen in East Asia (Rose et al. 2003). Identification of factors that affect the rate of progression would further increase understanding of myopia development and may facilitate advancement in the amelioration of myopia.

Myopia progression in children

Myopia progresses more rapidly in younger children (Parssinen & Lyyra 1993, Fulk et al. 2000). It increases by approximately 0.50 D per annum in myopic Caucasian children aged 8–13 years (Parssinen & Lyyra 1993), whereas Hong Kong Chinese children aged 5–16 years are reported to have a mean myopic progression of 0.63 D per annum (Fan et al. 2004). These studies were carried out on the general population and an optometrist in practice may see a different trend, due to self-selection (Pointer 2000). A 6-year longitudinal study analysed refractive error change in UK Caucasian children aged 7–13 years tested annually in optometric practice. Pointer (2001) found that, of the 41 children who attended all seven refractions, 73.2% showed an increase in myopic refraction (spherical equivalent refraction, SER) between visits one and seven: mean change –0.80 ± 0.80 D, equivalent to a myopic shift per annum of –0.13 D. If all children were taken into the analysis, a mean change in SER would equate to –0.54 ± 0.82 D (–0.09 D per annum). If only myopic children were considered, then a greater myopic shift in SER is observed: mean change –1.32 ± 0.99 D (–0.22 D per annum).

Myopia progression in young adults

Although it is generally accepted that coordinated biological growth of the eye ceases around 15 years of age (Sorsby & Leary 1970), there is a proportion of myopes, estimated between 8 and 15%, who have an onset of myopia between 15 and 18 years of age (Gilmartin 2004). This late-onset myopia has a slow progression (~0.16 D per annum) and rarely exceeds 2.00 D (Kinge et al. 1999).

Myopia progression in adults

In children and young adults, axial elongation, in particular vitreous chamber growth, accounts for the majority of myopia development and progression (Grosvenor & Scott 1993, Lin et al. 1996). In older adults, nuclear sclerosis of the lens may cause myopic shift due to changes in lenticular power; however, an increase in axial length with progression of myopia has also been found in this age group (McBrien & Adams 1997). A longitudinal study on the development of myopia in a specific occupational group (clinical microscopists) recorded that 45% (aged 21–63 years) became myopic (≥0.37 D) during the 2-year period (McBrien & Adams 1997).

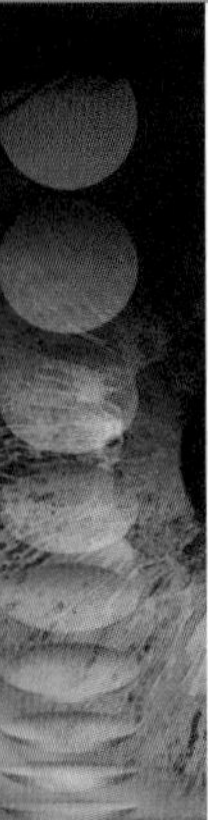

A retrospective study in adult contact lens wearers, aged 20–40 years, determined that approximately 20% had myopic progression of –1.00 D over 5 years, more common in subjects in their twenties (Bullimore et al. 2002). Unfortunately, no data on axial length were given for this subject cohort.

It is well known that there is significant individual variation in myopia progression, and although the onset of myopia in most people is abrupt, it is not instantaneous (Thorn et al. 2002).

CORRECTION FOR MYOPIA

In deciding the appropriate correction option for myopia, the efficacy, safety, comfort and convenience of the treatment modality should be considered. Whereas the primary mode for myopic correction is still spectacles, the principal alternatives are soft or rigid contact lenses and refractive surgery. Account should also be taken of whether the form of myopic correction exacerbates acceleration of the myopic progression.

CONTACT LENSES AND MYOPIA PROGRESSION

Soft contact lenses

Myopic progression associated with soft contact lenses was reported in the 1970s (Grosvenor 1975, Harris et al. 1975, Barnett & Rengstorff 1977). Harris and colleagues (1975) found a mean increase in myopia of –0.35 D in five randomly selected subjects who were followed for 9 months. Similarly, Grosvenor (1975) reported a small (–0.25 D) increase in myopia in ten soft lens wearers followed over a 12-month period. An average increase in myopia of –0.50 D was found in 40 subjects after only 3 months of soft lens wear (Barnett & Rengstorff 1977). All three studies also reported associated steepening of the cornea during the period of increasing myopia, suggesting that corneal oedema may be the cause of the increased myopia. The validity of these studies is limited as none had a control group to compare the myopia progression. In a long-term trial (average 5.4 years), 19 unilateral extended wear contact lens subjects were followed for 1 week after lens removal. The contralateral eye was used as a control (Rengstorff & Nilsson 1985). However, these eyes were emmetropic ($n = 11$), amblyopic ($n = 6$), had a cataract ($n = 1$) or had a prosthesis ($n = 1$), thus limiting the validity of use as a control eye. No significant change in refraction was found in the eyes that had worn the contact lens. Andreo (1990) retrospectively compared 37 teenage soft lens wearers (aged 14–19 years) with 19 teenagers wearing spectacles. After 1 year, no significant difference was found in the rate of myopia progression between the groups.

In order to overcome the limitations of previous studies, Horner et al. (1999) followed two randomized groups of 11–14-year-olds for 3 years. One group wore spectacles, the other soft lenses. No significant difference in the rate of myopia progression was found between the groups. The authors concluded that their findings should alleviate optometrists' concern about correcting myopic adolescents with soft contact lenses in terms of inducing additional myopia progression.

It is believed that the first-generation hydrogel lenses increased myopia by inducing corneal oedema as a consequence of hypoxia. This complication has been virtually eliminated with the emergence of silicone hydrogel lenses due to their high oxygen transmissibility (Dumbleton et al. 1999, Fonn et al. 2002).

To test the assumption that hypoxic changes were responsible for the increased myopia, studies have compared changes in refractive error with both high- and low-Dk hydrogel lenses (Dumbleton et al. 1999, Fonn et al. 2002). Myopia was not found to increase in a group of patients wearing high-Dk lotrafilcon A extended-wear lenses for 9 months compared with a group wearing low-Dk (etafilcon A) lenses (Dumbleton et al. 1999), whose average myopic increase was –0.30 D over the 9-month period. A subset of the low-Dk lens wearers was transferred to high-Dk lenses and the induced myopia was found to be reversible in the majority of these subjects over 3 months.

Another study (Fonn et al. 2002) compared the ocular effects of high-Dk balafilcon A silicone hydrogel lenses against low-Dk 2-hydroxyethyl methacrylate (HEMA) lenses. Twenty-four subjects, adapted to soft contact lens daily wear, wore the high-Dk lens in one eye and the low-Dk lens in the other eye on an extended-wear basis for 4 months. A significant difference in myopia increase was found in the eyes wearing the low-Dk (–0.50 D) compared to the high-Dk lens (–0.06 D).

Both these studies suggest that the induced myopia with low-Dk lenses resulted from a local corneal hypoxic effect that is essentially eliminated with the use of high-Dk lenses.

Table 30.3 summarizes the results found in the above studies on the effect of soft contact lenses on myopia progression.

Santodomingo-Rubido et al. (2005) reported data from an 18-month longitudinal study of neophyte contact lens wearers, aged between 18 and 25 years, and compared changes in ocular refraction and biometry induced by daily wear and continuous wear of two different silicone hydrogel (SiH) materials. Forty-five subjects were enrolled in the study and randomly assigned to wear one of two SiH materials – lotrafilcon A or balafilcon A – on either a daily or a continuous-wear basis. Measurements of objective refraction, axial length (using partial coherent interferometry), anterior chamber depth, corneal curvature and the rate of peripheral corneal flattening were carried out before and 1, 3, 6, 12 and 18 months after initial fitting. Mean spherical equivalent refractive error increased in the myopic direction in all contact lens groups across time ($p < 0.001$). Axial length was the main biometric contributor to the development of myopia. After 18 months of lens wear, subjects in the lotrafilcon A group showed the greater mean increase in myopia (i.e. –0.50 D). The study could not demonstrate, however, that SiH contact lens wear modified significantly those refractive changes that would usually be expected to occur in young normal adult non-contact lens wearers.

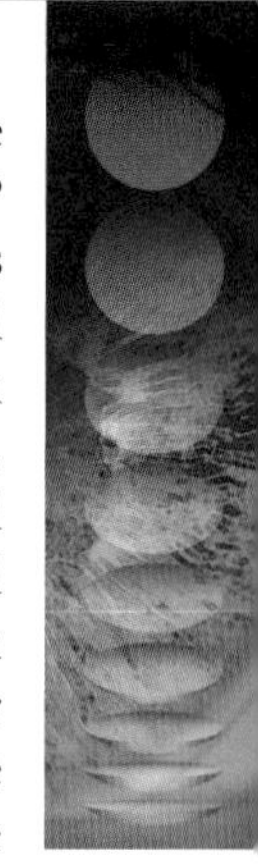

Table 30.3: Summary of the results found in previous studies on the effect of soft contact lenses on myopia progression

Study	No. subjects	Length of study	Myopia progression (spherical equivalent)
Harris et al. (1975)	5	9 months	0.35 D
Grosvenor (1975)	10	12 months	0.25 D
Barnett & Rengstorff (1977)	40	3 months	0.50 D
Rengstorff & Nilsson (1985)	19	5.4 years	<0.37 D*
Andreo (1990)	56	1 year	0.20 D
Horner et al. (1999)	175	3 years	<0.25 D*
Dumbleton et al. (1999)	62	9 months	0.30 D[1] and 0.00 D[2]*
Fonn et al. (2002)	24	4 months	0.50 D[1]and 0.06 D[2]*

*Not statistically significant; [1] lenses of low Dk; [2] lenses of high Dk.

Rigid gas-permeable contact lenses

Contrary to the original hypothesis regarding soft contact lenses and myopia progression, it has been suggested that wearing rigid lenses may actually reduce the progression of myopia in children. However, the results from published clinical trials are equivocal (Stone 1976, Grosvenor et al. 1991, Katz et al. 2003). Most of the evidence arises from studies using hard polymethylmethacrylate (PMMA) contact lenses (Morrison 1956, Kelly et al. 1975, Stone 1976). Morrison fitted over a thousand myopic patients, aged 7–19 years, with PMMA lenses. After 2 years, the myopic progression had ceased in all patients. Two later studies compared PMMA lens wearers with spectacle wearers (Kelly et al. 1975, Stone 1976). Kelly (1975) found that 38% of patients ($n = 57$) wearing PMMA lenses for 4 years ceased myopic progression compared with only 15% ($n = 86$) of spectacle wearers. The mechanical effect on the cornea is the most plausible theory to account for cessation of myopia progression with PMMA lenses. Stone's (1976) study over 5 years on 80 children wearing PMMA lenses showed a myopic increase of –0.10 D per annum compared to –0.35 D per annum in 40 children wearing spectacles. She concluded that the reduction in myopia progression could not be explained solely due to changes in corneal flattening as this effect was shown in both groups: 0.10 D for contact lens wearers and 0.20 D for spectacle lens wearers. Stone was the first to suggest that PMMA lenses may influence the axial growth of the eye; however, no measurements of axial length were taken in the study to confirm this hypothesis.

More recent studies have used rigid gas-permeable (RGP) lenses. The potential mechanisms of action of rigid contact lenses include transient flattening of the cornea and improved quality of the retinal image with reduction in blur for the peripheral image, possibly due to the aspheric design of RGP lenses. In a 3-year study, 100 myopic children aged 8–13 years were fitted with RGP lenses and matched for age and initial refractive error with a control group of 20 single vision spectacle wearers (Grosvenor et al. 1989, 1991, Perrigin et al. 1990). Fifty-six children wore their lenses on a regular basis and remained in the study for a period of 3 years. Myopia increased by –0.16 D per annum in the RGP lens wearers compared with –0.51 D per annum in the control group. Over the 3-year period, the mean increase in myopia was –1 D more in the spectacle wearers. After completing the study, 23 children wore their lenses for a further period of 8 months before discontinuing contact lens wear for 2–3 months, after which they resumed RGP lens wear. During the period that the children were not wearing contact lenses the mean increase in myopia was –0.27 D (equating to a myopic shift per annum of –1.30 D), with a corresponding mean corneal steepening of 0.25 D. One of the limitations of this study is that children were not randomly assigned to the control or treatment group. Approximately half the effect of reducing myopia progression with RGP lenses was due to transient corneal flattening.

The above studies were conducted on Caucasian populations, where the prevalence and rate of myopia progression is significantly lower than in Chinese populations (Zadnik et al. 1993, Fulk et al. 2002, Fan et al. 2004) who may yield different results. Khoo et al. (1999) matched two groups of 45 Singaporean children aged 10 years, one group wearing RGP lenses and the other spectacles. They found a slower rate of myopia progression among contact lens wearers compared with spectacle wearers. The mean increase over a 3-year period was –1.30 D for the contact lens wearers and –2.30 D for the spectacle wearers. The aetiology of myopia development, progression and retardation cannot be fully understood without examination of ocular biometric data such as axial length and corneal power. As previously mentioned, axial elongation and in particular an increased vitreous chamber depth, accounts for the majority of myopia progression in children and young adults (Grosvenor & Scott 1993, Lin et al. 1996). Khoo and colleagues (1999) used ultrasound to measure changes in axial length and found that the mean increase over 3 years was less for the contact lens wearers (0.22 mm) than for the spectacle wearers (0.31 mm).

The study concluded that the difference in myopia progression could not be fully explained by changes in corneal curvature: corneal flattening of 0.15 D in the RGP wearers and 0.07 D in the spectacle lens wearers. However, no alternative mechanism for the retardation of myopia progression was examined. Several factors limited the validity of this study:

- Children were not randomly assigned to the two groups.
- There was a significant difference in baseline myopia between the groups.
- There was a high drop-out rate of 47% among the contact lens wearers over the 3-year period.

Various factors limit the validity of these studies (Saw et al. 2002b):

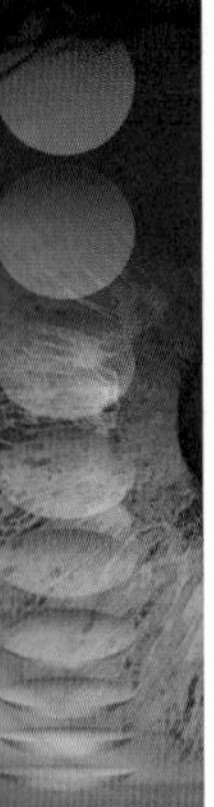

Table 30.4: Summary of the results found in previous studies on the effect of rigid gas-permeable contact lenses on myopia progression

Study	No. subjects	Length of study	Myopia progression (spherical equivalent)	Difference in myopia progression from control group
Grosvenor et al. (1989, 1991)	RGP 56 Sp 20	3 years	RGP –0.16 D Sp –0.51 D	0.35 D
Khoo et al. (1999)	RGP 45 Sp 45	3 years	RGP –1.30 D Sp –2.30 D	1.00 D
Katz et al. (2003)	RGP 105 Sp 192	2 years	RGP –1.34 D Sp –1.28 D	0.06 D*
Walline et al. (2004)	RGP 58 SCL 58	3 years	RGP –1.56 D SCL –2.19 D	0.63 D

*Not statistically significant; RGP, RGP lens group; Sp, spectacle lens group; SCL, soft contact lens group.

- High loss to follow-up.
- Inadequate control group.
- Inadequate or poorly selected entry criteria.
- Incomplete ocular component measurements.

To try to overcome these methodological problems, Katz and co-workers (2003) carried out a large randomized clinical trial to assess the efficacy of RGP lenses in retarding the progression of myopia in Singaporean children. Children of Chinese ethnicity, aged 6–12 years, with myopia between –1.00 and –4.00 D were randomly assigned to RGP or spectacle lens groups. After 2 years, 105 children remained in the RGP group and 192 in the spectacle group. No significant difference was found in myopia progression: –0.67 D per annum in the RGP group, –0.64 D per annum in spectacle group.

Findings to date suggest that it is unlikely that intervention with RGP contact lenses is a realistic method by which myopia progression can be slowed in Chinese children. Currently there is no evidence to suggest whether this finding also applies to Caucasian children.

More recently the US National Institutes of Health has completed the Contact Lens and Myopia Progression (CLAMP) study (Walline et al. 2004). This was a 3-year, single-masked, randomized trial that compared the effects on myopia progression of children wearing RGP lenses with those wearing disposable soft contact lenses. Of the 116 children aged between 8 and 11 years (mean 10.7) who took part in the study, 59 wore RGP lenses fitted on central alignment and 57 children wore 2-weekly disposable soft contact lenses (SCL).

Prior to the start of the CLAMP study children who met the study criteria were fitted with RGP contact lenses and enrolled in a run-in period to determine if they were able to adapt to RGP lens wear (Walline et al. 2001, 2003). Only subjects who successfully completed this run-in period were eligible to enter the study. The spherical component of presenting refraction ranged between –0.75 and –4.00 D and the primary outcome measure was 3-year change in spherical equivalent (SE) cycloplegic autorefraction.

The mean SE progressed to –1.56 ± 0.95 D for RGP wearers and –2.19 ± 0.89 D for SCL wearers, with most of the treatment effect occurring over the first year of the study. Although the difference between the two contact lens groups was significant, it was not attributable to a concomitant slowing of A-scan ultrasound measures of axial length in the RGP group. The difference was in part due to a relative flattening of the steeper corneal meridian over the 3-year period (i.e. RGP 0.62 ± 0.60 mm; SCL 0.88 ± 0.57 mm). Given that the treatment effect failed to accrue over the full treatment period, the lack of an axial length correlate and the likely transitory nature of contact lens-induced corneal flattening, the authors concluded that the data do not warrant the fitting of myopic children with RGP lenses solely for the purposes of significant myopia control.

Table 30.4 summarizes the results found in the above studies on the effect of RGP lenses and myopia progression.

CHANGING FROM SPECTACLES TO CONTACT LENSES

Most myopic children begin wearing spectacles between 9 and 11 years of age (Gilmartin 2004). However, by the age of 16 years, when the rapid phase of myopia progression usually ends (Goss & Winkler 1983), many choose to correct their myopia with soft contact lenses as an alternative to spectacles. What effect, if any, changing from spectacles to soft contact lenses has on myopia progression has been assessed by Fulk et al. (2003). At the end of the treatment phase of a randomized clinical trial to investigate the progression of myopia in children wearing bifocal spectacles compared to single vision spectacles (Fulk et al. 2000), subjects were allowed to select single vision spectacles, bifocal spectacles or soft contact lenses to correct their myopia. One year later their myopia was found to have progressed at an age-adjusted (mean age approximately 14 years) rate of –0.74 D in 19 children who switched to soft contact lenses compared with –0.25 D in 24 children who remained in spectacles (either single vision or bifocal). Although a greater increase in axial length growth was found in the children who opted to wear contact lenses, this increase in axial length only accounted for 41% of the myopia progression. Greater corneal steepening was found in the contact lens wearers and was responsible for 39% of the myopia progression.

Another interesting finding in this study was the significantly greater increase in near point exophoria (4.5 Δ) in the contact lens wearers compared to the spectacle wearers (1.4 Δ). These findings differ from a previous study by Horner et al. (1999), possibly because the children in Fulk's study were slightly older. Additionally, a different response may have occurred as all subjects had initially been selected to have a near point esophoria.

It has been suggested that an accommodative lag at near results in retinal blur, which drives myopia development (Gwiazda et al. 1995). The greater divergent shift in near phoria in the contact lens wearers may have resulted from an accommodative lag, and thus a greater stimulus for myopia development. Further research is required to clarify the effect on myopia progression of changing from spectacles to contact lenses.

Bifocal and multifocal contact lenses

Several recent studies suggest that it may be possible to retard myopia progression in children using bifocal and/or progressive spectacle lenses (Fulk et al. 2000, Edwards et al. 2002, Gwiazda et al. 2003). The rationale is that increased positive power at near reduces accommodative effort, improving accommodative accuracy and thus reducing the stimulus for ocular axial growth.

The trial by Fulk et al. (2000) investigated the effect of single vision versus bifocal spectacle lenses on myopia progression in 84 children with near point esophoria. A modest but significant slowing in myopia progression of 0.25 D was demonstrated over the 30-month test period.

Of three reports assessing the efficacy of progressive addition spectacle lenses (PALs) for myopia control in children (Shih et al. 2001, Edwards et al. 2002, Gwiazda et al. 2003), only the study of Gwiazda et al. (COMET: Correction of Myopia Evaluation Trial) was able to show a statistically significant, albeit small (0.20 ± 0.08 D; $p = 0.004$), slowing of progression. This retardation occurred during the first year of a 3-year trial and stabilized thereafter; however, these results were not clinically significant and do not warrant a change in the correction of myopic children in practice.

These studies suffered from the following limitations.

- No measurements of accommodative accuracy through the bifocal or progressive lenses were taken.
- No assessment was made of which part of the lens the child looks through when reading.

Of interest is the use of bifocal or progressive contact lenses, as they have the advantage that the near addition remains in the line of sight with eye movement and they are less likely to be removed during periods of near work.

Accommodative accuracy was measured objectively in 20 young adults (range of refractive error –5.50 to +3.50 D) while fully corrected with single vision (SV), bifocal (BIF) or progressive contact lenses (PA) (Hunt et al. 2004). The accommodative response to a 3.0 D stimulus was for SV 2.21 D, BIF 1.73 D and PA 1.83 D. The results suggest that the subjects accommodated less with progressive and bifocal contact lenses compared with single vision lenses. However, despite the lack of theoretical need, subjects wearing progressive contact lenses still exerted significant accommodation. The study examined accommodative response but there was no assessment of accommodative lag. Nevertheless, these findings warrant further research into progressive and bifocal contact lenses in children as a possible method to slow myopia progression.

Contact lenses as carriers for drugs to slow myopia progression

Clinical trials are attempting to arrest myopia progression by pharmacological intervention, with the majority of studies using the antimuscarinic drugs – atropine (Chua et al. 2003) or pirenzepine (Tan et al. 2003, Siatkowski et al. 2004). A reduction in myopia progression has been demonstrated with both drugs. Pirenzepine is thought to be a more selective antimuscarinic than atropine (although whether it is fully and solely selective for type 1 muscarinic receptors is equivocal) and, in terms of myopia control, the unwanted effects of mydriasis and cycloplegia are much less. Pirenzepine reduces myopia progression by approximately 50% (Tan et al. 2003, Siatkowski et al. 2004). The drugs are applied topically as a gel, causing some localized hyperaemia and the potential for variability in the amount of gel and the contact time.

Increased bioavailability and therapeutic efficacy of topically applied drugs may therefore be possible via delivery by contact lenses. The potential for soft contact lenses to deliver drugs to the eye was first described in 1965 by Sedlacek (cited in McDermott & Chandler 1989). A recent study has considered colloidal carriers (a nanostructure formulation) for the delivery of pirenzepine from hydrogel contact lenses (Punyamoonwongsa & Tighe 2004).

CONCLUSION

Further development in myopia research is likely to confirm that heredity predominates in the genesis of myopia. However, in terms of retardation of myopia progression, the potential for greater efficacy in clinical trials may result from a combination of therapies – for example, novel contact lenses that incorporate pirenzepine into the matrix of a bifocal or progressive contact lens or a contact lens that corrects for lower- and higher-order ocular aberrations (He et al. 2002).

References

Andreo, L. K. (1990) Long-term effects of hydrophilic contact lenses on myopia. Ann. Ophthalmol., 22, 224–229

Barnes, M., Williams, C., Lumb, R. et al. (2001) The prevalence of refractive errors in a UK birth cohort of children aged 7 years. Invest. Ophthalmol. Vis. Sci., ARVO E-abstract 2096

Barnett, W. A. and Rengstorff, R. H. (1977) Adaption to hydrogel contact lenses: variations in myopia and corneal

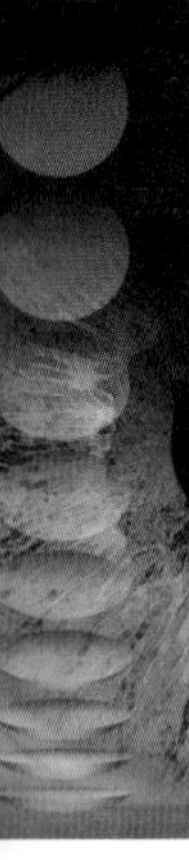

curvature measurements. Am. J. Optom. Assoc., 48, 363–366

Bullimore, M. A., Gilmartin, B. and Royston, J. M. (1992) Steady-state accommodation and ocular biometry in late-onset myopes. Doc. Ophthalmol., 80, 143–155

Bullimore, M. A., Jones, L. A., Moeschberger, M. L. et al. (2002) A retrospective study of myopia progression in adult contact lens wearers. Invest. Ophthalmol. Vis. Sci., 43(7), 2110–2113

Chua, W. H., Balakrishnan, V., Tan, D. et al. (2003) Efficacy results from the atropine in the treatment of myopia (ATOM) study. Invest. Ophthalmol. Vis. Sci., ARVO E-abstract 3119

Cook, R. C. and Glassock, R. E. (1951) Refractive and ocular findings in the newborn. Am. J. Ophthalmol., 34, 1407–1413

Curtin, B. J. (1985) The Myopias: Basic Science and Clinical Management. Philadelphia, PA: Harper and Row

Dandona, R., Dandona, L., Srinivas, M. et al. (2002) Refractive error in children in a rural population in India. Invest. Ophthalmol. Vis. Sci., 43, 615–622

Dumbleton, K. A., Chalmers, R. L., Richter, D. B. et al. (1999) Changes in myopic refractive error with nine months' extended wear of hydrogel lenses with high and low oxygen permeability. Optom. Vis. Sci., 76(12), 845–849

Edwards, M. H. (1998) Myopia: definitions, classifications and economic implications. In Myopia and Nearwork, pp. 1–12, eds. M. Rosenfield and B. Gilmartin. Oxford: Butterworth-Heinemann

Edwards, M. H., Li, R. W. H., Lam, C. S. Y., Lew, J. K. F. and Yu, B. S. Y. (2002) The Hong Kong progressive lens myopia control study: study design and main findings. Invest. Ophthalmol. Vis. Sci., 43(9), 2852–2858

Ellwein, L. B. (2002) Case finding for refractive errors: assessment of refractive error and visual impairment in children. Community Eye Health, 15, 37–38

Fan, D. S. P., Lam, D. S. C., Lam, R. F. et al. (2004) Prevalence, incidence and progression of myopia of school children in Hong Kong. Invest. Ophthalmol. Vis. Sci., 45(4), 1071–1075

Fonn, D., MacDonald, K. E., Richter, D. B. et al. (2002) The ocular response to extended wear of a high Dk silicone hydrogel contact lens. Clin. Exp. Optom., 85(3), 175–182

Fulk, G. W., Cyert, L. A. and Parker, D. E. (2000) A randomised trial of the effect of single vision vs. bifocal lenses on myopia progression in children with esophoria. Optom. Vis. Sci., 77, 395–401

Fulk, G. W., Cyert, L. A. and Parker, D. A. (2002) Seasonal variation in myopia progression and ocular elongation. Optom. Vis. Sci., 79(1), 46–51

Fulk, G. W., Cyert, L. A., Parker, D. E. et al. (2003) The effect of changing from glasses to soft contact lenses on myopia progression in adolescents. Ophthalmic Physiol. Opt., 23, 71–77

Gilmartin, B. (2004) Myopia: precedents for research in the twenty-first century. Clin. Exp. Ophthalmol., 32, 305–324

Goss, D. A. and Winkler, R. L. (1983) Progression of myopia in youth: age of cessation. Am. J. Optom. Physiol. Opt., 60(8), 651–658

Grosvenor, T. (1975) Changes in corneal curvature and subjective refraction of soft contact lens wearers. Am. J. Optom. Physiol. Opt., 52, 405–413

Grosvenor, T. and Scott, R. (1993) Three-year changes in refraction and its components in youth-onset and early adult-onset myopia. Optom. Vis. Sci., 68, 677–683

Grosvenor, T., Perrigin, J., Perrigin, D. et al. (1989) Use of silicone-acrylate contact-lenses for the control of myopia – results after 2 years of lens wear. Optom. Vis. Sci., 66(1), 41–47

Grosvenor, T., Perrigin, D., Perrigin, J. et al. (1991) Rigid gas-permeable contact lenses for myopia control – effects of discontinuation of lens wear. Optom. Vis. Sci., 68(5), 385–389

Gwiazda, J., Bauer, J., Thorn, F. et al. (1995) A dynamic relationship between myopia and blur-driven accommodation in school-aged children. Vis. Res., 35(9), 1299–1304

Gwiazda, J., Hyman, L., Hussein, M. et al. (2003) A randomised clinical trial of progressive addition lenses versus single vision lenses on the progression of myopia in children. Invest. Ophthalmol. Vis. Sci., 44(4), 1492–1500

Hammond, C. J., Snieder, H., Gilbert, C. E. et al. (2001) Genes and environment in refractive error: the Twin Eye Study. Invest. Ophthalmol. Vis. Sci., 42(6), 1232–1236

Harris, M. G., Sarver, M. D. and Polse, K. A. (1975) Corneal curvature and refractive error changes associated with wearing hydrogel contact lenses. Am. J. Optom. Physiol. Opt., 52, 313–319

He, J. C., Sun, P., Held, R. et al. (2002) Wavefront aberrations in eyes of emmetropic and moderately myopic school children and young adults. Vis. Res., 42, 1063–1070

He, M., Zeng, J., Liu, Y. et al. (2004) Refractive error and visual impairment in urban children in southern China. Invest. Ophthalmol. Vis. Sci., 45, 793–799

Horner, D. G., Soni, P. S., Salmon, T. O. et al. (1999) Myopia progression in adolescent wearers of soft contact lenses and spectacles. Optom. Vis. Sci., 76(7), 474–479

Hunt, O., Wolffsohn, J. S., García-Resúa, C. et al. (2004) Do progressive contact lenses negate ocular accommodation in pre-presbyopes – implications for myopia control? Cont. Lens Anterior Eye, 27, 98

Junghans, B. and Crewther, S. G. (2003) Prevalence of myopia among primary school children in eastern Sydney. Clin. Exp. Optom., 86(5), 339–345

Katz, J., Schein, O. D., Levy, B. et al. (2003) A randomized trial of rigid gas permeable contact lenses to reduce progression of children's myopia. Am. J. Ophthalmol., 136(1), 82–90

Kelly, T. S., Chatfield, C. and Tustin, G. (1975) Clinical assessment of the arrest of myopia. Br. J. Ophthalmol., 59, 529–538

Kempen, A. H., Mitchell, P., Lee, K. E. et al. (2004) The prevalence of refractive errors among adults in the United States, Western Europe and Australia. Arch. Ophthalmol., 122(4), 495–505

Khoo, C. Y., Chong, J. and Rajan, U. (1999) A 3-year study on the effect of RGP contact lenses on myopic children. Singapore Med. J., 40, 230–237

Kinge, B., Midelfart, A., Jacobsen, G. et al. (1999) Biometric changes in the eyes of Norwegian university students – a three-year longitudinal study. Acta Ophthalmol. Scand., 77(6), 648–652

Kleinstein, R. N., Jones, L. A., Hullet, S. et al. (2003) Refractive error and ethnicity in children. Arch. Ophthalmol., 121(8), 1141–1147

Lam, C. S. Y. and Goh, W. S. H. (1991) The incidence of refractive errors among school children in Hong Kong and its relationship with the optical components. Clin. Exp. Optom., 74(3), 97–103

Lam, C. S. Y., Goldschmidt, E. and Edwards, M. H. (2002) Prevalence of myopia in local and international schools in Hong Kong. 9th International Conference on Myopia, Hong Kong and Guangzhou

Lin, L. L. K., Shih, Y. F., Lee, Y. C. et al. (1996) Changes in ocular refraction and its components among medical students – a 5-year longitudinal study. Optom. Vis. Sci., 73(7), 495–498

Lin, L. L. K., Shih, Y. F., Hsiao, C. K. et al. (2001) Epidemiologic study of the prevalence and severity of myopia among school children in Taiwan in 2000. J. Formosan Med. Assoc., 100(10), 684–689

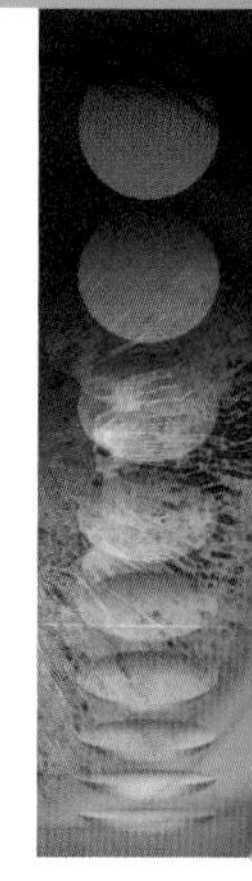

Matsumura, H. and Hirai, H. (1999) Prevalence of myopia and refractive changes in students from 3 to 17 years of age. Surv. Ophthalmol., 44, S109–S115

Maul, E., Barroso, S., Munoz, S. R. et al. (2000) Refractive error study in children: results from La Florida, Chile. Am. J. Ophthalmol., 129, 445–454

McBrien, N. A. and Adams, D. W. (1997) A longitudinal investigation of adult-onset and adult-progression of myopia in an occupational group. Invest. Ophthalmol. Vis. Sci., 38(2), 321–333

McDermott, M. L. and Chandler, J. W. (1989) Therapeutic uses of contact lenses. Surv. Ophthalmol., 33(5), 381–394

Midelfart, A., Kinge, B., Midelfart, S. et al. (2002) Prevalence of refractive errors in young and middle-aged adults in Norway. Acta Ophthalmol. Scand., 80(5), 501–505

Morrison, R. J. (1956) Contact lenses and the progression of myopia. Optom. Weekly, 47, 1487–1488

Murthy, G. V. S., Gupta, S. K., Ellwein, L. B. et al. (2002) Refractive error in children in an urban population in New Delhi. Invest. Ophthalmol. Vis. Sci., 43, 623–631

Naidoo, K. S., Raghunandan, A., Mashige, K. P. et al. (2003) Refractive error and visual impairment in African children in South Africa. Invest. Ophthalmol. Vis. Sci., 44, 3764–3770

Negrel, A. D., Maul, E., Pokharel, G. P. et al. (2000) Refractive Error Study in Children: sampling and measurement methods for a multi-country survey. Am. J. Ophthalmol., 129(4), 421–426

Pacella, R., McLellan, J., Grice, K. et al. (1999) Role of genetic factors in the etiology of juvenile-onset myopia based on a longitudinal study of refractive error. Optom. Vis. Sci., 76(6), 381–386

Parssinen, O. and Lyyra, A. L. (1993) Myopia and myopic progression among school children: a three-year follow-up study. Invest. Ophthalmol. Vis. Sci., 34, 2794–2802

Perrigin, J., Perrigin, D., Quintero, S. et al. (1990) Silicone-acrylate contact lenses for myopia control: 3-year results. Optom. Vis. Sci., 67(10), 764–769

Pointer, J. S. (2000) An optometric population is not the same as the general population. Optom. Pract., 1, 92–96

Pointer, J. S. (2001) A 6-year longitudinal optometric study of the refractive trend in school-aged children. Ophthalmol. Physiol. Opt., 21(5), 361–367

Pokharel, G. P., Negrel, A. D., Munoz, S. R. et al. (2000) Refractive error study in children: results from Mechi Zone, Nepal. Am. J. Ophthalmol., 129, 436–444

Punyamoonwongsa, P. and Tighe, B. (2004) Therapeutic applications of contact lenses: myopia and allergic eye disease. 28th BCLA Conference, Birmingham, UK

Rengstorff, R. H. and Nilsson, K. T. (1985) Long-term effects of extended wear lenses: changes in refraction, corneal curvature, and visual acuity. Am. J. Optom. Physiol. Opt., 62, 66–68

Robinson, B. E. (1999) Factors associated with the prevalence of myopia in 6-year-olds. Optom. Vis. Sci., 76(5), 266–271

Rose, K., Smith, W., Morgan, I. et al. (2003) The increasing prevalence of myopia: implications for Australia. Clin. Exp. Ophthalmol., 29, 116–120

Santodomingo-Rubido, J., Gilmartin, B. and Wolffsohn, J. S. (2005) Refractive and biometric changes with silicone hydrogel contact lenses. Optom. Vis. Sci., 82, 481–489

Saw, S. M. (2003) A synopsis of the prevalence rates and environmental risk factors for myopia. Clin. Exp. Optom., 86, 289–294

Saw, S. M., Carkeet, A., Chia, K. S. et al. (2002a) Component dependent risk factors for ocular parameters in Singapore Chinese children. Ophthalmology, 109, 2065–2071

Saw, S. M., Gazzard, G., Au Eong, K. G. et al. (2002b) Myopia: attempts to arrest progression. Br. J. Ophthalmol., 86(11), 1306–1311

Sedlacek, J. (1965) Possibilities of application of ophthalmic drugs with aid of gel-contact lenses. Cesk. Oftalmol., 21, 509–512

Shih, Y. F., Hsiao, C. K., Chen, C. J. et al. (2001) An intervention trial on efficacy of atropine and multi-focal glasses in controlling myopia progression. Acta Ophthalmol. Scand., 79, 233–236

Shimizu, N., Nomura, H., Ando, F. et al. (2003) Refractive errors and factors associated with myopia in an adult Japanese population. Jpn. J. Ophthalmol., 47(1), 6–12

Siatkowski, R. M., Cotter, S. A., Miller, J. M. et al. (2004) Pirenzepine 2% ophthalmic gel retards myopic progression in 8–12 year old children over 2 years. Invest. Ophthalmol. Vis. Sci., ARVO E-Abstract 2733

Smith, E. L. (1998) Environmentally induced refractive errors in animals. In Myopia and Nearwork, pp. 57–90, eds. M. Rosenfield and B. Gilmartin. Oxford: Butterworth-Heinemann

Sorsby, A. and Leary, G. A. (1970) A longitudinal study of refraction and its components during growth. Medical Research Council Special Report Series 309

Sperduto, R. D., Seigel, D., Roberts, J. et al. (1983) Prevalence of myopia in the United States. Arch. Ophthalmol., 101(3), 405–407

Stone, J. (1976) Possible influence of contact lenses on myopia. Br. J. Physiol. Opt., 31, 89–114

Tan, D. T., Lam, D., Chua, W. H. et al. (2003) Pirenzepine ophthalmic gel (PIR): safety and efficacy for pediatric myopia in a one-year study in Asia. Invest. Ophthalmol. Vis. Sci., ARVO E-Abstract 801

Tano, Y. (2002) Pathological myopia: where are we now? Am. J. Ophthalmol., 134, 645–660

Thorn, F., Held, R. and Gwiazda, J. (2002) The dynamics of myopia progression onset and offset revealed by exponential growth functions fit to individual longitudinal refractive data. Invest. Ophthalmol. Vis. Sci., ARVO E-abstract 2866

Villarreal, M. G., Ohlsson, J., Abrahamson, M. et al. (2000) Myopisation: the refractive tendency in teenagers. Prevalence of myopia among young teenagers in Sweden. Acta Ophthalmol. Scand. 78, 177–181

Walline, J. J., Mutti, D. O., Jones, L. A. et al. (2001) The contact lens and myopia progression (CLAMP) study: design and baseline data. Optom. Vis. Sci., 78(4), 223–233

Walline, J. J., Jones, L. A., Mutti, D. O. et al. (2003) Use of a run-in period to decrease loss to follow-up in the contact lens and myopia progression (CLAMP) study. Control. Clin. Trials, 24, 711–718

Walline, J. J., Jones, L. A., Mutti, D. O. and Zadnik K. (2004) A randomized trial of the effects of rigid contact lenses on myopia progression. Arch. Ophthalmol., 122, 1760–1766

Weale, R. A. (2003) Epidemiology of refractive errors and presbyopia. Surv. Ophthalmol., 48, 515–543

Wildsoet, C. F. (1998) Structural correlates of myopia. In Myopia and Nearwork, pp. 31–56, eds. M. Rosenfield and B. Gilmartin. Oxford: Butterworth-Heinemann

Wong, T. Y., Foster, P. J., Johnson, G. J. et al. (2003) Refractive errors, axial ocular dimensions, and age-related cataracts: the Tanjong Pagar Survey. Invest. Ophthalmol. Vis. Sci., 44(4), 1479–1485

World Health Organization (2002) Elimination of avoidable visual disability due to refractive errors. (WHO/PBL/00.79) Geneva: WHO. Online. Available: www.v2020.org

Zadnik, K., Mutti, D. O., Friedman, N. E. et al. (1993) Initial cross-sectional results from the Orinda longitudinal study of myopia. Optom. Vis. Sci., 70, 750–758

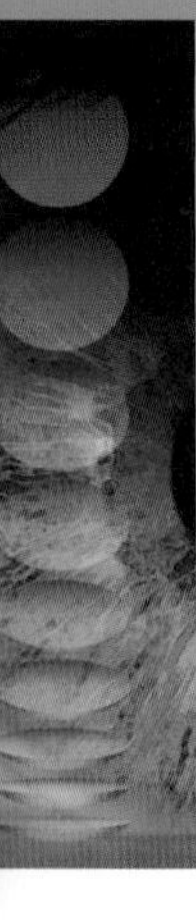

Zadnik, K., Manny, R. E., Yu, J. A. et al. (2003) Ocular component data in schoolchildren as a function of age and gender. Optom. Vis. Sci., 80(3), 226–236

Zadnik, K., Mitchell, G. L., Jones, L. A. et al. (2004) Factors associated with rapid myopia progression in school-aged children. Invest. Ophthalmol. Vis. Sci., 45, E-Abstract 2306

Zhao, J., Pan, X., Sui, R. et al. (2000) Refractive error study in children: results from Shunyi District, China. Am. J. Ophthalmol., 129, 427–435

Chapter 31

Contact lens standards

Tony Hough

CHAPTER CONTENTS

INTRODUCTION

In 1985, it was decided to use European standards to support the implementation of new European directives harmonizing national laws for health and safety; this became known as the 'new approach'. The standards work resulting from the new approach has been colossal. During the years 1985–2000, a work programme of more than 10,000 standards just for the European Committee for Standardization (CEN) was progressively built up, with approximately 2000 standards being mandated to support community legislation.

The sheer volume of work has resulted in the publication process appearing to go slowly because, not surprisingly, the build-up of work has caused considerable delays at the publishers.

The process of harmonization will go on for some time. In 1991, a cooperation agreement was signed between CEN and the International Organization for Standardization (ISO) to facilitate the alignment of European and global standards. At that time, the previously separate groupings of CEN and ISO committees came together, bringing on board the other trading groups, notably the USA, Japan and China and including Australia. The programme of work associated with developing contact lens standards became global rather than being perceived as just European. This harmonization process has been the spur, therefore, in the integration of current practice and protocols from the USA, Europe and Japan. The ultimate goal is 'mutual recognition', where products that are approved for sale in any one market automatically qualify for sale in others. The most important areas for mutual recognition are that lenses which carry the CE marking should be able to be sold freely in the USA and Japan, although restrictions by the Food and Drug Administration in the United States and by the Japanese Government may make this difficult to achieve in the short term.

The outcome of the harmonization process is that, since June 1998, contact lenses are required to carry the CE marking in order to be legally sold in the European Community, thereby achieving the objective of Europe-wide free trade. When one considers the scale of the task, to have achieved this level of free trade can fairly be regarded as good progress. The 'new approach' has now led the area of standardization within the field of contact lenses to a point where international, European and national standards are becoming indistinguishable.

The agreement between ISO and CEN (the 'Vienna Agreement') set out to eliminate unnecessary duplication of effort between ISO and CEN. It was agreed to adopt ISO (international) standards as European Standards (ENs) for contact lenses and to use a system of parallel approvals during the drafting, review and publication processes. The international committee work is carried out under the auspices of the ISO, with the European committees having been integrated to the equivalent ISO grouping.

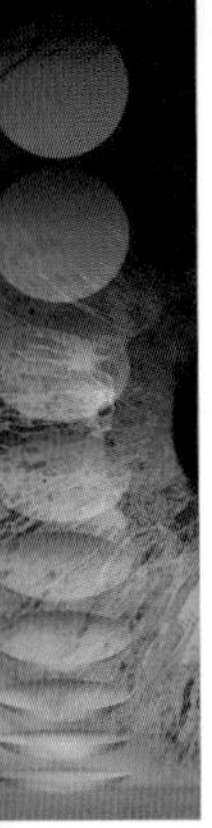

Duties of member countries of the European Union

As far as British or other national standards are concerned, for European Union (EU) member countries it is important to understand the difference between ISOs and ENs. At a national level, ISOs may be modified or qualified but as members of the EU, European Standards must be adopted verbatim. For this reason, the British Standards Institute (BSI), Association Française de Normalisation (AFNOR), Deutsches Institut für Normung (DIN) and other national standardization bodies urge their members and all contributing organizations to pay particular attention to developing European Standards.

WHAT MAKES A GOOD STANDARD?

In the words of the former British Standards Organisation's 'A standard for standards', a standard is:

> A technical specification or other document available to the public drawn up with the cooperation and consensus or general approval of all interests affected by it, *based on the consolidated results of science, technology and experience* [author's italics] aimed at the promotion of optimum community benefits and approved by a body recognized on the national, regional or international level.

At a practical level, there are three categories of standards that are useful as a basis for trade:

- *Terminology* – a collection of definitions that will enable everyone to 'speak the same language'.
- *Product specifications* – a list of the tolerances that are applicable to the dimensions of the products being dealt with.
- *Test methods* – a series of methods that are (preferably) widely available, well understood and which, if used according to carefully drawn protocols, will believably determine the dimensions of the products being dealt with.

There are other categories of standard, which are principally to provide information, but as far as commerce in the field of contact lenses is concerned, the three categories above encompass our specific area of interest.

In order to validate a test method it is subjected to a 'ring test' in which representative commercial samples are measured in a number of centres by independent operators using different instruments. The 'instrument' may, at times, be better described as an 'apparatus' – for example, in the determination of oxygen permeability for contact lens materials. This approach is described as an interlaboratory test conducted under 'conditions of reproducibility'.

ISO 5725, divided into six parts, describes statistical procedures that can be applied to the outcome of such ring tests to provide a statement of the 'believability' or 'credibility' of the method. Examples include how 'believable' a single measurement of the power of a soft lens was if measured on a focimeter in air, or how many measurements would be necessary to be reasonably confident ('reasonably confident' usually means 95% confident) that the result was credible at, say, the 0.25 D level. A ring test establishes these and other parameters of a particular method, and it has been agreed at ISO level that all contact lens test methods included in the standardization process will be assessed by means of an international ring test. Even with this approach, it is not always possible to have standards as well founded as one would like by comparison to the BSO definition.

The field of contact lenses is rapidly changing, with new products, materials and measurement technologies arriving continuously. Judgements are constantly needed between the desirability of only standardizing established technologies, and the pressure of the regulated marketplace where standards are used to help the implementation of directives that are intended to maintain and improve levels of health and safety by promoting fair competition. It is essential to publish standards that will benefit the manufacturing industry and the clinical profession in its widest sense while monitoring the performance of new and developing technologies in order to end up with standards that will stand the test of time.

An interesting example is the measurement of power of soft contact lenses while the lenses are immersed in saline. It is possible to reasonably determine the power of spherical soft lenses in air using the focimeter by blotting the lenses and measuring them carefully. However, if the same method is applied to toric soft lenses, the repeatability and reproducibility are too poor to be reliable. Again, if we wish to determine the power characteristics of either a multifocal or a progressively powered soft lens, the focimeter is not suitable.

It is generally agreed, therefore, that it is desirable to have an automated method for the determination of power-related parameters for soft lenses while they are immersed in saline, especially in the case of toric, multifocal and progressive lenses. In fact, the required measurements are the power-related parameters in air but they must be measured while immersed in saline so as to address the problems of drying and deformation which occur if we try to blot the lens and measure it on the focimeter.

In order to calculate the powers in air, it is then necessary to use intensive mathematical analysis, which is not really viable without a personal computer. Currently, there are two instruments available that measure soft lenses in saline. They are based on alternative methods and both originate in Israel. They have been assessed by international ring test and both produce 'suitable' power-related parameters that can be believably determined by means of relatively few replicate measurements. It is possible to structure a standard using either method but, under ISO rules, it is necessary to identify one of the methods as the 'reference method' in the event of commercial disputes. The rivalry between the suppliers of the competing technologies makes this difficult as is the task of obtaining a consensus at international level, both requiring patient diplomacy and firmness of purpose.

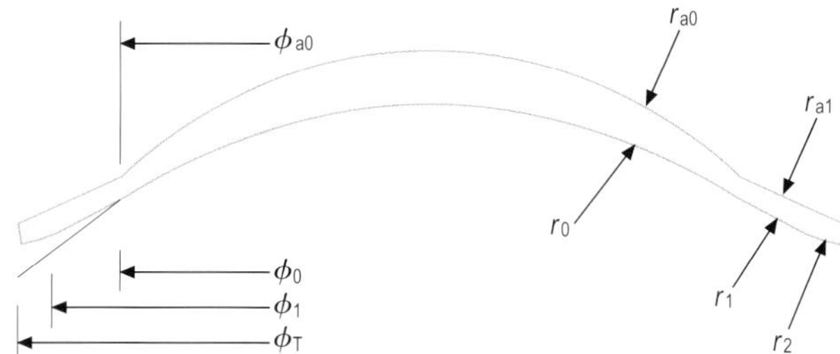

Figure 31.1 The symbols for radii and diameters, applied to a tricurve spherical rigid lens with a bicurve (lenticular) front surface

TERMINOLOGY AND SYMBOLS

The current ISO (also European and British standard) on contact lens terminology is ISO 8320-1:2003 *Contact lenses and contact lens care products. Vocabulary. Contact lenses.* Table 31.1 gives the key terms as defined in this standard while the symbols as applied to a spherical lens are shown in Figure 31.1. This standard is currently being redrafted to include a much wider range of terms on aspheric lenses and significantly enhanced sections on axial lift and thickness.

A completely new terminology standard on care products was published in 2001: ISO 8320-2:2001 *Contact lenses and contact lens care products. Vocabulary. Contact lens care products.* This sets out the terms and definitions that are required in the trade, as well as management of contact lens care products – their active ingredients, antimicrobial and disinfection activity, packaging and labelling requirements.

A note on abbreviations

There is an unfortunate tendency in the academic contact lens world to overuse initialization (abbreviations). This is particularly so in the lectures and publications of Australian, Canadian and US universities. The readability of many documents would be better if they avoided all but the most widely used abbreviations. Even though ISO 8320 was published in 1986, many authors still use Dk/L to denote oxygen transmissibility instead of the correct symbol of Dk/t. Where possible, abbreviations should be avoided and the ISO symbol used instead.

RIGID LENSES

Product specifications 1: rigid lenses

The dimensional and optical tolerances for rigid lenses are set out in ISO 8321-1:1991. The tolerances for rigid gas-permeable (RGP) and polymethylmethacrylate (PMMA) lenses are summarized in Tables 31.2 and 31.3.

Standardization: an imprecise art?

Many of the definitions and tolerances are unsatisfactory from a detailed technical standpoint. This is usually the result of the need to compromise on details in order to arrive at an international consensus. The definition of radial edge thickness is a case in point. In ISO 8320-1 radial edge thickness is defined as 'Thickness of the lens measured normal to the front surface at a specified point near the edge'. Instead of defining the radial edge thickness, this defines an infinite number of possible values and so begs the question. The position is shown in Figure 31.2. As epsilon moves, the value of edge thickness moves. Such a definition is of little use in the case, for example, of writing a computer program to calculate the edge thickness.

Table 31.1: Terms, symbols and abbreviations for contact lens dimensions

Dimension	Symbol[1]	Abbreviation[1]
Back optic zone radius	r_0	BOZR
Back peripheral radius	$r_1, r_2, \ldots$	
Front optic zone radius	r_{a0}	FOZR
Front peripheral radius	$r_{a1}, r_{a2}, \ldots$	
Back optic zone diameter	ϕ_0	BOZD
Back peripheral zone diameters	$\phi_1, \phi_2, \ldots$	
Total diameter	ϕ_T	TD
Front optic zone diameter	ϕ_{a0}	FOZD
Front peripheral diameters	$\phi_{a1}, \phi_{a2}, \ldots$	
Geometric centre thickness	t_c	tc
Carrier junction thickness	t_{a0}	
Radial edge thickness[2]	t_e	t_e
Axial edge thickness[3]	t_{ak}	
Axial edge lift	l_a	AEL
Radial edge lift	l_r	
Front vertex power	F_v	FVP
Back vertex power	F'_v	BVP
Oxygen flux	J	
Oxygen permeability	Dk	Dk
Oxygen transmissibility	Dk/t	Dk/t

[1] The terms and symbols are specified in ISO 8320-1986. The abbreviations are suggested by the author.
[2] Radial edge thickness is measured normal to the front surface at a (specified) point near the edge (see Fig. 31.2).
[3] The symbol for axial edge thickness depends on the number of curves on the front surface. In the case of a lenticular front surface, it is t_{a1} (see Fig. 31.2).

SOFT LENSES

A soft lens is defined as 'a contact lens which requires support to maintain its form'. The term 'soft lens' therefore includes hydrogel, silicone hydrogel and silicone elastomer (silicone

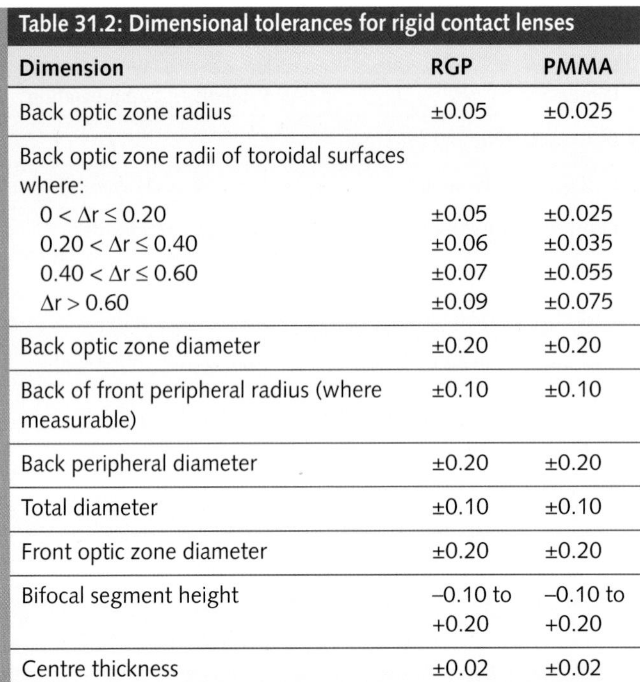

Table 31.2: Dimensional tolerances for rigid contact lenses		
Dimension	**RGP**	**PMMA**
Back optic zone radius	±0.05	±0.025
Back optic zone radii of toroidal surfaces where:		
$0 < \Delta r \leq 0.20$	±0.05	±0.025
$0.20 < \Delta r \leq 0.40$	±0.06	±0.035
$0.40 < \Delta r \leq 0.60$	±0.07	±0.055
$\Delta r > 0.60$	±0.09	±0.075
Back optic zone diameter	±0.20	±0.20
Back of front peripheral radius (where measurable)	±0.10	±0.10
Back peripheral diameter	±0.20	±0.20
Total diameter	±0.10	±0.10
Front optic zone diameter	±0.20	±0.20
Bifocal segment height	–0.10 to +0.20	–0.10 to +0.20
Centre thickness	±0.02	±0.02

Notes: Δr is the difference between the principal meridians. The tolerance applies to each meridian. These tolerances apply to lenses with spherical surfaces and distinct curves; they are for a finished lens and any blending may make measurement difficult.

Table 31.3: Optical tolerances for rigid lenses	
Dimension	**RGP & PMMA**
Back vertex power in the weaker meridian	
$\lvert F'_V \rvert \leq 5$ D	±0.12 D
$5\text{ D} < \lvert F'_V \rvert \leq 10$ D	±0.18 D
$10\text{ D} < \lvert F'_V \rvert \leq 15$ D	±0.25 D
$15\text{ D} < \lvert F'_V \rvert \leq 20$ D	±0.37 D
$\lvert F'_V \rvert > 20$ D	±0.50 D
Prismatic error, measured at the geometrical centre of the optic zone	
$\lvert F'_V \rvert \leq 6$ D	±0.25 cm/m
$\lvert F'_V \rvert > 6$ D	±0.50 cm/m
Prescribed prism	±0.25 cm/m
Cylinder power	
$\lvert F'_C \rvert \leq 2$ D	±0.25 D
$2\text{ D} < \lvert F'_C \rvert \leq 4$ D	±0.37 D
$\lvert F'_C \rvert > 4$ D	±0.50 D
Direction of cylinder axis	±5°

rubber) lenses. In practice, the use of silicone elastomer lenses is currently very small, so this category can be disregarded. While the standard was being developed, silicone hydrogel lenses were not commercially available so all the supporting work in relation to the measurement of lens dimensions was completed using hydrogel lenses, reflecting the marketplace at the time.

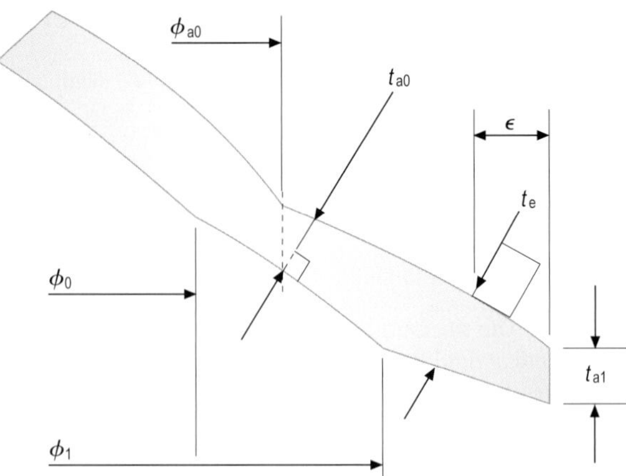

Figure 31.2 Symbols for axial and radial junction and edge thickness. Note that t_e depends on ε

Although silicone hydrogel lenses have been available since 1999 in Europe and Australia, they had not penetrated the market as effectively as the manufacturers had hoped up to the end of 2003. The growth of this material is now increasing dramatically but since the ISO system of material classification requires a minimum water content of 10% for the lens material to be assigned the *filcon* stem, silicone hydrogel is included and the published standards are applicable to this product type. For the purposes of setting out product dimension specifications, the term 'hydrogel lenses' is used to mean both traditional hydrogels and silicone hydrogels.

Product specifications 2: hydrogel (and silicone hydrogel) lenses

The current published standard for dimensional tolerances is limited to single-vision lenses due to the lack of suitable test methods for bifocal/varifocal lenses and the difficulties with validating such methods as were available. The dimensional and optical tolerances for single-vision hydrogel lenses given in Table 31.4 are as set out in ISO 8321-2:2000: *Optics and optical instruments. Contact lenses. Single-vision hydrogel contact lenses.* The material properties for hydrogels are regarded as being sufficiently important to have a dedicated tolerance section. The most important parameters are summarized in Table 31.5.

MATERIAL CLASSIFICATION

The new international standard method for the classification of contact lens materials is EN ISO 11539:1999 *Ophthalmic optics. Contact lenses. Classification and contact lens materials.*

Under this standard, each material is classified by a six-part code:

(prefix)(stem)(series suffix)(group suffix)(Dk range)(surface modification code)

The significance and application of each of these parts is described in Table 31.6.

Table 31.4: Dimensional and optical tolerances for hydrogel lenses (including silicone hydrogels)

Dimension	Tolerance
Back optic zone radius[1,2]	±0.20 mm
Sagitta at specified diameter[1]	±0.05 mm
Total diameter	±0.20 mm
Optic zone diameter	±0.20 mm
Centre thickness, where the nominal value is[3]: a) ≤ 0.10 mm b) > 0.10 mm	 a) ±0.01 mm + 10% b) ±0.015 mm + 5%
Back vertex power $\lvert F'_V \rvert \le 10$ D $10\text{ D} < \lvert F'_V \rvert \le 20$ D $\lvert F'_V \rvert > 20$ D	 ±0.25 D ±0.50 D ±1.00 D
Cylinder power $\lvert F'_C \rvert \le 2$ D $2\text{ D} < \lvert F'_C \rvert \le 4$ D $\lvert F'_C \rvert > 4$ D	 ±0.25 D ±0.37 D ±0.50 D
Direction of cylinder axis	±5°

[1] Use either the radius or sagittal height tolerance depending on how the lens manufacturer specifies the back surface curvature.
[2] This tolerance applies if the interval between successive BOZR in a range is ≥0.40 mm. If the interval is <0.40 mm, the tolerance is one-half the design step.
[3] Examples of centre thickness tolerance:

Nominal t_c	*Tolerance*
0.06 mm	±(0.01 + 0.006) = ±0.016 mm
0.20 mm	±(0.015 + 0.01) = ±0.025 mm

Table 31.5: Material property tolerances for hydrogel lenses

Dimension	Tolerance
Refractive index	±0.005
Water content	±2%
Oxygen permeability	±20%[1]

[1] The percentage tolerance applies to the nominal value of Dk.

Dk range

This part of the code is a numerical designation that categorizes the oxygen permeability in ISO Dk units at intervals considered significant in contact lens wear. For both lenses and materials the oxygen permeability is measured according to ISO 9913-1 or ISO 9913-2 and the Dk range is then denoted by a number as set out in Table 31.7.

Table 31.6: Material classification as set out in ISO 11539

Prefix	This is one of 2 parts of the code administered by USAN. Use of the prefix is optional for all countries other than the USA. For example, Etafilcon A has the USAN code 'Eta'; the use of this code is optional outside of the USA.	
Stem	**filcon** for soft lenses (hydrogel-containing lenses having at least 10% water content by mass) and **focon** for rigid lenses.	
Series suffix	Also administered by USAN, a capital letter added to the stem to indicate the revision level of the chemical formula: A is the original (first) formulation, B the second and so on. Can be omitted if there is only one formulation.	
Group suffix	**Rigid lenses**	**Soft lenses**
I	Does not contain either silicon or fluorine	<50% water content, non-ionic
II	Contains silicon but not fluorine	≥50% water content, non-ionic
III	Contains both silicon and fluorine	<50% water content, ionic
IV	Contains fluorine but not silicon	≥50% water content, ionic
Dk range	A numerical code which identifies the permeability in ranges which are considered significant in contact lens wear. Dk is expressed in ISO units: $(cm^2/s)\cdot[ml\ O_2/(ml \cdot hPa)]$.	
Modification code	A lower case **m** which denotes that the surface of the lens is modified, having different chemical characteristics from the bulk material.	

Table 31.7: Material classification: oxygen permeability (Dk range)

0	< 1 Dk unit
1	1 to 15 Dk units
2	16 to 30 Dk units
3	31 to 60 Dk units
4	61 to 100 Dk units
5	101 to 150 Dk units
6	151 to 200 Dk units
7, ...	add new categories in increments of 50 Dk units

Dk units are: $(cm^2/s) \cdot [ml\ O_2/(ml \cdot hPa)]$.

Example 1: The classification applied to a commercially available rigid lens material (Paragon HDS): Paflufocon B III 3

- *Paflu* – USAN prefix.
- *focon* – Stem indicates that this is a rigid lens material.
- *B* – USAN series suffix; B indicates that this is the second formulation of this polymer.
- *III* – Group suffix; III indicates that the material contains both silicon and fluorine.
- *3* – Dk range is 31–60 ISO units (the Dk in traditional units is 58, in ISO units 43.5).

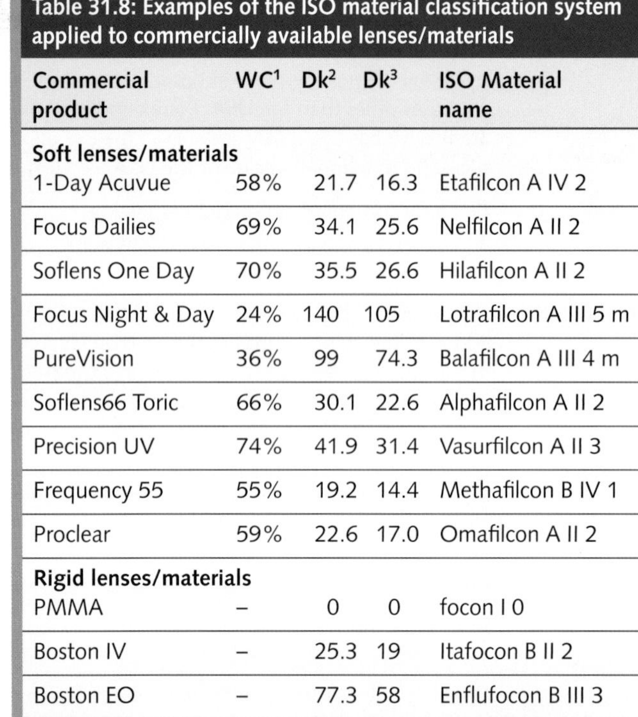

Table 31.8: Examples of the ISO material classification system applied to commercially available lenses/materials

Commercial product	WC[1]	Dk[2]	Dk[3]	ISO Material name
Soft lenses/materials				
1-Day Acuvue	58%	21.7	16.3	Etafilcon A IV 2
Focus Dailies	69%	34.1	25.6	Nelfilcon A II 2
Soflens One Day	70%	35.5	26.6	Hilafilcon A II 2
Focus Night & Day	24%	140	105	Lotrafilcon A III 5 m
PureVision	36%	99	74.3	Balafilcon A III 4 m
Soflens66 Toric	66%	30.1	22.6	Alphafilcon A II 2
Precision UV	74%	41.9	31.4	Vasurfilcon A II 3
Frequency 55	55%	19.2	14.4	Methafilcon B IV 1
Proclear	59%	22.6	17.0	Omafilcon A II 2
Rigid lenses/materials				
PMMA	–	0	0	focon I 0
Boston IV	–	25.3	19	Itafocon B II 2
Boston EO	–	77.3	58	Enflufocon B III 3
Boston XO	–	133	100	Hexafocon A III 4
Boston ES	–	24	18	Enflufocon B III 2
Paragon HDS	–	58	43.5	Paflufocon B III 3
FluoroPerm 30	–	30	22.5	Paflufocon C III 2

[1] Percentage water content.
[2] Dk in traditional units: $(cm^2/s) \cdot [ml\ O_2/ml \cdot mmHg)]$
[3] Dk in ISO units: $(cm^2/s) \cdot [ml\ O_2/(ml \cdot hPa)]$
Note – In the case of hydrogel materials, the permeability in traditional Dk units has been calculated using the Fatt formula $Dk = 2.0e^{0.0411W}$, where W is the percentage water content. In the case of silicone/hydrogel materials, the manufacturer's published value of traditional Dk is used.

Example 2: The classification applied to a commercially available soft lens (Acuvue 2, 58% water content): Etafilcon A IV 2

- *Eta* – USAN prefix.
- *filcon* – Stem indicates that this material contains ≥10% water by mass.
- *A* – USAN series suffix; A indicates that this is the first formulation of the polymer.
- *IV* – Group suffix; IV indicates that the water content is ≥50%, material is ionic.
- *2* – Dk range is 16–30 ISO units (the Dk in traditional units is 21.7, in ISO units 16.3).

Table 31.8 provides a number of examples of the classification system applied to a range of commercially available materials.

Units of oxygen permeability and transmissibility

Oxygen permeability is the oxygen flux under specified conditions through a contact lens material of unit thickness when subjected to unit pressure difference. It is denoted by the symbol Dk. Dk is stated in traditional units of: $(cm^2/s) \cdot [ml\ O_2/(ml \cdot mmHg)]$.

When the international standard unit of pressure, the hectopascal, is used instead of mmHg the units of Dk are: $(cm^2/s) \cdot [ml\ O_2/(ml \cdot hPa)]$.

To convert from traditional units to ISO units, multiply by the constant 0.75006. For example, 30 traditional Dk units is equivalent to 22.5 ISO units. Table 31.9 provides some examples of conversion from traditional to ISO units of Dk.

Table 31.9: Comparison of traditional and ISO units of Dk

Approximate reference material	Traditional units	ISO units
38% WC hydrogels	9.5	7.13
55% WC hydrogels	20	15
70% WC hydrogels	35	26.25
Silicone hydrogels	100	75
Many RGP materials	60	45

WC, water content.

Table 31.10: Examples of converting from traditional to ISO units for oxygen transmissibility (Dk/t)

Dk		*t* in mm	Dk/t	
Trad.	ISO		Trad.	ISO
9.5	7.13	0.06	15.83	11.88
20	15	0.08	25.00	18.75
35	26.25	0.15	23.33	17.50
60	45	0.15	40.00	30.00

Oxygen transmissibility (Dk/t)

Oxygen transmissibility is the oxygen permeability divided by the thickness (t), in centimetres, of the measured sample under specified conditions. It is denoted by the symbol Dk/t. Dk/t is stated in traditional units of: $(cm/s) \cdot [ml\ O_2/(ml \cdot mmHg)]$.

When the international standard unit of pressure, the hectopascal, is used instead of mmHg the units of Dk/t are: $(cm/s) \cdot [ml\ O_2/(ml \cdot hPa)]$

To convert from traditional units to ISO units, multiply by the constant 0.75006. For example, 175 traditional Dk/t units is equivalent to 131 ISO units. Table 31.10 provides some examples of conversion from traditional to ISO units of Dk/t (note that thickness is given in millimetres).

Chapter 32

Legal issues and contact lenses

Michael Mihailidis

CHAPTER CONTENTS

This chapter will endeavour to cover the necessary aspects of the legalities in fitting and prescribing contact lenses. To do this, an explanation of the tort of negligence (malpractice) is required with recent precedent case law. This is the basis of most claims in optometry that are 'negligence-based'.

Examples of the law in its application are given to emphasize certain contact modalities.

It is important for practitioners to understand the process in which litigation ensues and, if they can identify with the basic legal requirements and incorporate them into their mode of practice, this will ultimately diminish claims against them.

Legal issues with respect to contact lenses cover a wide spectrum and practitioners need to be acquainted with them.

Contact lenses are medical devices. The issues that pertain to contact lens practice are related to:

- Understanding the needs of each individual patient.
- Competence in fitting the lenses.
- The determination of the optimal visual correction.

By and large, the issues raised fall under the tort of negligence but other issues may instigate legal and ethical debate, including:

- The contact lens prescription.
- Its interpretation.
- Dispensing by third parties including online, internet sites.

Lastly, medical records are discussed as the starting point for medicolegal negligence litigation.

NEGLIGENCE

Negligence or malpractice is the term used to describe all possible civil liabilities a practitioner can incur as the end result of their professional services. Health professionals such as optometrists may be held liable if their patients suffer harm as a consequence of their health care.

There are two areas of law in which an optometrist can be held accountable: civil and criminal law. For the purposes of this chapter, we will concentrate on civil law, which encompasses tort law.

The area of tort law pertaining to optometric practice is negligence. An explanation of how negligence is determined is necessary in order to understand precedent case law. To make a

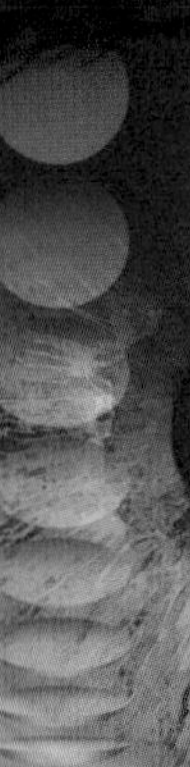

successful claim of negligence, a plaintiff (the patient) must be able to prove that:

- The defendant (the optometrist) owed the plaintiff a duty of care that the defendant breached by failing to exercise the necessary level of care.
- The plaintiff suffered damage that was inadequately met as a result of the defendant's breach.

'Duty' is defined as 'an obligation, recognized by law, to avoid conduct fraught with unreasonable risk of danger to others'.

On the issue of whether the optometrist (defendant) owed the patient (plaintiff) a duty of care, the plaintiff will need to establish forseeability of harm and the proximity between plaintiff and defendant. There is thus a duty to ensure that one's acts do not cause foreseeable harm to another.

The forseeability element will be established if the patient is a member of a class to whom damage was foreseeable. The forseeability element is only part of establishing the existence of a duty of care. It is also necessary to show that the relationship between the parties had the necessary degree of proximity. A patient has a proximal relationship with an optometrist because a patient would quite clearly be someone who would be injured by a failure on the part of the optometrist to take reasonable care.

STANDARD OF CARE

What is it and why is it applicable to everyday optometry? There has been a flurry of recent precedent law in favour of letting each patient remain an individual and to be treated as such. Prior cases emphasized the concept of paternalistic medicine whereby it was assumed that 'the doctor knew best'. The shift to treating the patient as an autonomous being allows them to make necessary decisions provided they have at their disposal all material facts.

The standard of care required by an optometrist is one of reasonableness. In determining a breach of duty, did the optometrist act with the level of care that one would expect of a 'reasonable person'? In the case of Bolam v Friern Hospital Management Committee (1957), the court considered the standard of care for doctors. Under the Bolam test, a medical practitioner or optometrist:

> ...would not be negligent if he or she has acted in accordance with a practice accepted as proper by a responsible body of medical men skilled in that particular art...a man is not negligent if he is acting in accordance with such a practice, merely because there is a body of opinion who would take a contrary view.

This test had the effect of embodying the 'reasonable man test' for the 'reasonable doctor' or 'reasonable optometrist'. It was an objective test. This principle was approved by the UK House of Lords in respect of diagnosis, treatment and information disclosure. The Bolam test was applied in the case of Sidaway v Board of Governors of Bethlem Royal Hospital (1985) in its consideration of the provision of information. This case involved a plaintiff suffering damage as a result of a spinal operation. The plaintiff alleged failure of the surgeon to fully disclose the risks associated with the operation. The trial judge rejected the plaintiff's claim on the basis that it had been established that a responsible body of neurosurgeons, at that time, had agreed that their colleague's standard of disclosure was acceptable.

Under the Bolam test, the professional practices and opinion against which an optometrist would be judged must be a 'responsible body', much like a 'peer review committee', but this need not be a substantial body of practitioners fitting contact lenses. For example, a small group of keratoconic fitting optometrists may be considered 'super-specialists' in fitting special/difficult gas-permeable lenses; hence, for the purpose of the Bolam test, the defendant's actions would be judged against the opinion of this group of practitioners rather than the whole group of practitioners who fit contact lenses generally.

However, the Bolam test has been criticized in subsequent cases in the United Kingdom, the United States and Australia.

In the Sidaway case above, Lord Scarman rejected the Bolam principle in respect of the provision of information stating that:

> ...English law must recognize a duty of the doctor to warn his patients of the risk inherent in the treatment in which he is participating...The critical limitation is that the duty is confined to material risk. The test of materiality is whether in the circumstances of the particular case, the court is satisfied that a reasonable person in the patient's position would be likely to attach significance to the risk.

Likewise, the Canterbury v Spence (1972) case involved a 19-year-old suffering damage as a result of a laminectomy. The judge in that case considered the scope of the disclosure required of the physician. The definition of 'scope' was in terms of the patient's rights to self-determination and therefore propounded the concept that *the degree of information depended on the needs of the particular patient and the particular procedure*. He said:

> A risk is thus material when a reasonable person, in what the physician knows or should know to be the patient's position, would be likely to attach significance to the risk or cluster of risks in deciding whether or not to forgo the proposed therapy.

Similarly, in Reibl v Hughes (1980), in which a patient suffered a stroke following a left carotid endarterectomy and where medical evidence estimated the incidence of the complication as 10%, the judge stated:

> To allow medical evidence to determine what risks are material and, hence should be disclosed and, correlatively, what risks are not material, is to hand over to the medical profession the entire question of the scope of the duty of disclosure, including the question whether there has been a breach of that duty...What is under consideration here is the patient's right to know what risks are involved in undergoing or forgoing certain surgery or other treatment.

In Australia, the rejection of Bolam came as a result of Rogers v Whitaker (1992) where the High Court considered the case of

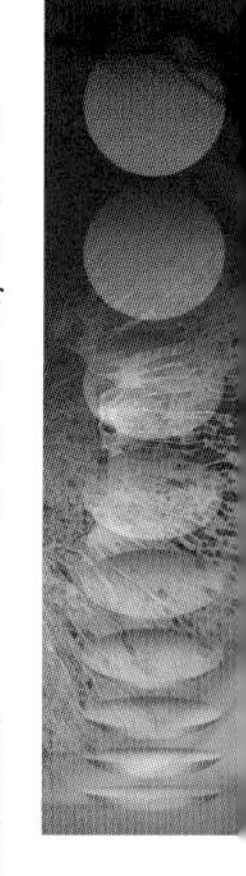

Maree Whitaker who had been blind in her right eye since childhood. She had been referred to Dr Rogers, an ophthalmic surgeon, who recommended an operation on her damaged eye to prevent the possible development of glaucoma. The surgery was claimed to be likely to improve the vision in her damaged eye and also to improve its cosmetic appearance. Postoperatively, she developed sympathetic ophthalmia – a rare condition with an incidence of about 1 in 17,000. The result was a loss of sight in her left eye and almost complete blindness. The plaintiff sued for negligence, alleging that Dr Rogers had failed to warn her of the possibility of sympathetic ophthalmia and the risk of loss of sight. She claimed that, had she been warned of this possibility, she would never have consented to the surgery. The High Court approached the task of the content of duty and its scope in these matters of 'failure to warn'. In defining the factors involved in a doctor's duty to warn, the High Court repeated:

> A doctor has a duty to warn a patient of a material risk inherent in the proposed treatment. A risk is material if, in the circumstances of the particular case, a reasonable person in the patient's position, if warned of the risk, would likely attach significance to it or if the medical practitioner is or should reasonably be aware that the particular patient, if warned of the risk, would be likely to attach significance to it.

The evolution from Bolam to Rogers was gradual and the courts came to hold the professions more accountable for adverse events arising out of their activities.

In Rogers, the High Court – in discussing 'material' risk – held that the subjective text was the model most appropriate when it stated: 'a particular patient, if warned of the risk would find it of significance'.

Medical ethicists have since endorsed this patient-orientated approach. They see the consent process as a change from a single event of paternalistic beneficence to an integrated process of information sharing and informed decision taking.

This standard is now *a consent, based on an autonomous patient making an informed decision based on understanding.*

Although the practitioner may in depth and comprehensively impart information, there is no guarantee that the patient will understand all they have been told. Patients may also be presented with hard copy data in the form of information sheets but the problem is that they may be too exhaustive and become incomprehensible. However, it is suggested that the provision of detailed brochures, as well as specific and detailed consent forms, is the minimum required in informing a group of patients for, say, an orthokeratology procedure. Patients may have unrealistic expectations of the result they would like to achieve and may be resistant to modifications or perceived compromises pre-discussed with the optometrist. On the other hand, the optometrist may be unreasonably optimistic in the portrayal of the outcomes. Many patients seeking to wear contact lenses are unrealistic in their appreciation of the visual outcome.

Likewise, a full appreciation of worst case scenarios should almost always be depicted to the patient as visual loss is the common denominator and generally why we look after these patients in preventative practice.

Since Rogers v Whitaker, cases of medical negligence have come to include allegations of 'failure to warn', almost always as a part of a claim. The application of this negligence metamorphosis is not confined to contact lens practice but to all aspects of patient care. In this change in determining standard of care, we can see how Rogers v Whitaker (at least in Australia but similarly in most other countries) can influence all duty of care situations.

FAILURE TO ADVISE ON THE CORRECT OR ALTERNATIVE MODALITIES

Current legal thinking emphasizes the critical role of patient autonomy in health care decision-making. This emphasis extends as far as creating an obligation for the optometrist to advise a patient about complementary and alternative visual corrections such as contact lenses.

The law imposes on the optometrist a duty to exercise reasonable care and skill, not only in examination, diagnosis and treatment but also in the provision of professional information and advice, being a 'single comprehensive duty'.

It is the patient who must make the decision but it is the optometrist who holds the information on which the decision must be made.

In Haughian v Paine (1987), it was ruled that 'one cannot make an informed decision to undertake a risk without knowing the alternatives to undergoing the risk'.

The area pertinent to the optometrist is the use of contact lenses as therapeutic devices rather than for simple cosmesis.

Consider the supply of spectacles to a moderate or severe keratoconic patient. In this case the practitioner may be considered negligent if they have not provided the optimal visual correction (contact lenses). The same would apply to an aphake or corneal graft recipient. Nevertheless this should be qualified by careful explanation about the trial of contact lenses, their effect, associated risks, complications of fitting, costs, time involved, etc. (which must all be given) and conveyed in such a way that the patient has all the facts at their disposal. Should they opt not to undergo any form of contact lens fitting then that is their decision, but the practitioner has at least satisfied the minimum legal requirements under Rogers v Whitaker.

It is incumbent on the optometrist to do what is necessary for their patient's ocular well-being. The practitioner has a duty to investigate what needs to be prescribed. They may also need to refer to someone more competent if their skill in a particular area is limited.

Keratoconus is a classic example where special expertise and advice is required. Practitioners should not assume that contact lens correction is automatically essential. If the visual acuities are, for example, 6/12 or better, the patient may be quite happy in a spectacle correction, and exposing them to the potential complications of contact lenses could leave the practitioner at risk. Similarly, they may be unable to attend for regular after-care when potential ocular damage could result and, where again, contact lenses should not be advised. How much information and trialling of the lenses should be conducted so

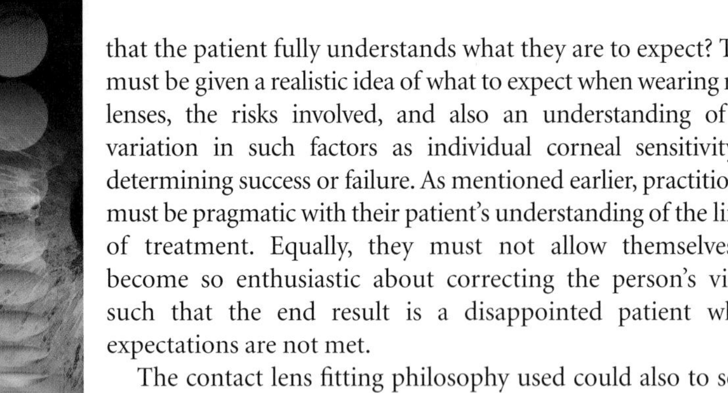

that the patient fully understands what they are to expect? They must be given a realistic idea of what to expect when wearing rigid lenses, the risks involved, and also an understanding of the variation in such factors as individual corneal sensitivity in determining success or failure. As mentioned earlier, practitioners must be pragmatic with their patient's understanding of the limits of treatment. Equally, they must not allow themselves to become so enthusiastic about correcting the person's vision such that the end result is a disappointed patient whose expectations are not met.

The contact lens fitting philosophy used could also to some extent determine possible future corneal scarring. Does the optometrist fit with apical clearance or apical touch, for example? What is important here is that whichever technique is used the practitioner must adhere to and become clinically competent at fitting the chosen philosophy. Under the Bolam principle the practitioner would not be required to explain the type of fitting design or the possibility of scarring as this would be considered clinically acceptable by an expert group of 'sub-specialists'. If we apply Rogers v Whitaker, the optometrist must explain possible and probable visual outcomes as well as the possibility of corneal scarring. Scarring would be considered a material risk in undergoing a keratoconic fitting, especially if, as mentioned earlier, the patient corrects to 6/12 with spectacles.

These examples are for therapeutic purposes; what of the situation where a contact lens wearer wears them for cosmetic reasons only? Does the optometrist have a duty to at least advise them of alternative lenses such as daily wear silicone hydrogels (as compared to conventional hydrogels), or does the practitioner say nothing? This situation would be harder to contest by a plaintiff patient as the long-term implications have not been quantified significantly to measure possible future harm or damage to the patient.

EXTENDED-WEAR LENSES

The development of silicone hydrogel lenses creates great opportunities for a whole new range of patients such as children and the elderly. The opportunity of wearing lenses for 30 days continuously may appeal to the patient as well as the practitioner in managing certain conditions or diseases without the need for lens insertion or removal, thereby reducing the risk of infection from lens handling. However, it increases the opportunities for negligence claims.

Follow-up and recall instructions for these patients is imperative, must be well documented and explained in detail to satisfy the requirements enunciated in Rogers v Whitaker, i.e. the patient must *at their level* understand what is involved in wearing lenses continuously, even if it is for a trial period. In this regard, proper record keeping is essential when managing those patients who may:

- Fail to keep appointments.
- Abuse their lenses.
- Disregard instructions such as not to wear lenses when swimming, etc.

Although these lenses are approved for 30-day continuous wear, what are the risks of microbial keratitis? Do we know enough about a particular microbe and its effect on the eye with these lenses? Similarly, what of the effects of contact lens peripheral ulcers? These, although relatively uncommon, are generally associated with continuous wear. Some patients are more predisposed than others. Could these factors be deemed 'material' for a patient who may be contemplating a corrective surgical procedure in the near future in terms of warning them of the relative risks involved? Again, the test of Rogers v Whittaker comes into place and the optometrist must always be conscious of the patient's long-term visual goals.

As another example, the practitioner may have a duty to inform the patient of newly available lens materials. If, for instance, the patient has been wearing a standard 2-weekly lens unremarkably in the past, but the optometrist notices minor corneal neovascularization, do they inform the patient and let them make a decision to change, say to a silicone hydrogel lens, or does the optometrist continue the status quo? A lot will depend on the particular patient and, as mentioned above, their opportunities to possibly undergo future corrective surgical procedures may be undermined if appropriate advice and action are not taken.

MONOVISION

This technique for correcting presbyopia has its limits. The patient must be made aware of reduced stereopsis and loss of contrast sensitivity, and that driving may be difficult, especially at night. Patients fitted this way must be informed of the risks they face, even in performing daily tasks – in particular, operating heavy or dangerous machinery or participating in sports. Patients must be advised to adapt to their lenses *first* before attempting any work, sport or driving.

If the practitioner feels that monovision poses a significant risk to the patient, then an alternative means of correction must be offered – for example, lenses that fully correct distance vision with associated over-spectacles for near work.

FITTING LENSES AND TRANSMISSIBLE DISEASES

In an era where it is understood that diseases may be transmitted by fluids, practitioners should be cautious for themselves, their patients and the actions of their patients.

Diseases such as new variant Creutzfeldt–Jakob disease (vCJD), human immunodeficiency virus (HIV), and others that can readily be transmitted by fluid, should always be a consideration in the fitting of contact lenses (see also Chapter 8). The safest is the usage of lenses that can be disposed of after a single trial.

A patient who attends for disposable soft lens fitting is the least at risk since the sterile trial lens is disposed of after the fit and vision have been checked. For those requiring conventional soft lenses, an experienced practitioner can still use an appropriate disposable diagnostic lens and then allow for the

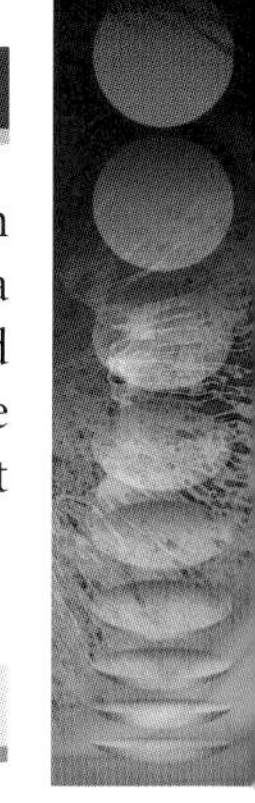

subtle differences in thickness and back optic zone radius (BOZR) when ordering the first patient lens.

In the UK, rigid lenses should be disposed of after a single patient use where possible. Complex rigid lenses that cannot easily be disposed of after a single use must be cleaned thoroughly and then soaked in a solution of 2% sodium hypochlorite for 1 hour at room temperature (www.college-optometrists.org/professional/cjd.pdf). There is no specific advice on cleaning soft trial lenses for reuse; single use is recommended wherever possible.

The first lens can be ordered empirically (see Chapter 9 and the CD-ROM) with an exchange warranty and the final lens parameters adjusted subsequently.

Lenses that pose the greatest risk are cosmetic lenses. Plano coloured lenses can be bought at unregistered outlets in many countries and may fit poorly. Friends often exchange them to try different 'looks'. Hence, when there is no regulation on their supply, it is difficult to control their use and the potential risk of serious infection.

THE CONTACT LENS PRESCRIPTION

What is it and what obligations are imposed on the practitioner for releasing such information?

In the UK, it is a legal requirement to provide the patient with their contact lens prescription once the practitioner judges the lenses to be satisfactory. In the United States, it is mandatory that a contact lens prescription be released immediately after the examination is completed.

To release a contact lens prescription, the practitioner must first determine the lens parameters for the patient, the suitability of wear schedules and the frequency of replacement.

The prescription must allow the patient to obtain lenses elsewhere (see below) but it should not be viewed as one-way traffic for so-called consumer rights. However, the practitioner must protect themselves from liability arising from incorrect dispensing and product liability.

A contact lens prescription should therefore contain the information necessary for the patient to have the prescription properly dispensed, including the following:

- Name of the lens manufacturer.
- Type of lens and mode of wear.
- Power.
- BOZR.
- Date the prescription was dispensed and its expiry date.
- Date of patient's last examination.
- Replacement frequency if applicable.
- Optometrist's signature and name (and registration number in the UK).

However, only the practitioner can determine when a contact lens examination is actually completed. Only then can the patient be handed a copy of their lens prescription.

Until the information from the trial fitting is determined with confidence, with an adaptation period completed while wearing the prescribed lens and the safety of lens wear ensured, there is no obligation to provide the patient with a contact lens prescription.

SAFEGUARDING THE PRACTITIONER

As mentioned earlier, a contact lens prescription should contain information such as the lens manufacturer. Therein lies a problem for online organizations that dispense their own brand or a substitute brand. Practitioners must therefore include in the patient release form (see below) that brand substitution is not appropriate and that this voids the contact lens prescription.

Expiry date

The practitioner must state the expiry date of the prescription, especially if it is for an extended-wear patient. If a patient is habitually wearing a silicone hydrogel lens for 30 continuous days and they purchase a 3-month supply, the optometrist is obliged to review them before the next supply. Hence continuous wear has given the practitioner greater leverage in prescription expiry dates. The expiry date should be limited to the minimum quantity of supply. For example, PureVision is supplied in 3-month units and hence should be given a 3-month expiry date if the practitioner feels that the patient requires it.

Expiry dates are therefore an effective way for the practitioner to safeguard themselves from non-compliant patients.

Wearing modality

The mode of wear must be stated; for example, 'for daily wear only'. This can be even if the type of lens is an extended-wear silicone hydrogel that has been determined as appropriate for daily wear only for a particular patient.

Similarly, although a manufacturer indicates that their lens is suitable for 30-day continuous wear, a particular patient may only be suitable for, say, not greater than 7 days of extended wear. This must be stated unambiguously on the release form that accompanies the contact lens prescription.

The contact lens release form

This should almost always accompany a contact lens prescription and may form an addendum to the prescription form.

The release form should contain information to the effect that if the contact lens prescription is not dispensed according to the specifications, the contact lens prescription is void.

The form should contain an obligation on the part of the third party supplier to assume liability for any complications that may arise (assuming the patient has had an uneventful adaptive trial period with the lenses).

RECORD KEEPING

Any starting point for medicolegal negligence litigation is the patient's record cards or other information.

Practitioners must, for their own protection, maintain a full history of the patient's contact lenses and trials. This is imperative to facilitate adequate management of the patient. Records should

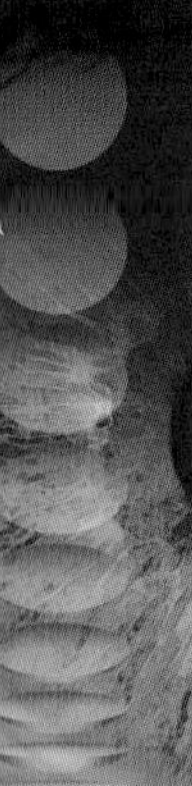

be legible and comprehensive, such that if another optometrist were to attend to the patient, they could easily follow the continuum of care, and practitioners should be aware of the legal implications if the records are incomplete.

What constitutes a record card?

A record card is a subjective and objective collection of information, signs and symptoms pieced together by a listening and observant practitioner about the patient who has, in their own words, indicated the reason for the consultation.

A full record of the patient's history, signs and symptoms should be completed at the time, as recollection at a later date would be nearly impossible. The subjective response(s) of the patient must therefore be documented, i.e. why they are being seen and what symptoms they report.

The history should include the main complaint, their ocular history and any past medical history, as well as any family ocular and general health history.

The examination should include all tests performed with clear and unambiguous results. What is important here is that when grading parts of the eye in question there must be an effort to be consistent with various clinical gradings that can be understood by other colleagues. Scales are usually numeric instead of the practitioner's subjective description. The two main scales commonly used are the IER grading scale (see Appendix B) or the Efron grading scale for contact lens complications.

Most records can be obtained under legal preliminary discovery, pre-trial discovery or under subpoena at hearing or shortly before. Hence the records (unless lost or destroyed) will come to the attention of the prospective plaintiff or the actual plaintiff.

Information must be meaningful, sufficient to allow evaluation and determination of key issues such as:

- Who examined the patient and why?
- What tests were performed and why?
- What information was given to the patient about the procedures?
- Did the patient give their consent, informed or passively, to any procedures?

Record keeping and litigation

Cases involving allegations of negligence against health care practitioners use the existence and quality of records as a key issue in the fact-finding process.

A patient-plaintiff is likely to remember more about the relevant details than the practitioner, as the practitioner sees many similar patients during the course of their day. Hence, unless detailed notes are made, it is likely that the practitioner's memories of a particular conversation will fade much more quickly than the patient's.

In order for an optometrist to prove or establish what may have happened a few years earlier they need to prove a general practice routine with respect to certain consultations; for example, a slit-lamp and topographical examination with resultant trial lens assessment for all new contact lens patients.

Records that the optometrist completes must be contemporaneous with the consultation. The following are examples of successful and unsuccessful 'compiled' record notes.

Successfully compiled notes

In Vale v Ho (1997) a patient alleged that his doctor failed to provide the kind of warnings mandated under the terms of Rogers v Whitaker (1992) of the risks involved in undergoing surgery. The defendant doctor was able to base his evidence on exclusive and detailed notes which he swore had been compiled contemporaneously. These notes contradicted much of the patient's evidence in relation to when and if warnings had been given, including what was said by the doctor to the patient. The judge found for the doctor as he based it on contemporaneity of the doctor's notes and the fact that they had been compiled before any allegations of impropriety had been made by the patient.

Ineffective notes

In Locher v Turner (1995) the plaintiff asserted that the doctor had failed unreasonably to investigate adequately the condition of the plaintiff's colon for some 12 months after his initial report of symptoms indicated significant problems with the colon.

The doctor's notes were in short-form style and were somewhat cryptic. In addition, the doctor purported to give evidence in court of her memories of her interaction with the patient, which were additional to what was found in her notes. The Court of Appeal stated that it could not decide the appeal on the basis of the doctor's verbal evidence which purported to fill in the gaps in her written notes.

In Hribar v Wells (1995), where the plaintiff sued her dentist, it was alleged that the dentist failed under the requirements articulated by the High Court in Rogers v Whitaker to properly warn her about the risks of an operation. The trial judge preferred the evidence of the plaintiff to that of the dentist who had few notes and relied upon his 'invariable practice' of providing verbal information to the patient prior to surgery.

The maintenance of contemporaneously produced, electronically secure, thorough, discreetly compiled records of practitioner–patient interactions is necessary to protect against litigation. It gives the practitioner a clear, convincing and highly probative account of what was done and said in respect of conversations and optometric interventions that may have been unremarkable at the time and may have occurred many years previously. Without such record keeping, litigation can ensue and be contested successfully, regardless of the practitioner's work and communication with the patient.

Long-term record keeping

Records need to be kept for several years after a patient has been discharged in case of future litigation. For any person over

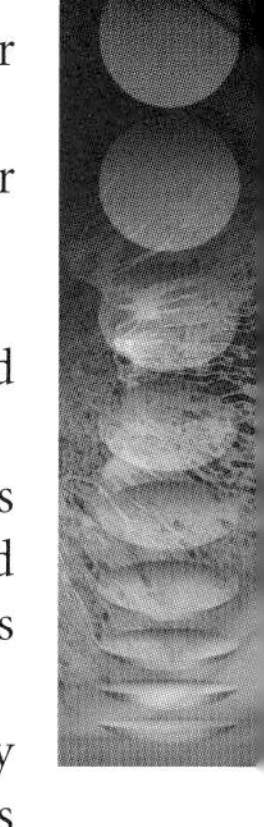

14 years old, records must be kept for 7 years; for children under 14 years, they should be kept for 30 years.

SUMMARY

It is well accepted that a practitioner *who is perceived by the patient* as competent and caring, and where there is a good interpersonal relationship between the practitioner and patient, is less likely to be sued. Nevertheless, prudent action by the optometrist during their time with the patient can significantly reduce the likelihood of future legal action.

- Ensure that your knowledge is current, comprehensive and adequate to deal with the specific patient.
- Offer all relevant modalities, even those that may fall outside your own scope of practice.
- Give detailed explanations of the pros and cons of each modality and the relative risks involved.
- Provide leaflets/brochures to back up verbal information and note that these have been issued.
- Refer the patient to another practitioner if it is in their interest.
- Note the patient's consent and understanding of your recommendations.
- Keep full and adequate records of all advice, tests and trials.
- Note the patient's understanding of the advice given and their acceptance or otherwise of your recommendations.
- Be prepared to issue a prescription for the final contact lens once you are satisfied that the lenses are of optimal fit and power and are safe for the patient. Give all the details relevant to the prescription as mentioned earlier.
- Issue a release form with the prescription to ensure that any third party dispensing the lenses does this exactly as prescribed and that they accept liability for the accuracy and safety of any lenses supplied.

Disclaimer

It should be stressed that advice given in this chapter is of a general nature only and may vary from country to country. Practitioners should always seek advice from their own professional body.

Legal cases referred to in this chapter

Bolam v Friern Hospital Management Committee (1957) 1 WLR 582 (English case)

Canterbury v Spence (1972) 464 F 2d 772 (US case)

Haughian v Paine (1987) 37 DLR (4th) 624 at 644 (Canadian case)

Hribar v Wells, Unreported, Supreme Court, Full Court, SA 8 June 1995 (Australian case)

Locher v Turner (1995) QCA 106 (Supreme Court of Queensland – Court of Appeals)

Reibl v Hughes (1980) 1 14 D.L.R. (3d) 1 (Canadian Supreme Court)

Rogers v Whittaker (1992) 67 ALJR 47 (Australian High Court)

Sidaway v Board of Governors of Bethlem Royal Hospital (1985) AC 871 at 887 per Lord Scarman (English case)

Vale v Ho (1997) CA 40331/95 (Supreme Court of New South Wales)

Chapter 33

Setting up a research project

Graeme Young

CHAPTER CONTENTS

There are several advantages to undertaking research in everyday practice rather than the academic setting.

- The full-time practitioner's depth of experience may be more attuned to clinical trends that deserve further investigation.
- Patients in a normal contact lens practice may be more representative of the real world and better motivated towards participating in a given study.
- Well-kept practice files can provide ready data for retrospective studies.

The equipment available to the practitioner may be less sophisticated than that at the disposal of the professional researcher. However, much research does not require more equipment than is available in a well-equipped practice. If additional equipment is needed, funding may be available from a variety of sources: professional organizations, companies or employers. Alternatively, arrangements might be made for equipment to be rented, borrowed or donated. Most companies, for instance, are willing to provide product samples for well-designed research projects, although potential sponsors do expect to see evidence of a carefully planned project.

In most countries, the clinical testing of unapproved, non-marketed contact lens products is subject to government regulation and, therefore, this type of research tends to be supervised by the manufacturer. These studies are often undertaken in a group of practices although the initiation, planning and analysis are usually outside the control of the individual practitioner. Nevertheless, participation in this type of research is more challenging than one might expect and most companies are receptive to approaches from competent, reliable investigators (Young et al. 1998). For those with a desire to supervise their own research project, the challenges are even greater but potentially more rewarding.

SELECTING A RESEARCH TOPIC

Finding the solution to a problem is relatively simple compared with finding the right question. Since resources are limited, it is important to find the topic best suited to one's capabilities and, most importantly, addresses a worthwhile problem. One recommendation is to consider the value of a given research question using the mnemonic FINER and judge it based on

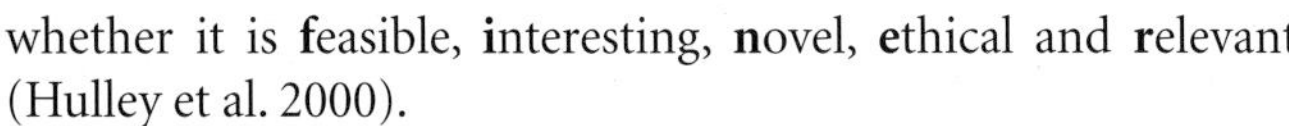

whether it is **f**easible, **i**nteresting, **n**ovel, **e**thical and **r**elevant (Hulley et al. 2000).

What areas are most suited to research by the clinician? In general, those questions that relate closely to everyday practice are more easily approached than basic scientific questions with no obvious clinical relevance. These can arise from the practitioner's own experience and are often prompted by questions and problems arising in the course of normal clinical practice.

- Does product A, for example, give better results than product B?
- Is a given category of patient more likely to exhibit a certain characteristic? The category might relate to age, sex or ametropia while the characteristic might be a sign, symptom, type of disorder or response to a given treatment.
- Does a certain new technique have advantages over a more conventional method?
- What are the success rates and limitations of a given product?

DEFINING THE OBJECTIVES

It is pointless to simply look at a problem. A clear statement of the reasons for undertaking the study and what the study hopes to achieve will direct the work at every stage. It will help in designing the experiment and deciding how the results should be analysed. The conclusions of the study should answer the questions posed by the objectives.

Defining the aims helps assess the feasibility and usefulness of a study. The objectives should not be too broad or too varied. For example, where the purpose is 'to determine whether contact lens A is better than contact lens B', it is unrealistic to attempt a broad assessment and therefore objectives need to be refined in order to consider selected aspects of lens performance. Where there is more than one objective, a potential conflict may become apparent. It may not be feasible, for example, to consider contact lens deposit resistance independently from physiological effects, as the two could be related.

With some studies it is appropriate to restate the research question as a hypothesis. In other words, phrasing the question as a simple but specific statement summarizing the theory under test; for example, 'Contact lens A provides better high-contrast visual acuity (VA) than contact lens B'. For the purposes of statistical testing, the hypothesis is often restated as a null hypothesis; for example, 'High-contrast VA is no better with contact lens A than with contact lens B'. By assuming no difference between data sets, the statistical test estimates the probability of the result happening by chance. If the statistics fail to confirm the null hypothesis, then the alternative hypothesis is accepted, in this case, that there is a difference in VA between the two lens types. Remember that scientific theories are not provable, only falsifiable.

RESEARCHING THE LITERATURE

By not properly understanding the background to a problem, there is a risk of any research being wasted through poor methodology or inappropriate study design. A survey of previous work helps to confirm that the proposed study is worthwhile as well as revealing gaps in current knowledge. If the subject has already been researched, a review of the literature may suggest alternative ways of approaching the subject or point to additional areas of research. It is usually helpful in developing the experimental method and selecting the techniques to use. If the subject turns out to have been researched already, this does not necessarily invalidate any further work, as there may have been deficiencies in the previous work. A study replicating the original results serves to add weight to the original findings but, of course, there is the possibility that the new study may produce entirely different results.

An internet literature search is an obvious good starting point. Medical databases such as PubMed (www.ncbi.nlm.nih.gov) allow online searches based on keywords, authors, etc. but tend to cover only refereed journals. The Bausch & Lomb/CCLR Reference Sight Database is useful as it covers the unrefereed contact lens literature (www.referencesight.com). The website provides abstracts of the articles, which can be downloaded, and these may provide enough information. However, it is usually necessary to see the full paper in order to have a good understanding of current knowledge and to derive the full benefit of previous work. Most journal publishers offer a download service, although a more economical method of obtaining papers is to order these from an institutional, university or national library – or better still, to arrange a visit.

DESIGNING THE STUDY

Having decided on the objectives of the study and reviewed how other people have tackled similar projects, the researcher will have a rough plan of how the study should proceed. At an early stage in the project, draft a summary of the key aspects:

- Objectives.
- Study design.
- Study products.
- Number of subjects.
- Entry criteria.
- Key variables, etc.

From this, a more detailed protocol can be prepared.

A wide range of ingenious study designs can be used in clinical research. However, most studies follow one of three fundamental designs (Table 33.1):

- *A case-control study* examines a given problem by comparing those who exhibit the problem with those who do not. This type of study helps to determine the risk factors associated with that problem. For instance, the habits and characteristics that predispose some patients to certain problems.
- *A cross-sectional study* involves measuring a wide range of variables at a given time and is particularly useful for measuring prevalence. The prevalence of a given problem is the proportion of patients who exhibit the problem at a given time as opposed to the incidence, which is the

Table 33.1: Advantages and disadvantages of main clinical study designs

Study design	Usage	Advantages	Disadvantages
Case-control	Comparing outcomes Risk factors	Small sample size Inexpensive Short duration	Potential sampling bias Potential survivor bias Limited to one outcome variable
Cross-sectional	Descriptive information Prevalence Correlates	Relatively short duration Control over selection of subjects Can study several outcomes	Potential measurement bias Potential survivor bias Does not yield incidence or risk
Cohort	Comparing treatments Incidence Risk factors Sequence of events	Avoids selection bias Avoids survival bias Can study several outcomes	Large sample sizes Long duration Expensive if prospective

Adapted from Hulley & Cummings (1988).

proportion who will exhibit the problem over a period of time.

- *A cohort study*, the largest and most complex type, involves assigning a given treatment (e.g. contact lens type) to a group of patients and then monitoring the outcomes over a period of time. This type of study may or may not include a control group and may be undertaken prospectively or retrospectively.

Taking 3 and 9 o'clock staining as an example, a retrospective cross-sectional study might be used to estimate the prevalence of the problem. This could be an evaluation of the records of all rigid lens-wearing patients seen for after-care over a given 6-month period. Causative factors could be determined using a case-control design comparing a group of patients showing 3 and 9 o'clock staining with a control group who show no corneal staining. If previous work has suggested a method for avoiding 3 and 9 o'clock staining, a cohort study might be undertaken to test the hypothesis that this results in a lower incidence of staining than existing methods.

A further categorization of clinical studies is whether they are:

- *Observational or non-interventional* – a study which does not modify the treatment that patients would normally receive.
- *Interventional or experimental* – a study that modifies some part of the treatment. These studies usually involve a control against which the treatment under test can be compared.

In some ways, the use of controls is easier in contact lens research than other areas of medical research:

- *Cross-over designs*, where test and control products are used in succession, are less likely to result in carry-over effects than with pharmaceutical trials.
- *Contralateral designs*, where different products are used simultaneously in opposite eyes, may be the most efficient method of comparing two contact lens designs or care products. However, there is some evidence of a sympathetic contralateral physiological response (Fonn et al. 1999) and a contralateral design may not be appropriate with some studies comparing physiology.

The number of subjects included in the study requires careful consideration. The main risk from using an inadequate sample size is failing to detect a significant difference where one exists; this is known as a Type II error (false-negative). Formulae exist for estimating the sample size required to demonstrate a statistically significant difference (Pocock 1983). These require:

- A determination of a clinically significant size difference.
- An estimation of the variance of the final results.

Because contact lens studies often examine a large range of variables and estimates of the outcomes are unavailable, sample sizes are frequently based on judgement rather than sample size calculations.

DEVELOPING THE STUDY PROTOCOL

The main function of the protocol is to ensure that the study is carried out in a consistent manner; for example:

- A measurement as basic as VA can be calculated in different ways, producing a variety of results.
- The responses from questionnaires can be influenced by the way the question is framed.
- Parameters that rely on a graded system of measurement can be open to varying interpretation.

The protocol, therefore, must clearly define the method and scale by which the parameter is evaluated. For example, if deposition on soft lenses is to be monitored, how is this first to be assessed: what method, what magnification – and how will degrees of spoilation be distinguished: number of spots, surface area or weight?

Where possible, it is preferable to use existing methodologies that have been described in the literature and validated by previous work. As well as being tried and tested, this allows the results to be more easily compared with previous findings. In evaluating contact lens-induced dry eye, for example, it would make sense to use an established definition for dry eye (Lemp 1995) and existing techniques for its assessment. Much work has already been done to determine the most effective

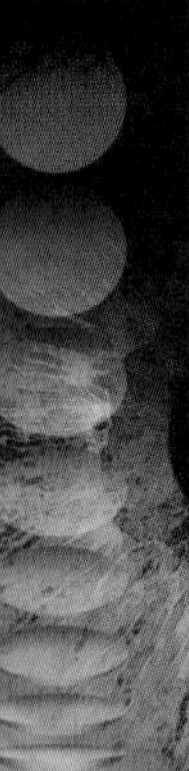

questionnaires (Nichols et al. 2002) and a number of grading scales exist for recording corneal and conjunctival staining (see Appendix B) (Bron et al. 2003).

A major difficulty with all clinical trials is the large number of possible variables influencing the final result. It is therefore necessary to be specific about the type of patient to be enrolled into the study; for example, age, astigmatism and previous lens wear history. The protocol should clearly define the entry criteria for the study. This is equally as necessary for retrospective studies as prospective studies.

The protocol should attempt to cater for all reasonable contingencies to ensure that problems can be dealt with in a way consistent with the aims of the study. How should lost or damaged lenses be considered? How should missed visits or other missing data be handled? In any long-term clinical study a proportion of patients will drop out for apparently non-clinical reasons; again, how should these be considered?

A pilot study may be relevant for clinical trials of long duration or large size:

- To help finalize the study design.
- To allow the researcher to check practical aspects of the protocol (e.g. the design of the record form).
- The results might help with sample size estimations.

UNDERTAKING THE STUDY

Once the study is underway, it is essential to adhere rigidly to the protocol. If shortcomings in the original protocol or the treatment or technique become apparent, it may be necessary to rewrite a section of the protocol. If so, this should be done with caution and with regard for the data already collected. With careful redesign it may be possible to avoid having to regather measurements.

The key concern during the clinical phase of the study is to collect quality data; in other words, data that are accurate, consistent and complete. Where the study involves more than one investigator, training is required to ensure consistency. For a simple study this might involve a meeting to compare notes and to ensure that the grading and measurements are being taken in a similar way. In a more complex study, it might be appropriate to train, test and certify investigators prior to their participation and to produce written instructions for some measurements to avoid confusion.

Missing data are inevitable with any sizeable study; however, if this is excessive, it weakens the data analysis. Investigators should be trained to check that record forms are completed at the end of each examination. Particularly at the start of a study, it can be helpful if the forms are checked by an assistant.

ETHICAL CONSIDERATIONS

The starting point for the ethical consideration of research involving human subjects is the Declaration of Helsinki (World Medical Association 2004). Most research likely to be carried out in contact lens practice is of a harmless nature. There are difficult ethical considerations, however, in combining research with professional care. The prime rule is that the interests of the patient should prevail over the interests of the research. Where treatment deviates from normal practice or where the patient's confidentiality is compromised, informed consent should be obtained. This includes advising the patient of the nature and procedures of the study, explaining the risks and benefits, and ensuring that they understand their rights as participants (ICH* 1997).

Non-interventional research that simply monitors normal practice routine does not require research ethics committee review provided the patients' right to confidentiality is not compromised. However, where the research involves deviating from normal treatment, it is usually appropriate to have the protocol reviewed by a research ethics committee (REC), the purpose of which is to ensure that the interests of the study subjects are protected. Although undertaking the same task, a variety of RECs exist, including many universities, hospitals and organizations that have their own committees. In addition, a number of commercial RECs exist primarily to serve the needs of industry.

- In North America, these are known as institutional review boards, which work in accordance with Food and Drug Administration (FDA) regulations.
- In the UK, all clinical trials undertaken within the National Health Service have to be submitted to an NHS REC (Central Office for Research Ethics Committees; www.corec.org.uk). The British Contact Lens Association is one example of an organization that has its own REC.
- In Australia it is a requirement that all research involving human participants is reviewed and approved by a Human Research Ethics Committee (HREC – www.nhmrc.gov.au/ethics/human). The Australian Clinical Trials Registry (ACTR – www.actr.org.au) was only set up in 2005; at present, registration of 'clinical trials' is voluntary but all those that do register must have HREC approval. Usually, HRECs operate within universities and hospitals.

ANALYSING THE RESULTS

Although there is a bewildering range of statistical tests, only a few are commonly used in contact lens research. However, it is important to appreciate when such tests may or may not be applied. Previously published work may provide a useful guide, although caution should be exercised as some tests have been inappropriately applied in the optometric literature. Care should also be taken in deciding whether to count eyes or subjects (Reading 1984, Glyn & Rosner 1992). It may be appropriate to average the results between eyes or to evaluate only one eye per subject.

The selection of the appropriate statistical test is governed by the type of data that have been collected (Table 33.2). Variables can be categorized in three ways:

* International Conference on Harmonisation of Technical Requirements for Registration of Pharmaceuticals for Human Use.

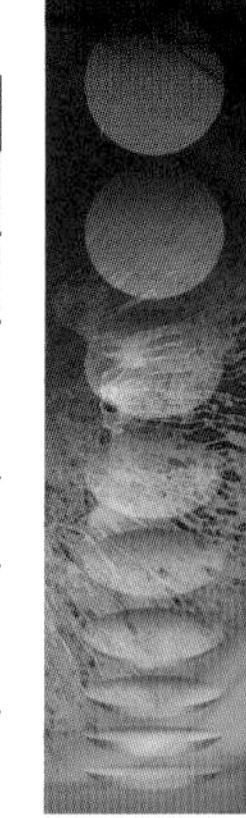

Table 33.2: Summary of commonly used statistical tests

Context	Type of data: Nominal	Ordinal	Interval (continuous)*
Two independent samples	N <20: Fisher's exact test N ≥20: Chi-square test	Mann–Whitney U test	Student's t-test
Paired sample	McNemar test	Wilcoxon signed rank test	Paired t-test
Three or more independent samples	Chi-square test	Kruskal–Wallis one-way ANOVA	One-way ANOVA
Three or more related samples	–	Friedman two-way ANOVA	Two-way (repeated measures) ANOVA
Correlation measurement	–	Spearman rank correlation coefficient	Pearson correlation coefficient

* In order to be suitable for parametric tests, the data should be normally distributed, measured using a scalar quantity and non-truncated.
ANOVA, analysis of variance.

- *Nominal* – the simplest type of variable places the sample into two or more categories (e.g. eye colour).
- *Ordinal* – the next level of data further classifies the variable by rank (e.g. according to slit-lamp grade).
- *Interval* – this is the most powerful type of measurement and uses a continuous scale. Assuming the data are normally distributed, these are evaluated using parametric statistical tests (see Further reading).

Although conventional spreadsheet software is capable of producing summary statistics (averages, variances, confidence intervals), current versions are able to undertake only a few statistical tests. A number of good user-friendly statistical packages are available (SPSS, Minitab, Systat); however, as noted earlier, it is important to have a working knowledge of when various statistical tests may be applied before using them.

DRAWING CONCLUSIONS

One of the functions of a clinical study is to attempt to draw conclusions from a necessarily limited clinical experience and relate this to the wider clinical situation. An obvious risk, therefore, is that the result may not truly represent the real situation. Again, using the example of a comparative contact lens trial, lens A may have performed significantly better than lens B under clinical trial conditions when perhaps only a single method of disinfection was used. However, lens A may later prove to perform worse when used in conjunction with all other disinfection systems. Experimental conclusions, therefore, should be applied to the broader situation with caution and, when presenting conclusions, reference should be made to any limitations that may apply.

Statistical significance, therefore, does not immediately imply clinical significance. Calculating the probability of results happening by chance determines whether differences in results are statistically significant. Commonly, a result is considered statistically significant if the probability of the result happening by chance is less than 1 in 20 ($p < 0.05$). However, this is an arbitrary cut-off point and is not appropriate in every situation. If a large number of tests are undertaken, at this level of significance, one experiment in 20 is likely to produce a false result. This is referred to as a Type I error (false-positive) and is avoided either by minimizing the number of tests performed or by using a lower cut-off point (i.e. lower p-value).

PUBLICATION

Having pushed back the barriers of contact lens research, it is only fair to publish one's findings to a wider audience. The preparation already done in researching the literature and writing the protocol will contribute a large amount to the final report, whether this is a poster, paper or presentation. The background literature and the study protocol usually need little modification to form the method section. The results section is a simple statement of the findings. The discussion section, however, requires more consideration but essentially covers four main areas:

- Clinical relevance of the findings.
- Comparison with previous work.
- Limitations or caveats.
- Possible further work.

The conclusions succinctly summarize the relevance of the findings and answer the questions posed by the study. The temptation to overstate the conclusions should be resisted.

CONCLUDING REMARKS

This introduction to clinical research is not meant to be a complete guide to the subject. Any practitioner embarking on a research project will wish to supplement their knowledge by referring to textbooks on the subject of research and statistics (see Further reading). In addition, mentoring advice

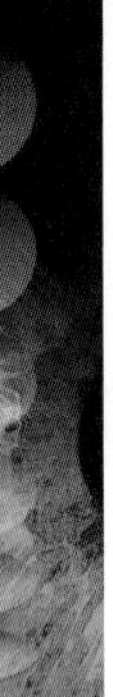

from a more experienced colleague can prove invaluable. However, the greatest insights do not always come from those with the most experience and the field is therefore open to newcomers with aptitude and enthusiasm.

References

Bausch & Lomb/Centre for Contact Lens Research Reference Sight Database. http://www.referencesight.com

Bron, A. J., Evans, V. E. and Smith, J. A. (2003) Grading of corneal and conjunctival staining in the context of the other dry eye tests. Cornea, 22, 640–650

COREC. http://www.corec.org.uk

Fonn, D., du Toit, R., Simpson, T. L., Vega, J. A., Situ, P. and Chalmers, R. L. (1999) Sympathetic swelling response of the control eye to soft lenses in the other eye. Invest. Ophthalmol. Vis. Sci., 40, 3116–3121

Glyn, R. J. and Rosner, B. (1992) Accounting for the correlation between fellow eyes in regression analysis. Arch. Ophthalmol., 110, 381–387

Lemp, M. A. (1995) Report of the National Eye Institute/Industry Workshop on the clinical trials in dry eyes. CLAO J., 21, 221–232

Nichols, J. J., Nichols, K. K., Puent, B., Saracino, M. and Mitchell, G. L. (2002) Evaluation of tear film interference patterns and measures of tear film break-up time. Optom. Vis. Sci., 70, 363–369

NIH PubMed. http://www.ncbi.nlm.nih.gov

Reading, V. M. (1984) Significance of the t-test applied to ocular measures. Am. J. Optom. Physiol., 61(2), 94–99

Wild, J. M. and Hussey, M. W. (1985) Some statistical concepts in the analysis of vision and visual acuity. Ophthalmic Physiol. Opt., 5(1), 63–71

World Medical Association (2004) Declaration of Helsinki. Online. Available: www.wma.net/e/policy/b3.htm

Young, G., Coleman, S. and Allsopp, G. (1998) How to be a good clinical research investigator. Optician, 215(5649), 36–37

Further reading

Altman, D. G. (1990) Practical Statistics for Medical Research. London: Chapman and Hall

Coggan, D. (1997) Statistics in Clinical Practice. London: BMJ Publishing Group

Hall, G. M. (ed). (1998) How to Write a Paper, 2nd edn. London: BMJ Books

Hulley, S., Cummings, S. R., Browner, W. S., Grady, D., Hearst, N. and Newman, T. B. (2000) Designing Clinical Research: An Epidemiologic Approach. Baltimore: Lippincott Williams and Wilkins

ICH (1997) ICH harmonised tripartite guideline for good clinical practice. Federal Register 62, 25691–25709. Online. Available: www.ich.org

Lang, T. A. and Secic, M. (1997) How to report statistics in medicine: annotated guidelines for authors, editors and reviewers. Philadelphia, PA: American College of Physicians

Pocock, S. J. (1983) Clinical Trials: A Practical Approach. Chichester: Wiley

Appendix A

Spectacle and ocular refraction, or effective power of spectacle lenses in air at various vertex distances

Body of table shows effective power at stated vertex distance (see Formulae *I* and *II*, on the attached CD-ROM)

Spectacle refraction or spectacle lens power (BVP)	Ocular refraction (D) for vertex distances (mm) of:														
(D)	6	7	8	9	10	11	12	13	14	15	16	17	18	19	20
–00.00	00.00–	00.00–	00.00–	00.00–	00.00–	00.00–	00.00–	00.00–	00.00–	00.00–	00.00–	00.00–	00.00–	00.00–	00.00–
+0.25	0.25	0.25	0.25	0.25	0.25	0.25	0.25	0.25	0.25	0.25	0.25	0.25	0.25	0.25	0.25
.50	0.50	0.50	0.50	0.50	0.50	0.50	0.50	0.50	0.50	0.50	0.50	0.50	0.50	0.50	0.51
.75	0.75	0.75	0.75	0.76	0.76	0.76	0.76	0.76	0.76	0.76	0.76	0.76	0.76	0.76	0.76
+1.00	1.01	1.01	1.01	1.01	1.01	1.01	1.01	1.01	1.01	1.02	1.02	1.02	1.01	1.02	1.02
.25	1.26	1.26	1.26	1.26	1.27	1.27	1.27	1.27	1.27	1.27	1.28	1.28	1.28	1.28	1.28
.50	1.51	1.52	1.52	1.52	1.52	1.52	1.53	1.53	1.53	1.53	1.54	1.54	1.54	1.54	1.55
.75	1.77	1.77	1.78	1.78	1.78	1.79	1.79	1.79	1.80	1.80	1.80	1.81	1.81	1.81	1.81
+2.00	2.02	2.03	2.03	2.04	2.04	2.04	2.05	2.05	2.06	2.06	2.07	2.07	2.07	2.08	2.08
.25	2.28	2.29	2.29	2.30	2.30	2.31	2.31	2.32	2.33	2.33	2.34	2.34	2.35	2.35	2.36
.50	2.54	2.54	2.55	2.56	2.56	2.57	2.58	2.58	2.59	2.60	2.60	2.61	2.62	2.62	2.63
.75	2.79	2.80	2.81	2.82	2.82	2.83	2.84	2.85	2.86	2.87	2.87	2.88	2.89	2.90	2.91
+3.00	3.06	3.06	3.07	3.08	3.09	3.10	3.11	3.12	3.13	3.14	3.15	3.16	3.17	3.18	3.19
.25	3.31	3.33	3.34	3.35	3.36	3.37	3.38	3.39	3.40	3.42	3.43	3.44	3.45	3.46	3.48
.50	3.58	3.59	3.60	3.61	3.63	3.64	3.65	3.67	3.68	3.69	3.71	3.72	3.74	3.75	3.76
.75	3.84	3.85	3.87	3.88	3.90	3.91	3.93	3.94	3.96	3.97	3.99	4.00	4.02	4.04	4.05
+4.00	4.10	4.12	4.13	4.15	4.17	4.18	4.20	4.22	4.24	4.26	4.27	4.29	4.31	4.33	4.35
.25	4.36	4.38	4.40	4.42	4.44	4.46	4.48	4.50	4.52	4.54	4.56	4.58	4.60	4.62	4.64
.50	4.63	4.65	4.67	4.69	4.71	4.73	4.76	4.78	4.80	4.83	4.85	4.87	4.90	4.92	4.95
.75	4.89	4.91	4.94	4.96	4.99	5.01	5.04	5.06	5.09	5.12	5.14	5.17	5.19	5.22	5.25
+5.00	5.15	5.18	5.21	5.24	5.26	5.29	5.32	5.35	5.38	5.41	5.43	5.46	5.49	5.52	5.56
.25	5.42	5.45	5.48	5.51	5.54	5.57	5.60	5.63	5.67	5.70	5.73	5.76	5.80	5.83	5.87

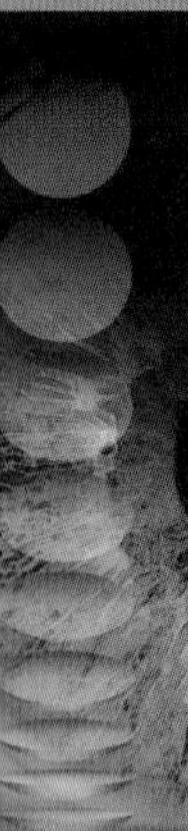

Appendix A (*cont'd*)

Spectacle refraction or spectacle lens power (BVP)	**Ocular refraction (D) for vertex distances (mm) of:**														
(D)	**6**	**7**	**8**	**9**	**10**	**11**	**12**	**13**	**14**	**15**	**16**	**17**	**18**	**19**	**20**
.50	5.69	5.72	5.75	5.79	5.82	5.85	5.89	5.92	5.96	6.00	6.03	6.07	6.11	6.14	6.18
.75	5.96	5.99	6.03	6.06	6.10	6.14	6.18	6.22	6.25	6.29	6.33	6.37	6.41	6.46	6.50
+6.00	6.22	6.26	6.30	6.34	6.38	6.42	6.46	6.51	6.55	6.59	6.64	6.68	6.72	6.77	6.82
.25	6.49	6.54	6.58	6.62	6.67	6.71	6.76	6.80	6.85	6.90	6.94	6.99	7.04	7.09	7.14
.50	6.77	6.81	6.86	6.91	6.95	7.00	7.05	7.10	7.15	7.20	7.26	7.31	7.36	7.42	7.47
.75	7.04	7.09	7.14	7.19	7.24	7.29	7.35	7.40	7.46	7.51	7.57	7.63	7.69	7.75	7.82
+7.00	7.30	7.36	7.41	7.47	7.52	7.58	7.64	7.70	7.76	7.82	7.88	7.94	8.01	8.07	8.14
.25	7.58	7.64	7.70	7.76	7.82	7.88	7.94	8.01	8.07	8.14	8.20	8.27	8.34	8.41	8.48
.50	7.86	7.92	7.98	8.05	8.11	8.18	8.24	8.31	8.38	8.45	8.53	8.60	8.67	8.75	8.83
.75	8.13	8.20	8.26	8.33	8.40	8.47	8.55	8.62	8.70	8.77	8.85	8.93	9.01	9.09	9.17
+8.00	8.40	8.47	8.55	8.62	8.70	8.77	8.85	8.93	9.01	9.09	9.17	9.26	9.35	9.43	9.52
.25	8.68	8.76	8.83	8.91	8.99	9.07	9.16	9.24	9.33	9.42	9.51	9.60	9.69	9.78	9.88
.50	8.96	9.04	9.12	9.21	9.29	9.38	9.47	9.56	9.65	9.75	9.84	9.94	10.04	10.14	10.25
.75	9.23	9.32	9.41	9.50	9.59	9.68	9.78	9.87	9.97	10.07	10.17	10.28	10.38	10.49	10.60
+9.00	9.51	9.61	9.70	9.79	9.89	9.98	10.09	10.19	10.30	10.41	10.52	10.63	10.74	10.86	10.98
.25	9.79	9.89	9.99	10.09	10.19	10.30	10.41	10.52	10.63	10.74	10.86	10.98	11.10	11.22	11.35
.50	10.07	10.17	10.28	10.38	10.49	10.60	10.72	10.83	10.95	11.07	11.20	11.33	11.45	11.59	11.72
.75	10.35	10.46	10.57	10.68	10.80	10.92	11.04	11.16	11.29	11.42	11.55	11.68	11.82	11.96	12.11
+10.00	10.64	10.75	10.87	10.99	11.11	11.24	11.36	11.49	11.63	11.76	11.90	12.05	12.20	12.35	12.50
.25	10.92	11.04	11.17	11.29	11.42	11.55	11.69	11.83	11.97	12.11	12.26	12.41	12.57	12.73	12.89
.50	11.21	11.33	11.46	11.60	11.73	11.87	12.01	12.16	12.31	12.46	12.62	12.78	12.95	13.12	13.29
.75	11.49	11.63	11.76	11.90	12.05	12.19	12.34	12.50	12.66	12.82	12.98	13.15	13.33	13.51	13.69
+11.00	11.78	11.92	12.06	12.21	12.36	12.51	12.67	12.84	13.00	13.17	13.35	13.53	13.72	13.91	14.10
.25	12.06	12.21	12.36	12.52	12.68	12.84	13.01	13.18	13.35	13.53	13.72	13.91	14.11	14.31	14.52
.50	12.35	12.51	12.66	12.83	12.99	13.16	13.34	13.52	13.71	13.90	14.09	14.29	14.50	14.71	14.93
.75	12.64	12.80	12.97	13.14	13.31	13.49	13.68	13.87	14.06	14.26	14.47	14.68	14.90	15.13	15.36
+12.00	12.93	13.10	13.27	13.45	13.64	13.82	14.02	14.22	14.42	14.63	14.85	15.08	15.31	15.54	15.79
.25	13.22	13.40	13.58	13.77	13.96	14.16	14.36	14.57	14.79	15.01	15.24	15.47	15.72	15.97	16.23
.50	13.51	13.70	13.89	14.08	14.29	14.49	14.71	14.93	15.15	15.38	15.62	15.87	16.13	16.39	16.67
.75	13.81	14.00	14.20	14.40	14.61	14.83	15.05	15.28	15.52	15.77	16.02	16.28	16.55	16.83	17.11
+13.00	14.10	14.30	14.51	14.72	14.94	15.17	15.40	15.64	15.89	16.15	16.41	16.69	16.97	17.27	17.57
.25	14.39	14.60	14.82	15.04	15.27	15.51	15.76	16.01	16.27	16.54	16.82	17.10	17.40	17.71	18.03
.50	14.69	14.91	15.14	15.37	15.61	15.86	16.11	16.37	16.65	16.93	17.22	17.52	17.83	18.16	18.49
.75	14.99	15.21	15.45	15.69	15.94	16.20	16.47	16.74	17.03	17.32	17.63	17.94	18.27	18.61	18.96
+14.00	15.28	15.52	15.77	16.02	16.28	16.55	16.83	17.11	17.41	17.72	18.04	18.37	18.72	19.07	19.44
.25	15.58	15.83	16.08	16.35	16.62	16.90	17.19	17.49	17.80	18.12	18.46	18.80	19.16	19.54	19.93
.50	15.88	16.14	16.40	16.68	16.96	17.25	17.55	17.87	18.19	18.53	18.88	19.24	19.62	20.01	20.42
.75	16.18	16.45	16.72	17.01	17.30	17.61	17.92	18.25	18.59	18.94	19.31	19.69	20.08	20.49	20.92
+15.00	16.48	16.76	17.04	17.34	17.65	17.96	18.29	18.63	18.99	19.35	19.74	20.13	20.55	20.98	21.43
.25	16.79	17.07	17.37	17.68	18.00	18.33	18.67	19.02	19.39	19.77	20.17	20.59	21.02	21.47	21.94
.50	17.09	17.39	17.69	18.01	18.34	18.68	19.04	19.41	19.79	20.19	20.61	21.04	21.50	21.97	22.46
.75	17.39	17.70	18.02	18.35	18.70	19.05	19.42	19.81	20.21	20.62	21.06	21.51	21.98	22.48	22.99
+16.00	17.70	18.02	18.35	18.69	19.05	19.42	19.80	20.20	20.62	21.05	21.51	21.98	22.47	22.99	23.53
.25	18.01	18.34	18.68	19.03	19.40	19.79	20.19	20.60	21.04	21.49	21.96	22.45	22.97	23.51	24.07
.50	18.31	18.65	19.01	19.38	19.76	20.16	20.57	21.01	21.46	21.93	22.42	22.93	23.47	24.03	24.63
.75	18.62	18.97	19.34	19.72	20.12	20.53	20.96	21.41	21.88	22.37	22.88	23.42	23.98	24.57	25.19
+17.00	18.93	19.30	19.68	20.07	20.48	20.91	21.36	21.82	22.31	22.82	23.35	23.91	24.50	25.11	25.76
.25	19.24	19.62	20.01	20.42	20.85	21.29	21.75	22.24	22.74	23.27	23.83	24.41	25.02	25.66	26.34

Appendix A (*cont'd*)

Spectacle refraction or spectacle lens power (BVP) (D)	**Ocular refraction (D) for vertex distances (mm) of:**														
	6	**7**	**8**	**9**	**10**	**11**	**12**	**13**	**14**	**15**	**16**	**17**	**18**	**19**	**20**
.50	19.55	19.94	20.35	20.77	21.21	21.67	22.15	22.65	23.18	23.73	24.31	24.91	25.55	26.22	26.92
.75	19.87	20.27	20.69	21.12	21.58	22.06	22.55	23.07	23.62	24.19	24.79	25.42	26.08	26.78	27.52
+18.00	20.18	20.59	21.03	21.48	21.95	22.44	22.96	23.50	24.06	24.66	25.28	25.94	26.63	27.36	28.12
.25	20.49	20.92	21.37	21.84	22.32	22.83	23.37	23.93	24.51	25.13	25.78	26.46	27.18	27.94	28.74
.50	20.81	21.25	21.71	22.20	22.70	23.23	23.78	24.36	24.97	25.61	26.28	26.99	27.74	28.53	29.37
.75	21.13	21.58	22.06	22.56	23.08	23.62	24.19	24.79	25.42	26.09	26.79	27.52	28.30	29.13	30.00
+19.00	21.44	21.91	22.41	22.92	23.46	24.02	24.61	25.23	25.89	26.57	27.30	28.06	28.88	29.73	30.65
.25	21.76	22.25	22.75	23.28	23.84	24.42	25.03	25.68	26.35	27.07	27.82	28.61	29.46	30.35	31.30
.50	22.08	22.58	23.10	23.65	24.22	24.82	25.46	26.12	26.82	27.56	28.34	29.17	30.05	30.98	31.97
.75	22.40	22.92	23.46	24.02	24.61	25.23	25.88	26.57	27.30	28.06	28.87	29.73	30.64	31.61	32.64
+20.00	22.73	23.26	23.81	24.39	25.00	25.64	26.32	27.03	27.78	28.57	29.41	30.30	31.25	32.26	33.33
−0.25	0.25	0.25	0.25	0.25	0.25	0.25	0.25	0.25	0.25	0.25	0.25	0.25	0.25	0.25	0.25
0.50	0.50	0.50	0.50	0.50	0.50	0.50	0.50	0.50	0.50	0.50	0.50	0.50	0.50	0.50	0.50
0.75	0.75	0.75	0.75	0.75	0.74	0.74	0.74	0.74	0.74	0.74	0.74	0.74	0.74	0.74	0.74
−1.00	0.99	0.99	0.99	0.99	0.99	0.99	0.99	0.99	0.99	0.99	0.98	0.98	0.98	0.98	0.98
.25	1.24	1.24	1.24	1.24	1.23	1.23	1.23	1.23	1.23	1.23	1.23	1.22	1.22	1.22	1.22
.50	1.49	1.48	1.48	1.48	1.48	1.48	1.47	1.47	1.47	1.47	1.46	1.46	1.46	1.46	1.46
.75	1.73	1.73	1.73	1.72	1.72	1.72	1.71	1.71	1.71	1.71	1.70	1.70	1.70	1.69	1.69
−2.00	1.98	1.97	1.97	1.96	1.96	1.96	1.95	1.95	1.95	1.94	1.94	1.93	1.93	1.93	1.92
.25	2.22	2.22	2.21	2.21	2.20	2.20	2.19	2.19	2.18	2.18	2.17	2.17	2.16	2.16	2.15
.50	2.46	2.46	2.45	2.44	2.44	2.43	2.43	2.42	2.42	2.41	2.40	2.40	2.39	2.39	2.38
.75	2.71	2.70	2.69	2.68	2.68	2.67	2.66	2.66	2.65	2.64	2.63	2.63	2.62	2.61	2.61
−3.00	2.95	2.94	2.93	2.92	2.91	2.90	2.90	2.89	2.88	2.87	2.86	2.85	2.85	2.84	2.83
.25	3.19	3.18	3.17	3.16	3.15	3.14	3.13	3.12	3.11	3.10	3.09	3.08	3.07	3.06	3.05
.50	3.43	3.42	3.40	3.39	3.38	3.37	3.36	3.35	3.34	3.33	3.31	3.30	3.29	3.28	3.27
.75	3.67	3.65	3.64	3.63	3.61	3.60	3.59	3.58	3.56	3.55	3.54	3.52	3.51	3.50	3.49
−4.00	3.91	3.89	3.88	3.86	3.85	3.83	3.82	3.80	3.79	3.77	3.76	3.75	3.73	3.72	3.70
.25	4.14	4.13	4.11	4.09	4.08	4.06	4.04	4.03	4.01	4.00	3.98	3.96	3.95	3.93	3.92
.50	4.38	4.36	4.34	4.33	4.34	4.29	4.27	4.25	4.23	4.22	4.20	4.18	4.16	4.15	4.13
.75	4.62	4.60	4.58	4.56	4.54	4.51	4.49	4.47	4.45	4.43	4.42	4.40	4.38	4.36	4.34
−5.00	4.85	4.83	4.81	4.78	4.76	4.74	4.72	4.69	4.67	4.65	4.63	4.61	4.59	4.57	4.55
.25	5.09	5.06	5.04	5.01	4.99	4.96	4.94	4.91	4.89	4.87	4.84	4.82	4.80	4.77	4.75
.50	5.32	5.30	5.27	5.24	5.21	5.19	5.16	5.13	5.11	5.08	5.06	5.03	5.01	4.98	4.96
.75	5.56	5.53	5.50	5.47	5.44	5.41	5.38	5.35	5.32	5.29	5.27	5.24	5.21	5.18	5.16
−6.00	5.79	5.76	5.72	5.69	5.66	5.63	5.60	5.56	5.53	5.50	5.47	5.44	5.41	5.39	5.36
.25	6.02	5.99	5.95	5.92	5.88	5.85	5.81	5.78	5.75	5.71	5.68	5.65	5.62	5.59	5.56
.50	6.26	6.22	6.18	6.14	6.11	6.07	6.03	6.00	5.96	5.92	5.89	5.85	5.82	5.79	5.75
.75	6.49	6.45	6.41	6.37	6.33	6.29	6.25	6.21	6.17	6.13	6.09	6.06	6.02	5.98	5.95
−7.00	6.72	6.67	6.63	6.58	6.54	6.50	6.46	6.41	6.37	6.33	6.29	6.25	6.22	6.18	6.14
.25	6.94	6.90	6.85	6.81	6.76	6.72	6.67	6.63	6.58	6.54	6.50	6.46	6.41	6.37	6.33
.50	7.18	7.13	7.08	7.03	6.98	6.93	6.88	6.84	6.79	6.74	6.70	6.65	6.61	6.57	6.52
.75	7.41	7.35	7.30	7.25	7.19	7.14	7.09	7.04	6.99	6.94	6.90	6.85	6.80	6.76	6.71
−8.00	7.63	7.58	7.52	7.46	7.41	7.35	7.30	7.25	7.19	7.14	7.09	7.04	6.99	6.94	6.90
.25	7.86	7.80	7.74	7.68	7.62	7.56	7.51	7.45	7.40	7.34	7.29	7.24	7.18	7.13	7.08
.50	8.09	8.03	7.96	7.90	7.84	7.78	7.72	7.66	7.60	7.54	7.49	7.43	7.37	7.32	7.27
.75	8.31	8.24	8.18	8.11	8.05	7.98	7.92	7.86	7.79	7.73	7.67	7.62	7.56	7.50	7.45
−9.00	8.54	8.47	8.40	8.33	8.26	8.19	8.12	8.06	7.99	7.93	7.87	7.81	7.75	7.69	7.63
.25	8.76	8.69	8.61	8.54	8.47	8.40	8.33	8.26	8.19	8.12	8.06	7.99	7.93	7.87	7.81

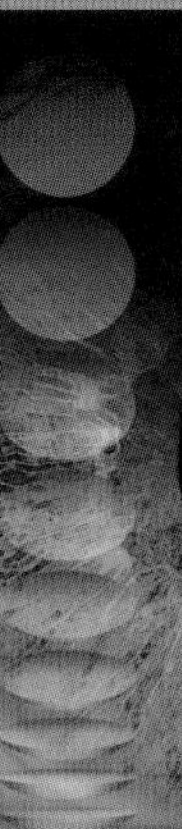

Appendix A (*cont'd*)

Spectacle refraction or spectacle lens power (BVP) (D)	**Ocular refraction (D) for vertex distances (mm) of:**														
	6	**7**	**8**	**9**	**10**	**11**	**12**	**13**	**14**	**15**	**16**	**17**	**18**	**19**	**20**
.50	8.98	8.90	8.83	8.75	8.67	8.60	8.53	8.45	8.38	8.31	8.24	8.18	8.11	8.05	7.98
.75	9.21	9.12	9.04	8.96	8.88	8.80	8.73	8.65	8.58	8.50	8.43	8.36	8.29	8.22	8.16
−10.00	9.43	9.35	9.26	9.17	9.09	9.01	8.93	8.85	8.77	8.70	8.62	8.55	8.47	8.40	8.33
.25	9.66	9.56	9.47	9.38	9.29	9.21	9.12	9.04	8.96	8.88	8.80	8.73	8.65	8.58	8.50
.50	9.88	9.78	9.69	9.59	9.50	9.41	9.32	9.24	9.15	9.07	8.99	8.91	8.83	8.75	8.68
.75	10.10	10.00	9.90	9.80	9.71	9.61	9.52	9.43	9.34	9.26	9.17	9.09	9.01	8.93	8.85
−11.00	10.32	10.21	10.11	10.01	9.91	9.81	9.72	9.62	9.53	9.44	9.35	9.27	9.18	9.10	9.02
.25	10.54	10.43	10.32	10.22	10.11	10.01	9.91	9.81	9.72	9.63	9.53	9.44	9.36	9.27	9.18
.50	10.76	10.64	10.53	10.42	10.31	10.21	10.11	10.00	9.90	9.81	9.71	9.62	9.53	9.44	9.35
.75	10.98	10.86	10.74	10.63	10.51	10.40	10.30	10.19	10.09	9.99	9.89	9.79	9.70	9.61	9.51
−12.00	11.19	11.07	10.95	10.83	10.71	10.60	10.49	10.38	10.27	10.17	10.07	9.97	9.87	9.77	9.68
.25	11.41	11.28	11.16	11.03	10.91	10.80	10.68	10.57	10.46	10.35	10.24	10.14	10.04	9.94	9.84
.50	11.63	11.49	11.36	11.24	11.11	10.99	10.87	10.75	10.64	10.53	10.42	10.31	10.20	10.10	10.00
.75	11.84	11.71	11.57	11.44	11.31	11.18	11.06	10.94	10.82	10.70	10.59	10.48	10.37	10.26	10.16
−13.00	12.06	11.92	11.78	11.64	11.50	11.37	11.25	11.12	11.00	10.88	10.76	10.65	10.54	10.43	10.32
.25	12.27	12.13	11.98	11.84	11.70	11.56	11.43	11.30	11.18	11.05	10.93	10.81	10.70	10.59	10.47
.50	12.49	12.34	12.18	12.04	11.89	11.76	11.62	11.49	11.35	11.23	11.10	10.98	10.86	10.74	10.63
.75	12.70	12.54	12.39	12.24	12.09	11.94	11.80	11.66	11.53	11.40	11.27	11.14	11.02	10.90	10.78
−14.00	12.91	12.75	12.59	12.43	12.28	12.13	11.99	11.84	11.71	11.57	11.44	11.31	11.18	11.06	10.94
.25	13.13	12.96	12.79	12.63	12.47	12.32	12.17	12.02	11.88	11.74	11.60	11.47	11.34	11.21	11.09
.50	13.34	13.16	12.99	12.83	12.66	12.50	12.35	12.20	12.05	11.91	11.77	11.63	11.50	11.37	11.24
.75	13.55	13.37	13.19	13.02	12.85	12.69	12.53	12.38	12.22	12.08	11.93	11.79	11.66	11.52	11.39
−15.00	13.76	13.57	13.39	13.22	13.04	12.87	12.71	12.55	12.40	12.24	12.10	11.95	11.81	11.67	11.54
.25	13.97	13.78	13.59	13.41	13.23	13.06	12.89	12.73	12.57	12.41	12.26	12.11	11.97	11.82	11.69
.50	14.18	13.98	13.79	13.60	13.42	13.24	13.07	12.90	12.74	12.58	12.42	12.27	12.12	11.97	11.83
.75	14.39	14.19	13.99	13.80	13.61	13.42	13.25	13.07	12.90	12.74	12.58	12.42	12.27	12.12	11.98
−16.00	14.60	14.39	14.18	13.99	13.79	13.61	13.42	13.25	13.07	12.90	12.74	12.58	12.42	12.27	12.12
.25	14.81	14.59	14.38	14.18	13.98	13.79	13.60	13.42	13.24	13.07	12.90	12.73	12.57	12.42	12.26
.50	15.01	14.79	14.58	14.37	14.16	13.96	13.77	13.59	13.40	13.23	13.05	12.88	12.72	12.56	12.41
.75	15.22	14.99	14.77	14.56	14.35	14.14	13.95	13.76	13.57	13.39	13.21	13.04	12.87	12.71	12.55
−17.00	15.43	15.19	14.97	14.74	14.53	14.32	14.12	13.92	13.73	13.55	13.37	13.19	13.02	12.85	12.69
.25	15.63	15.39	15.16	14.93	14.71	14.50	14.29	14.09	13.89	13.70	13.52	13.34	13.16	12.99	12.83
.50	15.84	15.59	15.35	15.12	14.89	14.68	14.46	14.26	14.06	13.86	13.67	13.49	13.31	13.13	12.96
.75	16.04	15.79	15.54	15.30	15.07	14.85	14.63	14.42	14.22	14.02	13.82	13.64	13.45	13.27	13.10
−18.00	16.24	15.98	15.73	15.49	15.25	15.02	14.80	14.59	14.38	14.17	13.97	13.78	13.59	13.41	13.23
.25	16.45	16.18	15.93	15.68	15.43	15.20	14.97	14.75	14.54	14.33	14.13	13.93	13.74	13.55	13.37
.50	16.65	16.38	16.12	15.86	15.61	15.37	15.14	14.91	14.70	14.48	14.28	14.07	13.88	13.69	13.50
.75	16.85	16.58	16.31	16.04	15.79	15.54	15.31	15.08	14.85	14.63	14.42	14.22	14.02	13.83	13.64
−19.00	17.06	16.77	16.49	16.23	15.97	15.72	15.47	15.24	15.01	14.79	14.57	14.36	14.16	13.96	13.77
.25	17.26	16.96	16.68	16.41	16.14	15.89	15.64	15.40	15.16	14.94	14.72	14.50	14.30	14.09	13.90
.50	17.46	17.16	16.87	16.59	16.32	16.06	15.80	15.56	15.32	15.09	14.86	14.65	14.43	14.23	14.03
.75	17.66	17.35	17.06	16.77	16.49	16.23	15.97	15.72	15.47	15.24	15.01	14.79	14.57	14.36	14.16
−20.00	17.86	17.54	17.24	16.95	16.67	16.39	16.13	15.87	15.62	15.38	15.15	14.93	14.71	14.49	14.29
.25	18.06	17.74	17.43	17.13	16.84	16.56	16.29	16.03	15.78	15.53	15.29	15.06	14.84	14.62	14.41
.50	18.25	17.93	17.61	17.31	17.01	16.73	16.45	16.19	15.93	15.68	15.44	15.20	14.97	14.75	14.54
.75	18.45	18.12	17.80	17.49	17.19	16.89	16.61	16.34	16.08	15.83	15.58	15.34	15.11	14.88	14.66
−21.00	18.65	18.31	17.98	17.66	17.36	17.06	16.77	16.50	16.23	15.97	15.72	15.48	15.24	15.01	14.79
.25	18.85	18.50	18.16	17.84	17.53	17.22	16.93	16.65	16.38	16.11	15.86	15.61	15.37	15.14	14.91

Appendix A (*cont'd*)

Spectacle refraction or spectacle lens power (BVP) (D)	**Ocular refraction (D) for vertex distances (mm) of:**														
	6	**7**	**8**	**9**	**10**	**11**	**12**	**13**	**14**	**15**	**16**	**17**	**18**	**19**	**20**
.50	19.04	18.69	18.34	18.01	17.70	17.39	17.09	16.80	16.53	16.26	16.00	15.75	15.50	15.26	15.04
.75	19.24	18.88	18.53	18.19	17.86	17.55	17.25	16.96	16.67	16.40	16.13	15.88	15.63	15.39	15.16
−22.00	19.43	19.06	18.71	18.36	18.03	17.71	17.40	17.11	16.82	16.54	16.27	16.01	15.76	15.51	15.28
.25	19.63	19.25	18.89	18.54	18.20	17.88	17.56	17.26	16.97	16.68	16.41	16.14	15.89	15.64	15.40
.50	19.82	19.44	19.07	18.71	18.37	18.04	17.72	17.41	17.11	16.82	16.54	16.30	16.01	15.76	15.52
.75	20.02	19.62	19.25	18.88	18.53	18.20	17.87	17.56	17.25	16.96	16.68	16.40	16.14	15.88	15.63
−23.00	20.21	19.81	19.43	19.06	18.70	18.36	18.02	17.71	17.40	17.10	16.81	16.53	16.27	16.01	15.75
.25	20.40	20.00	19.60	19.23	18.86	18.52	18.18	17.85	17.54	17.24	16.95	16.66	16.39	16.13	15.87
.50	20.60	20.18	19.78	19.40	19.03	18.67	18.33	18.00	17.68	17.38	17.08	16.79	16.52	16.25	15.99
.75	20.79	20.36	19.96	19.57	19.19	18.83	18.48	18.15	17.82	17.51	17.21	16.92	16.64	16.37	16.10
−24.00	20.98	20.55	20.13	19.74	19.35	18.99	18.63	18.29	17.96	17.65	17.34	17.04	16.76	16.48	16.22
.25	21.17	20.73	20.31	19.90	19.52	19.14	18.78	18.44	18.10	17.78	17.47	17.17	16.88	16.60	16.33
.50	21.36	20.91	20.48	20.07	19.68	19.30	18.93	18.58	18.24	17.91	17.60	17.30	17.00	16.72	16.44
.75	21.55	21.10	20.66	20.24	19.84	19.45	19.08	18.73	18.38	18.05	17.73	17.42	17.12	16.83	16.56
−25.00	21.74	21.28	20.83	20.41	20.00	19.61	19.23	18.87	18.52	18.18	17.86	17.54	17.24	16.95	16.67
.25	21.93	21.46	21.01	20.58	20.16	19.76	19.38	19.01	18.66	18.32	17.99	17.67	17.36	17.06	16.78
.50	22.12	21.64	21.18	20.74	20.32	19.91	19.52	19.15	18.79	18.44	18.11	17.79	17.48	17.18	16.89
.75	22.31	21.82	21.35	20.91	20.48	20.07	19.67	19.29	18.93	18.58	18.24	17.91	17.60	17.29	17.00
−26.00	22.49	22.00	21.52	21.07	20.64	20.22	19.82	19.43	19.06	18.71	18.36	18.03	17.71	17.40	17.11
.25	22.68	22.17	21.69	21.23	20.79	20.37	19.96	19.57	19.19	18.83	18.48	18.15	17.83	17.51	17.21
.50	22.86	22.35	21.86	21.39	20.95	20.52	20.10	19.71	19.33	18.96	18.61	18.27	17.94	17.62	17.32
.75	23.05	22.53	22.04	21.56	21.11	20.67	20.25	19.85	19.46	19.09	18.73	18.39	18.06	17.74	17.43
−27.00	23.23	22.71	22.20	21.72	21.26	20.82	20.39	19.98	19.59	19.22	18.85	18.50	18.17	17.84	17.53
.25	23.42	22.88	22.37	21.88	21.41	20.96	20.53	20.12	19.72	19.34	18.98	18.62	18.28	17.95	17.64
.50	23.61	23.06	22.54	22.04	21.57	21.11	20.68	20.26	19.86	19.47	19.10	18.74	18.40	18.06	17.74
.75	23.79	23.23	22.71	22.20	21.72	21.26	20.82	20.39	19.98	19.59	19.22	18.86	18.50	18.17	17.84
−28.00	23.97	23.41	22.88	22.36	21.87	21.41	20.96	20.53	20.11	19.72	19.34	18.97	18.62	18.28	17.95
.25	24.16	23.58	23.04	22.52	22.03	21.55	21.10	20.66	20.24	19.84	19.46	19.08	18.73	18.38	18.05
.50	24.34	23.76	23.21	22.68	22.18	21.70	21.24	20.79	20.37	19.96	19.57	19.20	18.84	18.49	18.15
.75	24.52	23.93	23.38	22.84	22.33	21.84	21.38	20.93	20.50	20.09	19.69	19.31	18.95	18.59	18.25
−29.00	24.70	24.11	23.54	23.00	22.48	21.99	21.51	21.06	20.63	20.21	19.81	19.43	19.05	18.70	18.36
.25	24.88	24.28	23.70	23.15	22.63	22.13	21.65	21.19	20.75	20.33	19.92	19.54	19.16	18.80	18.45
.50	25.06	24.45	23.87	23.31	22.78	22.27	21.79	21.32	20.88	20.45	20.04	19.65	19.27	18.90	18.55
.75	25.24	24.62	24.03	23.47	22.93	22.42	21.93	21.45	21.00	20.57	20.16	19.76	19.38	19.01	18.65
−30.00	25.42	24.79	24.19	23.62	23.08	22.56	22.06	21.58	21.13	20.69	20.27	19.87	19.48	19.11	18.75

Appendix B

IER Institute for Eye Research GRADING SCALES

Vision Cooperative Research Centre, Institute for Eye Research, University of New South Wales

APPLICATION OF GRADING SCALES

Patient management is based on how much the normal ocular appearance has changed. In general, a rating of slight (grade 2) or less is considered within normal limits for a population (except staining). A change of one grade or more at follow-up visits is considered clinically significant.

1. VERY SLIGHT	2. SLIGHT	3. MODERATE	4. SEVERE

BULBAR REDNESS

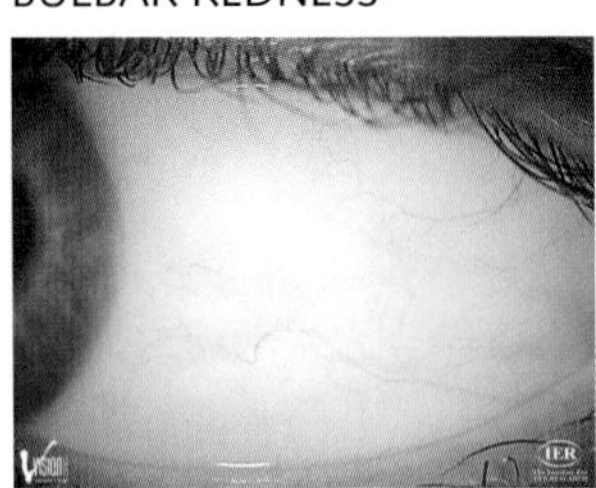
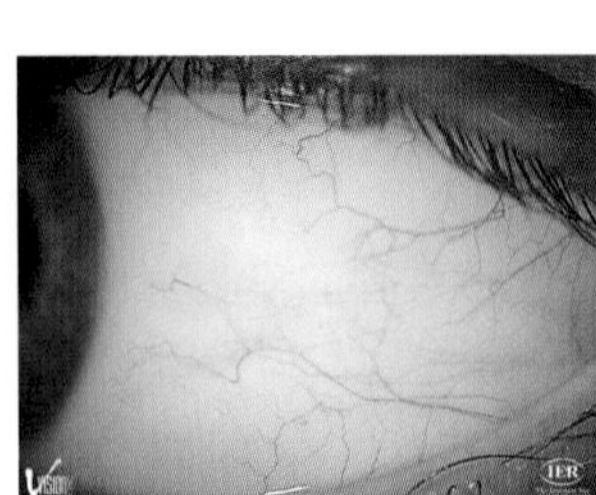
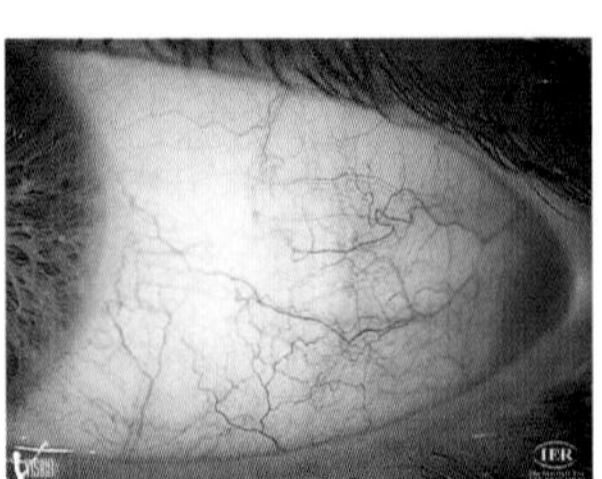
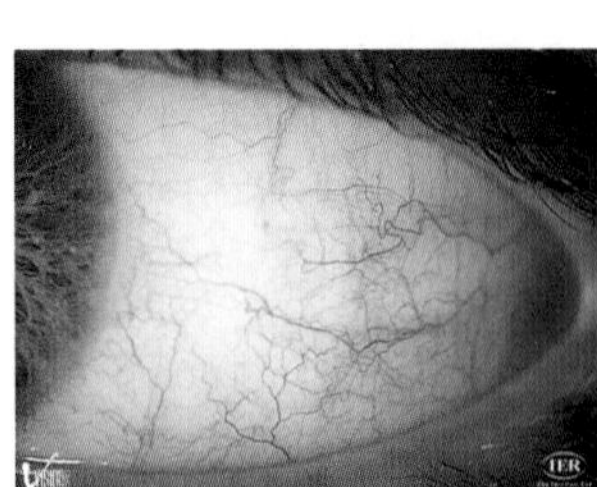

LIMBAL REDNESS

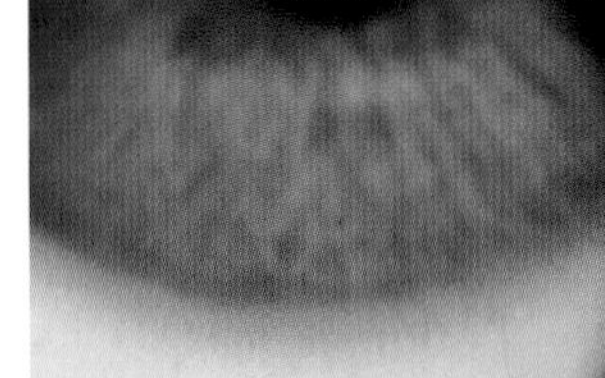
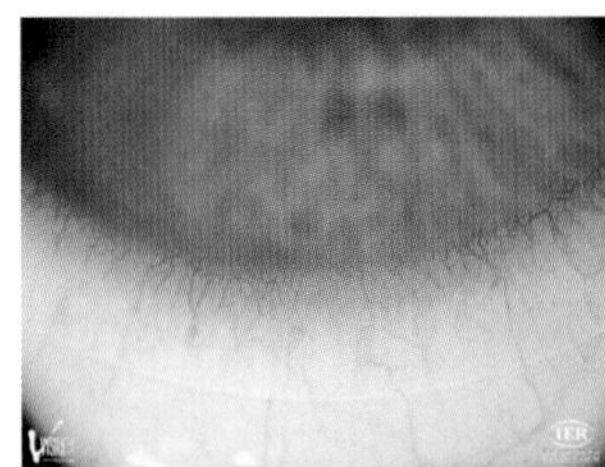
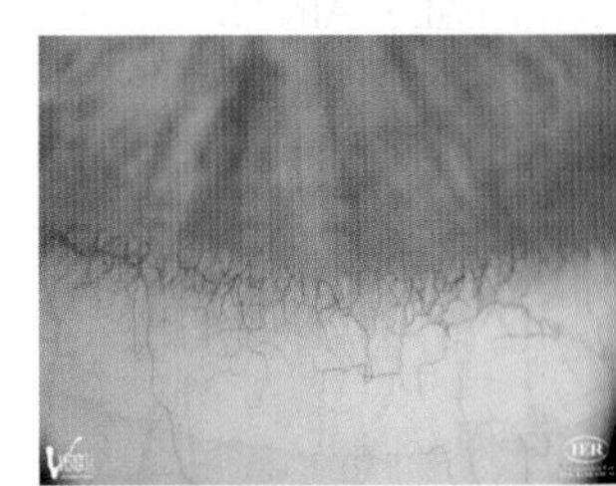

LID REDNESS (area 2)

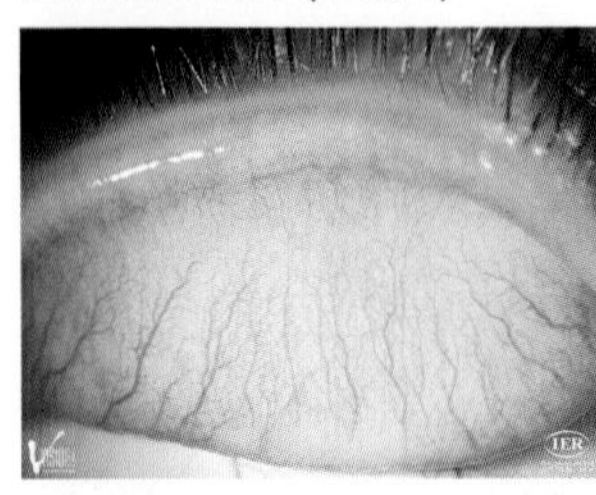
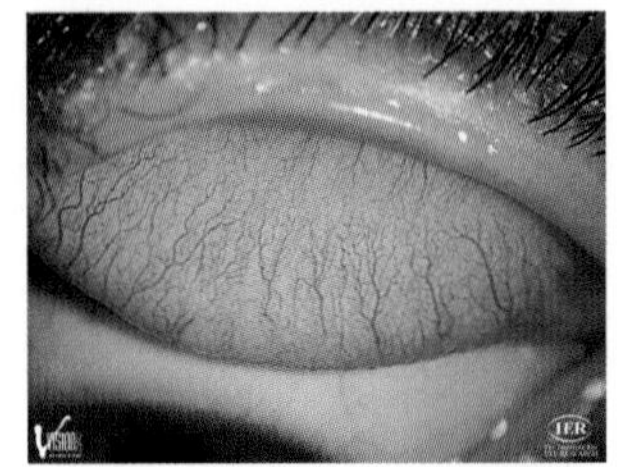
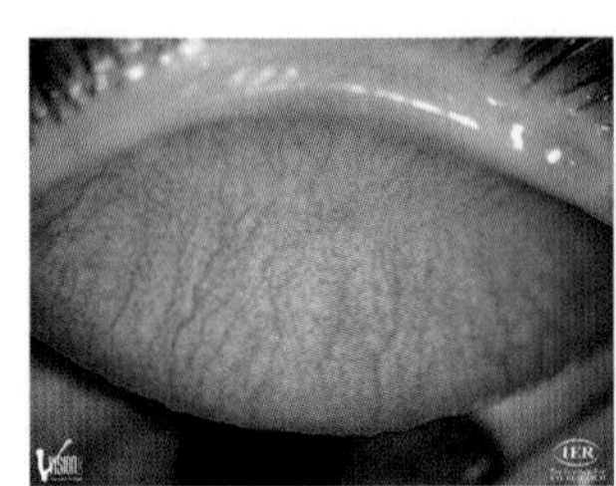
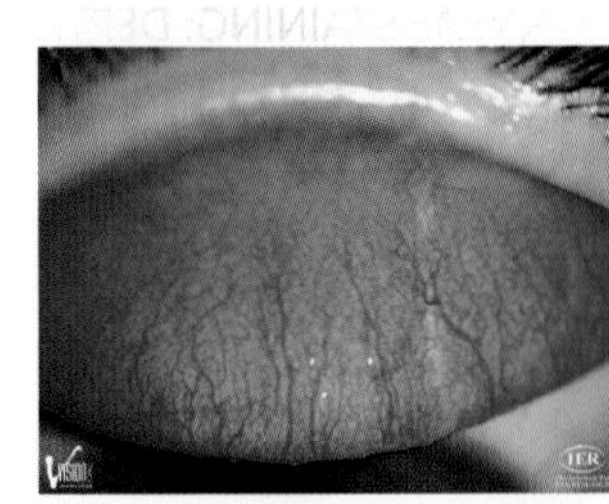

LID ROUGHNESS: WHITE LIGHT REFLEX (areas 1, 2)

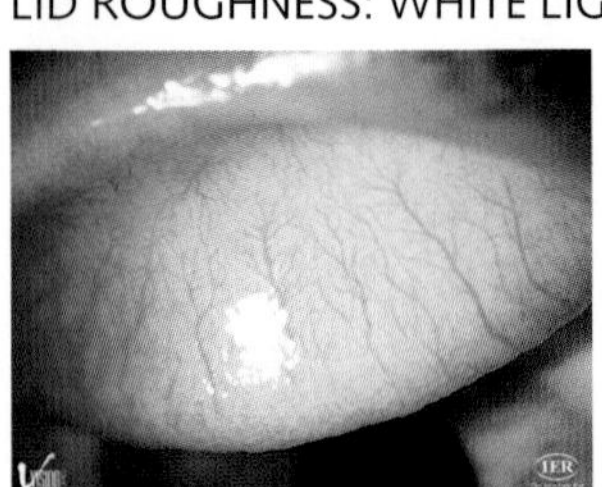
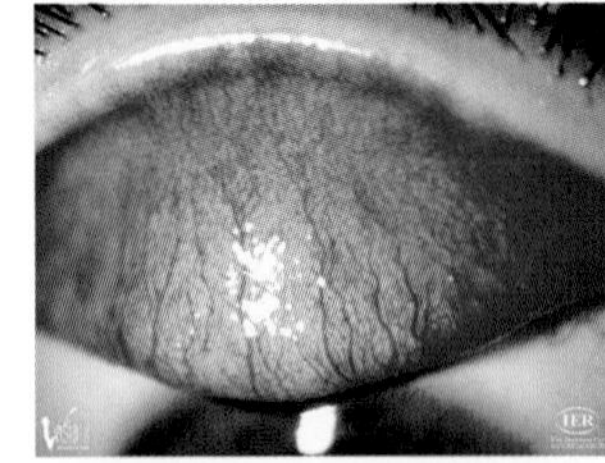
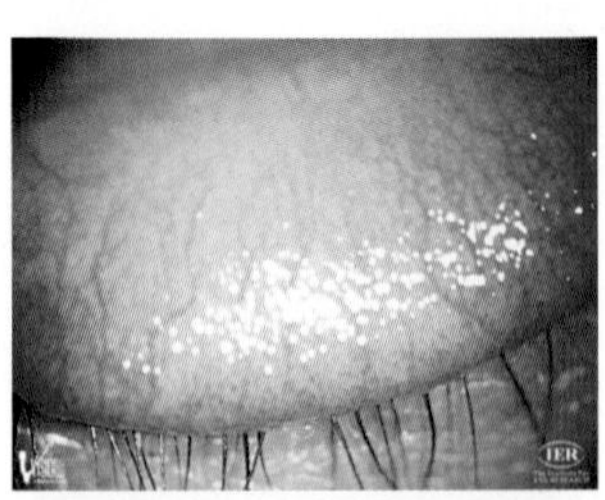
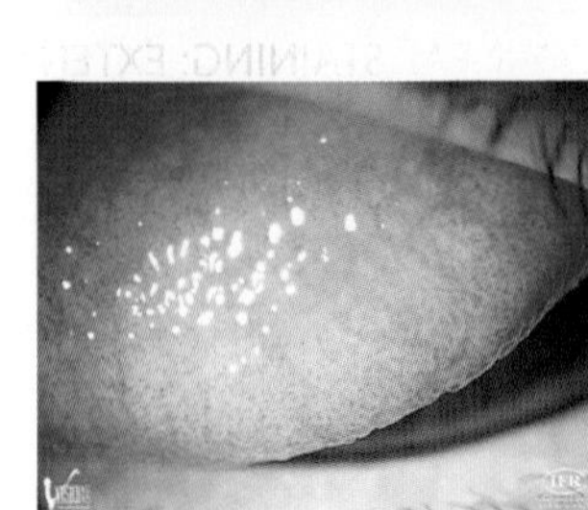

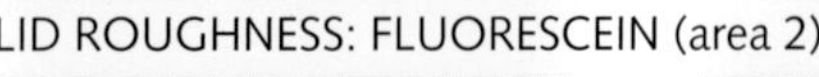

LID ROUGHNESS: FLUORESCEIN (area 2)

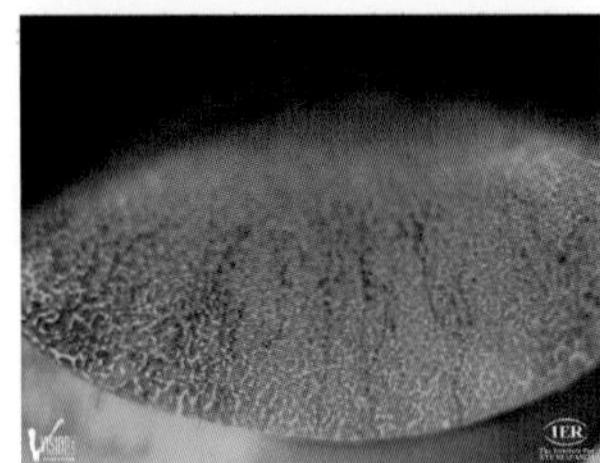
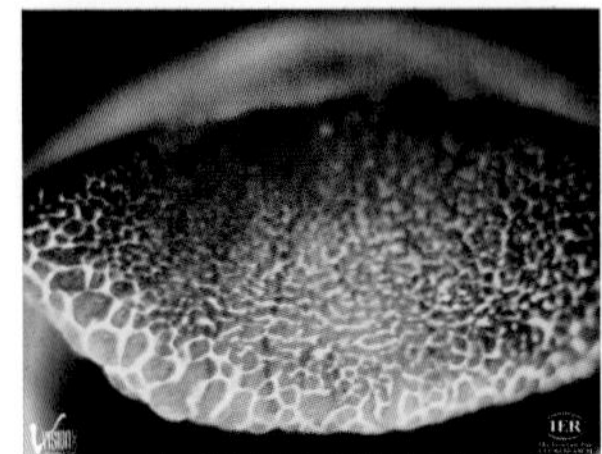
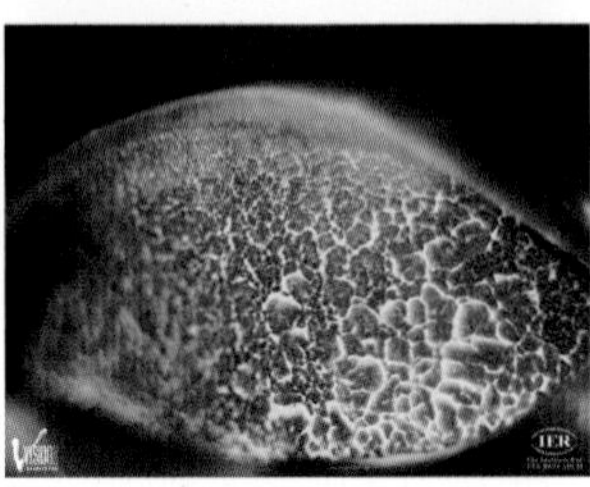

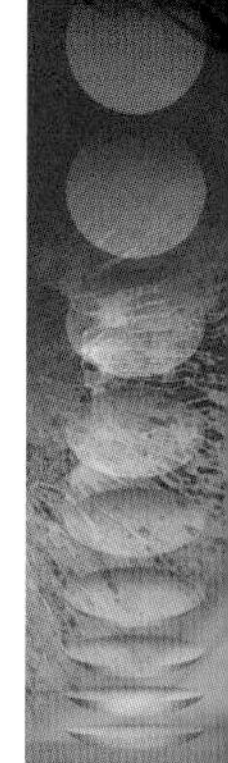

1. VERY SLIGHT	2. SLIGHT	3. MODERATE	4. SEVERE

POLYMEGETHISM

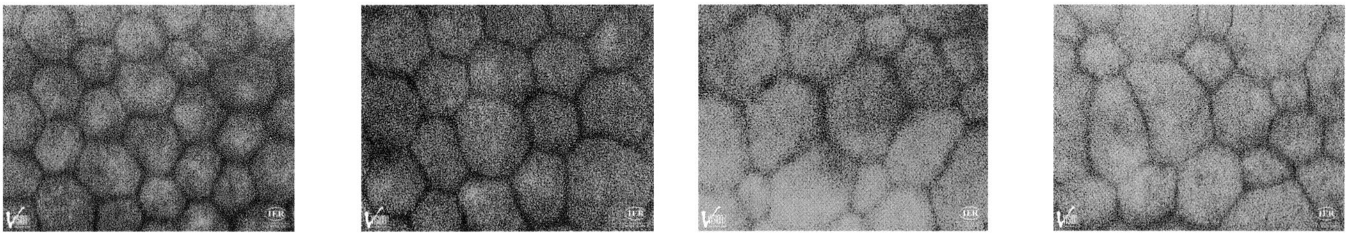

CORNEAL STAINING: TYPE

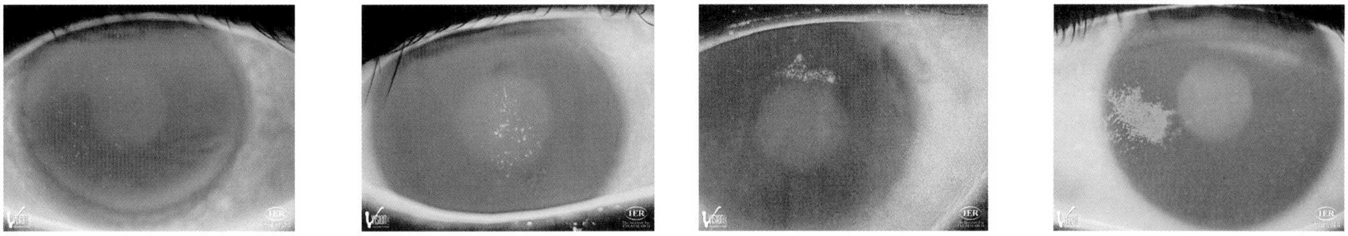

CORNEAL STAINING: DEPTH

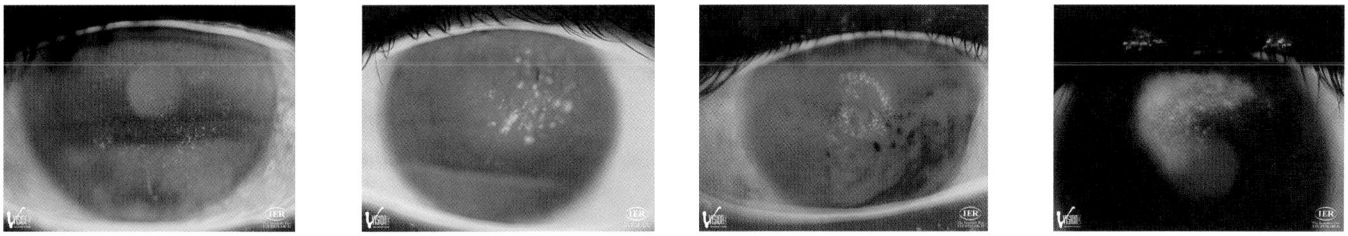

CORNEAL STAINING: EXTENT (area 5)

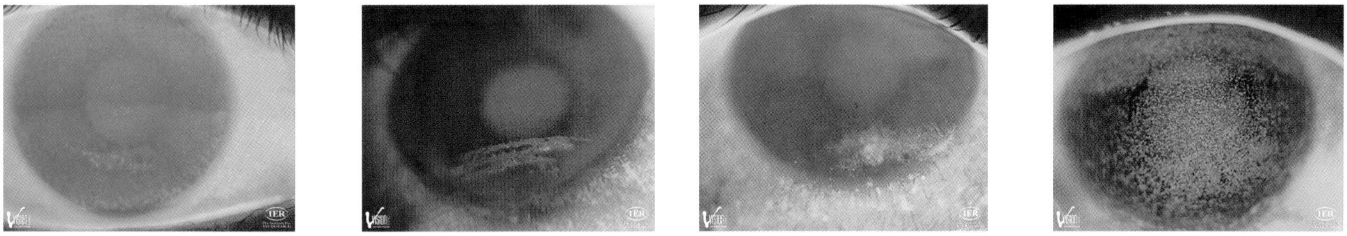

CONJUNCTIVAL STAINING

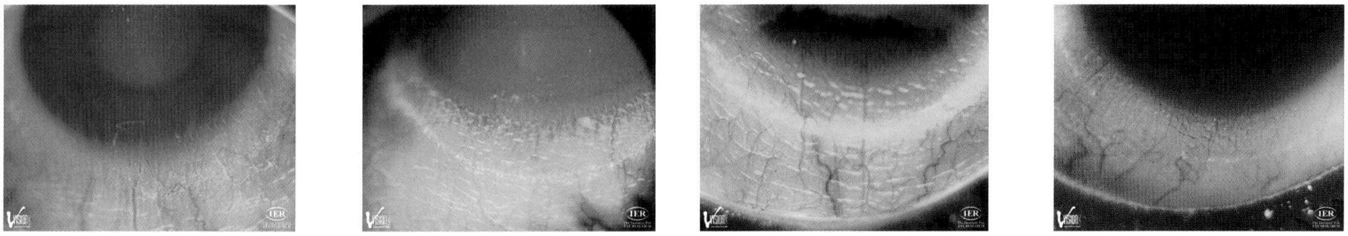

ADVERSE RESPONSES WITH CONTACT LENSES

INFILTRATES

Accumulation of inflammatory cells in corneal subepithelium or stroma

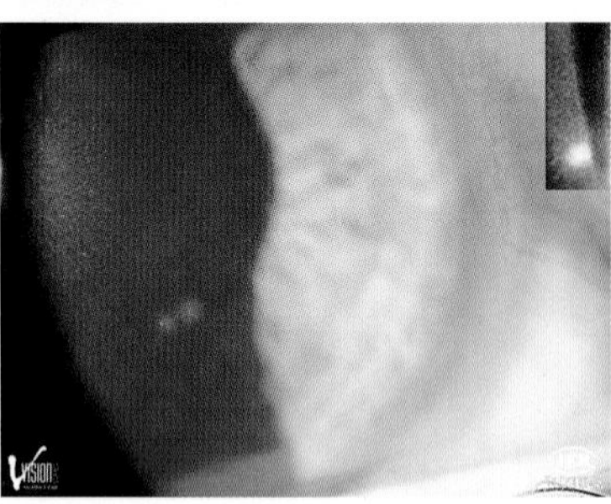

Signs:
- Whitish opacity (local) or grey haze (diffuse)
- Mostly 2–3 mm from limbus
- Localized redness

Symptoms:
- Asymptomatic or scratchy, foreign body sensation
- Redness, tearing and photophobia possible

CLARE CONTACT LENS ACUTE RED EYE

Acute corneal inflammation associated with overnight wear of soft contact lenses

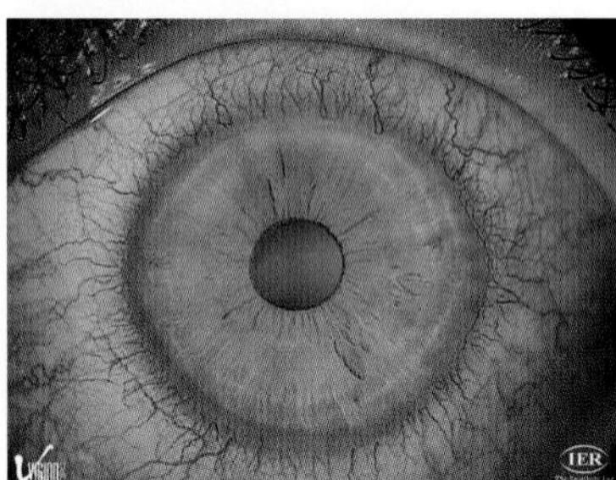

Signs:
- Unilateral
- Intense redness
- Inflltrates
- No epithelial break

Symptoms:
- Wakes with pain
- Photophobia
- Tearing

EROSION

Full-thickness epithelial loss over a discrete area

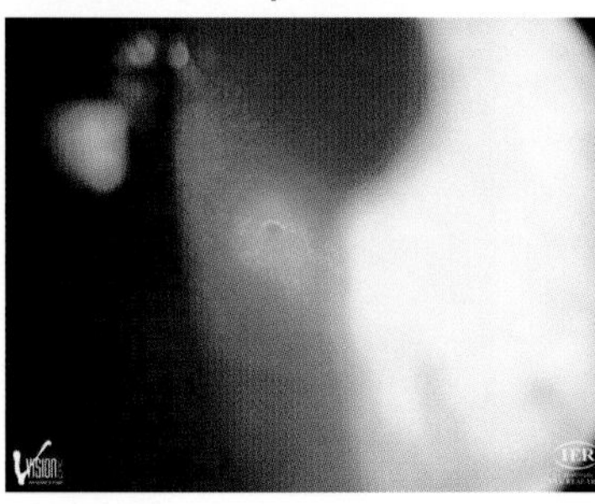

Signs:
- No stromal involvement
- Immediate spread of fluorescein in stroma

Symptoms:
- Pain
- Photophobia
- Lacrimation

CNPU CULTURE NEGATIVE PERIPHERAL ULCER

Full-thickness epithelial loss with stromal degeneration in corneal periphery. Inset: scar

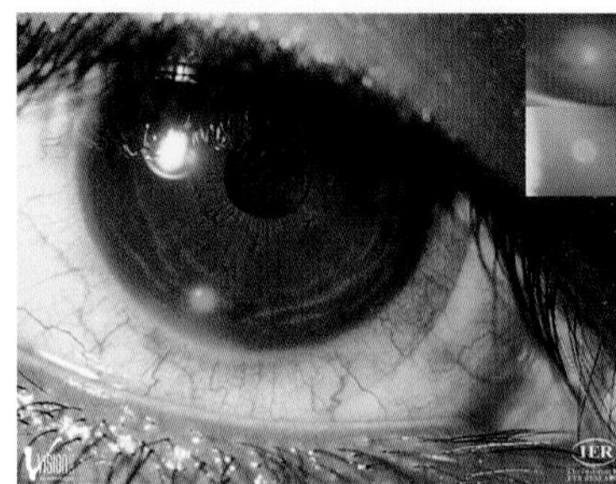

Signs:
- Unilateral
- Localized redness
- Infiltrates
- Post healing scar

Symptoms:
- Varies from mild to foreign body sensation to pain
- Tearing and photophobia may occur

INFECTED ULCER

Full-thickness epithelial loss with stromal degeneration, typically central or paracentral

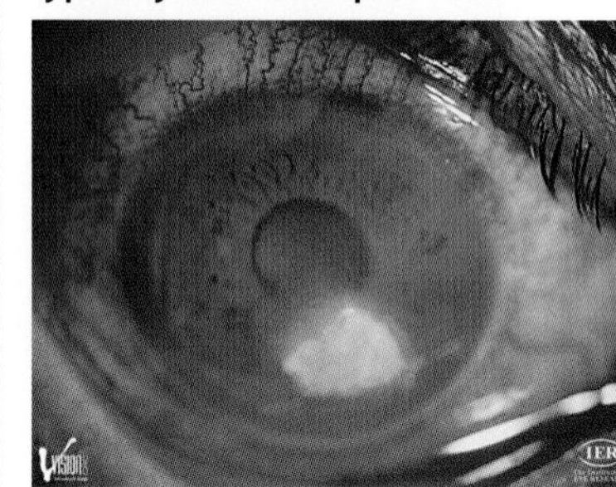

Signs:
- Intense redness
- Large white patch
- Infiltrates
- Epithelial and stromal loss

Symptoms:
- Pain
- Red eye
- Mucoid discharge
- Photophobia
- ↓VA (if over pupil)

CORNEAL STAINING GRADES (see p. 629)

- Staining assessed immediately after single instillation of fluorescein using cobalt blue light and Wratten 12 (yellow) filter over slit-lamp objective.
- The cornea is divided into five equal areas to grade the type, extent and depth of staining in each area.

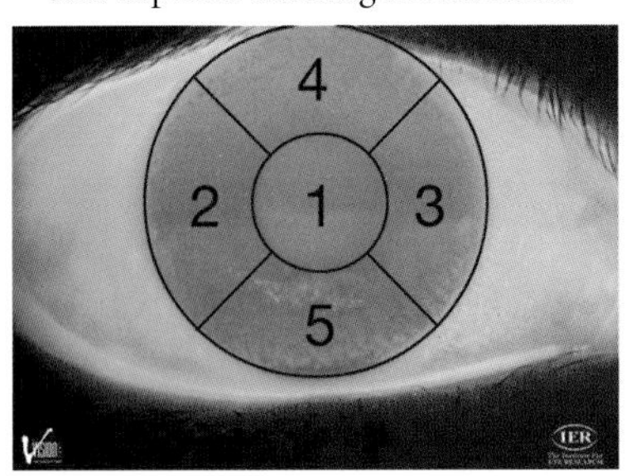

Type:

- Micropunctate
- Macropunctate
- Coalescent macropunctate
- Patch

Extent:	*Surface area*	*Depth**
1	1–15%	Superficial epithelium
2	16–30%	Deep epithelium, delayed stromal glow
3	31–45%	Immediate localized stromal glow
4	>45%	Immediate diffuse stromal glow

*Based on penetration of fluorescein and slit-lamp optic section.

LID AREAS (see p. 628)

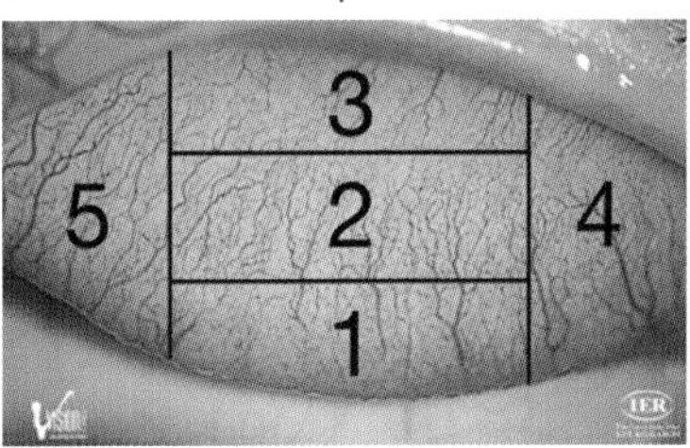

- The palpebral conjunctiva is divided into five areas to grade redness and roughness
- Areas 1, 2 and 3 most relevant in contact lens wear

VASCULARIZATION

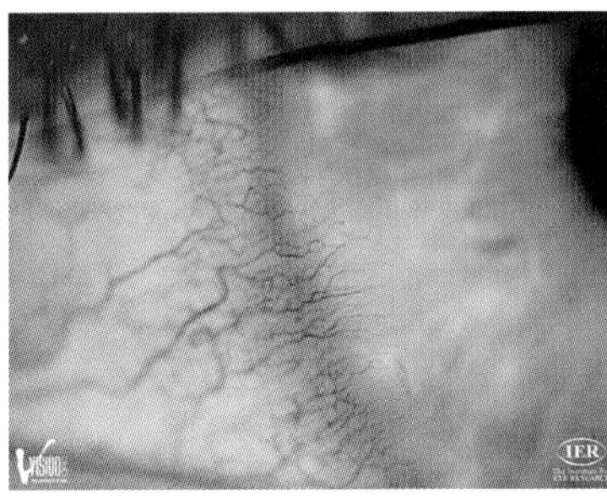

- Vessel extension beyond translucent limbal zone (mm)

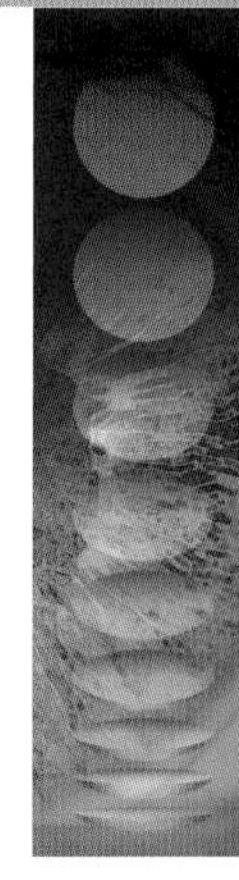

STROMAL STRIAE

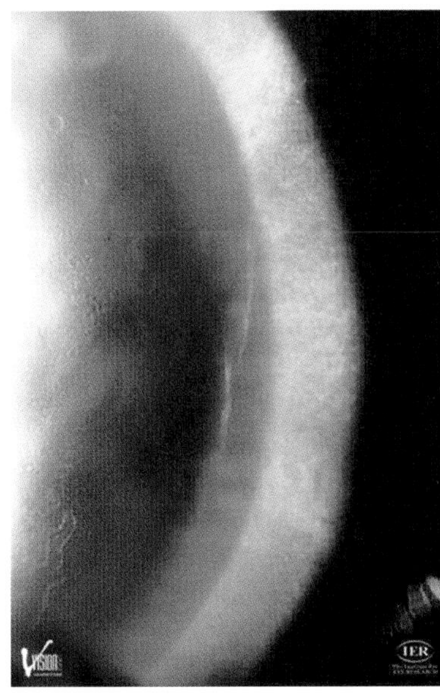

Record number
One stria = 5% oedema
One fold = 8% oedema
(each additional stria/fold is 1% more oedema)

STROMAL FOLDS

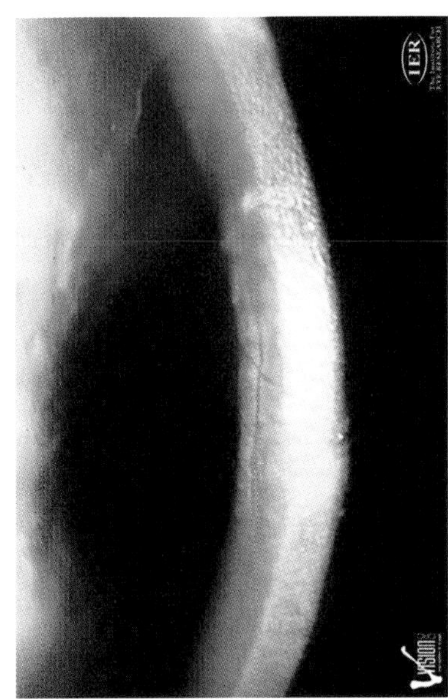

MICROCYSTS

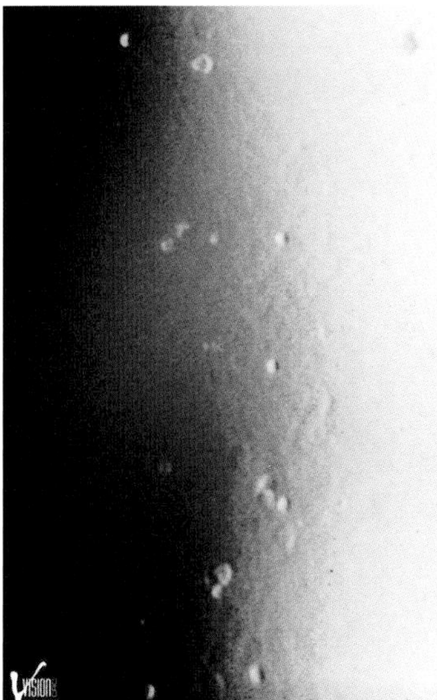

Identified by illumination
Microcysts = reversed
Vacuoles = unreversed
Recorded number
(>10 microcysts/vacuoles requires management)

VACUOLES

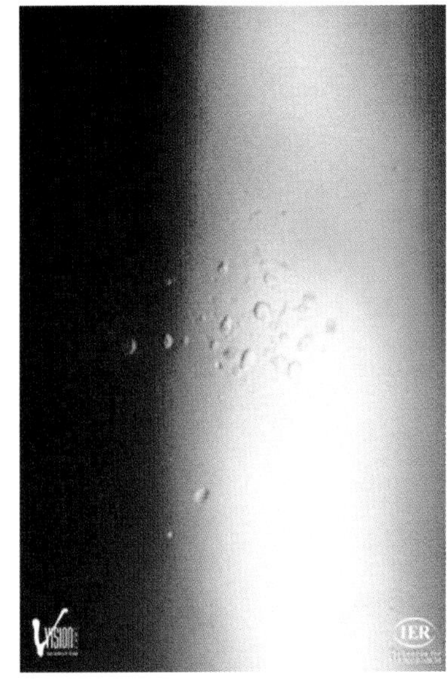

Appendix C

Instructions for the CD-ROM

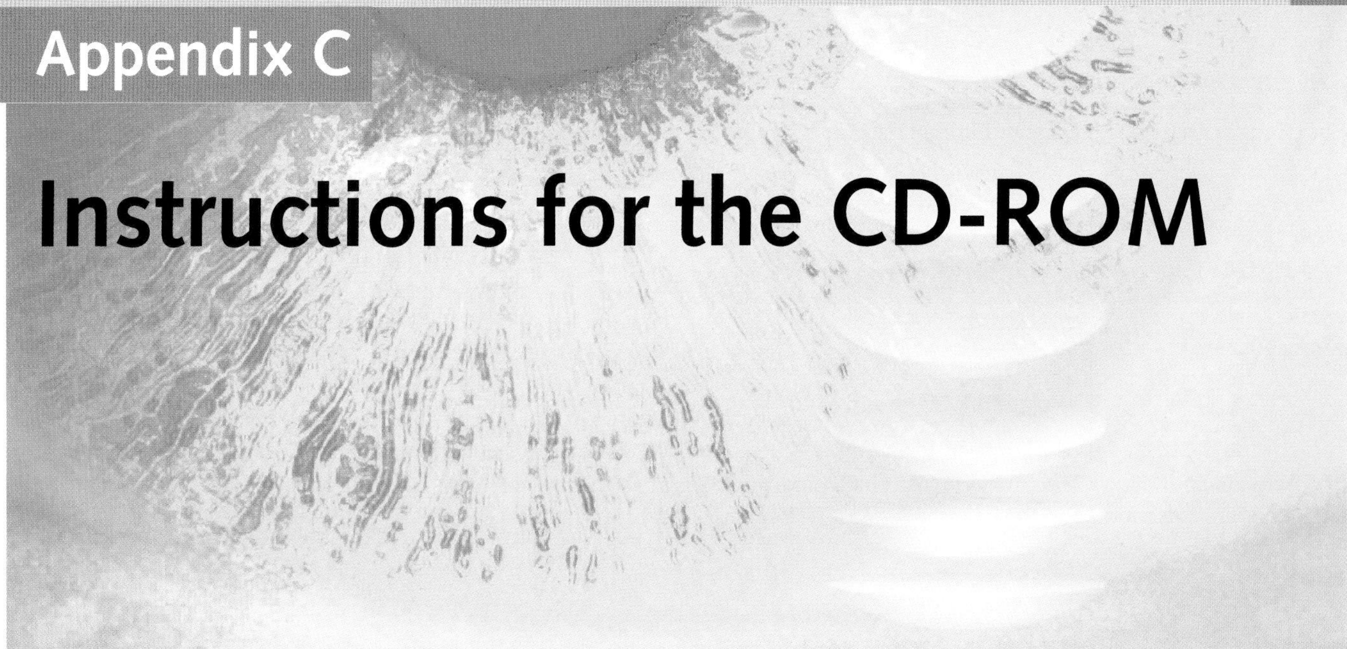

CD-ROM Purpose

1. To provide support for various sections of the book.
2. To provide a clinical Grading Scale with the facility to enlarge each picture for ease of viewing.
3. To provide practitioners and students with the facility to design RGP lenses and to assess the theoretical effect on lens fit and physiological performance.
4. To provide more detailed information on lens design that would be too space-consuming for inclusion in the book.

CD-ROM Contents

1. IER Grading Scales. Reproduced by kind permission of the Institute for Eye Research
2. Spherical RGP design
3. Advanced RGP design
4. Toric RGP design
5. Orthokeratology lens design
6. Tools/calculator
7. Chapter 6 Appendix *Aspects of Contact Lens Design* (Morley Ford and Janet Stone, revised by Ronald Rabbetts).

Installation/Getting started

SYSTEM REQUIREMENTS

Windows 98 SE or higher (Windows XP preferred), Pentium 366 or higher, 100 MB available disk space, CD-ROM drive.

Graphical displays and interface: Screen resolution

Graphics and interface layout will display correctly at 800 x 600 screen resolution but it is strongly recommended that the screen resolution is set to 1024 × 768 (XGA) or higher.

Windows 98 additional requirements

It is essential to have the Microsoft Windows components which handle ADO databases included in the host operating system. This will be guaranteed if any Microsoft Office 2000 or Microsoft Office XP component is installed (Word, Excel, PowerPoint, Access or Microsoft Works are the most obvious examples). If none of these products is installed on the host computer then it is essential to install the required database component management files by running the Microsoft file MDAC_TYP.EXE which can be downloaded from the Microsoft website (www.microsoft.com).

Installing the software

1. Insert the software CD in the CD-ROM drive.
2. The installation procedure should start automatically; if it does not, press Start on the taskbar and select Run.
3. In the Run command line, type: X:\SETUP (where X is the drive letter of the CD-ROM drive). Click OK.
4. Follow the on-screen instructions.

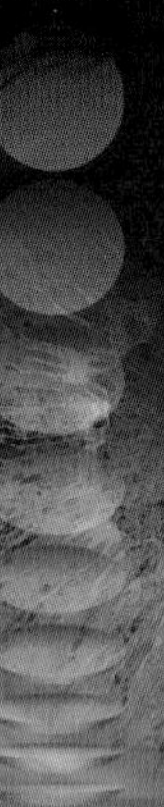

To run the software

Click **Start** > **Programs** > **Elsevier Limited** > **Contact Lenses 5**

Or

Double-click on the desktop program icon:

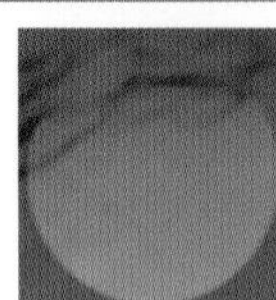

A UserGuide.pdf and Training Videos (including audio narration) are accessible from the CD-ROM.

Technical support

Technical support for this product is available between 7.30 a.m. and 7.00 p.m. CST, Monday through Friday.

Before calling, be sure that your computer meets the minimum system requirements to run this software.

Inside the United States and Canada, call 1-800-692-9010.
Inside the United Kingdom, call 0800-6929-0100.
Rest of World, call +1-314-872-8370.

You may also fax your questions to +1-314-523-4932, or contact Technical support via e-mail: technical.support@elsevier.com.

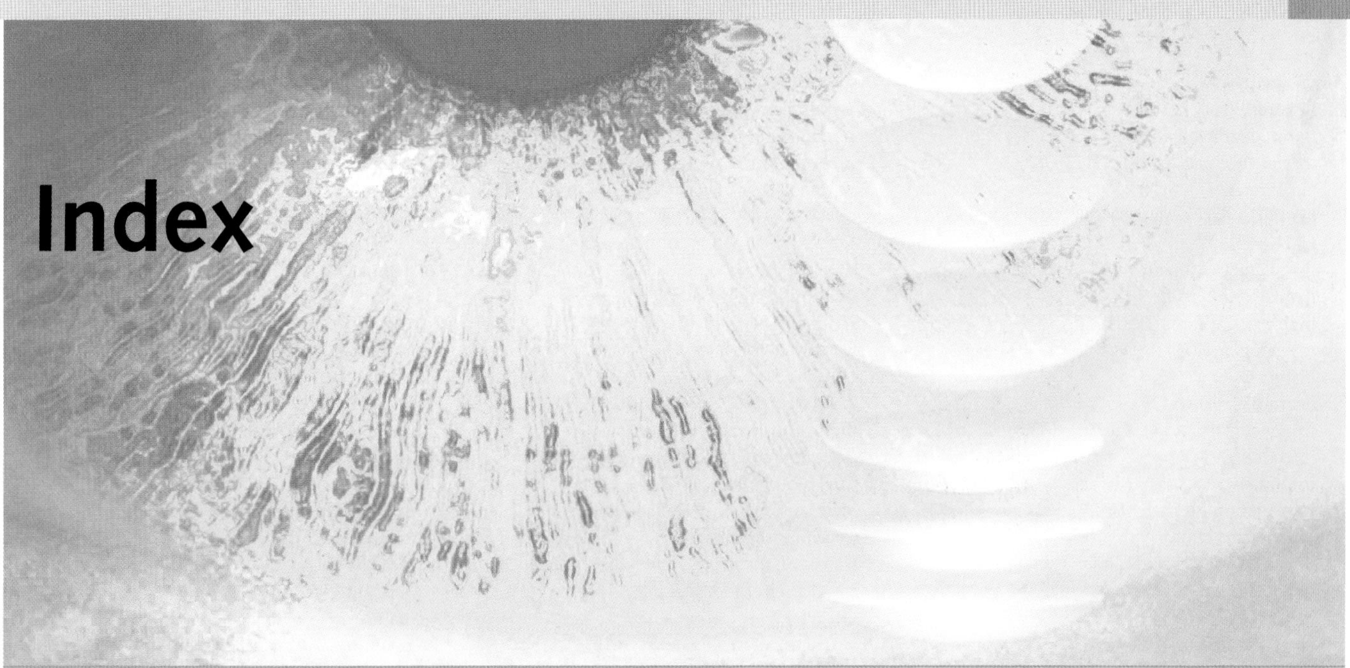

Index

A

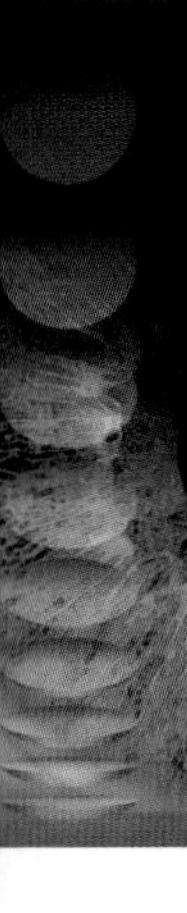

B

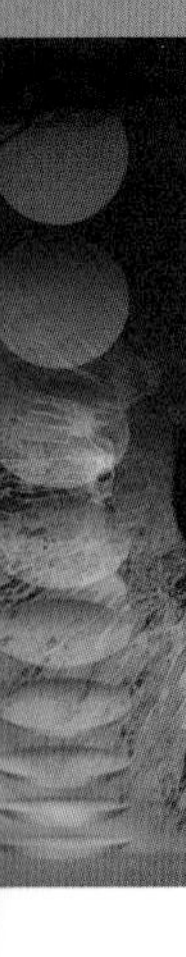

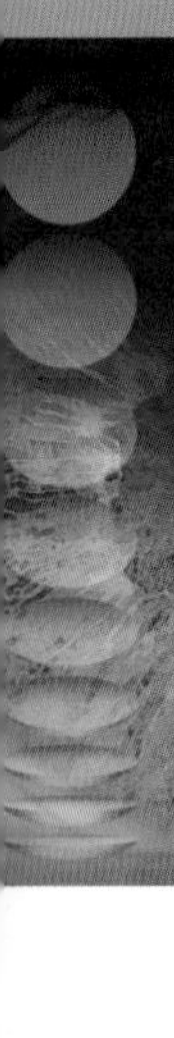

F

G

I

J

K

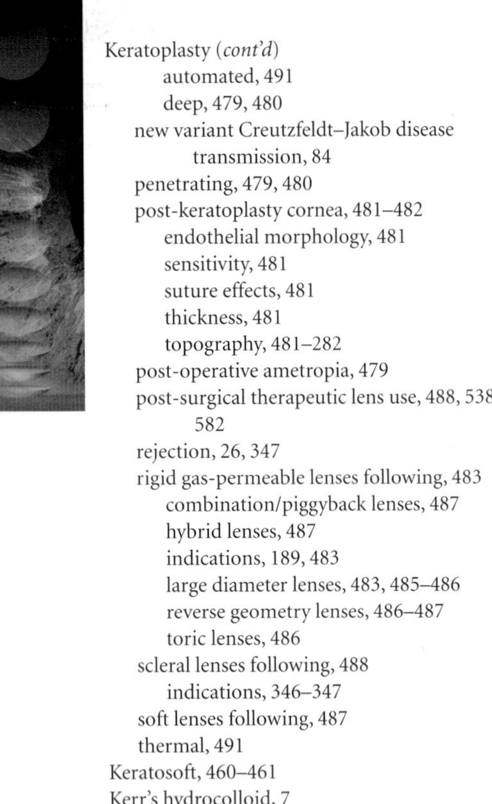

L

M

P

Q

R

S

T

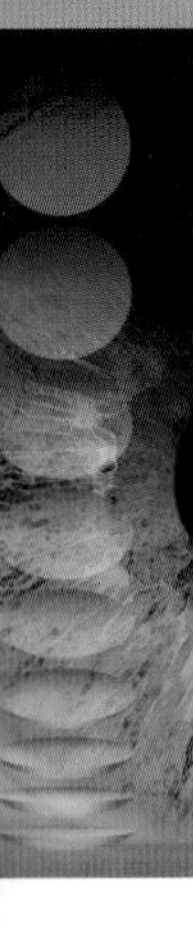

U

V

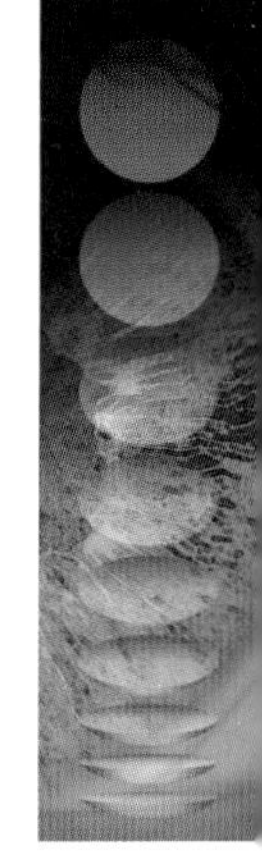

W

X

Y

Z